Y0-BEL-427

Second Edition

Pocket
Clinical &
Drug Guide

Paul DeBello M.D.

Acknowledgment
The encouragement and assistance of Clara Porter in preparing the manuscript is gratefully acknowledged.

Notice: The author has made every effort to verify the accuracy of information in this book, particularly in regards to drug use and dosage. However, because of the possibility of human error and because medical therapy including drug recommendations may change, the author cannot categorically guarantee the accuracy or currency of information contained in this book. The author and publisher disclaim responsibility for any adverse effects resulting from inadvertent errors in the text or from misunderstandings of the text. Therefore, readers are urged to consult the most recent reliable references in order to confirm that treatment recommendations are correct and consistent with current sound medical practice. In particular, readers should consult the product information included with each drug they plan to administer in order to verify drug indications, contraindications, and proper dosage. This is especially important with new or infrequently used drugs, and with dosages in elderly or pediatric patients. In short, it is the responsibility of the medical practitioner to ascertain the optimal therapy for each patient depending on the clinical setting and in accordance with the latest authoritative information. That this book is intended as a reference for trained health professionals is inherent in the foregoing comments.

Copyright 1991 by Tortoise Books, Inc.
All rights reserved. No part of this book may be reproduced, stored in a retrieval system, or transmitted by any means or in any form without written permission from the publisher. Printed in the United States of America.

Tortoise Books, Inc., 127 Victory Road, Henderson, Nevada, 89015.

ISBN 0 - 9627160 - 1 - 4

Contents of Clinical Section

Cardiovascular Disease

Pulmonary Disease

Renal Disease

Gastrointestinal Disease

Neurology

Endocrinology

Hematology

Rheumatoid and Autoimmune Disease

Skin Disease

Ear, Nose, Throat, and Mouth

Eye Disease

Obstetrics and Gynecology

Trauma

Miscellany

Bacterial and Viral Diseases

Note: A bacterial or viral disease primarily involving a specific organ system may be presented elsewhere in appropriate section.

Fungi

Protozoa

Metazoa

Cardiovascular Disease

Arrhythmias & Conduction Disturbances

VENTRICULAR FIBRILLATION (chaotic electrical activity of the ventricles) results in the cessation of cardiac output. It is most frequently due to myocardial ischemia or infarction. Other causes include electrocution; drug overdose (e.g. epinephrine, digitalis); drowning. **Treatment:** see appendix.

VENTRICULAR ASYSTOLE (the absence of electrical activity of the ventricles) may begin abruptly, follow ventricular fibrillation, or result from complete heart block. When complete heart block is the cause, the block is below the AV node and the ventricles are unable to act as escape pacemaker. **Treatment:** see appendix.

ELECTROMECHANICAL DISSOCIATION (EMD) is defined as the presence of organized EKG tracings in absence of effective myocardial contraction. **Treatment:** see appendix.

VENTRICULAR TACHYCARDIA (3 or more consecutive ventricular ectopic beats occurring at a rate of > 100—usually 150–220 beats/min). Rate is generally regular. The complexes are wide with a bundle branch pattern (usually left bundle branch pattern). This arrhythmia is often a complication of heart disease (especially myocardial infarction) but may also be due to drugs (e.g. digoxin, quinidine, procainamide, tricyclics). ●Ventricular tachycardia may be confused with supraventricular tachycardia with aberrant conduction. The latter can be excluded if the EKG discloses P waves that are dissociated from the QRS complexes. Carotid sinus massage may help reveal the P waves and may terminate supraventricular tachycardia. However, carotid sinus massage has no effect on ventricular tachycardia. Two other findings that may be observed with ventricular tachycardia include irregular cannon waves in the jugular veins and variation in intensity of the first heart sound while the patient holds his breath. **Treatment:** see appendix.

PREMATURE VENTRICULAR CONTRACTIONS (PVC's) are depolarizations that originate in the ventricles. They usually produce wide (> 0.12 sec) and bizarre QRS complexes that are generally followed by a T wave whose vector points away from the main QRS component. PVC's may be confused with supraventricular impulses with aberrant intraventricular conduction. The usual but not infallible way of distinguishing the two is to note that PVC's: (**1**) are not preceded by a P wave and (**2**) are usually followed by a full compensatory pause (interval between the QRS that precedes the PVC and the QRS that follows the PVC is exactly twice the usual QRS to QRS interval). The compensatory pause occurs because the PVC does not usually disturb the sinus node and therefore the next P wave appears on schedule. **Etiology:** PVC's commonly occur in normal persons. They are also associated with myocardial ischemia/infarction, cardiomyopathy, hypertensive cardiac disease, acute rheumatic fever, hypokalemia, hypocalcemia, hypoxia, acidosis. Drugs may be responsible: caffeine; catecholamines (epinephrine, amphetamines, isoproterenol, etc); tricyclic antidepressants; digitalis; quinidine; procainamide; tobacco. **Criteria for treatment:** Asymptomatic patients without evidence of cardiac disease do not require therapy. Patients with heart disease receive drug therapy if PVC's: are more frequent than 5 times/min, occur in runs of 2 or more in row, are multifocal, or fall on the preceding T wave. **Treatment:** see appendix.

SINUS BRADYCARDIA EKG shows normal P waves occurring regularly but at less than 60 times/minute. Sinus bradycardia may be normal (e.g. trained athlete, healthy elderly person). It may be due to the increased vagal nerve discharge associated with nausea, vomiting, pain, emotion, carotid sinus massage, ocular pressure, increased intracranial pressure, etc. Sinus bradycardia is often associated with acute myocardial infarction (especially inferior MI). Other causes: hypothyroidism; drugs (digitalis, morphine, methyldopa, propranolol or other beta–blockers, quinidine, reserpine); sinus node ischemia (e.g. coronary artery disease); rheumatic fever; cardiomyopathy; myocarditis; glaucoma; obstructive jaundice (effect of bile salts on sinus node); hyperkalemia; hypothermia. **Treatment:** see appendix.

SICK SINUS SYNDROME (SSS) refers to disease of the sinus node with the following possible consequences: severe sinus bradycardia, long sinus pauses, sinus arrest, sinoatrial block. There may be paroxysms of atrial tachycardia, atrial flutter, or atrial fibrillation (tachycardia–bradycardia syndrome). SSS is commonly due to ischemic heart disease and may transiently occur during acute myocardial infarction. Other causes include cardiomyopathy, cardiac surgery, inflammatory conditions, autoimmune conditions, amyloidosis. Drugs may be responsible (e.g. digitalis, quinidine, beta–blockers). **Treatment** is not required if the patient is asymptomatic. Treatment of symptomatic patient may be difficult. Digitalis may help but it may in some cases worsen the condition. Quinidine or procainamide is sometimes tried. A pacemaker may be necessary with digoxin as an adjunct to control the ventricular response should an atrial tachyarrhythmia occur.

PAROXYSMAL ATRIAL TACHYCARDIA (PAT) The atrial rate is 140–250/min. PAT usually begins suddenly, lasts variably (seconds to hours), and ends apruptly. The QRS complexes occur regularly and have a normal appearance, unless an associated intraventricular block causes QRS widening. In the latter case, PAT may be confused with ventricular tachycardia. A 2:1 AV block may be present if the atrial rate exceeds 200. The P waves are usually not visible since they are buried in the preceding T wave. **Etiology:** PAT is thought to be due to the presence of a re–entry pathway within the AV node or a retrograde pathway from ventricles to atria. In either case, a circulating wavefront (circus movement) is set up that results in PAT. PAT often occurs in otherwise normal patients. An inciting agent can sometimes be identified (e.g. exercise, caffeine, nicotine, catecholamines, alcohol). PAT may also accompany Wolff–Parkinson–White syndrome or myocardial infarction. **Treatment:** see appendix.

ECTOPIC ATRIAL TACHYCARDIA is due to enhanced automaticity of an ectopic focus in the atria. It may occur in otherwise normal patients. Pathologic causes include digitalis toxicity, COPD, or diseased atria. The foregoing historical clues may help differentiate this arrhythmia from PAT because the EKG may not clarify which is present. In the patient receiving digitalis, the presence of 2:1 AV block with atrial rates below 240 or the presence of higher AV conduction ratios (e.g. 3:1, 4:1) suggests ectopic atrial tachycardia. **Treatment** is directed toward the underlying cause (e.g. discontinuing digitalis, treatment COPD). Ectopic atrial tachycardia unrelated to digitalis toxicity or COPD may be treated with digitalis, beta–blockers, quinidine, disopyramide, or procainamide.

MULTIFOCAL ATRIAL TACHYCARDIA (MAT): P waves of varying configuration are seen because depolarizations (> 100/min) originate from changing atrial foci. The PR interval also varies. MAT is usually associated with severe lung or heart disease. **Treatment:** alleviate the causative lung or cardiac condition and correct any complicating factors (e.g. hypoxia, acidosis, electrolyte disturbances, etc).

ATRIAL FLUTTER There are aberrant atrial depolarizations occurring at a rate of 220–350 which usually have a "sawtooth" wave form that is best seen in leads 2, 3, and aVF. Except at slower rates, the AV node is not usually capable of conducting all the flutter waves. Consequently every 2nd, 3rd, ..., wave is conducted to the ventricles (i.e. atria–ventricle conduction ratios of 2:1, 3:1, etc). The most common situation is a 2:1 AV block with an atrial rate of about 300 and a ventricular response of about 150. The QRS complexes are generally normal. The T waves are not usually visible since they are buried within the flutter waves. ●Alarmingly high ventricular rates may ensue when certain drugs (e.g. quinidine, procainamide, disopyramide) that effect the AV node are administered and the atrial rate slows to about 200; for then the AV node is capable of conducting all the atrial impulses (i.e. 1:1 AV conduction). ●Carotid sinus massage may slow AV conduction and thereby increase the atrial–ventricle conduction ratio so that the flutter waves may be clarified. However, carotid sinus massage does not convert atrial flutter and the effect lasts only while pressure is applied. Atrial flutter often spontaneously converts to normal sinus rhythm or to atrial fibrillation. **Etiology:** Atrial flutter is observed in coronary artery disease, mitral or tricuspid valve disease, pulmonary embolism, cor pulmonale, hyperthyroidism. **Treatment:** see appendix.

ATRIAL FIBRILLATION (chaotic electrical and contractile activity of the atria) manifests as an irregular baseline on the EKG. Sometimes the irregular baseline is not discernible and atrial fibrillation is deduced by the absence of P waves and the irregular timing of the QRS complexes. The QRS complexes are generally of normal contour and duration although their amplitude may vary. The ventricular rate in untreated atrial fibrillation is usually 150–200. The cardiac rate heard at the apex exceeds the pulse rate because some atrial impulses penetrate the AV node only to depolarize ventricles that are still empty from the previous contraction. The pulse varies in amplitude, and the intensity of the first heart sound is variable. **Causes of atrial fibrillation** include mitral valve disease, left ventricular dysfunction, ischemic heart disease, hypertension, constrictive pericarditis, pulmonary embolism, atrial septal defect, thyrotoxicosis. **Treatment:** see appendix.

FIRST–DEGREE AV BLOCK is present when there is a delay in conduction thru the AV node (or sometimes thru the bundle of His or bundle branches) so that the PR interval exceeds 0.20 sec. The presence of normal QRS complexes confirms that the delay is confined to the AV node. First–degree AV block can occur in the normal heart and result from increased vagal tone, or be due to drugs that affect the conduction system (e.g. digitalis overdose). It may also be a sign of disease of the conduction system (e.g. inferior myocardial infarction, carditis of acute rheumatic fever) and may presage higher degrees of AV block. **Treatment** is not required, other than removal of the offending agent if any.

SECOND–DEGREE AV BLOCK, MOBITZ TYPE I (Wenckebach) is characterized by progressive widening of successive PR intervals until a P wave is not conducted and consequently not followed by a QRS complex. As the PR interval lengthens, the R to R interval shortens. The P to P interval does not change. The number of P waves conducted before a dropped beat occurs may vary. "Group beating" (QRS complexes in groups separated by pauses) is often obvious at a glance of the EKG. Wenckebach block is usually a manifestation of AV node dysfunction but it may be a normal physiologic phenomenom associated with tachycardia or increased vagal tone. Pathologic causes include myocardial ischemia or infarction, myocardial inflammation (e.g. acute rheumatic fever), digitalis intoxication. **Treatment** is usually not required since the condition is usually benign and transitory. If symptomatic bradycardia occurs, IV atropine is administered and if neccessary a temporary transvenous pacemaker is inserted.

SECOND–DEGREE AV BLOCK, MOBITZ TYPE II occurs when a P wave is not conducted and therefore not followed by a QRS complex. In contrast to Wenckebach block, the PR intervals are constant. Because the block usually occurs below the Bundle of His bifurcation, the QRS complexes generally have a bundle branch block pattern. This means that one of the bundle branches is blocked all of the time and that the dropped beats occur when the other branch is intermittently blocked. Mobitz type II block is a dangerous condition. It indicates extensive damage to the conduction system and it may progress to complete heart block. **Etiology** is the same as for 3rd degree AV block. **Treatment:** In the setting of anterior myocardial infarction, a permanent pacemaker is necessary and interim support with a temporary transvenous pacemaker may be required. ●If bradycardia occurs before a transvenous pacemaker can be inserted, administer IV atropine 0.5 mg and if neccessary give repeat 0.5–1.0 mg doses until a cumulative total of 2.0 mg given. If atropine fails to control symptomatic bradycardia, IV isoproterenol or an external pacemaker may be used until a transvenous pacemaker can be inserted. Patients with persistent or symptomatic block are candidates for permanent pacemaker.

THIRD–DEGREE AV BLOCK [complete AV block] (no atrial impulses reach the ventricles and consequently the atria and ventricles beat independently of each other). **Etiology:** include Lenegre's or Lev's disease, coronary artery disease, myocardial infarction, myocarditis, cardiomyopathy, cardiac surgery, congenital heart disease, syphilis, uremia, digitalis, quinidine, procainamide, propranolol. **Level of the block** may be inferred by the appearance and rate of the QRS complexes: (1) Normal appearing QRS complexes suggest disease of the AV node or the Bundle of His above its bifurcation, and the ventricular escape rate is usually 40–60. In most hearts the right coronary artery supplies the sinus node, AV node, Bundle of His, right ventricle, and inferior wall of the left ventricle. Consequently, inferior myocardial infarctions are frequently associated with AV block above the His bifurcation. (**2**) Wide and bizarre QRS complexes imply damage below the Bundle of His bifurcation and so the ventricular escape rate is often below 40. Anterior myocardial infarction is often associated with damage to both bundle branches and thus may present with this pattern of complete heart block. **Treatment:** In the setting of acute myocardial infarction, complete AV block above the His bifurcation is often transitory and the cardiac rate may be rapid enough to support adequate perfusion. If the cardiac rate should fall such that signs of cardiovascular compromise occur, IV atropine is administered and followed if necessary by a temporary transvenous pacemaker. A permanent pacemaker is indicated if symptomatic complete block persists or if the block has occurred in the His bundle or below. The patient may require interim support with IV isoproterenol initially and/or a temporary transvenous pacemaker.

AV DISSOCIATION is the condition in which the atria and the ventricles beat independently of each other (i.e. one pacemaker is controlling the atria and another pacemaker is controlling the ventricles). It is not to be confused with heart block, although it is true that complete AV block results in independent beating of atria and ventricles. In the case of AV dissociation, however, atrial impulses can penetrate the AV node and initiate ventricular impulses but do not consistently do so because usually the atrial pacemaker has slowed or the ventricular pacemaker has sped up. AV dissociation may occur when the SA node has slowed (e.g. increased vagal tone, digitalis) or when the AV node is made more irritable (e.g. myocardial ischemia or infarction, digitalis, acute infections, rheumatic fever). **Treatment:** None is required as long as the patient is asymptomatic with a sufficiently fast ventricular rate.

RIGHT BUNDLE BRANCH BLOCK (RBBB) is conveniently diagnosed in lead V1 (the QRS is > 0.12 sec and the terminal part of the QRS complex is positive). RBBB causes delayed contraction of the right ventricle, and therefore late closure of the pulmonic valve so that there is abnormally wide splitting of the 2nd heart sound. The anterior descending branch of the left coronary artery supplies the right bundle as it travels down the septum. Consequently, anteroseptal infarction often results in RBBB. **Etiology:** RBBB is occasionally seen in normal individuals. RBBB may result from the same causes listed under LBBB, and in addition RBBB may occur when the right side of the heart is stressed (e.g. pulmonary embolism, pulmonary hypertension, atrial septal defect). **Treatment:** A temporary pacemaker is advocated if RBBB occurs in the setting of acute anterior myocardial infarction. A permanent pacemaker is required if the left bundle is also impaired—e.g. RBBB with left anterior hemiblock, RBBB with left posterior hemiblock.

LEFT BUNDLE BRANCH BLOCK (LBBB) is conveniently diagnosed in lead V1 (the QRS is > 0.12 sec and the terminal part of the QRS complex is negative). The presence of LBBB may obscure EKG signs of myocardial infarction. LBBB causes delayed contraction of the left ventricle and therefore late closure of the aortic valve. This manifests as splitting of the 2nd heart sound on expiration (splitting of the 2nd heart sound normally occurs on inspiration). **Blood supply of left bundle:** The left bundle (before it divides into the anterior and posterior division) is supplied by both the right coronary artery and the left anterior descending coronary artery. The anterior division of the left bundle is supplied by the left anterior descending artery. The posterior division of the left bundle is supplied by branches of both right and left coronary arteries. **Etiology:** On rare occasions, LBBB is found in normal persons. Besides myocardial infarction/ischemia, LBBB may be due to Lenegre's disease (progressive fibrosis of the bundles), Lev's disease (sclerosis/calcification primarily of the left myocardium), trauma, congenital, cardiomyopathy, tumor, infection (e.g. syphilis). **Treatment:** A temporary pacemaker is advocated if LBBB occurs in the setting of acute anterior myocardial infarction. A permanent pacemaker is required if the right bundle is also impaired.

LEFT ANTERIOR HEMIBLOCK (LAH) is present when the anterior division of the left bundle is blocked. This causes left QRS axis deviation—usually to about minus 60 degrees. The QRS duration is normal except when (as is usually the case) RBBB is also present. Isolated LAH does not require insertion of pacemaker. However, a temporary pacemaker is indicated if there is a bifascicular block (e.g. LAH plus RBBB).

LEFT POSTERIOR HEMIBLOCK (LPH) is present when the posterior division of the left bundle is blocked. This causes right axis deviation—usually to about +120 degrees. The QRS duration is normal except when (as is almost always the case) RBBB is also present. LPH is much less common than LAH because the posterior division receives a dual blood supply. Both LAH and LPH can, by producing abnormal QRS patterns in various leads, mask or mimic myocardial infarction. Isolated LPH does not require insertion of pacemaker. However, a temporary pacemaker is indicated if there is a bifascicular block (e.g. LPH plus RBBB).

WOLFF–PARKINSON–WHITE (WPW) is an EKG diagnosis: PR interval < 0.12 sec, QRS > 0.1 sec, slurring of the upstroke of the QRS (delta wave). The P wave is normal. Most patients are male and the condition is usually benign. WPW syndrome is due to the presence of an accessory bundle (bundle of Kent) that allows atrial impulses to bypass the AV node and therefore circumvent the delay that normally occurs at the AV node. Some patients are prone to supraventricular arrhythmias— e.g. paroxysmal atrial tachycardia (most common), atrial fibrillation, atrial flutter. Rarely, sudden death occurs from atrial fibrillation because the accessory bundle allows a rapid ventricular response.

Treatment: Supraventricular tachycardia may sometimes be terminated with Valsalva maneuver or carotid sinus massage. A number of drugs may be effective in terminating SVT—e.g. verapamil, propranolol, lidocaine, procainamide. Electrical cardioversion is indicated if drug therapy fails or if the patient is unstable (e.g. hypotension, pulmonary edema). Overdrive pacing is an alternative. Preventitive agents that may be tried include propranolol and quinidine. Atrial fibrillation: Treatment/prevention of atrial fibrillation is with quinidine, procainamide, or disopyramide. Digitalis is generally contraindicated in patients with WPW (particularly in the setting of atrial flutter or atrial fibrillation) because it may decrease the refractory period of the accessory bundle. If this occurs, more atrial impulses reach the ventricles and a dangerously rapid ventricular rate may ensue. For the same reason, verapamil and lidocaine are also not recommended in WPW patients with atrial fibrillation or atrial flutter. A pacemaker or surgical transection of the accessory bundle may be indicated in those patients with tachyarrhytmias who do not respond adequately to conventional treatment.

STOKES–ADAMS ATTACK is the transient loss of consciousness that results from temporary loss of adequate ventricular activity. It may be due to transient episodes of asystole, ventricular fibrillation, ventricular tachycardia, or complete heart block with inadequate ventricular response. Bundle branch block, and 2nd or 3rd degree AV block are common predisposing factors. **Treatment:** Try precordial thump. If no response, begin CPR and the appropriate algorithm for the arrhythmia.

Angina Pectoris is defined as chest pain resulting from myocardial hypoxia.

Causes: Coronary artery disease: (**1**) atherosclerotic coronary artery disease— the most common cause; (**2**) coronary embolism arising from left atrial or left ventricular thrombus, from prosthetic valve thrombus, or from infective endocarditis; (**3**) syphilitic aortitis involving the coronary ostia; (**4**) dissecting aortic aneurysm involving coronary artery; (**5**) congenital coronary artery anomalies; (**6**) collagen–vascular disease. Myocardial hypoxia–induced angina in the absence of coronary artery disease: e.g. aortic stenosis, aortic regurgitation, mitral stenosis, anemia, thyrotoxicosis, tachycardia. Noncardiac conditions that may cause chest pain and may be confused with angina pectoris include musculoskeletal pain, esophageal spasm or reflux, peptic ulcer, pancreatitis, lung disease (e.g. pneumothorax, pneumonitis, pulmonary embolism).

Diagnosis: Angina is typically described as a squeezing pain/discomfort that is felt in the mid to upper sternal area. In some cases, the pain is felt over the lower sternum or both sides of the chest (mostly the left). The pain often radiates to the arms (mostly the left), neck, jaw, and sometimes to the left scapula. There may be a "heaviness" or tingling of the arms. Angina may be induced by exertion (including sexual intercourse), cold, emotions. Pain usually lasts for more than 30 seconds but less than 15 minutes (fleeting chest pain is not anginal). Angina does not present as pain localized to a small area about the left breast. The pain is nonpleuritic. It is alleviated by rest and nitrates. Physical exam during an anginal attack is often unremarkable. There may be tachycardia, S4 (due to hypoxic left ventricle), or a mitral regurgitant murmur (due to hypoxia of papillary muscle). Signs suggesting a musculoskeletal condition should be ruled out (e.g. tenderness chest wall, chest pain elicited by brief lifting or pulling). EKG typically reveals horizontal ST segment depression and T wave inversion that both revert to normal when angina subsides. Treadmill testing usually supports the diagnosis by inducing angina and typical EKG signs. However, patients with bona fide angina sometimes have a normal treadmill test. Furthermore, false positives are not unusual—particularly in those patients receiving digoxin or those with electrolyte or cardiac conduction disturbances. Thallium or technetium scan performed while exercising will also reveal myocardial hypoxia. This method is useful when interpretation of the exercise EKG would be difficult (e.g. cardiac conduction defect, digoxin therapy). Coronary arteriography is performed when the diagnosis of coronary artery disease is in doubt or when the patient is being evaluated for possible coronary artery bypass surgery or angioplasty.

Treatment of atherosclerotic coronary artery disease–associated angina: Nitrates: Sublingual nitroglycerin is generally the first drug employed. Long-acting nitrates (e.g. isosorbide dinitrate) or nitroglycerin paste may be needed in the patient with frequent angina. Beta blockers (e.g. propranolol, metoprolol, atenolol) are frequently prescribed and may be used in conjunction with nitrates. Calcium-channel blocker (nifedipine, verapamil, diltiazem) may alone control angina or may be used in conjunction with other drugs. Tranquilizer: Some patients benefit from drugs that relieve anxiety. Coronary angioplasty or coronary artery bypass surgery is considered in the following circumstances: angina intractable to medical therapy, left main coronary artery stenosis, or perhaps 3 vessel disease. Coronary angioplasty (introduction and inflation of a balloon catheter into a stenosed coronary artery) is most likely to be effective when the stenosis is noncalcified and proximal.

UNSTABLE ANGINA (preinfarction angina, crescendo angina) is defined as severe angina of new onset, or angina that has suddenly become worse. The patient may complain of pain that occurs at rest, is more severe, lasts longer, or is more frequent and/or requires more frequent use of nitroglycerin. **Treatment:** Patient should be hospitalized and aggressive medical therapy should be tried. Unless there is a contraindication, a beta-blocker (e.g. propranolol) is begun and the dose titrated to heart rate of 40–60. Transdermal nitroglycerin or an oral nitrate (isosorbide dinitrate) is begun concurrently with the beta blocker. A calcium channel blocker (e.g. nifedipine, diltiazem) is added if bouts of angina continue to occur at rest. Intractable cases may be candidates for coronary angioplasty or bypass.

PRINZMETAL'S ANGINA (variant angina) is a form of angina that results from coronary artery spasm. Spasm may occur in normal coronary arteries or in those with atherosclerotic stenosis. Angina occurs at rest. EKG may show ST segment elevation or depression. (This is in contrast to the usual angina patient who characteristically only has ST depression.) The ST elevations are often associated with heart block and/or ventricular arrhythmias. Not infrequently, ST elevation occurs in the absence of angina. Holter monitor is helpful in making the diagnosis since ST elevations may occur with or without angina, heart block, or arrhythmias. Coronary artery angiography is confirmatory. If spontaneous spasm does not occur during the procedure and if severe fixed stenosis is not present, spasm is induced with ergonovine maleate. **Treatment:** nitrates and a calcium channel blocker. **Other causes of ST elevation** include myocardial infarction, ventricular aneurysm, left bundle branch block, left ventricular hypertrophy.

Myocardial Infarction & Complications

Myocardial infarction usually results from obstruction of a coronary artery diseased by atherosclerosis. The risk of atherosclerosis and therefore of MI is increased by hyperlipidemia (particularly hypercholesterolemia), smoking, sedentary existence, hypertension. Circumstances other than atherosclerosis that may lead to MI include coronary artery spasm, coronary thrombosis as consequence of hypercoagulable condition (e.g. patient on oral contraceptive), coronary embolism (e.g. from endocarditis, from left atrial thrombus).

Signs/symptoms: Pain of MI is of similar character and radiation as angina, but differs from angina in that the pain generally lasts longer (usually > 1/2 hr to up to several hrs or even days), is often more severe, and is not alleviated by rest or nitroglycerin. An MI may occur in the absence of pain ("silent MI"), particularly in diabetics. Other manifestations may include: dyspnea, sweaty cool skin, tachycardia, distended neck veins (if there is right heart failure), pulsus alternans. The presence of nausea, vomiting, and bradycardia is common with an inferior MI, and is due to a parasympathetic reflex. Auscultation: (**1**) S1 and S2 may be soft, (**2**) S2 may be split if there is left bundle branch block, (**3**) an S4 is usually present, (**4**) an S3 may be heard if heart failure ensues, (**5**) apical pansystolic murmur may be present if there is mitral regurgitation secondary to papillary muscle dysfunction or dilation of left ventricle, (**6**) rales may heard if there is left heart failure with ensuing pulmonary edema, (**7**) pericardial friction rub is sometimes heard if pericarditis develops as a consequence of transmural MI.

EKG signs of a transmural MI: In a typical case the following sequence occurs: (**1**) ST elevation with upward convexity (representing myocardial injury) develops over minutes to hours in leads facing the infarct. There is reciprocal ST depression in leads opposite the infarct. (**2**) T wave inversion (representing myocardial ischemia) develops in the same leads as the ST elevations begin to return toward the baseline. Concurrently, there are reciprocal tall peaked upright T waves in leads opposite the infarct. (**3**) Q waves (representing myocardial necrosis) in leads facing the infarct develop within hours but sometimes take days to appear. As the Q wave in the QRS complex deepens, there is progressive reduction in the R wave. Q waves are usually permanent. ●Note that Q waves are normal in aVR, and small Q waves (1–2 mm deep and not exceeding 0.03 sec) are permitted in I, aVL, V5–6. Also QS complexes may be normal in V1–2. A Q wave in lead III may indicate an inferior MI but it is likely to be benign if it is < 0.03 sec, if it disappears or is substantially reduced with inspiration, and if it is not accompanied by Q waves in II and aVF. (**4**) ST segment returns to baseline soon after an MI unless a ventricular aneurysm develops. (**5**) Inverted T waves may take weeks or even months to return to normal upright position and as previously stated Q waves are usually permanent. Circumstances that may confuse EKG interptretation: A left bundle branch block produces QRS, ST, and ST changes which may make EKG diagnosis of an MI impossible. Also be aware that ST elevation may be a normal variant in individuals with early repolarization. Other causes of ST elevation include ventricular aneurysm, Prinzmetal's angina, left ventricular hypertrophy.

EKG signs of subendocardial MI (infarction of that portion of the myocardium nearest the ventricular cavity)**:** There is persistent (i.e. ≥ 48 hr) ST depression and T wave inversion in the limb or chest leads. Q waves are absent.

Identifying the site of an MI: The indicative changes (i.e. ST elevation, T wave inversion, Q waves) are found in leads facing the infarct and reciprocal changes (ST depression, tall R waves) are seen in leads away from the infarct. Thus an inferior MI is identified by indicative changes in the inferior leads (II, III, aVF) with reciprocal changes in I, aVL, V leads. High lateral MI is associated with indicative changes in leads I and aVL. An anterior MI is identified by indicative changes in leads facing the anterior surface (most of V1–6 as well as I and aVL) with reciprocal changes in the inferior leads (II, III, aVF). More localized anterior infarctions are identified as follows: anteroseptal MI (indicative changes in one or more of V1–4); anteroapical MI (indicative changes in V4–5); anterolateral MI (indicative changes in V4–6, I, aVL). ●Combinations of the foregoing often occur: e.g. inferolateral MI (indicative changes in II, III, aVF, V5–6); anteroinferior MI (indicative changes in II, III, aVF, V1–6); inferoapical MI (indicative changes in II, III, aVF, V4–5). ●Since there are no leads facing the posterior wall, posterior MI must be inferred from reciprocal changes (tall upright symmetical T waves, ST depression, tall R waves) in the anterior chest leads V1–2. Clinical significance of localizing the site of an MI lies in the prediction of certain complications. For instance, the right coronary artery supplies the inferior surface of the heart (most of the right ventricle and only a small portion of the left ventricle), sinus node, AV node, His bundle. Consequently, inferior MI's often result in sinus bradycardia, AV block, and right ventricular dysfunction. Anterior MI's frequently cause left ventricular dysfunction (e.g. pulmonary edema, cardiogenic shock) and bundle branch blocks.

Cardiac enzymes are released into the circulation when the heart muscle is damaged. The commonly measured enzymes are CK (creatine kinase), LDH (lactic dehydrogenase), and less frequently SGOT (serum glutamic–oxaloacetic transaminase). Creatine kinase (CK) is also present in skeletal muscle, brain, and lung; and may therefore be elevated with exercise, intramuscular injection, trauma, muscle disease, stroke, pulmonary infarction, hypothyroidism. To enhance specificity, the myocardial CK isoenzyme (myocardial band CK or MB–CK) is routinely measured. The MB–CK appears 4–6 hr after onset of an MI, peaks between 12–24 hr, and in the absence of complications returns to baseline in 36–48 hr. MB–CK is usually assayed on initial evaluation of a suspected MI and then 3–4 times at 8–12 hr intervals. Lactic dehydrogenas (LDH) is also present in tissues other than the heart (e.g. red blood cells, liver, kidney, brain, lung) and may therefore be elevated in conditions other than myocardial infarction or myocarditis (e.g. hemolysis, megaloblastic anemia, pulmonary embolism, malignancy). Specificity is improved by measuring LDH isoenzyme 1 (LDH 1). LDH becomes elevated within 12–48 hr, peaks in 2–6 days, returns to baseline in 8–14 days. LDH is generally assayed 3 times at 12 hr intervals.

WBC is elevated (up to 20,000) with a left shift and subsides in about a week. **ESR** is elevated for several weeks.

Technetium scan: Technetium–99m stannous pyrophosphate concentrates in damaged myocardial tissue. This test is useful when the EKG and/or cardiac enzymes leaves the diagnosis in doubt—e.g. left bundle branch block obscuring EKG interpretation, after cardiac surgery (cardiac enzymes and EKG are expected to be abnormal), several days after onset of an MI (when acute EKG signs are resolving and cardiac enzymes are returning to normal). Technetium scans are usually positive within 12–36 hrs and remain positive for 6–10 days. The scan is usually most sensitive at 36–48 hr but some patients may not have a positive scan until 5–7 days have elapsed. False–positive scans may occur in patients with pericarditis, aneurysm, calcified valves, healing rib fractures, breast tumors, or after electrical cardioversion. **Thallium scan** is another type of scan used to identify areas of infarction. In this test, however, thallium–201 concentrates in normal myocardial tissue leaving a "cold" infarcted area

Treatment uncomplicated acute MI: Activity: Initially, the patient is restricted to his bed almost all the time. However, even on the day of admission, the patient is generally allowed commode privileges and may sit in a chair for brief periods. Walking about the room is usually permitted by the 4–5th day. In the absence of complications, the patient leaves the CCU on the 5–7th day and is usually discharged from the hospital by day 14. Oxygen is administered via nasal cannulae at 2–4 liters/min so as to maintain PaO2 at not less than 80. Use face mask if the paO2 cannot be maintained above 80 with nasal cannulae at 4 liter/min. Note, however, that chronically hypoxic patients—who are dependent on hypoxic ventilatory drive—generally require less oxygen since the PaO2 must be maintained at a lower level. A Venturi mask may be used for more precise oxygen delivery. Continuous cardiac monitoring and an IV line are essential. Prophylactic lidocaine is administered for the first 24 hr even if PVC's or other arrhythmias are not present because ventricular fibrillation may suddenly occur in the absence of ventricular ectopy. Pain relief: Intravenous morphine or meperidine may be used to relieve pain during first 2 days. Meperidine may be advantageous in patients with inferior MI since it has an atropine–like effect that tends to oppose the vagally–mediated manifestations (nausea, vomiting, bradycardia) commonly associated with inferior MI. Some patients will obtain relief with sublingual or intravenous nitroglycerin. Nitrous oxide and oxygen administered together via a nonrebreathing mask is yet another analgesic option. Diazepam is commonly used for anxiety. Thrombolytic therapy (e.g. see "Tissue Plasminogen Activator" or streptokinase in drug section) is recommended to lyse an acute clot that might be occluding a coronary artery. To be effective, thrombolytic therapy must be initiated within 4–6 hr following onset of acute MI. Heparin and then warfarin anticoagulation follows thrombolytic therapy. In order to prevent venous thrombosis. patients who do not receive thrombolytic therapy should at least receive minidose heparin (8000 unit SC q8h) unless anticoagulation is contraindicated (e.g. pericarditis, severe hypertension, peptic ulcer, or bleeding diathesis). Diet: Keep the patient NPO for the first 4–24 hours until the paiient is judged to be stable. For 1–3 days, the diet is soft and bland with no added salt allowed (i.e. 4–5 gram-NaCl/day) and caloric intake of 1000–1500 calories/day. A diet low in cholesterol and saturated fats is advocated. Fluid intake is restricted to 2 liters/day. Stool softeners (e.g. Colace, Surfak) are routinely prescribed to prevent straining at stool. Laxatives are indicated for constipation. Beta blockers (e.g. metoprolol, timolol) reduce mortality and are administered for long-term prophylaxis. A beta blocker may be begun on the day that acute MI is diagnosed unless there are contraindications (e.g. severe heart failure, bradycardia, 2nd or 3rd degree block).

COMPLICATIONS OF MYOCARDIAL INFARCTION

MI–associated arrhythmias & conduction disturbances: Any number of types of arrhythmias (e.g. premature ventricular contractions, ventricular tachycardia or fibrillation, etc) and heart block may occur as a result of a MI. These are discussed in "Arrhythmias & Conduction Disturbances" chapter. ●The right coronary artery usually supplies the inferior surface of the heart (most of the right ventricle and only a small portion of the left ventricle), sinus node, AV node, and His bundle. Consequently, an inferior MI (in addition to causing right ventricular dysfunction) often results in sinus bradycardia; AV block (1st degree, Wenckebach, or complete). ●An anterior MI; in addition to causing left ventricular dysfunction (e.g. pulmonary edema, cardiogenic shock); often interrupts the conduction system below the His bundle with the following possible consequences: Mobitz II block, right or left bundle bundle branch block, complete block.

Anterior MI and left heart failure: Anterior MI results when there is occlusion of the left main coronary artery or its branches—the left anterior descending (which supplies the interventricular septum and the anterior wall of the left ventricle) and the circumflex (which supplies the lateral and posterior walls of the left ventricle). Consequently, anterior MI's frequently cause left ventricular dysfunction (e.g. pulmonary congestion/edema, cardiogenic shock) and bundle branch blocks. Refer to cardiogenic shock below and to "Congestive Heart Failure" chapter for further discussion of left heart failure, and its consequences and treatment. Bundle branch block is discussed under "Arrhythmias and Conduction Disturbances" chapter.

Cardiogenic shock occurs when ≥ 40% of the left ventricle has been infarcted. Mortality is 80%. It is said to be present when: (**1**) systolic pressure is < 80–90 mm Hg, or has fallen by over 30 mm Hg in a previously hypertensive patient; (**2**) there is compromised organ perfusion—e.g. urine output < 20–30 ml/hr, cool clammy skin, peripheral cyanosis, confusion; (**3**) the cardiac index is low (usually < 2.2 liter/min/square meter); (**4**) pulmonary capillary wedge pressure > 18 mm Hg (reflection of elevated left ventricular end–diastolic pressure). Treatment of cardiogenic shock: (**1**) Administer atropine if there is bradycardia. A pacemaker is required if significant bracycardia persists. (**2**) Start infusion of dobutamine or dopamine. (**3**) Insert arterial catheter, Foley catheter, and Swan–Ganz catheter. (**3**) If the pulmonary capillary wedge pressure (PCW) is < 15–18 mm Hg, hypovolemia may be causing or contributing to hypotension and shock. In this case, judicious fluid administration titrated to a PCW of 18 mm Hg may improve blood pressure and allow discontinuation of dobutamine or dopamine. (**4**) PCW > 18 mm Hg and cardiac index < 2.2 liter/min/square meter are indications for support with dobutamine or dopamine. (**5**) Thrombolytic therapy (e.g. see streptokinase or tissue plasminogen activator in drug section) may be tried if there has been an acute MI with onset within the last 4 hr. (**6**) Patients who are not responding to the foregoing measures and who are surgical candidates (e.g. coronary bypass, mitral valve replacement, repair of ruptured interventricular septum) may benefit from external counterpulsation or temporary insertion of an intraortic balloon pump. With the latter, the baloon (**1**) inflates during diastole when the aortic valve is closed thereby pumping blood to the periphery and to the coronary arteries, and (**2**) rapidly deflates at onset of systole thus reducing aortic systolic pressure and thereby facilitates left ventricular outflow so that left ventricular work is reduced.

Inferior MI and right heart failure: Inferior MI results when the right coronary artery is blocked. In most hearts, the right coronary artery supplies the inferior surface of the heart (i.e. most of the right ventricle and only a small portion of the left ventricle—the inferior wall), sinus node, AV node, His bundle. Consequently, inferior MI's often cause sinus bradycardia, AV block, and right ventricular dysfunction. If the right ventricle is damaged sufficiently; the right ventricle fails (see "Heart Failure" chapter), and so cardiac output falls, and hypotension may develop. Treatment: In contrast to left heart failure, where fluid restriction is the rule, the patient with decreased cardiac output and hypotension due to right heart failure may benefit from careful fluid administration (provided that left ventricular failure is not also present). Dobutamine may be added if necessary. ●The decision to administer fluids may be complicated by the fact that right heart failure commonly results from or coexists with left-sided failure. In the absence of overt left-sided failure (e.g. pulmonary edema) it may not be obvious whether right heart failure is a consequence of long-standing left heart failure or primarily due to right ventricular MI. Swan–Ganz catheterization may clarify the situation: (**1**) if only the right heart fails, the right atrial pressure and right ventricular end–diastolic pressure will be elevated while the wedge pressure will be normal or only slightly elevated; (**2**) if the left ventricle has also failed; the right atrial and right ventricular end–diastolic pressure, and wedge pressure will all be elevated.

Ventricular aneurysm may develop from days to months following an MI. The aneurysm increases the work of the heart and may therefore contribute to heart failure. There is increased risk of mural thrombi and embolization as well as ventricular arrhythmias. Diagnosis: (**1**) paradoxical movement of the anterior chest wall is sometimes seen or felt, (**2**) persistent ST elevations on the EKG weeks after an MI, (**3**) bulge of the left ventricular silhouette on chest x-ray, (**4**) paradoxical movement of the left ventricle on fluoroscopy, (**5**) echocardiography, (**6**) ventriculography, (**7**) cardiac catheterization—the only conclusive diagnostic method. Treatment: No specific treatment is required in asymptomatic cases. Surgical excision is indicated if there is CHF or arrhythmias not amenable to medical therapy.

Papillary muscle rupture is uncommon. It is most often associated with inferior or posterior MI. It usually occurs within 1–2 wk of an MI. Diagnosis: Findings vary according to whether there has been partial or complete rupture of the papillary muscle. Typical findings include: a loud apical pansystolic mitral regurgitant murmur which radiates to the axilla, a soft S1, a widely split S2. Often, there is evidence of left heart failure (e.g. S3, pulmonary edema and/or hypotension). Treatment: Diuretics, digoxin, and reduction of peripheral vascular resistance (e.g. hydralazine, captopril) may be tried if mitral regurgitation is not severe. However, most patients require mitral valve replacement. Medical management may also be tried in patients who are poor surgical candidates. Pending surgery, the unstable patient is managed as follows: (**1**) If the wedge pressure is > 20–25 mm Hg and the systolic pressure is normal, afterload reduction is indicated. Administer nitroprusside titrated to wedge pressure of 15–18 mm Hg while not allowing systolic pressure to fall below 100. (**2**) If the systolic pressure is < 100, administer dopamine (or dopamine plus nitroprusside) to support blood pressure, and insert an intra-aortic balloon pump. Clinical status allowing, coronary angiography is performed prior to surgery in order to assess whether coronary bypass should be performed in addition to valve replacement.

Papillary muscle malfunction may result from papillary muscle ischemia or infarction. Diagnosis: (**1**) pansystolic or late systolic murmur best heard at apex and occasionally heard at the lower left sternal border. If ischemia is the cause of the papillary muscle dysfunction, the murmur will disappear as the ischemia resolves. (**2**) In the case of papillary muscle infarction, the murmur persists and signs of left heart failure are usually present (e.g. S3, pulmonary edema), and shock may ensue. Treatment papillary muscle infarction: Need for surgery is dictated by the clinical course. Treatment guidelines are the same as for papillary muscle rupture (see above).

Ventricular rupture accounts for about 10% deaths from MI. Rupture is most likely to occur within the first 2 weeks following a transmural MI (i.e. before the infarcted myocardium can be replaced by fibrous tissue). Rupture of the interventricular septum typically presents with sudden onset of a loud systolic murmur and thrill at the lower left sternal border, together with pulmonary edema and/or other signs of CHF. Swan–Ganz catheterization reveals an increase in oxygen saturation when going from the right atrium to the right ventricle, elevated wedge pressure, and a left--to–right shunt. Treatment of interventricular rupture depends on the extent of left-to–right shunt. Surgery is indicated if shunting is > 2:1 but is delayed for 6 weeks if the patient is stable. Prior to surgery the unstable patient is managed in the same manner as the patient awaiting surgery following papillary muscle rupture (see above). Free ventricular wall rupture usually results in sudden cardiovascular collapse with absent pulse. Electromechanical dissociation is sometimes observed (see "Arrhythmias"). Free wall rupture is almost always fatal. Rarely, however, rupture presents as cardiac tamponade (the rupture is contained to some extent by the pericardium) and the patient survives long enough to undergo pericardiocentesis and surgery.

Pericarditis may occur 1–3 days following a transmural MI and generally resolves in 3–5 days (refer to "Pericardial Disease" chapter). Pericarditis may also occur several days to months following an MI as part of **Dressler's syndrome**: there is pericarditis together with pleuritis (sometimes with pleural effusion and/or pneumonitis). Other manifestations of Dressler's syndrome may include: fever, leukocytosis, elevated sedimentation rate, arthralgias and/or myalgias. An autoimmune etiology is suspected since antimyocardial antibodies have been found. Treatment: Aspirin (650 mg q4–6h) or some other nonsteroidal anti–inflammatory drug is used to treat either the early pericarditis or Dressler's syndrome. Corticosteroid therapy may be used in a severe case of Dressler's syndrome that does not respond to nonsteroidal agents. However, corticosteroids should be avoided in early pericarditis since they may delay healing. Unless essential, anticoagulants are contraindicated in either early pericarditis or Dressler's syndrome because anticoagulation increases the risk of hemorrhagic pericarditis with cardiac tamponade.

Shoulder–hand syndrome is rare. It develops weeks or months after an MI. Prolonged inactivity at the time of the MI and a localized activity of the sympathetic nervous system may play a role. Diagnosis: There is pain and limitation of movement of the left shoulder or both shoulders; pain and swelling of the arm(s) especially the hand(s). Furthermore, skin abnormalities may be evident in an affected extremity (e.g. atrophy, pigmentary effects, hypertrichosis, hyperhydrosis, nail changes). Contractures and osteoporosis (Sudeck's atrophy) may occur. Treatment: Mild cases may respond to exercise, local heat, and the injection of corticosteroid plus procaine into the shoulder joint. Severe cases require systemic corticosteroids (e.g. prednisone 60 mg/day for 2 wk, then tapered rapidly to 5–10 mg/day). Several months therapy is sometimes required.

Congestive Heart Failure

may be defined as failure of the heart to adequately eject blood so that there is inadequate cardiac output with (1) pulmonary venous congestion if the left heart fails and/or (2) systemic venous congestion if the right heart fails.

LEFT HEART FAILURE (left heart unable to adequately eject blood with consequent pulmonary venous congestion) may result from: (**1**) obstruction of outflow from the left atrium–e.g. mitral stenosis; (**2**) increased volume load–e.g. mitral regurgitation, aortic regurgitation, thyrotoxicosis, beri beri; (**3**) increased pressure load–e.g. systemic hypertension, aortic stenosis; (**4**) myocardial disease–e.g. cardiomyopathy, myocardial infarction. **Diagnosis:** symptoms; fatigue, dyspnea on exertion, orthopnea, paroxysmal nocturnal dyspnea; signs; tachypnea, tachycardia, rales, S3, pulsus alternans; chest x–ray; enlarged heart, pulmonary edema, pleural effusion, Kerley B lines. **Treatment mild–moderate left heart failure:** Salt restriction and a thiazide diuretic will suffice in mild cases. Furosemide is usually administered in more advanced failure. Digoxin is sometimes added but the response is variable. Digoxin is most likely to be effective in patients with CHF complicated by atrial fibrillation/flutter or ischemia, or in patients with CHF due to valvular heart disease (isolated mitral stenosis excepted) or congenital heart disease. Because of its tendency to precipitate arrhythmias, digoxin should not be administered if possible in the first few days following myocardial infarction. A vasodilator (e.g. captopril) may be tried if the response to diuretics and digoxin is inadequate. **Treatment severe left heart**

failure: Insert Swan–Ganz catheter to monitor wedge pressure. Wedge pressure and systemic blood pressure are used to help guide therapy. Administer IV atropine if the patient is bradycardic. A pacemaker is required if significant bradycardia persists. Furosemide 20 mg IV may benefit the patient by decreasing elevated wedge pressure. If the patient is normotensive or hypertensive, administer IV nitroprusside or IV nitroglycerin. Titrate to wedge pressure of 15–18 mm Hg while not allowing systolic blood pressure to fall below 90. If the patient is hypotensive, administer dobutamine or in more urgent cases, dopamine. Nitroprusside may be combined with dobutamine or dopamine in order to optimize wedge pressure and systemic blood pressure. PO vasodilator (e.g. captopril) may be beneficial if the wedge pressure is elevated upon discontinuation of IV therapy.

Acute cardiogenic pulmonary edema: Typical patient is markedly dyspneic, tachypneic, diaphoretic. Pink frothy sputum may be present. Diffuse rales are present. An S3 may be heard if it is not obscured by the breath sounds. Chest x-ray confirms pulmonary edema but there may be a lag before the x-ray becomes positive. **Treatment of acute cardiogenic pulmonary edema:** High flow 100% oxygen is administered via mask. Sit patient upright (preferably with legs dangling) provided that the patient is not hypotensive. The upright position is beneficial because it decreases venous return. Administer morphine sulfate 4–6 mg IV push if hypotension is not present. Morphine alleviates agitation, and reduces venous return by inducing venous dilation. Furosemide 40 mg IV. Larger dose may be required if the patient is already receiving furosemide. Diuretics must be administered cautiously in the patient who without a prior history of CHF and diuretic therapy suddenly develops acute cardiogenic pulmonary edema. This is because the patient may not be fluid overloaded and may therefore be prone to hypotension. For example, a patient with mitral stenosis may develop pulmonary edema in the absence of fluid overload. Antihypertensive therapy is indicated if the blood pressure is elevated and the patient has not responded to foregoing measures. Rotating tourniquets are sometimes helpful. Intubate if patient is obtunded or not responding to conventional measures. Phlebotomy of 300–500 ml is used as last resort and may be especially useful in renal failure patient who cannot respond to diuretics.

RIGHT HEART FAILURE (right heart unable to adequately eject blood so that systemic venous congestion ensues). Left ventricular failure is the most common cause of right heart failure. As the left ventricle fails, the pulmonary arterial pressure rises and the right heart is forced to work harder. Note that dysfunction of the interventricular septum may contribute to failure of right and/or left ventricles. Lung disease (e.g. emphysema) may provoke right heart failure because it may lead to increased pulmonary arterial pressure (see "Pulmonary Hypertension"). Other causes of right heart failure include: right ventricular MI (see "Myocardial Infarction" chapter), sundry congenital heart disorders, pulmonic stenosis or regurgitation, tricuspid regurgitation, tricuspid stenosis. The latter causes right atrial failure. **Diagnosis:** fatigue, jugular venous distension, pitting edema (generally most obvious in the lower legs), hepatomegaly due to hepatic venous congestion. Chronic hepatic venous congestion may in turn lead to cirrhosis and ascites. **Treatment right heart failure:** Remedy the underlying disorder if possible. Administer a diuretic and/or digoxin as indicated. Refer to "Pulmonary Hypertension" for the treatment of right ventricular failure in the setting of lung disease.

BIVENTRICULAR FAILURE most commonly occurs when left ventricular failure leads to right ventricular failure (see above). Cardiomyopathy may lead to biventricular failure but the initial signs are usually those of right heart failure. Constrictive pericarditis also presents as biventricular failure.

Pulmonary Hypertension

Definitions: Pulmonary hypertension (pulmonary arterial hypertension) is defined as pulmonary arterial pressure > 30/15 mm Hg. Chronic cor pulmonale is defined as right ventricular hypertrophy due to a lung disorder–provoked elevation of pulmonary arterial resistance. Definition therefore excludes pulmonary hypertension with right ventricular failure resulting from left heart dysfunction (e.g. left heart failure, mitral valve disease) or congenital heart disease (e.g. anomalies causing left–to–right shunting such as atrial or ventricular septal defect, patent ductus arteriosus). Acute cor pulmonale is defined as dilation and failure of the right side of the heart secondary to acute massive pulmonary embolism.

ACUTE PULMONARY HYPERTENSION WITH ACUTE COR PULMONALE: refer to "Pulmonary Embolism" chapter.

CHRONIC PULMONARY HYPERTENSION DUE TO RESPIRATORY DISORDERS:
Mechanisms: Pulmonary hypertension arises when the pulmonary vascular resistance increases secondary to (1) alveolar hypoxia and/or (2) obliteration or obstruction of pulmonary blood vessels. As pulmonary vascular resistance increases so does the pulmonary arterial pressure. The increased pressure load on the right heart leads to right ventricular hypertrophy (cor pulmonale) which may culminate in right heart failure. Alveolar hypoxia increases pulmonary vascular resistance by inducing pulmonary vasoconstriction. When hypoxia is chronic, the medial smooth muscle of pulmonary arteries/arterioles hypertrophies. Pulmonary vasoconstriction is also induced by acidosis (due to CO_2 retention) especially when hypoxia is present. Alveolar hypoxia may occur when the lungs are normal but ventilation is inadequate (e.g. kyphoscoliosis, decreased ventilatory drive, neuromuscular disease) or when there is disease of the lung itself (e.g. chronic bronchitis, emphysema, scleroderma, primary pulmonary hypertension, pulmonary fibrosis, sarcoidosis). Obliteration of pulmonary vessels (e.g. emphysema, lung resection) increases the pulmonary vascular resistance. However, obliteration alone seldom accounts for significant pulmonary hypertension because a large portion of the vascular bed can be lost without significantly increasing pulmonary vascular resistance. In emphysema (the most common cause of chronic cor pulmonale) for instance, loss of lung tissue reduces the size of the pulmonary capillary bed and does contribute to increased pulmonary vascular resistance. However, alveolar hypoxia is the major factor that induces pulmonary vasoconstriction leading to pulmonary hypertension and cor pulmonale. Obstruction of pulmonary vessels (e.g. pulmonary emboli, sickle cell disease, schistosomiasis, filariasis, interstitial fibrosis) increases pulmonary vascular resistance. Massive pulmonary embolism will cause acute cor pulmonale while recurrent small pulmonary emboli eventually lead to chronic cor pulmonale. Depending on clinical status, roughly 1/2 – 2/3 of the pulmonary vasculature must be occluded before cor pulmonale develops.
Diagnosis: Pulmonary hypertension in its early stages might only be suspected by a loud pulmonic component of S2, and a chest x–ray revealing prominent pulmonary arteries with diminished peripheral vascular markings. As right ventricular hypertrophy (cor pulmonale) develops other signs appear: (1) left parasternal heave, (2) early systolic pulmonic ejection click, (3) systolic ejection murmur that is best heard at the left 2nd interspace, (4) right–sided S4—distinguished from a left–sided S4 by being intensified with inspiration, (5) early diastolic murmur that is best heard on inspiration at the left 2nd interspace (the Graham Steell murmur due to pulmonic regurgitation), (6) EKG signs of right ventricular hypertrophy (e.g. right axis deviation, tall R wave with ST depression and T wave inversion in V1–2) and associated right atrial dilation (tall P waves in II, III, aVF). Note that In many cases of COPD, the EKG signs of right ventricular hypertrophy are obscured because the heart is rotated, and the lungs are hyperinflated with flattened diaphragms. And finally with development of right ventricular failure, additional signs appear : (1) As the right ventricle dilates so does the tricuspid ring. Consequently, there is a holosystolic tricuspid regurgitant murmur, best heard at the lower left sternal border on inspiration. Tricuspid regurgitation is also responsible for the systolic "v" waves that may be seen in the jugular veins and for systolic pulsations that may be felt over the liver. (2) Blood is backed–up in the systemic veins with the following possible consequences: jugular venous

distension, hepatomegaly, ascites, peripheral edema. (3) Chest x-ray: the transverse diameter of heart may be increased as a consequence of dilation of the right heart. This finding is often absent in COPD since the position of the heart is altered in many cases (see above).

Treatment: Treat the underlying disease if possible. Administer oxygen (to reduce pulmonary vasoconstriction) aiming for a PaO2 of $\geq$ 60 mm Hg. However, remember that the patient with chronic lung disease may be relying on hypoxia for his respiratory drive. If necessary, use a Venturi mask set to deliver oxygen at 24 or 28% with an oxygen flow rate of 4 liters/min. A diuretic is indicated if right failure is present. Digoxin is probably not useful in treating cor pulmonale.

PULMONARY HYPERTENSION DUE TO CARDIAC DISORDERS:

Congenital heart defects associated with left–to–right shunting (e.g. patent ductus arteriosus, atrial or ventricular septal defect) may lead to pulmonary hypertension. One or a combination of factors may be responsible for the elevated pulmonary arterial pressure—e.g. increased pulmonary blood flow, hypoxia–induced pulmonary vasoconstricton, hypertrophy of smooth muscle of media of pulmonary arteries, obstruction of pulmonary vessels due to injury–induced changes of intima and media.

Left heart dysfunction (e.g. left ventricular failure, mitral valve disorder) may lead to pulmonary hypertension. The left atrial pressure is elevated and this is reflected back so as to increase pulmonary capillary pressure. When the capillary hydrostatic pressure exceeds the oncotic pressure, fluid leaks into the interstitium leading to an increase in pulmonary vascular resistance by 2 mechanisms: (1) interstitial edema exerts perivascular pressure, (2) prolonged pulmonary interstitial edema leads to perivascular fibrosis. Furthermore, the intima and media of pulmonary vessels undergo alterations that obstruct normal pulmonary blood flow.

PRIMARY PULMONARY HYPERTENSION (pulmonary hypertension of unknown etiology) is a rare and nearly always fatal disease that is most common in females 20–40 yr of age. The diagnosis is made only after excluding other causes of pulmonary hypertension. As the disease progresses and pulmonary arterial pressure rises, cor pulmonale ensues with eventual right ventricular failure. Histology reveals occlusive changes in the arterioles and small pulmonary arteries—e.g. concentric intimal fibrosis ("onion skin" lesion). The pulmonary arterial pressure is elevated while the left atrial pressure and wedge pressure are normal. Some cases are associated with Raynaud's phenomenon and autoimmune disease.

Valvular Heart Disease

MITRAL STENOSIS is almost always due to rheumatic heart disease. Symptoms typically first develop about 20 years after the initial episode of rheumatic fever, and without appropriate therapy progress so that the patient is severely disabled about 7 years after the onset of symptoms. Dyspnea on exertion is usually the only initial complaint. Dyspnea at rest and orthopnea eventually develop and the patient is prone to pulmonary edema—especially with exertion. Dyspnea occurs because progressive mitral stenosis leads to an increase in left atrial pressure which in turn leads to pulmonary venous/capillary congestion. Congestion is made worse by lying flat and by exertion because both increase venous return, and also because exertion-induced tachycardia shortens diastole thereby reducing the time available for the left atrium to empty thru the stenotic mitral valve. Hemoptysis occurs mainly in the early stages of symptomatic mitral disease and is often precipitated by coughing. It is due to rupture of engorged bronchial veins that shunt blood from high pressure pulmonary veins to low pressure systemic veins. In later stages (as heart failure develops and the patient becomes bedridden), the patient is also predisposed to hemoptysis from pulmonary embolization with infarction. Chest pain is present in about 10% patients, usually those with severe pulmonary hypertension (see below). Peripheral cyanosis develops because of low cardiac ouput–induced vasoconstriction. A dusky malar appearance (mitral facies) may be noted. Pulse is characteristically of low amplitude. It is irregular if, as is often the case, atrial fibrillation has developed. Atrial fibrillation predisposes to systemic embolization from left atrial thrombi. Auscultation: (a) loud S1, (b) opening snap—a high pitched sound that occurs just after S2 and is not to be confused with an S3 or a split S2, **(c)** mid–diastolic rumble––a low pitched murmur that starts after the opening snap and is best heard at the apex with the bell of the stethoscope with patient in left lateral decubitus position, **(d)** presystolic murmur (absent if atrial fibrillation has developed). Pulmonary hypertension: Some patients are "protected" from increasing left atrial pressures and attendant pulmonary congestion by constriction of the pulmonary arteries/arterioles. Ensuing pulmonary hypertension leads to right ventricular hypertrophy, Consequ;ently, a heave may be felt at the lower left sternal border and an "a" wave may be seen in the jugular veins (latter also seen with tricuspid stenosis). Right ventricular failure ensues and may manifest as jugular venous distension, peripheral edema, hepatomegaly, and/or ascites. EKG findings: Unless atrial fibrillation has developed, there is usually evidence of left atrial enlargement—e.g. broad and notched P wave (P mitrale) or biphasic P wave. In the presence of severe pulmonary hypertension there will be right axis deviation and other evidence of right ventricular hypertrophy. Possible x–ray findings: ●evidence of left atrial enlargement—e.g. straightening of the left heart border, elevation of left mainstem bronchus, barium swallow showing posterior displacement of esophagus; ●calcified mitral valve occasionally seen; ●evidence of pulmonary arterial hypertension—e.g. enlarged pulmonary artery, right ventricle, and right atrium; ●dilated upper pulmonary veins; ●mottling of lung fields due to hemosideroris from repeated rupture of pulmonary vessels. Echocardiography is confirmatory. **Treatment mitral stenosis:** Anticoagulate if atrial fibrillation present and control ventricular rate as needed with digoxin. Treat right heart failure with diuretics. Symptomatic patients should undergo cardiac catheterization (pressure gradients across the mitral valve are used to determine the size of the valve orifice). Patients with noncalcified valves and without significant mitral regurgitation are candidates for closed valvotomy while others are considered for valve replacement. Surgical intervention is advised before pulmonary hypertension develops.

MITRAL REGURGITATION (mitral insufficiency) can result from: **(1)** rheumatic heart disease; **(2)** valve destruction–e.g. endocarditis; **(3)** myocardial infarction with papillary muscle rupture or dysfunction; **(4)** calcification of the valve ring or annulus (e.g. the elderly, Marfan's syndrome); **(5)** dilation of mitral valve ring secondary to congestive heart failure, hypertension, or aortic stenosis; **(6)** rupture of chordae tendineae—e.g. spontaneous, traumatic, endocarditis; **(7)** mitral valve prolapse syndrome—also known as floppy mitral valve, click–murmur syndrome, Barlow's syndrome, etc.

    Chronic mitral regurgitation (e.g. due to rheumatic heart disease) Symptoms usually evolve slowly over many years—first fatigue, then dyspnea on exertion, finally congestive heart failure. Auscultation: soft or absent S1, apical pansystolic murmur that typically radiates to axilla, widely split S2 due to early closure of aortic valve. Also, there is usually an S3 followed by a short mid–diastolic murrmur due to rapid flow into the left ventricle. Sustained apical ventricular heave is felt at the apex if regurgitation is severe. Chest x–ray reveals enlarged left atrium and ventricle, and sometimes mitral calcification. EKG: There is evidence of left ventricular hypertrophy. P mitrale demonstrates left atrial enlargement (assuming atrial fibrillation has not developed). Treatment: digoxin and reduction of the peripheral vascular resistance (e.g. hydralazine) are used to treat congestive heart failure but refractory cases are candidates for valve replacement.

    Acute mitral regurgitation (e.g. due to rupture of papillary muscle, valve cusp, or chordae) often results in sudden onset of pulmonary edema and shock. Surgery to replace valve is usually required. Refer to "Myocardial Infarction" chapter and find heading *papillary muscle rupture/malfunction*.

    Mitral valve prolapse is the most common cause of mitral regurgitation. It is usually benign. It is more prevalent in females (20% healthy females have echocardiographic evidence of mitral prolapse). Mitral prolapse may also be seen in Marfan's syndrome or may follow an MI. Symptoms: Most cases are asymptomatic but chest pain may occur. Dizziness, syncope, palpitations, or even sudden death may result from arrthythmias. Auscultation: During systole the mitral valve balloons into the left atrium so that there is a mid–systolic click that may or may not be followed by a late systolic murmur. Both the murmur and the click are heard later or may disappear when the left ventricle dilates as when squatting (squatting dilates ventricles by increasing venous return). Conversely, standing or the Valsalva maneuver causes the click and murmur to be heard earlier. Echocardiogram confirms the diagnosis. Treatment: Chest pain is treated with a beta–blocker (e.g. propranolol); nitroglycerin is not effective. Rarely, severe mitral regurgitation occurs and valve replacement is necessary. Endocarditis prophylaxis: There is increased risk of endocarditis. Antibiotic prophylaxis is required for dental or surgical procedures if mitral prolapse is causing mitral regurgitation.

AORTIC STENOSIS is most commonly the result of a congenital bicuspid valve. Aortic stenosis secondary to rheumatic heart disease is the next most common cause. Aortic stenosis may be seen in the elderly as a consequence of aortic sclerosis and calcification; there is a systolic ejection murmur but hemodynamically significant stenosis is not present. Note that systolic murmurs heard in the aortic area may also be due to dilation of the aorta (e.g. from hypertension, syphilis, atherosclerosis) or be due to idiopathic hypertrophic subaortic stenosis. Congenital bicuspid valve is present in about 1% population. Progressive fibrosis and calcification of the valve leads to significant stenosis and symptoms by about 4–5th decade. Rheumatic aortic stenosis is always associated with lesions of other cardiac valves—usually the mitral but occasionally the tricuspid valve. Aortic stenosis and aortic regurgitation frequently coexist. **Diagnosis of aortic stenosis:** Severe aortic stenosis may be present without symptoms but once symptoms develop there is, without surgery, progressive deterioration and death within 5 yr. The classic triad of manifestations are angina, syncope (especially with exertion), and left ventricular failure (e.g. orthopnea, dyspnea on exertion). Auscultation: There is a harsh systolic ejection murmur (accompanied by a thrill) that is best heard at the right 2nd intercostal space or left sternal border, and that radiates to the carotids. Squatting or inspiration, by increasing venous return, intensifies the murmur. Delayed closure of the aortic valve produces reverse splitting of S2 (aortic component follows the pulmonic component) and the aortic component may disappear as the aortic valve calcifies. An early systolic click (due to tension on the aortic cusps as the valve opens) may also be present if the valve is not calcified. An S4 may be heard (due to flow into a noncompliant left ventricle during atrial systole) and there may be an S3 if heart failure has developed. Other physical signs: The pulse is weak and prolonged and the pulse pressure is accordingly narrowed. The apex impulse may be displaced downward and to the left, and may be prolonged and heaving. EKG: There may be evidence of left ventricular hypertrophy. Left bundle branch block and/or nonspecific T wave inversion may be seen. Chest x–ray: Ascending aorta is usually dilated. Left ventricle is not enlarged unless left ventricular failure is present. A calcified aortic valve is often seen. Left heart catheterization: If the peak systolic pressure in the left ventricle exceeds the pressure in the aorta by less than 30 mm Hg, the stenosis is mild. A gradient > 80 mm Hg indicates severe stenosis. **Treatment aortic stenosis:** Angina is alleviated with nitrates. Heart failure may respond to diuretics and digoxin. Surgery is usually delayed until symptoms appear. However, young patients may have severe stenosis in the absence of symptoms, and therefore require catheterization to assess the need for surgery. Commisurotomy may suffice if the valve is not calcified but valve replacement is necessary if it is.

AORTIC REGURGITATION is most commonly due to rheumatic heart disease, congenital defect, endocarditis, aortic dissection. Aortic regurgitation may also be associated with hypertension, syphilis, Marfan's syndrome, trauma, Reiter's syndrome, ankylosing spondylitis, lupus, sinus of Valsalva aneurysm. In chronic aortic regurgitatiion the left ventricle adapts to the increased volume load by hypertrophy and dilation. The dilated ventricle contracts more vigorously as it is stretched (Starling's law) and the stroke volume is therefore increased. Peripheral vasodilation also helps ease the burden of emptying the left ventricle. Eventually these mechanisms fail and heart failure ensues. In acute aortic regurgitation, many of the signs mentioned below may not be present because the left ventricle does not dilate and the peripheral vascular resistance does not fall. Consequently, the volume of aortic regurgitation will not be as great nor will the pulse pressure be widened as much. **Diagnosis of aortic regurgitation:** Symptoms: Many patients with chronic aortic regurgitation (e.g. rheumatic heart disease) remain asymptomatic for years. Dyspnea on exertion is the first symptom to appear. Fatigue, dizziness, and angina may develop. Orthopnea and other manifestations of congestive heart failure are present in advanced cases. <u>Auscultation:</u> There is an early decrescendo diastolic murmur that is best heard at the left sternal border with the patient leaning forward while holding his breath in expiration. If the murmur is the result of dilation of the aortic root (e.g. syphilis, Marfan's, aortic dissection); the murmur may be best heard at the 2nd right intercostal space. ●Regurgitant flow thru the aortic valve may strike the anterior leaflet of the mitral valve causing a diastolic rumble that is best heard at the apex (Austin Flint murmur). This murmur may be confused with the murmur of mitral stenosis. However, the loud S1 and opening snap characteristic of mitral stenosis will be absent. ●A systolic ejection murmur may also be present and indicates either increased flow across the aortic valve, or (as in the case of rheumatic heart disease) coexisting aortic stenosis. ●With the bell of the stethoscope, a to–and–fro murmur is heard over the femoral artery (Duroziez's sign) and "pistol shot" sounds are also audible here. <u>Other physical signs:</u> There is a wide pulse pressure with an abnormally low diastolic pressure and an elevated systolic pressure. The rapid rise and fall in arterial pressure causes a collapsing or "water–hammer" pulse which can best be demonstrated by palpating the radial pulse with the patient's arm held overhead. The patient's head may nod with each heart beat and the arterial pulse may be visible on the neck. Capillary pulsations may be visible on transillumination of the nail-beds (Quincke's pulse). <u>Chest x-ray:</u> enlarged boot shaped left ventricle, dilated ascending aorta. <u>EKG:</u> signs of left ventricular hypertrophy. **Treatment aortic regurgitation:** A patient who is deteriorating rapidly (e.g. bacterial endocarditis) urgently requires valve replacement. Patient's with chronic aortic regurgitation who become symptomatic can sometimes be managed with diuretics and digoxin. However, valve replacement should be considered if more than mild diuresis is required to control heart failure. Without surgery, a poor prognosis is also likely if the pulse pressure exceeds 100 mm Hg or if chest x-ray reveals more than mild left ventriclar enlargement.

TRICUSPID REGURGITATION may result from dilation of the tricuspid ring secondary to dilation of right ventricle in patient with right ventricular failure. Tricuspid regurgitation is also a complication of bacterial endocarditis (usually resulting from IV drug abuse or IV catheter–induced septic phlebitis) or rheumatic heart disease. **Diagnosis:** A holosystolic murmur is present at the lower left sternal border; it is intensified by inspiration and squatting (both maneuvers increase venous return and thereby increase flow across the tricuspid valve). ●The murmur may be confused with mitral regurgitation. However, in the case of mitral regurgitation: (1) the murmur radiates to the axilla and is not intensified by inspiration, (2) systolic venous pulsations are not seen in the neck. ●A diastolic murmur (due to increased flow across tricuspid valve) may also be associated with tricuspid regurgitation. ●Systolic pulsations may be seen in the neck veins and felt over the liver. ●Jugular venous distension, hepatomegaly, ascites, peripheral edema, and/or pleural effusion may develop as the disease progresses. **Treatment:** Diuretics and/or digoxin may suffice. Valve replacement is necessary in severe cases or if drug therapy fails.

TRICUSPID STENOSIS is almost always due to rheumatic heart disease. There is usually concomitant disease of the mitral valve (particularly mitral stenosis) and/or aortic valve. **Diagnosis:** A mid–diastolic and a late diastolic murmur are heard at the lower left sternal border. Both are intensified with inspiration. An 'a' wave due to atrial contraction may be seen in the neck veins (not present if there is atrial fibrillation). As stenosis progresses; hepatomegaly, ascites, cirrhosis, and peripheral edema develop. EKG reveals tall P waves (indicative of right atrial enlargement) if atrial fibrillation has not developed. Chest x-ray demonstrates enlargement of the right atrium and superior vena cava. **Treatment:** Severe stenosis usually dictates valve replacement.

PULMONIC STENOSIS is usually congenital. Other causes include rheumatic heart disease, hypertrophic cardiomyopathy, carcinoid of the small intestine. **Diagnosis:** There is an early systolic ejection click followed by a mid–systolic murmur (accompanied by a thrill) best heard at the left 2nd interspace. The 2nd heart sound may be widely split. As the right ventricle hypertrophies, "a" waves are seen in the neck veins as a consequence of forceful atrial contraction. Right ventricular hypertrophy is demonstrated by a left parasternal heave and EKG signs. Chest x-ray may also reveal right ventricular enlargement as well as post-stenotic dilation of the pulmonary artery. **Treatment:** valvotomy if the stenosis is severe.

PULMONIC REGURGITATION is most often secondary to pulmonary hypertension. It may also be congenital or result from infective endocarditis. At the left 2nd interspace, one may hear an early diastolic murmur that is louder on inspiration (Graham Steel murmur).

Rheumatic Fever is an inflammatory disease that follows infection by

group A beta-hemolytic streptococci. The syndrome usually develops 10-20 days after the onset of the infection. It is a sequel to < 1% cases of streptococcal pharyngitis. It is most common between 5-15 yr (peak 8 yr, rare < 4 yr, uncommon > 18 yr).

Diagnosis is guided by the modified Jones criteria which designates major and minor criteria. The major criteria are carditis (endocarditis, myocarditis, and/or pericarditis); polyarthritis; chorea; subcutaneous nodules; erythema multiforme. Minor criteria include fever, arthralgia, history of rheumatic fever or rheumatic heart disease, prolonged PR interval, elevated sedimentation rate or C-reactive protein. Rheumatic fever is likely if there is evidence of a recent streptococcal infection together with (a) two of the major manifestations or (b) one of the major and 2 of the minor manifestations. Laboratory tests: Leukocytosis, elevated sedimentation rate, and elevated C-reactive protein are present but are nonspecific. Specific evidence of streptococcal infection is provided by a positive throat culture or specific antibody tests-e.g. antistreptolysin O (ASO), antistreptokinase, antihyaluronidase, anti-DNAase B. Migratory polyarthritis is common. The joints (usually the large joints) are often warm, red, swollen. Myocarditis characteristically manifests as tachycardia that persists after the fever subsides. The PR interval may be prolonged. Rarely, congestive heart failure occurs. Endocarditis may present with an apical mid-diastolic mitral regurgitant murmur (Carey Coombs murmur). Less often there is an aortic diastolic murmur. Tricuspid involvement is uncommon and pulmonic rare. Pericarditis sometimes occurs and a pericardial effusion can develop (refer to section on pericarditis). Erythema marginatum (nonpruritic evanescent rash of the trunk and limbs) is rare. Subcutaneous nodules are rare. They are painless and are usually seen on the extensor surfaces of the knees, elbows, and knuckles. Sydenham's chorea (nonrepetitive purposeless movements) is rare. Its appearance may be delayed up to 6 months after the streptococcal infection.

Treatment: Antibiotic: Once rheumatic fever is diagnosed, 1.2 million units of benzathine penicillin is administered IM to eradicate group A streptococci. A 10 day course of erythromycin is indicated if patient is allergic to penicillin. Aspirin: In the absence of carditis, aspirin is administered to control symptoms. Corticosteroids are indicated if carditis develops (e.g. prednisone 40 mg/day initially and subsequently titrated to effect). Prednisone may need to be continued for several weeks, then gradually tapered and discontinued. Neither aspirin nor corticosteroids alter the development of chronic valvular disease. Diuretics and/or digoxin are used if heart failure is present.

Prophylaxis against group A streptococcal infections is essential to prevent recurrences of rheumatic fever. The usual regimen is 1.2 million units (600,000 unit in child < 25 kg) benzathine penicillin IM monthly or penicillin VK 250 mg PO bid. Use erythromycin if patient is allergic to penicillin. Chronic prophylaxis is often discontinued at 18 yr of age, but continued prophylaxis is advised if there is cardiac damage. Also, patients with rheumatic valvular disease must receive antibiotic prophylaxis against bacterial endocarditis when they undergo dental, surgical, or certain other procedures (see "Infective Endocarditis" chapter).

Congenital Heart Disease (CHD)

VENTRICULAR SEPTAL DEFECT (VSD) is responsible for about 30% cases of CHD at birth. Blood is shunted from the left ventricle to the right ventricle. Large defects lead to heart failure and often cause death in infancy. Some may not become symptomatic until early adulthood; while small defects may remain asymptomatic and be compatible with a normal life span. **Diagnosis:** Infants with large VSD present with signs of heart failure. The adult initially complains of fatigue and dyspnea which then progresses to CHF. Auscultation: A pansystolic murmur is usually present and it is best heard at the lower left sternal border. The murmur is accentuated by squatting. A thrill is sometimes felt between the apex and the left sternal border. Increased flow thru the mitral valve may result in an apical mid-diastolic murmur. Chest x-ray, in the case of a large VSD, shows an enlarged left atrium and ventricles as well as prominent pulmonary vessels. Cardiac catheterization reveals, if the defect is sufficiently large, a step-up in oxygen saturation from right atrium to right ventricle. Injection of contrast dye confirms the VSD. Pulmonary hypertension develops in some patients. If the pulmonary vascular resistance is sufficiently high, the shunt reverses to right-to-left (Eisenmenger's syndrome) and cyanosis is usually present. **Treatment:** Some defects are clinically insignificant; some may close spontaneously. Surgery is indicated for large left-to-right shunts. However, surgery is not helpful once significant pulmonary hypertension has developed.

ATRIAL SEPTAL DEFECT (ASD) accounts for about 10% cases of CHD at birth. Blood is shunted from the left atrium to the right atrium. Two types of ASD: Ostium primum defects are located low in the atrial septum near the AV valves. The more common ostium secundum defect is located in the area of the fossa ovalis. **Diagnosis:** Auscultation: Delayed closure of the pulmonic valve causes wide splitting of the 2nd heart sound. The degree of splitting is not altered by respiration. Increased flow thru the pulmonic valve causes a systolic ejection murmur that is best heard at the left 2nd interspace. If the atrial septal defect is large, there is a mid-diastolic murmur (accentuated by inspiration) at the lower left sternal border due to increased flow across the tricuspid valve. With the ostium primum defect, there may be an abnormality of the mitral valve resulting in an apical systolic mitral regurgitant murmur. EKG shows evidence of right ventricular hypertrophy (rsR pattern in V1). There is right axis deviation with ostium secundum defects and left axis deviation with ostium primum defects. Chest x-ray shows slight cardiomegaly, small aortic knob, large pulmonary artery, and prominent pulmonary vasculature. Echocardiography reveals the location of the defect, abnormal motion of the ventricular septum, and an enlarged right ventricle and right atrium. Cardiac catheterization (usually not needed to confirm the diagnosis) shows oxygen saturation of right atrium > oxygen saturation of superior vena cava. Furthermore, the catheter may pass thru the ASD to the left atrium. Pulmonary hypertension is an uncommon development. If the pulmonary vascular resistance is sufficiently high, the shunt reverses to right-to-left (Eisenmenger's syndrome) and cyanosis is usually present. **Treatment:** surgery. However, surgery is contraindicated if right-to-left shunting has developed.

PATENT DUCTUS ARTERIOSUS (PDA) accounts for about 10% cases of CHD at birth. There is a left-to-right shunt: blood is shunted from the high pressure aorta to the low pressure pulmonary artery during both systole and diastole. **Diagnosis:** Auscultation: The murmur of PDA is termed continuous. However, it is usually not present throughout systole and diastole. For instance: it may start in systole, continue thru the 2nd heart sound, and end in diastole. The murmur is heard at the left sternal border 2nd interspace. The murmur will be absent if pulmonary hypertension has developed. Large shunts cause substantial increases in blood flow thru the lungs. This additional blood return to the left heart causes increased flow across the mitral valve which may be detected as an apical mid-diastolic murmur. Wide pulse pressure and a bounding pulse is characteristic if the shunt is large. Chest x-ray: Large shunts are associated with an enlarged aortic knob, pulmonary artery, and left ventricle. Pulmonary vessels are prominent. EKG is normal with small shunts. Signs of left ventricular hypertrophy may be seen with larger shunts. Signs of right ventricular hypertrophy may be present if pulmonary hypertension has developed. Echocardiography shows the shunt and reveals dilated left atrium, left ventricle, and aorta. Congestive heart failure may develop in infancy if the shunt is large. Pulmonary hypertension develops in some patients. This may eventually cause the shunt to reverse to right-to-left (Eisenmenger's syndrome) with ensuing cyanosis. However, in contrast to patients with ASD or VSD who develop Eisenmenger's syndrome, cyanosis is confined to the lower extremities since the right-to-left shunt is directed into the descending aorta (i.e. distal to the left subclavian artery). **Treatment:** Spontaneous closure may occur. Otherwise, surgical closure of ductus is generally advised unless Eisenmenger's syndrome has developed. In premature infants, surgery can sometimes be avoided if closure of the PDA can be achieved by IV injection of indomethacin.

PULMONIC STENOSIS accounts for about 7% cases of CHD at birth. Pulmonic stenosis is characterized by right ventricular hypertrophy and, if stenosis is severe, by right ventricular failure. **Diagnosis:** Symptoms: Depending on the degree of stenosis, the patient may be asymptomatic or be subject to dyspnea and/or syncope. Auscultation: There is a systolic ejection murmur—best heard at the left 2nd interspace. If stenosis is severe, the murmur is accompanied by a thrill in the same area. The murmur is sometimes preceded by a systolic ejection click. ●The 2nd heart sound varies according to the degree of stenosis: the more severe the stenosis—the more widely split the 2nd heart sound (wide splitting is due to delayed closure of pulmonic valve) and the softer the pulmonic component. In severe stenosis, it may not be possible to detect splitting of the 2nd heart sound because the pulmonic component is not audible. Other physical signs: Moderate-severe stenosis is associated with large presystolic jugular "a" waves and a parasternal right ventricular lift. EKG may be normal when stenosis is mild. With greater stenosis one may see evidence of right atrial enlargement (prominent P waves) and right ventricular enlargement. Chest x-ray demonstrates post-stenotic dilation of the pulmonary artery. Enlargement of the right atrium and right ventricle may also be seen with more stenotic valves. In severe stenosis, there is decreased pulmonary vascularity. Echocardiography reveals doming of the pulmonic valve leaflets into the pulmonary arterial trunk during systole. When stenosis is severe, right atrial dilation and hypertrophy of the right ventricle is also observed. Cardiac catheterization is used to assess the severity of obstruction by measuring the pressure drop across the pulmonic valve. **Treatment:** Mild stenosis may be left untreated. However, antibiotic prophylaxis against endocarditis is advised. Valvotomy or balloon valvuloplasty is indicated if the pressure drop across the pulmonic valve is > 50 mm Hg.

TETRALOGY of FALLOT is present in about 6% cases of CHD at birth. The main features are pulmonary stenosis and ventricular septal defect. There is also right ventricular hypertrophy and the aorta overrides the ventricular septal defect. Dyspnea and cyanosis results because pulmonary stenosis restricts blood flow to the lungs and because blood is shunted thru the ventricular septal defect (i.e. right-to-left shunt). In children, exercise-induced dyspnea is typically relieved by squatting. Squatting compresses the abdominal aorta and femoral arteries thereby increasing peripheral vascular resistance so that there is a decrease in right–left shunting. Depending on the severity of the pulmonary stenosis, cyanosis may develop soon after birth or be delayed until later in infancy or childhood. If pulmonary stenosis is not severe, blood may be shunted left-to-right and cyanosis will not be present. Syncope may occur. Arterial pulses are decreased in amplitude. Clubbing of the digits is common. Auscultation: There is a systolic ejection murmur (sometimes accompanied by a thrill) at the 2nd–3rd left interspace. With severe pulmonic stenosis, the 2nd heart sound has only one component because the pulmonic component is not audible. Chest x-ray reveals a boot-shaped cardiac silhouette due to the reduced size of the pulmonary artery. EKG: right axis deviation, right ventricular hypertrophy. Echocardiography shows pulmonic stenosis, ventricular septal defect, ventricular hypertrophy, and overriding aorta. Cardiac catheterization confirms the ventricular septal defect and pulmonic stenosis. Polycythemia ensues from chronic hypoxia. **Treatment** consists of fixing both the pulmonary stenosis and the ventricular septal defect. However, this procedure is often delayed until after infancy. In the meantime, if there is severe hypoxia, a shunt is created between the systemic and pulmonary circuits in order to increase blood flow to the lungs—e.g. Blalock (shunt between subclavian artery and pulmonary artery), Waterston (shunt between aorta and right pulmonary artery).

TRANSPOSITION of GREAT ARTERIES (the aorta arises from the right ventricle and the pulmonary artery arises from the left ventricle) is present in about 4% cases of CHD at birth and is the most frequent cardiac cause of cyanosis at birth. Signs of heart failure develop in the neonatal period. Transposition results in separate systemic and pulmonary circulations. Consequently, survival demands there be (and there usually is) a shunt between the two circulations (e.g. persistent foramen ovale, atrial septal defect, ventricular septal defect, patent ductus arteriosus). Echocardiography confirms the diagnosis. Treatment: Balloon septostomy to create a large atrial septal defect is a palliative measure performed when the anomaly is diagnosed. Definitive surgery is performed later.

COARCTATION of AORTA accounts for about 7% cases of CHD at birth (see discussion under "Hypertension" chapter).

CONGENITAL BICUSPID AORTIC VALVE See aortic stenosis in "Valvular Heart Disease" chapter.

Cardiomyopathy (disease of the heart muscle) by definition excludes the presence of the following: (a) heart disease involving the coronary vessels, cardiac valves, or pericardium; (b) systemic hypertension; (c) intracardiac shunt; (d) extracardiac arteriovenous fistula. There are 3 categories of cardiomyopathy: congestive, restrictive, and hypertrophic.

CONGESTIVE (DILATED) CARDIOMYOPATHY is characterized by both left and right heart failure. Both ventricles are dilated. The ventricles contract weakly. Consequently, cardiac output is low and the pulse is weak. There may be manifestations of both left heart failure (e.g. elevated left atrial pressure, dyspnea, orthopnea, pulmonary edema) and right heart failure (e.g. elevated right atrial pressure, peripheral edema, jugular venous distension). Auscultation: An S3 and/or S4 are often heard. Because the mitral and tricuspid rings dilate as the ventricles dilate, holosystolic mitral and/or holosystolic tricuspid regurgitatant murmurs are also often heard. EKG findings may include ectopic beats, atrial fibrillation, nonspecific ST and T wave abnormalities, Q waves, axis deviation. **Etiology:** idiopathic; familial; toxins (alcohol, doxorubicin, cobalt); radiation; infection (e.g. Coxsackie B, Chagas' disease); peripartum; hemochromatosis; sarcoidosis; neuromuscular disease (muscular dystrophy, Friedreich's ataxia, myotonia atrophica); beriberi; starvation; thyrotoxicosis; etc. **Treatment congestive cardiomyopathy:** (1) diuretics as needed, (2) digoxin is sometimes helpful, (3) anticoagulate—unless there is contraindication—in order to prevent pulmonary or systemic thromboembolism. Other recommendations: (1) Cardiomyopathy may resolve spontaneously if patient with alcoholic cardiomyopathy abstains from alcohol. (2) Patient with hemochromatosis will benefit from periodic phlebotomy. (3) Sarcoid cardiomyopathy may be helped by corticosteroids. (4) Peripartum cardiomyopathy patient should be warned against future pregnancies.

RESTRICTIVE CARDIOMYOPATHY in the U.S. is almost always due to primary amyloidosis. Other causes include endomyocardial fibrosis, Löffler's endocarditis, Fabry's disease, sarcoidosis.

    Primary amyloidosis Amyloid infiltration of the myocardium results in a clinical picture mimicking constrictive pericarditis. The ventricles are noncompliant. Consequently, filling of the ventricles during diastole is *restricted*. The left and right atrial pressures are high because the atria are not able to adequately empty into the non-compliant ventricles. This leads to pulmonary and systemic venous congestion. In contrast to congestive cardiomyopathy, the ventricles are not greatly dilated. **Diagnosis:** Physical exam is similar to constrictive pericarditis: distended neck veins that swell with inspiration (Kussmaul sign), hepatomegaly, ascites, peripheral edema, small-amplitude pulse. EKG abnormalities are common—e.g. low voltage QRS, left axis deviation, Q waves, bundle branch block, ectopic beats. Chest x-ray: Heart may be enlarged but not to the extent seen with congestive cardiomyopathy. The presence of pericardial calcification suggests constrictive pericarditis rather than amyloid cardiomyopathy. Catheterization discloses characteristic atrial (M-shaped waveform) and ventricular (square root sign) pressure recordings. Echocardiography demonstrates generalized thickening of the cardiac walls and cardiac valves as well as a characteristic "sparkling" detail to the myocardium. Rectal biopsy will usually confirm amyloidosis. Cardiac biopsy is seldom required.

Endomyocardial fibrosis is a form of restrictive cardiomyopathy that is not uncommon in equatorial regions. The endocardium and the inner portion of the myocardium are replaced by fibrous tissue. The ventricles become noncompliant as in amyloidosis. The fibrosis may be exuberant enough to fill the ventricles. Surgery is the only therapy.

HYPERTROPHIC OBSTRUCTIVE CARDIOMYOPATHY (idiopathic hypertrophic subaortic stenosis [IHSS]).

There is left ventricular hypertrophy. Hypertrophy may be particularly pronounced in the ventricular septum (asymmetric septal hypertrophy) or involve both septum and left ventricle free wall (concentric hypertrophy). There is impaired diastolic filling of the noncompliant left ventricle. There is obstruction of left ventricular outflow tract because during systole the mitral valve opens with the anterior leaflet moving against the septum. Histology: In patients with obstruction, bizarre and disorganized muscle cells are found, primarily in the septum. Histology of nonobstructed patients reveals similar findings in both septum and left ventricular free wall. Familial association is found in about 30% patients. Symptoms: Many patients are asymptomatic and a murmur or an abnormal EKG are the only clues. Other patients present with dyspnea, angina, palpitations, exertional syncope, sudden death. Auscultation: (**1**) There is a systolic ejection murmur best heard at the lower left sternal border. In contrast to aortic valvular stenosis, the murmur is heard poorly over the carotids. The obstruction and therefore the murmur is lessened by measures that dilate the left ventricle (e.g. squatting, fluid administration, hand grip) or decrease the force of contraction (e.g. propranolol). Conversely-standing, Valsalva maneuver, diuresis, hypotension, nitrates, digoxin, or isoproterenol intensify the murmur. (**2**) Often there is a holosystolic mitral regurgitant murmur. (**3**) An S4 is usually present due to atrial contraction against the noncompliant ventricle. Other physical signs: The pulse has an abrupt upstroke because of forceful contraction of the hypertrophied ventricle. Occasionally a thrill can be felt at the lower left sternal border. A jugular venous "a" wave may be seen—due to restricted filling of the right ventricle. EKG: signs of septal hypertrophy (deep Q waves in II, III, aVF, V5–6); signs of left ventricular hypertrophy. Echocardiography shows septal hypertrophy and systolic anterior motion of anterior leaflet of mitral valve. Cardiac catheterization: An elevated left ventricular end-diastolic pressure is often observed. A subvalvular pressure gradient is characteristic. **Treatment hypertrophic obstructive cardiomyopathy:** beta blockade (e.g. propranolol). Patients not improved by beta blockade are candidates for surgery. Avoid: digoxin or other inotropic agents, nitrates, vigorous diuresis or other measures that significantly reduce the blood pressure or intravascular volume. **Endocarditis prophylaxis** is advised. See "Infective Endocarditis" chapter.

Infective Endocarditis (infection of the endocardium—

primarily the heart valves) may be due to bacteria or fungi. Bacterial endocarditis is divided into 2 types: acute and subacute. Acute bacterial endocarditis (ABE) leads to rapid destruction of the involved heart valve(s) while subacute bacterial endocarditis (SBE) wreaks its effects over weeks to months. **Pathogens:** The most common agent causing ABE is Staphylococcus aureus (50–70% cases) while SBE is most commonly due to alpha–hemolytic streptococci (S. viridans). However, either is capable of causing ABE or SBE. Group D streptococci (e.g. S. faecalis, S. bovis) are also a common cause of endocarditis. Gram–negative aerobic (especially pseudomonas) and fungal endocarditis (e.g. Candida albicans, aspergilla) are common in IV drug abusers and in patients with prosthetic valves, but are otherwise rare. Staphylococcus epidermidis is rare except in patients with prosthetic valves. **Risk factors:** Both ABE and SBE are most likely to occur in patients with history of rheumatic valve disease; prosthetic heart valve; or congenital heart anomaly (e.g. ventricular septal defect, persistent ductus arteriosus, pulmonic stenosis, bicuspid aortic valve, coarctation of aorta, mitral valve prolapse). The majority of patients with either ABE or SBE have a pre–existing cardiac lesion (over 90% SBE patients have pre–existing lesion). The mitral and aortic valves are the most common targets of infection. However, there is an increased incidence of right heart endocarditis (usually of tricuspid valve) in the following circumstances: IV drug abuser, catheter–induced septic phlebitis, ventricular septal defect, patent ductus arteriosus.

Diagnosis: Consider the following to have endocarditis until proven otherwise: (1) unexplained fever in patient with pre–existing cardiac disease, (2) patient with fever and newly discovered or changing murmur, (3) patient with bacteremia due to S. aureus. Common manifestations include fever; malaise; murmur; petechiae (of skin, mucous membranes, conjunctiva, retina, or under fingernails [splinter hemorrhage]); splenomegaly; hematuria; albuminuria; arthralgia. Patients with SBE not infrequently present with only nonspecific complaints (e.g. fever, chills, sweats, weight loss). Uncommon manifestations include clubbing, Janeway lesions (painless hemorrhagic nodular lesions on palms and soles), Roth spots (hemorrhagic retinal areas with pale centers), Osler's nodes (tender red indurated nodes on the pads of fingers or toes). Complications of embolization: Emboli to the spleen, liver, or GI tract may lead to infarction of these organs, and so the presenting picture may be that of an acute abdomen. Kidney infarcts and abscesses are also common. Emboli to the brain may result in TIA, stroke (due to infarction or bleeding), brain abscess, meningitis, seizures. (Note that the latter may also result from high–dose penicillin therapy.) Septic emboli–induced mycotic aneurysms may rupture with ensuing intracranial bleeding. The increased risk of bleeding complications is the rationale for generally avoiding anticoagulation in setting of endocarditis. Myocardial invasion: Besides valvular destruction with ensuing heart failure, extension of the infection into the adjacent myocardium with abscess formation may interrupt the conduction system and cause bundle branch block (e.g. invasion of interventricular septum from aortic valve) or AV block (e.g. invasion of AV node or His bundle from mitral valve). Pulmonary embolization with pneumonia is a not uncommon complication of right heart endocarditis. Consequences of antibody response to infection: Formation of immune complexes may result in arthritis, glomerulonephritis (occasionally leading to renal failure), and possibly Osler's nodes and Janeway lesions. Laboratory: There is usually leukocytosis with left shift. There may be hematuria, albuminuria, elevated sedimentation rate, normochromic normocytic anemia, positive rheumatoid factor. Echocardiography may identify valvular vegetations down to 2 mm in diameter. Vegetations may persist for months or years after eradication of infection.

Treatment: Acute bacterial endocarditis: Obtain 3 sets of blood cultures at 15 minute intervals and then immediately start IV antibiotics. A set should include a culture for both aerobic and anaerobic bacteria as well as fungi. Incubate cultures for at least 14 days. The drugs of choice for acute bacterial endocarditis pending culture results are a combination of a penicillinase–resistant penicillin (oxacillin or nafcillin), penicillin G, and an aminoglycoside (gentamycin or tobramycin). Therapy is continued for 4–6 wk (e.g. 4 wk IV and 2 wk PO) with antibiotic choice modified according to therapeutic response and culture results. Subacute bacterial endocarditis: Prior to initiating antibiotics, obtain 3 sets of blood cultures (aeorbic, anaerobic, fungal) at intervals of 15 minutes or more. Start specific IV antibiotic therapy in 24 hr if cultures are positive. If cultures are negative after 24 hr, obtain 2 more sets of cultures and begin IV therapy with penicillin G combined with an aminoglycoside (gentamycin or tobramycin). Continue antibiotic for 6 wk (e.g. 4 wk IV and 2 wk PO) and modify as needed when culture results become available. Surgery is considered in following circumstances: progressive congestive heart failure and/or valve destruction, prosthetic valve endocarditis, uncontrolled infection, multiple embolic episodes, abscess or aneurysm of sinus of Valsalva.

Endocarditis prophylaxis is advised for patients undergoing surgery or certain other procedures if any of the following cardiac lesions are present: rheumatic or other acquired valve disease, prosthetic heart valve, most congenital heart anomalies, hypertrophic cardiomyopathy, prolapse mitral valve syndrome–associated mitral regurgitation. Note: (1) Patients with prosthetic heart valves, rheumatic valvular disease, or history of endocarditis should receive parenterally administered antibiotic. (2) Pediatric doses should not exceed recommended adult doses.
If there is no history of penicillin allergy, recommended options include:
●Amoxicillin 3 grams (50 mg/kg in child) PO 1 hour prior to procedure followed by 1.5 grams (25 mg/kg in child) PO 6 hours later.
●Ampicillin 2 gram (50 mg/kg in child) IV or IM 30 minutes prior to procedure plus gentamycin 1.5 mg/kg (2 mg/kg in child) IV or IM 30 minutes prior to procedure. A repeat dose of ampicillin and gentamycin is usually administered 8 hour later to patients undergoing GI or GU procedures, or otherwise considered to be at increased risk for bacteremia.
If there is a history of penicillin allergy and the patient is undergoing a dental or upper respiratory tract procedure, recommended options are:
●Erythromycin 1 gram (20 mg/kg in child) PO 2 hours prior to procedure followed by 500 mg (10 mg/kg in child) PO 6 hours later.
●Vancomycin 1 gram (20 mg/kg in child) IV infused over 60 min starting 1 hour before procedure.
If there is a history of penicillin allergy and the patient is undergoing a GI or GU procedure: Vancomycin 1 gram (20 mg/kg in child) IV infused over 60 min starting 1 hour prior to procedure plus gentamycin 1.5 mg/kg (2 mg/kg in child) IV or IM 30 minutes prior to procedure.

Pericardial Disease (acute pericarditis, chronic constrictive pericarditis, pericardial effusion/tamponade)

ACUTE PERICARDITIS **Causes:** infection (viral, bacterial, fungal, parasitic); rheumatic fever; autoimmmune (e.g. lupus, rheumatoid arthritis); neoplasia (usually metastatic, rarely primary mesothelioma); uremia; myxedema; mediastinal irradiation (pericarditis may ensue several months after radiation); allergic/hypersensitivity; blunt chest trauma. ●Transmural myocardial infarction–associated pericarditis may be responsible for chest pain that ensues 1–3 days after MI. Pericarditis may also develop weeks to months following an MI (Dressler's syndrome) or cardiac surgery.
Diagnosis: Pain of pericarditis is generally substernal and may radiate to the shoulders. It is usually sharp but may be aching. It may be aggravated by inspiration, coughing, lying flat, moving, or swallowing. Pain may be absent in uremic or tuberculous pericarditis. Friction rub is often present. Typically, it is best heard on expiration at the left lower sternal border with the patient leaning forward. The rub has a scratchy quality that results from movement of the inflamed visceral and parietal layers of the pericardium against each other. The rub may have 1, 2, or 3 components. When 3 components are heard (presystolic, systolic, diastolic); they are due respectively to atrial systole, ventricular systole, and ventricular diastole. When only 1 component is heard, it is due to ventricular systole. The rub may disappear if a pericardial effusion develops. History of fever and upper respiratory infection suggests viral pericarditis. EKG resembles that seen in an acute MI in some respects (ST segment elevation, T wave inversion) but is unlike an MI in that: (**1**) PR segments are often depressed, (**2**) ST elevations are widespread rather than in a few leads, (**3**) ST elevations are concave upward (lead III may be an exception) in contrast to concave downwards in an MI, (**4**) T wave inversion appears only after the ST segment returns to baseline, (**5**) Q waves are generally absent. Arrhythmias are common (usually supraventricular). Chest x-ray is obtained to rule out pneumonia, and

primary or metastatic lung tumor as the cause of pericarditis. An enlarged cardiac silhouette may suggest an associated pericardial effusion. Echocardiography will detect a pericardial effusion. Laboratory: As circumstances suggest, obtain tuberculin skin test, viral antibody tests, blood cultures, and/or ANA. **Treatment:** Viral pericarditis is usually brief and self-limited. Aspirin or some other nonsteroidal anti--inflammatory drug is administered. A short course of corticosteroid may be helpful if symptoms are prolonged. Dressler's syndrome or postsurgical syndromes are treated with aspirin or other nonsteroidal anti–inflammatory agent. A short course of a corticosteroid is sometimes necessary. Anticoagulants are avoided. Pericarditis that occurs within the first few days of MI is treated with aspirin or some other non-steroidal drug. Corticosteroids should not be used to treat this type of pericarditis. Anticoagulants are avoided. Bacterial pericarditis is treated with appropriate antibiotic. Surgical drainage of purulent fluid may be necessary. Uremic pericarditis usually resolves with dialysis. Lupus–associated pericarditis is treated with corticosteroids.

CHRONIC CONSTRICTIVE PERICARDITIS, the cause of which is often unknown, may be due to persistent inflammation by the same factors that cause acute pericarditis (e.g. infection, trauma, autoimmune, hemopericardium). The pericardium adheres to the myocardium forming a nondistensible capsule that prevents adequate filling of the ventricles during diastole and thus impedes venous return. The systemic venous pressure is elevated leading to peripheral edema, ascites (as liver becomes congested), protein losing enteropathy (as lymphatic return from the gut is impeded). Cardiac output is decreased but there is a compensatory tachycardia. Pulmonary edema is rare. Nephrotic syndrome may develop. **Diagnosis:** Kussmaul sign (distended neck veins that swell with inspiration), enlarged liver (may be obscured by associated ascites), peripheral edema, small–amplitude pulse, Auscultation; muffled 1st and 2nd heart sounds, S3 "knock" (early diastolic sound due to rapid ventricular filling that is best heard at lower sternal border). Chest x–ray usually shows a small or normal sized heart. However, the heart silhouette may be enlarged if there is pericardial effusion or myocardial disease. Chest x-ray reveals pericardial calcification in about half the cases (fluoroscopy reveals calcification in > 3/4th cases). EKG: P mitrale, atrial fibrillation (1/3 cases), low voltage QRS, flat or inverted T waves (the deeper the T wave inversion the more firmly adherent the pericardium to the myocardium). Echocardiography may show thickening of pericardium, and/or decreased size of ventricular chambers with enlarged atrial chambers. Cardiac catheterization may be diagnostically helpful but constrictive cardiomyopathy may demonstrate a similar pressure profile (i.e. elevated left and right atrial pressure, elevated right and left ventricular end diastolic pressure, elevated pulmonary artery pressure). **Treatment:** surgery to strip pericardium from myocardium.

PERICARDIAL EFFUSION may be due to heart failure or pericarditis. **Diagnosis:** Heart sounds may be muffled and a pericardial friction rub is sometimes heard. Signs and symptoms of pericardial tamponade may be present (see below). EKG may reveal low voltage QRS, ST segment elevation, electrical alternans, and sometimes total alternans. In the latter, alternate beats show decrease amplitude of P and QRS. Total alternans suggests a malignant effusion. Chest x-ray: Effusions > 250 ml enlarge the cardiac silhouette and may give it a globular outline. Echocardiography confirms diagnosis. Pericardiocentesis establishes the nature of the effusion.

PERICARDIAL TAMPONADE (compression of the heart from accumulation of pericardial fluid) results from blood in the pericardium (trauma, aortic dissection, neoplasia) or from effusions (see above). ●If there is sufficient pericardial fluid present to prevent the ventricles from filling adequately, the stroke volume falls (narrow pulse pressure and weak pulse) and venous return is impeded (distended neck veins). Cardiac output is maintained by a compensatory tachycardia. When this fails, hypotension and shock ensue. ●If the accumulation of pericardial fluid is slow, the parietal pericardium may stretch sufficiently so that tamponade is delayed or avoided. In this manner, large amounts of pericardial fluid are sometimes accomodated without causing tamponade. However, rapid accumulations of fluid may quickly lead to shock and require prompt treatment. **Diagnosis:** Signs may include muffled heart sounds, distended neck veins (absent if patient hypovolemic), tachycardia, weak pulse, narrow pulse pressure, hypotension, pulsus paradoxus (inspiratory fall in systolic pressure > 10 mm Hg). Echocardiography will show the effusion. However, this procedure should not delay emergency pericardiocentesis if that is clinically indicated. **Treatment:** pericardiocentesis via subxyphoid route. The V lead of the EKG is attached to the needle hub. ST segment elevation or QRS widening will occur if the myocardium is pricked. Removal of even small amounts of fluid sometimes results in dramatic improvement.

Hypertension in an adult may be defined as blood pressure exceeding the range 140/90 to 160/95 mm Hg. The upper range of normal is 140/90 for patient < 50 yr, 150/95 for patient 50–65 yr, and 170/95 for patient > 65 yr. ●Hypertension is said to be mild when the diastolic pressure is in the range 90–105, moderate when 105–115, and severe when > 115. ●See below for definition of isolated systolic hypertension. **Causes:** Over 95% patients have hypertension for which no cause can be found and are said to have essential (primary) hypertension. The remainder have secondary hypertension (hypertension with a specific identifiable cause). The most common causes of secondary hypertension are renovascular hypertension and disease of the renal parenchyma. Other causes of secondary hypertension include primary hyperaldosteronism, pheochromocytoma, coarctation of the aorta, Cushing's syndrome, renin–secreting tumors.

   Work–up of hypertension aims at excluding secondary causes and also assessing end–organ damage. Hypertension may suggest secondary causes: episodes of sweating, tremor, palpitations (? pheochromocytoma); pregnancy (? pre–eclampsia); birth control pills. Physical exam should not overlook careful fundoscopic exam. Look for arteriolar constriction (normal arteriole : venule ratio is 3:4 and decreases to 1: 2 with hypertension). There is arteriovenous nicking. In more severe cases, there is severe narrowing of arterioles with "copper wire" appearance progressing finally to signs of severe vascular disease (retinal hemorrhages, exudates). ●Signs of ventricular hypertrophy or failure should be sought. ●Decreased or absent femoral pulses suggest coarctation of the aorta. Initial laboratory screening includes CBC, urinalysis, serum electrolytes, serum creatinine, and EKG. Some would add the following in the initial screening: chest x–ray, fasting glucose, SMA–12 (the latter to assess serum uric acid, cholesterol, triglycerides, and calcium). In most cases the tests are normal and evaluation will stop here; the patient will be diagnosed as having essential hypertension and antihypertensive therapy will be started. Further screening is indicated if hypertension is severe or if any of the foregoing tests suggest secondary hypertension—e.g. hypokalemia (? primary aldosteronism), proteinuria or elevated serum creatinine (? disease of renal parenchyma). Further testing may also be prompted by new onset of hypertension in the young or the elderly. Clinical suspicion guides which of the following tests to perform: plasma aldosterone; plasma renin activity; rapid sequence IVP; 24 hr urine collection for catecholamines, metanephrine, and VMA; dexamethasone suppression test.

ESSENTIAL (PRIMARY) HYPERTENSION is present in about 1 in 5 adults. It is more prevalent in blacks than whites. It is asymptomatic until end–organ complications occur. Those complications are the same as those that might develop in any other form of hypertension and include: left ventricular hypertrophy/dilation, CHF, coronary artery disease/myocardial infarction, aortic dissection, renal failure, encephalopathy, stroke, retinopathy. **Treatment:** (**1**) Start with a thiazide or a thiazide--like diuretic and moderate salt restriction. Potassium supplementation is indicated if the serum potassium falls below 3 mEq/l, or falls below 3.5 mEq/l in the patient who is on digitalis or who has symptomatic hypokalemia. A potassium–sparing diuretic (e.g. spironolactone, triamterene) may be used in combination with a thiazide diuretic if potassium supplements are not tolerated. (**2**) If satisfactory reduction of blood pressure is not achieved in 3 weeks in spite of full dosage of a thiazide, add a beta blocker (e.g. propranolol) or clonidine. Other acceptable two–drug combinations are a thiazide diuretic plus one of the following: captopril, prazosin, or methyldopa. (**3**) If the response is still inadequate, a three–drug regimen may be tried by adding hydralazine or a calcium slow–channel blocker (e.g. nifedipine). The addition of prazosin is an alternative if it is not already part of two–drug regimen. (**4**) If hypertension persists, and assuming patient compliance is not in question, further screening for secondary causes of hypertension may be indicated. In stubborn cases, consider using minoxidil or guanethidine.

ISOLATED SYSTOLIC HYPERTENSION is said to be present when the systolic pressure exceeds 160 while the diastolic pressure remains ≤ 90. This finding is common in the elderly and is due to loss of elasticity of the arterial walls. This condition is associated with an increassed risk of cardiovascular complications. However, it is not clear that lowering the systolic pressure decreases the risk.

RENOVASCULAR HYPERTENSION (diastolic hypertension due to renal artery disease) is induced by the following mechanism: constriction of a renal artery induces the involved kidney to secrete an enzyme (renin) which in the blood stream acts upon an alpha–2 globulin (angiotensinogen) to release a decapeptide (angiotensin I). The latter is further converted, mainly in the lungs, to an octapeptide (angiotensin II). Angiotensin II induces hypertension in 2 ways: (1) it is itself a vasoconstrictor, (2) it induces the release of aldosterone from the renal cortex. Aldosterone in turn induces renal tubular sodium retention and therefore water retention. The latter leads to volume expansion with ensuing increase in blood pressure. Renovascular hypertension is most commonly due to atherosclerotic narrowing of the renal artery(s) in the elderly. The next most common cause is fibromuscular hyperplasia of the renal arterial wall (mostly females under 45 yr). Many other uncommon causes exist (e.g. renal tumor, renal cyst, renal aneurysm) but the common denominator is that they somehow constrict the renal arterial vessel(s) thereby inducing the ischemic kidney to secrete renin. **Diagnosis: (1)** Abdominal or flank bruit may be present. (**2**) Rapid sequence IVP often reveals the ischemic kidney to be reduced in size with delayed appearance and late persistence of dye. (**3**) Renal arteriography may visualize the stenosis. (**4**) A sample of blood from the renal veins of both kidneys is compared for plasma renin activity (PRA). The PRA from the affected kidney (if stenosis is not bilateral) should be at least 1.5–2 times as great as the uninvolved side (which should have a decreased PRA level) for functionally significant stenosis to be diagnosed and for there to be a reasonable chance of surgical cure. **Treatment:** Angiotensin converting enzyme–inhibitor therapy (e.g. captopril) may effectively reduce blood pressure. Transarterial balloon dilatation or surgery are options

RENAL PARENCHYMAL DISEASE can cause hypertension—e.g. chronic glomerulonephritis; chronic pyelonephritis; polycystic kidneys; obstructive uropathy; autoimmune disease (e.g. scleroderma, lupus). The hypertension is frequently attributed to sodium and water retention and/or increased renin.

PRIMARY HYPERALDOSTERONISM (Conn's syndrome) comprises ≤ 1% of all forms of hypertension. It is due to excessive production of aldosterone, usually by an adrenocortical adenoma. Excessive aldosterone secretion secondary to bilateral adrenocortical hyperplasia is sometimes responsible. Rarely, an adrenal carcinoma is the cause. Aldosterone induces renal tubular sodium retention and therefore water retention which in turn leads to volume expansion with increase in blood pressure. Rarely, malignant hypertension develops. **Diagnosis:** Symptoms: headache, muscle weakness, polyuria, polydipsia; hypertension—usually mild to moderate; Electrolyte abnormalities: There is hypokalemia (K< 3.5) in the absence of diuretic administration. Serum sodium may be normal or high. Hyperchloremia and metabolic alkalosis are characteristic. Aldosterone levels are elevated, or if normal are not suppressed by administration of normal saline 500 ml/hr for 4 hr (restore serum K levels to > 3.5 mEq/liter before administering saline). Plasma renin activity (PRA) is evaluated as follows: at 8 AM, obtain PRA blood sample and administer furosemide 1mg/kg PO; maintain upright posture and ambulate patient moderately until noon; repeat PRA at noon. Normally there is an increase in PRA of 1.5–4 times the 8 AM sample. In primary hyperaldosteronism, PRA remains low. **Treatment:** If primary hyperaldosteronism is confirmed, perform bilateral adrenal vein catheterization and sample aldosterone levels. If aldosterone levels are elevated on one side, an adenoma is present and unilateral kidney resection is curative. If unilateral aldosterone elevation is not found, bilateral adrenal hyperplasia is present and the aldosterone antagonist spironolactone is administered.

PHEOCHROMOCYTOMA (rare catecholamine–secreting tumor of chromaffin cells of adrenal medulla or sympathetic ganglia). 10% are bilateral adrenal tumors, 10% are ganglionic, 10% are familial, and < 10% are malignant. Most tumors of the adrenal medulla secrete epinephrine. Pheochromocytoma is sometimes associated with multiple endocrine neoplasia syndrome type 2. **Signs/symptoms:** ●Classically there is an episodic release of catecholamines resulting in paroxysms of hypertension, palpitations, sweating, pallor, headache, nausea, anxiety, tremor, abdominal pain. ●In some patients, hypertension persists between attacks while others are normotensive between attacks. Some have stable hypertension without paroxysmal symptoms. In some cases there is postural hypotension. ●Other potential manifestations include weight loss (due to increased metabolic rate), glucose intolerance, cardiomyopathy. **Diagnosis:** 24 hr urine collection for catecholamines, metanephrines, and vanillylmandelic acid (VMA). Ultrasound, CAT scan, and/or aortogram are used to locate the tumor. **Treatment:** Over 90% tumors are benign and surgery is curative. Preoperatively, the patient is treated with an alpha blocker (phenoxybenzamine or phentolamine) to control hypertension but aggressive hydration is needed to counteract the consequent drug-induced vasodilation. A beta blocker (e.g. propranolol) may be needed to control tachycardia. However, a beta blocker must not be administered until after alpha blockade has been effected or else hypertension will be made worse (beta blockers block epinephrine–mediated beta receptor vasodilation).

COARCTATION of AORTA (congenital narrowing of the aorta) usually occurs just distal to the left subclavian artery. Associated cardiac anomalies are common, particularly congenital bicuspid aortic valve. **Signs/symptoms:** ●Systolic pressure in the legs (using a thigh cuff) is less than that in the arms. The diastolic pressure (arms) usually does not become elevated until adulthood. ●Femoral pulses may be decreased or not felt. ●Since the amount of blood passing the coarctation is diminished, the arterial blood to the lower part of the body is shunted thru collateral vessels. These vessels become enlarged and pulsations can be felt and sometimes seen about the borders of the scapula and in the intercostal spaces. The collateral vessels may erode the underside of the ribs so that notching of the ribs is seen on x--ray and the coarctation may also be visible. There is usually a systolic murmur that is best heard on the back between the scapulae at the 4th intercostal space or at the left sternal border. **Possible complications** include left ventricular hypertrophy or failure, aortic dissection, cerebral hemorrhage, infection of the coarctation, cardiac failure in infancy. **Tests:** Echocardiography shows the coarctation and post-stenotic dilation of aorta as well as the enlarged left subclavian artery. Aortogram and intra–aortic pressure studies are also confirmatory. **Treatment:** surgery.

MALIGNANT (accelerated) HYPERTENSION is a severe form of hypertension (diastolic pressure usually > 130) characterized by widespread fibrinoid necrosis of the arterioles, especially the renal arterioles. It may develop in virtually any type of hypertension (e.g. essential, renal parenchymal, renovascular, etc). **Diagnostic** features may include: nephropathy (proteinuria, microcospic hematuria, urinary casts, elevated BUN and creatinine); microangiopathic hemolytic anemia; encephalopathy (headache, nausea, vomiting, somnolence, confusion, blurred vision, seizures, coma, focal neurologic abnormalities); retinopathy (papilledema, hemorrhages, exudates); cardiac abnormalities (left ventricular hypertrophy/dilation/failure, pulmonary edema). **Treatment:** Nitroprusside is the favored drug. Alternatives are diazoxide or hydralazine. Initially, the diastolic pressure should be reduced over several minutes to about 100. If feasible, oral hypertensives (e.g. diuretic plus clonidine) may be started at this point, and hopefully the parenteral antihypertensive will not be needed after a few hours.

HYPERTENSIVE ENCEPHALOPATHY is a common feature of malignant hypertension. However, the presence of hypertensive encephalopathy does not by itself imply that a patient has malignant hypertension. In order to make the diagnosis of malignant hypertension, the other clinical and histologic manifestations that define the syndrome of malignant hypertension must also be present. Furthermore, malignant hypertension may exist without encephalopathy. **Etiology:** Hypertensive encephalopathy results from an acute elevation of blood pressure of virtually any cause. Com-

mon causes are renal disease, eclampsia, abrupt discontinuation of clonidine.
Pathogenesis: Whatever the cause of hypertension, the common denominator of hypertensive encephalopathy is that he arterioles and capillaries are overcome by the increased pressure. The arterioles leak plasma and the brain swells. The blood pressure need not be severely elevated for hypertensive encephalopathy to occur. **Signs/symptoms** of encephalopathy include headache, nausea, vomiting, somnolence, confusion, blurred vision, seizures, coma, focal neurologic abnormalities. **Treatment** is as for malignant hypertension.

Aortic Aneurysm is usually secondary to atherosclerosis, and

most atheroslcerortic aortic aneurysms are located in the descending aorta distal to origin of the renal arteries. Aortic trauma or infection may result in aortic aneurysm. Syphilis is now an uncommon cause of aortic aneurysm (syphilitic aneurysm is usually of the ascending aorta or aortic arch). Aortic aneurysm may be associated with Marfan's syndrome, cystic medial necrosis (unassociated with Marfan's syndrome), Takayasu's aortitis. Some aortic aneurysms are congenital (e.g. aneurysm of sinus of Valsalva).
   Diagnosis: If the aorta is calcified, the diagnosis can often be made with a routine chest x-ray. Aortic aneurysms may also be seen with ultrasound, CAT scan, artography. The latter is used to visualize involvement of arterial branches of the aorta. Aneurysm of the ascending aorta may result in aortic regurgitation and left heart failure. Besides an early decrescendo diastolic murmur best heard at the 2nd right interspace, a pulsatile mass can sometimes be seen and felt on the upper chest or suprasternal notch. Erosion of the ribs and sternum causes pain. The aneurysm may obstruct the superior vena cava. Aneurysm of the aortic arch may compress the trachea or bronchus (and cause cough or wheezing), or recurrent laryngeal nerve (and cause hoarseness). Aneurysm of the abdominal aorta may cause pain in the epigastrium or lower back. Pain may be worse after meals. Pain may be felt in the legs (especially the left) or the testicles. Palpation of the abdomen above the umbilicus may reveal a widened aorta. Rupture may occur into the peritoneum, retroperitoneum (look for hematoma of flank or groin). Rarely, there is rupture into the duodenum (with GI bleeding) or inferior vena cava (with AV fistula).
   Treatment: surgery.

Dissecting Aortic Aneurysm
   Pathogenesis: There is a tear in the aortic intima, and so blood dissects along the aorta between the intima and adventitia. The media is usually diseased. Aortic dissection may culminate in one of 3 ways: (1) rupture into the pericardium, mediastinum, pleural cavity, or retroperitoneum; (2) again cut across the intima to reenter the aortic lumen forming a "double–barrel" aorta; (3) stabilize. **Risk factors:** Aortic dissection occurs most often in hypertensive middle–aged males. The risk is also increased in cystic medial necrosis, Marfan's syndrome, pregnancy, coarctation of aorta, aortic trauma.
   Type I dissection: The intimal tear is just distal to the aortic valve and dissection proceeds up the ascending aorta to involve the aortic arch or beyond, sometimes to the aortic bifurcation. Dissection may also proceed proximally. ●Type I dissection usually occurs in patients < 65 yr. Patients with cystic medial necrosis or Marfan's syndrome are particularly susceptible to type I dissection. ●Along its path, dissection may cause obstruction of: (**1**) aortic arch vessels and result in cerebral, spinal cord, or peripheral nerve ischemia; (**2**) renal arteries so that acute renal failure ensues; (**3**) mesenteric arteries with ensuing bowel infarction. ●If there is also proximal dissection, any of the following may ensue: (**1**) aortic regurgitation with possible left ventricular failure, (**2**) coronary artery occlusion with myocardial infarction, (**3**) hemopericardium with possible cardiac tamponade.
   Type II dissection is uncommon. It arises in and does not extend beyond the ascending aorta. Type II dissection is often associated with Marfan's syndrome.
   Type III dissection begins beyond the origin of the left subclavian artery and progresses down the descending aorta sometimes reaching the aortic bifurcation. Depending on the extent of dissection, there may be occlusion of renal and mesen-

teric arteries. If the dissection extends to the aortic bifurcation, the femoral artery(s) may be occluded. Type III dissection is most common in elderly hypertensive males with atherosclerosis.

Diagnosis: Pain: There is usually a sudden onset of severe sharp or tearing pain. The pain moves along with the dissection and the location of the pain may be a clue as to the site of dissection—e.g. chest pain: ascending aorta, neck pain: aortic arch, back pain: descending aorta. Pain–free intervals may occur. Pain may also be present in the arms or legs. If a coronary artery is occluded, the pain of myocardial infarction may be superimposed. Sometimes dissection occurs in the absence of pain. Pulses: Carotid, radial, or femoral pulses may be asymmetrical or absent. A pulsation is sometimes felt about the sternoclavicular joint(s). If the aortic valve is involved, there may be an aortic regurgitant murmur (early decrescendo diastolic murmur best heard at 2nd right intercostal space) and there may be signs of left heart failure. If there is leakage into the pericardial space, a pericardial friction rub may be heard and cardiac tamponade may ensue. Neurologic deficits may be present if the aortic arch vessels are occluded. Bloody diarrhea may result if there is occlusion of mesenteric arteries with supervening bowel infarction. Hematuria may indicate renal artery occlusion. There may be evidence of renal failure. Specific EKG signs are absent and cardiac enzymes are normal unless a coronary artery is occluded and myocardial infarction ensues. Chest x–ray may show a widened mediastinum. CAT scan with contrast dye will show the dissection. Aortography is confirmatory and shows the extent and details of involvement.

Treatment: Hypertension must be controlled. Trimethaphan is the drug of choice for initial treatment. It is administered while the patient is in the sitting position: add 500 mg trimethaphan to 500 ml D5W; start IV infusion at 3–4 ml/min and titrate to effect. ●Nitroprusside in combination with a beta blocker is an alternative way to manage hypertension. ●Proximal dissections require surgery. Distal dissections can (in the absence of unremitting pain or complications) sometimes be managed medically assuming there is no evidence of continuing dissection.

Pulmonary Disease

Respiratory Failure & Respiratory Support

Respiratory failure is present when the arterial PO_2 falls below 40–50 mm Hg. Reliance on the arterial PCO_2 as an indicator of respiratory failure is less clearcut and must be judged by the clinical setting. For instance, a patient with chronic lung disease may habitually have a $PaCO_2$ of 50 mm Hg and not be in distress while a "normal" $PaCO_2$ of 40 mm Hg in a patient undergoing an asthmatic attack indicates that the patient is tiring and that there is impending respiratory failure. Hypoxemia brings with it anaerobic metabolism which leads to accumulation of lactic acid with metabolic acidosis. Respiratory acidosis due to CO_2 retention may also be present and combine to further lower the pH.

Intubation: Refer to appendix for appropriate tube type and size.

Initial ventilator settings: Rate is initially set at 10–15 breaths/minute. Tidal volume is set at 10–15 ml/kg ideal body weight. Mode is set on control if patient is apneic. If spontaneous respirations are present, select assist control mode or IMV (intermittent mandatory ventilation) according to the patient's respiratory capability (see Mechanical Ventilator Modes below). Inspiratory—Expiratory ratio (ratio of duration of inspiration to expiration) is usually set at about 1: 2. Fl O_2 (fraction of inspired air that is O_2) is initially set at 90–100% to correct hypoxemia. Fl O_2 is later reduced in order to avoid oxygen toxicity (see Fl O_2 below). Arterial blood gas is checked 15–30 minutes after each adjustment in ventilation or oxygen concentration.

Ventilator rate is initially set at about 10–15 breaths/minute and subsequently adjusted in conjunction with the tidal volume to maintain arterial pH of 7.35–7.45. Increasing the ventilatory rate decreases the $PaCO_2$ and vice versa. The $PaCO_2$ adjusted to a normal of 40 mm Hg cannot be used as a guide to ventilatory rate unless there is a pure respiratory acidosis or pure respiratory alkalosis. The picture is often complicated by metabolic acidosis or metabolic alkalosis. Consequently, the ventilatory rate is adjusted according to the arterial pH not the $PaCO_2$.

Tidal volume (volume delivered/cycle) is normally set at 10–15 ml/kg *ideal* body weight. An inadequate tidal volume will decrease the PaO_2 thus impairing oxygen delivery to the tissues. An inadequate tidal volume by decreasing minute ventilation (minute ventilation = tidal volume x respiratory rate) also contributes to CO_2 retention and therefore increased $PaCO_2$.

Fl O_2 (fraction of inspired air that is O_2) is initially set at 90–100% to quickly correct hypoxemia. Once this is accomplished, the goal is to adjust the Fl O_2 to achieve an arterial PaO_2 of at least 60 mm Hg while keeping Fl $O_2 \leq 50\%$. Fl O_2 60–100% is safe for up to 24 hr or so, but will cause alveolar injury thereafter. Fl O_2 up to 50% can be tolerated for long periods. When in the intubated patient the Fl O_2 cannot be reduced below 60% without dropping the PaO_2 below 60 mm Hg, PEEP may improve the PaO_2 thereby allowing reduction in Fl O_2. Also check to see that the correct tidal volume (10–15 ml/kg ideal body weight) is being administered since an inadequate tidal volume will decrease the PaO_2.

PEEP (positive end–expiratory pressure) prevents alveolar collapse at end expiration. Hypoxemia is alleviated because right to left shunt is reduced. When the Fl O_2 cannot be reduced below 60% without dropping the PaO_2 below 60mm Hg, PEEP is instituted to hopefully improve the PaO_2 and thereby allow reductions in FlO_2. •Start at 5 cm H_2O and increase in 2–4 cm H_2O increments while monitoring blood pressure with intra-arterial line. PEEP of 5–15 cm H_2O is usually adequate. Sometimes PEEP must be increased to 20–25 cm H_2O for a satisfactory response in PaO_2. •PEEP increases the intrathoracic pressure and in so doing may impede venous return and thus lead to a fall in cardiac output. Swan–Ganz catheterization to monitor cardiac output, wedge pressure, and pulmonary shunting (Qs/Qt) is required if PEEP exceeds 10 cm H_2O so that PEEP–induced reductions in blood pressure and cardiac output can be avoided or relieved with judicious volume infusion to increase venous return. By adjusting PEEP and Fl O_2, a balance is hopefully achieved such that a $PaO_2 \geq 60$ mm Hg is realized while keeping Fl $O_2 < 60\%$. •PEEP–associated increase in alveolar pressure may rupture alveoli causing pneumothorax. PEEP must therefore be used with especial caution in patients with obstructive lung disease (COPD or uncontrolled asthma) because of the risk of pneumothorax in patients whose intra–alveolar pressure is already elevated. Pulmonary edema and adult respiratory distress syndrome are examples of situations in which PEEP may be useful.

Mechanical ventilator modes refers to the restrictions exerted by the ventilator over the intubated patient's breathing. There are 3 basic modes to choose from: (**1**) Controlled mode means that the patient has no control over his respirations. The ventilator delivers breaths at a predetermined rate and volume. The patient can neither initiate a breath nor control the volume inspired. This mode of ventilation is indicated for the apneic patient or for the patient that must be paralyzed to control his respirations. (**2**) Assist control mode means that the patient may initiate his own respirations but when he does the ventilator delivers a preset volume. The ventilator automaticallly takes over at a preset rate should apnea occur. Drawbacks are twofold: (a) respiratory alkalosis may occur if tachypnea is present; (b) the respiratory muscles lose their tone because the patient exerts no respiratory effort, and consequently weaning from the ventilator may be protracted. (**3**) Intermittent mandatory ventilation (IMV) delivers a preset number of ventilations/min. The patient breathes spontaneously between the mandatory ventilations. By encouraging the patient to breathe on his own, IMV helps maintain the tone of respiratory muscles. There is also less danger of compromising venous return and cardiac output if PEEP is used in conjunction with the mandatory ventilations. IMV is the preferred mode for most patients capable of spontaneous breathing. IMV facilitates weaning from a ventilator--as a patient improves, the number of mandatory ventilations/min is progressively decreased. A variation of IMV is synchronized IMV. In this mode the ventilator senses when the patient is initiating his own respiration and allows him to complete that respiration on his own before resuming as needed automatic ventilations.

Weaning from the ventilator and extubation: The approach to weaning depends on the clinical circumstances.

Patient without lung disease who only needed ventilator support for a short time (e.g. acute drug overdose): The ventilator is disconnected and the tracheal tube is connected to a T tube thru which humidified air/oxygen can be administered. The patient is observed, vital signs are monitored, and after a short period the patient is extubated (see instructions below) provided that the extubation criteria listed below are met.

Weaning patient recovering from hypoxemic respiratory failure (e.g. adult respiratory distress syndrome): Often in this situation, the patient has required PEEP in order to overcome lung stiffness and keep the small airways open. PEEP and FI O_2 are gradually decreased in stages. The goal is to reduce PEEP to $\leq$ 5 cm H_2O and to reduce FI O_2 to $\leq$ 50% while not letting PaO_2 fall below 60 mm Hg. An arterial blood gas is obtained 15–20 minutes after each adjustment. While making these adjustments—the ventilatory rate, mode, and tidal volume are adjusted as needed to maintain the arterial pH in the normal range.

Weaning patient recovering from ventilatory failure: One approach is to disconnect the patient from the ventilator for several 5–15 minute intervals each day, and then each subsequent day gradually increase the time the patient is allowed to breathe spontaneously. With the ventilator disconnected, the tracheal tube is connected to a T tube thru which humidified air/oxygen can be administered, and CPAP (continuous positive airway pressure) at 3–5 cm H_2O may be applied in order to keep small airways open. Extubation is considered when the patient is able to breathe for 1–4 hours without ventilator assistance. Some patients will require more gradual weaning with IMV before going to intermittent use of the T tube.

Extubation criteria: After 1–4 hours on the T tube without ventilator assistance, it is usually safe to extubate (while continuing supplemental oxygen) if the patient is alert, appears stable, and meets the following criteria: (**1**) while on FI O_2 < 50%, the PaO_2 is > 60 mm Hg with normal pH and normal $PaCO_2$ (or at least not elevated above 55 mm Hg if the patient usually has an elevated $PaCO_2$); (**2**) respiratory rate < 25/min; (**3**) vital capacity > 10–15 ml/kg; (**4**) able to generate on inspiration a negative pressure more negative than minus 25 cm H_2O; (**5**) minute ventilation is < 10 liters/minute and patient is able to voluntarily double this volume.

Extubation instructions: Monitor vital signs before and after extubation. Elevate the upper body to 45–90°, suction thoroughly, and administer 100% oxygen for about a minute. Deflate and remove the tracheal tube. Following extubation continue giving supplemental humidified oxygen but at a little higher FI O_2 than what was needed while intubated. Instruct patient to breathe deeply and cough. Suction as needed. Obtain arterial blood gas measurement about 15 minutes after extubation. Be prepared to re-intubate should the patient deteriorate.

PAO2 – PaO2 gradient: When as in pulmonary disease blood passes thru the lung but is not oxygenated, a right-to-left shunt is said to exist. This shunting results in a lower than normal PaO2 (partial pressure of O2 in the arterial blood) and therefore a large difference between it and the PAO2 (partial pressure of O2 in the alveoli). ●An arterial blood sample is measured for PaO2 and PaCO2. The PAO2 is then calculated as follows: PAO2 = (FI O2)(AT – 47) – (PaCO2/0.8) where AT = atmospheric pressure (760 mm Hg at sea level), FI O2 = fraction of inspired air that is O2 (expressed as a fraction not as per cent), PaCO2 = partial pressure of arterial CO2. ●The measured PaO2 is then subtracted from the PAO2. The normal PAO2 – PaO2 difference is < 15mm Hg. A PAO2 – PaO2 gradient = 65 mm Hg corresponds to a shunt of about 5%. A gradient of over 500 mm Hg means that shunting is over 50%.

Mixed venous partial pressure O2 (PmvO2) and mixed venous O2 saturation (SmvO2) are obtained by sampling the mixed venous blood from the distal port of Swan–Ganz catheter. A PmvO2 < 30 mm Hg or a SmvO2 < 50% indicate inadequate tissue oxygenation.

Shunt fraction (Qs/Qt) is the ratio of blood that passes through the lungs but is not oxygenated (Qs) to the total blood flow thru the lungs (i.e. cardiac output or Qt). Normally the shunt fraction is < 0.05. Ventilatory assistance with PEEP is often needed if the shunt fraction is > 0.2. Conditions that increase shunt fraction include adult respiratory distress syndrome; cardiogenic pulmonary edema; pneumonia; chemical pneumonitis (e.g. aspiration, smoke inhalation); atelectasis.

●When the PaO2 is less than 150 mm Hg, $Qs/Q_t =$

$$\frac{\{0.003 \times (AP - 40 - PaCO2 - PaO2)\} + \{(1.34 \times \text{hemoglobin}) \times (1 - SaO2)\}}{\{0.003 \times (AP - 40 - PaCO2 - PaO2)\} + \{(1.34 \times \text{hemoglobin}) \times (1 - SmvO2)\}}$$

●When the PaO2 is greater than 150 mm Hg, $Qs/Qt =$

$$\frac{0.003 \times (AP - 40 - PaCO2 - PaO2)}{0.003 \times (AP - 40 - PaCO2 - PaO2) + 0.003 \times (PaO2 - PmvO2) + (1.34 \times hb) \times (1 - SmvO2)}$$

Key: _AP_ is atmospheric pressure (760mm Hg at sea level), _Hb_ = hemoglobin concentration (gram/dl), _PaO2 and PaCO2_ are the respective partial pressures of O2 and CO2 obtained from an arterial blood gas sample, _SaO2_ is the oxygen saturation of arterial blood (*expressed as a fraction not as percent*) obtained from the arterial blood gas sample. _PmvO2_ (partial pressure oxygen of mixed venous blood) and _SvmO2_ (oxygen saturation mixed venous blood *expressed as a fraction not as percent*) are measurements of a blood sample obtained from central venous line if it is in the right atrium or preferably from the distal port of Swan–Ganz catheter.

Asthma is the condition in which there is reversible bronchospasm resulting

from increased responsiveness of the bronchial smooth muscle to certain stimuli. There are 2 types of asthma: allergic and nonallergic. In practice, however, a clear distinction cannot always be made since many asthmatics have characteristics of both. <u>Allergic asthma</u> typically begins in childhood and is precipitated by specific allergens (e.g. pollens, animal dander). Serum IgE levels are elevated. When specific allergens bind to IgE molecules attached to the surface of mast cells, the mast cells release mediators of bronchospasm—e.g. histamine, slow reacting substance of anaphylaxis (SRS–A), eosinophilic chemotactic factor of anaphylaxis (ECF–A). Seasonal exacerbations often occur. A family history of asthma, allergic rhinitis, or hives is often elicited. <u>Nonallergic asthma</u> begins in adulthood. Family history of atopy and seasonal exacerbations are absent. Bronchospasm is precipitated by nonallergenic stimulants—e.g. emotions, cold, exercise, respiratory infection, airborne pollutants. Aspirin and other nonsteroidal anti–inflammatory drugs may induce bronchospasm in some patients, particularly those with nasal polyposis and sinusitis. Serum IgE levels are normal. Bronchospasm, theory holds, is mediated by the vagus nerve in response to nonspecific irritation of the tracheobronchial tree.

Signs/symptoms: Typically there is dyspnea, cough, chest "tightness", and wheezing (both inspiratory and expiratory wheezing with a prolonged expiratory phase). In severe asthma there is pulsus paradoxus as well as supraclavicular and intercostal retractions. Wheezing may actually diminish or disappear as the bronchospasm increases. In severe cases, the patient may be unable to speak and eventually becomes obtunded and cyanotic as respiratory failure supervenes.

Laboratory: Arterial blood gases: The arterial blood gas reveals hypoxemia. Mild to moderate asthma is associated with respiratory alkalosis (pH > 7.4, pCO_2 < 35). As ventilation becomes progressively inadequate, there is CO_2 retention so that the pCO_2 and the pH may then return to the normal range and give the false impression of improvement. With further deterioration, respiratory acidosis (pCO_2 > 40, pH < 7.35) ensues. Spirometry can be used to monitor the severity of bronchospasm and the effectiveness of therapy, and thus lessen the need for frequent arterial blood gas measurements. The FEV_1 (forced expiratory volume in 1 sec) is the most commonly measured parameter. As bronchospasm increases, the FEV_1 decreases. With severe bronchospasm, the FEV_1 will be < 25% normal. CBC: Leukocytosis may suggest infection as the cause of the attack, and by the shift suggest whether a bacterial or viral agent is the culprit. However, the CBC must be drawn before drug therapy is initiated because catecholamines and corticosteroids induce leukocytosis. Eosinophilia is often but not invariably present. Sputum: If eosinophils predominate, respiratory infection probably did not incite the asthma attack. If neutrophils predominate, respiratory infection is likely.

Treatment of acute asthma attack (refer to drug section for drug doses)**:** Oxygen is administered—usually via nasal cannulae at 3–4 liter/min. Subcutaneous epinephrine, because of its cardiovascular effects, is usually reserved for patients < 40 yr without arrhythmias, hypertension, or other cardiovascular disease. However, SC epinephrine may be required regardless of age or complicating factors if there is severe bronchospasm and an adrenergic bronchodilator cannot be inhaled. If needed, subcutaneous epinephrine may be repeated twice at 20 minute intervals provided that excessive tachycardia does not occur. If a satisfactory response is achieved, a SC dose of sustain–action epinephrine suspension (Sus–Phrine) may be administered. Inhaled adrenergic bronchodilators (e.g. isoetharine) administered via nebulizer are as effective as SC epinephrine (unless inhalation is inadequate) and have the advantage of producing fewer side effects. Inhalation bronchodilator therapy may be used in children or adults and is particularly useful in patients over 40 yr and/or patients with hypertension, arrhythmias, or other cardiac disease. Intravenous aminophylline (added if the foregoing drugs are insufficient) is usually used in conjunction with nebulized adrenergic bronchodilator therapy. IV corticosteroid (e.g. methylprednisolone 1mg/kg IV q6h) is begun if a satisfactory response to the foregoing bronchodilators is not seen within 1 hr or if the patient has required high–dose corticosteroids within the last 12 months. After improvement occurs, IV corticosteroid therapy is replaced with prednisone (1–2 mg/kg/day PO initially) which can usually be tapered and discontinued (or reduced to previous maintenance level) over about a week. PO or IV fluids are administered to help mobilize bronchial secretions and to replace ongoing fluid losses (e.g. theophylline diuresis, evaporation from respiratory tract). If PO intake is inadequate, D5–1/2 NS or D5–1/4 NS at about 2 ml/kg/hr is usually sufficient initially. Avoid overhydration, especially in the elderly or in patients with cardiac disease. Serum electolytes are obtained periodically and imbalances corrected. Antibiotics should not be administered routinely but reserved for a clear indication such as pneumonia. Furthermore, most infections precipitating an asthma attack are viral, not bacterial.

Maintenance of remission: An inhaled adrenergic bronchodilator (e.g. albuterol, isoetharine) administered alone on a as needed basis may be sufficient. Cromolyn sodium may be effective in preventing asthma attacks but is ineffective and contraindicated during an acute attack. An inhaled corticosteroid (e.g. Beclovent) may be tried if necessary and may be used in conjunction with an inhaled adrenergic bronchodilator. Oral theophylline or an oral adrenergic bronchodilator (e.g. albuterol) may be needed in more stubborn cases. Oral corticosteroid (e.g. prednisone) therapy may be necessary for maintenance of remission in patients refractory to the foregoing measures. Adjunctive treatment with an inhaled corticosteroid may allow reduction of the dose of oral corticosteroid and thereby minimize the systemic side effects of chronic corticosteroid administration.

Chronic Obstructive Pulmonary Disease

(COPD) is the chronic and relatively irreversible obstructive lung disease that results from **emphysema** and/or **chronic bronchitis.** The two usually coexist but one may predominate over the other. Both chronic bronchitis and emphysema are obstructive. Forceful expiration is therefore impeded. Spirometry reflects this fact by showing a decreased FEV1 (forced expiratory volume for 1 second) and usually a decreased vital capacity (volume of air that can be exhaled from maximum inspiration).

Keeping in mind that emphysema and chronic bronchitis usually coexist and that the signs and symptoms of COPD are a function of the stage of the disease, **the following generalizations can be made:**

Emphysema is characterized by destruction of the alveolar walls with consequent enlargement of the air spaces distal to the bronchioles (hereditary alpha–1 antitrypsin deficiency is an example of a condition associated with emphysema alone). The typical patient with mainly emphysema (sometimes referred to as a "pink puffer") is underweight, has hypertrophic accessory respiratory muscles, and is dyspneic and tachypneic. There is generally little cough or sputum production. Breath sounds and heart sounds are "distant", and the chest wall is hypertympanitic. X–ray reveals hyperlucent and hyperinflated lungs with depressed diaphragm and small heart. Total lung capacity and residual lung volume are increased. Blood gases generally show mildly decreased PaO2 and PaCO2. Hematocrit is normal.

Chronic bronchitis is associated with excess mucus blocking the small airways. There is an increase in the size of mucous glands and the number of goblet cells. If chronic bronchitis is dominant ("blue bloater"), the typical patient contrasts with the "pink–puffer" described above in the following respects: there is a chronic productive cough, there may be cyanosis, and weight loss is not characteristic. Wheezing, rales, rhonchi are variably present. Blood gases show decreased PaO2 and elevated PaCO2. Chronic hypoxemia induces polycythemia. This may lead to pulmonary hypertension which in turn may result in right ventricular hypertrophy/failure (see "Pulmonary Hypertension"). Chest x–ray reveals prominent pulmonary arteries and the heart may be enlarged.

Treatment of COPD: Oxygen is administered to relieve hypoxemia and thus prevent pulmonary hypertension. Aim of therapy is to achieve a PaO2 of 60–80 mm Hg. Low-flow oxygen via nasal cannula at 1–3 liter/min usually achieves this goal. However, oxygen must be administered judiciously because exceeding a PaO2 of 60 mm Hg may cause those patients who are dependent on chronic hypoxia to stimulate ventilation to deteriorate. IV or PO theophylline preparations, and/or PO or inhaled adrenergic drugs are standard therapy (see "Asthma"). Corticosteroid therapy may be added when bronchodilators in full doses are not adequate. However, corticosteroids are not beneficial in many cases. Those who demonstrate eosinophilia in sputum or CBC, or who have a history of atopy are the ones most likely to improve with corticosteroid therapy. The effectiveness of corticosteroid therapy and justification for chronic administration is based on measurement of FEV1. While continuing bronchodilators in full doses, the patient receives a 3–4 wk trial of a corticosteroid (e.g. prednisone 30 mg once daily). If the corticosteroid is effective, there should be a significant increase in the FEV1. If this is the case, the corticosteroid is graduallly tapered and continued at the smallest effective dose. For chronic therapy, an inhaled corticosteroid (e.g. beclomethasone) may suffice or allow a reduction of the oral requirement. If the corticosteroid trial fails to significantly increase the FEV1, the corticosteroid is tapered and discontinued over 1–2 wk. Antibiotics are administered promptly whenever there is a purulent sputum or other signs of respiratory tract infection. Pneumococcus and Haemophilus influenza are the most commonly implicated organisms. Tetracycline or ampicillin is the usual antibiotic choice.

Adult Respiratory Distress Syndrome

(ARDS) is respiratory failure of abrupt onset due to the consequences of alveolar injury. **Causes:** Alveolar injury may result from diverse conditions—e.g. shock of any cause; trauma (pulmonary or nonpulmonary); postsurgical (particulary after cardiopulmonary bypass); gastric aspiration; drug overdose (e.g. heroin, barbiturates); sepsis; pneumonia; acute hemorrhagic pancreatitis; inhalation of toxic fumes; near-drowning; fat embolism. **Pathogenesis:** The pulmonary capillaries are excessively permeable and the injured alveoli leak and fill with fluid, protein, erythrocytes, and sometimes inflammatory cells. Hyaline membrane (derived from the fibrin which has leaked into the alveoli) covers the inside of the alveoli. These conditions cause right--to-left shunting with ventilation–perfusion mismatch. Hypoxemia results. In addition, the lungs become noncompliant since the pulmonary interstitium is also overcome with edema and inflammation.

Diagnosis: Signs/symptoms: progessive dyspnea, tachypnea, supraclavicular and intercostal inspiratory retractions, expiratory grunting, cyanosis. Arterial blood gas: There is hypoxemia. The PaO_2 is typically < 50 even with delivery of high oxygen concentrations (e.g. 100% oxygen via nonrebreather mask). Because of hyperventilation, the $PaCO_2$ may be normal or decreased. Consequently, the pH is typically normal or elevated as a reflection of respiratory alkalosis. $PAO_2 - PaO_2$ gradient: Shunting is demonstrated by an increased alveolar–arterial oxygen gradient. $PAO_2 - PaO_2$ (normally about 50 mm Hg or less) increases as ventilation–perfusion mismatch worsens. A $PAO_2 - PaO_2$ gradient = 65 mm Hg corresponds to a shunt of about 5%. A gradient of over 500 mm Hg means that shunting is over 50%. Refer to "Respiratory Failure and Respiratory Support" chapter for calculation of $PAO_2 - PaO_2$. Chest x-ray reveals pulmonary edema.

Treatment: ●Treat the underlying disorder. ●Most patients require intubation. ●PEEP (positive end–expiratory pressure) is instituted if inspired oxygen concentrations > 50% (FI O_2 > 50%) are required to achieve a PaO_2 of 60mm Hg. Remember that a prolonged FI $O_2 \geq 60\%$ can itself damage the lung. PEEP keeps the lungs expanded thereby preventing atelectasis. Shunt and mismatch are thus minimized which in turn minimizes hypoxemia. PEEP's drawback is that it may raise intrathoracic pressure and thus impede venous return with a consequent fall in cardiac output. A Swan-Ganz catheter is required in order to estimate the cardiac output and the shunt fraction so that optimal adjustments of PEEP can be made without compromising cardiac output and while not exceeding an FI O_2 of 60%. The goal is to achieve a PaO_2 of 60 mm Hg (or 90% O_2 saturation) while keeping FI O_2 < 60%. Refer to "Respiratory Failure and Respiratory Support" chapter.

Aspiration (inspiration of fluid or foreign matter into the airways) usually

occurs when there is a depressed level of consciousness and/or esophageal incompetence. ●Many aspiration incidents are unwitnessed and consequently must be suspected from the clinical setting (e.g. coma, debilitation, inebriation, cardiopulmonary resuscitation). ●The clinical course following aspiration is variable. It is a function of the volume of fluid or size of particles, acidity of aspirate, and presence of sterile or infected material.

Initial treatment: Prevention of further aspiration is paramount. If the patient is vomiting and conscious, position the patient head down and on right side in order to confine any aspiration to the right upper lobe. If the patient is unconscious and aspiration is suspected, intubate and suction immediately. ●Large objects obstructing the supraglottic airway may be dislodged by the Heimlich maneuver. Immediate cricothyroidotomy is required if this fails.

Diagnostic approach: Chest x-ray may reveal one or a combination of pulmonary infiltrate, empyema, or lung abscess. The location of a pneumonia or abscess may suggest aspiration. Since aspiration usually occurs with the patient supine and since the right mainstem bronchus is straighter than the left, the most vulnerable and likely area to find an infiltrate is the posterior segment of the right upper lobe. Other vulnerable regions include the superior segment ot the left upper lobe and the superior segments of the lower lobes. Sputum may be sent for gram stain and aerobic culture but anaerobic sputum culture is not useful since the specimen will be contaminated by anaerobes normally present in the oropharynx. Therefore, transtracheal aspirates should be obtained, gram stained, and cultured for both aerobes and anaerobes. Pleural effusions must be tapped and sent for gram stain, aerobic and anaerobic cultures, glucose, pH. Bronchoscopy is diagnostic and is useful for removing particulate material.

Aspiration of particulate matter: A large object (e.g. meat) may obstruct the upper airway and cause asphyxia. If a bronchus is occluded, a region of atelectasis or hyperinflation may sometimes be seen on x-ray. Particulate matter may have to be removed via bronchoscope.

Aspiration of gastric contents of sufficient volume with a pH < 2.5 provokes a severe chemical pneumonitis that may lead to adult respiratory distress syndrome. Treatment: Prevent further aspiration (see "Initial Measures" above). Intubate as clinical circumstances indicate and then suction. Neither steroids nor pulmonary lavage is advised. Antibiotic prophylaxis is usually recommended (see below). ●Also refer to "Adult Respiratory Distress Syndrome" chapter.

Aspiration–induced pulmonary infection: Infections may manifest as pneumonia, lung abscess (see "Lung Abscess" chapter), empyema (see also "Pleural Effusion"chapter). Pulmonary infection may follow directly from the aspiration of contaminated material or be the sequel to injury by sterile aspirates (e.g. highly–acid gastric aspirates). Pathogens: Sterile aspiration often leads to pulmonary infection by aerobes (e.g. pneumococcus, staphylococcus, streptococcus, gram–negative aerobes). Aspiration of contaminated material usually causes anaerobic (or mixed anaerobic and aerobic) lung infections that reflect aspiration of bacterial flora normally present in the mouth. Most community–acquired *anaerobic* pulmonary infections are due to aspiration. However, hospitalized patients often develop gram–negative aerobic infections following aspiration. Antibiotic prophylaxis: Opinion is divided but since so many aspirations result in infection, prophylactic penicillin is often routinely administered to cover anaerobes. Antibiotic therapy: Treat documented aspiration pneumonia infection as cultures dictate. Until cultures become available, penicillin is the drug of choice. Patients often respond to penicillin alone even when mixed aerobic and anaerobic infections are discovered or when penicillin–resistant Bacteroides fragilis is present as part of a mixed anaerobic infection. If aspiration occurs in a hospital setting, a cephalosporin plus an aminoglycoside are often administered pending culture and sensitivity results.

Lung Abscess

Etiology: Lung abscess usually results from aspiration of material contaminated with anaerobic bacteria from the oropharynx. Lung abscess is also not uncommonly the sequel to chemical pneumonitis following sterile aspiration (e.g. highly–acid gastric aspiration). See "Aspiration" chapter for information on regions most vulnerable to pneumonitis (and therefore lung abscess) following fluid aspiration. Other settings that may be associated with lung abscess include bronchogenic carcinoma; metastatic malignancy; septic pulmonary emboli (e.g. S. aureus, pseudomonas); pulmonary embolism with infarct and secondary infection; extension of a hepatic abscess (e.g. amebic abscess) thru the diaphragm; lung fluke infestation.

Natural history: In uncomplicated cases the following sequence occurs: (**1**) a necrotizing pneumonitis leads to a pus filled cavity; (**2**) the abscess subsequently ruptures into a bronchus leaving a partially filled cavity whose air–fluid level can be seen on x-ray; (**3**) with continued drainage and resolution of the infection, the cavity collapses and with time contracts and disappears. ●Occasionally an abscess erodes into pulmonary vessels and there is hemorrhage——sometimes massive and fatal (see "Hemoptysis" chapter). ●Empyema occurs abruptly if an abscess extends into the pleural space. A bronchopleural fistula may form.

Diagnosis: Signs/symptoms: Presentation may be that of a typical pneumonia with fever, chills, cough. Once the abscess has ruptured into a bronchus, there is usually copious sputum and it may be blood–stained. A foul sputum is consistent with anaerobic infection. Failure of a "pneumonia" to resolve promptly with antibiotics suggests the presence of an abscess and/or bronchogenic carcinoma. Chest x-ray reveals a consolidation which may have a globular appearance. An air–fluid level may be seen if rupture into a bronchus has occurred. Transtracheal aspirate: Specimens are obtained by transtracheal aspiration because sputum will be contaminated with anaerobes from the oropharynx. Culture the aspirate for aerobes, anaerobes, mycobacteria, and fungus; and obtain gram and acid–fast stain. <u>Blood culture</u> is usually negative in the case of anaerobic abscess because bacteremia is usually absent. Blood culture is usually positive in the case of lung abscess due to pseudomonas or S. aureus. <u>Bronchoscopy</u> is indicated if patient does not respond to antibiotic, or if a foreign body or bronchogenic carcinoma is suspected as the instigator of the abscess.

Treatment: <u>Postural drainage</u> is indicated. <u>Antibiotics:</u> ●Penicillin (IV or IM depending on the clinical severity) is the drug of choice pending culture results and/or clinical response. Switch to PO antibiotics when clinical improvement occurs and continue until the cavity closes—usually about 2–3 months. Fever may persist for weeks in spite of adequate antibiotic therapy. Patients often respond to penicillin alone even when mixed aerobic and anaerobic infections are discovered or when penicillin–resistant Bacteroides fragilis is present as part of a mixed anaerobic infection. ●Clindamycin is the drug of choice in penicillin–allergic patients. ●Antibiotic choice for lung abscess due to S. aureus, klebsiella, or pseudomonas is as for pneumonia secondary to these organisms (see "Pneumonia" chapter).

Hemoptysis

Etiology: <u>Infection</u> is the most common cause—e.g. bronchitis, pneumonia, lung abscess, bronchiectasis, tuberculosis. The latter 3 and lung carcinoma are the most common causes of massive hemoptysis (> 600 ml/48hr). Bronchitis is the most common cause of hemoptysis but is usually limited to blood–streaked sputum. <u>Trauma–related hemoptysis</u> (e.g. lung contusion or laceration, bronchial rupture) is also common. <u>Bronchogenic carcinoma</u> should be suspected in any smoker over 40 with hemoptysis. <u>Pulmonary hypertension</u> (e.g. primary pulmonary hypertension, secondary to congenital left–to–right shunt, secondary to high–altitude exposure) may provoke hemoptysis. <u>Pulmonary edema</u> may result in slight hemoptysis. <u>Pulmonary embolism with infarction</u> sometimes leads to hemoptysis. <u>Mitral stenosis</u> may cause hemoptysis but it is seldom severe. There is rupture of the engorged submucosal veins that shunt blood from the pulmonary veins to the systemic veins. <u>Coagulation disorders</u> (hereditary or iatrogenic) predispose to hemoptysis. <u>A foreign body</u> lodged in the tracheobronchial tree may precipitate hemoptysis. <u>Bronchlithiasis</u> may result in hemoptysis. <u>Rare causes of hemoptysis include:</u> bronchial adenoma; parasites (hookworm, strongyloides, ascaris, lung fluke); Goodpasture's syndrome; Wegener's granulomatosis; lupus; polyarteritis nodosa; pulmonary endometriosis; idiopathic pulmonary hemosiderosis; arteriovenous fistula; lung sequestration.

Diagnosis: History, physical exam, and chest x-ray generally point to the diagnosis, or narrow the diagnostic possibilities and suggest further diagnostic steps. Bronchoscopy is an important diagnostic procedure when the diagnosis is in doubt and may be a crucial therapeutic tool if bleeding is severe and the bleeding site needs to be identified and packed. <u>Bronchitis</u> is likely if there is a negative chest x-ray in the setting of a blood–streaked purulent sputum, cough, and/or history of preceding URI. <u>Pneumonia</u> may be associated with a purulent blood–streaked sputum along with fever, chills, pleuritic pain, and an infiltrate on chest x-ray. Sputum should be sent for gram stain and culture. <u>Bronchiectasis</u> is suggested by a history of chronic and often copious purulent sputum. Chest x-ray may reveal "honeycomb pattern". <u>Lung abscess</u> is accompanied by hemoptysis (sometimes massive) in over 30% cases. The typical patient is an alcoholic with poor oral hygiene and foul sputum. An air-fluid level may be seen on chest x-ray. <u>Tuberculosis</u> must be suspected if there is a history of Tb exposure or history suggesting Tb (e.g. night sweats, weight loss). See "Tuberculosis" chapter for work-up. <u>Lung carcinoma</u> must be excluded in any smoker over 40 who presents with hemoptysis (see "Lung Cancer" chapter). <u>Mitral stenosis</u> (see "Valvular Heart Disease"). <u>Pulmonary infarction</u> secondary to pulmonary embolism (see "Pulmonary Embolism"). <u>Aspergilloma</u> (fungus ball) usually develops in a cavity left by prior lung disease such as Tb. An aspergilloma may cause recurrent and sometimes severe hemoptysis. The fungus ball can be seen on upright chest x-ray and may change position within the cavity when a lateral decubitus view is obtained. The presence of precipitating antibodies to Aspergillus is diagnostically useful. <u>Goodpasture's syndrome and Wegener's granulomatosis</u> are suggested by the presence of infiltrates on chest x-ray together with evidence of glomerulonephritis.

Treatment of less than massive hemoptysis is directed toward treatment of the underlying disorder. Massive hemoptysis (> 600 ml in 48 hr) mandates rigid bronchoscopy to identify and possibly pack the bleeding site. To prevent aspiration into the uninvolved lung, the patient is positioned so that the normal lung is above the bleeding site. If significant respiratory embarrassment occurs, the uninvolved lung may be intubated. Unless there is a contraindication (e.g. widespread lung carcinoma, severe lung disease); massive hemoptysis mandates surgery.

Lung Cancer in the U.S. is the most common cause of cancer death

in both men and women. **Risk factors:** The leading risk factor is smoking. The risk is also increased in persons exposed to asbestos, uranium ores, nickel ores, chromates, arsenic, polycyclic aromatic hydrocarbons, chloromethyl, or methyl ether. **Four histologic types** of bronchogenic carcinoma are recognized: (**1**) squamous (epidermoid) cell carcinoma—arises from metaplastic squamous cells of the bronchial mucosa, tends to be centrally located, may cavitate, may obstruct bronchi; (**2**) small (oat) cell carcinoma—presumably arises from cells of bronchial glands, usually centrally located, usually metastasized by the time of diagnosis, not infrequently causes paraneoplastic endocrinopathies; (**3**) large cell carcinoma—usually peripheral and may cavitate; (**4**) adenocarcinoma—usually peripheral, may arise from a scar, may cavitate. Bronchoalveolar carcinoma is a subtype of adenocarcinoma which spreads along alveoli and may appear on chest x–ray as a pneumonia–like infiltrate. Association of histologic type with smoking is greatest for squamous cell carcinoma followed by undifferentiated small or large cell types. The association is less strong for adenocarcinoma and there is no apparent association with bronchoalveolar carcinoma.

SIGNS/SYMPTOMS: Cough (often productive) is the most common complaint. Hemoptysis is common but is usually limited to blood–tinged sputum. Copious hemoptysis due to erosion of a large vessel by the tumor is not common. Persistent localized chest pain may be due to invasion of the parietal pleura and chest wall. Fever and/or chest pain due to recurrent obstructive pneumomia is common. Localized wheezing may be present if the tumor partially obstructs a bronchus. Dyspnea may be the consequence of airway obstruction, pleural effusion, extensive pulmonary spread, stretching of pulmonary interstitial J receptors. Hoarseness may be due to a tumor of the left lung that involves the recurrent laryngeal nerve. Diaphragmatic paralysis is the consequence of involvement of the phrenic nerve. Pancoast syndrome may occur when a tumor of the lung apex (1) invades the brachial plexus resulting in shoulder and/or arm pain with weakness/paralysis of the arm or (2) involves the inferior sympathetic ganglion at the base of the neck resulting in Horner's syndrome (ptosis, miosis, enophthalmus). Superior vena cava syndrome may occur if the tumor invades or compresses the superior vena cava. There may be distension of the veins of the neck, fundi, and upper thorax as well as edema of the face, arms and upper chest. Orthopnea is common. Inadequate cerebral perfusion may result in headache, dizziness, vertigo, psychic abnormalities, or coma. This syndrome is an emergency usually requiring radiation. Chemotherapy is an option with radiation to follow if the chemotherapeutic response is inadequate.

Metastases: Hematogenous metastases to bone, liver, brain, adrenals, or opposite lung are common. The metastases are often asymptomatic—e.g most brain metastases are asymptomatic. Small cell carcinoma tends to metastasize early; metastasis has probably already occurred by the time of diagnosis. Of the nodes accessible to physical exam, the supraclavicular or cervical nodes are the most frequently involved.

Paraneoplastic consequences of lung cancer are common and include: ●Clubbing: soft tissue inflammation/enlargement of distal fingers and toes. ●Hypertrophic pulmonary osteoarthropathy (HPO) is an arthritis and proliferative periostitis (particularly of the distal long bones of the arms and legs) with pain, tenderness, and swelling. It is most often associated with tumor involvement of pleura. HPO is unusual with small cell carcinoma. ●Hypercalcemia is due to bone metastasis and/or tumor production of parathormone–like substances. ●Other endocrinopathies due to ectopic hormone production by a tumor include SIADH (ectopic ADH is usually due to a small cell carcinoma), Cushing's syndrome (ectopic ACTH is usually due to a small cell carcinoma), gynecomastia (from ectopic gonadotropin production), thyrotoxicosis (from ectopic TSH), carcinoid syntrome. ●Eaton–Lambert syndrome is a myasthenic syndrome (usually associated with small cell carcinoma) that, unlike myasthenia gravis, improves with activity and is unresponsive to acetylcholinesterase inhibitors. ●Neurologic syndromes unrelated to brain metastasis (e.g. cerebellar degeneration, encephalopathy, peripheral neuropathy). ●Migratory thrombophlebitis; ●Endocarditis that is unassociated with infection. ●Hematologic abnormalities (e.g. polycythemia, leukemoid reaction, anemia, thrombocytopenia). ●Acanthosis nigricans (hyperpigmentation and warty growths of axillae or groin).

DIAGNOSIS & METASTATIC WORKUP: Chest x-ray will reveal the tumor in 90% of symptomatic cases. The chest x-ray may also demonstrate involvement of hilar or mediastinal nodes. Sputum cytology is most likely to reveal malignant cells when a tumor is centrally located. The diagnostic yield is increased when repeated specimens are obtained. Positive cytology establishes the diagnosis since false positives seldom occur. Sputum cytology may be positive before a tumor is visible on x-ray. Bronchoscopy is the next step in the diagnosis of suspected lung cancer (e.g. suspicious lesion on chest x-ray, hemoptysis, hoarseness). It is also indicated if sputum cytology is positive. Bronchoscopy is not necessary if metastasis is evident. Furthermore, it is not required when sputum cytology reveals small cell carcinoma since in that case metastasis has very probably occurred by the time a lesion is detected on chest x-ray. Bronchoscopy not only enables one to obtain specimens (biopsy, brushings, washings) for diagnostic confirmation but also localizes the lesion for staging. The diagnosis will be confirmed about 90% of the time if the lesion can be seen with a bronchoscope. Bronchoscopic methods will fail to make the diagnosis in about half the cases of peripheral tumors that cannot be directly visualized. Percutaneous biopsy with fluoroscopic guidance is performed if there is a peripheral lesion and the diagnosis is still in doubt. There is a risk of pneumothorax or hemorrhage with this procedure. Biopsy suspicious palpable lymph nodes. Investigate pleural effusion; tap effusion and biopsy pleura. Bone scan is indicated if there is hypercalcemia, elevated alkaline phosphatase, or bone pain. Liver scan may be performed if the serum transaminases are elevated. CAT scan of the brain is indicated if there are neurologic abnormalities. Note: In the absence of clinical findings or chemical abnormalities suggesting metastases, the routine use of CAT scan, bone scan, or liver scan to detect metastases is not advised since the yield is low and false positives may occur. CAT scan of the thorax to assess extent of pulmonary spread, hilar node involvement, or spread to mediastinum may be justified if surgery is a consideration (see staging and treatment) Mediastinoscopy or mediastinotomy may sometimes be needed to provide staging information if surgery is a consideration.

SOLITARY PULMONARY NODULE (a well-demarcated rounded lesion < 6 cm in diameter encompassed by air-containing lung) is a not an uncommon incidental finding on chest x-ray. In most instances the lesion is benign—e.g. granuloma (tuberculoma, histoplasmona, coccidioidoma); hamartoma; bronchial adenoma; etc. A 4th to a 3rd of solitary nodules are malignant—mostly bronchogenic carcinomas, small percentage metastatic cancers, and rarely sarcomas. Lung cancer seldom occurs in a person < 35 yr. **Investigative steps:** (**1**) Compare with a previous x-ray if possible. The lesion is almost certainly benign if it has not enlarged over a period of at least 2 yr. (**2**) Tomography; A nodule with diffuse, central, or laminar calcification virtually always points to a benign lesion—e.g. central or laminar calcification is characteristic of granulomas, diffuse "popcorn" pattern of calcification is consistent with a hamartoma. (**3**) Sputum cytology is ordered (realizing that the yield is low for small peripheral neoplasms) if the foregoing do not rule out a malignant lesion. (**4**) Fiberoptic bronchoscopy (with brush biopsy and transbronchial biopsy), or percutaneous biopsy are the options if sputum cytology is negative. (**5**) Diagnostic thoracotomy is the next consideration (provided that there is no contraindication to surgery) if biopsy is negative or does not prove the lesion benign, particularly if the patient is over 40 or a heavy smoker. CAT scan of the thorax and/or mediastinoscopy is advised prior to thoracotomy in order to exclude mediastinal metastasis.

Note: The staging/treatment information presented below is extracted from National Cancer Institute PDQ State-of-the-Art Cancer Treatment Information 1/7/91. However, since cancer treatment is evolving, this information may not be current. The most up-to-date standard therapeutic options may be obtained by calling the National Cancer Institute Cancer Information Service at 1-800-4-CANCER. Inclusion of newly diagnosed patients in clinical trials of new therapeutic regimens is encouraged. Descriptions of these trials are also available.

STAGING/TREATMENT of SMALL CELL LUNG CANCER:

Limited stage (tumor confined to hemithorax of origin, the mediastinum, and/or the supraclavicular nodes encompassable within a "tolerable" radiotherapy port) is treated with combination chemotherapy ± chest irradiation ± prophylactic cranial irradiation. Combination chemotherapy is the cornerstone of therapy—e.g. CAV (cyclophosphamide + doxorubicin + vincristine), CAVP-16 (cyclophosphamide + doxorubicin + etoposide), VPP (etoposide + cisplatin ± other drugs such as vincristine, methotrexate, doxorubicin). Addition of chest irradiation to combination chemotherapy enhances the control of the primary tumor and may improve survival. Prophylactic cranial irradiation reduces the incidence of clinically evident brain metastases but does not appear to prolong life. Surgical resection may be considered in a small very select group of patients. Surgery is followed by combined chemotherapy ± prophylactic cranial irradiation. Prognosis; 2-year disease-free survival of treated limited stage disease is 15%.

Extensive stage disease is also treated with combination chemotherapy ± chest irradiation ± prophylactic cranial irradiation. In addition, patients may need palliative irradiation of metastatic sites that are unlikely to promptly respond to chemotherapy. Two-year disease-free survival of treated extensive stage disease is 2%.

STAGING/TREATMENT of NONSMALL CELL LUNG CANCER:

TNM classification: Primary tumor: **Tx**—malignant cells in bronchopulmonary secretions. **T0**—no x-ray or bronchoscopic evidence of primary tumor, or any tumor that cannot be assessed. **Tis**—carcinoma in situ. **T1**—tumor whose greatest diameter is ≤ 3 cm that is encompassed by lung or visceral pleura and which on bronchoscopy is no more proximal than a lobar bronchus. **T2**—tumor > 3 cm in greatest diameter; or tumor of any size that involves visceral pleura or is associated with atelectasis or obstructive pneumonitis reaching to hilum. Atelectasis or obstructive pneumonitis must not involve an entire lung. There must be no pleural effusion. The tumor's most proximal extension must be within a lobar bronchus and no closer than 2 cm from carina. **T3**—tumor of any size invading chest wall (including superior sulcus tumor), diaphragm, mediastinal pleura, or parietal pericardium. Or tumor within a main bronchus < 2 cm from the carina but sparing the carina (Note: a superficial tumor of any size whose invasive portion is restricted to the bronchial wall and which may reach proximal to a main bronchus is also designated T1). Or tumor associated with atelectasis or obstructive pneumonitis of entire lung. **T4**—tumor of any size invades mediastinum, carina, trachea, heart, great vessels, esophagus, or vertebrae. Or tumor associated with malignant effusion. Nodal involvement; **NX**—minimum requirements to assess regional nodes cannot be met. **N0**—no evidence of regional nodal involvement. **N1**—metastasis or direct extension to peribronchial and/or ipsilateral hilar nodes. **N2**—metastasis to ipsilateral mediastinal and/or subcarinal nodes. **N3**—metastasis to contralateral mediastinal or hilar nodes; or ipsi- or contralateral scalene or supraclavicular nodes. Distant metastasis; **MX**—minimum requirements to assess for distant metastasis cannot be met. **M0**—no known distant metastasis. **M1**—distant metastasis.

Occult stage (TX, N0, M0): Diagnostic measures aimed at locating the primary tumor are indicated—e.g. bronchoscopy, chest x-ray (monthly if necessary), tomography, CT thorax.

Stage 0 (Tis, N0, M0): surgical resection that spares as much normal lung tissue as possible (e.g. if feasible, segmentomy or wedge resection). Resection is limited because there is a high risk of 2nd lung cancers.

Stage I (T1–T2, N0, M0): standard treatment is surgery. The extent of resection is individualized. Radiation with curative intent may be employed if surgery is contraindicated.

Stage II (T1–T2, N1, M0) treatment is as for stage I.

Stage III A (T1–T2, N2, M0 or T3, N0–N2, M0): Small primary tumor (T1–T2, N2, M0): radiation alone. Selected patients may be considered for surgery with radiation. Surgery alone may be appropiate in highly selected cases. Superior sulcus tumor (T3, N0–N1, M0): radiation + surgery, radiation alone, or (in selected cases) surgery alone. Chest wall tumor (T3, N0–N1, M0): surgery ± radiation or radiation alone.

Stage III B (any T, N3, M0 or T4, any N, M0): radiation alone is standard treatment.

Stage IV (any T, any N, M1): palliative radiation as the need arises.

Pleural Effusion (accumulation of fluid in the pleural space) may

be a transudate or an exudate. The criteria for distinguishing between a transudate
and an exudate are presented below (see "Analyzing the data"). **Pleural
transudates** are generally low in protein and arise when a decrease in the plasma
oncotic pressure or a rise in the capillary hydrostatic pressure allows excessive
amounts of plasma solutes (mostly nonprotein solutes) with water to leak from pleural capillaries thru the pleural membrane into the pleural space. Transudates may be
the consequence of CHF (the most frequent cause), cirrhosis, hypoalbuminemia,
nephrotic syndrome, myxedema, peritoneal dialysis, acute atelectasis, Meigs'
syndrome. The latter is sometimes an exudate. **Pleural exudates:** Inflammatory
exudates are typically high in protein and arise when inflammation of the pleura
leads to an increase in permeability of the pleural capillaries so that protein–rich fluid
passes from the pleural capillaries thru the pleural membrane into the pleural space.
Inflammatory exudates may be due to neoplasia (the most common cause); infection
(the next most common); pulmonary infarction; pancreatitis; autoimmune disease
(lupus, rheumatoid arthritis); Dressler's syndrome; asbestosis; uremia; sarcoidosis;
chylothorax; etc. Obstructive exudate is the consequence of obstruction of lymphatic drainage (e.g. tumor of mediastinum). **Bacterial pneumonia–associated pleural exudates** are common and are one of 2 types: (**1**) parapneumonic effusion is a
sterile exudate (i.e. the fluid shows an elevated WBC count but bacteria are absent).
Sterile pleural effusions may be simple or loculated. (**2**) empyema is a purulent
bacteria–containing exudative effusion (stain and/or culture of the fluid is positive).
The pleural fluid pH and glucose concentration may further differentiate empyema
from a parapneumonic effusion (see below).

Diagnosis of effusion: Signs/symptoms may be absent. The patient may complain of a cough, pleuritic chest pain, or (if the effusion is large) dyspnea. Signs that
may be present include: decreased or absent breath sounds over the effusion, rales
adjacent to the effusion, friction rub above effusion, dullness to percussion and decreased tactile fremitus over the effusion, and egophony at the upper border of the
effusion. Chest x–ray: Standard upright PA and lateral chest x–ray will not reveal an
effusion unless there is at least 300 ml present while as little as 50 ml can sometimes be detected with a lateral decubitus view. Small effusions are revealed on upright chest x–ray as blunting of the costophrenic angles while larger effusions form a
concave upward meniscus along the lateral chest wall. If in doubt, comparison of a
lateral decubitus view with an upright view will confirm the presence of an effusion by
demonstrating a change in the position of free pleural fluid along the thoracic wall.

Establishing the cause of an effusion by thoracentesis is necessary unless
the cause is assured (e.g. straightforward CHF). Pleural fluid analysis should include: CBC with differential; protein; LDH; amylase; glucose; pH; cytology; gram and
acid–fast stains; cultures (aerobic and anaerobic bacterial, mycobacterial, fungal). A
serum glucose, serum protein, and serum LDH are simultaneously obtained. **Analyzing the data:** Gross examination of pleural fluid may suggest the diagnosis:
bloody fluid (e.g. trauma or traumatic tap, malignancy, pulmonary infarction, pancreatitis, uremia); anchovy color (amebiasis); foul odor (anaerobes); white milky (chylothorax); clear straw–colored (transudate, some exudates). Differentiating between
a transudate and an exudate narrows the diagnostic possibilities. Transudates are
generally low in protein and are defined by 3 criteria: (**1**) ratio of total pleural protein
to total serum protein < 0.5, (**2**) pleural fluid LDH < 200 IU/liter, (**3**) ratio of pleural
LDH to serum LDH < 0.6. Exudates are typically high in protein and are defined by
the reversal of any of the 3 criteria for transudates. Amylase: A pleural effusion that
results from pancreatitis, pancreatic pseudocyst, or esophageal rupture is
characteristically associated with a pleural fluid amylase > serum amylase. Cytology
and biopsy: Cytology reveals malignant cells in the pleural effusion of only 50–60%
cases of malignant effusion. Repeat tap and/or a Cope or Abrams needle pleural biopsy is indicated if cytology is negative and suspicion of malignancy still exists. Needle biopsy can be performed safely only when there is enough pleural fluid present to
separate the visceral and parietal pleural surfaces. Pleural biopsy is sometimes
necessary to diagnose a pleural effusion resulting from tuberculosis or rheumatoid
arthritis. Triglycerides are elevated in chylous effusions. Pleural WBC count: Only
generalizations can be made. Transudates typically contain < 1000 WBC/microliter
((mostly monocytes). Monocytes also predominate in pleural exudates due to tuber-

culosis, neoplasia, chronic rheumatoid pleurisy; however, the WBC count is > 1000. Empyemic, parapneumonic, and pancreatic effusions as well as effusions due to pulmonary infarction result in exudates with WBC count ≥ 5000—mostly neutrophils. Pleural fluid pH < 7.30 is typical for empyema, carcinoma, tuberculosis, autoimmune disease, esophageal rupture. The pleural fluid from a simple sterile effusion has a pH > 7.2 while the pH from either empyema or a loculated sterile effusion is usually < 7.2. Pleural fluid glucose: Empyema is usually associated with pleural fluid glucose < 60 mg/dl, or a pleural fluid to serum glucose ratio < 0.5. Carcinomatous and tuberculous effusion sometimes show a similar profile. Rheumatoid effusions are often associated with pleural effusion glucose < 30 mg/dl.

Treatment: Pleural effusions large enough to cause dyspnea or interfere with ventilation should be drained by thoracentesis or chest tube. To preclude development of ipsilateral pulmonary edema, drain no more than a liter at hourly intervals. Malignant effusions are drained via thoracentesis or chest tube. Recurrent malignant effusions require chest tube drainage and instillation of a sclerosing agent (e.g. tetracycline 500 mg in 50 ml normal saline). Empyema is treated with antibiotics and drainage (either thoracentesis with large-bore needle or with chest tube). Parapneumonic effusion (a pneumonia-associated sterile effusion) will generally resolve without drainage with treatment of the pneumonia per se. However, loculated sterile parapneumonic effusions require drainage.

Pulmonary Embolism and Venous Thrombosis

Pulmonary embolism (obstruction of pulmonary arteries by a transported thrombus, fat, air, etc) is almost synonymous with pulmonary thromboembolism since other types of pulmonary embolism are rare (see below). A pulmonary thromboembolus nearly always originates from deep veins in the legs (see Deep Vein Thrombosis below) and occasionally from pelvic veins. Fatal pulmonary embolism is usually due to thromboembolism from the femoral, iliac, or pelvic veins. Uncommonly, a pulmonary embolus originates from a mural thrombus of the right ventricle or right atrium in a patient with right heart failure, particularly if atrial fibrillation is also present. Left alone, nonfatal pulmonary thromboemboli are slowly lysed and resolve over 2–6 weeks.

Diagnosis of pulmonary *thrombo*embolism: Signs/symptoms: Dyspnea, tachypnea, and tachycardia may be the only indications of pulmonary embolism. If (as is often the case) pulmonary infarction results; there may be pleuritic chest pain, pleural friction rub, hemoptysis, low grade fever, and/or leukocytosis. Arterial blood gas: PaO_2 on room air is usually < 80 mm Hg. Pulmonary embolism is unlikely if the PaO_2 is > 90 mm Hg. PCO_2 is usually decreased. Presence of soluble fibrin complexes and fibrin degradation products are evidence of generation of a thrombus and its breakdown respectively. EKG: Unless acute cor pulmonale develops (see below), EKG signs are absent or limited to nonspecific ST and T wave abnormalities. Chest x-ray is often normal, especially in the absence of pulmonary infarction. Sometimes, the region of occlusion shows atelectasis or the pulmonary vasculature appears to be decreased. If pulmonary infarction has resulted, one may see a peripheral wedge-shaped infiltrate, a small peripheral effusion, and/or an elevated hemidiaphragm. Normal perfusion scan rules out pulmonary embolism. An abnormal perfusion scan, however, does not prove a pulmonary embolism since other conditions (e.g. pneumonia, tumors, emphysema) can cause abnormal perfusion scans. Ventilation scan is ordered If the perfusion scan is abnormal. If the ventilation scan is normal in an area where the perfusion scan is abnormal (i.e. ventilation–perfusion mismatch), it is likely that a pulmonary embolism has occurred. On the other hand, a *matched* ventilation–perfusion abnormality does not exclude pulmonary embolism since it is not uncommon for a pulmonary embolism to cause both perfusion and ventilation defects at the same site (i.e. bronchoconstriction frequently occurs in a region of inadequate perfusion). Note, however, that matched abnormalities may also occur in certain other lung diseases. Pulmonary angiography is performed if the diagnosis is still in doubt.

Acute cor pulmonale (acute dilation and failure of the right heart due to pulmonary embolism) occurs when the pulmonary arterial bed is occluded to such a degree as to impede right ventricular output. Occlusion of > 50% pulmonary arterial bed is generally required to provoke acute cor pulmonale. However, less extensive obstruction may suffice if cardiopulmonary disease is already present. <u>Signs/symptoms:</u> Patient is dyspneic, tachypneic; and in many cases is diaphoretic, cyanotic and syncopal. Shock may ensue (hypotension, cool clammy skin). There are signs that the right ventricle is having difficulty pumping against the increased pulmonary resistance—e.g. right ventricular heave, elevation of CVP with distended neck veins, accentuated pulmonic component of S2, systolic tricuspid regurgitant murmur, right-sided S3 and S4, and possibly EKG signs. <u>EKG signs</u> may include right ventricular strain (T wave inversion in V1–4); P–pulmonale (tall and pointed P waves in II, III, and aVF due to right atrial dilation); right axis deviation; right bundle branch block; S1Q3T3 pattern. A Q wave and an inverted T wave in lead III coupled with inverted T wave in V1–4 is sometimes confused with a combined inferior and anteroseptal MI. However, in contrast to an inferior MI, a Q wave is absent from lead II in acute cor pulmonale. <u>Chest x–ray</u> may be normal or it may show prominent pulmonary arteries proximal to the obstruction with decreased vasculature peripherally. Refer above for other chest x–ray signs that may be present with pulmonary embolism in general. <u>Ventilation/perfusion scan or pulmonary angiography</u> may be needed to make the diagnosis (see above).

Treatment of pulmonary *thrombo*embolism: (**1**) <u>Oxygen</u> is administered. (**2**) <u>Anticoagulation</u> is begun with IV heparin and continued for 7–10 days; the dose is adjusted to achieve a PTT of 1.5 to 2 times the control. Warfarin is started while the patient is still receiving IV heparin and both drugs are administered together for 3–5 days. Heparin is then discontinued if the prothrombin time (which is warfarin dependent) is adequately prolonged. Adjusting the warfarin dose to achieve a prothrombin time of 15 seconds with a control of 12 seconds should be an adequate level of anticoagulation while minimizing the risk of bleeding complications. Warfarin is continued for 2–4 months or indefinitely if significant risk of deep venous thrombosis or pulmonary thromboembolism persists. Refer to heparin and warfarin in drug section. (**3**) <u>Thrombolytic therapy</u> (e.g. streptokinase) may be considered in patients with massive pulmonary embolism. (**4**) <u>Emergency angiography followed by embolectomy</u> is the only recourse in the event of massive pulmonary embolism with persistent shock and hypoxemia in spite of IV fluids, vasopressors, mechanical ventilation, and/or thrombolytic therapy. (**5**) <u>Patients who experience recurrent emboli</u> despite anticoagulation or who cannot be anticoagulated safely may have clips placed on the inferior vena cava to prevent emboli from reaching the lung. Transvenous insertion of a inferior vena caval umbrella is an alternative in patients who are poor surgical risks.

OTHER TYPES OF PULMONARY EMBOLISM: <u>Amniotic fluid embolism</u> is a rare complication of labor and delivery that is lethal in many cases. Patient is treated supportively—i.e. oxygen, IV fluids, and if needed IV vasopressors. <u>Fat embolism</u> is an uncommon complication of long bone trauma. There may be evidence of systemic embolization (e.g. confusion from CNS embolization, petechiae) and/or pulmonary embolization (e.g. dyspnea, tachypnea, tachycardia, cyanosis, etc). The patient may be febrile. An elevated serum lipase and fat globules in the urine are diagnostic. <u>Air embolism:</u> Air may inadvertently enter the venous circulation thru a CVP line or occur during hemodialysis. It may be a complication of vaginal delivery. Two–three hundred ml of air can be fatal. The air blocks the right ventricular outflow tract and/or pulmonary artery and can precipitate acute cor pulmonale. Dyspnea, tachypnea, wheezing, cyanosis, hypotension, shock are characteristic findings. Air movement across the pulmonic valve causes a mill–wheel murmur to be heard over the precordium. The patient is placed in left lateral decubitus position. The air bubble then floats toward the apex of the heart and thereby clears the right ventricular outflow tract so that blood can flow thru the right ventricle. A needle or catheter can then be inserted into the right ventricle in an attempt to release the air.

DEEP VEIN THROMBOSIS (DVT): The presence of venous stasis, hypercoagulability, and/or vein wall damage (Virchow's triad) increases the risk of DVT. Conditions that therefore predispose to DVT include: prolonged bed rest, congestive heart failure, trauma, malignancy, polycythemia, COPD, fracture of lower limb, obesity, diabetes mellitus, pregnancy, possibly oral contraceptives. ●While the calf is the most common site of DVT, DVT of the calf is (unless propagation into the deep femoral veins occurs) less serious than DVT of femoral, iliac, or pelvic veins—the veins from which most fatal pulmonary emboli arise. **Diagnosis DVT:** Signs & symptoms may be absent or there may be warmth, redness, and tenderness over the involved vein. Calf vein DVT can cause swelling of the foot and ankle and possibly a positive Homan's sign (calf pain provoked by dorsiflexion of the foot). Swelling to the level of the knees suggests femoral vein thrombosis while swelling of the entire leg may occur with iliofemoral thrombosis. Because swelling may not be obvious, it is useful to measure the circumference of both legs for comparison. Venography confirms DVT and must be performed if long-term anticoagulation is anticipated. Doppler ultrasound and impedance plethysmography are less sensitive indicators of DVT that, in particular, may miss DVT of the calf or a partially occluding thrombus. **Treatment DVT:** (**1**) Bed rest with leg elevation for 1 wk and elastic support stockings. Ambulation is then permitted but the patient should be warned against prolonged sitting or standing. (**2**) Anticoagulation is begun with IV heparin and continued for 7–10 days. The dose is adjusted to achieve a PTT of 1.5 to 2 times the control. Warfarin is started while the patient is still receiving IV heparin and both drugs are administered together for 3–5 days. Heparin is then discontinued if the prothrombin time (which is warfarin dependent) is adequately prolonged. Adjusting the warfarin dose to achieve a prothrombin time of 15 seconds with a control of 12 seconds should be an adequate level of anticoagulation while minimizing the risk of bleeding complications. Warfarin is continued for 2–4 months or indefinitely if significant risk of deep venous thrombosis persists. Refer to heparin and warfarin in drug section. (**3**) Thrombectomy is indicated when iliofemoral thrombosis causes severe venous obstruction with cyanosis of the limb. (**4**) Patients who experience recurrent thromboembolism in spite of anticoagulation or who cannot be safely anticoagulated are candidates for insertion of an umbrella into (or a clip onto) the inferior vena cava. **Prophylaxis DVT:** Low–dose SC heparin (see drug section for dose) is advised for patients who are bedridden for prolonged periods and who are at risk for DVT (e.g. CHF, malignancy, COPD, fracture of lower limb, obesity, diabetes mellitus). Low-dose SC heparin is also indicated prior to and after major abdominal surgery (prostatic surgery excepted).

SUPERFICIAL THROMBOPHLEBITIS may result from trauma, IV therapy, or be associated with varicose veins, thromboangitis obliterans, abdominal malignancy (Trousseau's sign), systemic disease. **Diagnosis:** There is tenderness, erythema, and warmth along a superficial vein. The thrombosed vein can often be felt as a "cord". The limb as a whole is usually not swollen since edema is confined to the area about the involved vein. There may be fever and leukocytosis. The presence of chills and high fever suggests septic thrombophlebitis. Superficial thrombophlebitis may be confused with DVT, cellulitis, or lymphangitis. **Treatment:** (**1**) Heat, elevation, rest, elastic support stockings. (**2**) Anticoagulation is not indicated. (**3**) Aspirin or some other nonsteroidal anti–inflammatory drug such as indomethacin is prescribed for pain. (**4**) Administer antibiotics, if septic thrombophlebitis is present. Staph. aureus is the most common pathogen. (**5**) Venous stripping is considered in the event of recurrences. (**6**) If thrombophlebitis involves the saphenous vein near its juncture with the femoral vein, the saphenous vein is ligated to prevent pulmonary embolism.

Anaphylaxis & Anaphylactoid Reactions

Anaphylaxis is an IgE–mediated reaction (type I reaction) that occurs in a patient who has been previously exposed to an allergen (antigen). The allergen induces the production of IgE molecules which in turn bind to the surface of mast cells and basophils. On subsequent exposure, the allergen binds to IgE attached to the surface of mast cells and basophils and causes those cells to release substances (e.g. histamine, bradykinin, prostaglandins, ECF-A, etc.) that result in the clinical expression of anaphylaxis. Causes of anaphylaxis: A great variety of agents are known to induce anaphylaxis in susceptible individuals—e.g. hymenoptera venom (bees, wasps, hornets, yellow jackets, fire ants); pollens; foods (e.g. shellfish, eggs, nuts, grains, beans); antibiotics (e.g. penicillin, cephalosporin, sulfonamides, tetracyclines, aminoglycosides, amphotericin B, nitrofurantoin); local anesthetics (e.g. procaine [Novocain], lidocaine [Xylocaine]); animal serum or human serum (rarely).

Anaphylactoid reactions differ from anaphylaxis in that the reaction is not mediated by IgE. Therefore, prior exposure is not required. However, because mast cells and basophils are induced to release their contents, the clinical effect is the same and the treatment is the same. Causes of anaphylactoid reactions include nonsteroidal anti–inflammatory drugs (e.g. aspirin, indomethacin); mannitol; IV radiographic contrast dyes.

Clinical presentation is variable. The skin, respiratory tract, and/or cardiovascular system are commonly affected; the GI tract infrequently. Cutaneous expression may include itching, erythema, urticaria, angioedema. Submucosal angioedema may result in swelling of the lips, tongue, soft palate, and pharynx. Angioedema of the larynx or epiglottis causes hoarseness, and may lead to stridor and complete airway obstruction. Bronchospasm with wheezing may occur. Hypotension and shock may result from peripheral vasodilation and/or increased capillary permeability with decreased intravascular volume. Gastrointestinal symptoms (e.g. vomiting, diarrhea, abdominal cramping) are uncommon and are due to contraction of GI smooth muscle.

Treatment: see appendix.

Near-drowning
in most cases is not associated with aspiration of sufficient fluid to cause significant alteration of electrolyte balance. In fact, in 10–20% drowning accidents, laryngospasm effectively prevents aspiration of any water. The major deleterious effects of near–drowning are generally the consequence of (**1**) hypoxemia, (**2**) respiratory and metabolic acidosis, (**3**) chemical pneumonitis with possible subsequent development of adult respiratory distress syndrome, (**4**) pulmonary infection. Cardiac arrhythmias, cerebral edema and acute tubular necrosis are other potential complications.

Laboratory: Obtain arterial blood gas and chest x–ray. These may be normal at first, only to deteriorate later if pulmonary edema subsequently develops. Other labs: electrolytes, BUN, glucose, CBC, urinalysis, prothrombin time.

Treatment: If the patient is alert and breathing spontaneously, simply administer oxygen (via nonrebreather mask initially), apply cardiac monitor, and observe. If the patient is apneic, obtunded, or the PaO_2 remains < 50 despite 100% oxygen via nonrebreather mask: Intubate and mechanically ventilate. Acidosis, if present, will generally resolve with adequate ventilation. Sodium bicarbonate may be required in some cases. Cerebral edema: Hyperventilate the intubated patient to maintain the $PaCO_2$ at 25–30 mm Hg, and administer IV mannitol (see drug section). Hypotension, if present, usually resolves with correction of hypoxemia and acidosis, but intravenous crystalloid may be necessary. Dopamine may be needed if clinically significant hypotension persists. Aspiration of either water or stomach contents: Bronchoscopy may be indicated to assess pulmonary injury and to remove particulate material. Aspiration may result in ARDS. See "Adult Respiratory Distress Syndrome" chapter for treatment. Antibiotics are indicated if bacterial pneumonia develops but are not administered simply for prophylaxis. Corticosteroids: Whether or not they should be administered is unresolved.

Pneumonia (inflammation/infection of the alveoli)
Viral pneumonia is the most common type of pneumonia in children. Possible culpable viral agents include influenza, adenoviruses, parainfluenza viruses, respiratory syncytial virus, rhinoviruses, varicella–zoster, herpes simplex, cytomegalovirus, coxsackie, echovirus, rheovirus, measles. In adults, influenza virus is the most common pathogen; other viral pneumonias are unusual in adults. Signs/symptoms: Presentations vary. In a typical case, after an incubation period of 2–3 days, nonspecific viral symptoms develop (e.g. malaise, fever, chills, headache, myalgias) and there may be coryza and pharyngitis. This is followed by cough which is initially nonproductive and then becomes mucopurulent. Fever is usually present for 2–5 days and cough resolves over 1–2 wk or so. Chest x–ray reveals patchy infiltrates and sometimes a pleural effusion. Sputum gram stain is negative. WBC count is typically low or normal. Complications: Viral pneumonia is usually not a serious disease However, some high–risk patients (e.g. elderly or COPD patient with in-

fluenza pneumonia) are prone to progressive hypoxia and may succumb to respiratory failure. There is either progression of the viral pneumonia itself or a bacterial pneumonia ensues. Prophylaxis: Influenza vaccinations are recommended yearly in the following circumstances: persons over 65, diabetics, chronic pulmonary or renal disease, heart disease, chronic severe anemia, immunodeficiency.

Mycoplasma pneumonia is the most common cause of pneumonia in teenagers and young adults. However, ≤ 10% patients infected with Mycoplasma pmeumoniae develop pneumonia. Signs/symptoms: Incubation takes 1–3 wk and is followed by gradual onset of malaise, fever, headache, myalgia, nonproductive cough, and sometimes pleuritic chest pain. Fine rales may be heard. Pharyngitis with tender cervical nodes, and/or rash may also be present. Complications: Hemorrhagic or bullous myringitis is an uncommon finding. Occasionally, patients develop Stevens–Johnson syndrome, Raynaud's phenomenon, or hemolysis. Chest x–ray reveals patchy infiltrates, usually unilateral and usually in the lower lung(s). The x–ray often looks worse than what the physical signs would suggest. Laboratory: WBC count is generally normal; cold agglutinins are usually present; complement fixation confirms diagnosis. Treatment: Infection will almost always resolve without treatment. However, antibiotics will shorten the course of disease. Erythromycin for 7–10 days is the treatment of choice. Tetracycline is the alternative.

Pneumococcal pneumonia is due to Streptococcus pneumoniae. It is the most common pneumonia in adults. Signs/symptoms: Classically, there is sudden onset of fever, chills, pleuritic chest pain, and productive cough. Gradual onset of the syndrome is not uncommon. The patient may be tachypneic and dyspneic. Rales, decreased breath sounds, and perhaps a pleural friction rub may be heard over the area of pneumonia. With consolidation—there is dullness to percussion, vocal fremitus, and egophony. Sputum ranges from pink to rust–colored and becomes yellow mucopurulent as the infection resolves. Presumptive diagnosis is based on finding gram–positive lancet–shaped diplococci together with neutrophils in the sputum. Sputum culture (or culture of transtracheal aspirate) and blood cultures should be obtained even though they are often negative. Chest x–ray usually reveals lobar consolidation (most commonly of the middle and lower lobes) and a pleural effusion is not uncommon. Some patients do not show consolidation, but instead a bronchopneumonia with multiple patchy infiltrates. Emphysema patients may show patchy "honeycombed" infiltrates instead of consolidation. WBC count is generally elevated. A low count is not a good sign. Treatment: Penicillin is the drug of choice. Erythromycin or a cephalosporin are alternatives. Prevention: Immunization with polyvalent pneumococcal vaccine (Pneumovax) is advised for individuals over over 65 yr of age. It is also advised in patients over 2 yr of age who fall into the following categories: chronic cardiac or pulmonary disease, splenectomized or functionally asplenic patients, sickle cell anemia patients.

Staphylococcal pneumonia is usually a complication of a viral respiratory infection (e.g. influenza). Infants, the elderly, and immunocompromised or otherwise debilitated individuals are the most susceptible. Staph. pneumonia may also originate by hematogenous spread to the lung from another site (e.g. infectious endocarditis, septic thrombophlebitis, furuncle). Signs/symptoms: resemble pneumococcal pneumonia. Differentiating signs may include salmon–colored sputum (with diagnostic gram stain–see below) or furuncles (if there is bacteremia). Chest x–ray: Patchy pulmonary infiltrates with necrosis leading to lung abscess formation and cavitation are characteristic. However, lobar pneumonia may sometimes occur. Pleural effusions with empyema are common. Complications: Metastatic abscesses (e.g. to liver, brain, kidney) may ensue if there is bacteremia. Laboratory: Sputum gram stain may disclose gram–positive cocci in grapelike clusters. Sputum cultures are usually positive. Blood cultures are usually positive if there is bacteremia. Treatment: penicillinase–resistant penicillin (e.g. nafcillin) for at least 3–4 weeks.

Haemophilus influenza pneumonia is common in males with COPD or in alcoholics. It is also not uncommonly responsible for the bacterial pneumonia that complicates a viral pneumonia, especially influenza pneumonia. After viral pneumonia, H. influenza and pneumococcus are the most common cause of pneumonia in the 1 month–5 yr age group. Signs/symptoms: Fever, chills, cough, and possibly pleuritic pain are typical but the syndrome develops less rapidly than for pneumococcal pneumonia. Laboratory: Since H. influenza is normally found in the upper respiratory tract, gram stain or culture of the sputum is not diagnostic. Diagnosis is established by culture of blood or pleural fluid. Chest x-ray: Patchy infiltrates suggesting a bronchopneumonia is typical. Lobar consolidation is occasionally seen. Treatment: Ampicillin is the usual drug of choice but resistance occurs in about 20% cases. Resistant species are treated with cefaclor, cefamandole, trimethoprim–sulfamethoxazole, or chloramphenicol. Prophylaxis: Haemophilus b vaccine is recommended in children up to 5th birthday (see "Routine Immunizations" chapter).

Klebsiella pneumomia is most common in alcoholics and frequently occurs following aspiration. Diabetics and COPD patients are also susceptible. It is a necrotizing pneumonia that often results in abscesses with cavitation. Empyema is common. Chest x-ray: More than one lobe is usually involved. Involvement of the right upper lobe is common because aspiration is often the inciting mechanism. The inflammatory exudate may be voluminous enough to cause bulging of involved lobe(s). Hence, it is not uncommon to see outward bending of the interlobar fissures. Sputum is typically a blood–streaked gray–greenish or brick–red. Gram stain reveals encapsulated gram–negative bacilli. Sputum should also be sent for aerobic culture, or preferably a transtracheal aspirate is obtained for both aerobic and anaerobic cultures. Blood cultures should also be obtained. Treatment usually consists of cephalothin in conjunction with an aminoglycoside.

Pseudomonas aerugenosa pneumonia seldom occurs in the normal host even though P. aerugenosa is frequently found on the skin or in the GI tract of healthy persons. However, debilitated or immunocompromised patients not uncommonly develop pseudomonas infection. This organism is one of the most common causes of nosocomial infections. P. aerugenosa pneumonia may develop from bacteremic spread of the organism or as a primary pneumonia. Contamination from inhalation therapy equipment that employs reservoir nebulizers is a common source of primary pneumonia. A necrotizing pneumonia results when the pneumonia develops as a consequence of bacteremic spread; empyema is a common complication. Patients with cystic fibrosis are prone to chronic or recurrent pulmonary infection with P. aerugenosa. Treatment is with a combination of an aminoglycoside and carbenicillin (or ticarcillin). Piperacillin, mezlocillin, or azlocillin may be substituted for carbenicillin or ticarcillin.

Legionnaires' disease is due to the gram–negative rod Legionella pneumophila. Signs/symptoms: After an incubation period of 2–10 days, the patient typically develops malaise, fever, chills, headache, and myalgia. There is a nonproductive or a scantly productive cough. Pleuritic chest pain may be present. GI complaints (abdominal pain, vomiting, diarrhea) as well as neurologic findings (e.g. confusion, delirium, slurred speech, ataxia) are not uncommon. Heart rate is often lower (< 100) than would be expected from the high fever. Chest x-ray: Patchy infiltrates and then consolidation may be seen. Pleural effusions sometimes develop. Laboratory: ●WBC count ranges from 8000–10,000 with a left shift. ●There may be laboratory evidence of the effects of the infection on the kidneys (e.g. microscopic hematuria, azotemia) and/or liver (e.g. elevated transaminases). ●Gram stain of transtracheal aspirate shows neutrophils without bacteria (rarely, weakly–stained gram–negative rods are seen). Gimenez or Dieterle silver stain more consistently reveal the bacteria. ●Diagnosis is most rapidly established by direct fluorescent antibody testing of respiratory secretions. ●Because of special requirements, routine cultures are negative. Culture of respiratory secretions may be accomplished on charcoal yeast extract medium but this may take 10 days. Treatment: erythromycin for 3 weeks.

Pneunocystis carinii pneumonia is due to an opportunistic protozoan. Consequently, disease is most likely to occur in the immunocompromised (e.g. AIDS, corticosteroid or cancer therapy, malnourished infant). Signs/symptoms: Fever and dry cough is typical. Progressive respiratory embarassment occurs: dyspnea, tachypnea, cyanosis. Chest x-ray shows diffuse patchy infiltrates and then consolidation. Laboratory: Diagnosis is infrequently made by microscopic exam of sputum or transtracheal aspirates (e.g. with methenamine silver stain). The diagnosis is most often confirmed by staining specimens obtained via bronchoscopy (tracheobronchial brushings or transbronchial biopsy) or percutaneous lung biopsy. Treatment: trimethoprim–sulfamethoxazole for minimum of 14 days. Pentamidine is alternative.

Tuberculosis

is a granulomatous necrotizing disease that can cause disease in any organ but "favors" the lung. The cause is the acid–fast aerobic bacillus, Mycobacterium tuberculosis and rarely M. bovis. The usual sequence of events is as follows: The bacillus is inhaled into the alveoli and bronchioles, usually of the lower or middle lungs. The bacillus multiplies at this primary focus, spreads to hilar nodes, and disseminates via the bloodstream. With lymphohematogenous spread, the T lymphocytes become activated and typical granulomas and caseation necrosis develop at the primary focus of infection, hilar nodes, and other sites where the bacillus may have spread. Tuberculin skin sensitivity develops 4–10 weeks after acquiring the bacillus. The cell–mediated immune reaction arrests the growth of the bacillus (usually before symptoms develop) but some live bacteria remain for the life of the host. These dormant bacteria persist within granulomatous lesions with the potential to reactivate and produce disease at a later time. Reactivation is most likely when the immune system is compromised by illness or immunosuppressants such as corticosteroids. Most cases of clinical tuberculosis arise from reactivation of dormant bacteria within a primary site of infection—usually the upper lobe(s) of the lung where conditions favor proliferation. The bacteria arrive at this region by hematogenous spread during the primary infection. Occasionally the primary infection is not arrested but progresses with any of several consequences including: (1) progression at the primary pulmonary focus with caseation necrosis and possibly pneumonitis; (2) contiguous spread from the initial pulmonary focus to the pleura with ensuing pleurisy with effusion (not uncommonly in the absence x–ray signs of pulmonary parenchymal disease); (3) pericarditis from contiguous spread from infected hilar nodes; (4) hematogenous spread with ensuing miliary tuberculosis.

Diagnosis: Signs/symptoms: Onset is often insidious with malaise, anorexia, and weight loss being the only clues. With pulmonary involvement there is usually fever, productive cough (which may be blood–tinged), and night sweats. Tuberculin test: Intermediate strength PPD (5 TU) is injected intradermally. A positive test for Tb infection consists of > 10 mm induration at the injection site after 48 hr. A positive test does not prove active Tb, only that the patient is infected with the bacillus. Infection by atypical mycobacteria may also cause a positive PPD. Some patients with clinically active Tb have a negative PPD (i.e. anergy). Anergy may be ruled out by intradermal testing with mumps or Candida. Those patients being evaluated for Tb with a negative PPD (5 TU) should be tested with 250 TU. Anergy is most likely if there is disseminated Tb, viral illness, sarcoidosis, Hodgkin's or other lymphoreticular disease, or the patient is receiving a corticosteroid or some other immunosuppressive therapy. Faulty technique is often the cause of a false–negative PPD. PPD (1 TU) is used in children or other patients likely to be hypersensitive, and in patients with eye disease (e.g. choroidal tubercles on fundoscopic exam). Chest x–ray in an inactive case may reveal a Ghon complex (regional hilar lymph node calcification with a calcified peripheral granuloma). Active pulmonary Tb due to reactivation is nearly always seen in the upper lung as an infiltrate or cavitary disease. Sometimes, only a pleural effusion is present. Early in the course of miliary Tb, the miliary lesions may not be seen because they may be too small to be detected. Acid–fast stain of the sputum or any other suspicious site can provide presumptive evidence of tuberculosis pending culture results. However, a positive acid–fast stain does not conclusively prove tuberculosis since other mycobacteria have the same staining characteristics. Culture of M. tuberculosis (from sputum, gastric lavage, pleural fluid, CSF, tissue, ...) is the only conclusive method of proving tuberculosis. Furthermore, culture must be obtained so that antibiotic sensitivity can be established. Growth is slow; culture results usually take 2–6 weeks.

Extrapulmonary tuberculosis: Tuberculosis pleurisy produces an exudative effusion (see "Pleural Effusion"). Since acid–fast stain and culture of pleural fluid are often negative, diagnosis may depend on closed needle biopsy and culture of the pleura. Tuberculosis of the GU tract may be difficult to diagnosis since localizing signs and symptoms are often absent. Tuberculous pyelonephritis or cystitis may be suspected from the presence of "sterile pyuria" (i.e. urine shows WBC but routine urine culture is negative). IVP may reveal renal cavities and calcification. Involvement of the ureters may lead to obstructive hydronephrosis. Tuberculosis meningitis may occur when there is bloodstream dissemination to the meninges with subsequent rupture into the subarachnoid space, or when a CNS focus extends to the meninges. Typically, the CSF shows WBC count 100–600/cu mm with mononuclear predominance. Neutrophils may predominate early in the illness. The CSF glucose is usually less than half of simultaneously obtained serum glucose, and the CSF protein is elevated. A low CSF glucose with mononuclear pleocytosis is also encountered in fungal meningitis, or when a lymphoma or carcinoma invades the meninges. Sometimes CNS involvement presents as a brain mass (tuberculoma). Miliary tuberculosis can occur during the initial infection, or from reactivation of a latent focus. In either case, bacteremia results in widespread dissemination and any organ can be infected. Fever, night sweats, anorexia, weight loss are typical. An important diagnostic finding is the presence of choroidal tubercles on fundoscopy. PPD is often negative. Chest x–ray may reveal the miliary lesions; except early in the disease when they are too small to be seen. Cultures and acid–fast stain are obtained of sputum, urine, gastric fluid; and blood culture is obtained. Bone marrow involvement may cause anemia, thrombocytopenia, pancytopenia, or leukemoid reaction. Bone marrow biopsy with culture is sometimes required to make the diagnosis. Tuberculosis pericarditis may result from hematogenous spread but it is usually due to contiguous spread from infected hilar nodes. A pericardial effusion may be present and should be tapped for culture and acid–fast stain; pericardial biopsy is sometimes necessary. Prolonged pericardial involvement may lead to constrictive pericarditis (see "Pericarditis"). Tuberculosis of the GI tract may cause ulcerations of the GI mucosa at any site from the mouth to the anus but the cecum is the site most frequently involved. Sometimes, obstruction of the GI tract occurs and is usually thought to be a carcinoma until surgery proves otherwise. Fistulas and/or perforation may occur. Anorexia, weight loss, abdominal pain, and/or change in bowel habits are common presenting complaints. There may be GI bleeding. Tuberculosis peritonitis usually arises from contiguous spread (e.g. from intestines, regional nodes) and less often by hematogenous spread. Presentation is variable–e.g. fever, weight loss, abdominal pain, ascites. The peritoneal fluid is an exudate with mononuclear predominance. Since peritoneal fluid culture and acid–fast stain is often negative and evidence of pulmonary involvement may be absent, peritoneal biopsy may be required to make the diagnosis. Tuberculosis spondylitis (Pott's disease) results from tuberculous invasion of the vertebral bodies. There is back pain and sometimes a paraspinal abscess advances so as to present as a groin mass or supraclavicular mass. Compression of the spinal cord may result in neurologic deficits including paraplegia. X–ray reveals erosion of anterior vertebral bodies with anterior wedging, obliteration of intervertebral disc, and/or a paraspinal abscess. In the absence of active Tb in other organs, diagnosis may depend on biopsy with culture.

Treatment tuberculosis: Although the conclusive diagnosis awaits culture results, drug therapy should not be withheld if there is a presumptive diagnosis. Culture results may take 2–6 weeks and are often falsely negative.

Uncomplicated pulmonary and extrapulmonary tuberculosis: Isoniazid (INH) and rifampin are administered in combination. Sputum cultures are obtained at monthly intervals and both drugs are continued for at least 6 months after sputum culture converts from positive to negative. The minimum duration of therapy using this regimen is 9 months. Therapy can be shortened to 6 months if pyrazinamide is added to the regimen for the first 2 months.

Circumstances in which triple drug therapy is required initially: tuberculous meningitis, disseminated tuberculosis, AIDS and other immunosuppressive conditions, diabetes, silicosis, renal failure, gastrectomized patient, known exposure to drug–resistant strains of Tb, history of residence in regions where drug–resistant strains are common. The 3–drug regimen consists of isoniazid (INH), rifampin, and either ethambutol or pyrazinamide. In patients with tuberculous meningitis, the 3rd drug is usually pyrazinamide. Three drugs are usually administered for 2–3 months. Therapy is then continued with two drugs (INH plus rifampin) for a total duration of therapy of at least 12 months. ●Adding a 3rd drug for the first 2–3 months guards against the emergence of resistant strains.

Prophylaxis with INH is indicated in the following circumstances: **(1)** household or other close contacts of patient with active Tb. Prophylactic INH is discontinued at the end of 3 months if PPD is negative, and continued for additional 9 months if PPD is positive or if exposure to active case persists. **(2)** patient with positive PPD and x–ray evidence of prior pulmonary tuberculosis receives INH for 12 months; **(3)** person under 35 yr with positive PPD receives INH for 12 months; **(4)** person of any age who has within the last 2 years converted from negative to positive PPD receives INH for 12 months; **(5)** patient of any age with positive PPD who is at high risk for developing clinical disease receives INH for 12 months. High risk conditions include diabetes mellitus, silicosis, leukemia, lymphoma, postgastrectomy state, corticosteroid or other immunosuppressant therapy.

Influenza

Influenza is due to an RNA virus, specifically a myxovirus. <u>Antigenic components:</u> There are 3 distinct serotypes (A, B, and C) based on antigenic differences of internal proteins (matrix protein, nucleoprotein, polymerase). Influenza viruses have 2 kinds of glycoprotein projecting from their surface, hemagglutinin (H) and neuraminidase (N). H enables the virus to bind to a receptor site on the surface of cells being infected. H induces the production of neutralizing antibodies and is therefore the most important component in the development of immunity. N facilitates the release of newly formed virions from infected cells. Antibody to N impedes viral replication. <u>Antigenic shift and antigenic drift:</u> ●Influenza A is noteworthy in that the genes coding for H and N may change. New antigenic variants of H and/or N representing new strains of influenza A thus emerge and account for the recurrent epidemics of influenza. This phenomenon occurs less commonly with influenza B and probably does not occur with influenza C. ●A minor change in H and/or N is called antigenic drift while major change is referred to as antigenic shift. Pandemics occur when there is antigenic shift. ●Influenza A is divided into antigenic subtypes based on the major variants of H (of which there 3 known—H1, H2, and H3) and major variants of N (of which there are 2 known—N1 and N2). For instance, the influenza A virus causing the pandemic of 1968 is designated H3N2 while that of 1977, H1N1. <u>Seasonal occurrence:</u> Epidemics virtually always occur during the fall and winter. Two strains or subtypes of influenza A (or both influenza A and B) may sometimes be identified during an epidemic. <u>Transmission/pathogenesis:</u> Influenza is spread person-to-person, usually by inhalation of infected airborne droplets. Once in the respiratory tract, the virus invades and replicates within the columnar epithelial cells and these cells desquamate.

Signs/symptoms: Typically, after an incubation period of 1–3 days, there is an abrupt onset of fever and chills with headache, malaise, and myalgias. The temperature rises over the next 12–24 hr up to 39.5 C (103 F), sometimes higher. The temperature usually falls the next day. The fever, in the absence of complications, lasts 1–5 days (average 3 days). Headache is frequently accompanied by photophobia and there may be retrobulbar aching and pain with eye movement. The eyes may burn or tear, and the conjunctiva may be reddened. Coryza is present in many cases and nasal obstruction sometimes ensues. A sore and reddened throat is common but there is no exudate. Tender cervical nodes is a frequent finding. A nonproductive cough is often present from the outset and may worsen and become productive as the fever, headache, and myalgia resolve. Cough, weakness, fatigue may continue for a few weeks before the patient finally feels well. ●The foregoing are typical clinical findings. However, other syndromes are not uncommon. For example, influenza may cause the common cold, pharyngitis alone, or croup.

Treatment: <u>Amantadine</u> (100 mg PO bid x 3-5 days in adult) will reduce the severity and duration of illness. <u>Fever and pain</u> are treated with antipyretic analgesics. In patients < 16 yr, acetaminophen is recommended instead of aspirin because it is suspected that aspirin may induce Reye's syndrome in children with influenza. ●If necessary, codeine is combined with aspirin or acetaminophen to give added pain relief and also to alleviate cough (e.g. in adult: acetaminophen 325 mg plus codeine 30 mg at 4 hour intervals as needed).

Prophylaxis: <u>Influenza vaccines</u> are inactivated whole virus or viral subunits ("split virus") of influenza B and the most prevalent strains of influenza A. Whole or split vaccines are equally effective (about 80%) in preventing influenza but the split vaccine produces fewer side effects and is recommended for those under 13 yr. The composition of the vaccine is changed yearly to reflect the strains most likely to cause infection. Routine yearly vaccination is recommended for those over 65; for patients with chronic disease (e.g. diabetes mellitus, cardiac disease, severe chronic anemia, chronic pulmonary or renal disease); for medical personnel in contact with the latter; or for those who simply want to reduce the risk of infection. <u>Amantadine</u> may prevent influenza A but not influenza B. During an outbreak of influenza A, the drug is given until 2 wk after influenza vaccination, or until the outbreak is over if vaccination is not possible.

Complications: Viral pneumonia typically develops relatively early in the course of illness and may follow a fulminant course with hemoptysis, dyspnea, cyanosis. A fatal outcome is not uncommon in the elderly or patients with chronic pulmonary disease, cardiac disease, or other debilities. Secondary bacterial pneumonia should be suspected if fever persists beyond 5 days. Pneumococcus and H. influenza are the most common pathogens. S. aureus, Klebsiella, and streptococci are occasionally encountered. Other possible complications: Reye's syndrome, myositis with myoglobinuria and elevated CPK, myocarditis, pericarditis, encephalitis, Guillain–Barré syndrome.

Epiglottitis is an acute inflammation of the epiglottis and the aryepiglottic folds. It is almost always due to Haemophilus influenza B. Sometimes the aryepiglottic folds are mainly involved and so the syndrome may be more accurately termed supraglottitis. The subglottic structures (vocal cords, subglottic space, trachea) are spared. Epiglottitis is most common between 2 and 7 years of age, but it may occur at any age.

Diagnosis: Typically, with little prodrome there is abrupt onset and rapid development of full–blown syndrome which includes fever, sore throat, dysphagia with drooling, and inspiratory stridor with supraclavicular and subcostal retractions. Cyanosis and respiratory arrest may supervene. Diminished breath sounds on chest auscultation reflects decreased ventilation. The patient prefers to sit up and resists lying flat because it exacerbates the obstruction. Cherry–red epiglottis can sometimes be seen by simply having the patient open his mouth. However, unless prepared to intubate (or failing intubation to perform cricothyroidotomy), aggressive attempts to visualize the epiglottis are contraindicated because of the risk of provoking complete obstruction. In contrast to croup, a barking cough or hoarseness are absent. X–rays: Lateral and AP views of the neck, and chest x–ray are obtained with the patient sitting upright. The lateral view of the neck usually reveals an enlarged epiglottis. However, this finding may be absent if the aryepiglottic folds are mainly involved.

Treatment: A physician must remain in constant attendance in all suspected cases of epiglottitis, and must be prepared if necessary to intubate or to perform cricothyroidotomy. Intubation or possible cricothyroidotomy: If the diagnosis of epiglottitis is established, the patient should be intubated—preferably by an anesthesiologist in the operating room with an ENT surgeon standing by to handle complications. If the patient is in respiratory arrest or impending arrest (e.g. cyanosis), the patient can usually be initially ventilated with a bag–valve mask and 100% oxygen. Intubation should follow using an endotracheal tube that is 1–2 mm smaller than usual (see appendix for usual tube sizes). Failing intubation, a cricothyroidotomy should be performed until a more stable airway can be established. Cricothyroidotomy is perfromed with a 14 gauge plastic catheter–over needle. The catheter is subsequently connected via a 3–way stopcock to high–flow 100% oxygen. Once a stable airway is assured, blood and throat cultures are obtained, and IV chloramphenicol is begun. The patient can often be extubated in 24–48 hr.

Prevention: Haemophilus B vaccine is a routine part of the immunization schedule of infants and children.

Croup (acute laryngotracheobronchitis) is an acute inflammation of the larynx, trachea, bronchi, bronchioles, and lung parenchyma. The swelling leading to obstruction is most pronounced in the subglottic region. Croup is most often caused by parainfluenza viruses. Respiratory syncytial virus, influenza A & B, adenovirus, enterovirus, rhinovirus, or Mycoplasma pneumoniae are infrequently responsible. Croup is most common between 6 month and 3 year.

Diagnosis: Signs/symptoms: Barking cough with hoarseness is characteristic. With progression, there is inspiratory stridor with supraclavicular, intercostal, and subcostal retractions. Expiratory rhonchi and wheezing may be heard. Fever may be present. A history of an upper respiratory infection for the previous 1–3 days is often elicited. In contrast to epiglottitis, the patient does not resist lying flat, and drooling and dysphagia are absent. X–rays: AP and lateral views of the neck may reveal sub-glottic narrowing ("steeple sign"). If the diagnosis is in doubt and epiglottitis cannot be excluded, examination of the oropharynx may be attempted with extreme caution. Intubation and cricothyroidotomy equipment must be ready, and preferably an anesthesiologist standing by.

Differential diagnosis: epiglottitis, diptheria (has patient been immunized against diptheria?), foreign body, retropharyngeal abscess (palpation of the neck or lateral neck x–ray may reveal mass), angioedema of larynx (is there urticaria or swelling about eyes ?).

Treatment: Oxygen and nebulized mist may be all that is required in mild cases. A mist tent with oxygen is ordered if the patient is admitted. Racemic epinephrine 2.25% (0.5 ml in 3.5 ml normal saline delivered via nebulizer) is administered in more severe cases. Dexamethasone 0.3 mg/kg IM is given. Antibiotics are not indicated unless bacterial tracheitis is suspected. Intubation is indicated if (in spite of treatment with racemic epinephrine) there is progressive exhaustion, severe and worsening retractions, cyanosis, altered mental status, or carbon dioxide retention (pCO_2 > 40). Disposition: Patients who require racemic epinephrine should either be admitted, or observed for 4 hours to see that they do not subsequently deteriorate. Patients stable enough to be discharged should be treated with a vaporizer at home

Whooping Cough is due Bordetella pertussis, a small gram–negative coc-

cobacillus. The syndrome is also sometimes due to B. parapertussis or rarely to B. bronchiseptica. Infection is transmitted person–to–person via airborne droplets. Whooping cough may occur at any age. Neither vaccination nor infection confers lifelong immunity but the 2nd infection is usually mild or subclinical.

Signs/symptoms: Incubation is 1–3 wk. Symptoms last about 6 wk beginning with the catarrhal stage : sneezing, cough, conjunctival injection, lacrimation, and possibly a mild fever. The cough becomes more frequent and enters the paroxysmal stage 1–2 wk after onset of symptoms. During a paroxysm there are 5–20 short coughs rapidly following one upon the other and gathering in intensity. At the moment the coughing ceases there is a deep inspiration that causes the characteristic whoop. Viscid mucus may be expectorated during or following an attack, and frequently there is vomiting. Another paroxysm may occur after a short interval. Choking with apnea (rather than coughing paroxysms) may occur in infants, and may in some cases lead to asphyxia. Convalescent stage: the paroxysms gradually subside. However, even months after apparently complete recovery, paroxysms may again be provoked by an unrelated respiratory infection.

Complications: Pneumonia may develop. This is due to bacteria other than pertussis or to a virus. The presence of a fever may signal the onset of a secondary infection since a fever is not usually present with pertussis alone. Otitis media is common. Asphyxia may occur in infants. Interstitial or subcutaneous emphysema, or pneumothorax are uncommon complications that arise as a consequence of coughing–provoked increase in intrathoracic pressure. Bronchiectasis and/or atelectasis may be seen. Bleeding into the brain, eyes, or skin may result from the elevated venous pressure generated during paroxysms. Metabolic alkalosis and malnutrition may ensue from the vomiting.

Laboratory: Culture is the method of diagnosis prior to the paroxysmal stage. Culture is also the method of diagnosis in infants who may not have the classical coughing paroxysms. The most reliable way of culturing the organism is to pass a small sterile cotton swab (on the end of teflon or wire) thru the nares to the posterior nasopharynx and then immediately plate it on Bordet–Gengou medium. Over 80% cultures are positive in the catarrhal and early paroxysmal stages. Culture is much less reliable thereafter. WBC ccunt is usually 15,000–30,000 with 60–80% lymphocytes but the WBC count may range from normal to over 60,000.

Treatment: Antibiotic begun in the catarrhal or early paroxysmal stages may lessen the duration of illness. Antibiotic begun thereafter may not effect the illness but is administered so that the patient will become noncontagious. The drug of choice is erythromycin continued for 2–3 wk (refer to drug section for dose). The patient is isolated for the first week of antibiotic therapy.

Prophylaxis: Exposed children < 4 years of age should receive a booster pertussis vaccination and a 10 day course of erythromycin. Other contacts receive erythromycin alone for 10 days.
●Pertussis vaccination is recommended routinely as part of a triple vaccine (diptheria, pertussis, tetanus) at 2, 4, and 6 months of age with boosters at 1 yr and 5 yr. Pertussis vaccination is not advised beyond 6 yr of age because there is an increased risk of side effects and a decreased risk of symptomatic infection. Vaccination does not prevent B. parapertussis illness.

Renal Disease

Acute Renal Failure
Chronic Renal Failure
Interstitial Renal Disease
Glomerular Disease
Nephrotic Syndrome
Urinary Tract Infection
Epididymitis
Torsion of Spermatic Cord
Urinary Tract Obstruction
Nephrolithiasis
Prostatic Cancer
Renal Cell Carcinoma
Cancer of Bladder, Ureter, and/or Renal Pelvis/Calyces
Wilms' Tumor
Hyperkalemia
Hypokalemia
Hypernatremia
Hyponatremia
Acid–base Disturbances

Acute Renal Failure is the sudden loss of renal function with

decreased GFR, and increased serum creatinine and BUN. Oliguria is not a necessary feature since decreased GFR and azotemia can occur despite urine output >
500 ml/24hr. Acute renal failure is classified as prerenal, intrarenal, or postrenal.

Differentiating acute from chronic failure: See "Chronic Renal Failure" chapter.

Signs/symptoms: On initial presentation, it is not always obvious whether renal
failure is acute or chronic since azotemia is common to both, and uremic symptoms
may develop in either. However, a patient who presents with severe azotemia in the
absence of uremic symptoms is more likely to have chronic failure. The potential
signs/symptoms of renal failure are listed in the "Chronic Renal Failure" chapter.

PRERENAL FAILURE (renal failure due to inadequate perfusion of the kidneys) may
be the consequence of shock (e.g. hypovolemic, cardiogenic, septic); or bilateral
renal artery occlusion. ●The urine is concentrated (> 400 mOsm/liter and specific
gravity > 1.016), and the urine sodium is low (< 20mEq/liter). The BUN to serum
creatinine ratio is usually > 15:1.

POSTRENAL FAILURE (renal failure due to urinary tract obstruction). **Etiology:** The
most common cause is benign prostatic hypertrophy followed by prostate cancer or
urethral stricture. Uncommonly, ureteral obstruction from a stone or other lesion will
lead to postrenal failure when there is only one functioning kidney. Other causes include bladder and pelvic tumors, retroperitoneal fibrosis (e.g. due to methysergide
therapy for migraines), papillary necrosis (e.g. in diabetes mellitus, due to analgesic
abuse). **Diagnosis:** Hyaline and granular casts may be seen on urine microscopy.
History and/or physical exam often suggests the diagnosis (e.g. urinary hesitancy,
enlarged prostate on rectal exam, palpable bladder on abdominal exam). If necessary, ultrasound, CAT scan, or IVP may be needed to visualize/clarify an obstructing
lesion. Be aware that IVP or CAT scan with radiocontrast dye is risky in the presence
of diabetic nephropathy, multiple myeloma, or impaired renal perfusion. **Relief of
obstruction** is sometimes followed by a marked postobstructive diuresis that can
lead to hypovolemia and electrolyte disturbances.

INTRARENAL FAILURE in most cases ensues from **acute tubular necrosis (ATN)**.
ATN may result from: **(1)** renal ischemic insult—e.g. shock (hypovolemic, cardiogenic, septic); rhabdomyolysis with myoglobinuria; major trauma/surgery; pancreatitis;
vasopressors; **(2)** nephrotoxins—e.g. aminoglycosides, cephalosporins, amphotericin B, heavy metals, iodine-containing radiocontrast dye, carbon tetrachloride,
ethylene glycol, cyclosporin. The **remaining** minority of cases of intrarenal failure result from diverse conditions—e.g. acute glomerulonephritis; rapidly progressive
glomerulonephritis; interstitial nephritis (due to drug sensitivity—e.g. pencillins,
cephalosporins, sufonamides, rifampin, diuretics, phenytoin, allopurinal); renal tubular obstruction (e.g. from uric acid, sulfonamides, multiple myeloma); malignant hypertension; vasculitis; severe hypercalcemia; cortical or papillary necrosis; atheroem-
bolism, subacute bacterial endocarditis, systemic lupus.

   **Diagnosis of intrarenal failure and establishing the cause of intrarenal
failure:** As the preceding list suggests, the history may suggest the cause. Prerenal or postrenal failure must be excluded. Correction of concurrently abnormal
prerenal or postrenal conditions (e.g. relief of obstruction, correction of hypov-
olemia/hypotension) may not alter the eventual outcome of intrarenal failure. Acute
intrarenal failure of any cause is associated with an elevated BUN and serum
creatinine, usually with BUN to creatinine ratio < 10:1. Acute tubular necrosis
(ATN): Tubular damage leads to increased urinary sodium loss (urine sodium > 40–
50 mEq/liter) and compromised renal concentrating ability (urine osmolality < 400
mOsm/L). The urine contains renal tubular cells and pigmented granular casts.
Glomerular disease and not ATN as the cause of acute intrarenal failure is suggested by the presence of significant hematuria, proteinuria, and/or RBC casts. Allergic
interstitial nephritis may present with rash, eosinophilia, and urine disclosing eosinophils and renal tubular cells. An antibiotic is often implicated. Uric acid
nephropathy: Uric acid crystals in the urine suggests possibility that precipitation of
uric acid in the renal tubules has led to renal tubular obstruction. Severe hyperten-

sion–associated intrarenal failure may be the consequence of malignant hypertension, glomerulonephritis, or vasculitis. Renal biopsy may ultimately be needed to establish the etiology of intrarenal failure.

Course of acute tubular necrosis: Most patients intitially experience oliguria (urine output < 500 ml/24 hr) which usually lasts 7–14 days. However, > 20% patients are not oliguric. Oliguric or not the serum creatinine and BUN both rise because the glomerular filtration rate falls. In the oliguric patient, the recovery phase is signaled by an increased urine output. A decline in serum creatine and BUN follows when the urine output reaches 800–1000 ml/24 hr. BUN and serum creatinine are usually close to normal 1–2 weeks after onset of recovery phase. It may take several months to regain he ability to maximally concentrate and acidify the urine.

Guidelines in treatment of acute intrarenal failure: Record input and output: Record daily urine output, and any extrarenal losses of water taking into account the usual insensible water loss of about 400 ml/day. Record daily intake. Using the preceding data, replace daily fluid losses taking care to avoid fluid overload. The daily allowable fluid intake in an adult usually adds up to approximately half a liter plus the previous days urine output. Record daily weight. A weight loss of 0.25–0.5 kg/day is anticipated. Weight gain is usually attributable to excess fluid intake. Monitor serum electrolytes, BUN, serum creatinine; ●Serum sodium is an additional check of fluid status. Hyponatremia is usually dilutional and indicates excess fluid intake. Severe hyponatremia mandates dialysis. ●Serum potassium should be closely monitored. Potassium intake must be restricted. Do not add KCl to IV. Dialysis is indicated for severe hyperkalemia (K > 6.5), especially if there are EKG changes. EKG monitoring is essential. Refer to "Hyperkalemia" chapter for treatment. Furosemide: If the patient is oliguric, the judicious administration of fluids in conjunction with furosemide may convert oliguric to nonoliguric acute renal failure. This is advantageous because fluid management is simpler and mortality is reduced. However, an adequate furosemide–induced diuresis (> 40ml/hr) is unlikely to occur if urine output is < 200ml/24hr, if ARF has been present > 36hr, or if serum creatinine is > 5–6mg/dl. If successful, furosemide is repeated periodically as needed. The required dose in adults ranges from 80 to 400 mg. Diet: Protein ingestion is restricted to about 0.5–1.0 gram/kg/day. Emphasis is placed on proteins of highest biological value (e.g. eggs, fowl, meat). About 2000 calories/day of carbohydrate is recommended because the protein–sparing effect of carbohydrates helps minimize azotemia from protein catabolism. Salt is restricted to ≤ 2 gram/day. Dialysis can to some extent relieve these dietary constraints. Monitor CBC: Normochromic normocytic anemia is a common development in ATN. The anemia may be exacerbated by GI bleeding and/or hemolysis. GI bleeding is a major cause of mortality in ATN. Packed RBC are administered if anemia is severe. Infection is a common cause of death in acute renal failure. Therefore, avoid unnecessary IV lines and if possible avoid Indwelling urinary catheters or invasive procedures. Metabolic acidosis is usually present but does not require treatment unless the serum bicarbonate falls to < 15 mEq/liter. Sodium bicarbonate must be administered judiciously for it may contribute to fluid overload. Dialysis is required if serum bicarbonate falls below 10 mEq/liter despite bicarbonate administration. Dialysis is advised for severe acidosis; severe hyperkalemia; severe hyponatremia; severe hyperuricemia; severe azotemia (serum creatinine > 10, BUN > 100); CNS complications (e.g. coma, convulsions, somnolence, asterixis); cardiovascular complications (e.g. pulmonary edema due to fluid excess; dysrhythmias, severe hypertension); or when catabolism is significantly increased (e.g. fever, infection, major burns or trauma). Dialysis simplifies patient care and is often advocated even in the absence of the preceding indications, especially if the patient is oliguric. Peritoneal dialysis suffices in many cases. However, hemodialysis is advised when rapid reversal of abnormalities is required–e.g. severe hyperkalemia with EKG changes, severe uremic symptoms, certain poisonings (e.g. ethylene glycol, methanol). Hemodialysis is also advised if there is severe catabolism or severe tissue breakdown (e.g. severe trauma/burn, rhabdomyolysis, sepsis).

Chronic Renal Failure is the deterioration of renal function due to

gradual loss of nephrons. Azotemia refers to the accumulation of nitrogenous wastes that may ensue. The GFR does not begin to fall (and plasma creatinine to rise) until 70% of the nephrons are lost. Symptoms develop as nitrogenous wastes accumulate when over 90% of the nephrons are destroyed and the GFR falls to < 10-20 ml/minute.

ETIOLOGY: Some of the more common causes of chronic renal failure are glomerulonephritis, diabetes mellitus, hypertension, polycystic kidneys, analgesic nephropathy, urinary tract obstruction. **Glomerular disease** accounts for about half of all cases of chronic renal failure. The causes of glomerular disease are many and diverse. Some are confined to the kidney, are idiopathic, and have a diagnosis based primarily on histologic exam (e.g. focal glomerulosclerosis, membranous glomerulopathy, membranoproliferative glomerulonephritis). Others are the consequence of systemic diseases (e.g. diabetes mellitus, lupus, bacterial endocarditis, Wegener's granulomatosis, cryoglobulinemia, periarteritis nodosa, Henoch-Schönlein purpura, amyloidosis, Alport's syndrome, Goodpasture's syndrome, poststreptococcal glomerulonephritis). **Interstitial renal diseases** that may result in chronic renal failure include toxic nephropathy (e.g. analgesics, lead); diabetes mellitus; sickle cell disease; uric acid nephropathy; urinary tract obstruction; reflux nephropathy; kidney infection. **Cystic kidney disease:** Polycystic kidney disease is an inherited autosomal dominant disease. Renal cysts compress the renal parenchyma leading to progressive renal failure. Cysts of other intra-abdominal organs and/or intracranial aneurysms are also common. Medullary cystic disease (genetic or sporadic) leads to polyuria, salt wasting, acidosis, anemia, renal osteodystrophy.

Signs/symptoms (i.e. uremic syndrome): In most cases, azotemia is discovered before uremic manifestations have appeared (e.g. incidental finding on laboratory test). Furthermore, the syndrome may develop insidiously with nonspecific complaints (e.g. malaise, fatigue, anorexia). Neuromuscular; asterixis, cramps, muscle twitching, clonus, numbness, absent deep tendon reflexes, foot drop, paresthesias, impaired vibratory and pain sensation, impaired mentation, insomnia, drowsiness, encephalopathy, seizures. Cardiovascular: hypertension (usually due to hypervolemia); pericarditis; pericardial effusion/tamponade; congestive heart failure (due to one of or a combination of hypertension, hypervolemia, cardiomyopathy, anemia); arrhythmias (e.g. due to electrolyte or acid-base disturbances, due to metastatic calcification of cardiac conduction system); atherosclerosis. Pulmonary: pleuritis, pleural effusion. GI: anorexia, nausea, vomiting, hiccups, abnormal taste, stomatitis, gastroenteritis, GI bleeding. GU: nocturia, loss of libido, impotence. Blood: Decreased renal erythropoietin production leads to normochromic normocytic anemia. Bleeding with iron deficiency may contribute to the anemia. There is a bleeding diathesis due to platelet dysfunction, and consequently the bleeding time is increased. Ecchymoses may be present. Lymphopenia and impaired neutrophil function makes the patient susceptible to infection. Skin: pallor, yellow-brown discoloration, pruritis, excoriations, uremic frost (urea crystallizes from sweat), terry nails (brown arcs of distal nails). Calcium-phosphorus abnormalities: Phosphorus excretion is impaired. Excess plasma phosphorous causes hypocalcemia. This in turn leads to secondary hyperparathyroidism with ensuing development of renal osteodystrophy (osteoporosis, osteomalacia, osteitis fibrosa, metastatic calcification). There is impaired vitamin D metabolism leading to decreased GI absorption of calcium.

Differentiating acute from chronic failure: Uremic manifestations: On initial presentation, it is not always obvious whether renal failure is acute or chronic since azotemia is common to both, and uremic symptoms may develop in either. However, a patient who presents with severe azotemia in the absence of uremic symptoms is more likely to have chronic failure. Peripheral neuropathy or renal osteodystrophy are 2 features of the uremic syndrome that are not generally found in acute failure. Other findings suggestive of chronic failure (but which do not exclude acute failure) include anemia, hyperphosphatemia, hypocalcemia, severe but tolerable metabolic acidosis. History: An ischemic insult (e.g. shock), acute exposure to nephrotoxin (e.g. aminoglycoside), or some other historical fact can help simplify differentiation. Kidney size: Abdominal x-ray (or ultrasound) will usually reveal small kidneys in the case of chronic renal failure. However, chronic renal failure may be associated with enlarged kidneys in certain diseases (amyloidosis, diabetic nephrosclerosis, scleroderma, polycystic kidney disease). Urinalysis: Chronic failure is likely if broad casts are found in the urine.

Laboratory: Urine specific gravity and osmolarity: When the kidney is no longer capable of producing a concentrated urine, the specific gravity becomes fixed at about 1.010 with a fixed urine osmolarity 300-320 mOsm/liter (i.e. about the same as plasma osmolality). BUN and serum creatinine are elevated. Serum sodium may be normal or decreased (i.e. there may be sodium retention or sodium wasting). Hyperkalemia generally does not develop until GFR is < 5 ml/minute. Hyperphosphatemia develops as the GFR falls below 70% of normal because phosphate excretion is impaired. Hypocalcemia develops as the serum phosphate rises because the solubility product of calcium and phosphate is a constant. Furthermore, parathormone's ability to mobilize bone calcium is compromised, and there is impaired GI absorption of calcium. <u>Serum magnesium and serum uric acid</u> may be elevated when GFR falls below 30 ml/min. <u>In interstitial renal disease</u>, the primary insult is directed against the tubules and not the glomeruli. Consequently, proteinuria is usually < 2 gram/day. Furthermore, although there may be pyuria and sometimes hematuria, RBC casts suggesting glomerulopathy are absent. <u>In glomerular disease</u>, proteinuria is present and may exceed 2 gram/day. Hematuria and RBC casts are common. <u>Granular casts and waxy casts</u> may be seen with either glomerular or interstitial renal disease. <u>Anemia:</u> Decreased renal erythropoietin production leads to normochromic normocytic anemia. Hematocrit of 20–30% is a common finding. Hemodialysis brings the hematocrit back toward normal by improving RBC survival and by eliminating unidentified inhibitor(s) of erythropoietin activity. Iron deficiency frequently contributes to the anemia. Folate is lost with dialysis and may contribute to anemia unless it is replaced. <u>Acidosis:</u> Hyperchloremic (normal anion gap) acidosis develops because the decreased mass of renal tubular cells cannot produce enough ammonia (NH_3) to trap hydrogen ion within the tubular lumens for subsequent excretion as the ammonium ion (i.e. $NH_3 + H^+ \rightarrow NH_4^+$). Anion gap acidosis may ensue in later stages as the filtration of sulfate and phosphates becomes significantly impaired. <u>GFR is decreased.</u> The GFR closely approximates creatinine clearance.

Creatinine clearance =

$$\frac{\text{(urine creatinine concentration in mg/deciliter) x (24 hr urine volume in ml)}}{1440 \text{ X (plasma creatinine concentration in mg/deciliter)}}$$

The creatinine clearance can also be estimated by the formula:

creatinine clearance $= \frac{(140 - \text{age in yrs}) \times \text{ weight in kg}}{72 \times \text{ serum creatinine}}$

In women, multiply above result by 0.85.

A rough estimate of GFR is that each time the serum creatinine doubles the GFR is halved.

Treatment: <u>Correct/eliminate conditions contributing to renal failure</u>- e.g. hypovolemia, hypo- or hypertension, congestive heart failure, urinary obstruction, UTI, hypercalcemia, hypokalemia, nephrotoxic drugs. <u>Protein and carbohydrate intake:</u> Protein intake is restricted to 1 gram/kg/day when GFR has fallen to < 30ml/min. Further restriction is generally not recommended until symptoms appear. This can be expected to occur when the BUN has risen to > 75–100 and the GFR has fallen to < 5–10 ml/min. Protein is then restricted to about 0.5–0.75 gram/kg/day. Emphasis is placed on proteins of highest biological value (e.g. eggs, fowl, meat). However, milk products are restricted because of their high phosphate content. A high carbohydrate diet is necessary because carbohydrate has a protein-sparing effect that helps minimize azotemia due to protein catabolism. <u>Salt intake</u> is individualized. Sodium excess-induced hypervolemia is a common problem because the kidneys cannot excrete a sodium load. However, undue salt restriction is also avoided because the surviving tubules do not have the reabsorptive capacity to prevent sodium depletion in the face of reduced sodium intake. The hypovolemia that attends sodium depletion further compromises renal function by decreasing renal perfusion. Normally 4–6 gram salt/day (i.e. 1.6–2.4 gram sodium/day) will maintain salt balance. This can usually be achieved on a no-added-salt regimen that avoids highly salted foods. The patient can make adjustments in salt intake by weighing himself daily and noting daily fluctuations. The daily urine volume is relatively fixed and the kidneys are unable to conserve water if fluids are restricted, or to excrete excess water should volume overload occur. Physical signs (e.g. edema, jugular veins flat or distended, blood pressure) and the GFR can also be used to guide salt intake. When the GFR falls to < 10 ml/minute, the urine output may be significantly reduced and therefore sodium and water retention is more likely. Careful adjustments in dietary salt and fluid intake are needed to preclude hypervolemia with the attendant risks of hypertension, and congestive heart failure/pulmonary edema. <u>Hypertension</u> is often due to hypervolemia; salt intake should be carefully reduced. Antihypertensive medications are added as needed. <u>Potassium retention</u> is usually not a problem until the GFR is < 5 ml/min. Ingestion of excessive amounts of potassium-rich foods or use of potassium-sparing diuretics is contraindicated. Periodic administration of Kayexalate may be indicated in some patients. See "Hyperkalemia" chapter for specific treatment measures. <u>Hyperphosphatemia</u> develops when GFR falls to 70% of normal. Hyperphosphatemia in turn provokes parathyroid hyperplasia with hyperparathyroidism. Dairy products are restricted because of their high phosphate content. Antacids are given to prevent GI absorption of phosphates. Serum phosphorus should be maintained at 4–5 mg/dl. Aluminum–containing antacids (e.g. Amphogel) are preferred over magnesium–containing antacids because the latter may result in hypermagnesemia. However, aluminum–containing antacids may lead to aluminum–related brain disease and contribute to osteomalacia. Consequently, calcium carbonate 1 gram PO 4 times/day is begun (even though it is less effective) once the serum phosphate level is normal. Calcitriol (1,25-dihydroxy vitamin D) may be needed to enhance GI calcium absorption, and prevent hyperparathyroidism and bone disease. Renal failure–associated metabolic acidosis is treated only when the plasma bicarbonate falls below 15 mEq/liter. When the plasma bicarbonate reaches this level, acidosis may in part be due to other contributing factors (e.g. infection). Check serum calcium, potassium, and sodium levels before initiating bicarbonate therapy. Sodium bicarbonate (1 gram PO tid initially) is administered and titrated to a plasma bicarbonate of > 20 mEq/liter and to symptomatic relief (e.g. relief of dyspnea, anorexia, lethargy) but curtailed should signs of sodium overload appear. Congestive heart failure is treated with sodium restriction. Furosemide may be used and may be effective even when the GFR is < 10–20 ml/liter. Epoetin (a recombinant human erythropoietin preparation) is used to help correct chronic renal failure–associated anemia Iron and folate replacement: Patients on dialysis are prone to iron and folate deficiency. Iron deficiency should be corrected before starting epoetin. Pruritis may respond to dietary restriction of protein and phosphates. Other measures that may be tried are an antihistamine (e.g. diphenhydramine), activated charcoal, and/or ultraviolet irradiation.

Indications for dialysis or transplantation include: pericarditis; encephalopathy; seizures; motor neuropathy; refractory nausea/vomiting/anorexia/weight loss; refractory pruritus; severe hypertension or CHF due to refractory volume overload; life–threatening hyperkalemia; severe metabolic acidosis with volume overload that contraindicates sodium bicarbonate therapy; fluid/electrolyte/acid–base disturbances not amenable to conservative management; severe anemia; serious bleeding diathesis; osteodystrophy, diabetic complications (e.g. severe retinopathy, neuropathy, gastropathy). Glomerular filtration rate < 4 mg/minute is an indication for dialysis. At GFR ≥ 4mg/minute, the decision to begin dialysis or consider transplantation is based on clinical judgment since uremic manifestations appear at different GFR in different patients. However, anticipate that dialysis or transplantation will become necessary if the GFR is < 8 ml/min, the serum creatinine is > 10 mg/dl, and the BUN > 100 mg/dl.

Interstitial Renal Disease (renal disease primarily affecting the function and integrity of the renal tubules) is characterized by inflammation, fibrosis, atrophy, and/or necrosis of the tubules.

PRESENTATION: Tubular damage is revealed by; (**1**) *sodium wasting*—due to defective tubular reabsorption of sodium; (**2**) *polyuria*—due to inability to produce concentrated urine (urine concentration remains below 600mOsm even after withholding fluids for ≥ 12 hr); (**3**) *nonanion gap hyperchloremic acidosis*—due to tubular defect in hydrogen ion secretion with resultant loss of bicarbonate; (**4**) *impaired potassium excretion* with risk of hyperkalemia. Contrast with glomerular disease: The primary insult in interstitial disease is directed toward the tubules and not the glomeruli. Consequently, proteinuria is usually < 2 gram/day. Furthermore, although there may be pyuria and sometimes hematuria, RBC casts (suggesting glomerulopathy) are generally absent. Interstitial disease may manifest as papillary necrosis. Analgesic abuse, diabetes mellitus, and sickle cell disease are examples of conditions that may provoke papillary necrosis. Lumbar pain is typical and papillary tissue may be seen on urine microscopy. Acute renal failure may occur. For example, renal ischemia or nephrotoxins may cause acute tubular necrosis. Interstitial nephritis and papillary necrosis may also lead to acute renal failure. Refer to "Acute Renal Failure" chapter. Chronic renal failure may occur. Interstitial diseases resulting in chronic renal failure include analgesic nephropathy, diabetes mellitus, sickle cell disease, uric acid nephropathy, urinary tract obstruction. Refer to "Chronic Renal Failure" chapter.

EXAMPLES of INTERSTITIAL DISEASE: Analgesic nephropathy results from the chronic ingestion of analgesics. Phenacetin is the most commonly mentioned offender but others are implicated (e.g. chronic combined ingestion of aspirin and acetaminophen). The urine reveals RBC and WBC. Papillary necrosis may develop and papillary tissue may be seen in the urine. IVP may reveal papillary lesions. UTI is common. Chronic renal failure may develop. **Sickle cell disease** may lead to glomerulonephritis and/or interstitial disease. The latter may result in papillary necrosis and interstitial fibrosis. Impaired tubular function manifests as polyuria and renal tubular acidosis. **Diabetes mellitus**, while primarily associated with glomerular injury, may also result in interstitial disease with papillary necrosis. **Interstitial nephritis secondary to nephrotoxins:** Offenders include heavy metals (gold, mercury, lead); aminoglycosides; amphotericin B, outdated tetracyclines. Acute tubular necrosis may result. **Hypersensitivity interstitial nephritis** may present with fever, rash, eosinophilia, and urine disclosing eosinophils and renal tubular cells. Drugs are the usual incitants (e.g. penicillins, cephalosporins, sulfonamides, thiazide diuretics, furosemide, allopurinol, phenytoin). **Urinary tract obstruction:** refer to "Urinary Obstruction" chapter. **Vesicoureteral reflux** in the absence of obstruction may, like urinary obstruction, cause tubular injury and eventually lead to parenchymal atrophy. Reflux increases the risk of pyelonephritis which may also contribute to interstitial injury. Reflux is most often the consequence of a congenital defect at the ureterovesical junction. Neurogenic bladder is another common cause of reflux. Patients with recurrent episodes of pyelonephritis should be investigated for reflux—e.g. voiding cystourethrography. **Uric acid nephropathy:** Acute hyperuricemia (as occurs during cancer chemotherapy) may result in intratubular deposition of urates with ensuing tubular obstruction and acute renal failure. Increased fluid intake, alkalizing the urine, and allopurinol are preventative measures. Chronic hyperuricemia may result in chronic interstitial nephritis with ensuing chronic renal failure. Allopurinol and high fluid intake are advised. **Chronic hypercalcemia** can lead to calcification of the tubular basement membrane, and to calcium deposition within tubular cells and cortical interstitium. Inability to produce a concentrated urine is the initial functional impairment : there is polyuria secondary to tubular insensitivity to ADH (i.e. nephrogenic diabetes insipidus). The GFR progressively decreases and chronic renal failure eventually ensues. **Chronic hypokalemia** leads to polyuria because there is impaired responsiveness to ADH. Metabolic alkalosis develops as chloride is lost in the urine. Mild proteinuria may occur but azotemia does not. Normal renal function returns once hypokalemia is corrected. **Chronic nonobstructive pyelonephritis** may cause interstitial scarring but chronic renal failure seldom results.

Glomerular Disease   refers to renal disease that primarily affects the glomeruli while leaving tubular function/integrity relatively intact. The characteristic manifestations are proteinuria (due to altered glomerular capillary permeability), hematuria, pyuria, and RBC casts. As glomerular injury progresses and as functioning glomeruli are lost, the total filtration surface is diminished and the GFR falls.

PRESENTATION: Glomerular disease may present as the nephrotic syndrome (see "Nephrotic Syndrome" chapter), acute glomerulonephritis, rapidly progressive glomerulonephritis, chronic glomerulonephritis, or simply as asymptomatic proteinuria and hematuria.

Acute glomerulonephritis: Urinalysis: hematuria, RBC casts, and proteinuria. The urine may also contain some WBC and renal tubular cells. Oliguria, edema, and/or hypertension may be present. The latter two are primarily due to salt and water retention. GFR is usually decreased. Antibody titer: If infection is the incitant, it may be possible to detect a rise in a specific antibody titer (e.g. ASO titer in the case of poststreptococcal infection). C3 complement levels will be decreased. Histology reveals enlarged glomeruli with proliferation of endothelial, mesangial, and epithelial cells. Numerous WBC are seen. Immunofluorescence discloses immune complex deposition as demonstrated by the presence of "lumpy–bumpy" pattern over the glomerular capillaries and mesangium. Etiology: Streptococcal infection is the most common precipitant (acute poststreptococcal glomerulonephritis). Other infections that have the potential for inciting acute glomerulonephritis include pneumococcus, staphylococcus, enterococcus, mumps, rubella, varicella, coxsackie, infectious mononucleosis, viral hepatitis (especially type B), syphilis, malaria, toxoplasmosis. Noninfectious systemic diseases that may be associated with acute glomerulonephritis include systemic lupus; mixed cryoglobulinemia; vasculitides (e.g. Wegener's granulomatosis, periarteritis nodosa). Treatment is of the underlying disorder if possible. Antibiotics are indicated for bacterial infection. In the case of poststreptococcal infection, antibiotic therapy is advocated in order to eliminate antibody production. However, treatment of streptococcal infection does not appear to prevent poststreptococcal glomerulonephritis. Control hypertension (e.g. clonidine, methyldopa). Restrict salt if edema is present; this alone may control hypertension.

Rapidly progressive glomerulonephritis has many of the same features as acute glomerulonephritis (e.g. proteinuria, hematuria, RBC casts) but is distinguished by the rapid development of renal failure with uremia within 3–9 months. Histology reveals destruction of the glomeruli and proliferation of glomerular epithelial cells leading to the formation of characteristic "crescents" within Bowman's space. In many cases, IgG deposition may be demonstrated by immunofluorescence. Etiology is often unknown. Known associations include poststreptococcal glomerulonephritis, Goodpasture's syndrome, Wegener's granulomatosis, Henoch–Schönlein purpura, periarteritis nodosa, systemic lupus, mixed cryoglobulinemia, bacterial endocarditis. Treatment: There is no effective therapy to arrest the deterioration in renal function. Dialysis is eventually required.

Chronic glomerulonephritis is characterized by the gradual deterioration of renal function, sometimes over many years. The typical signs of glomerulonephritis are usually present (proteinuria, hematuria, RBC casts). Hypertension often develops. Anemia is common and is due to decreased renal erythropoeitin production. The patient may be asymptomatic until enough renal mass has been lost for uremia to develop (see "Chronic Renal Failure"). Histology may demonstrate glomerular sclerosis, interstitial fibrosis, and tubular atrophy. Treatment; see "Chronic Renal Failure" chapter.

EXAMPLES OF GLOMERULAR DISEASE:

Diabetic glomerulosclerosis: The first evidence of glomerular disease is proteinuria. Proteinuria may eventually become severe enough to produce the nephrotic syndrome. This portends progression to uremia within a few years. Diabetics may also develop: (1) urinary obstruction from papillary necrosis, or (2) neurogenic bladder. Neurogenic bladder–associated urine stasis increases the risk of UTI. Histology often demonstrates nodular glomerulosclerosis (Kimmelstiel–Wilson lesion) or diffuse glomerulosclerosis. There is hyaline thickening of the glomerular basement membrane.

Systemic lupus erythematosus (SLE) is associated with glomerular lesions in almost all patients, but up to a third of cases do not exhibit clinical signs or symptoms of renal disease. Various presentations are possible with SLE (i.e. nephrotic syndrome, acute rapidly progressive glomerulonephritis, chronic glomerulonephritis). Treatment: corticosteroids.

Goodpasture's syndrome is an uncommon disorder (most common in young adult males) that affects both the kidneys and the lungs. Most patients present with pulmonary symptoms first (e.g. severe hemoptysis, dyspnea) and then go on to develop glomerulonephritis (e.g. proteinuria, hematuria, RBC casts). Alveolar hemorrhage is seen on chest x–ray as bilateral diffuse infiltrates. There is pulmonary fibrosis and hemosiderin deposition. Iron deficiency anemia is present. There is rapid progression to renal failure, but without treatment pulmonary hemorrhage may be the preemptive cause of death. Renal biopsy demonstrates crescents and the other glomerular lesions typical of a rapidly progressive glomerulonephritis (see above). Immunofluorescence reveals linear deposition of IgG on the glomerular basement membrane and on the alveolar basement membrane. Also, there are antiglomerular basement membrane antibodies in the circulation. Treatment: High–dose corticosteroids and cytotoxics (e.g. cyclophosphamide) together with plasmapheresis are tried. The rationale for plasmapheresis is to reduce the levels of circulating antibody. If these measures fail, bilateral nephrectomy (to reduce the antigenic stimulus) may be needed to control life–threatening pulmonary hemorrhage. Bilateral nephrectomy is also advised if there is end–stage renal failure.

Wegener's granulomatosis is a granulomatous vasculitis that can affect multiple organs. Respiratory disease: There are lesions of both the upper respiratory tract (e.g. sinusitis, nasal mucosal ulcers, otitis media) and lower respiratory tract (e.g. cough, pleuritis, pneumonitis, hemoptysis). The pulmonary lesions may cavitate. Renal disease (absent in 20% patients) is a necrotizing glomerulonephritis which initially presents with proteinuria and hematuria and then progresses to renal failure. Other possible manifestations include skin ulcers, peripheral neuropathy, pericarditis, coronary arteritis. Definitive diagnosis is based on biopsy of the lesions. Treatment: Cyclophosphamide may induce remission.

Henoch–Schönlein purpura is more common in children. It is a chronic vasculitis that mainly affects the skin (e.g. palpable purpura, urticaria); joints (e.g. pain, effusions); GI tract (e.g. bleeding, vomiting, abdominal pain); and kidneys (glomerulonephritis in a 3rd of patients). Glomerulonephritis manifests as hematuria (sometimes gross) and proteinuria (sometimes severe enough to cause nephrotic syndrome). Glomerulonephritis in adults may sometimes progress to renal failure. Histology of glomeruli discloses mesangial deposits of IgA, IgG, and complement. IgA deposits are also seen on skin capillaries.

Periarteritis (polyarteritis) nodosa is more common in men. It is a vasculitis characterized by segmental inflammation and necrosis of small to medium–sized arteries. This disease process may result in small aneurysms which are commonly detected on angiography of renal, hepatic, or celiac arteries. Kidney disease occurs in 80–90% cases. There is vasculitis with aneurysms of arcuate and interlobar arteries, and/or focal glomerulonephritis with hematuria and proteinuria. Hypertension is common and chronic renal failure may ensue. Other organs: The disorder commonly affects the GI tract (abdominal pain, nausea, vomiting, diarrhea, bleeding); skin (ulcers, subcutaneous nodules, purpura, urticaria); heart (pericarditis, myocarditis, coronary arteritis); nervous system (peripheral neuropathy, headache, convulsions, psychosis). Laboratory: Elevated ESR, leukocytosis, anemia, and thrombocytosis are common. Hepatitis B antigen is present in about half the cases. Etiology: Drugs (e.g. penicillins, sulfonamides, thiazides, procainamide); viral infections (e.g. hepatitis B); bacterial infections (e.g. streptococci, staphylococci) have been implicated as possible causes of this disorder. Treatment: antihypertensive medication as needed; corticosteroids; cytotoxics (e.g. cyclophosphamide, azathioprine).

Amyloidosis is the extracellular accumulation of amyloid (a fibrillar protein that stains with Congo red dye to reveal green birefringence under polarizing microscope). Amyloid is of 2 main types. One type is derived from immunoglobulin light chain and its presence is often associated with multiple myeloma. The other type is the proteolytic derivative of a specific serum protein, and is associated with chronic inflammation—e.g. rheumatoid arthritis; systemic lupus; scleroderma; dermatomyositis; Reiter's syndrome; ankylosing spondylitis; ulcerative colitis, Crohn's disease; chronic infections (tuberculosis, osteomyelitis, leprosy, malaria, decubitus ulcers). And this type may also be associated with neoplasias—e.g. Hodgkin's, solid tumors. Any organ may be affected—e.g. heart (heart failure, arrhythmias); GI tract (bleeding, malabsorption). The liver, spleen, and kidneys are frequently enlarged. With kidney involvement, there is hematuria and proteinuria. Proteinuria may be severe enough to cause the nephrotic syndrome. Progressive renal failure is the rule. Hypertension is uncommon. Biopsy is required to make the diagnosis; the rectal mucosa is the usual site of biopsy. Treatment is directed at the underlying disorder in order that further accumulation of amyloid can hopefully be arrested.

Bacterial endocarditis–associated glomerulonephritis: Glomerular injury results when antigen–antibody complexes are deposited on the glomerular capillaries. Hematuria and proteinuria are present and the nephrotic syndrome may ensue. A similar picture is seen in patients who have ventriculoatrial shunts for treatment of hydrocephalus.

Nephrotic Syndrome is the condition in which there is

proteinuria exceeding 3–3.5 gram per 24 hr with ensuing hypoalbuminemia, hyperlipidemia/lipiduria, and/or edema.

Pathogenesis: Excessive urinary albumin excretion leads to hypoalbuminemia which in turn induces increased hepatic synthesis of albumin as well as other proteins. In particular, hepatic lipoprotein synthesis increases and is postulated to cause the hyperlipidemia (with elevated cholesterol, triglycerides, and phospholipids). Hyperlipemia may be sufficient to give the serum a milky appearance. Also, there is increased hepatic synthesis of protein procoagulants; this may in part explain the observed increased incidence of thromboembolic events. Edema results from the reduced plasma oncotic pressure that is secondary to hypoalbuminemia.

Etiology: 75% cases are idiopathic and are classified according to histopathologic findings (minimal change glomerulopathy, membranous glomerulopathy, membranoproliferative glomerulonephritis, focal sclerosis). Almost any disease that affects the glomeruli may be associated with the nephrotic syndrome. The most prevalent secondary causes are diabetes mellitus; systemic lupus; amyloidosis; lymphoma; solid tumor (breast, lung, GI). Other secondary causes include multiple myeloma; sickle cell disease; malaria; syphilis; toxins (gold, mercury, bismuth, probenecid, penicillamine, insect stings, snakebite, etc).

Presentation may include any of following: generalized edema; pleural effusion; pulmonary edema; pericardial effusion; ascites; hypovolemia with possible hypotension; thromboembolic phenomena (e.g. thrombophlebitis, pulmonary embolism, renal vein thrombosis, renal artery thrombosis).

Laboratory: •decreased serum albumin; •elevated serum cholesterol and triglycerides. •Urine sometimes reveals RBC's and RBC casts along with increased hyalin and granular casts. Fatty casts and oval fat bodies are typical of the nephrotic syndrome. Oval fat bodies are renal tubular cells filled with cholesterol esters. The latter are birefringent and appear as Maltese crosses under polarized light.

Treatment: Treat underlying disorder if possible. High protein diet is advised. Moderate salt restriction (2–4 gram salt/day) can usually be achieved by preparing meals without salt. Further salt restriction along with furosemide is indicated if effusions or marked symptoms occur. Corticosteroids: Some of the conditions listed above may respond to steroid therapy—e.g. minimal change glomerulopathy, lupus.

Urinary Tract Infection
UTI is divided into 2 categories, upper UTI (pyelonephritis) and lower UTI (cystitis, urethritis, prostatitis). Asymptomatic UTI is common. **Pathogens:** 80–90% of UTI are due to E. coli. Other aerobic gram–negative bacilli account for most of the rest (e.g. proteus, klebsiella, enterobacter, pseudomonas). Gram–positive bacteria (e.g. enterococci, staphylococci) are less common. Chlamydia trachomatis may be responsible for urethritis.

Laboratory: Obtaining urine specimen: A midstream specimen of the urine is collected for analysis. Urethral catheterization or suprapubic bladder aspiration are alternatives if a clean specimen cannot be obtained. Vigorous diuresis will temporarily dilute the urine and may thus give erroneously negative findings. Finding ≥ 10 WBC on a centrifuged specimen suggests presence of UTI. Significant bacteriuria is defined as a quantitative urine culture that shows > 100,000 bacterial colony forming units/ml. This indicates a > 80% likelihood of significant UTI if a clean-catch specimen is obtained and a 95% probability if the urine specimen is obtained by catheterization. Over 95% patients with significant bacteriuria as defined above will have significant findings on microscopic exam of UNSPUN urine (i.e. urine discloses WBC and gram stain reveals bacteria). White cell casts on spun or unspun urine suggests pyelonephritis. Alkaline urine suggests that UTI is due to urea–splitting bacteria (e.g. proteus). Persistent pyuria in the absence of demonstrable bacteriuria by gram stain and/or standard cultures suggests possibility of tubercular, fungal, or chlamydial infection.

CYSTITIS (infection of the bladder). The usual complaints are dysuria, frequency, urgency, and/or suprapubic pain. Differentiating cystitis from pyelonephritis: Some cystitis patients also present with signs and symptoms usually attributed to pyelonephritis–e.g. fever, chills, flank pain, costovertebral angle pain/tenderness. Thus, even though the latter manifestations make the diagnosis of pyelonephritis more likely, the distinction between pyelonephritis and cystitis cannot always be made with certainty on clinical findings. The presence of WBC casts on microscopic exam of the urine supports the diagnosis of pyelonephritis rather than cystitis. Testing for the presence of antibody–coated bacteria may provide further evidence for diagnosis of pyelonephritis. However, this test is not routinely performed nor is it completely reliable. Treatment: In the absence of pregnancy or urinary tract abnormalities, women with cystitis can be treated with: (1) single dose of amoxicillin 3 gram PO, or (2) single dose of two double–strength tablets of trimethoprim–sulfamethoxazole (Bactrim DS, Septra DS). Others (e.g. males, children, pregnant women, those with urinary tract abnormalities) require PO antibiotic for 10 days (e.g. amoxicillin, ampicillin, trimethoprim–sulfamethoxazole, cephalexin, or sulfisoxazole). A 2–3 day course of phenazopyridine (Pyridium) is often given concurrently to relieve dysuria. Cystitis patients are encouraged to increase fluid intake.

PYELONEPHRITIS (infection of the renal parenchyma) typically presents with fever, chills, flank pain, costovertebral angle pain/tenderness (bilateral if both kidneys are involved). There may be dysuria, frequency, urgency, and/or suprapubic pain. Anorexia, nausea, vomiting may also be present. <u>Laboratory:</u> Many WBC and perhaps WBC casts are seen on microscopic exam of a centrifuged unstained urine specimen. Urine gram stain and urine culture is usually positive (see "Laboratory" above). CBC and blood cultures should be obtained if systemic symptoms are present. <u>Treatment:</u> All pregnant patients must be hospitalized. The decision to hospitalize other patients requires good clinical judgment taking into account such factors as how "sick" the patient is, age, overall health, urinary tract abnormalities, reliability of patient. The safest approach is to admit the patient with pyelonephritis, treat with IV antibiotic initially, switch to PO antibiotic when clinical improvement occurs, and discharge with close follow–up when recovery is reasonably assured. Antibiotic should be administered for total of 10–14 days. The drug of choice is ampicillin for 10–14 days. Trimethoprim–sulfamethoxazole, cefadroxil, aminoglycosides are alternatives. ●If clinical improvement does not occur after 48 hour and urine gram stain is still positive, do a repeat urine culture and sensitivity. Addition of an aminoglycoside should be considered. ●If a patient is not admitted, realize that pyelonephritis can be a stubborn infection when treated with oral antibiotics. Therefore close follow–up with urinalysis, urine gram stain, and cultures is essential. ●All pyelonephritis patients require an urine culture 1–2 wk after completion of antibiotic therapy in order to assure that relapse has not occurred.

ASYMPTOMATIC BACTERIURIA is common. Pregnant women and patients with urinary tract abnormalities should be treated as for symptomatic cystitis with 10 day course of antibiotic. Preschool children should also be treated. Treatment of others is not necessarily required.

UTI in MALES: Unless the diagnosis is reasonably assured (e.g. straightforward prostatitis, urethritis), the investigation should attempt to rule out urinary tract abnormalities (e.g. stone, obstruction, congenital anomalies). Tests may include IVP, voiding cystourethrogram, ultrasound.

PROSTATITIS can be chronic or acute. Prostatitis, as for UTI in general, is usually due to gram–negative aerobes, especially E. coli.

    Chronic prostatitis: <u>Signs/symptoms:</u> Perineal and low back pain is characteristic. There may be urgency, frequency, dysuria. Symptoms may be the consequence of episodes of cystitis due to seeding of the bladder from the infected prostate. Rectal exam is often unremarkable, or may reveal a moderately tender prostate that may be boggy or indurated. <u>Diagnosis</u> is confirmed by obtaining urine specimens for quantitative culture as follows: (1) first 10 ml voided (urethral specimen), (2) midstream (bladder specimen), (3) perform prostatic massage collecting drops (prostatic specimen), (4) void again collecting first 10 ml for prostatic culture. <u>Treatment:</u> Chronic prostatitis is a stubborn infection requiring prolonged antibiotic therapy (e.g. trimethoprim–sulfamethoxazole for 12 weeks).

    Acute prostatitis: fever, chills, perineal and low back pain, dysuria, frequency, urgency. Rectal exam reveals a very tender, warm, and boggy prostate. <u>Laboratory:</u> Urine samples are collected (see *chronic prostatitis* above). However, because bacteremia may occur, prostatic massage to obtain specimen is contraindicated until adequate blood levels of antibiotic are achieved. Since cystitis often coexists, a standard midstream urine specimen is often satisfactory for revealing bacteria on gram stain and for providing for culture and sensitivity. <u>Treatment:</u> trimethoprim–sulfamethoxazole is usually administered because it yields high levels of antibiotic in the prostatic secretions. A different antibiotic may be subsequently chosen depending on results of culture and sensitivity, and clinical response. Treatment is continued for minimum of 30 days in order to prevent development of chronic prostatitis.

URETHRITIS may be due to gonorrhea (purulent urethral discharge) or Chlamydia trachomatis (typically a thin white mucoid discharge). There is burning on urination, frequency, urgency. <u>Laboratory:</u> ●In the case of gonorrhea, gram stain of the discharge discloses gram–negative intracellular cocci. Thayer–Martin culture is obtained if suspected gonocorrhea cannot be confirmed by gram stain. See also "Gonorrhea" chapter. ●Diagnosis of chlamydial infection is based on exclusion of gonorrhea on gram stain or culture. Also, immunodiagnostic slide tests are available for identifying chlamydia in the discharge. <u>Treatment:</u> Refer to "Gonorrhea" chapter for treatment of gonococcal urethritis. Chlamydial infection in nonpregnant adult is treated with tetracycline (500 mg PO 4 times/day for at least 7 days) or doxycycline (100 mg PO twice daily for at least 7 days).

Epididymitis is characterized by scrotal pain and swelling. There is in-
duration and exquisite tenderness along the spermatic cord. The testis may also be involved (epididymo–orchitis). With the patient standing, supporting the testis tends to relieve the pain. This finding contrasts with torsion of the spermatic cord in that support does not relieve pain due to torsion. Another distinguishing feature is that urinalysis in epididymitis typically reveals the presence of bacteria and WBC. Epididymitis is frequently the consequence of urine reflux thru the ejaculatory ducts, prostatitis, or urethral instrumentation. **Treatment:** tetracycline for 2–3 weeks. Sulfamethoxazole–trimethoprim (Bactrim, Septra) is an alternative. Prolonged antibiotic therapy may be required in patients with chronic epididymitis. ●Other recommended measures are rest, scrotal support, and analgesics as needed.

Torsion of Spermatic Cord Incidence is greatest in
adolescence. **Signs/symptoms:** There is abrupt onset of scrotal pain and swelling. The affected testis is exquisitely tender and swollen. The testis is typically displaced superiorly and may be misaligned. Sometimes a knot may be felt above the upper pole of the testis. With the patient standing, pain is not relieved by supporting the testis as is the case in epididymitis. The patient may give a history of previous episodes of testicular pain which resolved spontaneously. **Treatment:** A testicular scan may be obtained if the diagnosis is in doubt. However, there must be no unnecessary delay since emergency surgery is required to restore normal blood supply to the testis and thereby prevent gangrene. An urologist may attempt to manually untwist the spermatic cord. If successful, surgery for orchiopexy is still necessary to prevent recurrence. Orchiopexy of the opposite side is also performed since these patients have an increased risk of torsion of the uninvolved side.

Urinary Tract Obstruction
Consequences: Obstruction causes urine to accumulate. Consequently, pressure builds up proximal to the obstruction. There is hydronephrosis with elevated hydrostatic pressure in the ureters, renal papillae, and renal tubules. Pressure is initially exerted on the tubules such that neither a concentrated nor an acid urine can be produced. Pressure is then also exerted on the glomeruli so that reduced glomerular filtration ensues. There is tubular atrophy, and with time the renal medulla and then the cortex is obliterated. Renal function may to some extent be restored once obstruction is relieved. However, complete and irreversible loss of renal function is expected if complete obstruction persists over 6 weeks. Patients with partial or intermittent bilateral obstruction may develop progressive chronic renal failure, while acute complete and persistent bilateral renal obstruction results in acute renal failure. With unilateral obstruction, uremia is averted provided the patient has 2 functional kidneys and the function of the other kidney is not impaired. ●Once obstruction is relieved, there is a postobstructive diuresis as retained solutes are excreted. Rarely, the volume depletion that results can be severe.
Causes include: renal stone (most common cause); prostatic hypertrophy or carcinoma; pelvic tumor; pelvic inflammatory disease; endometriosis; postsurgical adhesions; Crohn's disease, retroperitoneal tumor or fibrosis; carcinoma bladder, ureter, or renal pelvis; papillary necrosis; bladder dysfunction (e.g. neurogenic bladder); ureteral irradiation; ureteral blood clot.
Diagnosis: <u>Signs/symptoms</u> depend on site, degree, and duration of obstruction. <u>History</u> may provide clue. For instance, recurrent UTI in males suggests possibility of an obstructive lesion. <u>Physical exam:</u> Perform thorough exam. Be sure to perform a rectal exam in males (an enlarged prostate is a common finding In older

men) and a pelvic exam in females. <u>Partial obstruction distal to the bladder outlet</u> results in frequency and dribbling. With progressive obstruction, the bladder distends with urine and is felt as a lower abdominal mass. There is considerable lower abdominal pain and tenderness. <u>Acute obstruction of an ureter</u>, usually causes renal colic (severe flank pain) that in many cases radiates to groin. <u>Chronic ureteral obstruction</u> may manifest as a dull flank pain or low back pain. Pain may be absent. <u>With partial obstruction,</u> there may be evidence of impaired tubular function— e.g. polyuria, nocturia. isosthenuria. Isosthenuria is the inability to produce a concentrated urine such that, regardless of fluid intake, the urine specific gravity becomes fixed at 1.010 (approximately that of protein–free plasma). Impaired tubular function may also manifest as an inability to produce urine with pH < 6.0; this is due to impaired function of the distal tubules. Other findings may include decreased GFR and a BUN to creatinine ratio > 15:1. The latter finding is due to the fact that the delay in urine excretion allows for more urea to be reabsorbed by the renal tubules. <u>Ultrasound</u> may reveal a dilated renal pelvis. <u>IVP</u> may also show dilated renal pelvis and calyces. When glomerular filtration is decreased, there is delayed visualization of the affected kidney(s). Remember that IVP contrast dye may precipitate renal failure when there is reduced renal perfusion, diabetic nephropathy, or multiple myeloma. <u>Additional studies</u> (e.g. cystoscopy, retrograde pyelography) may be needed once obstruction is confirmed in order to identify the site and etiology of the obstruction.

Treatment: Complete obstruction should if possible be corrected within 5 days (i.e. before irreversible pressure and ischemic atrophy begins to take its toll) because persistent obstruction will within a few weeks lead to permanently impaired renal function. Surgery is generally of no benefit once the renal cortex is lost unless there is a compelling reason (e.g. tumor, persistent urinary infection, ensuing uncontrolled hypertension). Clinical judgment dictates how to expeditiously deal with partial obstruction. Concurrent UTI makes relief of obstruction all the more urgent.

Nephrolithiasis (kidney stones)

Signs/symptoms: Renal colic is characterized by severe intermittent flank pain that typically radiates down the abdomen along the course of the ureter often to the groin and inner thigh. Nausea, vomiting, and abdominal distension (secondary to ileus) may be present. Chills, fever, hematuria, and frequency are also common.

Tests: <u>Urinalysis</u> usually reveals gross or microscopic hematuria. Hematuria may be absent if there is complete obstruction. <u>Plain abdominal x-ray</u> may reveal a stone (except pure uric acid stones which are radiolucent). The most common site for a stone to cause obstruction is at the ureterovesical junction folowed by the ureteropelvic junction and then the upper ureter. <u>IVP</u> may be needed to identify the stone. IVP also induces a diuresis that may help pass the stone. <u>Blood tests:</u> Obtain sodium, potassium, chloride, bicarbonate, calcium, uric acid, BUN, creatinine. <u>Instruct patient to strain urine</u> so that any stones thus obtained can be analyzed. <u>More extensive work–up</u> is advised in children or if there is a history of recurrent stones. Additional tests may include urine test for cystine; 24 hr urine collection for creatinine, uric acid, and calcium; 24 hr urine collection for oxalate in patients with impaired fat absorption or in pediatric patient.

Treatment in general: <u>Analgesia:</u> Renal colic is often so excruciating that *intravenous* narcotics are required. <u>Hydrate</u> patient adequately. <u>Surgery or lithotripsy:</u> Stones < 5 mm generally pass spontaneously. Stone must be eliminated if there is complete obstruction, unremitting pain, hydronephrosis, or degenerating kidney function.

Prevention: Drinking at least 2 quarts of fluid/day will reduce incidence of stone formation. Patient should remember to drink sufficient water at bedtime to be awakened to void during the night, at which time patient should drink additonal water. See below for specific preventive measures depending on the type stone.

CALCIUM STONES (65–75% cases) are composed of calcium oxalate, calcium phosphate, or a combination thereof. **Etiology:** Hypercalciuria, hyperuricosuria, and/or hyperoxaluria increase the risk of developing calcium stones, although many patients with calcium stones have none of these abnormalities. <u>Hypercalciuria:</u> Idiopathic hypercalciuria accounts for nearly half the cases of calcium stones. The diagnosis of

idiopathic hypercalciuria is made after ruling out identifiable causes of hypercalciuria-
-associated calcium stones: renal tubular acidosis (type 1), acetazolamide therapy,
medullary sponge kidney, or hypercalcemia–provoking conditions (e.g. primary hyperparathyroidism, hyperthyroidism, sarcoidosis, immobilization, hypervitaminosis D,
milk–alkali syndrome, Cushing's syndrome). Hyperuricosuria not only increases the
risk of pure uric acid stone formation but also predisposes to calcium stones (possibly because uric acid crystals act as nidus for precipitation of calcium oxalate and
phosphate). Hyperoxaluria may be due to increased dietary intake of oxalate or to
genetically determined overproduction of oxalate (primary hyperoxaluria). Usually,
however, hyperoxaluria is the consequence of conditions that compromise the intestinal absorption of fats—e.g. chronic pancreatitis, ileojejunal bypass, ileal resection,
inflammatory bowel disease. In these conditions, calcium binds to fat within the intestinal lumen instead of to oxalate. This leads to increased GI absorption of oxalate which in turn leads to increased urinary oxalate. **Calcium stone prophylaxis:**
Increase fluid intake—ingest at least 2 quarts/day. Patient should also remember
to drink sufficient water at bedtime to be awakened to void during the night, at which
time the patient should drink additional water. Prophylaxis idiopathic hypercalciuria-
-associated calcium stones: (**1**) Thiazide diuretics (e.g. hydrochlorothiazide 50 mg
1–2 times/day) decrease urinary calcium excretion thereby preventing stone
formation. A thiazide diuretic is suitable for treatment of *idiopathic hypercalciuria*,
but not for the clinically identifiable causes of hypercalciuria. Specifically, a thiazide
diuretic is contraindicated if there is hyperuricemia, hypercalcemia, or if
hypercalciuria is secondary to increased bone resorption (e.g. primary hyperparathyroidism, Cushing's syndrome, hyperthyroidism, immobilization, multiple myeloma,
bone metastases). (**2**) Low–calcium diet is an alternative approach to preventing idiopathic hypercalciuria–associated calcium stones. Milk products are eliminated
from the diet and the urine is later analyzed to verify that calcium excretion has been
reduced to < 4 mg/kg/24hr. One drawback of a low–calcium diet is that it may lead
to depletion of bone calcium, particularly in women. Prophylaxis hyperuricosuria-
associated calcium stone: Formation may be inhibited by low purine diet. If this
fails, allopurinol is usually effective. Prophylaxis hyperoxaluria–associated calcium
stones in which hyperoxaluria results from impaired fat absorption: low–oxalate
diet, low–fat diet, add medium–chain triglycerides to diet, avoid vitamin C supplements, use calcium supplements (titrated to normal urinary oxalate level). Cholestyramine is added if the preceding measures are inadequate. Prophylaxis primary
hyperoxaluria–associated calcium stone: low–oxalate diet, avoid vitamin C supplements, pyridoxine (400 mg/day), orthophosphates (Neutra–Phos, K–Phos), magnesium oxide (600 mg/day). Primary hyperparathyroidism–associated calcium
stones: parathyroid surgery. Type 1 renal tubular acidosis is treated with potassium supplementation and either sodium bicarbonate (5–10 gram/day) or sodium citrate (60–120 mEq/day). Potassium supplement should be begun first and then continued concurrently with sodium citrate or sodium bicarbonate. This is because the
latter medications given alone may correct the acidosis but in so doing may also
induce hypokalemia.

STRUVITE STONES (10–15% cases) result from UTI by urea–splitting bacteria. The
bacteria create an alkaline urine that favors precipitation of the constituents of struvite stones: struvite (magnesium ammonium phosphate), and calcium apatite (calcium carbonate and phosphate). Patients susceptible to chronic recurrent UTI (e.g.
chronic indwelling catheter, neurogenic bladder) are prone to struvite stones. Multiple courses of antibiotics for recurrent UTI often select out resistant urea–splitting
strains of proteus and pseudomonas. **Treatment:** (**1**) Acidify urine (e.g. cranberry
juice, high–protein diet). (**2**) Reduce dietary phosphate. Prescribe aluminum hydroxide antacid (e.g. Amphogel) to decrease GI absorption of phosphates. (**3**) Surgical
removal of stone may be necessary (e.g. ureteral obstruction, intractable pain). (**4**)
Treat acute UTI as they arise with appropriate antibiotic. (**5**) Prolonged suppressive
therapy with trimethoprim–sulfamethoxazole or methenamine mandelate is advised.

URIC ACID STONE (5–10% cases) **Etiology:** Excretion of an acid urine is the
most common condition leading to uric acid stones. Stones form, not because excessive uric acid is excreted in the urine (typically hyperuricosuria is not present), but
because uric acid has a low solubility and precipitates in acid urine. Excessive production of uric acid is the next most common reason for uric acid stone formation.

Hyperuricemia, hyperuricosuria, and gouty arthritis may be present. Excessive production of uric acid may be due to a primary metabolic abnormality (glycogen storage disease, Lesch–Nyhan syndrome); or to increased turnover of nucleic acids (e.g. leukemia, multiple myeloma, polycythemia vera, chronic hemolysis). Overexcretion of uric acid is an uncommon abnormality leading to uric acid stone formation. It may be due to uricosuric drugs (e.g. probenecid) or renal tubular abnormalities. The urinary concentration of uric acid may also be increased with dehydration. **Prevention:** (1) Generous fluid intake. (2) Sodium bicarbonate (e.g. 6–8 gram/day divided into 4 doses) or sodium citrate (e.g. 48–96mEq/day divided into 4 doses). The patient tests the urine with pH paper and the dose is adjusted such that a pH of 5.5–7.0 is achieved. (3) Allopurinol is added to the regimen if (a) urinary uric acid is > 1000 mg/24hr, or (b) urinary uric acid is 800–1000mg/24hr and alkali therapy is ineffective or contraindicated.

CYSTINE STONES (about 1% cases) form in patients with cystinuria, an uncommon autosomal recessive disease characterized by an abnormality in the renal tubular reabsoption of certain amino acids. Cystine is the least soluble and is liable to precipitate, especially if the urine is acid. **Prevention:** (1) Generous fluid intake is essential (≥ 3 quarts/day). (2) If fluid therapy is inadequate, try adding sodium bicarbonate (15–30 gram/day). (3) Penicillamine is used as last resort.

Prostatic Cancer
seldom occurs before age 60. It is, after lung and colon cancer, the 3rd most common cause of cancer in males. About 1 in every 20 males will develop prostate cancer. Over 95% are adenocarcinomas; others are squamous cell carcinoma, undifferentiated carcinoma, and sarcoma.

Signs/symptoms/diagnosis: Bladder outlet obstruction is often the first manifestation. Hematuria and/or urinary tract infection may be the presentation. Rectal exam: A prostate with hardened nodular lump(s) is characteristic. Since prostatic cancer typically progresses slowly, there may be no symptoms when the tumor is first discovered on rectal exam. With time, the prostate becomes diffusely hardened and irregular; the cancer spreads directly to the seminal vesicles and bladder neck; and the prostate becomes fixed to the rectum and lateral pelvic walls. Symptoms related to bone metastases are sometimes the initial complaint. For example, there may be bone pain or a pathologic fracture (e.g. vertebral fracture with paraplegia). The bones are most commonly involved by hematogenous spread. The pelvic bones and/or lumbar vertebrae are common sites of metastases. Other manifestations of metastases may include lymphadenopathy, nodular liver, signs of pulmonary metastasis on chest x-ray. Serum acid phosphatase and serum alkalkine phosphatase: Serum ACID phosphatase is usually elevated if there are bone metastases and may be elevated if the tumor has simply spread beyond the prostatic capsule. Also, the serum ALKALINE phosphatase may be elevated as a reflection of increased bone metabolism. Ultrasound may demonstrate tumor size and whether or not the tumor has spread beyond the capsule. Transrectal ultrasound may enhance visualization. Transrectal or transperineal needle biopsy is usually performed to confirm the diagnosis. Marrow biopsy at the iliac crest may sometimes confirm the diagnosis and demonstrate metastasis if needle biopsy of a small prostatic lesion is not successful. Chest x-ray, IVP, and bone scan are standard part of metastatic workup. Magnetic resonance imaging may be used if necessary to clarify local or distant lesions.

Note: The staging/treatment information presented below is extracted from National Cancer Institute PDQ State-of-the-Art Cancer Treatment Information 11/1/90. However, since cancer treatment is evolving, this information may not be current. The most up-to-date standard treatment options may be obtained by calling the National Cancer Institute Cancer Information Service at 1–800–4–CANCER. Patients may be considered for inclusion in clinical trials of new regimens. Descriptions of these trials are also available.

Staging: Stage A tumor is restricted to the prostate. The tumor is not palpable but is discovered as a result of prostatic surgery. Stage A is divided into two substages: stage A1—when there is a focal well-differentiated tumor and stage A2—when there is a multifocal or poorly differentiated tumor. Stage B (palpable tumor restricted to prostate) is divided into stage B1—when there is a solitary nodule within one lobe of prostate and stage B2—when there is more extensive involvement of one lobe or both lobes are involved. Stage C (tumor penetrates capsule and clinically involves periprostatic tissues and possibly the seminal vesicles). The tumor is designated stage C2 if the tumor causes obstruction of bladder outlet or ureter and stage C1 if it does not. Stage D is subdivided into 4 substages. Stage D0: the tumor appears clinically to be confined to the prostate but serum acid phosphatase is persistently elevated. Stage D1: there is metastasis to but not beyond the pelvic lymph nodes. Stage D2: metastases to distant lymph nodes, bones, and/or viscera. Stage D3 designates a stage D2 patient who has relapsed after adequate endocrine therapy.

Treatment of prostate cancer must be individualized. Many patients are aged and have other medical infirmities which would favor one form of treatment over another or even no treatment. Radical prostatectomy is usually only contemplated if the following criteria are met: (1) tumor confined to prostate—i.e. stage A or B, (2) < 70 yr of age, (3) otherwise in good health, (4) bone scan negative, (5) normal acid phosphatase. Pelvic node dissection is not necessary for well–differentiated nodules because positive nodes are found in < 5% of these cases. Pelvic node dissection is advised for larger, less well–differentiated tumors. If frozen section exam of the nodes is positive, the patient is stage D and radical prostatectomy is not performed and thus avoids the potential complications of radical prostatectomy (e.g. urinary incontinence, impotence). External beam radiation with curative intent may be employed in stages A2, B, C, and highly selected stage D1 patients. Candidates should have a negative bone scan. Clinical trials: With the exception of stage A1, patients may be considered for inclusion in clinical trials of new regimens.

Stage A: Most stage A1 patients do not require immediate treatment and may be followed carefully. However, stage A1 patients less than 60 are usually treated as for stage B unless compelling reasons dictate otherwise. Treatment of stage A2 is as for stage B.

Stage B standard therapeutic options are: (1) external beam radiation, Note: Because of the risk of stricture, patients who have undergone transurethral resection prostate should not receive external beam radiation until 4–6 wk postoperative. (2) radical prostatectomy, usually with pelvic lymphadenectomy. Patients who undergo radical prostatectomy are candidates for postoperative radiation if penetration of the capsule or involvement of the seminal vesicles is discovered at the time of surgery , or if PSA (prostate specific antigen) is detectable 3 wk after surgery. (3) observation in selected cases.

Stage C: External beam radiation with curative intent is the preferred treatment in most patients. However, because of the risk of stricture, patients who have undergone transurethral resection prostate should not receive external beam radiation until 4–6 wk postoperative. Radical prostatectomy is considered in highly selected cases. Patients who undergo radical prostatectomy are candidates for postoperative radiation if penetration of the capsule or involvement of the seminal vesicles is discovered at the time of surgery , or if PSA (prostate specific antigen) is detectable 3 wk after surgery. Palliative treatment may be necessary to relieve urinary symptoms. Palliation may entail radiation; transurethral resection of prostate; radical surgery; or hormonal therapy (see stage D).

Stage D: External beam radiation with curative intent is sometimes tried in highly selected stage D1 cases. However, because of the risk of stricture, patients who have undergone transurethral resection prostate should not receive external beam radiation until 4–6 wk postoperative. Hormonal manipulation is the principal mode of therapy for symptomatic stage D patients. The choices are estrogens (e.g. diethystilbestrol 1mg/day), leuprolide (a luteinizing hormone releasing hormone [LHRH] agonist), leuprolide + flutamide (the latter is an antiestrogen), or orchiectomy. Leuprolide appears to be as effective as diethystilbestrol and produces fewer adverse effects. Other palliative measures may be necessary—e.g. radiation to relieve pain of bone metastases, transurethral resection of prostate for obstruction.

Renal Cell Carcinoma (hypernephroma, Grawitz tumor) is

thought to develop from proximal tubular cells. It is the most common form of renal cancer in adults (about 85% cases). Transitional cell carcinomas of the renal pelvis account for most of the rest (see next chapter). Wilms' tumor is the most common kidney cancer in children (see "Wilms' Tumor" chapter). **Risk factors:** Males and those who smoke have the highest risk. Risk is also increased in those with adult polycystic kidney disease or von Hippel–Landau disease.

Signs/symptoms: Classic presentation consists of hematuria, flank pain, and an abdominal mass. However, all 3 findings are found in only about 10% cases. About 70% patients will have at least one of these manifestations. Other common manifestations include fever, weight loss, anemia, thrombophlebitis. Hormonal syndromes are common—e.g. hypercalcemia (due to parathormone or prostaglandins or bone metastases), polycythemia (due to tumor erythropoietin production), Cushing's syndrome (due to tumor ACTH production), hypertension. High–output congestive heart failure occasionally results when an AV fistula develops within the primary tumor or within a metastasis. Nonmetastatic liver function abnormalities may develop—e.g. prolonged prothrombin time, hypoalbuminemia, elevated alkaline phosphatase, elevated alpha–2 globulin. Metastases to lung, bone, liver, and brain are common.

Diagnosis: Plain x-ray may reveal a calcified tumor. IVP with tomograms is usually the first diagnostic test. Ultrasound follows if a renal mass is found on IVP or if IVP is equivocal. Investigation of a renal cyst: If a simple cyst (i.e. smooth margins with echo-free interior) is found on ultrasound, percutaneous cyst puncture with cytology is performed if the patient is symptomatic. Asymptomatic patients with a simple cyst on ultrasound generally do not require this procedure since a renal cell carcinoma is then unlikely. CAT scan (with and without contrast media) is indicated if (1) a solid or complex mass is seen on ultrasound, (2) the ultrasound is negative despite a positive or equivocal IVP, or (3) cyst puncture yields hemorrhagic fluid or equivocal cytology.

Note: The following staging, treatment, and prognosis information is extracted from National Cancer Institute PDQ State-of-the-Art Cancer Treatment Information 1/7/91. However, since cancer treatment is evolving, this information may not be current. The most up-to-date standard treatment options may be obtained by calling the National Cancer Institute Cancer Information Service at 1-800-4-CANCER. Patients may also be candidates for clinical trials of new therapeutic regimens. Descriptions of these trials are also available.

Staging/treatment: Stage I (tumor confined to kidney) is usually treated with simple or radical nephrectomy. Radical nephrectomy includes resection of adrenal, perinephric fat, and Gerota's fascia with or without regional node dissection. If surgery is contraindicated, palliative radiation or palliative arterial embolization may be used. In selected patients with bilateral tumor, partial nephrectomy may be recommended instead of bilateral nephrectomy. Stage II (tumor invades adrenal or perinephric tissue yet remains confined within Gerota's fascia) is usually treated with radical nephrectomy. Selected patients who undergo nephrectomy (particularly those with extensive tumor) may receive pre or postoperative external beam radiation although it is not definitely known whether survival is improved. If surgery is contraindicated, palliative radiation or palliative arterial embolization may be used. In selected patients with bilateral tumor, partial nephrectomy may be recommended instead of bilateral nephrectomy. Stage III (tumor invades regional nodes, renal vein, and/or inferior vena cava) may be treated with radical nephrectomy with lymph node dissection plus partial resection of the inferior vena cava if that is involved. Preoperative arterial embolization, or pre or postoperative radiation may be employed although it is of unproven value. If surgery is contraindicated or the tumor is inoperable, then palliative radiation or palliative arterial embolization are options. Nephrectomy may be performed simply for palliation. Stage IV (tumor involves adjacent organs not counting adrenal, and/or there are distant metastases) is treated with palliative measures—e.g. radiation, arterial embolization, palliative surgery. Progestins are sometimes palliative.

Prognosis (5 yr survival with treatment): stage I; 70%, stage II; 50%, stage III; 35%, stage IV; 5%.

Cancer of Bladder, Ureter, and/or Renal pelvis/Calyces

Etiology: Transitional cell carcinoma (TCC) is responsible for the great majority of cases. The malignancy arises from the transitional epithelial mucosal cells that line the urinary conduits from calyces to bladder. TCC is often multicentric and tends to recur. Risk of TCC is increased by smoking, chronic phenacetin ingestion, exposure to aromatic amines. Squamous cell carcinoma is uncommon. The risk is increased in patients with bladder infestation by Schistosoma haematobium or in patients with chronic nephrolithiasis. Adenocarcinomas occur rarely; they are usually derived from embryonic vestiges (e.g. urachus).

Signs/symptoms: Gross or microscopic hematuria is the most common manifestation of a TCC no matter where the tumor is located along the urinary collectiing system from calyces to bladder. Bladder TCC may also be associated with dysuria or frequency. A large bladder tumor is sometimes felt suprapubically or on bimanual rectal or vaginal exam. TCC of the ureter may present with colicky flank pain if there is ureteral obstruction.

Diagnosis: Urine cytology may reveal malignant cells. IVP is ordered. A "negative" shadow caused by the tumor protruding into the lumen of the renal pelvis, ureter, or bladder may be seen. IVP is often normal in the case of a bladder tumor. Retrograde urogram may be indicated if the IVP is inadequate or if the kidney is not functioning. Cytoscopy is performed. Bladder growths are biopsied. Ureteral brushings for cytology may be obtained. Additional tests may be ordered (e.g. ultrasound, CAT scan, chest x-ray, bone scan) to identify or further define the extent of a tumor and/or metastases.

Treatment of TCC of the calyces, renal pelvis, or ureter consists of nephrectomy with resection of the ureter. Postoperatively, because TCC is frequently multifocal and recurrent, periodic cytoscopy is necessary to exclude the development of bladder TCC.

Note: The following staging, treatment, and prognosis information is extracted from National Cancer Institute PDQ State-of-the-Art Cancer Treatment Information 1/7/91. However, since cancer treatment is evolving, this information may not be current. The most up-to-date standard treatment options may be obtained by calling the National Cancer Institute Cancer Information Service at 1–800–4–CANCER. Patients may also be candidates for inclusion in clinical trials. Descriptions of these trials are also available.

Staging/treatment of bladder cancer: Stage 0 (carcinoma in situ or nonivasive papillary carcinoma, lymph nodes not involved) is usually treated by transurethral resection with fulguration. Periodic cystoscopy is necesary since recurrences are common. Clinical trials have shown patients to benefit from postoperative intravesical chemotherapy (e.g. bladder instillation of thiotepa, doxorubicin, or mitomycin) or intravesical immunotherapy with bacillus Calmette–Guerin (BCG). Chemotherapy alone or immunotherapy alone is employed in some cases. Radical cystectomy may be necessary if there is extensive superficial disease unresponsive to intravesical chemotherapy. Stage I (invasion of subepithelial connective tissue, bladder muscle not involved, lymph nodes not involved, metastasis absent) may be treated similarly to stage 0. Additional options are: (1) external beam radiation for selected patients with extensive superficial disease; (2) interstitial radioisotope implantation with or without external beam radiation. Stage II (invasion of superficial muscle of bladder, nodes not involved, metastasis absent) may be managed in some cases by transurethral resection with fulguration. Clinical judgment must guide therapeutic decision. Other options are: (1) radical cystectomy ± pelvic node dissection, (2) radical cystectomy preceded by external beam radiation, (3) external beam radiation alone for patients who are not surgical candidates and selected patients, (4) interstitial radioisotope implantation preceded or followed by external beam radiation, (5) interstitial radioisotope implantation alone, (6) segmental cystectomy for highly selected patients. Stage III (invasion of deep muscle of bladder or perivesical fat, nodes not involved, metastasis absent) is usually treated with external beam radiation followed by radical cystectomy. Radical cystectomy ± pelvic node dissection is the principal alternative. Other options in selected patients are: (1) external beam radiation plus interstitial radioisotope implantation; (2) segmental cystectomy, or (3) external beam radiation with salvage cystectomy or transurethral resection should there be only local failure from radiation. Stage IV patient without distant metastasis: There is regional node (i.e. nodes within the true pelvis) involvement and/or there is invasion of the prostate, uterus, vagina, pelvic wall, or abdominal wall. Cures are seldom achieved. Treatment with curative intent consists of radical cystectomy ± preoperative radiation or pelvic node dissection. Palliative therapy is often necessary (e.g. cystectomy, urinary diversion, external beam radiation). Chemotherapy alone or as an adjunct may be beneficial (e.g. cisplatin + methotrexate + vinblastine ± doxorubicin). Stage IV with distant metastasis treatment is palliative—e.g. external beam radiation, palliative surgery (e.g. cystectomy, urinary diversion). Chemotherapy alone or as an adjunct may be beneficial.

Prognosis (5 year survival with treatment): stage 0: 90%, stage I: 75%, stage II: 55%, stage III: 35% if invasion is not beyond deep muscle of bladder, 20% if there is penetration thru the bladder wall into the perinephric fat; stage IV: < 5% without distant metastases, < 2% with distant metastases.

Wilms' Tumor (nephroblastoma). Most cases occur in children, usually children under 4 years of age. Tumors arise in both kidneys in 5–10% cases.

Signs/symptoms/diagnosis: Patients may present with abdominal pain, abdominal mass, hematuria, hypertension, and/or weight loss. IVP generally shows distortion of the kidney and calyces. Nonvisualization may be due to ureteral obstruction. CAT scan is indicated to further define the extent of the tumor, to reveal metastases, and to identify tumor in the opposite kidney. Chest x-ray is obtained to assess for pulmonary metastasis. Ultrasound and/or inferior venacavogram may be ordered for further clarification since the tumor not uncommonly invades or externally compresses the inferior vena cava.

Histopathology influences both the selection of the appropriate treatment regimen and the prognosis. Tumors with unfavorable histology are grouped as anaplastic or sarcomatous. The latter includes clear cell carcinoma of the kidney and rhabdoid carcinoma of the kidney.

Staging: Stage I: tumor confined to kidney and completely removed with surgery. Furthermore, the renal capsule is intact and the tumor is not ruptured before or during excision. Stage II: tumor not confined to kidney but is completely removed with surgery. Stage III: there is residual tumor following surgery but it is confined to the abdomen. Stage IV: hematogenous metastases—e.g. to lung, bone, brain, liver. Stage V: both kidneys involved.

Treatment is individualized according to both stage and histology of tumor. Surgical resection of all or as much of the primary tumor as possible or practical is the first step in almost all patients. If surgery is not initially possible (e.g. stage V patient with unresectable tumor), it may be possible to perform needle biopsy and defer surgery until after chemotherapy and/or radiotherapy shrinks the tumor. Chemotherapy is administered to all patients. Vincristine and dactinomycin are the cornerstone. Doxorubicin and perhaps cyclophosphamide may be added to the regimen depending on the stage and whether there is favorable or unfavorable histology. Radiation therapy may or may not be indicated depending on the stage and whether the histology is favorable or not.

Note: The most up-to-date standard treatment options according to stage and histology are outlined in National Cancer Institute PDQ State-of-the-Art Cancer Treatment Information. This information may be obtained by calling the National Cancer Institute Cancer Information Service at 1–800-4-CANCER. All Wilms' trials should be considered for inclusion in clinical trials. Descriptions of these trials are also available. Since optimal treatment requires the combined efforts of a pediatric surgeon and specialists experienced in pediatric oncology and radiotherapy, treatment is best administered as part of a clinical trial at a major medical center proficient in pediatric care.

Prognosis: Most patients can be cured. With favorable histology, the 4-year disease-free survival ranges from 91.8% for stage I to 77.9% for stage IV. Stage V 3-year survival is 84%. With unfavorable histology (about 10% of the cases), the 4-year disease-free survival ranges from 67% for stage I to 58.3% for stage IV. Stage V 3-year survival is 16%.

Hyperkalemia (serum potassium > 5.5 mEq/liter).

Etiology: Any oliguric condition will impair potassium excretion because potassium excretion is flow dependent. Hyperkalemia is therefore common in acute renal failure but is unusual in chronic renal failure until end-stage oliguria develops. Excessive parenteral or oral potassium may cause hyperkalemia, especially in the presence of renal insufficiency. Rhabdomyolysis (e.g. crush injury, arterial embolism) or hemolysis (e.g. GI bleed, burns) may release sufficient intracellular potassium to cause hyperkalemia. Potassium-sparing diuretics (e.g. aldosterone antagonist spironolactone) may induce hyperkalemia, especially in presence of renal insufficiency or excess potassium ingestion. Respiratory or metabolic acidosis can cause hyperkalemia (potassium moves out of cells while hydrogen ion moves into cells). The serum potassium increases by 0.6 mEq/liter for each 0.1 decrement in pH. Aldosterone deficiency (e.g. Addison's disease, adrenogenital syndrome) may lead to hyperkalemia because aldosterone acts at the distal tubules to promote potassium and hydrogen excretion as well as sodium retention. Low renin activity due to renal tubulointerstitial disease (e.g. diabetic nephropathy) may result in a decrease in aldosterone secretion with ensuing hyperkalemia. Hyperkalemic periodic paralysis is a rare autosomal dominant inherited disease characterized by release of intracellular potassium so that hyperkalemia-provoked paralysis ensues. Severe digitalis toxicity may be associated with hyperkalemia.
Pseudohyperkalemia; An erroneously elevated serum potassium measurement may occur when blood cells leak potassium after the blood sample is drawn (e.g. in vitro hemolysis, severe thrombocytosis, or severe leukocytosis). This erroneous reading can be avoided by measuring the PLASMA potassium without delay. Pseudohyperkalemia may also result from hemolysis of a blood sample taken from an extremity around which a tourniquet has been in place for a prolonged period, especially if that extremity has been exercised.

Signs/symptoms: Cardiovascular signs (e.g. bradycardia, heart block, arrhythmias, hypotension, cardiac arrest) are the most obvious. They are most likely to develop when serum K is > 6.5 mEq/liter. The EKG typically passes thru several stages with worsening hyperkalemia: tall peaked T wave → prolonged PR interval → widening QRS → disappearance of P wave → sine wave → ventricular fibrillation. However, severe hyperkalemia may sometimes present with only minimal EKG changes and yet precipitate cardiac arrest. Patients with conduction abnormalities are prone to 2nd and 3rd degree heart block even when hyperkalemia does not exceed 6.5 mEq/liter. Muscle weakness may occur and sometimes progress to paresthesias, hyporeflexia, paralysis (including respiratory paralysis).

Treatment of urgent cases (e.g. serum K > 6.5 with EKG abnormalities, serum K > 8.0): EKG monitor is essential. Calcium gluconate is promptly administered: 10 ml of 10% solution IV over 2–5 minutes. May repeat in 5 minutes if EKG signs are still present. Duration of effect is about 30–60 minutes. Use cautiously if patient is on digitalis. Sodium bicarbonate immediately follows: 1 mEq/kg IV push and repeated as needed in 10–15 minutes as EKG signs dictate. Sodium bicarbonate serves to drive potassium intracellularly. Onset < 1 hr, duration 1–2 hr. Glucose and insulin are also given to drive potassium intracellularly (25 gram 50% dextrose administered over 5 minutes along with 5–10 unit regular insulin IV). Dextrose alone will suffice if the patient has no other illness since his own endogenous insulin levels will rise in response to the glucose challenge. Onset of effect is about half hour, duration 2–4 hr. Kayexalate is administered to hasten elimination of potassium (see Kayexalate in drug section). Hemodialysis may be necessary in some cases—e.g. fluid overloaded patient in renal failure, ongoing release of intracellular potassium (e.g. severe catabolic state, rhabdomyolysis).

Treatment of nonurgent cases: If serum K < 6.5 mEq/liter; then correction of precipitating causes, restriction of potassium intake, and administration of Kayexalate will usually suffice.

Hypokalemia (serum K < 3.5 mEq/liter)

Etiology: insufficient potassium intake, vomiting or nasogastric suction, diarrhea, diuretics (excepting potassium–sparing diuretics), osmotic diuresis (e.g. diabetes mellitus, mannitol, urea); alkalosis; renal tubular acidosis; hypokalemic periodic paralysis; endogenous or exogenous mineralocorticoid excess; insulin administration; Bartter's syndrome; Liddle's syndrome; carbenicillin; amphotericin.

Signs/symptoms: Symptoms do not generally appear unless serum K is < 2.5 mEq/liter. Skeletal muscle abnormalities: muscle weakness (may be only complaint), ascending paralysis, tetany, muscle cramps. Muscle atrophy may develop with severe chronic hypokalemia. Sensory complaints: numbness, parasthesias. Gastrointestinal: Ileus may develop and ensuing vomiting may cause additional K depletion. Cardiac abnormalities: Arrhythmias are potentiated by digitalis therapy but can occur without digitalis. With worsening hypokalemia the EKG typically passes thru the following stages: flattening of T wave and appearance of U wave → T wave inversion → ST segment depression. Polyuria or decreased GFR may occur.

Treatment of urgent case (e.g. serum K < 2 mEq/liter, arrhythmias or other EKG abnormalities, digitalis intoxication, paralysis): Continuous EKG monitoring is essential and serum potassium should be measured every 2–4 hr. Potassium is administered intravenously via a peripheral vein. Because of the risk of provoking a fatal arrhythmia, IV potassium must never be given undiluted or IV push. Central venous or intracardiac administration is dangerous and should be avoided. Potassium infusion rate must not exceed 40mEq/hr. Concentration of potassium solution must not exceed 60mEq/liter. Concentrations > 40mEq/liter should not be given via a small vein because venous irritation with phlebitis may ensue. Administration of glucose is generally not advised because glucose can worsen hypokalemia by driving potassium intracellularly. For the same reason, bicarbonate administration is also avoided (unless serum pH is < 7.1 and serum bicarbonate is < 10mEq/liter) unless or until the serum potassium is > 2.5mEq/liter.

Treatment or nonurgent case: Unless a patient is receiving digitalis, the treatment of hypokalemia is generally not urgent if the serum K is > 2.0 mEq/liter. Oral potassium supplementation is the usual therapy (see drug section). Patients unable to tolerate oral potassium supplements may be given a potassium–sparing drug (e.g. spironolactone) or potassium–rich foods. If intravenous therapy must be used, the potassium infusion should be no faster than 10mEq/hr, the potassium concentration should not be > 40mEq/liter, and the total daily dose should not be > 200mEq. Choice of potassium salt: If hypokalemia is associated with metabolic acidosis; potassium bicarbonate or the potassium salt of a metabolic precursor of bicarbonate (potassium citrate, potassium gluconate, or potassium acetate) is generally recommended. However, in diabetic ketoacidosis, potassium chloride and/or potassium phosphate is usually used. In the case of hypokalemic hypochloremic metabolic alkalosis, potassium chloride must be used.

Hypernatremia (serum sodium > 145 mEq/liter)

Etiology: Thirst is such a potent stimulus that severe hypernatremia is unlikely unless: (a) water is not available, (b) thirst stimulus is compromised—e.g. hypothalamic lesion, (c) patient is comatose. Water depletion in excess of sodium loss: inadequate water intake; sweating; burns; diarrhea; respiratory evaporation; diabetes insipidus (nephrogenic or central); osmotic diuresis (e.g. diabetes mellitus, mannitol administration, urea). Administration of excess sodium: excessive hypertonic saline IV, ingestion large number salt tablets, oral administration of hypertonic sodium solutions to infants. Sodium retention: Cushing's syndrome, primary hyperaldosteronism.

Signs/symptoms: Thirst is generally present in the conscious patient. If hypernatremia is primarily due to water depletion, signs of dehydration may be present—e.g. decreased skin turgor; dry mucous membranes; hypotension; confusion; weakness; irritability; hemoconcentration (elevated sodium, elevated osmolality, elevated BUN, elevated hematocrit, etc). Also, the urine is concentrated (elevated specific gravity and osmolality) unless perhaps if hypernatremia is due to polyuria (e.g. diabetes insipidus, osmotic diuresis). Neurologic consequences of hypernatremia/hyperosmolality may be evident—e.g. lethargy, irritability, restlessness. In more severely affected patients, there may be tremor, muscle twitching, hyperreflexia, ataxia; and finally spasticity, convulsions, and death. The point at which various neurologic manifestations appear is not just a function of the absolute degree of hyperosmolality, but is influenced by the speed at which hyperosmolality develops and progresses, and the age of the patient (the elderly and infants are more sensitive).

Treatment overview: Treatment regimen depends on level of consciousness, severity of hypernatremia, and how hypernatremia developed. Correct the underlying problem if possible. Intravenous therapy is required in obtunded, comatose, or severely hypernatremic patients. Correct hypernatremia slowly; In general, safe correction of hypernatremia dictates that the serum sodium fall no faster than 1 mEq every 2 hr because otherwise cerebral edema may ensue. The mechanism leading to cerebral edema is as follows: (1) Hypernatremia causes movement of water out of brain cells. (2) So as not to shrink, the brain cells produce "idiogenic osmoles" which cause water to be retained by the brain cells. (3) If water is rapidly administered in order to quickly correct hypernatremia, water under the influence of the idiogenic osmoles enters the brain cells and cerebral edema ensues. If, on the other hand, hypernatremia is slowly corrected, cerebral edema is precluded because there is time for the idiogenic osmoles to be eliminated.

Treatment of hypernatremia with ECF excess: A diuretic (e.g. furosemide) is administered. As needed, 5% glucose solution is added to the therapy to replenish water loss and further correct hypernatremia slowly. Dialysis may be necessary in the setting of renal failure.

Treatment of hypernatremia in euvolemic patient: Therapy consists of PO water or intravenous 5% glucose solution.

Treatment of hypernatremia with ECF depletion:

●If volume depletion is severe enough to affect circulation (e.g. orthostatic hypotension, tachycardia, oliguria; first correct circulatory disturbance with intravenous normal saline. Then switch to hypotonic (0.45%) saline to slowly correct hypernatremia.

●If there is volume depletion in the absence of circulatory disturbance, proceed directly to treatment with intravenous hypotonic (0.45%) saline or 5% glucose solution to slowly correct hypernatremia. If 5% glucose solution is used, it must not be administered so rapidly as to provoke glucosuria. This would cause an osmotic diuresis that may itself make hypernatremia worse.

●If the serum sodium is < 160 mEq/liter and there is no evidence of circulatory disturbance, and the patient is sufficiently alert to safely take oral fluids, allowing the patient to drink water according to his thirst may suffice to correct hypernatremia.

●Amount of water needed to correct water depletion–induced hypernatremia is estimated by following equation:

$$\text{water deficit in liters} = \frac{0.6 \times (\text{weight in kg}) \times (140 - \text{serum sodium})}{140}$$

Hyponatremia (serum sodium < 135 mEq/liter) may occur in the

presence of excess total body water (I.e. hypervolemic/dilutional hyponatremia), normal total body water (normovolemic hyponatremia), or a deficit of total body water (hypovolemic dehydration). **Water intoxication** refers to the clinical manifestations of hyponatremia–associated hypotonicity (lightheadedness, weakness, lethargy, muscle cramps, nausea, vomiting, confusion, convulsions, coma). Water intoxication is due to hypotonicity; not hyponatremia per se. In clinical situations, hypotonicity is inevitably associated with hyponatremia. However, hyponatremia does not necessarily imply hypotonicity (e.g. see below "Hyponatremia with HYPERtonicity"). CNS symptoms are due to brain edema. The brain cells swell because water moves from the hypotonic extracellular space to the hypertonic intracellular space. When hyponatremia with hypotonicity develops slowly, the brain cells have time to compensate: sodium, potassium, and chloride leave the intracellular space thereby diminishing movement of water into the cells. Symptoms may be mild if hyponatremia with hypotonicity develops slowly over days to weeks (the serum sodium may reach 110 mEq/liter without severe manifestations). On the other hand, serious neurologic consequences may quickly ensue if hyponatremia with hypotonicity develops rapidly even when serum sodium does not fall below 125 mEq/liter.

Hyponatremia with ECF volume excess resulting in edema may be the consequence of heart failure, cirrhosis, nephrotic syndrome, or renal failure. Sodium is retained so that total body sodium is actually increased. However, dilutional hyponatremia ensues because there is proportionally greater retention of water. The excess extracellular water in turn leads to edema. In the case of renal failure–associated hyponatremia, impaired tubular function results in urine sodium concentration > 20mEq/liter. In the other conditions noted above, the tubules retain sodium to a greater extent and so the urine sodium is typically < 10mEq/liter provided that the patient is not on a diuretic. <u>Treatment:</u> Treat underlying condition. Restrict fluid intake. Administer furosemide if clinical condition is serious and provided that the kidneys are capable of responding. In urgent cases (e.g. seizures, coma); administration of 0.9% or 3% saline is combined with sufficient IV furosemide to prevent further edema. The goal is to achieve a serum sodium of 125 mEq/liter in about 6 hr and to thereafter achieve a normal serum sodium by fluid restriction.

Hyponatremia with normal ECF volume or with modest ECF excess without edema may be the consequence of hypothyroidism; glucocorticoid insufficiency; emotional stress (e.g. psychotic episode); physical stress (e.g. pain); SIADH; or drugs that induce ADH release or enhance its effects (e.g. acetaminophen, indomethacin, narcotics, barbiturates, carbamazepine, tricyclic antidepressants, clofibrate, tolbutamide, chlorpropamide, vincristine, cyclophosphamide). In these cases total body water may be increased but extracellular volume excess is characteristically insufficient to cause edema. <u>Treatment:</u> Correct underlying condition if possible. Fluid restriction alone usually suffices to resolve hyponatremia. In the severe symptomatic hyponatremia that may occur with SIADH, therapy consists of judicious administration of furosemide in conjunction with IV saline (0.9% or 3%) with enough KCl to replace urinary losses. Once neurologic symptoms are no longer present or the serum sodium has reached 125 mEq/liter, this mode of therapy is discontinued in favor of fluid restriction (1–1.5 liter/day). Rapid correction of the serum sodium to normal levels is discouraged because cerebral shrinkage may ensue. Demeclocycline may be employed in SIADH patients if fluid restriction is not tolerated or if SIADH is chronic. **SIADH (syndrome of inappropriate ADH secretion)** merits additional comment. <u>SIADH can result from</u> malignancy; CNS disease (e.g. meningitis, encephalitis, head trauma); pulmonary disease (pneumonia, tuberculosis, intermittent positive pressure breathing). <u>Diagnosis of SIADH should not be made unless all the following conditions are met:</u> (**1**) there is both serum hyponatremia and hypotonicity (typically < 260 mOsm/liter); (**2**) the urine, in view of the hypotonicity of the serum, is inappropriately concentrated (urine osmolarity is nearly always > serum osmolarity) and the urine sodium is elevated > 20 mEq/liter; (**3**) dehydration is not present; (**4**) there must be normal function of the kidneys as well as anterior pituitary, adrenal, and thyroid glands; (**5**) patient must not be receiving diuretics or receiving drugs that induce ADH release or enhance its effects; (**6**) absence of acute pain or severe emotional distress.

Hyponatremia with ECF volume depletion: Whenever sodium is lost, there is an obligatory loss of water. If sodium depletion proportionally exceeds water depletion, hyponatremia results. Hyponatremia may also sometimes occur when low–sodium or sodium–free solutions are used to replace fluid loss regardless of whether that loss be hypotonic, isotonic, or hypertonic. <u>Sodium depletion may be renal or nonrenal.</u> With renal depletion, the urine sodium is > 20 mEq/liter. With nonrenal depletion the urine sodium is < 10–15 mEq/liter. <u>Renal sodium loss</u> may result from diuretics; salt–losing nephritis; mineralocorticoid insufficiency; bicarbonaturia (metabolic alkalosis, renal tubular acidosis); ketonuria; osmotic diuresis (glucosuria, mannitol administration, urea). Examples of *osmotic* diuresis that may lead to hyponatremia are: (1) diabetes mellitus–related glucosuria and ketonuria (for each 100 mg/dl rise in serum glucose there is a 1.6 mEq/liter decrease in serum sodium); (2) urea diuresis that follows relief of urinary obstruction or accompanies the recovery phase of acute tubular necrosis. Note: Most hyponatremic conditions are associated with hypotonicity. However, in the case of osmotic diuresis, the excess plasma solute that causes *hyper*tonicity may at the same time draw intracellular water into the ECF and thus lead to *hypo*natremia. <u>Nonrenal sodium loss</u> may be due to vomiting; diarrhea; nasogastric suction; or third space loss (e.g. burns, pancreatitis, muscle trauma). <u>Treatment:</u> In urgent situations with neurologic manifestations (e.g. seizures, coma); administer 3% saline IV with the goal of achieving a serum sodium concentration of 125 mEq/liter in no less than 6 hr. Further correction should proceed much more slowly with isotonic (0.9%) saline. The number of mEq of sodium needed to achieve a serum sodium of 125 mEq/liter =

0.6 X (body weight in kg) X (125 – measured serum sodium).

Pseudohyponatremia results when plasma proteins (e.g. multiple myeloma) or lipids (e.g. hyperlipidemia) occupy an increased proportion of the plasma volume. The water fraction of the plasma (to which sodium is mostly confined) is therefore reduced. Consequently, while the sodium concentration of the total serum is reduced, the sodium concentration in the water fraction is normal. Fluid and electrolyte therapy is not required since there is no actual sodium abnormality and the serum osmolality is normal. Whether or not pseudohyponatremia occurs depends on the method used to determine serum sodium. The flame emission spectrometer method is susceptible to yielding a pseudohyponatremic result, while the ion selective electrode method will in the same circumstance give a true reading (provided that the serum sample is not diluted) because the latter method determines the serum sodium concentration of the serum water fraction, not the total serum.

Acid–base Disturbances

Henderson–Hasselbalch equation: $pH = pK + \dfrac{\log [HCO_3]}{(0.03 \times pCO_2)}$

The equation shows that (1) the bicarbonate concentration [HCO3] is directly proportional to the pH (i.e. when [HCO3] increases pH increases and conversely), and (2) the pCO2 is inversely proportional to the pH (i.e. when pCO2 increases the pH decreases and conversely).

The equation demonstrates the direction of compensation when there is a primary acid–base disturbance:

The larger arrows indicate the direction of the primary change; the smaller arrows indicate the compensatory changes.

With a primary decrease in [HCO3] (i.e. primary metabolic acidosis), the lungs compensate: ventilation increases thereby decreasing pCO2 (i.e. compensatory respiratory alkalosis) in order to drive the pH back towards normal.

$pH = pK + \dfrac{\log [HCO_3]\ \downarrow}{(0.03 \times pCO_2)\ \downarrow}$

With a primary increase in [HCO3] (i.e. primary metabolic alkalosis), the lungs compensate: ventilation decreases thereby increasing pCO2 (i.e. compensatory respiratory acidosis) in order to drive the pH back towards normal.

$pH = pK + \dfrac{\log [HCO_3]\ \uparrow}{(0.03 \times pCO_2)\ \uparrow}$

With a primary decrease in pCO2 (i.e. primary respiratory alkalosis), the kidneys compensate by increasing [HCO3] excretion (i.e. compensatory metabolic alkalosis) in order to drive the pH back towards normal.

$pH = pK + \dfrac{\log [HCO_3]\ \downarrow}{(0.03 \times pCO_2)\ \downarrow}$

With a primary increase in pCO2 (i.e. primary respiratory acidosis), the kidneys compensate by retaining [HCO3] (i.e. compensatory metabolic acidosis) in order to drive the pH back towards normal.

$pH = pK + \dfrac{\log [HCO_3]\ \uparrow}{(0.03 \times pCO_2)\ \uparrow}$

Estimating expected changes in pH, pCO2, and HCO3 concentration: (**1**) A change in the pCO2 of 10 mm Hg will cause a pH change of 0.08; (**2**) a change in [HCO3] of 10 mEq/liter will cause a pH change of 0.15. Examples: If a patient has a pCO2 of 50, the expected pH would be 7.32 if respiratory acidosis alone is present. However, if the actual pH is found to be 7.17, then the difference between the expected and actual pH (7.32 – 7.17 = 0.15) indicates a base deficit of 10 mEq/liter. The patient has therefore a respiratory acidosis combined with a metabolic acidosis.

If a patient with a pCO_2 of 50 has an actual pH of 7.47, the difference between the expected and the actual pH (7.47 − 7.32 = 0.15) would indicate a base excess of 10 mEq/liter. The patient would therefore have a respiratory acidosis combined with a metabolic alkalosis.

Normal arterial blood gas values (room air): pH 7.36–7.44, pCO_2 37–44 mm Hg, HCO_3 21–26 mEq/liter, base excess/deficit −2 to +2, pO_2 80–100 mm Hg, O_2 saturation > 85%.

Distinguishing the terms acidosis and alkalosis from acidemia and alkalemia respectively: The terms acidosis and alkalosis do not imply that the plasma is either acidic or alkaline respectively. For example, a patient could have a decreased $[HCO_3]$ (i.e. metabolic acidosis) combined with a decreased pCO_2 (i.e. respiratory alkalosis) resulting in an arterial pH is in the normal range. It is therefore best to use the terms acidemia or alkalemia when indicating the actual blood pH status.

METABOLIC ACIDOSIS is characterized by a primary decrease in serum bicarbonate $[HCO_3]$. If there is no respiratory compensation (i.e. pure metabolic acidosis), each 10 mEq/liter decrease in $[HCO_3]$ will cause the pH to fall by 0.15. For instance, a decrease in $[HCO_3]$ from a normal of 25 mEq/liter to 15 mEq/liter would be expected to lead to a fall in pH from 7.4 to about 7.25. If there is respiratory compensation (i.e. patient increases ventilation to eliminate more CO_2), the fall in pCO_2 will drive the pH up toward normal as predicted by the Henderson–Hasselbalch equation. In COMPENSATED metabolic acidosis, a convenient rule of thumb is that the pCO_2 will be about equal to the last two digits of the pH (e.g. pCO_2 of 30 implies pH of 7.30).

Metabolic acidosis is categorized as either high anion gap (normochloremic) acidosis or normal anion gap (hyperchloremic) acidosis. The anion gap is defined as $([Na] + [K]) − ([Cl] + [HCO_3])$. The normal range of anion gap is 12–16 mEq/liter. High anion gap (normochloremic) metabolic acidosis: When metabolic disturbances lead to an increase in UNMEASURED anions (e.g. lactic acidosis, diabetic ketoacidosis), HCO_3 is depleted and the anion gap increases. Normal anion gap (hyperchloremic) metabolic acidosis: If on the other hand, as in the case of hyperchloremic metabolic acidosis, HCO_3 depletion is offset by increase in chloride (e.g. renal failure, distal renal tubular acidosis), the anion gap remains in the normal range.

Causes of high anion gap (normochloremic) metabolic acidosis: ketoacidosis––e.g. diabetic ketoacidosis, alcohol–induced, starvation, rubbing alcohol–induced (increased lipolysis in these conditions generates increased ketoacids); lactic acidosis (e.g. hypoxemia, shock); renal failure (there is decreased excretion of inorganic acids–e.g. sulfates, phosphates); certain toxins (e.g. metabolism of methanol, ethylene glycol, salicylates, and paraldehyde produces organic acids).

Causes of normal anion gap (hyperchloremic) metabolic acidosis: GI bicarbonate loss (diarrhea, pancreatic fistula); potassium–sparing diuretics (e.g. spironolactone, triamterene) block the distal tubular reabsorption of Na in exchange for K and H ions so that there is increased urinary loss of $NaHCO_3$ with ensuing hyperkalemic hyperchloremic alkalosis; administration of acid salts (e.g. ammonium chloride, hyperalimentation); ureteral diversion (e.g. ureterosigmoidostomy): bicarbonate is lost neutralizing the acid urine entering the bowel and consequently GI absorption of chloride is increased in order to maintain electrical neutrality); decreased threshold for proximal tubular reabsorption of bicarbonate (proximal renal tubular acidosis, Fanconi syndrome, primary hyperparathyroidism); acetazolamide inhibits carbonic anhydrase thereby reducing the amount of sodium bicarbonate reabsorption at the proximal tubules; other (sulfamylon, amphotericin B).

RESPIRATORY ACIDOSIS is characterized by a primary increase in the serum pCO_2 owing to the retention of CO_2 that results from decreased ventilation. In the absence of metabolic compensation, each 10 mm Hg increase in pCO_2 leads to decrease in the pH of about 0.08. For instance, if the pCO_2 rises from 40 to 50, the pH will decrease from 7.40 to 7.32. If there is metabolic compensation (i.e. the kidneys retain HCO_3), the pH is driven up toward normal as predicted by the Henderson–Hasselbalch equation. **Causes** of decreased/impaired ventilation: CNS depression either from drugs (e.g. narcotics, sedatives) or a CNS lesion; neuromuscular disease (e.g. myasthenia gravis); abnormalities of the thorax (e.g. flail chest, kyphoscoliosis); airway obstruction (e.g. emphysema, chronic bronchitis, asthma, foreign body, croup, epiglottitis); other pulmonary lesions (massive pulmonary embolus, pneumothorax, acute severe pulmonary edema, severe pneumonia); metabolic (myxedema coma).

METABOLIC ALKALOSIS is characterized by a primary increase in serum bicarbonate [HCO_3]. If there is no respiratory compensation (i.e. pure metabolic acidosis), each 10 mEq/liter increase in [HCO_3] will cause the pH to increase by 0.15. For instance, an increase in [HCO_3] from a normal of 25 mEq/liter to 40 mEq/liter would be expected to result in a rise in pH from 7.4 to about 7.55. If there is respiratory compensation (i.e. the patient decreases his ventilation in order to retain more CO_2), the rise in pCO_2 will drive the pH down toward normal as predicted by the Henderson–Hasselbalch equation. In COMPENSATED metabolic alkalosis, a convenient rule of thumb is that the pCO_2 will be about equal to the last two digits of the pH (e.g. pCO_2 of 45 implies pH of 7.45).

Causes of saline responsive metabolic alkalosis (characterized by low urinary chloride, i.e.< 10 mEq/liter): gastrointestinal: vomiting, nasogastric suction, villous adenoma; renal: diuretics, carbenicillin, post–hypercapneic (example of the latter is when assisted ventilation in a COPD patient suddenly decreases the pCO_2 so that a high HCO_3 to pCO_2 ratio ensues); alkali administration: administration of bicarbonate or precursors (e.g. lactate, citrate, acetate); contraction alkalosis (i.e. extracellular volume depletion).

Causes of saline unresponsive metabolic alkalosis (characterized by high urinary chloride, i.e. > 10 mEq/liter): mineralocorticoid excess (e.g. hyperaldosteronism, Cushing's syndrome, Bartter's syndrome, Liddle's syndrome, hyperreninism); other (severe potassium depletion, nonparathryroid hypercalcemia).

RESPIRATORY ALKALOSIS is characterized by an decrease in pCO_2 owing to the depletion of CO_2 that results from increased ventilation. In the absence of metabolic compensation, each 10 mm Hg decrease in pCO_2 leads to an increase in the pH of about 0.08. For instance, if the pCO_2 decreases from 40 to 30, the pH will increase from 7.40 to 7.48. If there is metabolic compensation (i.e. the kidneys increase HCO_3 excretion), the pH will be driven down toward normal as predicted by the Henderson–Hasselbalch equation. **Causes** of increased ventilation: iatrogenic hyperventilation; anxiety; pain; hypoxemia; CNS lesion; pregnancy; hepatic insufficiency; hyperthyroidism; fever; gram–negative sepsis; mild pulmonary edema; pulmonary embolus; pneumonia; restrictive lung disease; drugs (e.g. salicylates, progestins, catecholamines).

Gastrointestinal Disease

Gastrointestinal Bleeding
Peptic Ulcer Disease
Hemorrhoids
Ulcerative Colitis
Crohn's Disease
Gastrointestinal Obstruction
Malabsorption
Microorganism-Mediated Diarrhea
Irritable Bowel Syndrome
Diverticulosis and Diverticulitis
Appendicitis
Gastroesophageal Reflux
Jaundice
Cirrhosis
Ascites
Alcoholic Liver Disease
Hepatitis A
Hepatitis B
Hepatitis C
Hepatic Abscess
Pancreatitis
Biliary Tract Disease
Pancreatic Cancer
Esophageal Cancer
Stomach Cancer
Colon Cancer
Rectal Cancer
Liver Tumors

Gastrointestinal Bleeding

ETIOLOGY: **Upper GI bleeding** is defined as bleeding from above the ligament of Treitz (a perintoneal fold at the duodenojejunal junction). It is most commonly due to duodenal ulcer, gastritis, gastric ulcer, varices, or Mallory-Weiss tear. Other causes include esophagitis, erosive duodenitis, ulcerated anastomosis, esophageal ulcer, hematobilia, Menetrier's disease. **Lower GI bleeding** (bleeding from below the ligament of Treitz) is most commonly due to hemorrhoids but this is seldom severe unless portal hypertension is present. The most common cause of massive lower GI bleeding is diverticulosis. Other causes of lower GI bleeding include infectious enterocolitis, anal fissure, inflammatory bowel disease, solitary colon ulcer, ischemic colitis, post–irradiation colitis, intussusception, Meckel's diverticulum, polyps. **Upper or lower GI bleeding:** neoplasia, hematologic disorders, angiodysplasia, vasculitis, AV malformation, aorto-enteric fistula, Osler-Weber-Rendu syndrome, CREST syndrome, blue rubber bleb disease, Ehlers-Danlos syndrome, pseudoxanthoma elasticum.

ESTABLISHING the CAUSE of GI BLEEDING:

Upper or lower GI bleeding? Bleeding stopped or ongoing? Severity of GI bleeding? : Hematemesis or blood in a nasogastric aspirate is consistent with upper GI bleeding. However, a negative gastric aspirate does not exclude upper GI bleeding distal to the pylorus because (1) upper GI bleeding may have stopped and blood has passed distally, (2) bleeding is slight and does not reflux into the stomach or (3) reflux is prevented by an abnormality of the pylorus (e.g. deformed pylorus consequent to peptic ulcer). Nevertheless, a gastric aspirate containing bile but not blood gives assurance that there is no ongoing UPPER GI bleeding. "Coffee grounds" emesis not tinged with fresh blood indicates that bleeding has stopped. Melena almost always indicates bleeding from above the ileocecal junction and is usually a sign of ≥ 500 ml blood loss. Hematochezia is usually associated with lower GI bleeding but massive upper GI bleeding (≥ 1000 ml) and/or a rapid transit time may have the same result.

History: recent episode of vomiting (Mallory-Weiss tear ?); history or symptoms suggesting peptic ulcer; alcoholism (varices or gastritis ?); heartburn (reflux esophagitis ?); altered bowel habits or stool diameter (colon cancer ?); aspirin or other nonsteroidal anti-inflammatory drug use (gastritis, ulcer ?); anticoagulant medication or bleeding disorder; epistaxis or hemoptysis; history of inflammatory bowel disease, hemorrhoids, GI surgery, or aorto-femoral bypass surgery.

Physical exam: evidence of liver disease ? : ascites, hepatomegaly, prominent abdominal collateral veins, palmar erythema, spider angioma); anorectal exam (external hemorrhoids ?; rectal masses ?; unusual mucocutaneous lesions ? : telangiectatic lesions of skin and mucous membranes (Osler-Weber-Rendu syndrome ?); cutaneous hemangiomas (blue rubber bleb disease ?); epidermal and sebaceous cysts (Gardner's syndrome ?); dark blue-black macules/papules (Kaposi's sarcoma ?); black-brown macules of lips, buccal mucosa, face, and/or hands (Peutz-Jeghers syndrome ?).

Diagnostic procedures for suspected upper GI bleeding: Endoscopy is the most accurate means of diagnosis but active bleeding may obscure the lesion. Arteriography is performed if bleeding continues and endoscopy fails to show the lesion. Arteriography also allows intra-arterial infusion of vasopressin. Upper GI series is not obtained while there is active bleeding as it will subsequently obscure both endoscopic and arteriographic visualization. Furthermore, it fails to reveal superficial lesions (e.g. gastritis, duodenitis, Mallory-Weiss tear), and although if may show a lesion, it cannot reveal whether that lesion is the source of the bleedng.

Diagnostic procedures for suspected lower GI bleeding: Anoscopy and proctosigmoidoscopy is performed. Arteriography of the superior and/or inferior mesenteric arteries is usually the next step if bleeding persists and the lesion has still not been identified. Time allowing, endoscopy may be performed prior to arteriography in order to rule out a postpyloric source of upper GI bleeding. Colonoscopy is sometimes attempted if bleeding has subsided. However, brisk bleeding makes colonoscopic visualization difficult. Barium enema is not obtained while there is active bleeding because it will interfere with subsequent arteriographic visualization. If bleeding stops, sigmoidoscopy is performed. If sigmoidoscopy is not diagnostic, the patient is observed for 48 hr. If bleeding does not recur, the bowel is cleansed and colonoscopy and/or barium enema are performed.

GENERAL TREATMENT GUIDE: ●Refer to "Hemorrhage" in the Trauma chapter for the treatment of shock. ●Type and crossmatch at least 3 units of blood. Obtain CBC, prothrombin time, partial prothrombin time, electrolytes, BUN, creatinine, glucose, arterial blood gas. ●Ice water lavage is begun if the nasogastric tube aspirate indicates active upper GI bleeding. A gastric aspirate containing "coffee grounds" untinged by red blood indicates bleeding has stopped.

SPECIFIC LESIONS & TREATMENT:

Peptic ulcer: see "Peptic Ulcer Disease" chapter.

Gastroesophageal varices are dilated collateral veins located submucosally in the lower esophagus and upper stomach that connect the portal and systemic veins. Varices develop as a consequence of portal hypertension, usually in the setting of alcoholic liver disease. The varices are fragile and prone to rupture. Ice water lavage is performed. Intravenous vasopressin infusion may be tried If bleeding persists in spite of ice water lavage. Sengstaken-Blakemore (SB) tube may inserted if the foregoing measures fail. The gastric balloon is inflated first (after verifying its position in the stomach with radiocontrast dye) and traction is applied. The esophageal balloon is inflated as well if bleeding persists. To preclude aspiration and/or airway obstruction, it is advisable to intubate prior to inserting an SB tube. The balloon(s) are deflated after 24 hr but remain in place for another 24 hr. Endoscopic sclerotherapy (injection of sclerosing agent into the varices) is yet another method used to control bleeding.

Mallory-Weiss tear is a tear in the gastric and/or esophageal mucosa. Often, there is a history of vomiting prior to the onset of hematemesis. Many patients are alcoholic. Bleeding usually stops spontaneously. If bleeding persists, endoscopic electrocoagulation or laser coagulation, intra-arterial infusion of vasopressin, or embolization with blood clot or gelfoam may be tried before resorting to surgery.

Gastritis-associated bleeding will usually stop spontaneously if the inciting agent is eliminated (e.g. alcohol, aspirin). Intra-arterial vasopressin infusion is tried if there is severe bleeding. Antacids and/or cimetidine may be useful in less severe cases. Surgery is the last resort because bleeding is often diffuse and therefore requires extensive gastric resection or gastrectomy.

Meckel's diverticulum (a congenital diverticulum of the ileum) is a rare cause of GI bleeding. Bleeding is intermittent. The lesion is often missed on barium x-ray. However, technetium scan may make detection possible because Meckel's diverticulum often contains ectopic gastric mucosa which takes up technetium-99m.

Diverticulosis: see "Diverticulosis".

Angiodysplasia (acquired lesion consisting of small dilated blood vessels, usually submucosal) may develop in the large or small bowel or stomach and is best visualized by endoscopy. Angiodysplasia is a frequent source of lower GI bleeding in the elderly (usually from the cecum or right colon). Upper GI bleeding is also possible. Bleeding may be intermittent or chronic and varies in severity. Endoscopic electrocoagulation or laser coagulation may be tried before resorting to surgery.

Ischemic colitis may be due to atherosclerosis, surgery, vasculitis, amyloidosis, colon cancer, or coagulation disorders. Signs/symptoms: Crampy abdominal pain of sudden onset, diarrhea (often bloody), and perhaps fever and/or vomiting are characteristic. Sometimes, symptoms have been intermittently present for weeks or months. There may be local or diffuse abdominal tenderness. Diagnosis: Sigmoidoscopy or colonoscopy sometimes reveals ulcers, blue-black submucosal blebs, or pseudomembrane. Symptoms often remit spontaneously allowing a barium enema study to be performed. There may be x-ray evidence of intramural edema and hemorrhage ("thumbprinting" and a narrowed irregular lumen). Mesenteric arteriography may show arterial occlusion. Treatment: Surgery is indicated if there are signs of bowel perforation or infarction, if symptoms persist, or if bowel stricture develops. The condition resolves spontaneously in many cases.

Bowel infarction may be the consequence of occlusion of the mesenteric ARTERIES by: an embolus, thrombosis (e.g. in the setting of atherosclerosis), aortic aneurysm, systemic vasculitis, or fibromuscular hyperplasia. Bowel infarction may also be the consequence of mesenteric VENOUS thrombosis. Bowel nfarction may result from low cardiac output. Signs/symptoms: Severe diffuse abdominal pain is characteristic. There may be GI bleeding, diarrhea, vomiting. Physical findings are often surprisingly unremarkable considering the severe abdominal pain. Peritoneal signs appear when transmural bowel necrosis develops. Diagnosis; Plain abdominal x-rays may show dilated bowel with air-fluid levels and thickening of the bowel wall. Angiography may demonstrate an occlusion. Treatment: surgery.

Intussusception (telescoping of one segment of bowel into another) is the most common cause of GI obstruction in patients < 2 years of age. The ileum is usually telescoped into the right colon but other large or small bowel sites of Intussusception are possible. Abdominal pain, vomiting, abdominal mass, and a "currant jelly" stool (blood mixed with mucus) are characteristic. Diagnosis is confirmed by barium enema. Barium enema will reduce the intussusception in over half the cases.

Hemorrhoids: see "Hemorrhoids" chapter.

Peptic Ulcer Disease
Over 75% of cases of symptomatic peptic ulcers are duodenal, and of those over 95% are at the duodenal bulb. Most gastric ulcers are found on the lesser curvature at the junction of the antrum and body. About 80% duodenal ulcer and about 60% gastric ulcer patients are male.

Symptoms/signs: Symptoms of ulcer disease are quite variable. Asymptomatic peptic ulcer disease is not uncommon. Most patients have epigastric pain. Pain is often severe but the character of the pain varies. Pain may or may not be relieved by food. In fact, in many cases food exacerbates the pain. In many patients, antacids do not relieve pain. Other nonspecific complaints variably present include anorexia, nausea, vomiting, bloating, belching. In the absence of a complication, physical exam is unremarkable, or in many cases there is epigastric tenderness.

Diagnosis is established by endoscopy or upper GI series, but the latter fails to reveal up to 20% ulcers. Special considerations in the case of a gastric ulcer: Because carcinoma-associated gastric ulcer is not uncommon, endoscopic biopsy and brush cytology is mandatory if x-ray identifies a gastric ulcer with malignant characteristics (e.g. ulcer entirely within gastric wall, ulcer within a gastric mass, nodular rather than smooth ulcer base, absence of rugae radiating from ulcer margin, large ulcer, absence of Hampton line). In those gastric ulcers that do not appear to be malignant, it is reasonable to forego immediate biopsy and start standard treatment. After 8–12 wk treatment an upper GI series is again obtained or endoscopy is performed to confirm gastric ulcer healing.

TREATMENT: General measures: Smoking (because it delays healing), alcohol (because it stimulates acid secretion and irritates the gastric mucosa), caffeine (because it stimulates acid secretion), aspirin and other nonsteroidal inflammatory agents (because they may cause gastric ulceration) are avoided. A special ulcer diet is not necessary.

Treatment of uncomplicated duodenal ulcer: The conventional treatment has been a magnesium-aluminum hydroxide antacid taken 7 times daily (15–30 ml 1 hr and 3 hr after meals and at bedtime). However, sucralfate or a H2-receptor antagonist (e.g. cimetidine [Tagamet], ranitidine [Zantac]) are as effective. Treatment with any of these options is continued for 4–6 weeks. Should a single agent fail to relieve symptoms after the recommended interval, the dose of a single agent may be increased or two drugs (e.g. antacid plus H2 antagonist) may be tried concurrently. If symptoms continue, endoscopy is performed to confirm the presence of an unhealed ulcer. If this is the case, surgery is considered after a fasting serum gastrin level is obtained to rule out Zollinger-Ellison syndrome. A popular surgical procedure is partial vagotomy (proximal gastric vagotomy). Partial vagotomy denervates the gastric parietal cells so that acid secretion is reduced, and yet leaves gastric motility and emptying unimpaired. The incidence of recurrent ulcers is about 10% with this procedure. Recurrence is only about 1% with the more drastic procedure: antrectomy with truncal vagotomy. However, the dumping syndrome, diarrhea, and weight loss are common consequences.

Treatment of gastric ulcer: Antacids or an H2 antagonist are equally effective. Treatment is continued for 8 wk. Because of the possibility that the gastric ulcer is secondary to gastric carcinoma, barium x-ray or endoscopy must be performed at the end of the treatment period in order to confirm healing. Endoscopic biopsy is obtained if healing has not occurred. If the biopsy is negative, medical therapy is continued for an additional 4–8 weeks: either increase the current medication or try 2 drugs concurrently (antacid plus H2-antagonist). Surgery is then performed if healing still has not occurred. Antrectomy without vagotomy is the usual surgical procedure in patients with benign gastric ulcer. Vagotomy, in most cases, is unnecessary since gastric ulcer is usually associated with low to normal gastric acid secretion.

COMPLICATIONS of PEPTIC ULCER:

Bleeding: Ulcers are the most frequent cause of upper GI bleeding. In about 20% patients, bleeding is the first indication that there is ulcer disease. The diagnostic approach to upper GI bleeding as well as general treatment measures for GI bleeding are discussed under "Gastrointestinal Bleeding". About 75% patients stop bleeding without surgery but 30-50% will eventually rebleed, sometimes years later. Patients who stop bleeding are usually managed with nasogastric suction, antacids, and H-2 antagonist (e.g. cimetidine, ranitidine). However, it is not certain that these measures prevent rebleeding. Bleeding is most likely to recur within 2 days after bleeding has stopped. Those with persistent or recurrent bleeding require surgery.

Obstruction: refer to "GI Obstruction" chapter.

Free perforation usually causes sudden onset of severe steady pain. At first, pain may be confined to the upper abdomen. Pain then spreads to involve the entire abdomen as diffuse peritonitis develops. With diffuse peritonitis, the abdomen is rigid and exquisitely tender and there is rebound tenderness. The abdomen becomes distended. Bowel sounds are usually decreased or absent. Nausea and vomiting are common. Other signs may include fever, leukocytosis, hemoconcentration (e.g. elevated hematocrit), hypotension, and eventually shock. The serum amylase is often elevated but the urinary amylase clearance is not (both are typically elevated in acute pancreatitis). Perforation is confirmed by finding free–air under the diaphragm on an upright x-ray. A left lateral decubitus film may also be used to detect free air. An upper GI series using water-soluble contrast is obtained if perforation is suspected but free–air is not seen on plain films. Treatment: surgery.

Penetration (ulcer perforation into a solid organ such as pancreas, liver, spleen). Posterior penetration of a duodenal ulcer is not uncommon; it is often associated with a change in ulcer pain (more persistent, radiates into the back, less consistently relieved by antacids or food). The serum amylase may be elevated If there is penetration into the pancreas but pancreatitis is unusual. Endoscopy or upper GI series may reveal the lesion. Medical treatment using the same drug regimen as for uncomplicated ulcer may be tried. Surgery is indicated if this fails.

Fistula is an infrequent complication of gastric or duodenal ulcer perforation. ●Duodenal ulcer fistula most commonly communicates with the common bile duct. Patient may be asymptomatic or develop cholangtitis. Diagnosis is made by finding (1) air in biliary tree on plain x-ray, or (2) barium in biliary tree on upper GI series. ●Gastrocolic or gastroduodenal fistulas are the most common types of fistula arising from gastric ulcer. Gastrocolic fistulas may cause diarrhea and malabsorption.

ZOLLINGER-ELLISON SYNDROME

is due to hypersecretion of gastric acid as a consequence of gastrin-secreting tumor(s). Z-E is more common in men. About a 4th of cases of Z-E are associated with multiple endocrine neoplasia type I (MEN I)–refer to endocrine section. **Suspect possibility of Z-E** if there is/are multiple ulcers or ulcers in uncommon locations (postduodenal bulb or jejunum), diarrhea, postoperative ulcer recurrence, failure of medical therapy, family history ulcers or presence of other endocrine disorders (? MEN I syndrome). **Diagnostic tests:** ●If Z-E is suspected, a fasting serum gastrin is obtained. If gastrin is elevated (i.e. > 200 pg/ml), then basal acid secretion is measured. A markedly elevated fasting serum gastrin (> 1000 pg/ml) with basal acid secretion > 15 mmole/hr is strong evidence for Z-E. With less pronounced elevations, Z-E is diagnosed by the secretin test (in Z-E the serum gastrin will rise by > 200 pg/ml within 2–10 minutes following IV injection of secretin 2 U/kg). ●CAT scan may locate tumor. ●Rarely, endoscopy reveals tumor at an unusual site (stomach or duodenum). **Treatment:** Surgery is performed to locate resectable pancreatic tumors. H-2 antagonist therapy (e.g. cimetidine, ranitidine) is employed if surgery fails to remove all gastrin-secreting tumor. Proximal vagotomy may also help reduce acid secretion if resectable tumor cannot be found.

Hemorrhoids (piles) are varicose dilations of the hemorrhoidal venous

plexus. They are the most common cause of rectal bleeding. <u>Internal hemorroids</u> are varicosities of the superior hemorrhoidal venous plexus located above the dentate line and are covered by mucosa. <u>External hemorroids</u> are varicosities of the inferior hemorrhoidal venous plexus located below the dentate line and are covered by skin. <u>Risk factors</u>: pregnancy, constipation, prolonged straining or standing, portal hypertension, or pelvic or abdominal tumors.

Signs/symptoms: <u>Bleeding</u>; bright red rectal bleeding. Bleeding is usually minor—ranging from small amounts noted on toilet tissue or coating stool to enough to discolor the toilet water. Chronic recurrent bleeding may cause anemia. <u>Pain and/or rectal urgency</u> are common complaints. <u>Mucoid discharge</u> may ensue from an internal hemorrhoid. <u>Anorectal exam</u>: External hemorrhoids can be seen on external exam. They may spontaneously resolve leaving a skin tag. Internal hemorrhoids, unlike external hemorrhoids, are not seen on external examination unless they are prolapsed. Furthermore, internal hemorrhoids are not felt on digital exam unless they are thrombosed or inflamed. An internal hemorrhoid is revealed as a protrusion as an anoscope is withdrawn.

Treatment may not be necessary in asymptomatic cases. <u>Conservative regimen</u> suffices in most patients: manual reduction if prolapsed, avoidance of straining, stools softeners (e.g. docusate), high-fiber diet and/or bulk-forming agents (e.g. Metamucil). <u>Excision</u> is considered f these measures fail or if symptoms are significant (e.g. severe pain, large protruding hemorrhoidal mass, severe bleeding). <u>Injection sclerosis</u> (for internal hemorrhoid only) or <u>rubber band ligation</u> are alternatives. <u>Treatment of thrombosed external hemorrhoid</u>: This condition will usually spontaneously resolve over a few days. Warm sitz baths, analgesics, and the conservative regimen outlined above are all that is normally required. However, the clot may be excised within the first 48 hours to relieve intolerable pain.

Ulcerative Colitis is an inflammatory disease of the colonic mu-

cosa and submucosa of unknown cause. Peak onset is in the 2nd–3rd decade. It is more common in females and in caucasians, particularly Jews. <u>Extent of disease varies</u>: The rectum is involved in almost all patients and in many cases the disease is restricted to the rectum (ulcerative proctitis). In 75% cases, disease does not extend beyond the left colon while the rest have pancolitis (entire bowel is affected). About 10% of patients with pancolitis have some ulceration of the distal ileum ("backwash ileitis") but aside from this finding, the remainder of the GI tract is not involved. The affected region of colon is continuously involved (i.e. there are no "skip" areas as is seen in Crohn's disease).

Signs/symptoms: diarrhea, bloody diarrhea in many cases, abdominal cramps, tenesmus, fever, weight loss. In severe cases there may be hypotension; shock may ensue. The presence of peritoneal signs (e.g. rebound tenderness) is an ominous indication that inflammation is no longer confined to the colonic mucosa/submucosa. A distended tender abdomen with diminished to absent bowel sounds is consistent with toxic megacolon.

DIAGNOSTIC PROCEDURES/TESTS: **Sigmoidoscopy** is a required diagnostic step. The mucosa is hyperemic, granular, friable (bleeds when touched with cotton swab), and edematous. The latter causes decreased visualization of the submucosal vascular pattern. In more serious cases, ulcers and pus are present. **Biopsy** is performed if the diagnosis is uncertain or may be used to exclude other causes of colitis (e.g. Crohn's disease, amebiasis, pseudomembranous colitis). One sees inflammatory cells in the lamina propria and microabscesses in the crypts of Lieberkuhn. Inflammation extends into the submucosa but the rest of the bowel wall is uninvolved except in fulminant cases. Biopsy may also identify dysplasia or carcinoma. **Colonoscopy** is indicated when the diagnosis is still uncertain after sigmoidoscopy and x-rays, but colonoscopy is discouraged during active disease for fear of causing hemorrhage or perforation. In patients with chronic disease, colonoscopy is useful for examining and obtaining biopsies of the proximal colon in order to detect carcinoma. **Laboratory:** At sigmoidoscopy, stool samples are obtained and examined for the presence of fecal leukocytes and amebae (E. histolytica). Cultures are sent for shigella, salmonella, and campylobacter. ●Anemia is common and is due to blood loss and/or chronic disease. There may be leukocytosis and an elevated sedimentation rate. Hypoalbuminemia may ensue from enteric protein loss. **X-ray evaluation:** Plain abdominal film may show diminished haustral markings. Severely ill patients are followed with serial plain abdominal x-rays in order to detect development of toxic megacolon. The diameter of midtransverse colon will exceed 6 cm if toxic megacolon develops. Upper GI series may be performed to exclude Crohn's disease but not until patient is in remission. Barium enema is obtained after remission is achieved in order to ascertain the extent of colon involvement and to detect other lesions (e.g. carcinoma). Findings may include shortened and narrowed colon, absent or diminished haustral markings, mucosal ulcers. Because of the risk of precipitating toxic megacolon, barium enema should not be performed while a patient is seriously ill. Furthermore, preparatory cathartics or enemas are contraindicated during any acute episode because they will exacerbate colitis.

TREATMENT:

Mild cases: Oral sulfasalazine alone may suffice. A corticosteroid is added if necessary (rectal suppository or enema if there is only rectal involvement, or PO if there is more extensive disease). As the disease remits, corticosteroids are tapered and discontinued, but sulfasalazine is continued because it reduces relapses. ●Low-residue diet and avoidance of milk products is also advised. Antidiarrhea agents (e.g. loperamide, diphenoxylate) may be used judiciously, but they are contraindicated in all but mild cases. ●Note: Mesalamine (Rowasa), also known as 5-aminosalicylic acid, is available as an enema. It is as effective as corticosteroid enemas for the treatment of mild to moderate proctitis/sigmoiditis. Mesalamine is the therapeutic hydrolytic component of sulfasalazine. The other component (sulfapyridine) often causes intolerable side effects. Therefore, mesalamine enemas are an alternative to sulfasalazine and/or corticosteroids in the treatment of mild to moderate distal ulcerative colitis.

Severe cases requiring hospitalization: NPO, IV fluids, IV corticosteroids (e.g. methylprednisolone 12 mg four times/day), IV antibiotics (e.g. ampicillin + gentamycin + metronidazole), and if necessary blood transfusion. Plain abdominal x-ray is ordered if development of toxic megacolon is suspected. If toxic megacolon does occur, physical exam is performed every few hours and an abdominal x-ray is obtained twice daily to assess the effects of medical therapy. If the patient with severe ulcerative colitis improves and stabilizes, clear fluids are allowed and subsequently advanced to a low-residue diet as tolerated. The patient is also started on sulfasalazine (continued chronically to reduce relapses) and prednisone 40 mg PO once daily. If the patient continues to improve, prednisone is tapered over a month's time to 20 mg/day; this dose is continued for 6–8 weeks and then gradually tapered before being discontinued. During the course of therapy, prednisone may be increased or restarted as clinical status dictates. In children, alternate day prednisone therapy is advised if possible in order to prevent growth retardation. Colectomy cures the disease. Severely affected patients still intractable after about a week of intensive medical therapy are candidates for colectomy. Emergency colectomy is necessary if toxic megacolon develops and is not relieved after 24–36 hours of intensive medical therapy. Colectomy is also mandated by perforation, massive bleeding, or colon carcinoma. Patients who despite medical therapy are chronically symptomatic or suffer frequent relapses are also surgical candidates.

COMPLICATIONS: Perforation may occur in severe cases, particulary if there is toxic megacolon. **Toxic megacolon** occurs when inflammation affects the muscular layer so that the colon dilates (diameter midtransverse colon $\geq$ 6 cm). Abdominal distension and tenderness with absent or decreased bowel sounds are characteristic. There may be fever, leukocytosis, hypokalemia, and evidence of dehydration. A surgery consult should be obtained in case intensive medical therapy fails or perforation occurs. **Risk of colon carcinoma** increases the longer ulcerative colitis has been present. Risk is also a function of the extent of disease. Patient with pancolitis has about 10% risk after 15 yr and about 40% risk after 25 yr. Adenomatous polyps are potentially malignant and must be excised. The presence of polyps should prompt thorough search to exclude colon carcinoma. **Other potential GI complications** include rectal prolapse, anal fissure, hemorrhoids, colon stricture, pararectal abscess. **Extraintestinal complications:** Both ulcerative colitis and Crohn's disease are often associated with extraintestinal complications—e.g. joints (peripheral arthritis, sacroiliitis, ankylosing spondylitis); hepatobiliary (fatty liver, hepatitis, cirrhosis, pericholangitis, sclerosing cholangitis, bile duct carcinoma, gallstones); renal (urate or calcium oxalate stones); ocular (conjunctivitis, iritis, episcleritis); skin (erythema nodosum, pyoderma gangrenosum); oral (aphthous stomatitis).

DIFFERENTIAL DIAGNOSIS includes Crohn's disease, amebiasis, shigellosis, salmonella, campylobacter, ischemic colitis, gonococcal proctitis, pseudomembranous colitis, histoplasmosis, lymphogranuloma venereum.

ULCERATIVE COLITIS AND CROHN'S DISEASE CONTRASTED: Except for "backwash ileitis", the only portion of the GI tract involved in ulcerative colitis is the colon. The affected region of colon is continuously involved (i.e. there are no "skip" areas as is seen in Crohn's disease). Ulcerative colitis also differs from Crohn's disease in that obstruction, fistulae, perianal disease, strictures are all uncommon. Furthermore, in contrast to ulcerative colitis, Crohn's disease affects the entire bowel wall from mucosa to serosa, and any portion of the GI tract (mouth to anus) may be involved. Rectal bleeding is less frequent and fulminant episodes are uncommon in Crohn's disease.

Crohn's Disease
is a chronic progressive disease that may involve any part of the GI tract. The ileum and/or colon are the most commonly involved regions. Over half the patients have disease affecting both the ileum and colon. In contrast to ulcerative colitis, there is transmural involvement of the bowel with thickening of the bowel wall. The mesentery is thickened as well and the mesenteric nodes are enlarged. Mesenteric fat is present on the serosa of affected bowel segments. Noncasseating granulomas may be present in the bowel wall and/or in mesenteric nodes. Adhesions and fistulas develop between adjacent bowel loops, and between bowel and other organs (e.g. stomach, bladder, gallbladder, vagina). The same process results in external fistulas that extend thru the perineal or abdominal skin.

Signs/symptoms: Diarrhea is a common complaint. Pain: Intermittent crampy abdominal pain aggravated by meals is characteristic. Patients with ileitis may develop pain and a mass in the right lower quadrant. Rectal bleeding occurs in about a third of those with colon involvement. Seldom is there severe hemorrhage like that seen with ulcerative colitis. Disease of the small bowel alone is usually not associated with hematochezia. Systemic signs (weight loss, fever) may be present. Anal fissure or pararectal abscess may occur. Fistulas may develop (e.g. perianal fistulas, fistulas thru the abdominal wall, or into the vagina). Signs/symptoms of GI obstruction may be present (see "GI Obstruction" chapter).

X-ray signs: Upper and lower GI series are obtained. Characteristic findings include: discontinuous involvement (diseased bowel separated by normal bowel called skip areas); thickened bowel wall; bowel narrowing and strictures (the narrow longitudinal barium outline of the bowel lumen at a stricture is referred to as the "string" sign); fistulas (e.g. from bowel to bowel, or from bowel to stomach, skin, bladder, gallbladder, or vagina); mucosal ulcers (transverse and longitudinal ulcers together result in a "cobblestone" pattern); absence of haustra.

Laboratory findings vary according to the severity and location of disease. With involvement of the ileum, the absorption of bile salts and B-12 is impaired; steatorrhea and macrocytic anemia are the respective consequences (refer to "Malabsorption" chapter). Anemia may be due to the combined effects of iron, B-12, and folate deficiency. Hypoalbuminemia is the consequence of malnutrition and/or enteric loss. Malabsorption may result in hypocalcemia and hypomagnesemia.

Treatment: There is no cure. A low residue diet may be helpful. Vitamin supplements are recommended. Patients with lactose intolerance benefit from avoidance of milk and milk products. Neither prednisone nor sulfasalazine appear to be effective prophylaxis against exacerbations. Exacerbations of Crohn's disease involving the colon are treated with sulfasalazine preferably. A corticosteroid (e.g. prednisone) is the alternative but the combination of prednisone plus sulfasalazine is no more effective than prednisone alone. Exacerbations of Crohn's disease confined to the small bowel are treated with a corticosteroid (e.g. prednisone 40-60 mg once daily initially). Metronidazole 10 mg/kg daily in divided doses may also be effective for controlling exacerbations of Crohn's disease. Surgery is indicated in cases of obstruction, perforation, fistulas between the bowel and extraintestinal organs, massive unmanageable hemorrhage, or toxic megacolon unresponsive to medical therapy. Unlike ulcerative colitis which is cured by colectomy, recurrence of Crohn's disease is almost inevitable despite surgery.

Extraintestinal complications are the same as ulcerative colitis (see above).

Differential diagnosis: ulcerative colitis, appendicitis, intestinal lymphoma, carcinoma, nongranulomatous jejunoileitis, eosinophilic gastroenteritis, intestinal tuberculosis, amebiasis, campylobacter, Yersinia enterocolitica.

Gastrointestinal Obstruction may be the consequence of impaired peristalsis (adynamic [paralytic] ileus) or mechanical obstruction.

ADYNAMIC (PARALYTIC) ILEUS: **Causes** include abdominal surgery/trauma; spinal trauma; peritonitis (e.g. from bacterial infection, from bile, from blood, or from pancreatic juices); severe electrolyte abnormalities (particularly hypokalemia); uremia; bowel infarction; sepsis; pneumonia; pancreatitis. **Signs/symptoms:** Bowel sounds are absent or infrequent. There is steady noncramping generalized abdominal pain. The abdomen is diffusely painful and tender, but not severely so unless there is associated peritonitis. **Plain x-rays** reveal uniform distension of both small and large bowel. **Postsurgical paralytic ileus** following intra-abdominal operations lasts from 12 to 24 hours with relatively minor surgery, and up to 4 days after major surgery.

GASTRIC OUTLET OBSTRUCTION: **Causes:** The most common cause is a duodenal ulcer. Edema, spasm, and scarring are the mechanisms by which an ulcer causes obstruction. Obstruction due to a gastric ulcer close to the pylorus is less common. Other causes of gastric outlet obstruction include antral carcinoma, gastric lymphoma, pancreatic carcinoma, pancreatitis, annular pancreas, hypertrophic pyloric stenosis, Crohn's disease, caustic ingestion–associated stricture, antral polyp, eosinophilic gastritis. The stomach may also fail to empty because of atony (e.g. diabetic gastroparesis) or vagotomy. **Signs/symptoms:** early satiety, epigastric fullness/pain, vomiting (especially vomiting of undigested food several hours after a meal), weight loss. Other findings may include: signs of dehydration, upper abdominal tenderness, succussion splash heard over the stomach. Peristalsis is sometimes seen on the abdomen of a slender patient. **Diagnosis:** Saline load test: Insert a nasogastric tube and empty the stomach. Infuse 750 ml of normal saline via the nasogastric tube and clamp the tube. The stomach is suctioned 30 minutes later. Removal of more than 300-400 ml is consistent with gastric obstruction. X-rays: Plain abdominal film may reveal a dilated stomach with an extensive fluid level. An upper GI series performed after the stomach is emptied confirms gastric retention (some barium should leave the stomach within 30 min and almost all by 4–6 hr). Endoscopy will also confirm the diagnosis and may help exclude gastric malignancy. **Laboratory:** Vomiting causes loss of electrolytes (HCl, Na, K) with ensuing development of hyponatremia and hypokalemic hypochloremic metabolic alkalosis. The kidneys in an attempt to correct the alkalosis compound the electrolyte losses. With dehydration comes hemoconcentration and prerenal azotemia (BUN : creatinine ratio > 10: 1). **Treatment:** Continuous nasogastric suction for a minimum of 48–72 hours can relieve edema and spasm. The saline load test may be repeated periodically to monitor possible improvement. IV cimetidine will reduce the loss of HCl. Intravenous fluids: Establish an IV line, and correct dehydration and electrolyte abnormalities. Subsequently administer the necessary maintenance requirements and replace any other ongoing losses (e.g. from nasogastric suction). Serum electrolytes must be monitored. A suitable starting IV solution might be D5 1/2 NS with 20-30mEq KCl added per liter. Make subsequent adjustments according to clinical and serum electrolyte status. Restart diet once the saline load test signals improvement. Begin with a liquid diet and advance to a regular diet if there is continued improvement. Surgery is advised if relief is not obtained after 3–7 days.

MECHANICAL SMALL BOWEL OBSTRUCTION **Causes:** The most common cause is adhesions followed by incarcerated external hernia (e.g. inguinal, femoral, umbilical). Other causes include internal hernia (i.e. bowel incarcerates in an internal anatomic defect); volvulus; neoplasm; gallstone (stone passes thru cholecystoenteric fistula to block small intestine); stricture (e.g. Crohn's disease); intussusception. **Signs/symptoms** vary according to the level of obstruction. High obstruction is associated with early and frequent vomiting, mild distension, and intermittent relatively mild crampy pain in epigastrium or midabdomen. With more distal obstruction there is more pronounced abdominal distension but less vomiting and the emesis is increasingly likely to be feculent. Mid to distal small bowel obstruction causes periumbilical or poorly localized intermittent crampy abdominal pain. Bowel movements: Constipation and absence of flatus are characteristic of complete bowel obstruction but a small amount of stool may be passed in the early stage of obstruction. Bowel movements, usually diarrhea, may continue if the obstruction is partial or intermittent. Bowel sounds are characteristically hyperactive, high-pitched, tinkling with gurgles and rushes. Peristalsis proximal to the obstruction is sometimes visible on the abdomen of thin patients. Dehydration, electrolyte and acid-base disturbances are due to the combined effect of (1) vomiting, (2) impaired GI absorption of water and electrolytes, (3) unreabsorbed digestive secretions. Eventually, if obstruction persists, there is leakage of plasma protein and water from the injured GI mucosa into the GI lumen. The accumulation of extracellular water in the GI lumen is an example of "third spacing". Dehydration manifests as thirst, dry mouth, decreased skin turgor, hypotension, and ultimately shock. Fever and peritoneal signs appear if there is perforation and/or strangulation. **Laboratory:** Hemoconcentration and leukocytosis is the consequence of dehydration. Electrolyte abnormalities vary according to the level of obstruction. For instance, more proximal obstruction is typically associated with more vomiting and this would tend to cause hypochloremia with alkalosis. **X-ray:** Plain films show dilated small bowel. Small bowel is identified by the valvulae conniventes which are seen as transverse lines that extend completely across the bowel lumen. This contrasts with the large bowel where the transverse haustral lines do not extend completely across the diameter of the colon. Dilated loops of small bowel are often seen in a stepladder arrangement. Upright or decubitus views may reveal air-fluid levels on uneven planes. These signs may be absent in early obstruction, closed loop obstruction, or if the obstructed bowel contains fluid but no gas. **Treatment:** nasogastric suction, IV fluids to correct dehydration and electrolyte deficits. Surgery if obstruction does not resolve. Antibiotics are started if there is evidence of peritonitis.

MECHANICAL COLON OBSTRUCTION **Causes:** The most common cause is colon carcinoma followed in order by diverticulitis and volvulus. Less common causes include inflammatory bowel disease, benign tumor, fecal impaction, intussusception (unusual in adults), adhesions (rare). **Signs/symptoms:** With complete obstruction there is obstipation (except that evacuation of the colon distal to the obstruction may occur at an early stage) and flatus is generally absent. With partial obstruction there may be frequent small stools. Pain: There is usually an insidious onset of intermittent crampy lower abdominal pain. Constant severe pain is consistent with strangulation or peritonitis. Abdominal exam: Abdomen is distended and tympanitic. Bowel sounds are typically hyperactive and high-pitched with gurgles and rushes. The presence of a tender mass suggests that there is strangulated closed loop. If rupture occurs, there may be local or diffuse peritoneal signs. Late in the course of colon obstruction in a patient with an INCOMPETENT ileocecal valve (10-20% cases): Since the valve allows reflux into the small intestine, there may be feculent vomiting as one might see with a distal small bowel obstruction. A COMPETENT ileocecal valve on the other hand results in a closed loop obstruction (i.e. occlusion both proximally and distally) with progressive distension of the colon proximal to the obstruction. This is because the ileum continues to discharge its contents into the cecum but the competent valve prevents reflux which would otherwise relieve pressure. The cecal wall is thinner and weaker than the rest of the colon, distends to greater extent, and is therefore the most likely segment of the colon to perforate. Obstruction at the ileocecal valve itself manifests as a distal small bowel obstruction. **X-rays:** Plain films show dilated colon (differentiated from small bowel by the presence of transverse haustral lines which do not completely cross the diameter of the colon). Barium enema confirms and clarifies the obstruction but, because of the risk of precipitating perforation, should not be performed if the cecal diameter is ≥ 10 cm or if there is clinical evidence of strangulation. PO barium studies are contraindicated as they may exacerbate a colon obstruction. **Treatment** is usually surgical. Intussusception is frequently reduced by a barium enema. A sigmoid volvulus is sometimes relieved by gently passing a soft tube into the obstructing segment with the aid of a sigmoidoscope.

STRANGULATION is most commonly due to hernia, volvulus, or intussusception. Strangulation causes vascular occlusion (first venous then arterial) with ensuing ischemia, gangrene, and ultimately perforation. **Diagnosis:** Strangulation is often difficult to diagnose; the signs and symptoms are often similar to an uncomplicated mechanical obstruction. Clues may include (1) presence of a tender mass or simply localized tenderness, (2) change in character of pain from a cramping intermittent pain to a severe constant pain, (3) hematemesis or rectal bleeding. Eventually peritonitis develops (absent bowel sounds, rebound tenderness, rigid abdomen, fever, leukocytosis more elevated than would be accounted for by hemoconcentration). **Treatment:** emergent surgery.

Malabsorption

Measurement of fecal fat (steatorrhea defined): Feces are collected for 72 hours while the patient is eating 75–100 gram fat/day. Normally, ≤ 6 gram fat should be collected/24 hour. Steatorrhea is present if > 6 gram fat/day is excreted. This is the single most important screening test for malabsorption because steatorrhea is present in almost all cases of malabsorption. Primary mucosal disorders (e.g. lactase deficiency, sucrase deficiency, congenital glucose-galactose malabsorption) are the exception to the rule that steatorrhea is a necessary feature of malabsorption. Sudan stain of a stool sample detects fat globules and so can also demonstrate steatorrhea This method is simpler and more convenient than the 72 hour collection method and will usually detect steatorrhea in patients excreting > 20 gram fat/day. However, milder steatorrhea may not be detected by the sudan stain method. Serum carotene may be low if there is impaired fat absorption, but this is an insensitive test since low dietary intake will cause low serum levels and certain diseases (hypothyroidism, hyperlipidemia, diabetes mellitus, anorexia nervosa) may be associated with high levels of serum carotene.

GI series is usually the next step if measurement of fecal fat reveals steatorrhea. GI series may identify an abnormality leading to bacterial overgrowth as the cause of malabsorption (e.g. blind loop, diverticula, fistula, stricture). Other x-ray findings (e.g. small intestine dilation, thickening of mucosal folds, scattering or fragmentation of barium) may be consistent with such disorders as celiac disease, Whipple's disease, Crohn's disease, eosinophilic gastroenteritis, amyloidosis.

D-xylose absorption test is performed if the GI series is normal or equivocal. Test presumes that there is normal renal function, absence of dehydration, and absence of gastric retention or vomiting. Urine is collected for the 5 hours following ingestion of 25 gram of d-xylose. Normally, > 5 gram is excreted in the urine over 5 hours. Explanation of test: D-xylose is absorbed in the small bowel (mainly the jejunum) by active mucosal cell transport. However, d-xylose is not metabolized quickly and therefore significant amounts are excreted in the urine if GI absorption is not impaired. The absorption of d-xylose is not dependent on normal pancreatic function. D-xylose absorption test is abnormal in following conditions: (1) diseases affecting the mucosa of the small intestine (e.g. adult celiac disease, tropical sprue, Whipple's disease, amyloidosis, eosinophilic gastroenteritis, intestinal ischemia, Crohn's disease); (2) extensive resection of the small bowel; (3) GI bacterial overgrowth (e.g. fistulas between segments of bowel, gastrectomy, partial obstruction, scleroderma).

Secretin test is the next test if GI series and d-xylose test are normal in a patient with documented steatorrhea. The test measures pancreatic exocrine function. A double lumen tube is inserted PO into the duodenum. A 20 minute aspirate is measured for volume and bicarbonate concentration. Secretin is administered IV and then several more 20 minute aspirates are measured. A normal response to secretin is the production in a 20 minute aspirate of a 2 ml/kg volume with a bicarbonate concentration of 85 mEq/liter.

Jejunal biopsy is indicated if the d–xylose test is abnormal. It is also indicated if a patient has documented steatorrhea but GI series, d–xylose, and secretin test are normal. Biopsy may help diagnose a variety of disorders (e.g. celiac disease, tropical sprue, Whipple's disease, lymphoma, amyloidosis, eosinophilic gastroenteritis, nongranulomatous ileojejunitis, abetalipoproteinemia, giardiasis).

Lactose tolerance test is usually an unnecessary test since lactose intolerance is suggested by history of diarrhea, abdominal cramps, and/or bloating following ingestion of milk. The serum glucose is measured serially after ingestion of 50–100 gram lactose (2 g/kg in child). Serum glucose should normally rise $\geq$ 20 mg/ml.

Bile acid breath test is used to detect bacterial overgrowth as a cause of malabsorption. Under normal conditions, bile salts are reabsorbed (mostly by the terminal ileum) and are resecreted in the bile (enterohepatic circulation). When there is bacterial overgrowth in the small intestine, anaerobic bacteria deconjugate bile salts releasing taurine and glycine. Radiolabeled 14C glycine-cholate is administered PO and the breath is measured for radiolabeled carbon dioxide over the next 4–8 hours. Normally, only traces of radiolabeled carbon dioxide are detected. However, increased levels are detected if there are bacteria in the small bowel to deconjugate radiolabeled bile salt (For in this case, radiolabeled glycine is absorbed and metabolized to 14C labeled carbon dioxide). Besides bacterial overgrowth, an abnormal result may also occur if the ileum is diseased or has been resected.

Schilling test: Vitamin B-12 is absorbed in the terminal ileum. Gastric parietal cells secrete a glycoprotein (intrinsic factor) which binds to B-12 and is necessary for ileal absorption of B-12. 1–2 mcg of radiolabeled vitamin B-12 is administered PO at the same time that 1000 mcg of unlabeled vitamin B-12 is given IM (the latter to saturate the body with B-12 and therefore enhance urinary excretion of B-12). The urine is collected over the next 24 hours. Normally > 7 % of the radiolabeled PO dose of B-12 is excreted in the urine. If the test is abnormal, pernicious anemia must be excluded by repeating the test with the addition of intrinsic factor. If the test is still abnormal, there is probably bacterial overgrowth or a diseased ileum.

EXAMPLES OF MALABSORPTION

PANCREATIC INSUFFICIENCY causes steatorrhea because the absence of lipase impairs the hydrolysis of triglycerides to fatty acids and beta-monoglycerides. Protein malabsorption occurs because of a deficiency of pancreatic proteases. Patients may develop deficiencies of fat soluble vitamins or B-12. Generally, the d–xylose test is normal but the secretin test is abnormal. Causes: The most common cause of pancreatic insufficiency is chronic pancreatitis. Other causes include pancreatic carcinoma, surgical resection pancreas, cystic fibrosis. Treatment: pancrelipase (see drug section) is prescribed. Cimetidine is recommended 1 hour before meals to reduce the acidity that would otherwise inactivate the exogenous enzymes.

Zollinger-Ellison syndrome may be associated with malabsorption because the large amount of acidic gastric fluid reaching the duodenum may overwhelm the alkaline secretions of the pancreas and inactivate them (pancreatic lipase is inactive in an acidic environment and bile salts precipitate).

BILE SALT ABNORMALITIES: Impaired bile secretion: cholestasis, biliary cirrhosis, biliary duct obstruction. **Resection or disease of the distal ileum**. Bile salts are normally reabsorbed in the distal ileum and resecreted in the bile (enterohepatic circulation). If bile salts are not reabsorbed, the amount available for secretion is depleted because the liver cannot synthesize sufficient bile salts to keep up with amount lost in the feces. Treatment of bile acid deficiency–associated malabsorption: Short of correcting the underlying condition, the patient may benefit from a diet which includes medium-chain triglycerides (they are absorbed without the aid of bile salts). Vitamin A, D, K, and calcium supplementation is advised if there is chronic cholestasis. **Bacterial overgrowth:** Anaerobic bacteria deconjugate bile salts yielding glycine or taurine and free bile acids. Fat absorption is impaired because the unconjugated bile acids are incapable of forming micelles with free fatty acids and beta-monoglycerides. Vitamin B-12 deficiency develops because the bacteria ultilize this vitamin. Conditions causing bacterial overgrowth include surgical blind loop, multiple jejunal diverticuli, fistulas, stasis (e.g. scleroderma), obstruction. Treatment of bacterial overgrowth—associated malabsorption: chronic or intermittent antibiotic therapy (e.g. ampicillin, tetracycline).

SPECIFIC MUCOSAL CELL DEFICIENCIES: Lactose intolerance is due to a deficiency of lactase in the microvilli of the mucosa of the small intestine. Causes: Congenital lactase deficiency is rare. The most common form of lactase deficiency develops for unknown reasons later in life (infancy to adulthood). Blacks are most commonly affected followed by orientals and then whites. Lactose intolerance may also be due to mucosal disease (see below); intestinal infection (e.g. infectious gastroenteritis, giardiasis); or extensive small bowel resection. Diagnosis: Diarrhea ensues soon after an affected person ingests milk or milk products because water is retained in the bowel lumen as a consequence of the osmotic effect exerted by the undigested lactose. Bloating, abdominal cramps, flatulence may also be present. Steatorrhea is not present. Lactose tolerance test is usually unnecessary since the diagnosis of lactose intolerance can usually be made by the history and the response to milk avoidance. Treatment of the nonpathologic form of lactose intolerance: none except avoidance of milk or milk products. **Sucrase** deficiency and congenital glucose-galactose malabsorption are rare deficits of sugar absorption. **Amino acid absorption** deficits are rare: e.g. cystinuria (impaired absorption of cystine, lysine, arginine, ornithine); Hartnup disease (impaired absorption of neutral amino acids—tryptophan, phenylalanine, leucine, etc). **Imerslund's syndrome** is a rare abnormality of the ileal mucosa resulting in impaired vitamin B-12 absorption.

NONINFECTIOUS MUCOSAL DISEASE: Celiac disease (nontropical sprue) is due to injury to the small intestinal mucosa by gluten (a protein found in wheat and other cereal grains). There may be a familial predisposition; an association with histoincompatibility antigens HLA-DW3 and HLA-B8 is common. Symptoms (e.g. diarrhea, abdominal discomfort) usually begin at 6–18 months of age after wheat products are introduced into the diet. Often, there is a clinical remission in older children. Clinical expression may resurface as an adult. Tests: Steatorrhea is present. D-xylose test is abnormal. Vitamin B-12 absorption is sometimes impaired. Upper GI series frequently shows nonspecific abnormalities. Jejunal biopsy reveals villous atrophy. Treatment: avoid gluten (i.e. avoid all cereal grains except rice and corn). **Eosinophilic gastroenteritis** is sometimes an allergic response to certain foods (e.g. milk, fish, meat). Patients often have a history of allergic disorders (asthma, hay fever, eczema). There is blood eosinophilia and eosinophils are also seen in the small intestinal mucosa. There may be steatorrhea, diarrhea, abdominal cramps, vomiting, GI bleeding, and/or fever. Protein-losing enteropathy may ensue and possibly lead to hypoproteinemia with edema and ascites. Treatment: avoid foods that might be responsible. Some patients require prednisone therapy. **Other mucosal diseases:** amyloidosis; nongranulomatous ileojejunitis; Crohn's disease (see "Inflammatory Bowel Disease"); intestinal ischemia (e.g. from atherosclerosis, lupus, periarteritis nodosa, Henoch-Schönlein purpura, Behçét's disease, Degos' disease).

INFECTION: Tropical sprue is a disease endemic to the tropics that is associated with bacterial overgrowth in the small intestinal. It does not occur in temperate climates unless a patient has previously lived in the tropics. Diarrhea, weight loss, megaloblastic anemia, steatorrhea, abnormal d-xylose test are characteristic findings. Jejunal biopsy reveals villous atrophy similar to celiac disease. Treatment: tetracycline, balanced diet, oral vitamin supplements, and (at first) monthly intramuscular vitamin B-12 injections. **Whipple's disease** is a very rare disease occurring mostly in males over 40. Characteristic manifestations are arthritis, lymphadenopathy, diarrhea, weight loss, steatorrhea, abnormal d-xylose test, anemia, elevated sedimentation rate. Diagnosis is confirmed by performing jejunal biopsy to reveal PAS positive macrophages in the lamina propria. An infectious cause is likely because bacilli can be seen on electron microscopy of biopsy specimen, and the disease responds to antibiotics. However, the organism has not been isolated. Treatment: oral antibiotics indefinitely (penicillin, ampicillin, or tetracycline). **Giardiasis** in most instances is asymptomatic, but it not uncommonly causes diarrhea with malabsorption (Giardiasis is discussed in more detail elsewhere in this volume). **Viral or bacterial gastroenteritis** may temporarily cause malabsorption. **Worm infestations** (e.g. tapeworm, hookworm, strongyloid) may impair GI absorption.

INTESTINAL LYMPHATIC OBSTRUCTION: lymphoma, tuberculosis, primary intestinal lymphangiectasia, retroperitoneal fibrosis, metastasis to mesenteric nodes or intestinal lymphatics.

OTHER POSSIBLE CAUSES OF MALABSORPTION: gastrectomy, ileal resection, radiation injury, hypoparathyroidism, hypogammaglobulinemia, carcinoid.

Microorganism-Mediated Diarrhea

Bacteria, viruses, or protozoa may cause diarrhea. The mechanism by which diarrhea is induced varies—e.g. some bacteria produce an enterotoxin, others invade the intestinal mucosa.

Narrowing the diagnosis: History may be helpful–e.g. recent travel, antibiotic therapy, family or other contacts with similar complaints, ingestion of undercooked foods. Watery stools are most likely with viral gastroenteritis, enterotoxin-producing bacteria, or Giardia. Blood and/or mucus is commonly associated with invasive bacteria or amebae. Fecal leukocytes on microscopic exam of methylene blue stain of specimen suggests infection by invasive bacteria (e.g. salmonellae, shigella).

Fluid therapy: Patients who are not seriously ill and who are not significantly dehydrated may be treated with oral fluids. A suitable solution for oral ingestion is prepared as follows: to each liter of water add 2.5 gram NaCl, 2.5 gram NaHCO3, 1.5 gram KCl, and 20 gram glucose. In an adult, a quarter of a liter of fluid may be ingested every 15 minutes initially. The patient according to his thirst will usually judge the amount required. Severely dehydrated patients or those unable to drink are initially treated with intravenous Ringer's lactate; 100 ml/kg if patient is in shock and 50–80 ml/kg in less severe cases. Half of this amount is infused as quickly as possible and the remainder over 2–4 hours. Another approach is to rapidly administer intravenous Ringer's lactate until a normal pulse pressure (40 mm Hg) or a strong radial pulse is obtained, and then reduce the rate of infusion and guide further fluid administration according to vital signs, urine output, neck veins, skin turgor. With either approach, potassium chloride is added to the IV bottle after the initial rapid infusion of Ringer's lactate. KCl infusion should not exceed 10 mEq/hr and the concentration of KCl in the solution should not exceed 40 mEq/liter. The total KCl administered should be about 15 mEq for each liter of Ringer's lactate administered. The patient is switched to oral fluids as soon as is feasible.

VIRAL GASTROENTERITIS: Viruses are a very common cause of acute watery diarrhea—e.g. rotavirus, Norwalk agent, adenovirus, coronavirus, parvovirus. Rotavirus is particularly common in children and is in fact the most frequent cause of infant diarrhea in winter. Suspicion of a viral etiology is enhanced when families or other closely associated groups present with the same symptoms. Watery diarrhea is induced upon viral invasion of the epithelial cells of the GI mucosa. Signs/symptoms: Watery diarrhea is often accompanied by fever, nausea, vomiting, abdominal cramping, headache, myalgias, and/or malaise. The latter three are suggestive of a virally-induced diarrhea. Symptoms usually resolve after 1–2 days, although diarrhea may sometimes persist for a few days after the other symptoms have disappeared. Fecal leukocytes are not a characteristic finding in viral gastroenteritis.

ENTEROTOXIN-PRODUCING BACTERIA:

Staphylococcus aureus food poisoning is due to a heat-stable enterotoxin that is produced when the bacteria grow in sundry foods. The enterotoxin is thus ingested preformed and bacterial colonization of the intestine does not occur. Signs/symptoms: Vomiting, watery diarrhea, and abdominal cramps begin 2–6 hours following ingestion, subside within 12 hours with recovery usually within 24 hours. Fever is absent. Laboratory: In many cases it is not possible to recover S. aureus from the stool. Fecal leukocytes are not present.

Bacillus cereus food poisoning, like staph food poisoning, is due to ingestion of a preformed enterotoxin produced when the bacteria grow in contaminated food. Depending on which of 2 types of enterotoxin is produced, one of two syndromes is possible—one is like that produced by S. aureus enterotoxin, the other like that of C. perfringens. Illness resolves within 24 hours.

Clostridium perfringens food poisoning. Undercooked food (e.g. meat, poultry) allows heat-resistant clostridial spores to survive and subsequently germinate. In the small intestine, the ingested bacteria produce an enterotoxin. Signs/symptoms: Watery diarrhea and cramping begins 8–14 hours following ingestion. Fever, nausea, or vomiting is less common. Illness resolves spontaneously within 2–4 hours of onset. <u>Laboratory:</u> Anaerobic stool culture may recover the bacteria. Fecal leukocytes are not present.

Vibrio cholerae is spread via water contaminated by human feces. In the U.S., sporadic outbreaks of cholera occur along the Gulf of Mexico. The ingested bacteria multiply in the small bowel elaborating an enterotoxin that acts on the intestinal mucosa to induce a watery diarrhea. The bacteria do not invade the mucosa. Consequently, there is no blood or mucus, and fecal leukocytes are not present. Infection may be asymptomatic, or cause mild to severe diarrhea. Diarrhea may be profuse and, without adequate fluid replacement, lead to hypovolemic shock. Treatment: fluid therapy and tetracycline 500 mg (10 mg/kg) PO every 6 hours for 48 hours.

Toxigenic E. coli is a frequent cause of travelers' diarrhea. Like cholera, the ingested bacteria multiply in the small intestine where they elaborate an enterotoxin that acts on the intestinal mucosa to induce a watery diarrhea devoid of gross blood, mucus, or fecal leukocytes. This presentation contrasts with invasive E. coli (see below). <u>Prophylaxis:</u> doxycycline 100 mg PO once daily.

Clostridium difficile causes pseudomembranous colitis, an illness that results from clostridial overgrowth in the colon. In nearly all cases, the patient has been treated with an antibiotic (e.g. clindamycin, lincomycin, ampicillin, cephalosporin). C. difficile elaborates an enterotoxin which injures the colonic mucosa. <u>Signs/symptoms:</u> Watery diarrhea sometimes with mucus and/or blood, abdominal cramps, fever, and leukocytosis are characteristic. The symptoms usually begin 4–9 days after starting an antibiotic but the syndrome may sometimes be delayed as long as 2–10 weeks after completing antibiotic therapy. <u>Diagnosis:</u> Sigmoidoscopy discloses plaques (pseudomembrane) on the mucosal surface consisting of fibrin, inflammatory cells, and epithelial debris. Diagnosis is confirmed by demonstrating C. difficile toxin, usually by immunologic methods. <u>Treatment:</u> Diarrhea usually resolves upon discontinuing the antibiotic. Oral vancomycin is administered If diarrhea does not stop, or if the syndrome begins after antibiotic therapy is completed.

INVASIVE BACTERIA:

Shigella is most often spread person-to-person via fecal-oral route. Fecally-contaminated food or water is another source of infection. <u>Signs/symptoms:</u> Incubation is 2–4 days. Bacteria first multiply in distal jejunum, ileum, and colon to initially produce a watery diarrhea. The bacteria then invade and multiply within the colonic mucosal cells. The resulting inflammation (which is confined to the mucosal layer) is associated with large numbers of neutrophils which, along with numerous erythrocytes, are found in the stool. In the more severely affected patient, the diarrheal stool contains mucus and is grossly bloody. Abdominal cramps and tenesmus are common complaints. Fever, myalgias, and/or vomiting are occasionally present. <u>Laboratory:</u> Microscopic exam (e.g. methylene blue stain) reveals neutrophils and erythrocytes. Stool culture confirms the diagnosis. <u>Treatment:</u> The illness is usually self-limited, lasting 3–8 days. However, a 5 day course of oral ampicillin or trimethoprim-sulfamethoxazole is advocated to speed recovery and to curtail fecal excretion of shigellae.

Invasive E. coli cause a syndrome similar to shigella.

Campylobacter jejuni infection is spread via the feces of man or animal. Contaminated dairy products are a common source of infection. The organism multiplies in both the small and large bowel where it invades the mucosa and often provokes a syndrome similar to shigellosis. <u>Treatment:</u> fluid therapy. Erythromycin 250 mg PO qid for 5 days is sometimes advocated to eradicate bacteria from stool and prevent relapse but the effect on the illness is uncertain.

Vibrio parahaemolyticus is transmitted via contaminated undercooked shrimp or shellfish. Incubation is 12–36 hours. Bacteria invade the intestinal mucosa provoking an inflammatory response so that neutrophils along with erythrocytes may be found in the stool. There is watery diarrhea (sometimes grossly bloody) often with vomiting and abdominal cramping. Fever is sometimes present. Illness resolves spontaneously within 3 days.

Yersinia enterocolitica is spread by the feces of man or animals via fecally contaminated food or water. The organism invades the intesinal mucosa (small intestine mainly), and secondarily the mesenteric lymph nodes to cause mesenteric lymphadenitis. There is diarrhea and it may be bloody. Typically, there is abdominal pain and fever. In some cases there is right lower quadrant pain and the syndrome is mistaken for appendicitis. Illness usually resolves spontaneously.

Nontyphoidal salmonella infection. Salmonellae may be found in the feces of infected man or animals. The most common source of infection in man is contaminated food (e.g. eggs, poultry, meat, milk products) and sometimes fecally contaminated water. Gastrectomized patients and sickle cell patients are particularly susceptible to salmonella infection. Signs/symptoms/laboratory: Incubation is 12–72 hours and the illness lasts 2–7 days. The organisms invade the mucosa of the ileum and colon. There is diarrhea (usually watery), abdominal cramps, nausea, and sometimes vomiting. Fever (usually without leukocytosis) is common. The stools contain leukocytes, but mucus and blood (except for trace amounts) are rarely present. Diagnosis is confirmed by stool culture. Treatment: Antibiotics are not indicated in uncomplicated gastroenteritis because they may prolong the carrier state. However, antibiotic is recommended for very sick patients, infants, and the elderly or otherwise debilitated patients. Treatment is with oral ampicillin for 3–5 days. Alternatives are trimethoprim-sulfamethoxazole or chloramphenicol for 3–5 days. Complications: Salmonella bacteremia sometimes occurs amd may be associated with a focal infections (e.g. bones, joints, GU, CNS, lungs, cardiac valves). Some species of salmonella besides S. typhi can cause a prolonged febrile bacteremic illness similar to typhoid fever and require antibiotic therapy.

Typhoid fever is due to S. typhi. Carriers (usually asymptomatic carriers) spread the organism by fecally contaminating food or water. Carriers often have preexisting gallbladder disease. Signs/symptoms: Incubation is 3–25 days and the illness typically lasts about a month. Patient gradually develops fever, malaise, anorexia, constipation, abdominal pain/distension, headache, body ache, sore throat. Other signs that my develop in the course of the illness include diarrhea, diagnostic "rose spots" on chest and abdomen, relative bradycardia considering the fever, leukopenia, splenomegaly, delirium. Potential complications include intestinal hemorrhage or perforation, pneumonia, acute cholecystitis, pyelonephritis. Diagnosis is confirmed by positive stool, urine, or blood culture, and the Widal test. Treatment is with ampicillin or chloramphenicol for at least 14 days.

Staphylococcal enterocolitis is a rare, often fatal condition. It usually occurs in aged debilitated patients. It is due to the intestinal overgrowth of staphylococcus and antibiotic therapy is frequently responsible. Signs/symptoms: Typically, there is a sudden onset of severe and often bloody diarrhea with abdominal pain/distension, ileus, and fever. Dehydration and shock ensue. Laboratory: Many neutrophils are found in the stool and gram-positive cocci are seen on gram stain. Treatment: oral vancomycin.

PROTOZOA:

Giardia lamblia is a protozoan spread: (1) by water contaminated by feces of man or animal (e.g. dogs), or (2) directly from person-to-person. Cysts are ingested and excyst in the stomach. The trophozoite form subsequently proliferates in the small bowel where it may adhere to the mucosa of the small bowel to induce a watery diarrhea. Diarrhea may be accompanied by fever, abdominal cramping/distention, flatulence. Chronic diarrhea with malabsorption may develop. Many infections are asymptomatic. Diagnosis is established by finding trophozoites or cysts in the stool, or trophozoites in a duodenal sample (string test or biopsy). Neither blood nor neutrophils are present in the stool. Treatment: metronidazole. A clinical trial of metronidazole is justified if the diagnosis is suspected but not proven.

Entamoeba histolytica (amebiasis) is a protozoan that is spread by ingestion of cysts in fecally contaminated food or water, or by direct contact (e.g. unwashed hands, sexual activity). Trophozoites multiply in the colon. Signs/symptoms: Most infections are asymptomatic. Symptoms develop when the mucosa is invaded: diarrhea, constipation, abdominal cramping, flatulence. The stools may contain mucus and blood. Complications: Sometimes the amebae are carried via the portal circulation to the liver and a liver abscess develops (see "Liver Abscess"). Other organs may be infected—e.g. lungs, brain. Laboratory: Indirect hemagglutination assay is usually positive in active cases. However, elevated titers may persist long after infection has resolved. Serologic tests are usually negative in asymptomatic carriers. Finding trophozoites or cysts in the stool may be difficult. Specimens are placed in preservatives if exam cannot be performed promptly. Treatment: metronidazole.

Irritable Bowel Syndrome (functional bowel syndrome)

is a diagnosis of exclusion—i.e. the patient has GI symptoms but workup fails to identify an organic lesion. Typically there is abdominal pain that in many cases is associated with meals. There may be constipation and/or diarrhea. Bloating, excessive flatus, belching are also common. The disorder often seems to be related to stress or emotional problems. **Diagnosis** is made by excluding other possibilities. To do this the following studies are obtained: barium enema, proctosigmoidoscopy, stool test for occult blood, stool exam for ova and parasites, serologic test for amebiasis. Also a sample of jejunal contents (obtained by passing a string or by aspiration) may be examined for giardia. Routine blood tests are also obtained. **Treatment:** Laxatives are avoided. A high fiber diet (e.g. bran) and/or psyllium (e.g. Metamucil) is recommended for constipation. An anticholinergic (e.g. propantheline—refer to drug section) may relieve spasm. Loperamide or diphenoxylate may be prescribed if diarrhea is a significant problem.

Diverticulosis and Diverticulitis

A **diverticulum** of the colon is a herniation of the colonic mucosa thru the muscular layer. The outpocketing therefore consists of mucosa and serosa. The presence of diverticula in the absence of inflammation is called **diverticulosis**. **Diverticulitis** is said to be present when a diverticulum perforates and a small localized abscess forms.

DIVERTICULOSIS is most prevalent in Western society and is attributed to the increased intraluminal pressure that results from a diet low in fiber. Most diverticula form where a blood vessel penetrates the muscular layer (a weak point in the bowel wall). About 95% patients with diverticula will have them in the sigmoid colon and 50% will have them only in the sigmoid. Diverticula are progressively less prevalent in the more proximal segments of the colon. Diverticulosis incidence increases with age and is uncommon in those under 40. In the US, 10% of persons over 40 will have diverticulosis with a prevalence of 40% by age 70. **Signs/symptoms:** Diverticulosis is usually asymptomatic. There may be left lower quadrant pain/tenderness, constipation, and/or diarrhea. These manifestations are probably not due to the diverticula per se but instead represent spasm of the colon. ●Fever and leukocytosis are <u>not</u> present. ●GI bleeding may occur and may be massive. **Treatment diverticulosis:** Uncomplicated diverticulosis is treated with a high residue diet (e.g. bran, fruits, vegetables, whole grains). ●Bleeding secondary to diverticulosis usually subsides spontaneously. Intra-arterial vasopressin infusion may stop the bleeding. Surgery is indicated for massive bleeding.

DIVERTICULITIS: Diagnosis: <u>Fever with leukocytosis</u> is present. The temperature is usually < 39° C in uncomplicated cases. <u>Pain/tenderness</u> is usually left lower quadrant (as would be expected since most diverticula are of the sigmoid) but sometimes the pain is suprapubic, right lower quadrant, or bilateral lower quadrant. There may be signs of peritoneal irritation—e.g. local rebound tenderness. <u>A Mass</u> is sometimes felt in the left lower quadrant. <u>With frank perforation,</u> characteristic findings include generalized rebound tenderness, absent bowel sounds, high fever, abdominal distension/rigidity. <u>Rectal exam:</u> Occult blood is commonly detected on rectal exam. However, gross blood is uncommon and hemorrhage is rare. Rectal exam may also reveal a tender mass if an abscess has formed. <u>Frequent loose bowel movements or constipation</u> is common. Nausea and/or vomiting may occur. <u>Possible urinary tract manifestations:</u> Dysuria may occur if the inflammatory process involves the bladder. A few WBC and RBC in the urine is consistent with irritation of the urinary tract. However, many WBC and RBC in the urine suggests more significant involvement. Sometimes a fistula to the bladder develops, and so fecaluria and pneumaturia ensue. <u>Plain flat and upright x-rays</u> are obtained. Free-air under the diaphragm indicates free perforation of a diverticulum. Dilated bowel and/or airfluid levels are signs of obstruction/ileus. Plain x-ray may also detect an abscess. <u>Barium enema</u> is not advised early in the course of diverticulitis but may be attempted when the attack has abated. Barium enema will show the presence of diverticulosis and possibly reveal an abscess, obstruction, or a fistula (e.g. in communication with bladder, ureter, small bowel, cecum, vagina, or uterus). <u>Ultrasound</u> may detect an abscess or show thickening of the involved bowel wall. <u>Sigmoidoscopy</u> is performed to help rule out other lesions. However, the sigmoidoscope often cannot be advanced past the rectosigmoid junction because of spasm, angulation, and fixation at that point. **Differential diagnosis:** appendicitis, Crohn's disease, ulcerative colitis, ischemic colitis, colon carcinoma, retroperitoneal tumor, ovarian tumor, pelvic inflammatory disease, endometriosis, **Treatment diverticulitis:** NPO, nasogastric suction, IV fluid, broad spectrum antibiotics (e.g. ampicillin). Combination antibiotic coverage (e.g. aminoglycoside + clindamycin) is advised if there is a high fever or if there is a complication. Surgery is indicated if the patient fails to improve or if there is a complication (i.e. large abscess, generalized peritonitis, free perforation, GI obstruction, fistula).

Appendicitis
in about two thirds cases follows obstruction of the lumen of the appendix (e.g. by fecalith, fibrous bands, tumor, parasites, foreign body, lymphoid hyperplasia) while no evidence of obstruction is found in the remainder. Whatever the inciting mechanism, there is bacterial infection with inflammation that leads to edema which in turn compresses the blood supply to the appendix. The ensuing ischemia may result in gangrene with perforation.

Signs/symptoms: Appendicitis may present in a variety of ways. This is in part due to the fact that the appendix may occupy any one of several anatomic positions. <u>Usual position</u> (adjacent to the right anterior pelvic wall): At first there is steady discomfort/pain and cramping in the midepigastrium or periumbilical area due to distension or spasm of the appendix. Anorexia, nausea, and sometimes vomiting follow. Mild fever (<102) is common. There may be constipation and the patient may have tried laxatives but without relief. After a number of hours the pain shifts to the right lower quadrant as the inflamed appendix begins to irritate the overlying parietal peritoneum. The pain in this area will be aggravated by walking. Typically, there is localized tenderness at McBurney's point (1/3 distance from anterior superior iliac spine to umbilicus) and often there is rebound tenderness referred to the same region. Bowel sounds are normal or slightly diminished. <u>Retrocecal position:</u> The initial manifestations may be the same as above; however, the pain does not usually shift to the right lower quadrant because the inflamed appendix is not lying against the anterior abdominal wall. Consequently, there may be little or no tenderness in the right lower quadrant. However, the psoas muscle may be irritated and cause (1) the patient to keep his right hip flexed and (2) a positive psoas sign—pain with hyperextension of the right hip. An inflamed appendix adjacent to an ureter may cause dysuria with pain radiating to the groin and perhaps hematuria. <u>Pelvic position:</u> In this case also, there is typically no shift in pain/tenderness to the right lower quadrant. Nausea, vomiting, and diarrhea may be more pronounced so that the patient is thought to have gastroenteritis. Diarrhea may be the consequence of irritation of the sigmoid colon by the inflamed appendix. Tenderness is sometimes noted on the right side on rectal or vaginal exam. The obturator sign may be present (internal and external rotation of the thigh with the thigh flexed at 90° elicits pain). <u>Other possibilities:</u> (1) congenital malrotation may find the cecum and appendix on the left side, (2) cecum and appendix may be in the right upper quadrant, (3) pregnancy also pushes the cecum and appendix toward the right upper quadrant, (4) an unusually long appendix may result in any number of clinical manifestations.

Laboratory: <u>Leukocytosis with a left shift</u> is typical. However, about 10% patients do not have leukocytosis. <u>Urinalysis</u> is usually normal or there may be a few WBC and RBC. <u>Plain x-rays:</u> Chest x-ray, and flat and upright abdominal x-rays are obtained. Possible findings include an appendolith, obscured right psoas margin, mass right lower quadrant, sentinel loop (single dilated loop of small bowel containing air–fluid levels on about the same plane), isolated dilated cecum. Free–air indicates that perforation has occurrred. Both large and small bowel will be distended should generalized peritonitis develop. <u>Barium enema:</u> In the absence of complications (e.g. evidence of perforated viscus, peritonitis), a barium enema may be obtained if the diagnosis is in doubt. Appendicitis is unlikely if the appendix fills normally with barium. However, an unfilled appendix does not prove appendicitis.

Differential diagnosis includes gastroenteritis, cholecystitis, pancreatitis, peptic ulcer, mesenteric adenitis, Crohn's disease, ureteral colic, pyelonephritis, ectopic pregnancy, pelvic inflammatory disease, ruptured ovarian follicle, twisted ovarian cyst, adnexal torsion.

Perforation and its consequences: ●Perforation may lead to a localized abscess if the omentum and/or adjacent organs contain the infection. A mass is sometimes felt in the right lower quadrant. ●Free perforation results in generalized peritonitis (distended and rigid abdomen, diffuse rebound tenderness, vomiting, ileus) and septic shock may ensue.

Gastroesophageal Reflux (GER) is the consequence

of diminished tone and/or abnormal relaxation of the lower esophageal sphincter. Reflux esophagitis is said to be present when the reflux of gastric contents irritates/injures the esophageal mucosa and/or provokes symptoms characteristic of GER.

Symptoms: Heartburn (epigastric and retrosternal burning sensation) frequently occurs after eating. Heartburn is typically provoked or aggravated by lying down or bending forward, and is often relieved by standing or antacids. Aspiration: Regurgitation of gastric contents into the mouth may occur, especially when the patient is recumbent. Sometimes gastric contents enter the respiratory passages and cause hoarseness or respiratory difficulty. Dysphagia is common but does not necessarily indicate the development of a stricture.

Diagnostic tests: Barium swallow is obtained although reflux is demonstrated in < 20% patients with GER. A hiatal hernia may be seen but does not prove GER since hiatal hernias are present in many patients without GER, and conversely some patients with GER do not have a hiatal hernia. Barium swallow may disclose an esophageal stricture or ulceration. Upper GI series is performed in order to identify other lesions that might be causing the symptoms. If x-rays are unremarkable, a trial of medical therapy is reasonable (see below). Bernstein test: If medical treatment fails, the Bernstein test may be performed to ascertain whether the infusion of acid into the esophagus reproduces the patient's symptoms. Via a tube inserted to the body of the esophagus, normal saline and 0.1 N HCl are alternately infused into the esophagus at a rate of 6 ml/minute. If reflux is the cause of the symptoms, the patient's discomfort should correlate with the HCl infusion and not with the saline infusion. False postive results may be obtained in peptic ulcer disease and gastritis. Monitoring esophageal pH and lower esophageal pressure: ●If the Bernstein test is positive, gastric acid reflux may be confirmed by monitoring the pH of the esophagus. A pH probe connected to a manometry catheter is inserted to 5 cm proximal to the lower esophageal sphincter (lower esophageal sphincter pressure is usually measured at the same time and the catheter facilitates proper positioning of the pH probe). Infusion of 300 ml of 0.1 N HCl into the stomach via the manometry catheter may facilitate the study and the patient may be asked to perform various maneuvers to help induce reflux (e.g. lie flat, lean forward, Valsalva, deep breathing, cough). The esophageal pH may be monitored for 30 minutes to 24 hours. Normally, the esophageal pH should not fall below 4. ●A lower esophageal sphincter pressure < 11 mm Hg is found with GER but about a fourth of patients without GER will be found to have decreased pressure. GER is very likely if the pressure is ≤ 2 mm Hg. Esophageal manometry may also be used to diagnose abnormal esophageal peristalsis. Endoscopy is performed if there is hematemesis, if there is dysphagia, if barium swallow shows a stricture or other suspicious lesion, or if medical therapy fails.

Differential diagnosis includes angina pectoris, achalasia, peptic ulcer, gallstones, diverticulosis.

Treatment: Avoid substances that relax the lower esophageal sphincter (coffee, tea, alcohol, anticholinergic drugs). Minimize reflux: more frequent small meals instead of widely spaced larger meals, avoid food or drink at bedtime, elevate head of the bed with 4–6 inch blocks, weight reduction if obese. Antacids may be taken 1 and 3 hr after meals and bedtime. H2 antagonist (e.g. cimetidine, ranitidine) may be tried if the foregoing measures fail. Bethanechol may also help by increasing the tone of the lower esophageal sphincter. Surgery is considered in refractory cases.

Jaundice

(icterus) is the yellow discoloration of the skin, sclerae, and mucous membranes that results from the accumulation bilirubin. Jaundice becomes evident when the total serum bilirubin exceeds 2–4 mg/100ml. **Source and metabolism of bilirubin:** 80–90% bilirubin is formed in the reticuloendothelial system from the breakdown of aged RBC's as the heme component of hemoglobin is catabolized to bilirubin. The remainder of the bilirubin is derived from the breakdown of erythrocyte precursors in the bone marrow, and from the degredation of heme–containing cytochromes, catalases, peroxidases. Bilirubin is released into the circulation unconjugated where it binds to albumin and is then transported to the liver. In the liver, bilirubin is conjugated to glucoronic acid, and is then secreted in the bile. In the gut, conjugated bilirubin is catabolized by bacteria to colorless urobilinogens and thence to colored urobilins. Some of the urobilinogen is absorbed by the gut and is then secreted in the bile (enterohepatic circulation) while a smaller proportion of the absorbed urobilinogen is excreted in the urine. **Unconjugated bilirubin**, being rather tightly bound to albumin, is not filtered by the glomerulus and hence does not appear in the urine. It is not water–soluble and is therefore not excreted in the bile. It is fat–soluble however, and can therefore cross the placenta and the blood–brain barrier. Normally, all the bilirubin in the blood is unconjugated. **Conjugated bilirubin** is water–soluble and is therefore readily excreted in the bile. It is not tightly bound to albumin and can therefore be filtered by the glomerulus. Consequently, conjugated bilirubin may be found in the urine when the plasma conjugated bilirubin level is elevated.

CAUSES OF UNCONJUGATED HYPERBILIRUBINEMIA:

Overproduction of bilirubin: increased hemolysis (e.g. sickle cell anemia, spherocytosis, immune–mediated) or ineffective erythropoiesis (e.g. pernicious anemia); **impaired hepatic uptake:** Gilbert syndrome, neonate, sepsis, or administration of certain drugs (e.g. radiorapic dyes); **inadequate conjugation:** Gilbert syndrome, Crigler–Najjar syndrome, neonate, hepatocellular disease, sepsis, or administration of certain drugs (chloramphenicol, novobiocin).

Gilbert syndrome is inherited (autosomal–dominant). It is a benign disorder that affects 3–7% of the population. The condition is most likely to surface in males, especially during the 2nd and 3rd decade. Jaundice is intermittent and is aggravated by fasting or infection. Both impaired hepatic uptake and a defect in bilirubin conjugation are responsible for the disorder. Liver enzyme levels are normal. No therapy is required.

Crigler–Najjar syndrome is a rare inherited disorder. Manifestations begin in infancy. There is severe unconjugated hyperbilirubinemia due to absence or deficiency of glucoronyl transferase.

CAUSES OF CONJUGATED HYPERBILIRUBINEMIA:

Defective hepatic excretion of conjugated bilirubin: ●Dubin–Johnson syndrome, Rotor syndrome. ●Intrahepatic cholestasis—e.g. pregnancy; primary biliary cirrhosis; hepatitis; cirrhosis; drugs (e.g. phenothiazines, oral contraceptives, methyltestosterone). **Extrahepatic obstruction:** from gallstone; carcinoma (e.g. of bile duct, pancreas, ampulla of Vater); bile duct stricture; biliary atresia.

Dubin–Johnson syndrome is autosomal recessive disorder characterized by impaired excretion of conjugated bilirubin as well as some organic anions (e.g. cholangiographic dyes). Consequently, the gallbladder is not usually seen on intravenous or oral cholecystogram. Bile salts are excreted normally. The serum conjugated bilirubin is elevated and conjugated bilirubin is present in the urine. Bilirubin accumulates in the hepatocytes and is grossly visible on liver biopsy. Subjecting the liver to certain stresses may induce jaundice (e.g. pregnancy, estrogens, alcohol, infection). The disorder is benign and therapy is not required.

Rotor syndrome is benign cause of conjugated hyperbilirubinemia similar to Dubin–Johnson syndrome. One difference is that bilirubin does not accumulate in the liver as in the Dubin–Johnson syndrome.

ESTABLISHING THE CAUSE OF JAUNDICE:

History and physical exam serves as a guide to further workup. Question as to: exposure to hepatitis; IV drug abuse; alcohol abuse; drugs (e.g. oral contraceptives, phenothiazines); pregnancy; dark urine (suggests conjugated hyperbilirubine-mia); pale stools with pruritis (suggests cholestasis or biliary obstruction); family history of jaundice.

Testing for bilirubin and urobilinogen: Determining whether hyperbilirubinemia is primarily conjugated or unconjugated will help narrow the diagnostic possibilities. Van den Bergh reaction test performed in an acqueous medium measures conjugated bilirubin (direct fraction). Addition of methanol to the sample allows measurement of both conjugated and unconjugated bilirubin thus giving the total bilirubin. The concentration of unconjugated bilirubin (indirect fraction) is then obtained by subtracting the direct fraction from the total bilirubin. Normally, all the bilirubin in the plasma is unconjugated. However, because measurement of the direct fraction is only approximate, conjugated bilirubin may be reported in a healthy person. The normal reported laboratory range for direct (conjugated) bilirubin is 0.0–0.2 mg/dl while the total bilirubin is normally < 1.5 mg/dl. Detecting bilirubin in the urine: Since only conjugated bilirubin can appear in the urine and since bilirubin is not normally found in the urine, detection of conjugated bilirubin in the urine demonstrates that the plasma conjugated bilirubin is elevated. Dipstick tests are available to detect conjugated bilirubin in the urine. The foam test may also be used: the presence of persistent yellow foam after shaking a tube of urine is a positive test. Urobilinogen is normally found in the urine (< 4 mg/day). Elevated levels occur when there is increased breakdown of RBC's (hemolytic anemia, GI bleed) or when there is hepatocellular disease. Urine urobilinogen may be absent when the enterohepatic circulation of urobilinogen is impaired (e.g. common bile duct obstruction).

Further laboratory testing: Serum transaminases are > 10–15 times normal if there is hepatocellular injury. With extrahepatic biliary obstruction, the transaminases may be normal or elevated. If elevated, they are < 10–15 times normal. The transaminases are generally normal in other disorders causing jaundice. The SGPT is more specific for liver disease than is SGOT. Serum alkaline phosphatase is > 3 times normal with bile duct obstruction. With hepatocellular injury, the alkaline phosphatase is normal or elevated (if elevated, it is less elevated than with bile duct obstruction). Serum cholesterol is elevated with bile duct obstruction. It may be normal or elevated in cases of cholestasis. Serum tests for viral hepatitis may be indicated.

Additional diagnostic procedures may be needed to establish the cause of jaundice if history, physical exam, and/or the foregoing tests are not conclusive. The following procedures may be considered: ultrasound (e.g. may reveal gallstones or dilated bile ducts); CAT scan (may disclose dilated bile ducts, abdominal tumor); percutaneous transhepatic cholangiography or endoscopic retrograde cholangiography (to visualize bile ducts); liver biopsy.

Cirrhosis

Alcoholic cirrhosis (see "Alcoholism and its Consequences").

Chronic active hepatitis. Hepatitis viruses that cause chronic active hepatitis (hepatitis B virus or non–A non–B virus) may ultimately lead to cirrhosis. In contrast to alcoholic cirrhosis, the histologic findings are that of macronodular cirrhosis (i.e. the areas of regenerating hepatic nodules are > 3 mm). The clinical consequences of this form of cirrhosis (postnecrotic cirrhosis) are the same as for alcoholic cirrhosis.

Wilson's disease (hepatolenticular degeneration) is rare. It is an autosomal recessive inherited disease. Apparently, the defect is an inablility to excrete copper in the bile. Copper accumulates in the liver, CNS, kidneys, and elsewhere. Hepatic disease: Chronic hepatitis ensues and may go on to cirrhosis. Sometimes the initial presentation is like viral hepatitis or there is fulminant hepatic failure. CNS disease: Accumulation of copper in the CNS causes injury to the basal ganglia with ensuing tremor, ataxia, rigidity, choreoathetosis. Other possible complications include hemolytic anemia and renal disease (aminoaciduria, uricosuria, phosphaturia). Copper accumulates in the cornea so that eventually the diagnostic Kayser–Fleischer rings become evident. Laboratory: Serum ceruloplasmin (copper–binding protein) is low or low normal, urinary copper is increased. Liver biopsy discloses an increase in hepatic copper. Treatment: copper chelation with penicillamine.

Hemochromatosis is an inherited disease in which there is enhanced GI absorption of iron. About 80% patients are male. Iron accumulates in the liver and this eventually leads to cirrhosis. The liver is enlarged, firm, and in many cases tender. Iron also accumulates in other organs—e.g. heart (may result in heart failure, heart block, arrhythmias), pancreas (possibly leading to diabetes), gonads (testicular atrophy and impotence), skin (pigmentation), joints (arthritis, pseudogout). The risk of developing hepatocellular carcinoma is markedly increased. <u>Diagnosis</u> : serum iron > 250 mcg/dl, serum iron–binding capacity > 80%, serum ferritin > 1000 ng/ml (ferritin level reflects total body iron store), liver biopsy. <u>Treatment</u>: weekly phlebotomy (500 ml/wk) while periodically following laboratory parameters. Patients may have accumulated 20–60 gram of iron and therefore require phlebotomy for 1–2 years (500 ml whole blood contains 250 mg iron). Successful therapy is associated with decrease in liver size and resolution of pigmentation. Liver biopsy is eventually performed to assess effectiveness of therapy. In anemic patients, chelation therapy is sometimes employed instead of phlebotomy.

Primary biliary cirrhosis is a disease of insidious onset that is most likely to afflict women (about 90% cases)—mostly those between 30 and 65. An autoimmune etiology is probable since antimitochondrial antibodies are found, and the disorder is often associated with rheumatoid arthritis, Sjögren's syndrome, scleroderma, CREST syndrome, or thyroiditis. <u>Signs/symptoms</u>: Pruritis (due to accumulation of bile salts in the skin) appears first and there may be no other complaints for a few years. Jaundice follows months to years later. Other findings may include dark urine, hepatomegaly, splenomegaly, xanthomas, pigmentation, osteopenia/bone pain, steatorrhea. Eventually the consequences of cirrhosis and portal hypertension become evident. <u>Liver biopsy</u> reveals portal inflammation, damaged bile ductules, bile stasis. Periportal fibrosis and cirrhosis are found at a later stage. <u>Laboratory</u>: Most patients have antimitochondrial antibodies and elevated serum IgM. Other lab findings may include serum elevations of alkaline phosphatase (nearly always), bilirubin, cholesterol, bile acids, SGOT, and/or SGPT. The prothrombin time may be prolonged and the serum calcium decreased. <u>Treatment</u>: There is no cure. Pruritis and xanthomas respond to cholestyramine. Monthly intramuscular vitamin K is indicated if the prothrombin time is prolonged. Vitamin D therapy is advised if there is osteomalacia.

Secondary biliary cirrhosis The following conditions may obstruct the outflow of bile and lead to periportal fibrosis and ultimately to cirrhosis: bile duct stricture (e.g. due to surgery), chronic pancreatitis, gallstone, pancreatic or bile duct tumor, cystic fibrosis, biliary atresia, sclerosing cholangitis. <u>Clinical consequences</u> may include jaundice, pruritis, steatorrhea, osteoporosis, xanthomas. <u>Laboratory</u> findings may include elevations of alkaline phosphatase, bilirubin, transaminases, prothrombin time, cholesterol, and/or bile acids.

Obstruction of hepatic venous outflow causes dilation of the hepatic venules and the sinusoids surrounding them. If the congestion is chronic, cirrhosis and possibly ascites may result. ●The most common cause of this type of cirrhosis is right side heart failure followed by constrictive pericarditis, and rarely the Budd–Chiari syndrome (hepatic vein thrombosis).

Alpha–1–antitrypsin deficiency is an inherited disorder (autosomal codominant) characterized by deficiency in alpha–1–antitrypsin, a serum glycoprotein that inactivates trypsin and other proteases. Affected patients may develop emphysema and are susceptible to sundry liver diseases (e.g. cirrhosis, chronic active hepatitis, neonatal hepatitis, hepatocellular carcinoma).

Other causes of cirrhosis include drugs (e.g. methotrexate, isoniazid, methyldopa); sarcoidosis, jejunoileal bypass, glycogen storage disease.

Ascites is the accumulation of fluid in the peritoneal cavity.

There are **3 categories of ascites:** transudative, exudative, and chylous ascites.

Causes of transudative ascites (ascitic fluid protein content < 3 gram/dl): Cirrhosis, especially alcoholic cirrhosis, accounts for over 90% cases of ascites. Cirrhosis–induced ascites appears to result from a combination of factors: (**1**) There is *hypoalbuminemia* due to decreased hepatic albumin synthesis. The consequent decrease in intravascular osmotic pressure leads to increased movement of fluid into the interstitium and peritoneal cavity. (**2**) There is *portal hypertension*. The elevated pressure in the intrahepatic sinusoids favors movement of fluid out of the sinusoids and subsequently thru the hepatic capsule into the peritoneal cavity. Furthermore, portal hypertension may also foster movement of fluid into the peritoneal cavity from the splanchnic vascular bed. (**3**) There is *increased hepatic and splanchnic lymph formation* with transudation into the peritoneal cavity. (**4**) There is *renal salt and water retention* due to inappropriately increased proximal tubular and aldosterone–mediated distal renal tubular sodium reabsorption. Antidiuretic hormone–mediated decrease in free–water clearance may also possibly contribute to water retention. Obstruction of hepatic venous outflow may lead to ascites: e.g. right heart failure, tricuspid insufficiency, constrictive pericarditis, Budd–Chiari syndrome (hepatic vein thrombosis), obstruction inferior vena cava. Portal vein obstruction leads to movement of fluid into the peritoneal cavity from the splanchnic vascular bed. Hypoalbuminemia (e.g. nephrotic syndrome, malnutrition, protein–losing enteropathy) reduces the intravascular osmotic pressure and thus leads to transudation of fluid into the interstitium with generalized edema and movement of transudate into the peritoneal cavity. Other conditions associated with ascites: Meig's syndrome (ovarian fibroma or cystadenoma with ascites and hydrothorax), granulomatous disease involving the liver (e.g. sarcoid), myxedema.

Causes of exudative ascites (ascitic fluid protein content > 3 gram/dl): pancreatic ascites (e.g. chronic pancreatitis, leaking pancreatic pseudocyst, leaking pancreatic duct); tuberculous peritonitis; spontaneous bacterial peritonitis; bile peritonitis (e.g. ruptured gallbladder); GI rupture (e.g. of peptic ulcer, diverticulitis–associated, appendicitis–associated); tumor metastasis to liver or peritoneum; hepatocellular carcinoma; cholangiocarcinoma.

Transudative or exudative ascites: Liver tumor, lymphoma involving the liver, or myeloid metaplasia may lead to a transudative or exudative ascites.

Chylous ascites may be the consequence of lymphatic obstruction (e.g. from thoracic duct trauma, mediastinal tumor, filariasis, tuberculosis, cirrhosis). Chylous ascites may also follow rupture of abdominal lymphatics with subsequent leakage into the peritoneal cavity.

Conditions sometimes confused with ascites: ovarian, pancreatic, or mesenteric cyst; intraperitoneal leakage of urine following urinary tract rupture.

SIGNS/SYMPTOMS of ASCITES: Abdominal exam: Less than 1–2 liter of ascitic fluid is not easily demonstrated by physical exam. A puddle sign is sometimes present (dullness to percussion of dependent abdomen with patient on hands and knees). When ≥ 2 liters accumulates in the peritoneal cavity, there is usually dullness to percussion at the flanks and shifting dullness. When a large volume has accumulated the abdomen may become tense with the umbilicus flat or everted. Furthermore, a fluid wave may be demonstrated. **Pain/discomfort:** Ascites may be uncomfortable but is not painful per se until the abdomen becomes tense with massive ascites. **Early satiety** may occur when a large amount of peritoneal fluid has accumulated. **Dyspnea** may result when there is sufficient peritoneal fluid to impede movement of the diaphragm. **Scrotal edema** may be present.

DIAGNOSTIC TESTS/PROCEDURES:

X–rays: Chest x–ray may reveal an associated pleural effusion. Plain x–rays of the abdomen may suggest presence of ascitic fluid—e.g. diffuse hazy appearance, unclear soft tissue anatomy, separated bowel loops.

Ultrasound or CAT scan is sensitive and may detect small accumulations of ascitic fluid.

Diagnostic paracentesis is advised to exclude neoplasia or infection even when the cause of ascites appears established. The prothrombin time and platelet count must be measured before paracentesis in order to assure that the procedure is not likely to precipitate intra-abdominal bleeding. If need be, fresh frozen plasma and/or platelet transfusion are administered before paracentesis. The patient should void prior to paracentesis. A 20-22 gauge needle is used; large gauge needles may lead to persistent seepage. <u>Ascitic fluid should be examined for clarity and the following tests performed</u>: protein concentration, CBC with differential, gram stain, acid-fast stain, cytology, cultures. <u>In uncomplicated cirrhosis</u>, the ascitic fluid is a clear straw-colored transudate (protein count < 3 gram/100ml) with WBC < 500/cu mm. <u>Gross or microscopic blood</u> may be due to a traumatic tap, or may indicate tuberculosis or a tumor. <u>Cloudy appearance</u> is consistent with infection, neoplasia, pancreatic ascites, or chylous ascites. <u>Milky appearance</u> indicates chylous ascites. <u>Elevated ascitic fluid amylase</u> is most often associated with pancreatic ascites. However, ovarian or intestinal disease may also cause an elevated amylase. <u>Protein content</u> helps narrow the diagnostic possibilities-. A transudate contains < 3 gram/dl while an exudate contains > 3 gram/dl.

TREATMENT:

Cirrhotic ascites: <u>Bed rest and salt restriction</u> is tried. In severe ascites, restrict NaCl to 1 gram/day; in moderate ascites 1-3 gram/day is allowed. <u>Fluid restriction</u> is not advised unless the serum sodium is < 130 mEq/liter. <u>Diuretics</u>: Spironolactone (refer to drug section) is included in the regimen if there has been no weight loss after 2 days. Furosemide may be used concurrently with spironolactone if the latter is not effective. The aim of therapy is to achieve no more than 1/3 kg/day weight loss in the patient without edema, and no more than 2/3 kg/day weight loss in the patient with edema. The rationale is that no more than a liter of ascites fluid can be mobilized/day. More aggressive diuresis will only deplete the intravascular compartment and risk the development of hypovolemic shock. Patients undergoing diuresis should have periodic measurement of eledtrolytes and BUN. <u>Paracentesis</u>: A cirrhotic patient with a painfully tense abdomen or ascites-induced respiratory compromise may obtain relief if 1-2 liters of fluid is slowly removed by paracentesis. <u>Shunt</u>: Selected patients with cirrhosis-induced ascites may benefit from a permanently implanted LeVeen shunt (peritoneal-jugular shunt).

Malignancy-induced ascites may respond to diuretics. In many cases, however, relief is not obtained without paracentesis.

Alcoholic Liver Disease may consist of one or a combination of fatty liver, hepatitis, or cirrhosis.

Fatty liver is the most common hepatic consequence of alcoholism. It is due to deranged fat metabolism (e.g. increased hepatic uptake fatty acids, increased hepatic synthesis triglycerides, decreased oxidation fatty acids, decreased lipoprotein synthesis). Histology discloses hepatocytes filled with fat. <u>Signs/symptoms</u> may be absent or there may be an enlarged and/or tender liver. <u>Laboratory</u>: Serum bilirubin and transaminases may be slightly elevated and the serum albumin decreased. <u>Treatment</u>: Fatty liver resolves in 4-6 weeks with abstention and a nutritious diet.

Alcoholic hepatitis is recognized histologically by the presence of hepatocellular degeneration/necrosis, neutrophil infiltrate, and Mallory bodies (hyaline deposits within hepatocytes). Cirrhosis may also be evident. <u>Signs/symptoms</u> may be absent or there may be nausea, vomiting, abdominal pain, enlarged tender liver, and/or jaundice. There may be fever and/or leukocytosis in the absence of infection. <u>Laboratory</u> findings commonly include hyperbilirubinemia, elevated SGOT and SGPT, hypoalbuminemia, prolonged prothrombin time, leukocytosis. <u>Treatment</u>: Alcoholic hepatitis may resolve with abstention and proper nutrition. However, some patients (especially those who continue to drink) go on to develop cirrhosis.

Alcoholic cirrhosis develops in only a minority of alcoholics (≤ 12%), usually after 5-15 years of excessive alcohol ingestion. Poor nutrition is often associated with and may hasten the development of cirrhosis. However, since cirrhosis may also occur in well-nourished alcoholics, it is evident that the toxic effect of alcohol is the key factor. <u>Histology</u>: Alcoholic cirrhosis usually takes the form of micronodular (Laennec's) cirrhosis: histologic exam discloses multiple small nodules of regenerated hepatocytes surrounded by bands of fibrous tissue. Evidence of alcoholic hepatitis and fatty infiltration are superimposed on this picture if there is continued alcohol consumption. Liver size and consistency: The cirrhotic liver is firm. The size varies. It may be enlarged in early stages because of fat infiltration. In later stages, the liver becomes progressively scarred and shrunken.

Clinical consequences of hepatic cirrhosis: Cirrhosis is not uncommonly asymptomatic. In clinically evident cases, the presentation is a function of the: (1) degree to which scarring impairs portal venous flow, and (2) extent of loss or dysfunction of hepatocytes. Effects of scarring: Scarring sufficient to significantly impair portal venous flow causes portal hypertension. Portal hypertension in turn may result in varices, splenomegaly and hypersplenism. The latter manifests as thrombocytopenia, anemia, and leukopenia. Portal hypertension is a major contributing factor in the development of ascites. Insufficiency of portal venous flow also compromises hepatocyte function. Loss and dysfunction of hepatocytes. Continued alcohol ingestion compromises the metabolic function of hepatocytes, and perpetuates the deleterious consequences of alcoholic hepatitis. When enough hepatocytes are lost or dysfunctional: (**1**) serum bilirubin rises (jaundice may develop), (**2**) hepatic protein synthesis declines (there is hypoalbuminemia and ascites may ensue, there is a deficiency of clotting factors so that PT is prolonged and there may be evidence of bleeding diathesis–e.g bruising), (**3**) BUN decreases (due to impaired hepatic urea synthesis), and (**4**) nitrogenous compounds accumulate (encephalopathy may ensue). Other signs of hepatocellular failure include spider angiomas, palmar erythema, gynecomastia, testicular atrophy, clubbing, Dupuytren's contractures, enlarged parotid glands, anemia. The serum transaminases may be elevated if there is ongoing alcoholic hepatitis.

Transudative ascites is a common sequel to advanced alcoholic cirrhosis. Refer to "Ascites" chapter.

Hepatorenal syndrome may develop in any case of advanced liver disease but it is most commonly seen in the cirrhotic patient with ascites. It has the characteristics of prerenal failure in that intrarenal vasoconstriction causes a fall in the GFR so that oliguria and azotemia and ensue. However, tubular function is preserved—the small amount of urine excreted is concentrated (urine osmolality > plasma osmolality) and has a low sodium concentration (< 10 mEq/liter) indicating that the tubules are capable of concentrating urine and retaining solutes. Moreover, renal histology is normal. In fact, the kidneys of patients with this syndrome have been used successfully as donor transplants. The prognosis is poor although some patients have been saved by LeVeen shunt (peritoneal–jugular shunt). Other causes of renal failure must be excluded before concluding upon diagnosis of hepatorenal syndrome. For instance, renal failure in a cirrhotic patient with ascites is frequently due to diuretic-induced hypovolemia with ensuing underperfusion of the kidneys.

Hepatic encephalopathy is the consequence of liver failure (e.g. fulminant viral hepatitis, alcoholic cirrhosis). The exact agent(s) causing hepatic encephalopathy is debated. Ammonia, amino acids or their derivatives, short chain fatty acids, or combinations of the foregoing are suspect. Encephalopathy may be precipitated by excessive protein intake, GI bleeding, constipation, infection, azotemia, sedating drugs. Aggressive diuretic therapy in a cirrhotic patient with ascites may also be a precipitant because: (1) hypovolemia with underperfusion of the liver may result, (2) hyponatremia and/or hypokalemic alkalosis may ensue. Patients are sensitive to these electrolyte disturbances. Furthermore, alkalosis increases the dissociation of NH_4^+ to NH_3 and the latter easily crosses the blood–brain barrier. Signs/symptoms: depressed consciousness ranging from sleepiness to coma, restlessness, reversal of sleep pattern, irritability, slow thinking, impaired handwriting, confusion, forgetfulness, asterixis (flapping tremor—best elicited by having patient extend the pronated arms with the wrists extended), myoclonus, hyperreflexia, positive Babinski. Treatment consists of (**1**) correction of precipitating causes, (**2**) protein restriction—no more than 40 gram/day in mild cases and complete restriction until improvement occurs in more serious cases, (**3**) lactulose to reduce GI absorption of ammonia (see "Laxatives" in drug section).

OTHER CONSEQUENCES OF ALCOHOLISM: Neurologic: polyneuropathy, cerebral atrophy, cerebellar degeneration, withdrawal syndromes (e.g. delirium tremens), Werniche's encephalopathy, Korsakoff's psychosis. The latter three are discussed in "Neurologic Consequences of Alcoholism" chapter. **Blood:** The hematologic picture is often confused by the superimposition of two or more of the following abnormalities: **(1)** macrocytic anemia due to folate deficiency, **(2)** microcytic hypochromic anemia due to GI blood loss, **(3)** normocytic normochromic anemia, **(4)** thrombocytopenia and neutropenia in patient with hypersplenism secondary to cirrhosis, **(5)** thrombocytopenia and neutropenia resulting from ethanol–induced bone marrow suppression, **(6)** prolonged prothrombin time due to impaired hepatic synthesis of coagulation factors, **(7)** spur and target cells due to abnormal cholesterol metabolism secondary to alcoholic liver disease. **Gastrointestinal** (in addition to liver complications already discussed): gastritis, malabsorption, pancreatitis, increased risk of esophageal cancer. **Metabolic:** Hypoglycemia may result from **(1)** depletion of hepatic glycogen in an alcoholic whose chief or sole carbohydrate source is alcohol, and/or **(2)** inhibition of hepatic gluconeogenesis by alcohol. Hypoglycemia should be considered in any comatose or stuporous patient even when the patient's condition is apparently due to ethanol. Diabetes–independent ketoacidosis is most likely to occur in the starved dehydrated alcoholic. The mechanism is unknown. Administration of fluids usually corrects the problem. Hyperlipidemia. **Cardiac:** cardiomyopathy, arrhythmias. **Other:** myopathy, hypophosphatemia, hypocalcemia, hypomagnesemia, fetal alcohol syndrome.

Hepatitis A virus (HAV) is an RNA enterovirus. It s transmitted
by fecal–oral route or via contaminated water/food. It is not transmitted parenterally (e.g. blood transfusion, contaminated needles). Incubation and duration of infectivity: The incubation period is 15–40 days. The virus is excreted in the feces and viremia is present during the latter 1–2 weeks of the incubation period, during the prodrome, and during the early icteric period. Fecal excretion of virus is almost over by the time jaundice appears. The patient is no longer contagious thereafter. Antibody response: Anti–HAV IgM (IgM antibody directed against hepatitis A virus) appears about the time symptoms develop and disappears within a few months. The presence of anti–HAV IgM is therefore indicative of active or recent infection. Anti–HAV IgG develops later in the course of illness and persists, thereby providing long–term immunity.

Symptoms: Hepatitis A is usually a mild self–limited illness. Many cases are asymptomatic. Symptoms may include malaise, fatigue, headache, myalgia, weakness, headache, anorexia, nausea, vomiting, fever. Alteration in taste or smell is common (e.g. aversion to cigarettes or some foods). Jaundice may develop 2–5 days after the onset of illness, although most patients do not become jaundiced. With jaundice, there is hyperbilirubinuria and so the urine turns dark. Stools are pale. Right upper quadrant pain may be present. Pruritis may occur.

Physical exam may reveal (in addition to jaundice) an enlarged and sometimes tender liver. The spleen is enlarged in a small percentage of cases.

Laboratory: Bilirubin: Serum total bilirubin is elevated (almost always < 15–20 mg/100ml) with elevation of direct (conjugated) bilirubin fraction. Conjugated bilirubin is detected in the urine with qualitative dipstick test. Serum transaminases (SGPT, SGOT) are elevated (often > 10–15 times normal) but the degree of elevation is not indicative of the severity of the illness. Serum alkaline phosphatase is mildly elevated in many cases. WBC count is normal or low. Antibodies: The presence of anti–HAV IgM confirms the presence of active or recent hepatitis A infection. The presence of anti–HAV IgG alone is evidence of past HAV infection.

Treatment consists of rest, high–calorie high–protein diet (unless hepatic encephalopathy develops), avoidance of alcohol and drugs. Small amounts of an antiemetic (e.g. diphenhydramine, hydroxyzine) may be prescribed if necessary. Hospitalization is required if there severe nausea and vomiting, or if liver function is significantly compromised as evidenced by hepatic encephalopathy, prolonged prothrombin time, and/or hypoalbuminemia.

Prognosis: The patient is usually well in 2–3 weeks. Massive hepatic necrosis and death are rare. Chronic hepatitis or the carrier state does not occur.

Prophylaxis with immune serum globulin (ISG) is recommended for close contacts of patients and for travelers to endemic areas where sanitation is poor.

Hepatitis B virus (HBV) is a double stranded DNA virus. It is

present in nearly all the body fluids (blood, urine, semen, feces, saliva, bile, milk) of
infected persons and may therefore be transmitted via blood transfusions, contaminated needles, kissing, sexual intercourse, etc. Incubation period is 50–180 days.

Components and serology of HBV: The complete HBV (Dane particle) has a lipoprotein
outer coat which contains the HBV surface antigen (HBsAg)–the Australian antigen. The inner
core of the virus consists of DNA, DNA polymerase, core antigen (HBcAg), "e" antigens (HBeAg),
etc. HBsAg induces anti–HBs antibodies. HBsAg appears 2 weeks–2 months before symptoms
develop and disappears about the time the acute or icteric phase of the illness is resolving. Typically, a few weeks after HBsAg disappears, antibody to surface antigen (anti–HBs) appears and provides long–term immunity. The patient is usually not contagious by the time HBsAg disappears and
is certainly not by the time anti–HBs appears. If anti–HBs production is not induced, HBsAg persists. Persistence of HBsAg for > 3–6 months usually marks a chronic carrier, or a patient who is
likely to develop chronic hepatitis. However, in some uncomplicated cases in which chronic infection does not develop, HBsAg can remain for a year or so before disappearing. HBV core antigen
(HBcAg) induces anti–HBc antibodies. Anti–HBc appears shortly after the surface antigen
(HBsAg) appears–at about the time the patient is becoming symptomatic and the serum transaminases (SGOT, SGPT) are increasing. The presence of high titers of anti–HBc indicates active viral
replication. Anti–HBc may be the only serologic evidence of HBV infection during the "window" period (the interval between the disappearance of HBsAg and the appearance of anti–HBs). Consequently, patients who are HBsAg negative but anti–HBc positive may be contagious. Anti–HBc does
not confer immunity. Anti–HBc is present during both acute and chronic infection and is detectable
for several years after acute hepatitis has resolved. Thus, anti–HBc positivity together with HBsAg
negativity means either (1) test serum was taken during the window period, or (2) past hepatitis B
infection. In the latter case, anti–HBs is usually present since it persists indefinitely. Note that
hepatitis B infection is ruled out if anti–HBc does not appear. The e antigen (HBeAg), another
component of the core, appears about the same time HBsAg appears. HBeAg is usually transient
(< 3 months) but may persist if chronic infection develops. The presence of HBeAg indicates ongoing viral replication and high infectivity. With the development of anti–HBe (antibody against e antigen), infectivity is significantly diminished. Anti–HBe usually disappear after convalescence but
may persist in chronic cases. The delta virus is an incomplete RNA virus that uses HBV as a
helper. It may cause infection coincident with acute HBV infection or cause infection after chronic
HBV infection is established. Antibody to delta virus is present in either case.

Symptoms and physical exam in *acute* HBV infection are essentially the
same as presented above under Hepatitis A. Hovever, HBV is more likely to result in
severe disease. The prodrome may last a month. Many patients are asymptomatic.
A serum sickness reaction due to the deposition of HBV antigen–antibody complexes
sometimes develops with HBV infection. Manifestations may include arthritis, urticaria, angioedema, and/or a diffuse maculopapular rash.

Laboratory: Aside from serology, the laboratory parameters are the same as presented under Hepatitis A. The serum transaminases (SGOT, SGPT) rise and then fall
in concert with the appearance and disappearance of symptoms.

Prophylaxis: HBIG (hepatitis B immune globulin) is recommended for HBV seronegative individuals following exposure to HBV contaminated materials (e.g. needle
stick, mucosal exposure, oral ingestion). The dose is 0.06 ml/kg IM administered
as soon as possible after exposure (preferably within 7 days). The usual adult dose
is 3–5 ml. A repeat dose is given in 30 days. HBIG is also given to infants born to
HBV infected (HBsAg positive) mothers: 0.5 ml as soon as possible after birth (preferably within 24 hours) with repeat doses at 3 and 6 months. HBIG may possibly be
useful following sexual contact or other close contact. Hepatitis B vaccine is recommended for HBV seronegative persons at increased risk of HBV infection (e.g. health
and lab personnel, hemodialysis patients, institutionalized patients, household or intimate contacts of patients with HBV infection, patients requiring frequent transfusions or clotting factor concentrates, users of illicit injectable drugs, sexually promiscuous persons). The vaccine may also be used in conjunction with HBIG (e.g. following accidental exposure to contaminated materials, infants born to infected mothers). Either of two equally effective preparations may be used: formalin–inactivated
preparation derived from HBsAg positive individuals, or recombinant DNA vaccine.
The regimen with either preparation consists of a series of 3 IM injections (2nd and
3rd doses 1 and 6 months after the first dose).

Treatment of uncomplicated HBV infection is as outlined under hepatitis A.

COMPLICATIONS OF HBV HEPATITIS:

Chronic hepatitis B (persistent hepatitis for more than 3–6 months) may take
one of 3 forms: chronic persistent hepatitis, chronic lobular hepatitis, chronic active
hepatitis. Chronic persistent hepatitis (CPH) patients may experience fatigue

and/or right upper quadrant discomfort but they are usually asymptomatic. HBsAg is often detected and liver enzymes (SGPT, SGOT) are mildly elevated. Histology demonstrates lymphocytic portal inflammation with preservation of normal lobular architecture. CPH is self-limited. Chronic active hepatitis is a serious disease that may have a fatal outcome. The presentation is variable—asymptomatic to very ill with jaundice and hepatosplenomegaly. Spider angiomas, indicating chronic liver disease, may be seen. Histology discloses portal and periportal inflammation (lymphocytes and plasma cells), hepatocellular necrosis (sometimes with bridging necrosis), and fibrosis. Laboratory findings may include elevated transaminases (SGPT, SGOT), hyperbilirubinemia, prolonged prothrombin time, hypoalbuminemia (the latter two are consistent with decreased hepatic protein synthesis), elevated serum gammaglobulin, persistent HBsAg. Treatment is supportive; corticosteroids are not recommended. Outcome is unpredictable. Cirrhosis with its attendant complications may occur. Some patients progressively deteriorate; others have a fluctuating course—sometimes with transient remissions. Chronic lobular hepatitis is an uncommon and usually benign condition. Histology reveals focal areas of hepatocellular necrosis along with portal inflammation.

Fulminant hepatitis is an uncommon complication of hepatitis B infection (< 1% cases) that is rapidly fatal in over 75% cases. There is massive hepatocellular necrosis leading to liver failure with ensuing encephalopathy. Manifestations include hyperbilirubinemia; jaundice; shrunken liver; encephalopathy (e.g. confusion, coma); prolonged bleeding time (due to impaired hepatic synthesis clotting factors). Other common findings are hypoglycemia (due to compromised gluconeogenesis), hypokalemia, hyponatremia, respiratory alkalosis, metabolic acidosis, bleeding, cerebral edema, renal failure. **Treatment of fulminant hepatitis:** Close monitoring of vital signs, serum glucose, electrolytes, pH, prothrombin time, urine output, and perhaps central venous pressure. Intravenous fluids/electrolytes are administered with composition and rate guided by electrolyte and hemodynamic status. Intravenous glucose (10% dextrose) infusion is necessary and additional IV glucose (50% dextrose) is administered should hypoglycemia ensue. Protein intake is stopped and lactulose is administered in order to reduce the accumulation of nitrogenous products. Oral antacids or IV cimetidine may be administered to reduce likelihood of gastric stress ulcers and GI bleeding. Vitamin K is administered to enhance synthesis of clotting factors. Fresh frozen plasma is administered if serious bleeding occurs. Mannitol infusion may be required If there is evidence of cerebral edema with increased intracranial pressure.

Other complications of HBV infection include glomerulonephritis, vasculitis (polyarteritis nodosa is often associated with HBV infection), cryoglobulinemia, pancreatitis, cholestasis. Cholestasis is characterized by elevated alkaline phosphatase, elevated direct bilirubin, and pruritis (the latter results from accumulation of bile salts).

Hepatitis C

Hepatitis non-A non-B has been shown to be usually due to a virus now known as hepatitis C virus (HCV). The virus has been cloned and anti-HCV antibody can now be detected in the serum of infected individuals. **Transmission** has been shown to be the same as for HBV in many cases (e.g. blood transfusion, contaminated needle, sexual or other close contact). Transfusion accounts for only 5–10% of HCV infections. At least 40% cases result from exposure to contaminated needles. About 10% appear to be acquired by sexual or other close contact. The mode of transmission for the remainder is unknown. **Detection of anti–HVC antibody:** An enzyme–linked assay and a radioimmunoassay have been developed to detect anti–HCV antibody. In transfusion–acquired infection, anti–HCV antibody is not detected until nearly 6 months after transfusion and nearly 4 months after the development of hepatitis. In nontransfusion–acquired infection, anti–HCV antibody may be detected from within 6 weeks of illness onset, or be delayed for up to as long as 6 months. **Consequences of infection:** About half of HCV–infected patients develop chronic hepatitis with elevated serum levels of liver enzymes. About 20% of those who develop chronic hepatitis will go on to develop chronic active hepatitis with cirrhosis. Fulminant hepatitis may also occur.

Hepatic Abscess

PYOGENIC ABSCESS   Risk factors: Pyogenic abscess is most likely to occur when there is biliary tract disease (e.g. obstruction with cholangitis). Other predisposing conditions include abdominal trauma, infection in regions drained by portal vein (e.g. diverticulitis, appendicitis); subphrenic abscess; septicemia (e.g. bacterial endocarditis). **Common pathogens:** anaerobes; gram–negative aerobes (e.g. E. coli, Klebsiella); streptococci; Staphylococcus aureus. Mixed aerobic and anaerobic abscesses are common. **Multiple abscesses** occur in about half the cases. **Signs/symptoms** may be minimal or nonspecific (e.g. fever, chills, malaise, anorexia, weight loss). Other manifestations may include right upper quadrant pain/tenderness, hepatomegaly, friction rub over the liver, mild jaundice, cough, rales. **Diagnosis:** <u>Laboratory:</u> Alkaline phosphatase and serum bilirubin may be elevated. Anemia and/or leukocytosis may be present. Blood cultures are often positive. <u>Possible x–ray findings:</u> elevated right hemidiaphragm, right pleural effusion, right–sided atelectasis. A gas–filled hepatic cavity may be seen if the abscess is due to gasforming bacteria (e.g. clostridia). <u>CAT scan</u> is the most sensitive method of detection and may be used to assess the success of therapy. <u>Ultrasound</u> may also reveal the abscess. <u>Radionucleotide scan</u> may be employed but may miss a small abscess. <u>Percutaneous needle aspiration</u> may be used to confirm the diagnosis if the lesion is accessible. Samples are sent for gram stain as well as aerobic and anaerobic culture and sensitivity. Antibiotics are begun before needle aspiration (see treatment). Aspiration may be therapeutic and the clinician may elect to leave a percutaneous drain in place. **Treatment:** Until culture results become available, the patient is treated with an aminoglycoside (usually gentamycin or tobramycin) plus one of metronidazole, chloramphenicol, or clindamycin. Therapy is continued for a minimum of 4–6 wk. Treatment is individualized. Some patients will do well with antibiotic therapy alone or cannot be treated otherwise (e.g. multiple small abscesses). For other patients, percutaneous catheter or surgical drainage may be necessary and possible.

AMEBIC LIVER ABSCESS is due to the protozoan, Entamebae histolytica. The organism presumably reaches the liver from the infected colon via radicles of the portal vein. Amebic dysentery and liver abscess are common in geographic regions with poor sanitation. Most patients are male. Amebiasis is umcommon in the U.S. **Signs/symptoms** are similar to pyogenic abscess. There may or may not be clinical evidence of colon infection (diarrhea, abdominal cramps, flatulence, mucus or blood in stools). Patient may recall an episode of dysentery. **Diagnosis:** <u>Alkaline phosphatase and serum bilirubin</u> may be normal or elevated. <u>Moderate leukocytosis</u> may be present. <u>CAT scan, ultrasound, or radionucleotide scan</u> will detect the lesion but will not distinguish it from a pyogenic abscess. <u>Indirect hemagglutination assay</u> (titer $\geq 1{:}128$) or gel difusion precipitin test is positive in over 90% cases. <u>Stool</u> is examined but the organism is usually not found since colon infection is no longer present in many cases. <u>Needle aspiration of the liver abscess</u> is not necessary if serology and epidemiology support the diagnosis of amebiasis. Moreover, the aspirate frequently does not reveal amebae. That portion of the aspirate from the periphery of the abscess (where the amebae are present) is most likely to be positive. The aspirate consists of necrotic liver and RBC's. Unless there is a coexisting pyogenic abscess, there are few WBC's and bacteria are absent. The semi–fluid yellow to chocolate–colored aspirate is often described as resembling "anchovy paste". <u>In doubtful cases, a therapeutic trial</u> with dehydroemetine and chloroquine combined may help make the diagnosis of amebic abscess. A trial of metronidazole is not diagnostic because it is also effective against anaerobic bacteria. **Treatment:** metronidazole in conjunction with diiodohydroxyquin (the latter to insure eradication of the intestinal infection). Refer to metronidazole in drug section for the regimen. Surgical drainage is indicated if the abscess ruptures into the pleural, pericardial, or peritoneal cavity.

Pancreatitis

ACUTE PANCREATITIS The pathogenetic mechanism is debated. Apparently, pancreatic juices are released into and digest the pancreatic tissue. In mild cases, the pancreas becomes edematous and there may be small foci of parenchymal necrosis accompanied by inflammatory cells. In severe cases, bleeding into the pancreatic parenchyma occurs (hemorrhagic pancreatitis). Hemorrhagic pancreatitis is fatal in > 50% cases. **Etiology:** alcohol; biliary tract disease (e.g. gallstone); familial; pancreatic ischemia (e.g. shock, vasculitis); abdominal trauma/surgery; viral infection (e.g. mumps, coxsackie); drugs (e.g. corticosteroids, thiazide diuretics, sulfonamides, oral contraceptives, isoniazid, azathioprine); hypertriglyceridemia; hyperparathyroidism; posterior penetration of duodenal ulcer; tumor or other condition obstructing pancreatic ducts; idiopathic.

Signs/symptoms: Pain: A steady severe epigastric pain radiating to the back is characteristic. Pain may be lessened by flexion at the waist or leaning forward, and is aggravated by movement. Pain generally persists for 3–7 days. Nausea and vomiting are common. Tenderness may be confined to the epigastrium but in some cases it is more diffuse. Rebound tenderness is usually not present. Abdominal guarding and rigidity are generally not prominent. Bowel sounds are usually normal but sometimes decreased. Fever (≤ 102) is not uncommon. Signs of dehydration may be present and sometimes hypotension and shock develop (large amounts of fluid may accumulate retroperitoneally). Ecchymosis of the flank (Grey Turner sign) or about the umbilicus (Cullen sign) may occur with hemorrhagic pancreatitis. Tender subcutaneous nodules may develop (presumably due to effects of lipase released into the circulation). Tetany and/or positive Trousseau or Chvostek signs are occasionally seen as a consequence of hypocalcemia.

Laboratory: Serum amylase typically becomes elevated within 6–12 hours after the attack begins, peaks at about 24 hours, and then returns to normal over the next 3–5 days as the pain resolves. Occasionally the serum amylase is normal because (1) there is rapid renal clearance of amylase, (2) the blood sample is drawn after the plasma level has fallen, or (3) pancreatitis–associated hyperlipidemia may influence the measurement. Conditions other than pancreatitis that may be associated with elevated serum amylase include peptic ulcer, perforated bowel, intestinal infarction, small bowel obstruction, cholecystitis, peritonitis, ruptured ectopic pregnancy, renal failure, burns, diabetic ketoacidosis, macroamylasemia, slow renal clearance of amylase, salivary gland inflammation or trauma, certain metastatic tumors. Urinary amylase clearance is more sensitive and specific than the serum amylase. The basis for this test is that proximal renal tubular reabsorption of amylase is decreased in pancreatitis and amylase is therefore more quickly excreted in the urine. Thus, it is possible for a patient with pancreatitis to have a normal serum amylase because of enhanced urinary excretion of amylase. A random specimen of urine is obtained and the ratio of amylase clearance to creatinine clearance is calculated: (urine amylase/plasma amylase) ÷ (urine creatinine/plasma creatinine) x 100%. A value > 5% is consistent with pancreatitis. Serum lipase is commonly elevated. Serum total bilirubin may be elevated but is usually not > 2 mg/dl. Hyperglycemia is not uncommon. Hypocalcemia commonly develops after 36–48 hours. It is thought to be due to the formation of calcium–fatty acid salts (saponification) following release of fatty acids in the peri–pancreatic tissue. An aberrant response to parathyroid hormone is also postulated to account for hypocalcemia. WBC count may be elevated (12,000–20,000). Plain abdominal x-rays may reveal a sentinel loop (a dilated isolated segment small bowel or colon) or colon cut–off sign (air–filled ascending and transverse colon that stops sharply at the mid to left transverse colon).

Treatment acute pancreatitis: NPO and nasogastric suction. The rationale is to reduce the the stimulus for pancreatic secretion. Nasogastric suction is not required in mild-moderate cases. Intravenous fluids are administered. Electrolyte abnormalities are corrected. Intravenous colloids and/or blood transfusion are administered if hypotension or shock develops. Analgesia: IV or IM narcotics may be needed for pain relief. Meperidine is commonly used because it does not contract the sphincter of Oddi. IV calcium gluconate is administered if hypocalcemia is present.

Complications acute pancreatitis: Pancreatic pseudocyst is suspected if pain persists over a week. The serum amylase continues to be elevated in many cases. There may be a palpable abdominal mass. Ultrasound or CAT scan will reveal the lesion. A pseudocyst is an encapsulated cyst (containing pancreatic juice) that is formed by inflammatory fibrosis of the peritoneum and the serosal surfaces of the abdominal organs. It is termed a PSEUDOcyst because the walls of the cyst are not lined by epithelium as true cysts are. The decision to surgically drain a pseudocyst is individualized according to: (1) size of the pseudocyst, (2) presence of symptoms, (3) whether or not pseudocyst is enlarging. Pancreatic abscess is suspected when symptoms persist and there is a rising temperature with continued leukocytosis. A tender epigastric mass may be present. Gas bubbles about the pancreas are sometimes seen on plain x-ray. Ultrasound or CAT scan are obtained. Surgical drainage is the treatment. Other complications of acute pancreatitis include pancreatic ascites, left pleural effusion, pulmonary atelectasis, adult respiratory distress syndrome.

CHRONIC PANCREATITIS is usually the consequence of alcoholism. It may be idiopathic or hereditary. It may be due to cystic fibrosis, malnutrition, trauma, hyperlipidemia, hyperparathyroidism, biliary tract disease. In contrast to acute pancreatitis, irreversible damage has occurred.

Signs/symptoms: Pain ranges from severe to mild, and an occasional patient may be pain–free in spite of significant disease. Like acute pancreatitis, the pain is usually located in the epigastrium and often radiates to the back. In some cases, there is diffuse abdominal pain Pain may be intermittent (chronic relapsing pancreatitis) with acute attacks clinically similar to acute pancreatis followed by pain–free interval lasting weeks or months. This picture is frequently observed in alcoholics who experience attacks in association with drinking binges. Other patients may have more or less continuous pain that may fluctuate from day to day, and is therefore sometimes confused with ulcer disease, gastritis, or biliary tract disorders. Diabetes mellitus may develop in advanced cases. Malabsorption appears when 90% of pancreatic parenchyma is destroyed. Weight loss and greasy stools are characteristic.

Laboratory: Serum amylase may or may not be elevated. A low or normal serum amylase during an acute exacerbation may be explained by the fact that the pancreas has diminished reserves as a consequence of parenchymal loss. Evidence of diabetes mellitus may be present. If exocrine pancreatic insufficiency is suspected further tests may be indicated (see "Malabsorption" chapter). **Further exams** are obtained if the diagnosis of chronic pancreatitis is uncertain: plain x–ray often reveals pancreatic calcification; CAT scan may provide further clarification, identify a pseudocyst, and exclude pancreatic tumor; ERCP (endoscopic retrograde cholangiopancreatography) is sometimes necessary.

Treatment chronic pancreatitis: Acute attacks are treated in the same manner as acute pancreatitis. Alcohol is discouraged and other inciting conditions are corrected if possible (e.g. surgery for gallstones or obstructed duct). Pain relief: Analgesics are prescribed as needed. In some cases, pain is alleviated with administration of large doses of pancreatic enzymes PO. Surgery may be recommended for intractable pain. Pancreatic enzymes (refer to pancrelipase in drug section) in large doses are administered if there is evidence of malabsorption. Antacids or an H2–antagonist (e.g. cimetidine, ranitidine) are administered along with the enzymes in order to prevent inactivation of enzymes by stomach acid. Diabetes is treated. Patients who develop diabetes are ketosis–prone.

Biliary Tract Disease

BILIARY COLIC is the characteristic pain that results from increased pressure within and distension of the gallbladder or bile ducts. The most common cause of biliary colic is a stone obstructing the cystic duct or common bile duct. Typically, there is rapid development of right upper quadrant pain (sometimes epigastric or left upper quadrant) which gathers in intensity to reach a steady level. It is emphasized that the pain is usually steady, not colicky (i.e. not waxing and waning). Frequently, there is also referred pain in the right scapular region.

GALLSTONES About 10% general U.S. population and 30% patients over 65 have gallstones. There are 2 kinds of gallstones: mainly cholesterol (75% cases in the U.S.) and mainly pigment stones. **Cholesterol stones** form when the bile contains an excess concentration of cholesterol in relation to bile salts and phospholipids. The likelihood of developing gallstones is greater with/in: increasing age, females, multiparity, obesity, American Indians, prolonged fasting, parenteral hyperalimentation, oral contraceptives. Cholesterol stones are radiolucent in 80% cases. **Pigment stones** are composed of calcium bilirubinate and bile acids chiefly. Predisposing conditions are chronic hemolysis, cirrhosis, elevated concentration of unconjugated bilirubin in the bile. The latter condition is not uncommon in the orient in patients with worm infestations of the biliary ducts and may be due to the associated presence of E. coli in the biliary tree (E. coli produces an enzyme capable of deconjugating conjugated bilirubin). More than half of gallstones in Japan are pigment stones. In the U.S., only 25% are pigment stones. About 80% of pigment stones are radiopaque. **Asymptomatic gallstones:** From 30 to 50% patients with gallstones are asymptomatic. Surgery is recommended in diabetics (because of the increased risk of complications and mortality should acute cholecystitis develop), and in patients with calcified gallbladder (because of the common association with carcinoma).

CHRONIC CHOLECYSTITIS: Histologic appearance of the gallbladder may be essentially normal or there may be obvious evidence of inflammation and fibrosis. **Diagnosis:** Pain: Patients have typical attacks of biliary colic due to transient obstruction of the cystic duct by a gallstone. The pain may last for several hours before abating. Episodes may occur frequently or not recur for years. Meals, particularly fatty meals, appear to induce attacks in some cases. Chronic cholecystitis is differentiated from acute cholecystitis in that chronic cholecystitis is not associated with fever or leukocytosis nor is there right upper quadrant guarding/spasm. Furthermore, a palpable tender gallbladder is not present as is often the case with acute cholecystitis. Ultrasound is the most reliable method of demonstrating gallstones. **Treatment:** Analgesics are administered during an acute attack. Elective surgery is the standard definitive treatment. Dissolution of the gallstones with ursodeoxycholic acid (ursodiol) is an alternative method of treatment for patients with radiolucent noncalcified gallstones < 20 mm in diameter who refuse surgery or who are poor surgical risks. Dose is 8–10 mg/kg/day divided into 2–3 daily doses PO with meals.

ACUTE CHOLECYSTITIS (acute inflammation of the gallbladder) in about 95% cases is the consequence of a stone obstructing the cystic duct. The remaining cases (acalculous cholecystitis) may be incited by conditions such as: tumor obstructing cystic duct; ischemia (e.g. cystic artery occlusion); prolonged fasting (e.g. following an operation, parenteral hyperalimentation); primary bacterial infection (e.g. Salmonellae typhi).

Signs/symptoms: Biliary colic is present. Not uncommonly, pain is also referred to the right scapula. Abdominal exam: There is tenderness in the right subcostal area with a positive Murphy's sign (patient resists taking a deep breath while this area is palpated because it worsens the pain). An enlarged tender gallbladder can be palpated in many cases. Nausea and vomiting are common. Jaundice is present in 10–20% cases. Fever is usually present but typically remains ≤ 101. High fever and chills should arouse suspicion of a complication (e.g. empyema, gangrene, perforation) or some other diagnosis (e.g. cholangitis).

Tests: WBC count ranges from normal to 15,000 with a left shift. Elevated serum total bilirubin up to 4 mg/dl is not uncommon and is probably the result of associated edema of the common duct. Higher levels suggest obstruction of the common duct. Serum amylase and alkaline phosphatase may also be elevated. Plain x-rays reveal gallstones in the 15% of patients with radioopaque stones. Ultrasound will detect stones and dilated biliary ducts. Technetium–99m radionuclide scan confirms the diagnosis: the bile ducts will be seen but the gallbladder will not (i.e. the gallbladder will not fill with contrast agent). On the other hand, acute cholecystitis is improbable if the gallbladder is visualized.

Treatment acute cholecystitis: NPO, IV fluids, NG suction, parenteral analgesia. Meperidine is the preferred analgesic because it does not cause spasm of sphincter of Oddi. An attack of acute cholecystitis will in most cases resolve with this therapy. <u>IV antibiotics are advised in the following circumstances</u>: sepsis or other complications, symptoms are severe or have been present for over 3 days, and/or if the patient is over 60 or a diabetic. Ampicillin or a cephalosporin are the drugs of choice. An aminoglycoside is added in the event of sepsis or complication. <u>The timing of surgery is individualized</u>: **(1)** Emergency operation is mandated in the presence of temp > 102, chills, and WBC > 15,000. Other indications for urgent surgery are hypotension, peritoneal signs (gallbladder perforation ?), evidence of clinical deterioration or failure to improve despite the medical therapy outlined above. **(2)** Patients in less serious condition than the foregoing who do not have the diagnostic tender palpable gallbladder should, in order to confirm the diagnosis, undergo intravenous cholangiography prior to surgery. Surgery should not be long delayed in diabetics experiencing an attack of acute cholecystitis because they are particularly prone to complications and mortality. **(3)** If an attack resolves with medical therapy, surgery is usually delayed for several days to up to 1–2 months. Dissolution of the gallstones with ursodeoxycholic acid (ursodiol) is an alternative to surgery for patients with radiolucent noncalcified gallstones < 20 mm in diameter who refuse surgery or who are poor surgical risks. Dose is 8–10 mg/kg/day divided into 2–3 daily doses PO with meals. **(4)** Patients who are poor surgical risks pose a special challenge. Attempts to improve the patient's general condition and medical therapy aimed at resolving the acute attack of cholecystitis may be advisable first. If the attack of acute cholecystitis resolves or appears to be abating, surgery is considered for a later time. Dissolution of gallstones with ursodiol (see above) may be an alternative if the acute attack resolves and the patient has radiolucent noncalcified stones < 20 mm in diameter. If one is forced to resort to emergency surgery, the treatment of choice may be cholecystostomy (with local anesthesia) instead of cholecystectomy.

Complications of acute cholecystitis: <u>Gallbladder empyema</u> (pus in gallbladder) is associated with chills, fever > 102, WBC > 15,000. <u>Pericholecystic abscess</u> is a localized abscess associated with gallbladder perforation. <u>Free perforation</u> may result in bile peritonitis (mortality > 50%) if the obstructing stone is dislodged, or purulent peritonitis (mortality 20%) if it is not dislodged. <u>Cholecystenteric fistula</u> occurs when the gallbladder adheres to stomach or bowel and then perforates.

CHOLEDOCOLITHIASIS (stone in the common bile duct). Common bile duct stones usually originate in the gallbladder. In fact, 15% patients with gallstones will also have stones in the bile ducts. In some cases, stones form de novo within the intrahepatic or extrahepatic ducts. Stones often pass into the duodenum from the common duct without causing clinical difficulty. Up to 50% individuals with common duct stones are asymptomatic. Temporary obstruction of the common duct by a stone produces attacks of biliary colic identical to that caused by transient obstruction of the cystic duct.

CHOLANGITIS (inflammation of the bile ducts) is due to bacterial infection of the biliary tree when it is obstructed by either a stone in the common duct or a tumor. **Signs/symptoms:** Charcot's triad (biliary colic, fever and chills, jaundice) and right upper quadrant tenderness are typical findings. **Laboratory:** leukocytosis (usually 15,000–20,000 or above), elevated serum bilirubin (usually 2–4 mg/dl but seldom > 10 because obstruction is rarely complete), elevated alkaline phosphatase, elevated SGOT and SGPT, elevated amylase. **Treatment:** <u>If the patient is severely ill</u> (septicemia, shock) suggesting suppurative cholangitis; IV fluid resuscitation and IV antibiotics (clindamycin + aminoglycoside) are begun without delay and emergency surgery is performed. <u>Relatively stable patients</u>, on the other hand, are treated with IV fluids and IV antibiotics. Improvement is usually seen within 1–2 days. Diagnostic tests are obtained as indicated—e.g. ultrasound, CAT scan, percutaneous transhepatic cholangiography, ERCP (endoscopic retrograde cholangiopancreatography). The latter two tests must not be performed until infection is brought under control. Surgery is scheduled once the attack has resolved. Patients who fail to improve or who deteriorate within 2–4 days of initiating antibiotic therapy should undergo surgery without further delay.

GALLBLADDER CARCINOMA is usually an adenocarcinoma. It is primarily a disease of the elderly and is more common in women. Most patients have a history of gallstones. Patients often present with recurrent attacks of biliary colic as in chronic cholecystitis. Sometimes the clinical picture is that of acute cholecystitis. Jaundice develops if there is involvement of the common bile duct and it becomes obstructed. In many cases, a right upper quadrant mass is felt. Ultrasound and CAT scan may show the lesion.

BILE DUCT MALIGNANCY is usually an adenocarcinoma. Typically, there is a gradual development of jaundice, often with pruritis. Right upper quadrant discomfort or pain is common. The gallbladder is often found to be distended as a consequence of common duct obstruction. The combination of a enlarged palpable nontender gallbladder and obstructive jaundice is very suggestive of neoplastic involvement of the common duct. Jaundice tends to be severe (serum total bilirubin >15 mg/dl). Obstruction of the common duct leads to (as revealed by ultrasound and CAT scan) dilation of the intrahepatic ducts. Transhepatic cholangiography or ERCP (endoscopic retrograde cholangiopancreatography) may further clarify the lesion.

Pancreatic Cancer is the 4th most common cause of cancer

death after cancer of the lung, colon, and breast. **Types:** About 90% of cases are adenocarcinomas (i.e. derived from pancreatic duct cells). The remaining pancreatic cancers include islet cell carcinomas, acinar cell carcinoma, adenosquamous, cystadenocarcinoma, undifferentiated. **Location:** About two thirds of the tumors are located in the head of the pancreas; the rest in the body or tail. **Risk factors:** smoking, coffee, chronic hereditary pancreatitis, and perhaps diabetes mellitus. Males are twice as likely to develop pancreatic cancer.

Signs/symptoms: Jaundice may occur when a tumor of the head of the pancreas encroaches upon and obstructs the common bile duct. The obstructive nature of the jaundice is revealed by the fact that it is chiefly the *direct* bilirubin fraction that is elevated. Abdominal pain—often a gnawing epigastric pain that in many cases radiates to the back. Characteristically, the pain is relieved by leaning forward and aggravated by lying supine. Abdominal exam: An abdominal mass is sometimes felt. A palpable nontender gallbladder accompanied by jaundice is very suggestive of cancer of the head of the pancreas (Courvoisier's law). Common bile duct neoplasia is another possibility. Hepatomegaly may indicate liver metastases. Weight loss, anorexia, and/or nausea are common. "Bad taste" is a frequent complaint. A distaste for certain foods (particularly meat) is common. Vomiting, hematemesis, or melena may occur if the cancer invades the stomach or duodenum. Cancer of the tail of the pancreas tends to remain clinically silent until it is far advanced and has extended to adjacent structures—commonly the spleen. Other associated conditions that may develop include migratory thrombophlebitis (Trouseau's sign); diabetes mellitus; paraneoplastic endocrinopathies (e.g. Cushing's syndrome, hypercalcemia).

Diagnosis: Elevated serum bilirubin (mainly direct fraction) may result if the common bile duct becomes obstructed. Elevated alkaline phosphatase reflects common bile duct obstruction and/or liver metastases. Carcinoembryonic antigen is elevated in most patients but is not specific for pancreatic cancer. Ultrasound or CAT scan will detect 80-90% of pancreatic tumors > 3 cm in diameter. Tumors < 1–2 cm will not be detected by either method. Percutaneous fine needle aspiration biopsy under ultrasonic or CAT guidance may be used to confirm the diagnosis If ultrasound or CAT scan reveals a large accessible uncalcified pancreatic mass and the bile ducts are not dilated. ERCP (endoscopic retrocholangiopancreatography) is often the next diagnostic step (1) if ultrasound or CAT scan are equivocal or negative and suspicion still lingers, (2) if a small pancreatic mass is seen, or (3) if there is pancreatic calcification. ERCP has diagnostic accuracy of about 90% in pancreatic cancer. Percutaneous transhepatic cholangiography with a Chiba needle is a more easily performed alternative to ERCP that can be used if the bile ducts are dilated. Upper GI series may reveal encroachment by the tumor on the stomach or duodenum.

Note: The treatment information presented below is extracted from National Cancer Institute PDQ State-of-the-Art Cancer Treatment Information 6/1/90. However, since cancer treatment is evolving, this information may not be current. The most up-to-date standard treatment options may be obtained by calling the National Cancer Institute Cancer Information Service at 1–800–4–CANCER.

Because patients are rarely cured, and because, except for stage I, standard therapy is only pallia-tive, all patients should be considered for inclusion in clinical trials of new regimens. Descriptions of these trials are also available.

Treatment: Stage I (i.e. tumor confined to the pancreas; or tumor with limited direct extension to duodenum, bile ducts, or stomach that would allow tumor resection): Surgery with curative intent is attempted. The Whipple procedure (removal of distal stomach, entire duodenum, common bile duct, gallbladder, proximal pancreas to midbody) is performed for tumors of the head of the pan-creas. The procedure must also include total pancreatectomy if a sufficiently wide margin cannot be achieved with the standard Whipple procedure. Distal pancreatectomy may be adequate treat-ment for small tumors of the tail of the pancreas. The value of adjunctive radiation therapy is being investigated. The 3 yr survival with surgery for stage I tumors confined to the wall of the pan-creas is 15%; for other stage I cases, 3 yr survival is 1%. Standard treatment of stages II–IV is palliative—e.g. surgery, radiation, and/or chemotherapy. Obstructive jaundice may be palliated by percutaneous transhepatic stenting of the bile duct, percutaneous transhepatic external drainage, cholecystojejunostomy, or choledochojejunostomy. The 3 yr survival of stages II–III is 2 %., and of stage IV is 1%. Stage II–IV patients should be considered for inclusion in clinical trials (e.g. radi-osensitizers, particle beam radiation, chemotherapy).

Esophageal Cancer is more common in males and in blacks.

Other risk factors include smoking, alcohol consumption, history of ionizing radiation, esophageal stasis (e.g. achalasia), esophageal lye injury, history of squamous cell cancer of head or neck, Barrett's epithelium (see below). **Cellular types:** Squamous cell carcinoma accounts for about 60% of esophageal cancer cases. This is not surprising since most of the lumen of the esophagus is lined with strati-fied squamous epithelium. Adenocarcinomas are responsible for nearly all the rest. Adenocarcinomas are derived from gastric tissue or from Barrett's epithelium in the distal 1/3 of the esophagus. Patients with severe chronic reflux esophagitis are prone to develop Barrett's epithelium. It is a glandular epithelium that has arisen from the transformation of normal stratified squamous epithelium. Barrett's epitheli-um is a fertile field from which adenocarcinoma may develop (about 10% patients with Barrett's epithelium will develop adenocarcinoma). Esophageal sarcomas and melanomas are rare.

Signs/symptoms: Progressive dysphagia is the chief complaint. Patient initial-ly has difficulty swallowing solid food and may eventually have difficulty with fluids. Weight loss with inanition is almost inevitable. Chest pain usually means the can-cer has spread to adjacent mediastinal structures. Occult bleeding with ensuing anemia is common but severe bleeding is uncommon. Cough and/or aspiration pneumonitis may result if there is reflux from an obstructed esophagus, or if a fistu-la develops between the esophagus and trachea. Other potential complications include: (1) invasion of adjacent great vessels with ensuing hemorrhage, (2) arrhythmias due to invasion of pericardium, (3) hoarseness due to involvement of re-current laryngeal nerve.

Diagnosis/metastatic workup: Barium swallow is performed. This is followed by esophagoscopy with biopsy and cytology. ●If there is a positive diagnosis, evalua-tion for metastases is necessary: physical exam (? suspicious nodes), chest x-ray, bronchoscopy (? tracheal invasion), CAT scan thorax (? mediastinal spread), ultrasound, liver scan, liver function tests, serum calcium. The most common sites of metastases are the liver, lung, bone, and brain.

Note: The following information is extracted from National Cancer Institute PDQ State-of-the-Art Cancer Treatment Information 12/3/90. However, since cancer treatment is evolving, this infor-mation may not be current. The most up-to-date standard treatment options may be obtained by calling the National Cancer Institute Cancer Information Service at 1–800–4–CANCER. All newly di-agnosed patients should be considered for inclusion in clinical trials of new therapeutic regimens. Descriptions of these trials are also available.

TNM classification: Primary tumor: **TX** (primary tumor cannot be assessed), **T0** (evidence of primary tumor absent), **Tis** (carcinoma in situ), **T1** (tumor invades lamina propria or submucosa), **T2** (tumor invades muscularis propria), **T3** (tumor invades adventitia), **T4** (tumor invades adjacent structures). Regional lymph nodes: **NX** (regional nodes cannot be assessed), **N0** (regional node metastasis absent), **N1** (regional node metastasis present). Distant metastasis: **MX** (presence of metastasis cannot be assessed), **M0** (distant metastasis absent), **M1** (distant metastasis).

Staging: Stage 0: Tis, N0, M0. Stage 1: T1, N0, M0. Stage 2A: T2-T3, N0, M0. Stage 2B: T1-T2, N1, M0. Stage 3: T3, N1, M0 or T4, any N, M0. Stage 4: any T, any N, M1.

Prognosis (5 yr survival with treatment): Stage 0: excellent. Stage 1: > 50%. Stage 2A: 15%. Stage 2B: 10%. Stage 3: < 10%. Stage 4: rare.

Treatment modality is influenced by such factors as the location of the tumor, whether or not there is obstruction, whether or not there is partial or complete obstruction, the stage of the tumor, and the cellular type. Surgical resection is usually recommended if there is complete obstruction and clinical evidence of systemic metastases is absent. Radiation may be recommended to mitigate partial obstruction, particularly if there is tumor of the proximal 1/3 of the esophagus—which is more difficult to resect surgically. Other measures may be needed to relieve obstruction and permit swallowing or feeding—e.g. bougienage, placement of intraluminal plastic tubes, or laser therapy. Clinical trials of investigational regimens should be considered in all new cases. For instance, clinical trials employing adjuvant combination chemotherapy that includes cisplatin are in progress. However, some cases of adenocarcinoma may not be as sensitive to chemotherapy as squamous carcinoma. Furthermore, adenocarcinoma may be less sensitive to radiation. With the foregoing comments in mind, the **standard treatment options according to stage are as follows:** Stage 0 is seldom diagnosed in the U.S. However, in Asia success is achieved with surgery. Stage 1: surgery or radiation are equivalent alternatives. Stage 2: (a) surgery or (b) radiation ± intraluminal intubation and dilation. Stage 3: radiation ± intraluminal intubation and dilation. Palliative surgical resection is an alternative for T3a lesions. Stage 4: radiation ± intraluminal intubation and dilation.

Stomach Cancer

incidence has dropped markedly in the U.S. over the last 3–4 decades. Other Anglo–Saxon countries and Western Europe have also seen a decline. For unknown reasons, this decline has been accompanied by a rise in the incidence of colon cancer. The incidence of gastric cancer is still high in Eastern Europe, Japan, and certain regions of Latin America. **Risk factors** include male sex (twice as common as women), black race, chronic atrophic gastritis, prior partial gastrectomy for benign peptic ulcer, gastric adenomatous polyps, type A blood. Diets high in certain foods (e.g. salted fish, pickled foods) are suspected of increasing the risk. Stomach cancer seldom occurs before age 40. Incidence is highest in the 50s and 60s. **Types of stomach cancer:** Over 90% of stomach cancers are adenocarcinomas; lymphomas account for about 5%; sarcomas (e.g. leiomyosarcoma) are unusual. Benign tumors are uncommon. ●Adenocarcinoma may express itself as an ulcerating carcinoma, polypoid carcinoma, superficial spreading carcinoma (involves the mucosa and submucosa only), or linitis plastica (involves all layers and is associated with a fibrotic nonpliable stomach). **Location:** Gastric cancer is found in pyloric area in 60% cases, body 30%, cardia 5%, diffuse 5%.

Signs/symptoms may include weight loss, epigastric distress/pain/tenderness, palpable epigastric mass, vomiting (? obstruction), anorexia (aversion to meat notably), early satiety, dysphagia (perhaps due to tumor invasion in region of gastroesophageal junction), symptoms of anemia, hemoccult positive stools, severe gastric bleeding (seldom), perforation (unusual). Evidence of metastasis may include lymphadenopathy (e.g. Virchow node—a palpable left supraclavicular node suggesting spread via thoracic duct), hepatomegaly, obstructive jaundice, enlarged ovaries (Krukenberg tumors), ascites due to peritoneal metastases, Blumer shelf (shelf–like perirectal mass felt on rectal exam). Paraneoplastic findings occur rarely—e.g. acanthosis nigricans, migratory thrombophlebitis (Trousseau's syndrome), neurologic disturbances.

Diagnosis/metastatic workup: First step is usually an upper GI series with double–contrast technique to enhance accuracy. This is followed by gastroscopy with brushings for cytology and multiple biopsy. Evaluation for metastasis may include liver function tests, liver scan, chest x-ray, ultrasound or CAT scan of abdomen, biopsy of suspicious nodes, laparoscopy. The most common sites of hematogeous metastasis are the lungs, liver, bone, and brain.

Note: The following information is extracted from National Cancer Institute PDQ State–of–the–Art Cancer Treatment Information 11/1/90. However, because cancer treatment is evolving, this information may not be current. The most up-to-date standard treatment options may be obtained by calling the National Cancer Institute Cancer Information Service at 1–800–4–CANCER. Patients may also be candidates for clinical trials of new therapeutic regimens. Descriptions of these trials are also available.

TNM classification: Tumor; **TX** (minimum requirements to assess primary tumor cannot be met), **T0** (no evidence of primary tumor), **Tis** (tumor confined to mucosa without invading lamina propria); **T1** (tumor invades lamina propria or submucosa), **T2** (tumor invades muscularis propria or subserosa, and the tumor may even invade the gastrocolic or gastrohepatic ligaments or greater or lesser omentum so long as the visceral peritoneum [serosa] covering these structures is not perforated either grossly or microscopically); **T3** (tumor penetrates serosa, and may invade gastric ligaments or omenta with perforation of visceral peritoneum [serosa] covering these structures, but other adjacent structures are not invaded); **T4**: tumor penetrates serosa and invades adjacent structures (e.g. small intestine, transverse colon, pancreas, retroperitoneum, kidney, adrenals, diaphragm, spleen, liver, abdominal wall) or spreads intramurally to involve the esophagus or duodenum. Regional node involvement refers to involvement of left or right gastric, perigastric NOS, periesophageal, splenic, hepatic, or celiac nodes. Involvement of other nodes is categorized as distant disease (M1). **NX** (minimum requirements to assess regional nodes cannot be met); **N0** (nodes negative); **N1** (positive perigastric nodes < 3cm from edge of primary tumor); **N2** (positive perigastric nodes ≥ 3cm from edge of primary tumor, or positive nodes along left gastric, splenic, celiac, and common hepatic arteries). Distant metastasis: **MX** (minimum requirements to assess for distant metastasis cannot be met), **M0** (no known distant metastasis), **M1** (metastasis present).

Staging: Stage 0; Tis, N0, M0; Stage IA; T1, N0, M0; Stage IB; (Tl, Nl, M0) or (T2, N0, M0); Stage II; (T1, N2, M0) or (T2, N1, M0) or (T3, N0, M0); Stage IIIA; (T2, N2, M0) or (T3, N1, M0) or (T4, N0, M0); Stage IIIB; (T3, N2, M0) or (T4, N1, M0); Stage IV; (T4, N2, M0) or (any T, any N, M1).

Treatment: Stage 0; gastrectomy with lymphadenectomy. Stage I treatment consists of surgical resection including lymphadenectomy. If the cancer does not involve the stomach diffusely nor involve the cardioesophageal junction, radical distal subtotal gastrectomy is advised. If the cardia is involved, perform proximal subtotal gastrectomy or total gastrectomy (either procedure should include resection of a sufficient part of distal esophagus). If there is diffuse gastric involvement, total gastrectomy is indicated. Gastric resection procedures should at a minimum include resection of regional nodes, and the greater and lesser omentum. Stage II is treated similarly to stage I but with extended lymphadenectomy. If the tumor grossly or microscopically invades the serosa, the patient may also be included in clinical trials employing adjuvant chemotherapy and/or radiation. Stage III; Radical surgery is standard therapy. However, surgical resection is performed with curative intent only if nodal involvement is not found to be extensive at the time of surgery (the increased operative mortality makes palliative total gastrectomy inadvisable). All newly diagnosed stage III patients may also be considered for inclusion in clinical trials. In particular, clinical trials employing adjuvant chemotherapy and/or radiation are suitable in stage III cases in which there is gross or microscopic invasion of the serosa. Stage IV may be treated with palliative combination chemotherapy or (if feasible) by surgical resection. The latter generally prolongs life more than other measures, and precludes obstruction and bleeding. Endoscopic destruction may be used to relieve obstruction by a tumor blocking the gastric inlet. Palliative combination chemotherapy options include FAM (fluorouracil + doxorubicin + mitomycin C), FAP (fluorouracil + doxorubicin + cisplatin). In a recent trial, EAP (etoposide + doxorubicin + cisplatin) produced a response in over half the cases, and the tumor may even regress sufficiently to make a previously demonstrated stage IV (T4, N3) patient a candidate for surgical resection with curative intent. All newly diagnosed stage IV patients should be considered for inclusion in a clinical trial if possible.

Prognosis (5 yr survival with treatment): stage 0; > 90%, stage I; 52-85%, stage II (T1-T2, N1-N2, M0); > 20%, Stage II (T3, N0, M0); < 20%, stage III; 17%, stage IV; < 5%.

Colon Cancer in the U.S. is the 2nd most common cause of cancer death in men, and the third most common in women.

Risk factors include familial polyposis, Gardner's syndrome, Peutz–Jeghers syndrome, ulcerative colitis, immunodeficiency, history of female genital cancer, previous colon cancer, history of adenoma of colon (particularly villous adenoma). Patients with familial polyposis or Gardner's syndrome nearly all develop colon cancer by age 40; preemptive colectomy is therefore advised.

Geographic incidence: In general, the incidence of colon cancer is greatest in developed countries (Japan is an exception). Dietary factors are postulated to account for the difference; diets high in fiber and low in animal fats/protein are thought to exert a protective effect. Vitamin C and E may also be protective.

Signs/symptoms: Rectal tumors often present with bleeding, mucoid discharge, tenesmus, and/or feeling of incomplete evacuation. Most rectal tumors can be felt on digital exam. Tumors of the left colon, where the feces is semisolid and the lumen smaller than the right colon, tend to cause alterations in bowel habits and bowel obstruction. History of constipation, increased frequency of defecation, and/or small caliber stools may be elicited. There may be bright red or dark blood in the stool but bleeding is seldom severe. Symptoms of obstruction may develop—e.g. cramping abdominal pain, distension. The right colon has a large lumen and contains fluid feces. Consequently, obstructive symptoms with changes in bowel habits characteristic of tumors of the left colon are unusual. Instead, the diagnosis tends to be delayed until the patient presents with a palpable abdominal mass, pain, weight loss, and/or symptoms of anemia. Evidence of metastasis should be sought. ●The lymph nodes are the most common site of metastases. Examine the supraclavicular and inguinal regions carefully. ●Hematogenous spread to the liver via the portal circulation is the next most common site of metastasis. Check for hepatomegaly, distended veins on the abdomen (? portal obstruction). ●Other findings of metastasis may include enlarged ovaries, Blumer shelf (a shelf-like mass is felt on rectal exam). Vaginal and rectovaginal exam is important.

Laboratory: CBC (iron deficiency anemia is common), alkaline phosphatase, SGOT, bilirubin, calcium, creatinine. Serum carcinoembryonic antigen (CEA) is elevated in many cases but it is not specific. However, CEA may be useful in detecting cancer recurrence following surgery.

Diagnosis: Hemoccult testing of stool is a valuable screening method. Rectal exam: From 10 to 15% colon tumors may be palpable on digital rectal exam. Proctosigmoidoscopy will reach as many as 50% colon tumors. Double-contrast barium enema is ordered. It is ordered even if rectal or sigmoidoscopic exam is positive because it must be determined if there are more proximal synchronous tumors. However, caution must be exercised in the presence of a distal tumor because an overly aggressive barium enema may cause perforation. Upper GI series is contraindicated because this may precipitate bowel obstruction. Fiberoptic colonoscopy is indicated (1) if barium exam is equivocal or if there is lingering suspicion, and (2) to obtain biopsy specimen of lesions not within reach of proctosigmoidoscope. Chest x-ray is obtained to rule out lung metastasis.

Note: The following information is extracted from National Cancer Institute PDQ State-of-the-Art Cancer Treatment Information 12/3/90. However, since cancer treatment is evolving, this information may not be current. The most up-to-date standard treatment options may be obtained by calling the National Cancer Institute Cancer Information Service at 1–800–4–CANCER. Patients may also be candidates for clinical trials of new therapeutic regimens. Descriptions of these trials are also available.

Dukes staging: Dukes A (tumor confined to bowel wall); Dukes B (thru entire bowel wall to adjacent tissues, nodes negative); Dukes C (regional nodes positive); Dukes D (distant metastases or extensive local spread precluding surgical resection).

TNM definitions: Primary tumor: TX: minimum requirements to assess primary tumor cannot be met, TO: no evidence of primary tumor, Tis: carcinoma in situ, T1: tumor invades submucosa, T2: tumor invades muscularis propria, T3: tumor penetrates muscularis propria to invade subserosa or nonperitonealized pericolic tissues, T4: tumor perforates visceral peritoneum, or directly invades other organs or structures. Invasion of other segments of colon/rectum by way of serosa counts as a direct invasion of other organ or structure. Regional lymph nodes: NX: minimum requirements to assess regional nodes cannot be met, N0: regional lymph node metastases absent, N1: metastases to 1–3 pericolic lymph nodes, N2: metastases to 4 or more pericolic nodes, N3: metastases to any lymph node along course of a named vascular trunk. Distant Metastasis: MX: minimum requirements to assess for distant metastasis cannot be met, M0: distant metastasis absent, M1: distant metastasis present.

Staging: Stage 0; carcinoma in situ (Tis, N0, M0); Stage I; T1–T2, N0, M0; Stage II; T3–T4, N0, M0; Stage III; any T, N1–N3, M0; Stage IV; any T, any N, M1.

Treatment: Stage 0 (tumor confined to mucosa without invasion of lamina propria): (1) local resection or simple polypectomy, (2) wedge resection for larger lesions that cannot be resected by local excision. Stage I or Dukes A; wide resection and anastomosis. Stage II or Dukes B; wide resection and anastomosis. Cases in which there is tumor adherence/fixation to adjacent structures, perforation, and/or obstruction are considered for adjuvant therapy. For instance, postoperative radiotherapy may improve local control if there is tumor adherence/fixation to adjacent structures. Patient may be considered for inclusion in a clinical trial (e.g. postoperative chemotherapy or radiotherapy, biological therapy). Stage III or Dukes C; Standard therapy is wide resection and anastomosis plus postoperative chemotherapy, preferably as part of a clinical trial. Postoperative treatment with fluorouracil/levamisole should be considered if the patient is not a trial candidate. A variety of clinical trials are underway (e.g. adjuvant chemotherapy, radiotherapy, biological therapy). Stage IV patients may require palliative surgery (e.g. for obstruction, bleeding, perforation) and/or may benefit from palliative radiotherapy and/or chemotherapy. Resection of isolated metastases (liver, lung, ovaries) may be considered. Inclusion in a clinical trial employing biological or chemotherapy regimen is also a possibility.

Prognosis (5 yr survival with treatment): stage 0; > 95%, stage I; 75–100%, stage II; 50–75%, stage III; 30–50%, stage IV; less than 10%.

Rectal Cancer

For other than treatment information, refer to the applicable "Colon Cancer" chapter above.

Note: The following information is extracted from National Cancer Institute PDQ State-of-the-Art Cancer Treatment Information 9/28/90. However, since cancer treatment is evolving, this information may not be current. The most up-to-date standard treatment options may be obtained by calling the National Cancer Institute Cancer Information Service at 1–800–4–CANCER. Patients may be candidates for inclusion in clinical trials. Descriptions of these trials are also available.

Treatment:

Stage 0 (tumor confined to mucosa without invasion of lamina propria): (1) local resection or simple polypectomy, (2) wedge resection for larger lesions that cannot be resected by local excision.

Stage I standard options are: (1) wide surgical resection——with anastomosis if adequate resection leaves sufficient distal rectum, (2) wide surgical resection with abdominoperineal resection. Selected patients may be candidates for endocavitary radiation, electrofulguration, or local transanal resection.

Stage II and III standard options are: (1) wide surgical resection with anastomosis if feasible followed by chemotherapy and radiation, preferably as part of a clinical trial; (2) wide surgical resection with abdominoperineal resection plus adjuvant chemotherapy and postoperative radiation, preferably as part of a clinical trial; (3) preoperative radiation with surgery that attempts to preserve sphincter function followed by chemotherapy. Pelvic exenteration + chemotherapy + radiotherapy may be necessary if the bladder or prostate is invaded.

Stage IV options are: (1) palliative resection of primary tumor in selected cases with radiation of locally unresectable disease; (2) surgical resection of isolated metastases, (3) palliative systemic chemotherapy.

Liver Tumors

METASTATIC MALIGNANCY accounts for the great majority of cases of malignant liver tumors in the U.S. Cancer of the lung, colon, pancreas, stomach, melanoma, and lymphoma frequently metastasize to the liver.

HEPATOCELLULAR CARCINOMA is uncommon in the U.S. and Europe. However, it is very common in some regions of Africa and the Orient—regions where there is high incidence of hepatitis B infection.

Risk factors: (**1**) chronic hepatitis B infection; (**2**) cirrhosis (50–85% patients with hepatocellular carcinoma have cirrhosis. Risk is greatest in those patients with cirrhosis resulting from chronic active hepatitis B or hemochromatosis, and less so for alcoholic cirrhosis.); (**3**) male sex (males outnumber females by at least 4 to 1); (**4**) chronic ingestion of foods containing aflatoxins (e.g. grains contaminated by the mold Aspergillus flavus) is suspected of increasing the risk .

Signs/symptoms may include epigastric or right upper quadrant pain and/or mass, hepatomegaly, obstructive jaundice, arterial bruit and/or friction rub heard over the liver. **Possible complications include:** bloody ascites, liver failure, rupture into the peritoneum with hemorrhagic shock, portal hypertension. The latter may be associated with splenomegaly or lead to varices with GI bleeding.

Diagnosis: Serum alkaline phosphatase and bilirubin are often elevated. Serum alpha–fetoprotein elevated in 50–70% U.S. cases. However, alphafetoprotein may also be elevated in certain other malignancies—e.g. testicular tumor. Uncommon laboratory findings: erythrocytosis, hypercalcemia, hypoglycemia, elevated serum cholesterol, porphyria, dysfibrinogenemia. Liver scan, ultrasound, CAT scan (with contrast media), and arteriography are the choice of tests that may be used to diagnose and locate the tumor. Biopsy may also be employed but there is a risk of serious bleeding.

Note: The following treatment information is extracted from National Cancer Institute PDQ State-of-the-Art Cancer Treatment Information 9/28/90. However, since cancer treatment is evolving, this information may not be current. The most up-to-date standard treatment options may be obtained by calling the National Cancer Institute Cancer Information Service at 1–800–4–CANCER.

Treatment hepatocellular carcinoma: Localized resectable tumor; Surgical resection is the treatment of choice. However, because of high mortality, generally no more than a wedge resection is usually attempted in patients with cirrhosis or chronic active hepatitis. Because the incidence of relapse following surgical resection is high, patients may be considered for inclusion in clinical trials of adjuvant therapy (e.g. systemic chemotherapy or regional arterial infusion chemotherapy). If the tumor is not resectable, the patient should be included in a clinical trial (e.g. systemic chemotherapy, hepatic artery infusion chemotherapy, radiosensitizers, external beam radiation, surgical resection of dominant liver mass + radiotherapy and chemotherapy). **Childhood liver cancer** is rare. All patients should be considered for inclusion in a clinical trial. The tumor is resected if possible and this is followed by systemic combination chemotherapy. If the tumor is unresectable, chemotherapy and radiotherapy may render the tumor amenable to subsequent surgical resection. Other regimens undergoing evaluation as part of clinical trials include adjuvant iodine 131 antiferritin, nonoperative arterial embolization, various systemic combination chemotherapy regimens, intrahepatic arterial infusion chemotherapy.

OTHER PRIMARY MALIGNANT LIVER TUMORS are uncommon or rare—e.g. cholangiocarcinoma (the 2nd most common after hepatocellular carcinoma), mixed hepatocellular cholangiocarcinoma, cystadenocarcinoma, angiosarcoma, squamous carcinoma.

BENIGN TUMORS

Hepatocellular adenoma is virtually restricted to women and most cases are associated with oral contraceptives. Most adenomas are solitary. Malignant degeneration rarely if ever occurs. <u>Signs/symptoms:</u> Many cases are asymptomatic. In symptomatic patients, there is pain in the right upper quadrant and frequently there is a palpable liver mass. <u>Tests:</u> Liver scan may show a focal defect. Angiography may also reveal the tumor but may not distinguish it from a malignant hepatoma. However, serum alpha–fetoprotein level is usually normal with benign adenomas. <u>Treatment:</u> Sometimes there is acute onset of right upper quadrant pain with rupture into the peritoneum. Emergency surgery is required because hemorrhagic shock may ensue. Because of the risk of rupture, surgery is also advised for less urgent symptomatic cases and also for asymptomatic patients. In the asymptomatic patient on oral contraceptives, the adenoma may sometimes regress spontaneously upon discontinuation of the pills. In this case, therefore, one may elect to discontinue the pills and follow the patient with periodic liver scans.

Hemangioma is the most common benign liver tumor. It is more common in women. Most are asymptomatic, small, and solitary. With larger tumors there may be a palpable mass or abdominal pain. Sometimes rupture with hemorrhage occurs. Angiography or CAT scan with contrast is diagnostic. Symptomatic hemangiomas are resected. Asymptomatic tumors are not biopsied or resected because of the risk of provoking uncontrollable bleeding.

Focal nodular hyperplasia is a benign tumor without malignant potential. It is more common in women. In contrast to hepatocellular adenoma, it is not associated with oral contraceptives, it is usually asymptomatic, and it seldom hemorrhages.

Other uncommon benign liver tumors include bile duct adenomas, fibromas, leiomyoma, lipoma.

Neurology

Coma

Coma is said to be present when a patient cannot be aroused. **For coma to be present at least one of the following conditions must be met: (1)** lesion of that part of the reticular activating system located in the pons-midbrain-diencephalon **(2)** impairment of both cerebral hemispheres (e.g. extensive bilateral cerebral infarct), **(3)** diffuse CNS impairment (e.g. toxic or metabolic derangement). ●Lesions of the spinal cord or medulla alone do not cause coma. Neither does an unilateral cerebral hemisphere lesion result in coma unless its presence affects the brainstem or contralateral hemisphere. For instance, a patient with an uncomplicated stroke of one cerebral hemisphere is not rendered comatose. However, a patient with an expanding epidural or subdural hematoma may become comatose if pressure is exerted on the opposite cerebral hemisphere and/or on the brainstem. A posterior fossa lesion can similarly cause coma if it compresses the brainstem. **Structural lesions causing coma** are divided into <u>supratentorial lesions</u> (e.g. epidural or subdural hematoma, cerebral hemorrhage or infarct, brain tumor or abscess) and <u>subtentorial lesions</u> (e.g. brainstem trauma/infarct/hemorrhage/tumor, cerebellar hemorrhage/tumor). **Other causes of coma** include uremia, hepatic coma, hyper or hypoglycemia, hyper or hyponatremia, hyper or hypokalemia, hyper or hypocalcemia, acidosis or alkalosis, hyper or hypotension, myxedema, Addison's disease, Wernicke's encephalopathy, alcohol or drug overdose, meningitis, encephalitis.

Initial treatment of coma and diagnostic tests: <u>Airway and ventilation</u> must be assured. <u>Immobilize cervical spine</u> if there is any possibility of head or neck injury. <u>Establish IV immediately</u> and treat hypotension as clinical circumstances dictate. <u>Administer glucose</u> immediately after drawing blood sample for blood glucose in case hypoglycemia is the cause of coma: 50 ml of 50% (25 gram) dextrose IV push in adult (0.5–1.0 gram/kg in child). <u>Thiamine</u> 50–100 mg IV is also given if alcoholism is suspected. Otherwise the glucose infusion could induce Wernicke's encephalopathy. <u>Naloxone</u> 0.4 mg IV is administered in suspected drug overdose in order to reverse the effects of opiates. Dose may be repeated at 5 minute intervals as needed. <u>Laboratory:</u> blood glucose, electrolytes, BUN, creatinine, calcium, CBC, prothrombin time, partial thromboplastin time, alcohol, arterial blood gas and urinalysis. <u>Additional tests</u> as circumstances dictate: EKG, CAT scan, blood and urine toxicology screen, lumbar puncture, chest x-ray.

Assessment of coma: <u>History</u> of diabetes, seizures, alcoholism, drug addiction, trauma, cardiac disease ? <u>Movement of extremities:</u> Is there movement ? Is it spontaneous or only in response to painful stimuli ? Is there movement of all extremities and is it symmetrical ? Is there decorticate or decerebrate posturing ? <u>Reflexes:</u> Are deep tendon relflexes present and are they symmetrical ? Is there a Babinski reflex ? Assess pupillary and corneal reflexes (see below). <u>Response to stimuli:</u> Responds to verbal stimulus, to painful stimulus, or not at all? <u>Breath:</u> Smell of alcohol, acetone, etc ? <u>Signs of elevated intracranial pressure:</u> papilledema ?, slowed pulse or respirations ? <u>Signs of head trauma;</u> hemotympanum, Battle sign, CSF leakage from ears or nose ? <u>Respiratory pattern:</u> see below. <u>Eyes:</u> pupils (see below), eye movements (see below), corneal reflex (see below). <u>Fever</u> ? <u>Hypo- or hypertension</u> ?

Assessment of pupils: The pupillary light reflex is mediated by a pathway that leads from the retina via the optic nerve and optic tract to the midbrain and thence from the midbrain to the iris via the 3rd cranial nerves. The presence, therefore, of pupils that react to light is indicative of a functioning midbrain and 3rd cranial nerves. <u>Midposition pupils that do not react to light</u> indicates midbrain injury. The pupils may spontaneously constrict or dilate however. <u>Unilateral fixed and dilated pupil</u> indicates involvement of the 3rd cranial nerve. A space-occupying lesion is most likely displacing the ipsilateral temporal lobe so that the inferomedial segment (the uncus) herniates over the tentorium and compresses the ipsilateral 3rd cranial nerve. <u>Pinpoint pupils that react to light</u> may indicate injury to the pons or diencephalon. Drugs such as opiates, pilocarpine, anticholinesterases (e.g. physostigmine, neostigmine, organophosphates) or metabolic derangements may also provoke miosis. <u>Dilated pupils that do not react to light</u> may be due to anoxia, anticholinergics (e.g. atropine, scopolamine); glutethimide (Doriden). <u>Metabolic derangements</u> generally do not eliminate pupillary reactivity although the pupils may react sluggishly. Anoxia and certain drugs such as those just mentioned that dilate the pupils are exceptions.

Corneal reflex: Touching the cornea with a wisp of cotton will normally cause the eyelids to close. The sensory component of this reflex arc is carried by the ophthalmic division of the 5th cranial nerve while the motor component of the 7th cranial nerve mediates closure of the eyelid.

Eye movements in a comatose patient may yield information on the integrity of the brainstem and may indicate the possible location of a CNS lesion. <u>Deviation of the eyes:</u> The eyes may deviate laterally ("point") to the side of a destructive cerebral lesion or away from an irritative cerebral lesion. Thalamic or upper midbrain lesions may result in downward deviation of the eyes. <u>Oculocephalic reflexes</u> (doll's eye movement): If the brainstem is intact, rapidly turning the head of a comatose patient to one side is accompanied by conjugate movement of the eyes in the opposite direction. Of course, this maneuver should not be attempted if there is any question of injury to the cervical spine. <u>Oculovestibular reflex</u> (ice-water caloric test): If the ear of an alert patient is irrigated with ice water, horizontal nystagmus will be elicited with the slow component directed toward the irrigated ear. If the brainstem is intact, the fast component is progressively lost with deteriorating level of consciousness; and with deep coma, the eyes remain conjugately deviated toward the irrigated ear. When performing this test, the patient should be inclined with the head end 30° to the horizontal and the ear should be checked to see that the tympanic membrane is intact. In deep coma, both the oculocephalic and oculovestibular reflexes may be absent.

Respiratory pattern: <u>Cheyne-Stokes respiration</u> (periodic breathing) is characterized by a gradual increase in the depth of respirations followed by gradually shallower breathing leading to an apneic interval; cycle then starts over again. This can occur with metabolic disorders (e.g. uremia), a diencephalic lesion, dysfunction of both cerebral hemispheres, or congestive heart failure; or in a normal person at high altitude. The presence of Cheyne-Stokes respirations means that the brainstem is intact. <u>Central neurogenic hyperventilation</u> (respirations are deep and rapid) is associated with lesions of the midbrain and upper pons. Rapid deep breathing is also seen with hypoxia or metabolic acidosis. <u>Apneustic breathing</u> (inspiratory gasping alternating with expiratory hiatus) is seen with lesions of the lower pons. <u>Ataxic breathing</u> (irregular breathing) is associated with lesions of the medulla.

Posture: <u>Decorticate rigidity</u> (arms *flexed* at the elbow, legs extended and plantar-flexed) is due to lesions affecting the motor pathways above the midbrain (i.e. cerebral white matter, internal capsule, thalamus). <u>Decerebrate rigidity</u> (arms *extended* at elbow and internally rotated, legs extended and plantar-flexed) may result from a specific lesion of the midbrain but is usually seen with transtentorial herniation. Metabolic disturbances may also be responsible. In some comatose patients, a provocative stimulus such as sternal pressure may be needed to elicit these postures.

Elevated Intracranial Pressure

Causes: intracranial masses (tumor, abscess, hematoma, parasites); spinal cord tumor; obstruction of CSF outflow with ensuing hydrocephalus; subarachnoid or intracerebral bleeding; brain infarction; meningitis; encephalitis; infectious polyneuritis (Guillain-Barré syndrome); jugular venous obstruction; cerebral or jugular venous occlusion; anoxia; hypercapnia; COPD; CHF; pericardial effusion; Reye's syndrome; pseudotumor cerebri (see below for discussion of latter).

CSF pressure is normally 65-195 mm H_2O. This is the pressure that would normally be obtained by lumbar puncture with the patient lying flat, or measured from the level of the foramen magnum if the patient is sitting. Remember, however, that the lumbar pressure may not be elevated despite elevated intracranial pressure if there is proximal CSF obstruction (e.g. noncommunicating hydrocephalus).

Signs/symptoms: <u>History</u>: headache? lethargy? personality change? confusion? altered level consciousness? nausea? vomiting? If there is vomiting, is it projectile? <u>Headache:</u> Elevated intracranial pressure–associated headache is often aggravated by straining or coughing. It is frequently worse when lying down and therefore worse in the morning and alleviated by upright position. The quality of the headache is not a dependable diagnostic feature: in some cases there is a deep dull nonpulsatile headache while others report a throbbing pain. Headache may be generalized or local. Headaches that have become progressively worse and more frequent, especially in a patient who is not prone to headaches, is a clue that there may be an expanding intracranial lesion. Headache is absent in some cases. <u>Papilledema</u> is a characteristic sign but is not always present. Furthermore, papilledema may occur in the absence of elevated intracranial pressure. The finding of retinal venous pulsastions indicates that the intracranial pressure is normal or only mildly increased. <u>6th nerve palsy with diplopia</u> may occur. <u>Systolic hypertension, bradycardia, and slowed respirations</u> may appear. <u>With pressure from an unilateral supratentorial mass,</u> the ipsilateral uncus may herniate across the tentorium and compress the ipsilateral 3rd cranial nerve so that ipsilateral pupil dilation results. Contralateral hemiplegia commonly follows. With further increase in pressure, ipsilateral hemiplegia develops as well. Central neurogenic hyperventilation as well as decerebrate posturing may ensue. Eventually there is ataxic breathing, bilateral dilated pupils, and negative response to Doll's eye maneuver or calorics. <u>When increased intracranial pressure is not exerted from one side</u> as just described, lateralizing signs are generally absent. However, pressure exerted against the brainstem may provoke decreased level of consciousness, aberrations in respiratory pattern, eventual dilation of both pupils, bilateral Babinski reflex, decorticate and then decerebrate posturing, and negative response to Doll's eye maneuver or calorics. <u>Additional signs in infants and children may include</u> abnormal increase in head circumference, delay in closure of anterior fontanelle beyond 18 months of age, separation of cranial sutures, skull that transilluminates (e.g. hydrocephalus, subdural fluid, cyst). Note that when the sutures are open, papilledema is usually absent despite elevated intracranial pressure.

Laboratory: Clinical circumstances dictate the approach. CAT scan is usually obtained. Lumbar puncture is generally contraindicated.

Treatment: Treat underlying disorder if possible. **In emergencies** with worsening neurologic status, the following temporizing measures may need to be employed to reduce intracranial pressure: (**1**) <u>Intubate, and hyperventilate</u> to maintain the pCO_2 between 30 and no less than 25mm Hg. Reducing the CO_2 reduces intracranial pressure by decreasing cerebral blood flow. (**2**) <u>Osmotic diuresis:</u> IV mannitol is frequently used in urgent cases because of its rapid effect (see mannitol in drug section). Glycerol has slower onset but it is safer, can be used for longer periods, and can be administered PO or IV. (**3**) <u>Dexamethasone</u> 10 mg IV initially followed by 4 mg at 6 hour intervals IV, IM, or PO.

PSEUDOTUMOR CEREBRI (benign intracranial hypertension) is the condition in which an alert patient presents with elevated intracranial pressure in the absence of intracranial masses, hydrocephalus, or CSF abnormalities. Most patients are obese females of reproductive age. **Causes:** Most cases are idiopathic. A variety of conditions have been implicated—e.g. pregnancy, menarche, oral contraceptives, head trauma, cerebral venous sinus obstruction, hypoparathyroidism, Addison's disease, prolonged corticosteroid administration, corticosteroid withdrawal, hyper or hypovitaminosis A, tetracycline, sulfonamides, phenothiazines. **Signs/symptoms:** ●Bilateral papilledema is nearly always found. ●Patients may be asymptomatic or develop any of the following: headache, nausea, vomiting, vertigo, orbital pain, diplopia, decreased visual acuity, blurred vision, scotomas. **Tests:** Lumbar puncture is performed to verify that the CSF pressure is elevated <u>but only after</u> obtaining a CAT scan or NMR scan to exclude dilated ventricles or an intracranial space-occupying lesion. **Treatment** consists of elimination of possible inciting factors. Specific treatment is controversial since spontaneous remissions are common. In order to protect against visual impairment, some authorities will advocate lowering the intracranial pressure with diuretics (e.g. furosemide, acetazolamide) and/or removal of CSF fluid with weekly lumbar puncture. Sometimes, as a last resort, a ventricular shunt is introduced.

Seizures and Epilepsy

Seizure is a paroxysmal depolarization of a group of neurons that results in involuntary motor activity, abnormal sensation, abnormal behavior, and/or altered consciousness. **Epilepsy** is said to be present when seizures recur chronically. A patient may have one or even a few seizures without being an epileptic. For instance, a patient undergoing a seizure simply because of a temporary condition such as hypoglycemia does not have epilepsy. Epilepsy affects 0.5–2.0% general population. About 30% have more than one type of epilepsy.

SEIZURE WORK-UP: Age considerations: Convulsions occuring before the age of 2 yr are most often due to infection (e.g. fever, meningitis); congenital/developmental abnormalities; trauma; birth injury; metabolic derangements. Idiopathic epilepsy (e.g. petit mal, some grand mal) usually appears by 18 years of age. Stroke–provoked seizures are primarily seen from middle age on. Neoplasia–induced seizures are most common in adults as are alcohol and drug-related seizures. **History:** Birth trauma? Head trauma resulting in loss of consciousness, especially within the last 2 years? Stroke history? Meningitis or other CNS infection? Drug or alcohol history? Diabetes or other metabolic disease? Family history of epilepsy? **Obtain a description of the seizure if possible:** focal signs, incontinence, tonic-clonic activity, loss of consciousness? Was there a premonitory aura? Was there postictal confusion and lethargy after regaining consciousness? Was there actually a convulsion or merely syncope? **Physical exam:** Hypertension? Incontinence? Tongue bite? Neck bruits? Stiff neck—suggesting meningitis or subarachnoid hemorrhage? Are there any focal signs either during the seizure or subsequently—e.g. Todd's paralysis (temporary postictal paralysis) or other lateralizing signs (e.g. positive Babinski, asymmetrical reflexes)? **Laboratory:** Obtain appropriate tests as circumstances suggest—e.g. serum glucose, serum electrolytes, serum calcium, BUN, CBC, urinalysis, lumbar puncture, EEG, CAT scan, EKG, chest x-ray, toxicology screen, serum anticonvulsant level (if anticonvulsants have been prescribed).

PRIMARY GENERALIZED SEIZURES:

Primary (idiopathic) generalized epilepsy may manifest as a tonic or tonic-clonic (grand mal) convulsion. There is immediate loss of consciousness and focal clinical signs are not observed prior to, during, or after the seizure. While it is true that a patient with primary (idiopathic) generalized convulsive epilepsy does not experience a premonitory aura, there may be an "epigastric rising" feeling as the convulsion begins. Furthermore, in some cases, there is a foreboding (e.g. uneasiness, poor appetite, difficulty sleeping) or the patient may experience myoclonic episodes prior to the seizure. See Grand Mal Seizure below for description and treatment of grand mal. ●NOTE: (**1**) Generalized convulsions are more often an expression of focal epilepsy with secondary generalization (see Focal Seizures below). (**2**) Even when closely observed, it is not always possible to discern whether a generalized convulsion is focal (partial) with secondary generalization or primary generalized. (**3**) Generalized convulsions often occur in nonepileptics (see Convulsions in Nonepileptics below).

Petit mal epilepsy is associated with absence seizures. There is a brief loss of consciousness (generally < 10 seconds) wherein the patient abruptly stops what he is doing. There may be flickering of the eyelids, movements of the mouth, generalized jerking movements. During an attack, the EEG typically reveals a generalized symmetrical regular 3 cycle/sec spike-and-wave pattern. Following the attack, the patient becomes immediately alert and the EEG simultaneously reverts to normal. Many episodes may occur each day in some cases. Hyperventilating for 1–3 minutes may sometimes induce an absence attack. Onset of petit mal epilepsy is usually between 2 and 12 years, and petit mal usually disappears by age 20.

Atypical absence seizures differ from the classic petit mal type in that the absence attacks often last longer than 10 seconds and there may be postictal confusion with persistent postictal or interictal EEG abnormalities. Furthermore, the EEG lacks the symmetrical and regular pattern seen in classic petit mal. Lennox-Gastaut syndrome is an example of an epileptic disorder that is associated with atypical absence seizures. These patients may evince other neurologic stigmata including mental retardation and other kinds of generalized seizures.

Juvenile (bilateral) epileptic myoclonus is an uncommon childhood syndrome associated with repetitive bilateral symmetrical myoclonic jerks, particularly of the arms and shoulders.

Akinetic seizures (drop attacks) are generalized seizures occuring in children. There is a brief loss of consciousness associated with a loss of postural muscle tone so that the child falls to the ground.

Infantile spasms occur in children ≤ 3 yr and are usually associated with brain damage. There may be facial twitching or generalized spasms (e.g. brief flexion of the arms and trunk with extension of the legs).

Progressive myoclonic epilepsy refers to an assortment of degenerative brain syndromes associated with myoclonic and other convulsive manifestations as well as progressive neurologic and mental impairment.

FOCAL (PARTIAL) SEIZURES are initiated by depolarization of neurons within a localized area of one cerebral hemisphere. The focal cerebral abnormality responsible for inducing the seizure(s) may be idiopathic or due to an identifiable brain insult (e.g. trauma, tumor, infarct, hemorrhage). Focal (or nonfocal) seizures can also occur in patients without a specific CNS abnormality—e.g. hypoglycemia, alcohol or sedative drug withdrawal (see below Convulsions in Nonepileptics). Focal neurologic signs depend on the area of the brain affected—e.g. muscle twitching of a region on one side of the body (motor cortex of the contralateral frontal lobe), local numbness/tingling (sensory cortex of contralateral parietal lobe), chewing or lip smacking (anterior temporal lobe), olfactory hallucination (posterior temporal lobe), vivid scenes (temporal lobe), flashing lights on one side of visual field (contralateral occipital lobe).

Simple partial seizure is a focal seizure that remains confined to a discrete region of the cortex, and therefore results in a localized sensory or motor disturbance such as one of those just described. Furthermore, the level of consciousness is not altered.

Complex partial seizure is said to be present if the abnormal discharge spreads so that other signs and symptoms appear and/or there is loss of consciousness. The initial focal (partial) symptoms are called the aura. Jacksonian seizure is an example ot a complex partial seizure originating from the motor cortex. It often starts with a twitching on one side of the face, or hand or foot. As the abnormal discharge spreads, clonic movements progress (e.g. "march" up an extremity and subsequently involve one side of the body). The head and eyes may tonically turn to one side. In many cases, seizure activity spreads to the other hemisphere whereupon the patient becomes unconscious and a generalized tonic-clonic (grand mal) convulsion ensues. Even when closely observed, it is not always possible to discern whether a generalized convulsion is focal (partial) with secondary generalization or primary generalized. This is because a focal motor seizure may spread rapidly to the diencephalon (or emanate from a "silent" area of the brain) so that a grand mal convulsion supervenes without an antecedent aura. The patient's postictal exam may provide clues that the seizure was focal in origin—e.g. transient postictal (Todd's) paralysis, aphasia, asymmetrical reflexes, asymmetrical Babinski. Signs of focality should be assiduously sought because focal seizures may reflect a correctible underlying brain lesion. An EEG may establish the focal origin of the seizures and other tests (e.g. CAT scan) may possibly identify the lesion.

Psychomotor epilepsy (temporal lobe epilepsy) is a type of complex partial (focal) epilepsy characterized by purposeless movements ("automatisms")—e.g. chewing, lip smacking/licking, head turning. There may be tonic spasm of the extremities. The patient may stagger, utter unintelligble sounds, and some patients become violent. The seizure may be preceded by hallucinations of taste, smell, or vision. During an attack the patient is confused and does not understand when spoken to. Confusion persists for a few minutes afterward and there is no recollection of the seizure.

GRAND MAL (TONIC-CLONIC) SEIZURES may be the consequence of (1) primary (idiopathic) generalized epileptic disorder, (2) focal epileptic disorder with secondary generalization, or (3) convulsion-provoking conditions in a nonepileptic person.

Signs/symptoms of grand mal: There is loss of consciousness and a brief generalized muscular spasm (tonic phase) followed by generalized jerking movements (clonic phase). There may be urinary or fecal incontinence, tongue biting, cyanosis. The patient remains unconscious for several minutes following the seizure. After regaining consciousness, the patient is usually confused, sleepy, and may complain of a headache and muscle soreness. If the grand mal is focal in origin there may be an antecedent aura with focal signs as the seizure develops and/or postictal signs (see Focal Seizures above). **Grand mal status epilepticus** is defined as a generalized tonic-clonic convulsion lasting longer than 15 minutes, or repetitive tonic-clonic convulsions between which the patient does not regain consciousness. Note that the term status epilepticus (continual or rapidly repetitive seizures) does not just refer to *grand mal* status epilepticus. Other examples of status epilepticus are petit mal status, partial (focal) motor status, partial complex status.

Treatment grand mal (see drug section for dose of individual drugs): Assure airway, establish IV, and obtain blood for tests (glucose, electrolytes including calcium). Administer IV dextrose (50 ml of 50% dextrose in adult, 1ml/kg of 50% dextrose in child, 2 ml/kg of 25% dextrose in infant). Next administer IV diazepam: In adult, administer 5 mg/minute until seizure stops or until maximum of 20 mg is reached (see drug section for pediatric dose). Diazepam may stop seizure but will not prevent recurrence. IV phenytoin (see drug section) is subsequently administered to prevent seizure recurrence and may be effective if diazepam has failed. IV phenobarbital is the drug of 3rd choice followed by paraldehyde. General anesthesia may be required in refractory cases. Treatment must of course be directed against and modified according to conditions that may have precipitated the convulsions—e.g. fever, electrolyte abnormalities, CNS infection, brain tumor, toxic or metabolic disturbances.

SEIZURE TREATMENT SUMMARY (see drug section for dose of individual drugs)**:** If a seizure is the consequence of an correctible condition (e.g. hypoglycemia, hypocalcemia, fever), treat that. If grand mal status epilepticus is present, see above.
Drug treatment guidelines: Start with a single drug. Do not add a 2nd drug until the maximum recommended dose of the first drug has been tried and a serum level has been checked to confirm adequate therapeutic level and compliance. Substitute another drug if one has proved ineffective. If a drug is partially effective, add a 2nd drug. To preclude exacerbating seizures, a drug should not be stopped suddenly unless serious side effects occur or the drug has failed to lessen the frequency of seizures.

Major motor epilepsy (generalized tonic-clonic) or **focal motor epilepsy:** Phenytoin or carbamazepine are the drugs of first choice. Phenobarbital or primidone are alternatives. (Phenobarbital is the drug of first choice in infants.) Primidone may be effective alone but is often used in conjunction with phenytoin if single agents have failed. Valproic acid is yet another possible option if other drugs have failed.

Complex partial epilepsy (e.g. psychomotor epilepsy): Phenytoin is usually the drug of first choice but carbamazepine (Tegretol) may be preferred in children. Phenytoin and primidone are usually tried in combination if single agents fail. Phenobarbital or primidone (Mysoline) are drugs of 2nd choice.

Petit mal epilepsy: Ethosuximide (Zarontin) is the drug of choice. Valproic acid is recommended if ethosuximide fails and is the drug of first choice if the patient is also afflicted with primary generalized tonic-clonic seizures. Clonazepam or trimethadione are alternatives if the foregoing drugs are ineffective. Patients undergoing petit mal status epilepticus are initially treated with IV diazepam. **Juvenile (bilateral) epileptic myoclonus** is treated in the same manner as petit mal.

CONVULSIONS IN NONEPILEPTICS may be provoked by a variety of conditions—e.g. alcohol or sedative withdrawal; fever; hypoglycemia; hypocalcemia; hyponatremia; uremia; stroke; head trauma; meningitis; encephalitis; cerebral hypoxia; eclampsia; hypertensive encephalopathy; overdose certain drugs (e.g. phenothiazines, tricyclic antidepressants, amphetamines). ●The patient may have one or several seizures without being classified as an epileptic. However, some of the foregoing precipitants (e.g. head trauma, stroke, meningitis) may cause brain scarring and consequently lead to chronic recurrent seizures (i.e. epilepsy). ●Nonepileptic convulsions may be focal or nonfocal.

Febrile seizures in children: About 4% children will have a febrile seizure by the age of 7. The temperature should be reduced quickly by sponging with tepid water, and acetaminophen administered. Ongoing seizure is treated with IV phenobarbital. Lumbar puncture to rule out meningitis should be performed (unless there is evidence of increased intracranial pressure) if any of the following prevail: (**1**) child is ≤ 2 years of age, (**2**) there is clinical evidence of meningitis, (**3**) seizure lasts > 15 minutes, (**4**) there are focal neurologic findings. Phenobarbital to prevent recurrence of febrile seizures is *not* indicated unless: (**1**) seizure lasts over 15 minutes, (**2**) seizure is focal, (**3**) there are post-seizure neurologic abnormalities, (**4**) there is family history of nonfebrile seizures. Phenobarbital is continued for at least 2 years and then slowly withdrawn over 1–2 months.

Headache (cephalalgia)

TENSION HEADACHE (muscle contraction headache) presumably results from prolonged contraction of the scalp or neck muscles. Depression may be a factor. **Signs/symptoms:** Headache is usually bilateral and most often arises in the occipital or bifrontal region. In many cases headache then spreads to involve entire scalp in a "tight band". Pain is typically constant with a dull non-throbbing pressure-like quality. There may be tenderness of scalp and posterior neck muscles. Headaches tend to occur during times of stress, and usually start or become more severe toward the end of the day. Headache may in some cases last for days or weeks. **Treatment:** Relief of stress, massage, and aspirin or its equivalent are usually adequate treatment. If headaches are frequent or unrelenting, an antidepressant (e.g. amitriptyline) may be prescribed if depression is implicated or a benzodiazepine (e.g. diazepam) may be tried if the headaches are related to anxiety. Regular exercise, good sleeping habits, adequate nutrition, and avoidance of alcohol or stimulants may all be helpful in reducing the frequency of headaches.

MIGRAINES are vascular headaches; the headaches are attributed to dilation of arteries in the distribution of the carotid arteries. Dilation incites nerve endings attached to those arteries. **Types of migraine:** Common migraine accounts for about 90% of migraines; about 10% are classic migraines. Both types may occur in the same patient. Unusual types of migraine include basilar migraines, ophthalmoplegic migraine, and hemiplegic migraine.

Common migraine may appear without warning, or the headache may develop slowly preceded by psychic abnormalities or GI complaints. The common migraine tends to last longer than the classic migraine, sometimes many hours or even days. The headache can affect either side; it can also begin on one side and become bilateral or vice versa. Nausea, vomiting, and light sensitivity commonly accompany the headache. Possible precipitants of common migraine are fatigue, excessive sleep, tension or relief of tension, hunger, alcohol, foods containing vasoactive substances (chocolate, certain cheeses, red wine); estrogens (including birth control pills); reserpine; nitroglycerin; menstruation; high altitude. Other distinguishing characteristics of common migraine: Common migraines are more common in females. There is usually a family history. They can start at any age but typically begin in the teens, become less frequent after 30, and sometimes remit after 50. Menopause may be associated with aggravation or mitigation of migraines.

Classic migraine differs from common migraine in that there is a clearly defined prodrome (aura) that typically lasts a few minutes to half an hour. The aura (attributed to intracerebral vasoconstriction with neurologic consequences) usually consists of homonymous visual effects (e.g. flashing lights, zigzag lines, scotomas). Uncommon auras include hemianopsia, impaired speech, unilateral paresthesias or sensory impairment, or unilateral weakness. Typically as the aura disappears, an unilateral throbbing headache (presumably due to dilation of cranial arteries) emerges that is contralateral to the side of the neurologic prodromal symptoms. In some cases, the aura continues with the headache. Pain is usually felt over the frontotemporal area and ranges from mild to severe. Untreated the headache usually lasts 4-6 hours, although it may persist for days in unusual cases. Autonomic signs (e.g. nausea, vomiting, diarrhea, sweating, pallor, coldness) often accompany the migraine. Vomiting often mitigates the headache and sleep frequently relieves it.

There is often a sensitivity to light or noise so that the patient prefers a quiet dark environment. Succeeding migraines can occur on either side.

Treatment of common or classic migraine: Some migraines are mild and aspirin or the equivalent suffices. Sleep can provide relief; sedatives may therefore help. Ergotamine (see drug section) taken at the first sign of an attack can often abort or lessen the severity of a migraine (and relief is diagnostic of migraine). The earlier the medication is given, the more likely the patient will benefit. Once a severe migraine is in progress however, one can resort to a narcotic. A sedative is customarily administed concurrently.

Migraine prophylaxis: The need for prophylaxis varies since attacks may occur daily or (as is commonly the case with classic migraine) be separated by months. Propranolol is usually the first prophylactic agent to be tried. If propranolol fails, other prophylactics to consider include slow calcium channel blockers (e.g. verapamil); antihistamines (e.g. cyproheptadine); Fiorinal (butalbital + aspirin + caffeine); tricyclic antidepressants (e.g. amitriptyline); methysergide. Methysergide may have dangerous side effects including retroperitoneal fibrosis. If migraine is associated with menstruation, a diuretic taken for the 3–5 days prior to the anticipated menses is sometimes helpful (e.g. acetazolamide 250 mg 3 times/day). Regular exercise may be helpful.

CLUSTER HEADACHE is another type of vascular headache that also presumably results from dilation of extracerebral cranial arteries. It is more common in males, and clusters typically occur between 20 and 60 yr of age. As the name suggests, headaches occur repetitively for several weeks and then may not appear for months. Alcohol ingestion can sometimes precipitate the headache. Cluster headaches recur on the same side. One or a few headaches may occur daily. Headaches tend to occur at the same time of the day, and in many cases the patient is awakened at night by a headache. There is no prodrome and the headache usually lasts 1/2 to 2 hours. Sleep does not bring relief. The pain is unilateral behind the eye or at the side of the face and has a severe knife-like quality. Typical signs on the affected side include facial flushing; tearing red eye; nasal stuffiness or rhinorrhea; ipsilateral Horner's syndrome (ptosis, miosis, anhidrosis). **Treatment:** ergotamine (see drug section). **Prophylaxis:** If, as is often the case, the headaches occur at the same time each day, ergotamine can be given 1 hour prior to the anticipated attack. Methysergide is an alternative in other cases. Prednisone may help.

CRANIAL ARTERITIS is uncommon cause of headache that chiefly affects persons over 60. There is unilateral or bilateral inflammation of internal carotids, temporal, retinal, ophthalmic, or vertebral arteries. Depending on the arteries affected, the headache may be localized over the eye, temple, occiput, or frontal region. The patient may present with impaired vision or loss of vision on the affected side if there is inflammation/occlusion of the retinal artery. With temporal arteritis, there is tenderness over that artery and biopsy of the temporal artery may disclose giant cell arteritis. Fever, malaise, anorexia, weight loss are characteristic. The erythrocyte sedimentation is elevated. Treatment is with high–dose corticosteroids. See Giant Cell Arteritis under "Vasculitides" chapter for further discussion.

OTHER CAUSES OF HEADACHE: See the following: "Subarachnoid Hemorrhage", "Meningitis", "Elevated Intracranial Pressure", "Glaucoma", "Sinusitis".

Dizziness/Vertigo
Vertigo is the illusion that the environment or oneself is turning or rotating. Other illusions of movement may be experienced (e.g. to-fro, rocking). Dizziness is a more general term that is variously used to mean vertigo, lightheadedness, faintness, unsteadiness. Vertigo is categorized as peripheral if the lesion causing the vertigo involves the labyrinth (inner ear apparatus—i.e. semicircular canals, vestibule, cochlea); or central if the lesion involves the 8th cranial nerve, brainstem, or cerebellum.

WORKUP of DIZZINESS and VERTIGO:
History: Does the patient experience a rotational or undulating sensation, or does he feel unsteady or unbalanced ? Does he ever faint or feel he is about to?

Do certain positions or movements precipitate the symptoms? Is there tinnitus or hearing loss?

General physical exam is important with emphasis on the cardiac exam. Do not overlook neck bruits. Is there visual impairment?

Neurologic exam: Check cranial nerves carefully. Check for signs of cerebellar dysfunction—e.g. intention tremor (perform finger-to-nose test), difficulty performing rapid alternatiing movements or heel-to-shin test. Does the patient walk with broad-based gait or is there difficulty tandem walking? Check for nystagmus: vertical nystagmus suggests a brainstem lesion but certain medications can be responsible. Rotatory nystagmus suggests a peripheral lesion.

Hearing and ear exam: Can patient hear a ticking watch? Examine tympanic membrane for evidence of middle ear disease. Is earwax occluding the external auditory meatus?

Head turning: Have patient turn head to one side for 10–15 seconds; repeat in opposite direction. Also ask patient to walk and then suddenly turn. Do these maneuvers provoke symptoms or elicit nystagmus?

Nylen test (positional test): Patient sits on a table. Then, while turning his head to one side, the patient (with support from the examiner) quickly lies back to the supine position so that his head (supported by the examiner) overhangs the table at about 30° to the horizontal. The test is then repeated with the head turned to the opposite side. If there is a peripheral lesion causing vertigo, there will be a few seconds delay after performing the maneuver before the onset of nystagmus and vertigo. Furthermore, nystagmus and vertigo will becomes more difficult to provoke with repeated testing. In contrast, if there is a central lesion: nystagmus begins immediately upon performing the maneuver and repeated testing does not diminish the response.

Caloric testing is used to assess the sensitivity of the vestibular apparatus. Cold or warm water irrigation produces convection currents of the endolymph within the semicircular canal and this in turn induces nystagmus. The endolymph flows in the same direction as the slow component of nystagmus and this is the same direction as the hallucination of movement of the environment that the patient experiences. The patient lies supine with the head flexed at 30° (this angle is chosen so that one pair of the semicircular canals lies in the horizontal plane). One ear is irrigated with cold (30° C) or warm (43° C) water and the response is noted. After 5 minutes the other ear is similarly irrigated. Normally, cold water irrigation produces horizontal nystagmus with the fast component away from the irrigated ear. Warm water has opposite effect. The magnitude and duration of nystagmus should be the same when both sides are compared. When a *CNS* lesion is responsible for vertigo, caloric testing will usually elicit a normal response. With an acoustic neuroma, however, nystagmus will be absent or diminished when the affected side is irrigated because tramsmission of vestibular signals to the brainstem via the 8th cranial nerve is impaired. In vestibular neuronitis, there is a decreased response on the affected side. Ménière's disease may also be associated with decreased response on involved side. If vestibular dysfunction is secondary to ototoxic drugs, both sides typically exhibit a diminished response.

Blood pressure: Take BP in the supine position, and then immediately upon standing, and then again a few minutes later. Note any orthostatic changes, and whether or not the patient experiences lightheadedness or dizziness.

Carotid sinus stimulation is performed to rule out a hyperactive carotid sinus as the cause of dizziness. Carotid sinus pressure initiates a reflex (mediated thru the vasomotor and cardioinhibitory centers of the medulla) increase in parasympathetic and decrease in sympathetic outflow that leads to vasodilation and decreased cardiac rate. Gentle pressure is applied to the carotid sinus on the right for 20 seconds with the patient supine and on a cardiac monitor. Asystole for 3 seconds or a 50 mm Hg drop in systolic and diastolic pressure is considered significant. The test is repeated on the left. Test is repeated in the sitting position if the response is negative.

Hyperventilation: Patient hyperventilates for 3 minutes to see if this reproduces symptoms.

Laboratory: CBC, urinalysis, chemistry panel, and chest x-ray are routine. As clinical circumstances suggest, additional tests may be needed (e.g. EKG, Holter monitor, Barany rotation test, audiology, EEG, electronystagnography, CAT scan).

DIFFERENTIATING CENTRAL FROM PERIPHERAL LESION is important because a central lesion is more likely to have grave implications. **Findings suggestive of a peripheral lesion include:** severe vertigo, tinnitus and/or hearing loss, rotatory nystagmus, abnormal caloric test, Nylen test indicative of a peripheral lesion (see above). **Findings suggestive of a central lesion include:** relatively mild vertigo (frequently out of proportion to the pronounced nystagmus); absence of tinnitus and/or hearing loss; presence of other neurologic abnormalities (e.g. cranial nerve deficits, cerebellar signs); vertical nystagmus (indicates a brainstem lesion); normal calorics; Nylen test outcome characteristic of central lesion (see above). **Cerebellopontine angle tumor** may initially evince features of a peripheral lesion, and then with central encroachment go on to develop central lesion characteristics (see below).

CENTRAL CAUSES OF VERTIGO: **Cerebellopontine angle tumor** is most often an acoustic neuroma derived from the Schwann cells of the 8th cranial nerve. Other possibilities include meningioma, cholesteatoma, metastatic tumor, aneurysm. Tinnitus and hearing loss are the initial symptoms. Vertigo and/or unsteadiness may be present. As the tumor grows, it encroaches on the cerebellum (often leading to ataxia) and the cranial nerves emanating from the brainstem (e.g. facial numbness/weakness, absent corneal reflex). Pyramidal signs are not present. There is a decreased response to caloric stimulation on the involved side. CAT scan may reveal the tumor. **Multiple sclerosis** patients not infrequently develop vertigo with nystagmus (often vertical nystagmus). Lesions of the pons and/or medulla are responsible. Other CNS signs and symptoms are usually present (or have previously occurred) to help make the diagnosis but sometimes vertigo is the initial complaint. MS usually begins between 20 and 40 yr, and seldom after 50 yr. Other brainstem signs may be present (e.g. bilateral internuclear ophthalmoplegia, lateral gaze–provoked ataxia of eye movements). Vertigo is usually not severe and is usually temporary. **Vertebrobasilar artery insufficiency** occurs in the elderly, usually those with atherosclerosis. The patient is subject to brief episodes of vertigo upon turning the head abruptly. **Other central disorders that may cause vertigo** include cerebellar lesions (e.g. tumor, infarction, degenerative disease); brainstem lesions (e.g. tumor, syringobulbia, ischemia); temproral lobe epilepsy; basilar migraine; encephalitis; meningitis; metabolic disorders (diabetes mellitus, hypothyroidism); Arnold-Chiari malformation; neuropathy of 8th cranial nerve (e.g. herpes zoster).

PERIPHERAL CAUSES OF VERTIGO: **Benign Positional Vertigo** is the most common vertigo disorder. The cause is uncertain. The patient experiences vertigo that is precipitated by changes in position (e.g. lying down, sitting up, turning head suddenly). Episodes of vertigo usually last less than a minute. Nystagmus is observed during an attack and there may be nausea and vomiting. Nylen test (see above) supports the diagnosis: when the patient lies down so that the affected ear is lowermost and the eyes are turned toward that ear, rotatory nystagmus will be elicited after a delay of several seconds (clockwise if the left is the affected and lowermost positioned ear and counterclockwise if the right is the affected and lowermost positioned ear). Rotary nystagmus in the reverse direction may occur upon sitting up. Caloric testing is normal. Hearing is typically unimpaired. Neurologic exam is otherwise normal. Treatment: Antihistamines may help (see below) but basically the patient learns to avoid positions or actions that precipitate an attack. The condition usually resolves spontaneously within several weeks. **Ménière's disease** (a disorder of the vestibular and cochlear apparatus of the inner ear) is distinguished by the triad of vertigo, tinnitus, and hearing loss. The disease affects both ears in 15-20% patients. Onset is between 30 and 60 years. The patient is subject to attacks of vertigo that may last from several minutes to hours. Attacks occur abruptly without premonition, or may be heralded by a full sensation and tinnitus in the affected ear. Nystagmus accompanies the vertigo; and there is usually nausea, vomiting, and/or sweating. Tinnitus and hearing loss (which may have been present for some time before the onset of vertigo) is worsened during an attack and returns to baseline after the attack. Caloric testing shows a decreased response in the affected ear. **Acute labyrinthitis** is associated with abrupt onset of vertigo and nystagmus (rotatory or horizontal with fast component away from the affected side) that is frequently accompanied by nausea and/or vomiting. Hearing is sometimes impaired on the involved side but caloric testing is normal. The precipitant is uncertain in many cases, possibly a viral labyrinthitis. Sometimes bacterial labyrinthitis or otitis media is implicated. If the middle ear is involved, pressing on the outer ear over the external auditory meatus may elicit the symptoms. Symptoms usually relent over 2–3 days. Some patients experience unsteadiness and recurrent bouts of vertigo for several months. An attack may be treated with bed rest and an antivertigo agent (e.g. meclizine). An antibiotic is indicated if a bacterial infection is diagnosed. **Vestibular neuronitis** is a neuronitis of the vestibular division of the 8th cranial nerve. It is possibly due to a viral infection. Signs and symptoms are similar to acute labyrinthitis except that there is a decreased response on caloric testing of the involved side. **Drug toxicity:** Aminoglycosides may injure the labyrinth. Toxicity is potentiated by furosemide or ethacrynic acid. The toxic effects may not be reversible. Findings may include tinnitus, hearing loss, vertigo, impaired balance, ataxia, abnormal Romberg sign. Vertigo may be present without nystagmus, and furthermore the Barany rotation test may fail to induce nystagmus. The response to caloric stimulation is decreased or absent. ●Phenytoin and phenobarbital can cause vertigo, nystagmus, and ataxia; but hearing is not impaired and caloric testing is normal. Symptoms resolve upon discontinuation or reduction of the dose. **Other causes of peripheral vertigo include** cervical spondylosis, post head trauma, blood dyscrasia with bleeding into the labyrinth.

TREATMENT: Definitive treatment of dizziness/vertigo depends on the etiology. Symptomatic relief is sometimes achieved with antihistamines. For mild attacks, PO antihistamines are used—e.g. meclizine (Antivert), cyclizine (Marezine), dimenhydrinate (Dramamine), diphenhydramine (Benadryl), promethazine (Phenergan). Prochlorperazine (Compazine) suppositories may be administered if there is vomiting. For severe attacks, IV or IM diphenhydramine or dimenhydrinate is commonly used. Parenteral scopolamine (0.6–1.0 mg) is also effective. Transdermal scopolamine patches may be used to prevent motion sickness.

Transient Ischemic Attack (TIA) is a transient focal
neurologic abnormality that results from impaired blood flow along the internal carotid artery distribution or vertebral-basilar arterial distribution. The neurologic deficit may last from minutes to hours but as a rule < 24 hours. There is complete recovery of neurologic function. ●About a third of patients with TIA's will eventually have a thrombotic stroke, and up to 2/3 patients with thrombotic strokes have prior history of TIA.

Causes: Occluding emboli are responsible for many TIA's. The emboli originate from (**1**) the heart (e.g. from mural thrombi in patient with myocardial infarction, from atrial thrombus in patient with atrial fibrillation); or (**2**) the aorta or large arteries in the neck (e.g. from atheromatous lesions of the walls of these vessels). Emboli originating from the heart or aorta are most likely to travel up the carotid arteries. Therefore, emboli-induced TIA's are most common in the internal carotid artery distribution—primarily the ophthalmic or middle cerebral artery tributaries and rarely the anterior cerebral arteries. Stenotic lesions of either cervical or intracranial arteries may account for TIA. Stenosis is usually due to atherosclerosis. The carotid artery must be more than 80% occluded before ischemic symptoms appear. A carotid artery is most often occluded at the common carotid artery bifurcation. Atherosclerotic obstruction is more common in the vertebral and basilar arteries than in the carotid distribution. In some cases, a TIA is precipitated when an embolus arrives at a stenosis. Subclavian steal syndrome is a rare cause of TIA. There is stenosis of the subclavian artery proximal to the origin of the vertebral artery. If the left subclavian artery is stenosed for example, some blood may reach the distal left subclavian by reversed flow via the left vertebral artery. When the patient exercises his left arm, there may not be sufficient blood flow in the right vertebral artery to accomodate the required flow for both the basilar artery and the left subclavian artery. Consequently, the patient may develop signs of basilar artery insufficiency. Other conditions that may provoke TIA include arterial spasm (e.g. migraine); cardiac arrhythmias; orthostatic hypotension; inflammatory arteritis (e.g. giant cell arteritis, collagen vascular disease, syphilis); fibromuscular hyperplasia; polycythemia; thrombocytosis; sickle cell anemia; hypercoagulable conditions (e.g. DIC, TTP, pregnancy, oral contraceptive–induced).

Differential diagnosis: ●Vertigo/dizziness, tinnitus, or deafness may represent disease of the labyrinth (e.g. benign positional vertigo, Ménière's syndrome) rather than TIA. ●Syncope, lightheadedness, dizziness may be cardiac–related. ●Other conditions that may cause transient neurologic abnormalities include postictal (Todd's) paralysis, brain tumor, subdural hematoma, multiple sclerosis.

Signs/symptoms: Ischemia in the internal carotid artery distribution accounts for the majority of TIA's. Most of these are due to ischemia in regions supplied by the ophthalmic or middle cerebral arteries. TIA's in the distribution of the anterior cerebral arteries are rare. ●Before bifurcating into the anterior and middle cerebral arteries, each internal carotid artery gives off an ophthalmic artery. A TIA in the distribution of an ophthalmic artery might manifest as amaurosis fugax (ipsilateral monocular blindness) and/or partial Horner's syndrome (ipsilateral ptosis and miosis). ●The anterior and middle cerebral arteries supply the frontal, parietal, and part of temporal lobes. The potential neurologic deficits associated with ischemia of these regions is outlined in the "Stroke" chapter that follows. Vertebral-basilar artery distribution supplies the brainstem, cerebellum, and parts of the occipital and temporal lobes. A diverse array of neurologic abnormalities are possible with ischemia in this distribution—see "Stroke" chapter that follows. Contrasts between TIA's in the carotid artery distribution and those in the vertebrobasilar artery distribution; (**1**) TIA's in the vertebrobasilar distribution often differ from one episode to another, while those in the carotid distribution often demonstrate the same neurologic abnormalities on successive episodes; (**2**) vertebrobasilar artery TIA's are often associated with bilateral motor and sensory deficits, or unilateral motor or sensory impairment with signs of cranial nerve nuclei involvement, while TIA's in the carotid distribution tend to be more limited (e.g. weakness with sensory loss in a single extremity); (**3**) TIA in the distribution of the anterior cerebral artery is rare and so recurrent temporary weakness or paresthesias isolated to a lower extremity are more likely to be due to a TIA in the vertebrobasilar distribution.

Work-up: follow the guidelines in the "Stroke" chapter.

Treatment depends on such factors as cause (e.g. thrombotic or embolic occlusion), location (e.g. carotid or vertebrobasilar distribution), and whether or not there is a correctible underlying condition. Carotid endarterectomy or bypass may be possible for certain lesions (revealed by cerebral angiography) in the internal carotid system. Anticoagulation is advocated (unless there is a contraindication) for patients with thrombotic TIA who have: (**1**) lesions in the internal carotid distribution and who are not surgical candidates, (**2**) vertebrobasilar lesions. Anticoagulate with heparin initially. Switch to warfarin and continue for 3 months. Finally switch to aspirin 325 mg once daily. Warfarin is reinstituted if TIA's recur. CBC, platelets, coagulation parameters are checked, and CAT scan and lumbar puncture are performed prior to starting anticoagulation in order to exclude intracranial bleeding or other contraindications to anticoagulation. If TIA is due to emboli, treat as outlined under *Embolic Stroke* in the "Stroke" chapter that follows.

Stroke (cerebrovascular accident [CVA]) is usually due to thrombosis (the most common cause), emboli, or hemorrhage. Aortic arch dissection is an uncommon cause.

STROKE WORK-UP: Premonitory signs? Transient ischemic attacks often precede thrombotic strokes. When did neurologic symptoms appear? Thrombotic stroke tends to occur during sleep or periods of inactivity while other types of stroke tend to occur when the patient is active. Was the full neurologic deficit present from the outset? That would suggest embolic stroke. In hemorrhagic strokes the neurologic syndrome tends to evolve over several minutes to hours. In thrombotic stroke the full clinical picture typically takes hours or even days to emerge. Evaluate cardiac status: Are there irregularities in rhythm, or evidence of mitral or aortic valve disease? Obtain EKG. Cardiac monitor, Holter monitor, and/or echocardiogram are obtained as clinical circumstances suggest. Embolic strokes are often cardiac in origin (see *Embolic Stroke* below). Carotid pulse—diminished or absent? If so, is the pulse of branches of the external carotid artery (which may serve as collateral circulation) stronger on the side of the affected carotid artery? This may be ascertained by checking the pulse at the superficial temporal artery and supertrochlear artery (palpable at the superior orbit rim). Neck bruits? When evaluating neck bruits be aware that: (1) stenosis may be present without a bruit and vice versa, (2) a neck bruit may be the consequence of a transmitted heart sound. However, if the bruit is due to carotid stenosis, the bruit should disappear below the stenosis. Femoral and pedal pulses—present and symmetrical? Asymmetry may indicate aortic dissection. Neck stiffness is consistent with subarachnoid hemorrhage. Blood pressure should be taken in both arms (e.g. BP will be lower on the affected side in patients with subclavian steal syndrome). Is there orthostatic hypotension? Neurologic exam, In particular, try to ascertain whether the findings support a lesion in the internal carotid or the vertebrobasilar distribution (see diagram below). CBC, platelets, PT, and PTT, Evaluate results before lumbar puncture if that procedure is anticipated. CAT scan: Blood appears as area of increased density on CAT scan. Intracerebral bleeding is detected within an hour after onset of symptoms. Subarachnoid hemorrhage may be detected as interhemispheric blood. The infarct that results from thrombotic or embolic stroke appears as an area of decreased density after 24–48 hours. Lumbar puncture; Unless contraindicated, lumbar puncture is performed if: (1) intracranial bleeding cannot be excluded and anticoagulative therapy is contemplated, (2) CAT scan is negative and diagnosis is uncertain, or (3) CAT scan is not available and intracerebral bleeding or subarachnoid hemorrhage is suspected. In subarachnoid hemorrhage, the CSF is grossly bloody (usually > 25,000 RBC/cu mm) and the CSF pressure is elevated (i.e. > 195 mm CSF). Intracerebral bleeding is typically associated with over 1000 RBC/cu mm CSF and an elevated CSF pressure, but a normal CSF is found in about 10% cases. RBC's are usually absent from the CSF in thrombotic or embolic stroke unless the infarcted region hemorrhages (however, WBC and protein may be slightly increased). A traumatic lumbar puncture may confuse the picture but the following findings suggest a traumatic tap: (1) there is progressively less blood in sequential samples of CSF, (2) the blood clots in the tube, (3) xanthochromia is absent in the supernatant of centrifuged CSF. Cerebral arteriography is indicated if the diagnosis is uncertain, or if surgery is contemplated—e.g. for berry aneurysm, for arteriovenous malformation, endarterectomy.

THROMBOTIC STROKE most often occurs in patients with atherosclerosis, particularly if there is also hypertension or diabetes mellitus. Additional risk factors include coagulation disorders or vascular inflammation (e.g. polyarteritis nodosa, systemic lupus).

   Distinguishing characteristics of thrombotic stroke: Episodes of TIA precede thrombotic stroke in 1/2–2/3 patients. The onset of thrombotic stroke often occurs while the patient is asleep or inactive. Neurologic deficits tend to develop in stages, over hours sometimes days (stroke in evolution), and may be punctuated by intervals of transient improvement. The patient usually presents conscious and may have a headache. Neurologic impairment may resolve to a varying extent over a period of days to weeks. CAT scan is initially negative but usually becomes positive after 24–48 hours. The infarct appears as an area of decreased density that can be further delineated with contrast agent. CSF is negative for RBC's, but protein and WBC may be slightly increased. See Stroke Work–up above for indications for lumbar puncture.

   Neurologic deficits depend on the site of occlusion (see schematic diagram).

   Treatment of thrombotic stroke: Anticoagulant therapy for thrombotic stroke is controversial. Anticoagulation does not benefit a patient with completed (nonprogressing) stroke. Anticoagulation is advocated if the stroke is continuing to evolve—i.e. signs of worsening neurologic function or onset of additional neurologic abnormalities. Be aware that anticoagulation increases the risk of bleeding from a brain infarct. Anticoagulation is started only after excluding conditions contraindicating anticoagulation—e.g. bleeding diathesis, uremia, diastolic pressure > 100. Intracranial bleeding must also be excluded by lumbar puncture and CAT scan (arteriography if CAT scan not available). ●If the above conditions are met, IV heparin may be begun after waiting a minimum of 2 hours following lumbar puncture. Heparin dose is adjusted to achieve a PTT of 1.5 to 2 x control (see heparin in drug section). Within 3–5 days a decision is made whether or not to continue anticoagulation. Heparin is discontinued if (1) focal neurologic deficits resolve completely, (2) there is no further progression since admission, (3) patient appears to have undergone a major completed stroke with extensive brain infarction. If neurologic deterioration is arrested while receiving heparin, heparin is continued and warfarin is added to the regimen. Both drugs are administered together for 3–5 days. Heparin is then discontinued when the prothrombin time (which is warfarin dependent) is adequately prolonged. Adjusting the warfarin dose to achieve a prothrombin time of 15 seconds with a control of 12 seconds should provide an adequate level of anticoagulation while minimizing the risk of bleeding complications. Warfarin is prescribed only if the patients clinical status and the prothrombin time can be adequately monitored. Warfarin is discontinued after 2–3 months and aspirin therapy is begun. The optimum aspirin dose is uncertain (80 mg a day to 325 mg 4 times/day). Endarterectomy may sometimes be justified in order to prevent further strokes in patients with stenotic lesions of the carotid arteries who have only mild neurologic impairment. The cerebral edema that follows 2–3 days after an extensive cerebral infarction may be severe enough to cause transtentorial herniation. If signs of brainstem dysfunction develop, the patient is intubated and hyperventilated to achieve an arterial pCO_2 of about 25–30 mm Hg, and IV mannitol is administered. The edema associated with cerebellar infarction may compress the brainstem and require surgical decompression. Blood pressure: It is dangerous to acutely lower the blood pressure in the setting of thrombotic stroke since blood flow thru a stenotic vessel may be further compromised.

EMBOLIC STROKE in many cases occurs without premonition while the patient is awake. Typically, there is a sudden onset of neurologic deficit. Substantial recovery of neurologic function often occurs over the next few days.

Source of emboli: Emboli often originate (1) from a thrombus in the left atrium of patients with atrial fibrillation, or (2) from a mural thrombus of the left ventricle in cases of CHF, dilated cardiomyopathy, or myocardial infarction. Emboli originating from the left heart are also seen in patients with prolapsing mitral valve, prosthetic valve, or endocarditis. An atherosclerotic plaque (e.g. of carotid or vertebral artery) may be the source. Rare culprits include atrial myxoma, fat from a long bone fracture, and paradoxical embolus (a venous clot passing thru an intracardiac shunt). Recurrent cerebral emboli are common when the heart is the source, and in this case embolization to other organs (e.g. kidney, spleen) is also common.

Neurologic deficits depend on the site of occlusion (see schematic diagram).

Tests: CAT scan, as in cerebral thrombosis, is initially normal but may show a region of decreased density after 24–48 hours. CSF is generally clear but may be bloody if there is subsequent bleeding of the infarct site with rupture into the cerebral ventricles. CSF protein and WBC may be slightly increased. See *Stroke Workup* above for indications for lumbar puncture.

Treatment of thromboembolic stroke: Anticoagulation may be considered (see *Thrombotic Stroke* above for details of heparin and warfarin anticoagulation). In some cases when the heart is the source of embolism (e.g. atrial fibrillation, prosthetic heart valve); warfarin may have to be continued indefinitely. If the source of embolism is a myocardial infarction–associated mural thrombus, warfarin is generally discontinued after 8 weeks.

Occlusion of the internal carotid artery (usually by thrombosis) may produce neurologic deficits typical of occlusion of the middle and/or anterior cerebral arteries since these two arteries form the bifurcation of the internal carotid artery. Because of the anastomoses provided by the circle of Willis and external carotid distribution, complete obstruction of one internal carotid artery can sometimes occur without producing any neurologic deficit, especially if the obstruction develops slowly. Ischemia in the distribution of the internal carotid artery does not impair consciousness unless ischemia results in a seizure. This is because the anatomic region that governs consciousness (the reticular activating system) resides in the brainstem which is supplied by the vertebrobasilar circulation and not the internal carotid arterial distribution.

Ophthalmic arteries (which supply the retina and optic nerves) arise from the internal carotid arteries prior to the anterior cerebral—middle cerebral artery bifurcation. Consequently, obstruction of an internal carotid artery or an ophthalmic artery (or its branch--the central retinal artery) can cause amaurosis fugax (blindness in ipsilateral eye) and/or partial Horner's syndrome (ipsilateral ptosis and miosis).

Anterior cerebral arteries supply segments of the frontal and parietal lobes. Occlusion of an anterior cerebral artery leads to contralateral leg weakness/paralysis and sensory impairment. Additional signs may include urinary incontinence, perseveration, grasp reflex, suck reflex, behavioral abnormalities. The patient may suffer no neurologic derangement if an anterior cerebral artery is obstructed proximal to the anterior communicating artery because then there may be adequate blood flow from the opposite anterior cerebral artery thru the anterior communicating artery to preclude cerebral ischemia.

Middle cerebral arteries supply large parts of the frontal, parietal, and temporal lobes as well as the basal ganglia and internal capsule. Occlusion of middle cerebral artery (usually by embolus) may produce contralateral hemiparesis and contralateral hemisensory impairment (with motor and sensory deficits more severe in the face and arm than in the leg), contralateral homonymous hemianopia, aphasia (if there is lesion of dominant hemisphere), slurred speech, apraxia or anosognosia (if non—dominant hemisphere is affected). There may be conjugate deviation of the eyes toward the side of occlusion.

Posterior cerebral arteries supply the upper brainstem, thalamus, hippocampus, occipital lobes, and part of the temporal lobes. Occlusion of a posterior cerebral artery compromises blood flow to an occipital lobe with ensuing contralateral homonymous hemianopsia or contralateral superior quadrantanopsia. Other deficits may include sensory impairment of contralateral extremity, alexia (but not agraphia) if the dominant temporal hemisphere is affected, loss of recent memory (hippocampus lesion), thalamic pain with hyperpathia, hemiballism (due to contralateral subthalamic nucleus lesion), hemichoreoathetosis.

Occlusion of the basilar artery is usually catastrophic (e.g. quadriplegia, persistent coma).

Obstruction of one of the vertebral arteries may result in little or no neurologic impairment if there is sufficient collateral flow from the other vertebral artery. However, if the posterior inferior cerebellar artery branch is included in the obstruction, the lateral medullary syndrome will ensue: ipsilateral ataxia of arm and leg, ipsilateral facial numbness, ipsilateral Horner's syndrome, ipsilateral eye pain, loss of pinprick and temperature sense in contralateral extremities, hoarseness, dysphagia, hiccups, vertigo, nausea.

anterior cerebral artery
internal carotid artery
middle cerebral artery
anterior commun. artery
circle of Willis
posterior commun. artery
posterior cerebral artery
superior cerebellar artery
basilar artery
anterior inferior cerebellar art.
Posterior inferior cerebellar artery
vertebral artery
anterior spinal artery

SUBARACHNOID HEMORRHAGE (bleeding into subarachnoid space)

Causes: Head trauma is the most common cause. Rupture of a berry aneurysm is the next most common cause. Berry aneurysms are typically located at branch points of the Circle of Willis, branch points along the anterior or middle cerebral arteries, or sometimes at branch points of the basilar or vertebral arteries. They are thought to develop because of a congenital weakness of the arterial media. Berry aneurysms are more likely to develop in persons with chronic hypertension, and they are more common in patients with polycystic kidneys or coarctation of the aorta. Berry aneurysms most often rupture between 40 and 60 years of age. When spontaneous subarachnoid hemorrhage occurs in a young patient, it is often found to be due to a ruptured berry aneurysm. Intracerebral hemorrhage with subsequent rupture into the subarachnoid space sometimes occurs. A patient on anticoagulants or with hereditary coagulation deficiency is particularly susceptible to this development. Less common causes of subarachnoid hemorrhage include rupture of CNS arteriovenous malformation, rupture of arteriosclerotic or mycotic aneurysm, hemorrhage from brain tumor.

Signs/symptoms: Headache; Typically, while the patient is active there is an abrupt onset of a severe and constant headache. Headache may be diffuse, occipital, or frontal and may radiate to the neck and back. Photophobia is common. Transient loss or decreased level of consciousness, seizure, dizziness, vomiting, and/or changes in pulse and respiratory rate may occur and are provoked by subarachnoid bleeding—induced elevation of intracranial pressure. Unremitting coma suggests transtentorial herniation, or that bleeding has eroded into the brain substance. Signs of meningeal irritation (stiff neck, positive Kernig and/or Brudzinski's sign) develop within 12–24 hours if there is sufficient bleeding. The irritation is due to the noxious effects of bile pigments from lyzed erythrocytes. Stiff neck is not present at first unless bleeding is substantial enough to exert pressure to force the cerebellar tonsils downward. Fundoscopic findings: Retinal bleeding may be evident. It is subhyaloid (i.e. anterior to the retina). Bleeding results from impaired flow in the central retinal vein which in turn is the consequence of elevated CSF pressure. The optic nerve sheath is an extension of the meninges, and the subarachnoid layer with its contained CSF envelops the optic nerve. Elevations in CSF pressure are therefore exerted on structures lying within the optic nerve sheath—e.g. the central retinal vein. Elevated CSF pressure transmitted within the optic sheath to the back of the eyeball may also lead to papilledema. Focal neurologic signs are usually absent. The presence of focal signs from the outset suggests that a jet of leaking arterial blood has eroded into the brain or cranial nerves. Neurologic derangements that develop later are due to: (**1**) ischemic cerebral infarction from arterial vasospasm. Vasospasm is provoked by the presence of subarachnoid blood. Vasospasm and its consequences usually begin a few days after the hemorrhage. (**2**) mass effects of a hematoma—e.g. pressure on cranial nerves or brainstem, transtentorial compression; (**3**) recurrent bleeding. This may be signaled by the resurgence of severe headache. (**4**) communicating hydrocephalus—a late development. Catecholamine effects; Subarachnoid hemorrhage stimulates release of considerable amounts of catecholamines and this may result in fever, hyperglycemia, leukocytosis. Furthermore, the elevated levels of catecholamines may cause myocardial micronecrosis with EKG findings suggestive of myocardial infarction. SIADH is a common consequence of subarachnoid hemorrhage.

Diagnostic studies: CAT scan may reveal blood in the subarachnoid space, and possibly within the ventricles and/or brain parenchyma. CAT scan with contrast enhancement may identify aneurysms > 5 mm in diameter. CAT scan may be negative if bleeding is slight or if the study is delayed a few days. Lumbar puncture is performed if CAT scan is negative and there are no contraindications. Be sure to check CBC, platelets, PT, and PTT before performing lumbar puncture. The CSF pressure is typically increased. The CSF is hemorrhagic and the ratio of RBC to WBC is initially the same as the blood; later there is a preponderance of WBC as meningeal irritation ensues. A traumatic lumbar puncture is suspected if progressively less blood is found as the sequential samples of CSF are obtained. The supernatant of centrifuged CSF becomes xanthochromic 6 hours or so after subarachnoid hemorrhage. Cerebral arteriography is performed only if surgery is anticipated or if the diagnosis is uncertain. Berry aneurysms and AV malformations may be identified. Cerebral vasospasm may also be revealed by arteriography.

Treatment berry aneurysm-associated subarachnoid hemorrhage: bed rest, sedation, control of hypertension, stool softener. Because rebleeding is frequent (particularly within the first 2 weeks) and mortality is high with rebleeding, surgery is advised if the patient is a good surgical candidate (e.g. absence of coma, obtundation, or dire neurologic abnormality). ●Many neurosurgeons, however, delay surgery for 10–14 days until cerebral edema and vasospasm have subsided. ●In the meantime, some authorities advocate aminocaproic acid (Amicar) to prevent clot lysis and rebleeding. ●Nimodipine (Nimotrop) is a calcium-entry blocker that appears to decrease the incidence of permanent neurologic damage and death following subarachnoid hemorrhage. It presumably acts by preventing cerebral vasospasm. Treatment is for 21 days (60 mg PO every 4 hours) beginning within 96 hours of bleeding. ●Cerebral arteriography is performed prior to surgery in order to exclude vasospasm before proceeding. ●Surgery usually consists of ligating the neck of the aneurysm (e.g. with a metal clip). If this is not feasible, the artery proximal to the aneurysm is sometimes ligated. This may be preceded by temporal artery to middle cerebral artery anastomosis if the aneurysm is in the carotid arterial distribution.

INTRACEREBRAL HEMORRHAGE (bleeding into the brain substance) usually involves a branch of the middle cerebral artery. Consequently, the basal ganglia (putamen, globus pallidus, caudate nucleus, amygdala); internal capsule; thalamus; and cerebrum are often involved. The cerebellum and brainstem are less common sites of intracerebral bleeding.

Etiology: Hypertension, particularly in the setting of arteriosclerosis, is the most common condition leading to intracerebral hemorrhage. Intracerebral hemorrhage may also be the consequence of rupture of congenital aneurysm, rupture of mycotic aneurysm, brain infarct (e.g. following cerebral thrombosis or embolism), rupture of arteriovenous malformation, trauma, anticoagulation, blood dyscrasia, hemorrhage from brain tumor.

Signs/symptoms/locating site of intracerebral bleeding: The typical patient is awake and active when there is sudden onset of headache followed by progressive neurologic dysfunction over several minutes to hours. Coma often occurs; it may be present at the outset or develop slowly. Nausea, vomiting, or convulsions (focal or generalized) are common. Patients who survive usually gradually regain some lost neurologic function. Bleeding in the region of the putamen causes contralateral hemiplegia. The eyes may deviate ("point") to the side of the bleeding. Thalamic bleeding manifests as a pronounced contralateral sensory deficit. If there is involvement of the internal capsule there may be contralateral hemiplegia or hemiparesis. Involvement of the ipsilateral optic radiation in the posterior segment of the internal capsule results in contralateral homonymous hemianopsia. Consequences of ongoing supratentorial hemorrhage with elevated intracranial pressure: Pressure on the midbrain may cause a variety of eye abnormalities—e.g. defective upward gaze so that the eyes are directed down and may point toward the tip of the nose, nystagmus, miosis, unequal and/or unreactive pupils. Other possible consequences of increasing pressure on the brainstem, and ensuing uncal and brainstem herniation include: systolic hypertension, bradycardia, slowed respirations, unilateral dilated pupil progressing to bilateral dilation, aberrations in respiratory pattern, hemiplegia and then quadriplegia, unilateral or bilateral Babinski's, decorticate and then decerebrate posturing, absence of response to Doll's eye maneuver or calorics. Pontine hemorrhage is characterized by coma, quadriplegia, pinpoint pupils that react to light (seen under magnification), absence of Doll's eye phenomenom, no response to caloric testing, irregular breathing, and/or decerebrate posturing. Cerebellar bleeding is characteristically associated with occipital headache and vomiting. Inability to walk despite the fact that strength and sensation are generally preserved may sometimes be observed. Slurred speech is common. The expanding hematoma may exert pressure on the brainstem with several possible consequences—e.g. diplopia with difficulty looking toward the side of the bleeding (due to effects on the medial longitudinal fasciculus or on cranial nerves III, IV, and VI); ipsilateral facial weakness; nystagmus; vertigo; extremity weakness; coma; pinpoint pupils.

Diagnostic tests: CAT scan will usually reveal the site of bleeding within 1 hour of onset of clinical signs (blood appears as area of increased density). Lumbar puncture is therefore unnecessary. The CSF is positive for blood in about 90% cases because blood usually gains access to the subarachnoid space. Consequently, the

CSF pressure is usually increased (> 200 mm CSF). If CAT scan is not available, lumbar puncture may be performed provided that there is no evidence of elevated intracranial pressure—e.g. papilledema, signs or transtentrorial herniation (e.g. unilateral dilated pupil).

Treatment of intracerebral bleeding: Treat hypertension. Assess PT, PTT, platelets and correct deficiencies. Surgery is indicated if there is (**1**) cerebellar hemorrhage with neurologic signs, (**2**) CAT scan evidence of brainstem compression or hydrocephalus, (**3**) nondominant putamen bleeding resulting in transtentorial herniation and brainstem herniation.

LACUNAR STROKE: Lacunes are small cavities within the brain due to thrombosis–associated infarcts in the distribution of small arteries. Lacunes are not seen on CAT scan (unless adjacent lacunes coalesce to form larger cavities) or by arteriography. They are identified at autopsy. **Examples of lacunar syndromes include:** (**1**) pure hemiplegia secondary to a lacune in the internal capsule or pons; (**2**) weakness and ataxia of one leg secondary to lacune of internal capsule or pons; (**3**) pure sensory deficit secondary to lacune of the thalamus; (**4**) clumsy weak hand with slurred speech secondary to lacune of pons. **Treatment:** No specific therapy is indicated except that hypertension be controlled should it be present.

Meningitis is an inflammation of the meninges. Specifically, there is inflammation of the pia and arachnoid covering of the brain and spinal cord.

ETIOLOGY:
Bacterial meningitis: Pneumococcus is the most common cause of bacterial meningitis in adults (30-50% cases) and is not uncommon in children (10-20% cases). In many cases, there is a pneumococcal–associated pneumonia, otitis media, sinusitis, or mastoiditis. Pneumococcal meningitis is a not uncommon sequel to closed head injuries. Meningititis in children with sickle cell anemia is often pneumococcal. Meningococcal meningitis is the next most common meningitis in adults. The incidence of meningococcal meningitis is greatest in adolescents and young adults. Epidemics of meningococcal meningitis occur in closed populations (e.g. military recruits) and are often traced to asymptomatic carriers. Haemophilus influenza meningitis is the most common type of bacterial meningitis in children under 4 years and is uncommon thereafter. It is rare in adults but can occur with head trauma or immunocompromise. Gram-negative bacilli are the most frequent cause of neonatal meningitis (particularly E. coli followed by Klebsiella and Enterobacter). Gram-negative meningitis is most often associated with immunocompromise, or penetrating head injury or surgery. Staphylococcal meningitis should be part of the differential if meningitis occurs in the setting of penetrating head injury or surgery, infected ventriculo-atrial shunt, or immunocompromise. Listeria monocytogenes meningitis is most often seen in the setting of immunocompromise. Tuberculous meningitis is more common in adults. Summary of the principal causes of bacterial meningitis according to age: Neonatal meningitis is most often due to gram-negative bacteria (particularly E. coli) followed by group B streptococci. From then to 15 years, the most common cause is Haemophilus influenza followed by meningococcus with pneumococcus a distant 3rd. After 15 years, pneumococcus is the most common cause followed by meningococcus.

Fungal meningitis is most common in the immunocompromised.

Aseptic meningitis is said to present if all three of the following criteria are met: (**1**) CSF leukocytosis, (**2**) normal CSF glucose, (**3**) absence of CSF bacteria (e.g. negative CSF culture and smear). Viruses are the most frequent cause of aseptic meningitis—e.g. mumps, herpes simplex, herpes zoster, ECHO virus, Coxsackie, polio, lymphocytic choriomeningitis, arboviruses. Other infections that may have an aseptic presentation include fungi, mycoplasma, tuberculosis, syphilis, leptospirosis, partially treated bacterial meningitis. Noninfectious meningitis: neoplasia, intrathecal injections, stroke, lead poisoning, sarcoid, etc.

SIGNS/SYMPTOMS: Stiff neck is common and the patient resists neck flexion. The spinal cord nerve roots are irritated by the surrounding inflamed meninges. Consequently, the patient typically resists neck flexion because this puts tension on the nerve roots and thus provokes pain. Two signs demonstrating meningeal inflammation with avoidance of nerve root tension are: (**1**) Brudzinski's sign—passive flexion of the neck causes the patient to flex his legs, (**2**) Kernig's sign—with the thigh flexed the patient resists knee extension. Other findings may include fever; headache; vomiting; photophobia; confusion; lethargy; stupor; coma; seizures; focal cerebral signs (e.g. hemiparesis); cranial nerve dysfunction (e.g. Bell's palsy, oculomotor palsy); unilateral or bilateral deafness (may be sensorineural and/or conduction deafness); communicating or noncommunicating hydrocephalus. Papilledema is unusual even though the CSF pressure is typically elevated. One should suspect a space-occupying lesion (e.g. brain abscess, subdural abscess, epidural abscess) if papilledema is seen. Purpura or petechiae suggests meningococcal meningitis. In infants, irritability, poor feeding, fever, seizure, or a bulging fontanel are typical signs. Stiff neck is commonly absent. In the elderly, confusion or altered level of consciousness are often the only signs.

LABORATORY: Note appearance of the CSF and obtain opening and closing pressures when performing the LP. Normal CSF is clear and colorless. A CSF protein > 100 mg/dl imparts a slight yellow color while cloudiness is present with > 200–300 WBC/cu mm. Normal CSF pressure is 100–200 mm CSF. Order the following CSF tests: CSF cultures (bacteria, tuberculosis, fungi); CSF stains (gram, acid-fast, India ink); CSF cell count with differential; CSF protein; and CSF glucose (blood glucose is simultaneously obtained). Also obtain CBC with differential, blood cultures, throat culture, urine culture, serum electrolytes. **Additional lab** may be indicated as clinical circumstances suggest: Immunologic tests: Countercurrent immunoelectrophoresis (CIE) or latex agglutination tests of the CSF for detecting bacterial antigens may be useful in identifying pneumococcus, Haemophilus influenza, meningococcus. These tests are reserved for cases in which the gram stain is negative or fails to identify the bacteria that are seen. Gram stain of the blood buffy coat can sometimes detect bacteremia. If viral meningitis is suspected, obtain viral cultures (CSF, throat, rectal, vesicular skin lesions) and blood for viral antibody titers. Work-up of suspected tuberculous meningitis includes (in additon to the routine CSF tuberculosis culture and CSF acid-fast stain) sputum and urine culture for acid-fast bacteria, sputum acid-fast stain, PPD skin test. Work-up of suspected fungal meningitis: (**1**) fungal culture of CSF, blood, urine, and sputum; (**2**) India ink preparation and latex agglutination test for cryptococcus; (**3**) coccidioidomycosis and histoplasmosis serology test. VDRL may be indicated.

INTERPRETING CSF LAB:

Normal: (**1**) CSF WBC < 5/cu mm—all mononuclear; (**2**) CSF glucose 50–100 mg/dl or 50–60% of simultaneously obtained blood glucose; (**3**) CSF protein 20–40 mg/dl.

Bacterial meningitis: CSF WBC count 100–10,000 with over 80% neutrophils. WBC may be 0–100 in the early stages, in leukopenic patients, or in severely debilitated patients who are unable to mount a response. CSF glucose < 50% of simultaneously obtained blood glucose or CSF glucose < 40 mg/dl. CSF protein 100–1000 mg/dl.

Partially treated bacterial meningitis: CSF can be difficult to interpret and can give the picture of a viral meningitis—e.g. WBC 100–500 with either mononuclear or neutrophilic predominance, CSF glucose < 50, CSF protein 50–100.

Parameningeal infection (e.g. brain abscess, subdural or epidural abscess): CSF WBC 0–1000 with either mononuclear or neutrophilic predominance, CSF glucose < 40–80, CSF protein 50–100 or sometimes greater. Bacteria are usually absent from the CSF.

Syphilis meningitis: CSF WBC 100–500 usually with mononuclear predominance, CSF glucose 20–40, CSF protein 50–400.

Viral meningitis is suggested by: CSF WBC 10–2000. Neutrophils predominate early in the infection followed by mononuclear predominance later. CSF glucose is normal or at least not < 40 mg/dl. CSF protein is 50–100 mg/dl.

Tuberculous meningitis: CSF WBC 20–1000 with mononuclear predominance, CSF glucose 20–80, CSF protein 50–1000.

Fungal meningitis: CSF WBC 25–500 with mononuclear predominance, CSF glucose 20–40, CSF protein 25–500.

TREATMENT should not be delayed when meningitis is suspected. Promptly perform lumbar puncture and begin antibiotic therapy. If for some reason the lumbar puncture should not or cannot be immediately performed, begin drug therapy and then do the lumbar puncture as soon as possible. Delaying therapy can have disasterous consequences.

Antibiotic choice while awaiting culture/sensitivity results when organisms are not seen or cannot be positively identified on microscopic exam of CSF smear: In adults, high-dose IV penicillin G and IV chloramphenicol are administered concurrently. IV ampicillin plus IV chloramphenicol is an alternative. A suitable 3rd generation cephalosporin (e.g. ceftriaxone, cefotaxime) may be substituted for chloramphenicol. A 3rd generation cephalosporin would be the usual choice if the gram stain revealed gram-negative bacilli. In children, the standard regimen has been IV ampicillin combined with IV chloramphenicol. IV ceftriaxone or IV cefotaxime alone is also suitable. In infants < 2 months, the usual choice is IV ampicillin plus gentamycin.

Pneumococcal or meningococcal: Standard treatment is with high-dose IV penicillin G. Chloramphenicol is administered if the patient is penicillin allergic. Treatment is continued for at least 10 days and until patient has been afebrile for 5 days. Close contacts of patients with meningococcal meningitis should receive rifampin prophylaxis for 2 days.

Haemophilus influenza: Administer ampicillin and chloramphenicol while awaiting culture results. Continue ampicillin if the bacteria are ampicillin-sensitive. Continue both ampicillin and chloramphenicol if the bacteria are not ampicillin sensitive. If the patient is allergic to penicillins, chloramphenicol can be administered alone. A suitable 3rd generation cephalosporin (e.g. ceftriaxone, cefotaxime) is an alternative but caution is advised since penicillin-allergic patients are not uncommonly allergic to cephalosporins as well. Trimethoprim-sulfamethoxazole is yet another option in the penicillin-allergic patient. Antibiotic treatment is continued for at least 10 days and until patient has been afebrile for 5 days.

Gram-negative bacilli excepting Pseudomonas (e.g. E. coli, proteus, klebsiella): cefotaxime, cefotriaxone, or ceftizoxime. Ampicillin, chloramphenicol, or trimethoprim-sulfamethoxazole are possible options as culture results indicate.

Pseudomonas aeruginosa and Acinetobacter: Treatment consists of an extended spectrum penicillin (e.g. ticarcillin, carbenicillin) plus an aminoglycoside (e.g. gentamycin). Both intravenous and intrathecal gentamycin may be needed since aminoglycosides do not easily enter the CSF by the intravenous route.

Staphylococcus aureus: nafcillin or oxacillin. Alternative is IV vancomycin (which may need to be supplemented with intrathecal vancomycin).

Stapylococcus epidermidis: vancomycin.

Listeria monocytogenes: IV ampicillin and gentamycin concurrently.

Tuberculosis: refer to "Tuberculosis" chapter.

Fungal meningitis: amphotericin B. Add flucytosine when treating cryptococcosis.

Brain Abscess
may be the consequence of direct extension from an infection within the skull (e.g. infection of the ear, nasal sinuses, mastoid); hematogenous spread from distant site (e.g. lung infection, endocarditis); or contamination from penetrating head trauma/surgery.

Pathogens: Brain abscess may be due to bacteria, fungi, or parasites. The most common pathogens are aerobic or anaerobic streptococci. Bacteroides and other enteric bacteria are the next most common nontrauma-related pathogens and these are mixed infection in many cases. Staph. aureus brain abscess may follow penetrating head injury or be introduced hematogenously. Uncommon pathogens include pneumococcus, clostridia, Nocardia, fungi.

Signs/symptoms: Evidence of elevated intracranial pressure may be present (see "Elevated Intracranial Pressure" chapter). A diverse array of focal neurological abnormalities are possible depending on the site of the abscess. Signs of systemic infection (fever, chills, leukocytosis) are usual but may be absent if the abscess is encapsulated. A search should be made for the original site of infection (e.g. sinus, ear, lung, heart).

Tests: <u>CAT scan with and without contrast</u> is the diagnostic study of choice. Typically, the abscess appears as a radiolucent lesion with a dense border which is itself enclosed by a lucent margin. <u>Brain scan</u> is the alternative if CAT scan is unavailable. <u>Lumbar puncture is generally contraindicated</u> since the intracranial pressure is usually elevated. If lumbar puncture happens to be performed, see *Interpreting the CSF Lab—parameningeal infection* in the "Meningitis" chapter.

Treatment: <u>Antibiotic therapy</u> is begun without delay. In the adult, IV penicillin G 10–20 million units a day divided q4–6h will cover the culpable pathogen in most cases. IV penicillin G and IV chloramphenicol are commonly administered concurrently if the pathogen(s) is uncertain. A penicillinase–resistant penicillin (e.g. nafcillin) is administered if staphylococcal brain abscess is suspected. <u>Serial CAT scans</u> are used to follow progress of therapy. <u>Surgical drainage/excision</u> may be necessary.

Subdural Abscess (subdural empyema) may result from (1) contiguous spread of infection (e.g. brain abscess, meningitis, otitis media, sinusitis, osteomyelitis), (2) hematogenous spread; or (3) contamination from penetrating head trauma/surgery. **Pathogens:** Aerobic or anaerobic streptococci are the most common pathogens. Gram–negative enteric bacteria (e.g. bacteroides) and staphylococci are also common.

Signs/symptoms: The patient is febrile, may complain of headache, is usually confused and obtunded or has lapsed into coma. Tapping the skull over the abscess area may be painful. Signs of meningeal irritation may be evident (stiff neck, Kernig's sign). Focal neurological abnormalities may be apparent. These neurological abnormalities may be due to pressure effects on the underlying brain, cerebral thrombophlebitis, cerebral infarction, or elevated intracranial pressure with herniation.

Tests: <u>CAT scan with contrast</u> is obtained. <u>Cerebral arteriography</u> is the next best test if CAT is unavailable. <u>Lumbar puncture is generally contraindicated</u> because of the risk of herniation from elevated intracranial pressure. Moreover, the CSF is usually sterile; although CSF pressure, WBC count, and protein are typically elevated.

Treatment: <u>Antibiotic therapy</u> is begun without delay. In the adult, IV penicillin G 10–20 million units a day divided q4–6h will cover the culpable pathogen in most cases. However, the choice of antibiotic is guided by clinical judgment. <u>Surgical drainage</u> is performed as soon as possible.

Neurologic Consequences of Alcoholism

ALCOHOL WITHDRAWAL SYNDROMES: In practice, the following syndromes do not usually occur in a neatly arranged and sequential manner as the descriptions suggest. For instance, delirium tremens may develop in the absence of preceding or concurrent hallucinosis or seizures, or two or more syndromes may occur concurrently. Abstention from alcohol is not necessarily a prerequisite for the development of symptoms; merely a reduction in blood ethanol level below the habitual level may be sufficient to provoke an alcohol withdrawal syndrome.

Tremulousness may begin within 8 hours of the last drink, not uncommonly before blood ethanol level returns to zero. Anorexia, nausea, tachycardia, sweating, anxiety, insomnia may also be present. The alcoholic is prompted to drink again in order to reverse these symptoms.

Hallucinosis may occur within the first 24 hours of abstinence. The syndrome may continue for a week or longer but usually resolves within 48–72 hours. Hallucinations may be auditory or visual. The patient is agitated and complains of nightmares and insomnia.

Withdrawal seizures are generalized seizures that tend to occur within 12–36 hours of abstinence. Often, there are several brief seizures over a short interval. Focal seizures are the exception and merit a CAT scan to exclude a CNS lesion. In the absence of idiopathic or post–traumatic epilepsy, the EEG will be normal after the postictal period. With continued abstinence, about a third of patients who experience withdrawal seizures will go on to develop delirium tremens.

Delirium tremens (DT's) is a potentially fatal condition. In most cases DT's begin 2–5 days following cessation or reduction in alcohol intake and runs its course over 1–6 days. The syndrome is sometimes delayed for up to 10–14 days. It is characterized by marked tremor; confusion; agitation; hallucinations; anxiety; insomnia; and signs of autonomic hyperactivity (e.g. fever, sweating, tachycardia, hyperventilation, hypertension, mydriasis, incontinence).

Treatment of alcohol withdrawal syndromes: A benzodiazepine is administered to control tremor/agitation. In mild cases, an orally administered benzodiazepine may suffice (e.g. diazepam 10 mg PO 3–4 times/day). Intravenous administration is necessary in more severe cases—e.g. diazepam 10 mg IV and then 5–10 mg IV every 5–10 minutes until the patient is adequately sedated (over 200 mg has been used to control severe agitation). Diazepam 5–10 mg IV may be subsequently repeated prn at 1–4 hour intervals. IV diazepam must be administered cautiously since apnea, hypotension, or cardiac arrest can occur. Oversedation must be avoided, especially in the elderly or patients with compromised liver function because diazepam is metabolized by the liver and the half-life of the major active metabolite is 50–100 hours. With clinical improvement the patient can be switched to oral diazepam and tapered over about a week. Intravenous diazepam is administered to stop a seizure in progress. However, prophylactic anticonvulsants (e.g. phenytoin) are not recommended in uncomplicated alcohol withdrawal seizures. Thiamine (100 mg IV or if necessary IM) is administered to prevent development of Wernicke's syndrome or Korsakoff's psychosis. Other B complex vitamins are also routinely added to the IV bottle. Fluid and electrolyte replacement: Dehydration is common because ethanol suppresses ADH secretion and is an osmotic diuretic. Patients requiring intravenous fluids receive IV dextrose solutions (e.g. D5 NS if there is hypotension, D5 1/2NS otherwise). Serum glucose, and electrolytes including potassium, sodium, chloride, bicarbonate, magnesium, calcium, and phosphorus are determined and abnormalities corrected. Magnesium sulfate (see drug section) is usually routinely administered because ethanol–induced magnesium depletion is common in alcoholics.

WERNICKE'S ENCEPHALOPATHY and KORSAKOFF'S PSYCHOSIS:

Wernicke's encephalopathy is the result of thiamine deficiency, a deficiency that many malnourished alcoholics are prone to. The principal signs are confusion; paresis of extraocular muscles (diplopia, nystagmus); and ataxia. Lethargy and peripheral neuritis may also be present.

Korsakoff's psychosis is another alcoholism and thiamine deficiency–associated neurologic syndrome that may follow Wernicke's encephalopathy. The patient is unable to remember recent events and may compensate by confabulating.

Treatment of either syndrome is principally with thiamine (100 mg IV or IM initially). Glucose must not be administered until after thiamine has been given because otherwise encephathopathy may be acutely exacerbated. Wernicke's encephalopathy is more likely to respond to thiamine treatment than Korsakoff's psychosis. Eye weakness usually resolves but some patients are left with permanent ataxia. Other alcohol–associated disorders are treated, thiamine and other B complex vitamins are continued, and a nutritious diet and abstinence are encouraged.

HEPATIC ENCEPHALOPATHY is the consequence of liver failure (e.g. fulminant viral hepatitis, alcoholic cirrhosis). The syndrome is discussed in "Alcoholic Liver Disease" chapter.

OTHER NEUROLOGIC CONSEQUENCES OF ALCOHOLISM include polyneuropathy, cerebral atrophy, cerebellar degeneration.

Parkinsonism

Parkinsonism is a chronic CNS disease associated with degeneration of the basal ganglia and substantia nigra. In particular, there is a deficiency of dopamine in the nigrostriatal pathway—i.e. neurons with axons projecting from the substantia nigra to the basal ganglia (specifically the putamen and caudate nucleus). Parkinsonism may be idiopathic (Parkinson's disease) or secondary. <u>Secondary causes</u> include postencephalitis; head trauma; tumor in proximity to basal ganglia; toxins (e.g. carbon monoxide, manganese); drugs (e.g. phenothiazines, haloperidol, reserpine); CNS diseases (e.g. arteriosclerosis, Wilson's disease, Huntington's disease, Shy–Drager syndrome, olivopontocerebellar degeneration, progressive supranuclear palsy). <u>Idiopathic parkinsonism (Parkinson's disease)</u> almost always begins after age 40 (patients under 30 with parkinson symptoms are more likely to have secondary parkinsonism). Males account for about 60% cases. Onset is insidious with slow deterioration over a period of years.

Signs of parkinsonism: <u>Resting tremor</u> that improves or disappears with voluntary movement is a key manifestation. Tremor in one hand is often the initial presentation. The tremor is made worse by emotional stress or fatigue. It is absent during sleep. <u>Muscular rigidity</u> is characteristic. This rigidity is perceived by the examiner on passive movement of a patient's extremity as an uniform resistance ("lead–pipe rigidity") or ratchet–like sensation ("cog–wheel rigidity"). <u>Bradykinesia (movements slow and deliberate) and akinesia (voluntary movement diminished)</u> are characteristic. There may be difficulty in starting, stopping, or continuing movements. Facial expression is diminished, eyes unblinking, and mouth slightly ajar. Speech is slow and soft. Patient walks bent forward with a slow, shuffling, and unsteady gait with the arms flexed and unswinging. <u>Micrographia</u> is often present. <u>Depression and dementia</u> are common.

Treatment: Mild parkinsonism may not require drug therapy. <u>An anticholinergic</u> drug is usually the first step if drug therapy becomes necessary—e.g. benztropine (Cogentin), trihexyphenidyl (Artane), diphenhydramine (Benadryl). <u>Amantadine</u> (Symmetrel) can be used as the initial drug if an anticholinergic is contraindicated or not tolerated. Furthermore, amantadine and an anticholinergic can be used concurrently. <u>Sinemet</u> (levodopa combined with carbidopa) is the next step for patients with more severe symptoms. If necessary, amantadine and/or an anticholinergic may be administered concurrently with Sinemet. Concurrent therapy may become necessary when the dose of Sinemet must be reduced because of intolerable side effects. <u>Bromocriptine</u> (Parlodel) is a dopaminergic agonist that is usually used as an adjunct to Sinemet when the latter is not sufficiently effective. It may also allow a reduction in the dose of Sinemet when intolerable side effects are present. Furthermore, it may be tried instead of Sinemet if Sinemet is contraindicated or ineffective.

Multiple Sclerosis

Multiple Sclerosis (MS) is characterized by demyelination of scattered areas of the brain and spinal cord. MS usually presents between 20 and 40 years of age (mean 33, range 10–early 50s). <u>Geographic distribution:</u> MS is uncommon in the tropics but becomes progressively more common in more temperate latitudes. An individual who migrates from the tropics to a temperate region after the age of 15 retains the same low risk as one who remains in the tropics. However, a person who makes the same move before age 5 increases his risk of developing MS. These observations support the theory that pre-pubertal exposure to an as yet unidentified virus, particularly in a temperate latitiude, may be the cause of MS. <u>Genetic predisposition:</u> Incidence is increased in first degree relatives and there is a 50% concordance in identical twins. Furthermore, there is a frequent association with specific HLA haplotypes. MS rarely occurs in Orientals.

Diagnostic considerations and disease course: MS is often suggested (**1**) by the presence of divergent neurologic abnormalities due to scattered CNS lesions and (**2**) by exacerbations followed by periods of remission. For this reason, it is often said that MS is characterized by CNS lesions "separated in both space and time". MS is unpredictable: the array of neurologic deficits is variable and the duration of remissions is variable. Some patients, paticularly those with onset after age 40, may have a progressive downhill course without remissions while others may have remissions lasting years. A common pattern is that of progressively shorter remissions with progressive neurologic deterioration. It is usually not possible to make a firm diagnosis of MS on the initial presentation, especially if there is a single focal neurologic deficit. However, suspicion is enhanced by the history of a neurologic impairment that has since abated or disappeared. In order to make the diagnosis of MS, there must be (**1**) two or more neurologic abnormalities attributable to disparate regions of the CNS and (**2**) some of the neurologic abnormalities must make their appearance separated by more than a month.

Neurologic findings: Temperature sensitivity is characteristic. Neurologic disturbances tend to worsen when the temperature is elevated. Muscular weakness and spasticity nearly always develop. One or more limbs may be affected. Hyperreflexia, clonus, and/or positive Babinski reflex are usually found. Gait ataxia and intention tremor are common. Dysarthria or scanning speech develops in about half the cases. Paresthesias (e.g. extremity tingling, numbness, heaviness, pain) are common. Focal sensory impairment (decreased touch, pain, temperature, vibratory, and/or position sense) is often evident. Urinary dysfunction (e.g. retention, frequency, incontinence, impotence) occurs in about 80% cases. Constipation is a common complaint. Vertigo, hearing loss, and/or tinnitus may develop. Optic neuritis is a common occurrence. There is temporary unilateral impairment of vision—e.g. decreased acuity, central scotoma, blindness. The affected eye may be painful. The optic disc is pale. The visual evoked response time is prolonged. Internuclear ophthalmoplegia develops when a brainstem lesion interrupts the medial longitudinal fasciculus (MLF)—the link between the 3rd and 6th cranial nerves. If the right MLF is interrupted and the patient looks to the left, the right eye is unable to or only partially able to turn nasally (because fibers of the right MLF leading to the right 3rd cranial nucleus are interrupted) while the left eye ABducts and exhibits nystagmus. The MLF is often involved bilaterally. Lesions of the MLF do not affect convergence because the pathway for convergence is different from that of conjugate gaze. Seizures may occur. Psychiatric disturbances (e.g. emotional lability, euphoria, apathy, poor judgment, dementia) may emerge. Lhermitte's sign (neck flexion provokes an electric shock-like sensation in the limbs) may be present.

Tests may support but do not alone make the diagnosis. CSF analysis: CSF protein and lymphocytes are sometimes slightly increased. The gamma globulin fraction of CSF protein is > 13% in over 75% cases and oliclonal bands are detected within the gamma region in about 90% cases. VDRL should be obtained to rule out neurosyphilis. Screening tests for autoimmune disease (e.g. ANA) are advised. CBC is obtained to exclude pernicious anemia. Visual evoked response is prolonged in most patients. CAT scan may help exclude other CNS lesions. CAT scan may reveal hypodense areas but an NMR scan is more sensitive in this regard.

Differential diagnosis: spinal cord compression, intracranial tumor or abscess, stroke, cerebral AV malformation, syringomyelia, pernicious anemia, amyotrophic lateral sclerosis, hereditary ataxias, neurosyphilis, autoimmune disease, platybasia.

Treatment: No cure is available. Some authorities advocate prednisone or other corticosteroid for acute exacerbations. Otherwise therapy is supportive—e.g. physical therapy, prevention/treatment of urinary infections or decubiti.

Amyotrophic Lateral Sclerosis

ALS is a degenerative disease affecting both upper and lower motor neurons.

Signs/symptoms: Degeneration of the upper motor neurons (i.e. corticobulbar tract, lateral corticospinal tract) contributes to weakness, hyperreflexia, spasticity, and positive Babinski reflex. Degeneration of lower motor neurons (i.e. anterior horn cells, cranial motor neurons) also results in weakness and is responsible for muscle atrophy and fasciculations. Extremity weakness and atrophy is initially noticed distally with subsequent progression proximally—e.g. first the hands, then the forearms, and so forth. Weakness may begin in any limb or limbs—symmetrically or asymmetrically and the pattern of progression differs from patient to patient. Corticobulbar tract involvement may be evident (tongue atrophy with fasciculations, progressive difficulty swallowing and chewing) but the extraocular muscles are not affected. Bowel and bladder function is not affected. Sensory derangements are rare. Cremasteric and superficial abdominal reflexes are not impaired. Anal sphincter tone and anal "wink" reflex are normal.

Tests: CSF is normal. EMG abnormalities characteristic of lower motor neuron involvement are found: (1) spontaneous fibrillations and fasciculations at rest, (2) mainly large motor unit discharges with voluntary contraction. However, nerve conduction velocity is normal.

Treatment: There is no treatment to prevent progression of the disease or the fatal outcome in 2–7 years.

Poliomyelitis is caused by one of the picornaviruses (small nonencapsulated ether-resistant RNA viruses). It is an enterovirus (i.e. propagates in the GI tract and is spread by fecal contamination). Polio may also be caused by other enteroviruses (see "differential diagnosis" below). There are 3 immunological subtypes of poliovirus. <u>Spread:</u> Man is the only natural host. Spread is person-to-person by fecal-oral route or mouth-to-mouth. <u>Dissemination within the host:</u> After exposure, the virus invades and replicates within lymphoid cells in the walls of the pharynx and intestines. Viremia ensues. Subsequent spread to the CNS is probably via the bloodstream although the virus may also reach the CNS along neural pathways from the GI tract. Poliovirus can be found in the pharynx, feces, and blood 3–4 days following exposure, and can be recovered from the throat for up to 2 weeks and from the feces for 3 to over 6 weeks. Viremia is abolished in a matter of days as the virus–specific antibody level rises. <u>Risk of developing serious paralytic disease</u> increases with increasing age and with pregnancy. Exercise during the asymptomatic period or early phase of CNS involvement increases the risk of paralysis of those extremities exercised. Recent tonsilectomy predisposes to brainstem involvement. Recent inoculation predisposes the injected limb to paralysis.

Signs/symptoms: Poliovirus infection is usually inapparent. <u>Minor illness:</u> Of those that do become symptomatic, the majority have a mild 2–3 day illness beginning 3–5 days after exposure. Manifestations may include the following: fever, malaise, headache, sore throat, anorexia, nausea, vomiting, and/or diarrhea. <u>Major illness:</u> Of the small minority that do develop CNS disease, a few first experience the minor illness. CNS disease usually begins 1–2 weeks after exposure and is heralded by fever, headache, stiff neck, myalgia, muscle cramps, and perhaps fasciculations. Paralysis may ensue in a matter of hours, or there may be progressive weakness over days such that the full paralytic consequences may not be realized for 4–5 days. There may be parasthesias or hypersthesias, but sensory loss is unusual. Paralysis is asymmetric in most cases. There is a flaccid paralysis with loss of deep tendon reflexes in the affected region. The legs and trunk are most often affected. There may be quadriplegia. Involvement of the brainstem nuclei may result in facial paralysis, dysphagia, laryngeal paralysis. However, the oculomotor nuclei are not usually involved. Brainstem involvement may also lead to autonomic dysfunction with hypertension, pulmonary edema, tachycardia, and/or arrhythmias. Respiratory impairment may occur because of (1) laryngeal/pharyngeal paralysis with airway obstruction, (2) paralysis of respiratory muscles, (3) involvement of respiratory center in the medulla, and/or (4) pulmonary edema. Urinary retention is common.

Laboratory: <u>CSF analysis:</u> WBC count is usually elevated (range 10–1000/ml), mostly lymphocytes. Neutrophils may predominate in early phase. The cell count is occasionally normal. Typically, the protein count is mildly elevated. Glucose level is normal. <u>Blood:</u> CBC may be normal or there may be leukocytosis.

Differential diagnosis: <u>Guillain-Barré syndrome</u> is distinguished from poliomyelitis by the absence of fever and the presence of symmetrical paralysis—often with sensory deficits. Furthermore, the CSF reveals a normal WBC count with elevated protein. <u>Enterovirus other than poliovirus</u> may cause poliomyelitis—e.g. coxsackie, echovirus, enterovirus 70 (the agent causing acute hemorrhagic conjunctivitis). <u>Epidemic neuromyasthenia</u> is distinguished from poliomyelitis by the presence of *spastic* paralysis with *hyper*reflexia. Furthermore, the CSF is nearly always normal.

Treatment is supportive. Bed rest for several days is advised. Aspirin or other mild nonnarcotic analgesics are administered as needed. Patients with impaired respiration may need airway suction to remove secretions, intubation, artificial ventilation, tracheostomy, etc. Hypertension and cardiac arrhythmias are handled in the usual manner. Catheterization may be necessary if there is urinary retention. Physical therapy for paralytic disease is begun after the acute illness subsides.

Prognosis: Recovery from paralysis is complete in many cases and many others are not seriously disabled. Recovery is most likely in partially disabled muscle regions. Of the muscle function that is restored, most can be expected to occur within the first 6 months, although there may be continued improvement for up to 2 years. Fatal paralytic disease occurs in 1–4% cases, mostly adults and patients with brainstem involvement.

Polyneuropathy (disease affecting many peripheral nerves simultaneously and symmetrically) has many possible precipitants: postinfectious; malignancy; diabetes mellitus; uremia; hypothyroidism; amyloidosis; vitamin B complex deficiency (e.g. alcoholism, malabsoption, beri beri, pernicious anemia); drugs (e.g. isoniazid, sulfonamides, nitrofurantoin, chloramphenicol, vincristine, cis-platinum, lithium, pyridoxine); toxins (e.g. heavy metals, carbon monoxide, cyanide, sundry industrial products). The Guillain-Barré syndrome is distinguished by the presence of motor deficits mainly with relatively mild sensory findings. It is discussed in more detail in the following chapter.

Signs/symptoms may vary according to the etiology. Paresthesias (e.g. numbness, tingling, burning) usually begin in the hands and feet. Sensory loss: As the disease progresses, there is loss of vibratory sense and proprioreception. Pain, pressure, and touch sensations are often lost in a glove and stocking distribution. Deep tendon reflexes are decreased. Gait may be impaired secondary to loss of sensation in general or loss of proprioreception in particular. Muscle weakness is usually minimal. Autonomic dysfunction may occur (e.g. orthostatic hypotension, impotence, urinary or bowel incontinence, diarrhea).

Guillain-Barré Syndrome is a polyneuropathy that in many cases follows a febrile (often viral) illness. The peripheral nerve fibers are affected by an inflammatory reaction with segmental demyelination.

Signs/symptoms: Motor disturbances: Muscle weakness often begins in the legs, ascends to the arms, and then to the face. Other patterns of progression may occur. Weakness may progress to paralysis—a flaccid paralysis. The muscles are tender. There may be cramping. Tendon reflexes are decreased or absent. The extent of weakness/paralysis varies from case to case. Quadriplegia may ensue. The muscles of respiration may be affected and the patient may require assisted ventilation. Swallowing or speaking may become difficult or impossible. Even eye movement may be impaired. Sensory disability, in contrast, is relatively mild. The patient may complain of numbness, tingling, or other paresthesias, especially of the hands or feet. However, there is usually only slight objective sensory impairment (decreased pinprick, vibration, and position perception). Autonomic nervous system may be affected. Consequently, there may be hyper or hypotension, brady or tachyarrhythmias, T wave abnormalities, sweating, urinary retention, ileus, etc.

Laboratory: CSF protein is elevated (notably the IgG fraction) although the level may be normal initially. The CSF cell count is not elevated.

Differential diagnosis: botulism, arsenic or organophosphate poisoning, tick paralysis, porphyria, autoimmune disease, post-diptheria, polio.

Treatment: Provide respiratory support as needed. ●Treat hypotension with IV fluids. Use vasopressors only as last resort. ●Control significant hypertension—cautiously. ●Cardiac monitor. Treat arrhythmias. ●Nasogastric feeding if patient is unable to swallow. Because of the risk of aspiration, nasogastric feeding should be done with upper body elevated and the patient should remain so positioned for about an hour.

Prognosis: Usually, there is progressive weakness for 1–4 weeks. As a rule, improvement begins 2–3 weeks after the patient stops deteriorating and there is usually complete recovery. However, some patients are left with permanent weakness.

Reye's Syndrome is characterized chiefly by cerebral edema

with encephalopathy, and fatty degeneration of the liver. Children, particularly those from 6 to 11 years, are the most common victims. Adult cases are rare. A viral illness precedes the syndrome. Influenza B or varicella-zoster infection are often implicated but many other viruses have been associated (e.g. influenza A, parainfluenza, herpes simplex, Ebstein-Barr, Coxsackie, adenovirus, reovirus, measles, rubella). Aspirin ingestion may be a contributing precipitating factor. Histology: Electron microscopy reveals mitochondrial injury in the liver, brain, kidneys, pancreas, heart, and skeletal muscle. Lipid accumulates in hepatocytes.

Signs/symptoms: Typically, as the viral illness begins to resolve, the patient starts to vomit (often severely) and there is lethargy. Delirium, hyperventilation, and/or hyperreflexia may ensue. In still more severe cases, coma develops and one may observe seizures, decorticate and then decerebrate posturing, areflexia, fixed dilated pupils, irregular respirations, respiratory arrest. Papilledema is usually absent. The liver is often enlarged and may be tender.

Tests: Blood ammonia must be elevated to make the diagnosis. The arterial ammonia may need to be measured since the venous ammonia may be normal in the early stage. Serum total bilirubin *less than* 2.5 mg/100ml. The serum bilirubin is characteristically normal. Bilirubin > 5 mg/100ml or jaundice is very unusual in Reye's syndrome. Liver enzymes (SGPT, SGOT) are typically elevated > 3 times normal. Prothrombin time and partial thromboplastin time may be prolonged. CPK is characteristically elevated. The myocardial and skeletal fractions are increased but the brain fraction remains normal. Hypoglycemia is common. Hypoglycemia is most likely in patients < 5 years old, particularly those < 1 year. Acid-base abnormalities are common—e.g. metabolic acidosis with compensatory respiratory alkalosis. There may be lactic acidemia. Electrolyte disturbances may develop—e.g. hypokalemia, hypernatremia. Serum free fatty acids (e.g. dicarboxylic acid) are elevated. Serum amylase is occasionally elevated. EKG abnormalities may be seen if myocarditis ensues. CBC, differential, platelet count are typically normal. CSF analysis: CSF pressure is usually elevated. CSF is otherwise normal. Lumbar puncture is performed to rule out meningitis but one should be wary of performing lumbar puncture if there are signs of elevated intracranial pressure. CAT scan reveals cerebral edema with ventricles narrowed to slits. Liver biopsy for histology is seldom required to confirm the diagnosis.

Treatment: If the patient is comatose, steps must be taken to relieve elevated intracranial pressure; elevate head and torso to 30°, intubate and ventilate to achieve a pCO2 of 20-25 (paralyze with pancuronium if necessary to control ventilation), The following drugs may be administered to help reduce intracranial pressure: furosemide 1mg/kg/day divided q6-8h, mannitol (see drug section), dexamethasone 0.5 mg/kg/day in 4-6 divided doses. In patients with liver failure, reduce GI absorption of ammonia with lactulose or neomycin. Administer intravenous dextrose and correct electrolyte disturbances; Electrolyte solutions containing 10% dextrose are advised. Administer dextrose bolus if hypoglycemia develops. Give sufficient fluids to achieve urine output of at least 0.5 ml/kg/hr. Administer vitamin K 5 mg IV q12h if coagulation is impaired. Fresh frozen plasma may be needed, particularly if invasive procedures are to be performed. Antacids or IV cimetidine may be administered to reduce risk of GI ulcers and bleeding.

Myasthenia Gravis is an autoimmune disease that results from

the presence of circulating antibodies directed against post-synaptic acetylcholine receptors at the myoneural junction. The disease may develop at any age including the newborn. In children and the aged, the incidence in males is about the same as females. In between, women are afflicted more often than men.

Signs/symptoms: The characteristic finding is that affected muscles become progressively weaker with repetitive or persistent contraction, and that there is some recovery of strength with return to baseline after resting. Myasthemia gravis may progress to severe incapacitation—e.g. unable to walk, respiratory compromise due to respiratory muscle weakness. Weakness is most common in muscles innervated by the cranial nerves, particularly the eye musculature. Common findings therefore include ptosis, diplopia, dysarthria, dysphagia. Having the patient look up for several minutes may elicit progressive drooping of the upper eyelids. The voice may become hoarse and fade after talking for a while. Chewing and swallowing may become dif̶ficult during the course of a meal. Sensory function is unimpaired; There are no sensory complaints and sensory exam is normal.

Diagnosis: Edrophonium (Tensilon) is a short-acting anticholinesterase that reverses muscle weakness in about a minute if myasthenia gravis is present. The effect lasts about 5 minutes. See "Anticholinesterases" in drug section. Electromyogram is confirmatory.

Treatment: Anticholinesterase treatment is begun: neostigmine or the slightly longer–acting pyridostigmine (Mestinon). Thymectomy benefits about 85% patients. The decision to perform thymectomy is individualized. Thymectomy is generally not advocated if weakness is confined to the extraocular muscles, and there may be misgivings about performing thymectomy on children or the aged. Plasmapheresis nearly always leads to rapid improvement. Unfortunately, improvement is only temporary (days to weeks) and the procedure must therefore be repeated periodically. Immunosuppression with prednisone or azathioprine is yet another often effective approach.

Muscular Dystrophy refers to a group of hereditary diseases

characterized by muscle weakness due to degeneration of muscle fibers in the absence of disease of the central or peripheral nervous system.

Duchenne dystrophy is the most common type of muscular dystrophy. It is a sex-linked recessive form and therefore almost always afflicts boys. Disease starts between 2 and 6 years of age. Muscle weakness begins first in the pelvic girdle and thighs; the patient has a waddling walk and trouble walking up stairs. The shoulder muscles are less conspicuously affected. Weakness of the back muscles causes difficulty in going from lying to standing position—the patient may use his hands to "walk" up his legs in order to stand (Gower's sign). Loordosis is characteristic. The muscles are pseudohypertrophic—i.e. they are weak but are large (calves in particular) because of fat and fibrous infiltration. The serum CPK is elevated. With time the patient becomes too weak to walk. Muscle and tendon contractures develop. Breathing is eventually affected, and the patient becomes susceptible to pulmonary infections and succumbs in his 20s.

Becker dystrophy is a sex-linked recessive form of dystrophy similar to Duchenne dystrophy. In contrast, the disease begins later in childhood and may progress more slowly.

Emery–Dreyfus dystrophy is yet another X-linked recessive type of dystrophy that begins later than and is less severe than the Duchenne type. Also, in contrast, pseudohypertrophy is absent and serum CPK is normal or only mildly elevated. Patients are susceptible to potentially fatal cardiac arrhythmias.

Limb–girdle muscular dystrophy (autosomal recessive) typically begins between 15 and 20 years of age. Females are afflicted as often as males. As in Duchenne dystrophy, there is progressive weakness—usually beginning in the pelvic girdle muscles with weakness of the shoulders developing subsequently. Serious disability occurs within 10 years. In contrast to Duchenne dystrophy, pseudohypertrophy is absent and the serum CPK is normal or only mildly elevated.

Facioscapulohumeral muscular dystrophy (autosomal dominant) begins between 10 and 20 years of age. In contrast to the other types of dystrophy, weakness of the shoulders is usually the initial complaint. Another distinguishing feature is the subsequent development of facial weakness. The patient also develops weakness and wasting of the muscles of the pelvic girdle and trunk. "Winged" scapulas result from weakness of the latissimus dorsi. There may be pronounced weakness of the anterior tibial muscles so that gait is affected. The pectoralis muscles develop an unusual appearance because atrophy is more pronounced at the sternal head than the clavicular head. The serum CPK is normal or only mildly elevated. A normal life-span is expected.

Intervertebral Disc Rupture & Herniation

When the vertebral column is subjected to acute or repeated traumatic vertical force, the anulus fibrosus of an intervertebral disc may rupture and thus allow the nucleus pulposus to herniate posteriorly into the cord or spinal roots.

LUMBAR DISC HERNIATION, in about 90% cases, occurs between vertebrae 4 and 5 or between 5 and the sacrum. The next most common site of lumbar herniation is at L3–4. Posterolateral herniation is most likely to compress the nerve root proceding to the intervertebral foramen just below—e.g. L3–4 disc compressing L4 nerve root, L4–5 disc compressing L5 root, L5–sacrum disc compressing S1 nerve root (and/or not infrequently L5 nerve root).

Signs/symptoms: Local pain/spasm: There is usually low back pain and there may be spasm of the paravertebral muscles. Sciatica (sensory abnormality in the sciatic nerve distribution L4–S3) is characteristic. Sciatic pain is usually felt down the buttock, posterior/lateral thigh, and/or calf. There is considerable individual variation in sensory distribution. However, compression of L5 nerve root typically results in pain that radiates down to the great toe, while compression of S1 nerve root is associated with pain that radiates along the lateral aspect of the foot. L4 root compression is typically felt along the anterior thigh. Numbness or other paresthesias may be present in the sciatic nerve distribution. Pain is aggravated by movement, particularly in extending the back. Sitting typically aggravates the pain; standing less so. Lying down tends to lessen pain. Valsalva maneuver (e.g. straining at stool, coughing) characteristically aggravates pain because it increases subarachnoid pressure which is transmitted to the herniated disc. Passive straight leg raise: With the patient in supine position, the examiner lifts the leg (with the knee straight) on the symptomatic side. This maneuver stretches the nerve roots and should therefore increase low back and radicular pain. A positive *crossed* straight-leg raise sign (i.e. passive straight–leg raise on the asymptomatic side provokes sciatica on the symptomatic side) lends additional support to the diagnosis of herniated disk. Muscle weakness/depressed reflexes: Compression of L5 root may cause weakness of dorsiflexion of the foot and therefore difficulty walking on the heels. S1 root compression may cause weakness of plantar flexion, and therefore difficulty walking on the toes and depressed/absent ankle jerk. L4 compression may result in quadricep weakness with depressed knee jerk. Muscle atrophy and fasciculations of the involved muscle region may develop with time. Cauda equina syndrome: Large midline posterior herniations may compress the cauda equina so that urinary retention/incontinence, bowel dysfunction, and/or bilateral leg weakness may ensue.

Tests: Lumbosacral spine x-rays may reveal narrowing of the intervertebral spaces, but this is not diagnostically useful since aymptomatic individuals just as often have this finding. Spasm of the paraspinal muscles may cause lumbar scoliosis that is concave toward the side of the spasm. A large herniated disc may sometimes be seen on plain x-ray. CAT scan or myelography is diagnostic. Electromyography or nerve conduction velocity may be used to document deterioration/loss of nerve function in the distribution of the lumbar roots.

Treatment: Bed rest on a firm mattress for 1–2 weeks benefits many patients. Local heat (e.g. hydrocolator packs) may be soothing. Analgesia: A nonsteroidal anti-inflammatory drug is usually prescribed (e.g. ibuprofen). If pain is severe, a narcotic (e.g. oxycodone) may be necessary for 1–2 days. Other conservative measures: After the period of bed rest, physical therapy is begun and the patient may be fitted with a low–back corset. Overweight patients are encouraged to lose weight. Surgery is necessary if (**1**) a midline herniation squeezes the cauda equina so that there is bladder or bowel dysfunction, (**2**) there is progressive neurologic impairment, (**3**) there is intractable disabling pain. Intradisc enzyme injections of chymopapain to dissolve the disc is advocated by some authorities.

CERVICAL DISC HERNIATION The most vulnerable cervical discs are between vertebrae 5 and 6, and between 6 and 7. Usually, the nucleus pulposus herniates posterolaterally so that there is compression of a nerve root with pain down an arm. Rarely, there is posterocentral herniation so that the cord is compressed and quadriplegia results.

THORACIC DISC HERNIATION is rare but is particularly dangerous because here the relatively narrow vertebral canal makes cord compression more likely.

Endocrinology

Posterior Pituitary Disease

The precursors of oxytocin and antidiuretic hormone (vasopressin) are produced in the hypothalamus within neurons whose axons extend into the posterior pituitary. These prohormones move down the axons where they are stored and converted to the nonapeptides oxytocin and ADH prior to being released from the posterior pituitary. Oxytocin stimulates uterine contractions during labor and mediates the release of milk in response to suckling. Antidiuretic hormone (ADH) regulates water excretion in response to blood osmolality. Osmoreceptors in the hypothalamus sense when the blood osmolality is elevated, and this stimulates increased ADH synthesis and release. ADH in turn acts on the distal renal tubules and collecting ducts to increase the permeability of these structures to water. Water reabsorption is thereby increased and the urine becomes more concentrated. In contrast, when the serum osmolality falls below 280 mOsm/kg water, ADH secretion stops and the distal renal tubules and collecting ducts become impermeable to water. Water excretion is increased and the urine becomes dilute. ●Hypovolemia also induces ADH release but, unless hypovolemia is pronounced, blood osmolality is the main factor controlling ADH secretion.

DIABETES INSIPIDUS

Central diabetes insipidus (excretion of large volume of dilute urine due to inadequate secretion of ADH). Etiology is unknown in about a third of cases. Most of the remainder are secondary to head trauma; pituitary surgery; or intercranial neoplasm (e.g. craniopharyngioma, metastatic tumor). ●It should be noted that destruction or removal of the posterior pituitary, or transection of the pituitary stalk only results in temporary diabetes insipidus. The hypothalamus itself must be affected if diabetes insipidus is to be permanent. ●Uncommon conditions leading to central DI include anoxia; histiocytosis; granulomatous disease (e.g. sarcoid, Tb); aneurysm; thrombosis; encephalitis; meningitis; familial (e.g. Lawrence–Moon–Biedl syndrome). ●Some drugs (e.g. alcohol, phenytoin) may provoke a mild and transient diabetes insipidus by suppressing ADH secretion. Signs/symptoms: There is polyuria and polydipsia. The typical patient craves cold water. The patient with complete central diabetes insipidus (i.e. hypothalamus incapable of secreting any ADH) may excrete > 15 liter urine/24 hour. As long as thirst induces the patient to replenish water lost; hyperosmolality and hypernatremia, dehydration, or other adverse consequences do not occur. However, if for some reason the patient is unable to drink water, dehydration with hypotension and/or hypernatremia with encephalopathy will result. Treatment: vasopressin or vasopressin analogs by injection or intranasally (refer to drug section). Patients with *partial* central DI may sometimes be managed with chlorpropamide, a drug that induces ADH secretion. However, there is danger of inducing hypoglycemia with this drug. ●In emergencies (e.g. serum sodium > 160 mEq/liter with encephalopathy, severe volume depletion with hypotension), patients are initially treated with acqueous vasopressin 5–10 units IM q4–6h and intravenous normal saline. See "Hypernatremia" for details of fluid therapy.

Nephrogenic diabetes insipidus is the inappropriate excretion of large volumes of dilute urine due to impaired responsiveness of the renal tubules to ADH. Etiology: May be hereditary (rare) or be the consequence of acquired renal disease secondary to sundry conditions—e.g. sickle cell anemia; hypercalcemia; hypokalemia; drugs (e.g. lithium, amphotericin B, demeclocycline, fluorocarbon anesthesia); analgesic nephropathy; multiple myeloma; severe protein deficiency. Treatment: Treat the underlying disorder or remove the offending agent if possible. In some cases, nephrogenic DI may be mitigated by sodium restriction and administration of a thiazide diuretic (e.g. hydrochlorothiazide 50–100 mg/day). The resultant sodium depletion means that less sodium and therefore less water reaches the collecting tubules. Consequently, proportionally more water is reabsorbed by the proximal tubules. ●In emergencies (e.g. serum sodium > 160 mEq/liter with encephalopathy, severe volume depletion with hypotension), patients are initially treated with intravenous normal saline. See "Hypernatremia" for details of fluid therapy.

Psychogenic polydipsia (compulsive water drinking) may be confused with central or nephrogenic diabetes insipidus. Patients may consume and excrete > 20 liter water/day. In contrast to diabetes insipidus, however, nocturia is typically not present nor are patients awakened by thirst.

Differentiating central DI, nephrogenic DI, and psychogenic polydipsia: Clinical circumstances often suggest the diagnosis. Confirmation rests on the results of water deprivation and vasopressin administration: Obtain patient weight, serum sodium, serum osmolality, urine osmolality. Under close supervision, body weight and urine osmolality is measured hourly and the patient is deprived of fluids for 12 hours or until: (**1**) there is loss 3–5% body weight, (**2**) postural hypotension or tachycardia ensues, or (**3**) the change in osmolality of urine samples obtained an hour apart is < 30 mOsm/kg. After the period of water deprivation; serum sodium, serum osmolality, and urine osmolality are again measured and then acqueous vasopressin 5 units is administered subcutaneously. The urine osmolality is again measured an hour later. **Test interpretation:** (**1**) Normal subject: urine osmolality > 800 mOsm and serum osmolality < 295 mOsm after the period of water deprivation. And there is little or no change in urine osmolality after vasopressin administration. (**2**) Psychogenic polydipsia: urine osmolality 500–800 mOsm after water deprivation with little or no change after vasopressin injection. (**3**) Nephrogenic DI: urine osmolality < 600 mOsm after water deprivation and no change after vasopressin injection. (**4**) Complete central DI: urine osmolality < 250 mOsm and serum osmolality may be > 320 mOsm after water deprivation. And the urine osmolality increases to 350–500 mOsm or by over 50% after vasopressin injection. (**5**) Partial central DI: urine osmolality > 350 mOsm after water deprivation with 10–25% increase after vasopressin injection.

SYNDROME OF INAPPROPRIATE ADH SECRETION (SIADH) is characterized by hyponatremia (hypoosmolality) in the presence of a paradoxically hypertonic urine. Urine sodium is typically > 15–20 mEq/liter. Urine osmolality is usually > plasma osmolality. The total body sodium is normal. Total body water is increased but edema rarely occurs. **Diagnosis** is confirmed by restricting fluids and noting the return to a normal serum osmolality and serum sodium. The condition generally recurs if the patient is allowed 2–3 liter fluid per day. ●SIADH cannot be diagnosed if the patient (1) is dehydrated; (2) has renal, adrenal, or anterior pituitary disease; (3) is receiving diuretics. **Causes:** SIADH may be the consequence of head trauma; intracranial tumor; subarachnoid hemorrhage; meningitis; encephalitis; pulmonary disease (e.g. pneumonia, tuberculosis); intermittent positive pressure ventilation; acute intermittent porphyria. ●Drugs that either stimulate pituitary ADH release or potentiate the effect of ADH on the renal tubules may be responsible (e.g. amitriptyline, phenothiazines, carbamazepine, barbiturates, clofibrate, chlorpropamide, tolbutamide, cyclophosphamide, vincristine). ●SIADH may also result from ectopic ADH production (e.g. lung carcinoma—particularly oat cell). **Treatment:** Correct underlying condition if possible. If SIADH is the result of a temporary and nonemergent condition, then fluid restriction to 1–1.5 liter/day is the only treatment required. If SIADH is expected to be chronic, then demeclocycline may mitigate the condition by blocking the effect of ADH on the renal tubules. In hyponatremic emergencies (e.g. coma, convulsions), therapy consists of judicious administration of IV 3% saline along with IV furosemide. KCl is added to the IV bottle as needed to maintain normal serum potassium. Once neurologic signs are no longer present or the serum sodium reaches 120–125 mEq/liter, this mode of therapy is discontinued in favor of fluid restriction.

Space-occupying Lesions Pituitary Fossa

PITUITARY TUMORS may manifest by one or a combination of mechanisms: First, an enlarging tumor may compress surrounding structures and produce: (**1**) headache; (**2**) visual field defects due to compression of the optic chiasm (e.g. bitemporal hemianopsia, sometimes culminating in complete blindness); (**3**) oculomotor palsies (e.g. diplopia, ptosis) with lateral involvement of 3rd, 4th, or 6th cranial nerves; (**4**) hydrocephalus due to compression of the 3rd ventricle; (**5**) hypothalamic dysfunction due to compression of hypothalamus (e.g. impaired satiety with ensuing obesity, disordered temperature regulation, altered consciousness, retarded sexual development, diabetes insipidus); (**6**) CSF rhinorrhea as consequence of anterior erosion into the sphenoid sinus. Second, an enlarging tumor may compress normal pituitary tissue provoking pituitary hormone deficiencies. The destructive effects of pituitary apoplexy may also cause hypopituitarism (see below). Third, the tumor may be functional and result in a pituitary hormone excess. **Diagnostic tests:** Skull x-rays may reveal an enlarged or eroded sella turcica. CAT scan of the pituitary may reveal the tumor and may even detect tumor smaller than 10 mm. Serum prolactin is an useful screening test because not only is it elevated when there is a prolactin-secreting tumor, but it is also elevated when any pituitary tumor (functional or non-functional) prevents transport of dopamine from the hypothalamus to the pituitary (e.g. by compressing pituitary stalk). This is because dopamine normally inhibits the secretion of prolactin; the absence of dopamine therefore allows prolactin levels to rise. Visual field testing and/or visual evoked response may be abnormal if there is compression of optic chiasm.

EMPTY SELLA is the condition in which a defect in the diaphragma sellae permits the arachnoid membrane and CSF to push into the pituitary fossa so that there is compression of the pituitary gland and perhaps ensuing enlargement of the sella turcica. It is a common and usually benign condition occurring most often in obese hypertensive females. Patients may complain of headache but other complaints are rare (e.g. visual field defects, pseudotumor cerebri–papilledema, CSF rhinorrhea). Furthermore, compression of the pituitary gland rarely causes pituitary hormone deficiencies. Skull x-rays may reveal an enlarged sella. CAT scan following intrathecal injection of dye may delineate the lesion. Corrective measures are usually only required if visual field defects ensue.

PITUITARY APOPLEXY (hemorrhage into a pituitary tumor) is an unusual and potentially disasterous event. Presentation may include (**1**) manifestations of subarachnoid hemorrhage (headache, stiff neck, nausea, vomiting, depressed consciousness); (**2**) blindness due to compression of the optic chiasm; and (**3**) dilated pupil(s) and deviated eyes due to cranial nerve compression. **Treatment:** Emergency transphenoidal surgery is often necessary. Glucocorticoids are begun at the time of diagnosis since ACTH secretion is likely to be compromised. Panhypopituitarism and hypothalamic impairment are common sequelae.

Hypopituitarism (Anterior Pituitary Insufficiency)

Growth hormone insufficiency in adults produces no significant disturbance. In children, dwarfism results; and there is poor muscular development, delayed puberty, and sometimes fasting hypoglycemia. Growth hormone is the therapy. However, therapy must be begun before the epiphyses have closed if it is to promote bone growth.

Thyroid stimulating hormone (TSH) deficiency results in hypothyroidism (refer to "Hypothyroidism" chapter).

Adrenocorticotrophic hormone (ACTH) insufficiency results in a deficiency of cortisol. However, in contrast to primary adrenal insufficiency, aldosterone secretion by the adrenal continues because ACTH has minimal influence over aldosterone production. Also in contrast to primary adrenal insufficiency, the skin is pale because the melanocyte stimulating effects of ACTH and MSH are absent. For further discussion of ACTH deficiency, refer to *Secondary Adrenal Insufficiency* in "Adrenocortical Insufficiency" chapter.

Gonadotropin (FSH, LH) insufficiency: In males gonadotropin insufficiency beginning in adulthood results in testicular atrophy, decreased sex interest, decreased spermatogenesis and infertility, decreased hair growth on face and body. In adult females there is secondary amenorrhea, breast atrophy, decreased axillary and pubic hair. Gonadotropin insufficiency in childhood in females results in primary amenorrhea, retarded breast development, decreased–absent axillary and pubic hair. Gonadotropin insufficiency in childhood in males leads to small testes, small penis, and scant body hair. Growth in children: Children with isolated gonadotropin deficiency grow relatively taller than those with multiple anterior pituitary hormone deficiencies. If the disorder is not treated before growth is complete, eunuchoid habitus may develop (e.g. arm span exceeds the height).

PANHYPOPITUITARISM (deficiency of all anterior pituitary hormones) The exact presentation depends upon the patient's age, sex, and the amount of pituitary tissue remaining FSH and LH levels are usually the first to decrease followed by growth hormone, ACTH, and lastly TSH. Panhypopituitarsm may lead to life-threatening hyponatremia even though aldosterone secretion is normal. Severe hypoglycemia may also occur since patients are unusually sensitive to insulin.

Causes of panhypopituitarism include Sheehan's syndrome (postpartum pituitary necrosis); pituitary adenoma; craniopharyngioma; pituitary apoplexy; metastatic tumors; parasellar tumors; hypophysectomy; head trauma; granuloma (e.g. sarcoid, histiocytosis); hemochromatosis; internal carotid artery aneurysm; radiation; infection. ●Lesions involving the hypothalamus may also cause panhypopituitarism by impairing production and secretion of hypothalamic releasing factors—e.g. gonadotropin releasing hormone (GnRH), thyrotropin releasing hormone (TRH). ●When there is uncertainty as to whether the lesion is hypothalamic or pituitary, hypothalamic releasing hormones may be administered to test pituitary reserve: TRH to stimulate TSH release, GnRH (gonadotropin releasing hormone) to stimulate FSH and LH release, metyrapone to stimulate ACTH release, TRH or chlorpromazine to stimulate prolactin release.

Treatment panhypopituitarism: Thyroxine and hydrocortisone supplements are necessary. In addition, (**1**) children require growth hormone, (**2**) men require testosterone for maintenance of secondary sex characteristics, and HCG (human chorionic gonadotropin) with FSH to become fertile, (**3**) women require estrogens to maintain secondary sex characteristics. Women with panhypopituitarism secondary to pituitary disease who wish to become fertile receive cyclical FSH and LH with addition of HCG to induce ovulation. Women with infertility secondary to hypothalamic dysfunction are treated with gonadotropin releasing hormone (GnRH).

Hyperpituitarism (anterior pituitary hormone excess)

practically speaking refers to excessive secretion of growth hormone, prolactin, or ACTH. Excessive secretion of TSH, FSH, or LH is rare.

ACTH EXCESS (Cushing's disease): See "Adrenocortical Excess" chapter.

GROWTH HORMONE EXCESS before the epiphyses have closed causes gigantism. Growth hormone excess beginning in adulthood results in acromegaly.

Signs/symptoms: Bone enlargement: Cortical thickening and periosteal overgrowth leads to wider thicker bones. As a consequence there is enlargement of the hands and feet, enlargement of the head, protrusion of the jaw with malocclusion and separation of the teeth. Arthritis is due to hypertrophic involvement of joints. Soft tissue enlargement (e.g. tongue, heart, kidneys, liver, spleen) may be evident. Soft tissue overgrowth may compress the median nerve provoking carpal tunnel syndrome. Coarsening of facial features is due to soft tissue growth as well as bone growth. Other common manifestations: fatigue, myalgia, hypertension, hyperglycemia, glucose intolerance, heat intolerance, exessive sweating, hypertrichosis in women, galactorrhea. Expansion and encroachment of the pituitary tumor may lead to headaches, visual field defects (e.g. bitemporal hemianopsia). Compression of the remaining pituitary gland may lead to deficiencies of the other pituitary hormones (see "Hypopituitarism" chapter).

Diagnostic tests: Serum growth hormone: Fasting recumbent serum growth hormone level is usually elevated (> 5–10 ng/ml). However, because stress alone can induce growth hormone secretion, the response to glucose administration is used as a confirmatory test: 1–2 hours after administering 100 gram glucose PO, the serum growth hormone level will normally be suppressed to < 5 ng/ml in women and to < 2 ng/ml in men. However, growth hormone remains elevated in acromegaly. Serum somatomedins are elevated. Possible x-ray findings: enlarged sella turcica and frontal sinuses, increased heel pad thickness (> 20 mm in nonobese patient) due to soft tissue overgrowth, enlarged fingers. CAT scan may identify tumor.

Treatment is usually transphenoidal surgery.

PROLACTIN HORMONE EXCESS: Etiology: Lesion of hypothalamus, pituitary stalk, or pituitary gland: Prolactin excess may be due to a prolactin–secreting pituitary tumor. A lesion of the hypothalamus or pituitary stalk that eliminates the influence of dopamine may also lead to prolactin excess (dopamine is secreted by the hypothalamus and normally inhibits pituitary prolactin secretion). <u>Drugs</u> that may induce hypersecretion of prolactin include methyldopa, reserpine, phenothiazines, estrogens, heroin, morphine. <u>Other conditions</u> known to induce prolactin secretion and possibly galactorrhea include breast stimulation, chest surgery, cirrhosis, hypothyroidism.

Signs/symptoms: <u>In males,</u> prolactin excess sometimes leads to gynecomastia, galactorrhea, and/or inpotence. <u>In women,</u> there may be amenorrhea, galactorrhea (see "Galactorrhea" chapter), and infertility. <u>Local effects:</u> A large tumor may cause headache, visual field defects, oculomotor deficits, or may compress the remaining pituitary gland so that deficiencies of other pituitary hormones develop.

Laboratory: The normal serum prolactin is < 20 ng/ml in males and < 30 in females. A prolactin level > 200 ng/ml is indicative of a prolactin–secreting tumor. A less elevated prolactin level does not differentiate a prolactin–secreting tumor from other causes of prolactin elevation.

Treatment: Treat underlying disease or remove offending agent if possible. ●Many prolactin–secreting pituitary tumors may be managed with bromocriptine. The drug suppresses prolactin secretion and shrinks the tumor. ●Large tumors require resection. Preoperative bromocriptine therapy may be used to shrink the tumor.

Adrenocortical Insufficiency

PRIMARY ADRENOCORTICAL INSUFFICIENCY (ADDISON'S DISEASE)   Most cases are due to autoimmune injury to the adrenal cortex. Antiadrenal antibodies are found and the adrenal cortex is infiltrated with lymphocytes and plasma cells. Moreover, Addison's disease is not uncommonly associated with other autoimmune diseases (e.g. diabetes mellitus, Hashimoto's thyroiditis, Graves' disease, hypoparathyroidism, pernicious anemia). Besides autoimmune disease, Addison's disease may result from adrenal involvement by tuberculosis, histoplasmosis, sarcoidosis, amyloidosis, metastatic carcinoma.

Signs/symptoms Addison's disease: <u>Nonspecific symptoms:</u> fatigue, weakness, weight loss, anorexia, nausea, vomiting, diarrhea. <u>Electrolyte and fluid abnormalities and consequences:</u> Aldosterone influences the distal renal tubules to reabsorb sodium. Consequently, a decrease in aldosterone leads to hyponatremia. There is also hyperkalemia due to concurrent impairment of renal potassium excretion. Sodium loss is associated with water loss. Consequently, there may be dehydration with hypovolemia. This may manifest as hypotension and a small heart may be evident on x-ray. <u>Hyperpigmentation</u> develops because negative feedback inhibition of pituitary ACTH and MSH secretion is removed as the serum cortisol falls. The elevated ACTH and MSH levels that ensue are a stimulus to increased synthesis of melanin. <u>Loss of body hair in females</u> is due to decreased production of adrenal androgens.

Laboratory: <u>Routine laboratory findings:</u> There is hyponatremia with hyperkalemia. Dehydration leads to elevated BUN and creatinine. Eosinophilia is characteristic. <u>Serum ACTH</u> level is elevated (> 250 pg/ml) and <u>serum cortisol</u> is low. <u>24 hr urinary 17-hydroxycorticosteroids</u> are decreased. <u>Cosyntropin test</u> helps confirm the diagnosis. Synthetic ACTH (cosyntropin) is administered. In adult, inject cosyntropin 0.25 mg IM (0.1mg in infant < 1 yr, 0.15 mg in child 1–5 yr). Blood samples for serum cortisol determination are obtained prior to the injection and 30 and 60 minutes following the injection. Adrenocortical insufficiency (adrenal, pituitary, or hypothalamic) is ruled out if the 30 minute serum cortisol level is > 18 mcg/ml and is ≥ 10 mcg/ml above the basal cortisol level. Also normally, the serum cortisol will rise to approximately twice that of the basal level. An abnormal cosyntropin test together with an elevated serum ACTH is diagnostic of *primary* adrenocortical insufficiency.

Treatment Addison's disease: Chronic primary (Addison's) adrenocortical insufficiency is treated with prednisone (7.5 mg PO once daily) and fludrocortisone (0.05–0.1mg PO once daily). Patient will require additional prednisone or IV hydrocortisone during periods of stress (e.g. febrile illness, gastroenteritis, surgery).

SECONDARY (PITUITARY) ADRENAL INSUFFICIENCY (adrenal insufficiency resulting from deficiency of pituitary ACTH) may occur in association with panhypopituitarism (see "Anterior Pituitary Disease") or occur as an isolated ACTH deficiency.
Adrenal insufficiency secondary to exogenous glucocorticoid suppression of pituitary ACTH: Isolated ACTH deficiency is virtually always the consequence of suppression of pituitary ACTH secretion by exogenous glucocorticoid administration. Large doses of glucocorticoids given for ≤ 3 days do not suppress the hypothalamic-pituitary-adrenal axis and neither does prolonged administration of 5 mg prednisone once daily in the morning. However, 20–30 mg or more of prednisone or the equivalent a day for ≥ 5 days will suppress the hypothalamic-pituitary-adrenal axis. The patient who is receiving suppressive doses of glucocorticoids is most likely to get into trouble (see *adrenal crisis* below) when glucocorticoids are abruptly discontinued or sharply reduced. The patient is then particularly vulnerable to stress (e.g. febrile illness). After glucocorticoid therapy is discontinued or substantially reduced, it may be many months before the pituitary gland fully regains its ability to adequately secrete ACTH in response to stress. Therefore, unless glucocorticoid therapy has been brief, glucocorticoid therapy must be discontinued only after a period of gradual tapering (refer to Corticosteroids in drug section for withdrawal schedules).

    Signs/symptoms/laboratory: Nonspecific symptoms: fatigue, weakness, weight loss, anorexia, nausea, vomiting, diarrhea. Hyperpigmentation is absent (in contrast to primary adrenal insufficiency) because ACTH and MSH are decreased. Serum ACTH is typically ≤ 50 pg/ml in secondary adrenocortical insufficiency. Electrolyte abnormalities: Also in contrast to primary adrenal insufficiency, hyperkalemia does not occur because adrenal aldosterone secretion is not dependent on ACTH stimulation. However, hyponatremia may occur because decreased levels of cortisol result in decreased free-water clearance. If ACTH deficiency is part of panhypopituitarism, there may also be signs and symptoms of thyroid and gonadal insufficiency due to depressed levels of TSH, LH, or FSH. Cosyntropin test (see Primary Adrenal Insufficiency above) is nearly always abnormal in patients with secondary adrenal insufficiency. However, the test may be normal in a patient whose pituitary is still secreting some ACTH. If this happens and the diagnosis is uncertain, a prolonged cosyntropin stimulation test, a metyrapone test, or an insulin tolerance test may be diagnostic.

    Treatment: Panhypopituitarism is treated with glucocorticoids (e.g. prednisone), thyroxine, and sex steroids. Children also require growth hormone.

ACUTE ADRENAL INSUFFICIENCY (adrenal crisis) is a potentially life-threatening condition that may occur with either primary or secondary adrenal insufficiency. The syndrome is usually precipitated by a stressful situation—e.g. infection, trauma, surgery, fasting, excessive sweating. Adrenal hemorrhage secondary to sepsis or anticoagulant therapy may also precipitate the syndrome.

    Signs/symptoms: The patient is profoundly weak and may complain of pain in the abdomen, lower back, and/or legs. Nausea, vomiting, diarrhea may be present. Hypotension, shock, and coma may ensue unless treatment is instituted promptly.

    Treatment: Hydrocortisone 100 mg IV over 30 seconds. Subsequent doses (100 mg every 6 hours for 24–48 hours) may be diluted in D5NS and administered IV over 1–4 hours. Dehydration may be profound and adults may require 4 liters of D5NS over the first 4 hours to treat shock and hyponatremia. After 2 days most patients can begin oral prednisone therapy. Prednisone is subsequently tapered as clinical circumstances suggest (refer to Corticosteroids in drug section for further discussion on tapering). Patients with primary (Addison's) insufficiency are also started on a mineralocorticoid (fludrocortisone 0.05–0.1 mg daily).

Adrenocortical Excess

CUSHING'S SYNDROME (glucocorticoid excess syndrome) may be the consequence of chronic glucocorticoid therapy, excess ACTH production (pituitary or ectopic), or adrenal neoplasia.

Signs/symptoms: <u>central obesity</u> (e.g. truncal obesity, moon face, buffalo hump); <u>skin lesions</u> (e.g. atrophic skin with purple striae & easy bruising; poor wound healing); <u>muscle</u> wasting/weakness; <u>osteoporosis; hypertension; peripheral edema; psychiatric abnormalities</u> (e.g. depression, euphoria). <u>Women</u>, because of increased output of adrenal androgens, often complain of menstrual irregularities, acne, hirsutism. <u>Men</u> may, because of cortisol inhibition of pituitary gonadotropins, complain of decreased libido, impotence, gynecomastia.

Laboratory: <u>Hypokalemia</u> may occur. <u>Laboratory evidence of diabetes mellitus</u> may be found. <u>Plasma cortisol</u> normally has a diurnal variation (10–25 mcg/dl at 6–8 AM and decreasing to < 10 mcg after 6 PM). In Cushing's syndrome the evening cortisol remains elevated. <u>The 24 hour urine free-cortisol</u> is usually elevated in Cushing's syndrome. However, physical or psychological stress may in the absence of Cushing's syndrome result in elevated 24 hour urine free-cortisol. <u>Overnight dexamethasone suppression test</u>: Dexamethasone 1 mg PO is given at 11 PM and a serum cortisol is obtained at 8 AM following morning. Normally, the morning cortisol is < 5 mcg/dl and this together with a 24 hour urine free-cortisol in the normal range usually rules out Cushing's syndrome. However, false positives may occur with obesity, chronic renal failure, estrogen therapy, phenytoin administration, great physical or emotional stress, etc. <u>Two day low-dose dexamethasone suppression</u> may help establish or exclude Cushing's syndrome in equivocal cases. A baseline serum cortisol or a baseline measurement of urinary steroids (urinary free-cortisol or urinary 17-hydroxysteroids) is first obtained. Then, dexamethasone is administered for two days (0.5 mg PO every 6 hours for total of 8 doses). On day 2 of dexamethasone administration, a 24 hour urine collection for urinary steroids is obtained. A blood sample for serum cortisol is obtained 6 hours after the last dexamethasone dose. Normally, the serum cortisol should be suppressed to < 50% of the baseline or to < 5mcg/ml. Also normally, the urine free cortisol should be suppressed to < 25 mcg/24hr and the urine 17-hydroxysteroids should be < 4 mg/24hr. <u>High-dose dexamethasone test</u> is performed if Cushing's syndrome is diagnosed: At 11 PM, obtain a blood sample for serum cortisol and administer 8 mg dexamethasone PO. At 8 AM the following morning, obtain another serum cortisol. If pituitary overproduction of ACTH (i.e. Cushing's disease) is the cause of Cushing's syndrome, the serum cortisol will usually be suppressed by more than half of the baseline level. Failure to suppress suggests ectopic ACTH production or an adrenal tumor. <u>Plasma ACTH levels</u> may also help identify the cause of Cushing's syndrome. In Cushing's disease, the plasma ACTH is often elevated but usually does not exceed 200 pg/ml. With ectopic ACTH production, the plasma ACTH often exceeds 200 pg/ml. In the case of Cushing's syndrome secondary to an adrenal tumor, the plasma ACTH is often low or undetectable. <u>Administration of synthetic ACTH</u> (cosyntropin 25 units) may help distinguish adrenal adenoma from carcinoma. A normal response is a doubling or more of the serum cortisol. A normal response may occur with an adrenal adenoma but over 90% of adrenal carcinomas fail to respond.

CONDITIONS LEADING TO CUSHING'S SYNDROME:

Cushing's disease is the disorder in which excess ACTH production by a pituitary adenoma causes bilateral adrenal cortical hyperplasia that in turn leads to Cushing's syndrome. Incidence of Cushing's disease is greatest in females of reproductive age. In addition to the usual stigmata of Cushing's syndrome, there may also be ACTH–induced hyperpigmentation. The pituitary adenoma can sometimes be seen on CAT scan. Hypophysectomy is the usual treatment.

Ectopic ACTH: The most common source is a lung carcinoma but many other tumors have been implicated. If surgical removal of the tumor is not feasible, inhibitors of corticosteroid synthesis (e.g. metyrapone, mitotane, aminoglutethimide) may be needed to control symptoms and correct metabolic abnormalities (e.g. hypokalemia).

Adrenal cortical tumors (adenocarcinoma or more commonly a benign adenoma) may produce excess cortisol and inhibit pituitary ACTH release. The adrenal cortex, aside from the tumor itself, is therefore bilaterally atrophic. The tumor is sometimes felt on exam or revealed by CAT scan, angiography, or IVP. Treatment: resect the tumor. Glucocorticoids are required following surgery because the hypo-thalamic-pituitary-adrenal axis is suppressed.

Chronic glucocorticoid administration-induced Cushing's syndrome differs from Cushing's syndrome resulting from other causes in that there is generally no evidence of excessive adrenal androgens (e.g. hirsutism, acne). Furthermore, some of the side effects of glucocorticoid administration (e.g. cataracts, glaucoma, benign intracranial hypertension, pancreatitis) are seldom seen in Cushing's syndrome re-sulting from other causes.

HYPERALDOSTERONISM:

Aldosterone and the renin-angiotensin system: Aldosterone is produced by the adrenal cortex. It acts on specific receptor sites of the distal renal tubules to induce sodium retention and potassium loss. The secretion of aldosterone is regulated by the renin-angiotensin system. Hypokalemia also induces aldosterone secretion by directly stimulating adrenal aldosterone production. ACTH to a lesser extent may stimulate aldosterone production. ●The source of renin is the juxtaglomerular cells of the afferent renal arterioles. Renin release is mediated by the intra-arteriolar pressure adjacent to the juxtaglomerular cells, and by the macula densa (that portion of the distal convoluted tubules lying adjacent to the juxtaglomerular cells which senses the amount of sodium reaching the distal tubule). ●When the intra-arteriolar pressure decreases at the juxtaglomerular cells or the amount of sodium reaching the macula densa decreases, the juxtaglomerular cells release renin. Renin is a pro-teolytic enzyme that acts on angiotensinogen (a circulating alpha–2 globulin) to pro-duce angiotensin I which in turn is converted to angiotensin II. Angiotensin II stimu-lates the production of aldosterone by the zona glomerulosa of the adrenal cortex.

Primary hyperaldosteronism (Conn's syndrome) is the excessive secretion of aldosterone due to autonomous overproduction by the adrenal gland (i.e. an extra–adrenal stimulus is not present). Conn's syndrome may result from bilateral adrenal hyperplasia (85%), adrenal adenoma (15%), or adrenal carcinoma (rare). **Presentation:** Patients present with mild to severe hypertension and there is usual-ly hypokalemia. Hypokalemia may manifest as muscle weakness, fatigue, nocturia. ●Hypokalemia may be accompanied by metabolic alkalosis and sometimes hypo-magnesemia. ●Sodium retention leads to an increase in extracellular volume but pa-tients seldom exhibit edema because sodium retention has an upper limit so that at some point the "escape phenomenon" comes into play (i.e. at some point sodium excretion increases because proximal renal tubular reabsorption of sodium does not increase further). The serum sodium is seldom < 140 mEq/liter unless the patient has been receiving diuretics. **Diagnosis:** Hypokalemia in absence of diuretic therapy is found in most cases. If the patient with primary hyperaldosteronism is normokalemic, hypokalemia will be induced in by sodium chloride adminstration (e.g. 2 gram PO 3 times/day for 5 days). A normal or elevated serum potassium following sodium chloride loading rules out primary hyperaldosteronism. Plasma renin activity (PRA) is usually low in primary hyperaldosteronism. The reliability of this test is en-hanced by obtaining the blood sample after the patient has been upright for 5 hours following administration of furosemide 60 mg PO. It should be noted that 25% pa-tients with essential hypertension will also have decreased PRA. A 24 hour urine aldosterone is obtained if the PRA is low. The urinary aldosterone is usually > 17 mcg/24 hr in primary hyperaldosteronism. Serum aldosterone may be elevated, particularly if an adenoma is present. Furthermore, in patients with primary hyperal-dosteronism, the serum aldosterone will not be suppressed by salt loading (e.g. 2 liter normal saline IV over 4 hours may be administered unless there is a contraindi-cation). The level of serum aldosterone and/or posture–mediated changes in serum aldosterone may help identify the cause of primary hyperaldosteronism: (**1**) An ade-noma is usually associated with serum aldosterone > 20 ng/dl after being recum-bent overnight and there is no increase after a period of assuming upright position. (**2**) In contrast, a patient with bilateral adrenal hyperplasia will usually have a serum aldosterone < 20 ng/dl after overnight recumbency and there will be an increase after a period of assuming upright position. **Treatment:** ●Bilateral adrenal hyperpla-sia is treated with the aldosterone antagonist, spironolactone 400–600 mg/day. A normal blood pressure and serum potassium is often restored after 4–6 weeks treat-ment. In many patients, however, complete blood pressure control is not achieved without concurrent treatment with other antihypertensive(s). ●Adenomas are resected.

Secondary hyperaldosteronism (hyperaldosteronism due to increased renin activity as a consequence of an extra–adrenal stimulus). **Etiology:** Edematous conditions (e.g. congestive heart failure, cirrhosis, and nephrotic syndrome) may be associated with elevated aldosterone & renin in the absence of hypertension. In Bartter's syndrome, the patient is hypo– or normotensive with elevated aldosterone & renin. Malignant hypertension is associated with elevated aldosterone & renin. Renovascular hypertension is associated with normal to high aldosterone & renin. Estrogen therapy induces an increase in renin substrate. Other: renin–secreting tumor, renal salt–wasting disorders.

DOC (11–DEOXYCORTICOSTERONE) EXCESS SYNDROMES: DOC is a precursor of aldosterone. It is a potent mineralocorticoid that (like aldosterone) causes sodium retention with fluid retention, and may therefore provoke hypertension. The DOC excess syndromes, like primary hyperalderostism, are associated with hypertension, hypokalemia, and low plasma renin levels. In contrast, however, plasma aldosterone levels are usually low in DOC excess syndromes.

Elevated ACTH (e.g. Cushing's disease, ectopic ACTH) stimulates adrenal production of DOC.

DOC-secreting adenoma is a rare cause of DOC excess.

Congenital adrenal hyperplasia (CAH) is due to a defect in glucocorticoid synthesis (11-beta-hydroxylase or 17-alpha-hydroxylase deficiency) so that cortisol synthesis is impaired. With cortisol deficiency, negative feedback inhibition of ACTH secretion is absent. Increased ACTH secretion in turn causes adrenal hyperplasia so that DOC production is increased. The 11-beta-hydroxylase deficiency (in addition to provoking increased DOC production) is associated with virilism because adrenal testosterone production is increased (urinary 17-ketosteroids are elevated). In contrast, the 17-alpha-hydroxylase deficiency causes hypogonadism because neither the gonads nor the adrenals are capable of producing sufficient testosterone or estradiol. Treatment of CAH is with glucocorticoids to suppress ACTH production. A mineralocorticoid may also be needed.

Note: There are other rare conditions *not* associated with mineralocorticoid excess that may nevertheless result in hypertension with hypokalemia and low plasma renin activity—e.g. Liddle's syndrome, licorice ingestion. Licorice contains glycyrrhizic acid which, while not a mineralocorticoid, acts like one because of its action on renal tubular aldosterone sites.

Diabetes Mellitus

Criteria for diagnosis of diabetes mellitus (at least one of the following): Unequivocal elevation of a random plasma glucose together with classic symptoms of diabetes **or** fasting plasma glucose > 140 mg/100 ml on at least two separate days **or** positive oral glucose tolerance test. Oral glucose tolerance test is performed as follows: (**1**) patient is allowed unrestricted diet and activity for 3 days prior to the test and then fasted for at least 10 hours prior to the morning of the test, (**2**) 75 gram glucose PO is administered in the morning, (**3**) a blood sample is obtained 30, 60, 90, and 120 minutes after glucose ingestion. Diabetes is diagnosed if the plasma glucose exceeds 200 mg/100ml on at least one of the 30, 60, or 90 minute samples, and also on the 120 minute sample.

Signs/symptoms: Acute symptoms of diabetes occur when the plasma glucose exceeds 300 mg/100ml. There may be polyuria, polydipsia, polyphagia, weight loss, fatigue, blurred vision. Other signs and symptoms are presented below (see diabetic ketoacidosis, nonketotic hyperosmolar coma, chronic complications).

Treatment: Any diabetic with a pancreas not capable of secreting insulin is treated with insulin. Diabetic ketoacidosis and nonketotic hyperosmolar coma mandates insulin therapy. Insulin therapy is discussed in the next chapter. Obese type II diabetics with mild hyperglycemia may not need insulin, but may respond to weight reduction by diet and judicious exercise. If these measures fail in type II diabetes, an oral hypoglycemic drug (see "Sulfonylureas" in drug section) is sometimes tried before resorting to insulin therapy.

THREE CATEGORIES OF DIABETES MELLITUS ARE RECOGNIZED:

Type I diabetes (insulin–dependent diabetes) is sometimes called juvenile onset diabetes because the disease usually begins during youth. However, type I diabetes may start at any age. The onset is usually before 30–40 years of age; peak age of onset is 11–13 years. ●There is a severe deficiency or absence of endogenous insulin, and patients require insulin to prevent ketoacidosis and to survive. Cause is unknown. However, an autoimmune mechanism is suggested by the fact that many cases are associated with antibodies directed against islet cells. Family history of diabetes is common and there is a common association with the presence of certain HLA antigens. A "honeymoon" interval sometimes ensues after the disease has surfaced. Endogenous insulin levels increase significantly and insulin therapy may not be needed. After 2–6 months remission, however, endogenous insulin levels again fall so that lifelong insulin therapy is required.

Type II diabetes (non-insulin–dependent diabetes) usually begins after age 40, obesity is usually present, A family history is common. However, unlike type I diabetes, an association with certain HLA antigens is absent. ●The islet cells are capable of secreting insulin and insulin levels may range from low (although greater than type I diabetes) to normal, or in some cases it may even be elevated. Diabetes in the face of normal or elevated insulin level is explained by the fact that there is resistance to the effects of insulin. Insulin resistance is attributed in part to a defect in cell membrane insulin receptors. ●In contrast to type I diabetics, there is generally sufficient endogenous insulin to protect against ketoacidosis; although stress (e.g. infection, trauma) may precipitate ketoacidosis.

Secondary diabetes (diabetes resulting from a known cause) may be due to pancreatic disease (e.g. pancreatitis; pancreas–associated neoplasia, hemochromatosis, amyloidosis, or transfusion hemosiderosis); hormones that oppose the effects of insulin (e.g. corticosteroid therapy, Cushing's syndrome, acromegaly, gluconoma, pheochromocytoma); drugs (e.g. thiazides, beta-blockers, clonidine, tricyclics); insulin receptor defects (e.g. acanthosis nigricans, congenital lipodystrophy); genetic syndromes (e.g. Turner's, Klinefelter's, Werner's, Laurence-Moon-Biedl, Down's, Friedreich's ataxia); autoimmune disorders.

DIABETIC KETOACIDOSIS (DKA): Pathogenesis: Lack of insulin provokes hyperglycemia because there is decreased peripheral utilization of glucose (e.g. by fat tissue and muscle), and there is increased gluconeogenesis (primarily by the liver and kidneys). Lack of insulin also provokes ketoacidosis because, in the absence of insulin, the adipose tissue increases lipolysis and releases free fatty acids into the circulation. The free fatty acids are transported to the liver where, under the influence of increased levels of glucagon, there is enhanced uptake of fatty acids into the hepatic mitochondria. Here, fatty acids are metabolized to keto acids (acetoacetate, beta-hydroxybutyrate) which are responsible for the acidosis.

Signs/symptoms of DKA may include polyuria; polydipsia; anorexia; nausea; vomiting; abdominal pain; acetone breath; Kussmaul respirations; headache; myalgia; altered mental status; signs of dehydration (e.g. dry mucous membranes, soft eyeballs, tenting of skin, neck veins flat in recumbent position, orthostatic hypotension). DKA–provoked abdominal pain is attributed to acidosis, gastric distension, or swelling of liver capsule. However, care must be exercised in not overlooking other causes of abdominal pain.

Laboratory: plasma glucose is usually 300–800 mg/100ml; arterial blood gas: pH < 7.2 with bicarbonate < 15 mEq/liter; plasma osmolality increased up to 340 mOsm/kg. Serum ketones are elevated. However, the nitroprusside test (e.g. Acetest, Keto-Diastix) measures acetoacetate mainly and does not detect beta-hydroxybutyrate. The nitroprusside test may therefore be an unreliable indicator of the severity of ketosis. For instance, during insulin therapy there may be proportionally more acetoacetate than beta-hydroxybutyrate even though ketonemia may be resolving overall. The nitroprusside test may also give an erroneous impression if there is concomitant lactic acidosis because lactate favors formation of beta-hydroxybutyrate over acetoacetate. Because of the shortcomings of the nitroprusside test, the best serial method of following ketoacidosis is to obtain serum electrolytes and calculate the anion gap which is = (Na + K) − (Cl + HCO3). Normal gap is 12–16 mEq/liter.

Serum potassium may be low, normal or elevated. Whatever the reading, the body's store of potassium is depleted in DKA. Normal or elevated serum potassium levels may occur despite potassium depletion because acidosis promotes hydrogen ions to enter the cells in exchange for potassium. As acidosis resolves, potassium enters the cells and so the plasma potassium falls. Serum sodium concentration is unpredictable. It may be low, normal, or elevated even though the body is sodium depleted. ●The serum sodium concentration may be elevated because of dehydration. ●The serum sodium may be decreased because lipemia (which is frequently present in DKA) causes the serum sodium to be underestimated. This is because sodium is confined to the water fraction of the plasma but the measurement itself is relative to the water and lipemic fractions combined. ●Elevated blood glucose and ketones may contribute to lowering the serum sodium concentration because under their influence water leaves the cells and thus tends to dilute the plasma sodium. BUN and creatinine may be elevated. This is usuallly due to the prerenal effect of volume depletion. Leukocytosis is common even though infection may or may not be present. Serum amylase may be elevated in the absence of pancreatitis. Blood glucose and electrolytes are usually measured at least every 2 hours for the first 6–8 hours. A flow sheet should be maintained to include glucose, electrolytes, BUN, creatinine, urine output, fluid input, insulin administered, cardiovascular status, mental status. **Additional investigation:** It is important to ascertain what precipitated an episode of DKA (e.g. failure to take insulin, myocardial infarction, stroke, trauma, pregnancy). Infection is a particularly common precipitant. However, one should not depend on the WBC count as an indicator of infection since leukocytosis is often present in the absence of infection. Nor should one depend on the temperature as an indicator of infection since fever is often absent in the presence of infection. Hypothermia is in fact common in DKA. If infection is suspected, the appropriate tests are obtained (urinalysis, blood and urine cultures, chest x-ray) and anitbiotics are begun promptly.

Treatment of DKA: see next chapter.

NONKETOTIC HYPEROSMOLAR COMA occurs in patients whose pancreas is capable of secreting some insulin (e.g. type II diabetes). ●This syndrome most often develops in the elderly type II diabetic and is often brought on by an illness (e.g. infection, myocardial infarction) that has been present for several days in association with symptoms of worsening hyperglycemia (polyuria, polydipsia).

Signs/symptoms/laboratory: Severe hyperglycemia: blood glucose 600–2000 mg/100ml or more. Hyperosmolarity is present. The serum osmolality may be estimated by following: $2 \times (Na + K) + (glucose/18)$. Ketoacidosis is absent, in contrast to DKA, presumably because there is sufficient endogenous insulin to prevent lipolysis (see mechanism of ketone production under DKA above). Neurologic consequences: Hyperglycemia induces an osmotic diuresis that leaves the patient markedly dehydrated. Mental status deteriorates as the serum osmolarity rises. Stupor and coma only develop when the serum osmolarity exceeds 340 mOsm/kg. Focal neurologic signs are often present despite the absence of a stroke. Hemoconcentration, however, does make the patient susceptible to stroke. There may be seizures and they may be resistant to anticonvulsant medication. Renal consequences: The intravascular volume is progressively depleted with worsening dehydration. Consequently, renal perfusion is impaired, and so the GFR decreases and the BUN increases. Hyperglycemia is exacerbated because the capacity for renal excretion of glucose is compromised. Contrast with DKA: Nonketotic hyperosmolar coma shares some of the manifestations of DKA (e.g. polyuria, polydipsia, dehydration). However, because ketosis does not occur, acidosis is absent or there is at most a mild acidosis with a slight decrease in serum bicarbonate. Furthermore, the clinical manifestations of ketoacidosis are not present—e.g. Kussmaul respirations, acetone breath. Hypernatremia develops, in spite of marked urinary sodium loss, when the hyperglycemia—induced osmotic diuresis has progressed to the stage that substantial dilutional shifts of water from the intracellular space are no longer possible. Serum potassium: There is substantial urinary potassium loss. However, because of dehydration, the serum potassium concentration is generally normal or sometimes may be elevated. Elevated hematocrit is a reflection of dehydration–induced hemoconcentration.

Treatment: see next chapter.

CHRONIC COMPLICATIONS OF DIABETES:

Retinopathy: Nonproliferative (background) retinopathy is the first manifestation of retinopathy. Fundoscopy may disclose microaneurysms, retinal hemorrhages, exudates, and/or macular edema. These lesions are very common but vision is usually not affected except in the case of macular edema. Proliferative retinopathy, in contrast, is less common but visual impairment/blindness often ensues. There is neovascularization of the retina with subsequent vitreous hemorrhages and possibly retinal detachment. Proliferative retinopathy is treated with laser photocoagulolation.

Renal disease is heralded by the presence of significant proteinuria (> 500 mg/24hr) so that the nephrotic syndrome sometimes ensues. The GFR gradually decreases and azotemia usually develops 1–3 years after the onset of persistent proteinuria. End-stage renal failure follows the onset of azotemia by about 3 years on the average. Histology may reveal nodular glomerulosclerosis (Kimmelstiel-Wilson disease) or diffuse glomerulosclerosis. These histologic findings are academic since biopsy to confirm renal disease is seldom necessary. Papillary necrosis is an uncommon development. Neurogenic bladder may develop and lead to frequent urinary infections. Diabetics have an increased risk of acute renal failure following radiographic dye studies.

Atherosclerosis is more common in diabetics. Consequently, there is increased risk of coronary artery disease, stroke, and peripheral vascular disease. The latter is most noticeable in the lower extremities where there may be intermittent claudication, absent dorsalis pedis pulse, cool feet, thin skin.

Neuropathy may become apparent in sundry ways. There may be evidence of autonomic dysfunction—e.g. impotence, neurogenic bladder, orthostatic hypotension, gastroparesis, constipation or diarrhea, abnormal sweating (anhydrosis or hyperhydrosis), silent myocardial infarction, decreased variation of R–R interval. Mononeuropathy may be present: dysfunction (usually temporary) of cranial nerve 3, 4, 6, or 7; motor or sensory peripheral mononeuropathy (e.g. foot drop, pain in the distribution of a nerve); muscle wasting (e.g. interosseous muscle atrophy in hands, atrophy of thenar muscles). Peripheral symmetric polyneuropathy presents with bilateral distal paresthesias (particularly of the lower extremities) often with decreased sensastion (e.g. impaired pin prick & vibratory sense) and susceptibility to neuropathic foot ulcers. Knee & ankle reflex may be absent. Charcot joints may develop.

Treatment of Diabetes Mellitus

DIABETIC KETOACIDOSIS in ADULT: Prepare two IV lines, one to restore fluid and electrolytes (line A) and the other (line B) for insulin administration.

Line A: Administer isotonic saline (0.9% NaCl) at rate of 1 liter/hr until intravascular volume depletion has been relieved (e.g. normotension with absence of postural changes). More rapid infusion may be necessary initially if patient is in critical condition. Caution is advised in the elderly, or patients with renal insufficiency or borderline cardiac reserve (a CVP line may be inserted to guard against fluid overload). If the patient presents with a blood glucose of less than 400 mg/dl, the intravenous infusion should include dextrose. Switch to 0.45% NaCl (half–normal saline) when it appears that the intravascular volume has been replenished, and run IV at 150–250 ml/hr. Diabetic ketoacidosis patients usually present with fluid deficit $\geq$ 10% of body weight (i.e. $\geq$ 7 liter in 70 kg patient). One half the deficit is administered in the first 8 hours and the remainder in the next 16 hours. The rate of infusion is adjusted so that the urine ouput is at least 30 ml/hr. Switch to 5% dextrose and 0.45% NaCl (D5-1/2 NS) when blood glucose falls to 300 mg/dl and adjust infusion rate so that blood glucose does not fall below 250 mg/dl during first 12 hours of therapy. This is to preclude hypoglycemia and/or cerebral edema. Continue D5-1/2 NS until patient is eating. Overly rapid correction of fluid deficit is to be avoided since this may contribute to cerebral edema (the osmotic gradient resulting from idiogenic osmoles generated within brain cells during the throes of diabetic ketoacidosis may lead to swelling of brain cells as fluid correction occurs). Replenishing potassium stores: In the absence of hyperkalemia and once adequate urine output has been verified, 10–40 mEq potassium chloride is added to each liter of IV fluid so that the patient is receiving about 10 mEq potassium per hour (up to maximum 40 mEq/hr with EKG monitoring if there is hypokalemia). Sodium bicarbonate is administered if pH falls to 7.1 or less (e.g. add 1 mEq/kg sodium bicarbonate to IV fluid and infuse over 1 hour, repeat as needed).

Line B: Intravenous insulin therapy: First administer an IV bolus of 20 units regular insulin. The continuous IV insulin infusion that follows is prepared by mixing 100 units regular insulin in 500 ml of half–normal saline (0.45 % NaCl). Flush the tubing and volutrol discarding the first 100 ml in order to saturate insulin binding to the plastic (this maneuver insures more complete delivery of insulin to patient). Using an infusion pump, initially run IV at 50–75 ml/hr (10–15 units insulin/hr). Subsequently adjust infusion rate so that blood glucose falls by 75–100 mg/dl/hr, but do not allow the blood glucose to fall below 250 mg/dl during first 12 hours of therapy. Switching to subcutaneous insulin: After dehydration and acidosis have been corrected, and on the first morning the patient is able to feed, subcutaneous insulin therapy can be started. The patient who has previously been on intermediate--acting insulin is given his usual morning dose of NPH or lente; while the patient who has not been on insulin prior to onset of this illness is given a 10–20 unit subcutaneous dose of NPH or lente. Later that morning, the IV insulin infusion can usually be stopped. Supplements of regular insulin are administered subcutaneously as needed at 4–6 hour intervals according to blood glucose measurement or preprandial double–void urine testing:

urine glucose	urine ketones	insulin
0–2+	0	0
3+	0	5 unit
4+	0	10 unit
4+	small	15 unit

Check anion gap and serum bicarbonate if there is more than small urine ketones. Further adjustments of the intermediate-acting insulin (NPH or lente) and regular insulin doses are made until an optimal amount and proportion of intermediate and regular insulin are being administered. The goal in patients previously requiring insulin is to hopefully achieve control with the insulin and diet regimen that was successful prior to this illness. In newly diagnosed patients, the approach to optimizing insulin therapy presented below under the heading *Insulin Therapy in Symptomatic but Uncomplicated Diabetes* is generally applicable.

Monitoring progress of therapy: Initial laboratory tests include arterial blood gas, blood glucose, electrolytes, BUN, creatinine, serum osmolality, serum ketones, serum calcium, serum phosphorus. Unless the specific incitant leading to DKA is known, the patient also merits CBC, urinalysis, blood and urine culture, chest x-ray, and EKG. Antibiotic therapy is initiated if infection is suspected as the underlying precipitant of diabetic ketoacidosis. Ongoing laboratory tests: The blood glucose, electrolytes, and anion gap are determined every 1–2 hours during the initial stages of therapy and then less frequently as the patient is stabilized. If treatment is proceeding smoothly, measurement of glucose and electrolytes at 1, 2, 3, 5, 8, 12 hours following initiation of therapy and then at 4–6 hour intervals should be adequate surveillance. The degree of ketoacidosis is best followed by the anion gap and the serum bicarbonate. Serial testing for serum ketones is not a reliable method of assessing ketosis because a major portion of the ketones is beta-hydroxybutyrate which is not detected by standard testing. A flow sheet should be kept showing the ongoing results of laboratory tests, fluid input, urine output, vital signs, and mental status.

DIABETIC KETOACIDOSIS in CHILDREN:
Prepare two IV lines, one to restore fluid and electrolytes (line A) and the other (line B) for insulin administration.

Line A: In moderate to severe diabetic ketoacidosis the total water deficit is assumed to be 100 ml/kg (10% dehydration). Also calculate the usual daily maintenance requirements (see "Intravenous Fluids" in drug section) which should be administered in addition to correcting the fluid deficit. As far as the deficit is concerned, half the deficit is administered in the first 8 hr and the remainder over the next 16 hr. Begin by administering isotonic saline (0.9% NaCl) 20 ml/kg over 1–2 hr. Then switch to 0.45% saline (half-normal saline). Switch to 5% dextrose and 0.45% NaCl (D5-1/2NS) when blood glucose falls to 300 mg/dl. Replenishing potassium stores: After adequate urine output is confirmed and in the absence of hyperkalemia, add 20–30 mEq KCl per liter IV fluid (up to maximum 40 mEq/liter if hypokalemia is present). KCl must never be administered faster than 1 mEq/kg/hr and continuous EKG monitoring is necessary if the rate exceeds 0.5 mEq/kg/hr. The total potassium deficit is usually 5–10 mEq/kg. Administer sodium bicarbonate only if pH is 7.1 or less. Add 1–2 mEq to IV fluid and infuse over 1–2 hr. Repeat if necessary.

Line B: Intravenous insulin therapy: First administer an IV bolus of regular insulin 0.2 units/kg. The continuous IV insulin infusion that follows may be prepared by adding 50 units regular insulin to 250 ml isotonic saline (0.9% NaCl). Flush the tubing and volutrol discarding the first 50 ml in order to saturate insulin binding to the plastic (this maneuver insures more complete delivery of insulin to patient). Using an infusion pump, initially run IV at 0.5 ml/kg/hr (0.1 unit insulin/kg/hr). Subsequently adjust infusion rate so that blood glucose falls at 75–100 mg/dl/hr but do not allow the blood glucose to fall below 250 mg/dl during first 12 hr therapy. When blood glucose falls to 300 mg/dl, slow but do not stop the insulin infusion (e.g. 0.02–0.06 unit insulin/kg/hr is usually appropriate). Also change line A to D5-1/2 NS to prevent hypoglycemia. Switching to subcutaneous insulin: When acidosis resolves and on the first morning the patient is able to feed, the patient's usual insulin dose is administered subcutaneously. If the patient has not been on insulin prior to this illness, inject 0.5 unit/kg subcutaneously (2/3 as NPH and 1/3 as regular). Later that morning the IV insulin infusion may be stopped. Supplements of regular insulin can then be administered subcutaneously at 4–6 hour intervals as needed according to blood glucose measurements or preprandial double-void urine testing.

| | Insulin dose in units/kg | |
urine glucose	urine ketones absent	urine ketones present
0–1+	0	0
2+	0.03–0.10	0.05–0.12
3+	0.07–0.20	0.10–0.25
4+	0.15–0.40	0.20–0.50

Check anion gap and serum bicarbonate if there is more than small urine ketones. Further adjustments of the intermediate-acting insulin (NPH or lente) and regular insulin doses are made until an optimal amount and proportion of intermediate and regular insulin are being administered. The goal in patients previously requiring insulin is to hopefully achieve control with the insulin and diet regimen that was successful prior to this illness. In newly diagnosed patients, the approach to optimizing insulin therapy presented below under the heading *Insulin Therapy in Symptomatic but Uncomplicated Diabetes* is generally applicable.

Monitoring progress of therapy: as for adult. See above.

TREATMENT of NON-KETOTIC HYPEROSMOLAR COMA: Therapy is similar to that of diabetic ketoacidosis. Keep in mind, however, that dehydration and electrolyte losses usually exceed those seen in DKA. Furthermore, patients are often quite sensitive to insulin and generally require less insulin to achieve an equivalent rate of fall in blood glucose.

INSULIN THERAPY in SYMPTOMATIC but UNCOMPLICATED DIABETES (i.e. absence of ketosis, significant dehydration, or other complications requiring intensive fluid and insulin therapy):

Adult: In a ketosis–prone diabetic (e.g. type I diabetic), insulin therapy should be initiated in the hospital with regular monitoring of blood glucose. Dosing must be individualized and the following comments are given only to suggest one approach to insulin therapy. In the patient whose pancreas is still able to secrete some insulin (as is usually the case in a newly diagnosed diabetic), the insulin requirement is usually 0.2–0.5 units/kg/day. Two daily subcutaneous insulin injections are usually needed to achieve adequate control. In the initial regimen 2/3 of the daily insulin requirement is given 30 minutes before breakfast, and 1/3 is given 30 minutes before dinner. Both the pre–breakfast injection and the pre–dinner injection are usually divided into 2/3 intermediate–acting insulin (NPH or lente) and 1/3 regular insulin. Subsequent tuning of the insulin dosage is made gradually in 2–3 unit/day increments as follows: **(1)** If there is late morning hyperglycemia, add regular insulin to the pre–breakfast NPH injection. **(2)** If there is pre–dinner hyperglycemia, increase the amount of NPH in the pre–breakfast dose. Conversely, if there is pre–dinner hypoglycemia, reduce the amount of NPH in the pre–breakfast dose (or take an afternoon snack). **(3)** If there is late evening hyperglycemia, add regular insulin to the pre–dinner injection. **(4)** If there is pre–breakfast hyperglycemia, increase the amount of NPH in the pre–dinner injection (or reduce the amount of the bedtime snack). In a patient who requires insulin but is not ketosis-prone, one can usually start with 10–20 units of intermediate–acting insulin (NPH or lente) as a single subcutaneous injection 30–60 minutes before breakfast. This dose is gradually increased as needed at 2–3 day intervals by 3–5 unit increments until the pre–dinner glucose level (when NPH and lente activity usually peaks) is acceptable. If there is late morning hyperglycemia, regular insulin is added to the pre–breakfast dose of intermediate–acting insulin. If late evening to next morning glucose levels are unacceptably high, a split–dose regimen as outlined above for the ketosis–prone diabetic will be necessary.

   Pediatric diabetics are often ketosis–prone (e.g. type I diabetic). Consequently, two daily subcutaneous insulin injections are usually needed to achieve adequate control and prevent ketoacidosis. The approach is as outlined above for adults. The total daily insulin requirement depends in part on how much (if any) insulin the pancreas is capable of secreting. The usual inital dosage range is 0.5 to 1.5 units/kg/day. Treatment must be initiated in the hospital with regular monitoring of blood glucose.

Thyroid Function Tests

Preliminary remarks on thyroid hormone biosynthesis and regulation: Thyroid hormone synthesis: Iodide is extracted from the circulation by the thyroid gland against a 50 :1 concentration gradient. Iodide is then oxidized and subsequently bound to tyrosine residues of thyroglobulin thus forming the precursors monoiodotyrosine (MIT) and diiodotyrosine (DIT). Coupling of the precursors leads to the formation of T3 (3,5,3' triiodothyronine) and T4 (thyroxine), both of which are still incorporated into the thyroglobulin sequence. The thyroid gland produces 10–15 times more T4 than T3. Before secretion into the circulation, T3 and T4 are cleaved from thyroglobulin. Free versus bound thyroid hormone: Once in the circulation only a small fraction (0.3% of T3 and 0.02% of T4) is free; the remainder is bound to plasma proteins—mostly thyroid-binding globulin (TBG), some to thyroid–binding pre-albumin (TBPA) and albumin. The free fraction is the metabolically active portion and T3 is more metabolically active than T4. About 80% of plasma T3 is derived from the extrathyroidal deiodination of T4. Reverse T3: In serious chronic disease or starvation, deiodination of T4 may lead to increased formation of rT3 (reverse T3) which is inactive. Despite decreased levels of T3 at the expense of increased rT3, T4 levels are normal and these patients are euthyroid. Hypothyroidism is associated with low levels of both T3 and rT3 as well as T4. Pituitary and hypothalamic influences: Thyroid gland activity (i.e. growth, iodine uptake, thyroid hormone synthesis/secretion) is stimulated by pituitary TSH (thyroid stimulating hormone). The secretion of TSH is itself stimulated by hypothalamic TRH (thyrotropin-releasing hormone). Elevated levels of free thyroid hormone inhibit the secretion of TSH and perhaps TRH, while low levels of free thyroid hormone lead to increased TSH and TRH secretion.

THYROID FUNCTION TESTS:

   Total serum T4 (normal 5–12mcg/100ml) is often simply called serum T4 or plasma T4. Most of the blood thyroxine is bound to thyroid–binding globulin (TBG) while only a small fraction is free. The unbound T4 is the metabolically active portion, and it is therefore that portion which must be estimated when evaluating thyroid disease (e.g. see free T4 index below). Total serum T4 cannot by itself be used to assess thyroid function because conditions not associated with thyroid disease can increase or decrease the amount of thyroid-binding globulin (TBG) without changing the amount of metabolically active unbound T4. For instance, an increase in TBG may lead to an increase in bound T4 (and therefore total T4) without changing the amount of the metabolically active unbound (free) T4. Similarly, a decrease in TBG may lead to a decrease in total T4 without a changing the amount of free T4. TBG is elevated by/in estrogen therapy (e.g. pregnancy, oral contraceptives); acute hepatitis; chronic heroin or methadone use; neonate. TBG is decreased with increased androgens, chronic glucocorticoid administration, cirrhosis, nephrotic syndrome, severe illness, hereditary TBG deficiency.

Free T4 index (normal 5.8–10.6) is obtained by measuring the serum total T4 and by performing the resin T3 uptake test. The free T4 index = (total serum T4) X (T3 uptake ratio) where the T3 uptake ratio = (measured T3 uptake) / (normal mean T3 uptake). The normal mean T3 uptake is 30%. T3 uptake test is performed by incubating a sample of the patient's serum with radioactive T3 and a T3-binding resin. In hyperthyroidism, TBG sites are relatively saturated and so larger amounts of radiolabeled T3 bind to the resin than would if the patient were hypothyroid. The T3 uptake test does not measure the serum T3 but instead is an indirect estimate of TBG concentration. In hyperthyroidism, both total serum T4 and T3 uptake are elevated and consequently free T4 index is high. In hypothyroidism, both total serum T4 and T3 uptake are decreased and consequently free T4 index is low. Free T4 index may be normal and the patient euthyroid in the following circumstances: (1) both total T4 and T3 uptake in the normal range, (2) elevated total T4 combined with a decreased T3 uptake due to elevated TBG, (3) decreased total T4 combined with an elevated T3 uptake due to low TBG.

Free T4 concentration (normal 1.0–2.0 ng/100ml). Free T4 concentration = (total serum T4) X (percent free T4). The percent free T4 is obtained by adding tracer amount of radioactive T4 to sample of the patient's serum and measuring the % of radioactive T4 that is dialyzable. The free T4 parallels the free T4 index and therefore provides essentially the same information as the free T4 index. However, the free T4 is more costly and is more likely to be falsely elevated in severe nonthyroidal illness.

Serum TSH (normal 2–10 microU/ml) is measured by radioimmunoassay. In primary (thyroidal) hypothyroidism, TSH is elevated because feedback inhibition of pituitary TSH secretion by thyroid hormone is absent. The TSH level is especially helpful in establishing primary hypothyroidism when the free T4 index or free T4 are in the low normal range. TSH levels may also be used to assess adequacy of (and to titrate) thyroid hormone therapy in hypothyroidism. In secondary (pituitary) or hypothalamic hypothyroidism, TSH levels are low or undetectable. TSH level should be obtained before starting thyroid hormone therapy in any case of hypothyroidism so that pituitary or hypothalamic causes of hypothyroidism can be excluded.

TRH (thyrotropin-releasing hormone) test: A sample of blood is obtained for measurement of serum TSH before and 30 minutes after the intravenous injection of 400 microgram TRH. TRH test is used to confirm primary hypothyroidism when the serum TSH level is only borderline elevated: If primary hypothyroidism is present, the injection of TRH will cause a marked increase in TSH. TRH test may differentiate pituitary from hypothalamic hypothyroidism: In pituitary TSH deficiency, TSH levels are undetectable and there is no increase following TRH injection. In hypothalamic deficiency, a TSH response to TRH is present but the response may be delayed or prolonged. In hyperthyroidism there may be no response to TRH or the response may be blunted.

Caveats in the interpretation of thyroid function tests: Caution must be exercised in interpreting thyroid tests in patient with nonthyroidal illness since the tests may suggest hyper- or hypo-thyroidism when in fact the patient is euthyroid. Nonthyroidal conditions that cause increased or decreased TBG with consequent respective elevations or depression of the total serum T4 have already been mentioned (see "total serum T4" above). In most of these cases the unbound fraction of T4 is normal (and the patient is euthyroid), and consequently the free T4 index and free T4 are normal. Examples of nonthyroidal conditions that may cause aberrations of thyroid function tests not necessarily attributable to alterations in TBG levels include: severe illness (decreased total T4, free T4 index, free T4, & T3); nonspecific illness especially in elderly (elevated total T4 & free T4 index); starvation (decreased total T4); acute psychiatric condition (elevated total T4, free T4 index, & T3); chronic liver disease (unpredictable results); chronic renal disease; inherited disorders of thyroid hormone resistance (elevated total T4); phenytoin therapy (decreased total T4 & free T4, elevated TSH); propranolol therapy (decreased T3 with increased rT3); amphetamine use (elevated total T4).

Hyperthyroidism (thyrotoxicosis)

Signs/symptoms may include nervousness, restlessness, overactivity, tremor, heat intolerance, sweating, increased frequency bowel movements, weight loss despite increased appetite, muscle weakness, hyperactive reflexes, onycholysis (separation at distal nailbed), increased pulse pressure, tachycardia, atrial fibrillation, systolic flow murmur, stare, lid lag, exophthalmos, pretibial myxedema. The latter two signs are restricted to Graves' disease. Apathetic hyperthyroidism: The elderly may have an atypical presentation: "apathetic hyperthyroidism". The syndrome is so-called because many of the usual signs of increased sympathetic activity are absent. These patients may be depressed and have decreased appetite with weight loss. Tachycardia, atrial fibrillation, or congestive heart failure may be present.

THYROID STORM (thyrotoxic crisis) is an emergency in which the manifestations of hyperthyroidism are markedly heightened. The patient is febrile, very diaphoretic, and is markedly tachycardic. There may be agitation, confusion, arrhythmias, heart failure. Stress (e.g. surgery, infection) precipitates the syndrome in many cases. **Treatment:** Propylthiouracil 400 mg every 6 hours orally or via nasogastric tube. Propranolol 40–60 mg PO every 6 hours. Unusually, IV propranolol is required. Up to 5 mg IV may be adminstered cautiously (no faster than 1 mg/minute) with EKG and blood pressure monitoring. IV dose may be repeated as needed in 4–6 hours. Propranolol should be avoided in presence of congestive heart failure (unless CHF is secondary to a supraventricular tachyarrhythmia) and used with caution if there is a history of CHF or asthma. Hydrocortisone 100 mg IV 3 times/day is administered because the stress of this condition induces a relative adrenal insufficiency. Sodium iodide 250 mg IV or PO every 6 hours. Iodine blocks release of thyroid hormone but initiation of therapy is delayed until a few hours after the initial dose of propylthiouracil. Fever is treated with acetaminophen and external cooling (e.g. sponging, cooling blanket). Aspirin is contraindicated since it may increase serum free–T3. Hypotension, if present, is treated with IV fluids. Vasopressors may be added if necessary.

GRAVES' DISEASE (toxic diffuse goiter), the most common cause of hyperthyroidism, is more common in women. It is an autoimmune disease that is associated with a TSH–like immunoglobulin. That immunoglobulin binds to the TSH receptor sites of the thyroid gland, and thereby stimulates the thyroid gland to increase production and release of thyroid hormone. **Signs/symptoms:** Any of the manifestations described above for hyperthyroidism in general. Thyroid gland: Typically, the gland is diffusely enlarged bilaterally. A bruit is sometimes heard over the gland. Exophthalmos (proptosis): The majority of patients with Graves' disease will develop ophthalmopathy. However, exophthalmos (which is diagnostic of Graves' disease) may not be present and when present may not be striking. When it does occur, exophthalmos may develop before or coincident with hyperthyroidism, or it may sometimes develop after hyperthyroidism has subsided. Occasionally, exophthalmos–associated Graves' disease occurs without ever developing hyperthyroidism. Eye protrusion is due to edema of the extraocular muscles, and the accumulation of fat and mucopolysaccharides behind the globe. The condition is sometimes unilateral. Other eye findings (stare, lid lag) are not unique to Graves' disease but may occur in other hyperthyroid disorders. Pretibial myxedema (infiltrative dermopathy) occurs in < 5% of Graves' patients, and like exophthalmos does not occur in other types of hyperthyroidism. It manifests as a violaceous nonpitting thickening of the skin in the pretibial region, ankles, and/or feet. It is due to dermal infiltration by mucopolysaccharide.

Treatment: If thyroid storm occurs, the patient is treated according to the protocol outlined above. In uncomplicated cases, antithyroid medication is begun— propylthiouracil [PTU] or methimazole. After signs and symptoms have subsided, the mode of treatment may be individualized. The options are surgery, radioiodine therapy, or continued antithryroid drug therapy. The disadvantage of surgery or radioiodine therapy is that the patient may later become hypothyroid. Antithyroid drug therapy may be tried for 6–18 months since remission occurs in a substantial number of cases. The patient should be followed with periodic measurements of the serum T3, free T4 index, and TSH.

TOXIC NODULAR GOITER (Plummer's disease) occurs mostly in the elderly, usually in patients with longstanding nontoxic nodular goiter. Toxic nodular goiter is said to be present when the nodule(s) begins to function autonomously and hyperthyroidism ensues. However, the majority of patients with nodular goiters are euthyroid and never develop hyperthyroidism. Sometimes hyperthyroidism is provoked by the administration of iodides (Jod-Basedow phenomenon). **Diagnosis** may not be suspected since, as previously stated, elderly patients do not always evince the usual clinical signs associated with hyperthyroidism. The total T4 and free T4 are usually elevated, although in some cases these levels are normal and it is the serum total T3 that is high (T3 toxicosis). **Treatment:** Propylthiouracil is administered until euthyroidism is achieved. Most patients are subsequently treated with radioactive iodine.

T3 TOXICOSIS (hyperthyroidism associated with elevated levels of T3 and normal T4) does not differ clinically from hyperthyroidism that is associated with elevation of both T3 and T4. The patient who seems to be thyrotoxic but who has normal T4 values should have the serum T3 checked and a free T3 index determination. T3 toxicosis may develop in Grave's disease, toxic nodular goiter, or from an autonomous thyroid adenoma.

SUBACUTE GRANULOMATOUS THYROIDITIS (de Quervain's thyroiditis) is probably due to viral infection. Histology reveals giant cells and granulomas. The gland is very tender (in contrast to Graves' disease) and may be diffusely enlarged. Sedimentation rate is increased. Radioactive iodine uptake by the thyroid gland is decreased. The patient may be transiently hyperthyroid, and this may be followed by transient hypothyroidism. **Treatment/prognosis:** Aspirin or other nonsteroidal antiinflammatory drug to relieve pain. In severe cases, prednisone 20 mg PO twice daily may be needed for short period. Propranolol 40 mg PO 3 times/day may be used to mitigate symptoms of hyperthyroidism. The disease resolves spontaneously over weeks to months regardless of therapy. Permanent hypothyroidism is a rare sequel.

Hypothyroidism   that is present from infancy results in the syndrome called cretinism. Severe hypothyroidism in adults is called myxedema.

Etiology: Cretinism is rare. It may be the consequence of thyroid dysgenesis, inborn errors thyroid hormone synthesis, severe iodide deficiency. Acquired hypothyroidism: Hashimoto's thyroiditis; idiopathic atrophic; iatrogenic (thyroid surgery, radioiodine therapy, lithium, iodides). Pituitary disease–provoked hypothyroidism—e.g. pituitary surgery/radiation, postpartum pituitary necrosis (Sheehan's syndrome), neoplasia, granulomatous disease. Hypothalamic disease–provoked hypothyroidism—e.g. radiation, neoplasia, granulomatous disease.

Signs/symptoms: hypoactivity, lethargy, cold intolerance, hypothermia, constipation, weight gain despite decreased appetite, myalgia, arthralgias, abnormal taste/smell, bradycardia. Hair is dry and coarse. There may be hair loss. Skin is dry, scaly, coarse, cool. and may have a yellow tinge due to decreased conversion of carotene to vitamin A. In severe cases, there may be nonpitting edema due to subcutaneous infiltration of mucopolysaccharide. This is most noticeable in the face, particularly about the eyes. Tongue may be thickened. Neurologic/psychiatric: delayed relaxation phase of deep tendon reflexes, paresthesias due to nerve entrapment (e.g. carpal tunnel syndrome), deafness due to nerve entrapment, slow thinking, slow speech, depression, confusion, psychosis. Gynecologic complaints are common (e.g. amenorrhea, irregular menses). Exudative effusions may develop --e.g. pleural effusion, pericardial effusion, joint effusion, ascites.

Laboratory: Thyroid function tests: Serum total T4 and free T4 are decreased. TSH is elevated unless hypothyroidism is due to hypothalamic or pituitary dysfunction, in which case TSH will be low. EKG abnormalities: low voltage complexes, bradycardia, heart block. Other lab abnormalities may include hyponatremia (due to decreased free-water clearance), elevated CPK, elevated serum cholesterol, elevated CSF protein, mild proteinuria, anemia (usually normocytic normochromic).

Treatment: Levothyroxine is administered in doses sufficient to return TSH to normal (see levothyroxine in drug section).

MYXEDEMA COMA is an emergency complication of hypothyroidism. Stress (e.g. cold, infection, trauma, surgery) may precipitate the syndrome which includes stupor or coma, hypothermia, hypoventilation with respiratory acidosis, hypotension, hyponatremia, bradycardia. **Treatment** is begun immediately. Ventilatory assistance may be needed to treat hypoventilation and reverse respiratory acidosis. Administer IV fluids as needed to correct hypotension or electrolyte abnormalities. Administer sodium levothyroxine 500 mcg IV (refer to drug section) after drawing blood for thyroid function tests including a TSH. Thyroid hormone therapy must not be delayed for results of thyroid function tests. Also administer hydrocortisone 100–300 mg IV once daily. Treat any underlying infection.

HASHIMOTO'S (chronic lymphocytic) THYROIDITIS is an autoimmune disease. It is more common in women and usually develops in the 20s–40s. The thyroid gland is firm, nontender, and may have a nodular consistency. The gland is usually enlarged although it may be shrunken in later stages of the disease. **Diagnosis:** Antithyroid antibodies can be detected (e.g. antithyroglobulin, antimicrosomal). Histologic exam of needle biopsy specimen reveals lymphocytic infiltration, eosinophilia, fibrosis. Patients may be euthyroid, hypothyroid, or even hyperthyroid rarely. **Treatment:** ●Hypothyroid patients require thyroid hormone medication for life (see levothyroxine in drug section). ●Thyroid hormone medication may also be advocated for euthyroid patients with enlarged thyroid gland in order to suppress pituitary TSH secretion and thereby reduce the stimulus for further thyroid enlargement.

IATROGENIC HYPOTHYROIDISM: Radioactive iodine therapy may depending on the dose cause hypothyroidism. Hypothyroidism may not appear until years later. **Neck irradiation or thyroid surgery** are also obvious causes. **Wolff-Chaikoff effect:** Sometimes, thyroid hormone synthesis and release may be severely curtailed by administering large doses of iodine to susceptible patients (e.g. patient with history of Hashimoto's thyroiditis, thyroid surgery, or radioactive iodine treatment). Common sources of large amounts of iodine are radiologic dyes and SSKI (saturated solution potassium iodide) for thinning bronchial secretions. **Antithyroid drugs** (propylthiouracil, methimazole) in excess can lead to hypothyroidism. **Lithium** may inhibit the synthesis and release of thyroid hormone so that goiter results. However, clinical hypothyroidism seldom ensues.

SEVERELY ILL PATIENTS WITHOUT THYROID DISEASE are not infrequently found to have a low serum total T4 and free T4 index. However, the serum free T4 concentration is normal. The serum T3 may be low with elevation of reverse T3. The serum TSH is usually normal indicating that primary (thyroidal) hypothyroidism is not present. The TSH response to TRH administration is sometimes blunted. These patient do not require thyroid hormone therapy.

Goiter (enlargement of the thyroid gland not resulting from neoplasia) may be

associated with hyperthyroidism (e.g. Graves' disease, toxic nodular goiter), euthyroidism (e.g. simple goiter due to iodine deficiency), or hypothyroidism (e.g. Hashimoto's thyroiditis). **Mechanisms of thyroid enlargement:** The stimulatory effects of increased pituitary TSH secretion is responsible for thyroid enlargement in many cases. For instance, whenever thyroid hormone secretion decreases, thyroid hormone feedback inhibition of pituitary TSH secretion is reduced. TSH levels rise and the stimulatory effects of TSH may lead to hyperplasia of the thyroid gland. The hyperplastic thyroid gland increases both uptake of iodine and synthesis of thyroid hormone. In the euthyroid patient this compensatory mechanism is sufficient to maintain an adequate thyroid hormone level while in hypothyroidism it is not. In Graves' disease, thyroid enlargement is thought to be due to the stimulatory effects of a TSH–like immunoglobulin. Inflammation (e.g. subacute granulomatous thyroiditis) may cause the thyroid to be enlarged.

ENDEMIC GOITER is said to be present when a significant proportion of the population of an area have similar enlargement of the thyroid gland. Endemic goiter is usually due to iodine deficiency in areas where food sources of iodine are scarce (e.g. Andes, Himalayas). The decreased availability of iodine tends to cause a decrease in thyroid hormone synthesis. TSH levels rise and thyroid enlargement supervenes (see mechanisms of thyroid enlargement above). Hyperplasia of the thyroid gland enhances iodine uptake and thus serves to compensate for iodine deficiency. The incidence of endemic goiter has been reduced with iodine supplementation (e.g. iodized salt). Goitrogenic substances in the food or water in some areas may also be responsible for endemic goiter. **Treatment** is with levothyroxine 150–200 mcg/day if goiter is due to iodine deficiency. Thyroid hormone administration suppresses TSH secretion and should over a period of months result in diminution of the thyroid gland. The serum T4 should be followed. If the T4 level increases disproportionately, then autonomous production of thyroid hormone should be suspected (e.g. euthyroid Graves' disease, nontoxic multinodular goiter). If a goitrogen is responsible for the goiter, simply discontinue ingestion of the culpable substance.

SPORADIC GOITER may be the result of a congenital defect in thyroid hormone synthesis or to ingestion of goitrogens (e.g. lithium, cabbage, large doses of iodine).

Thyroid Carcinoma is divided into the following categories:
papillary, follicular, mixed papillary–follicular, anaplastic, and medullary. The first 3 categories together account for about 75–85% of all cases while about 10–15% are anaplastic and 5–10% medullary.

Papillary carcinoma is the most common type of thyroid carcinoma and has the best prognosis. Majority patients are women. Older persons are no more likely to develop papillary carcinoma than young adults. The cancer is slow–growing. When metastasis occurs, it is typically via lymphatics to regional nodes.

Follicular carcinoma, like papillary carcinoma, is typically slow-growing and is more common in women. However, in contrast, the risk of developing follicular carcinoma increases with age, and the prognosis is not as good if there has been local invasion or distant metastasis. Furthermore, even though lymphatic spread to regional nodes may occur, hematogenous metastasis is more likely. The lungs, bone, liver, or brain are the most common metastatic sites.

Anaplastic carcinoma almost always occurs in persons over 50. There is local invasion (e.g. trachea, muscle, neurovascular structures). Consequently; pain, hoarseness and dysphagia are common. There may be metastases to regional nodes or distant metastases (e.g. lungs). Prognosis is poor.

Medullary carcinoma is derived from parafollicular C cells (the cells that produce calcitonin). Cases may occur sporadically or be familial with autosomal dominant inheritance. Familial cases are frequently associated with multiple endocrine neoplasia syndrome (type 2). Calcitonin levels are elevated but patients are not hypocalcemic. In suspected familial cases, relatives at risk should be tested with an IV infusion of calcium or pentagastrin. An exaggerated calcitonin response is indicative of cancer in preclinical stage.

INVESTIGATION of a SOLITARY THYROID NODULE: Besides history and physical exam, the three basic diagnostic tools are radioiodide uptake (RAIU) test, ultrasound, and fine needle aspiration biopsy. A serum calcitonin is also obtained to exclude medullary carcinoma. **The chance that a solitary nodule is malignant is increased if: (1)** there is history of head or neck radiation as a child (however, the risk is not increased by I-131 therapy for Graves' disease); **(2)** nodule is "cold" on RAIU test (over 99% of "warm or hot" nodules are not malignant while about 10% of "cold" nodules are malignant); **(3)** lesion is solid as opposed to a cystic (ultrasound will disclose whether the lesion is cystic); **(4)** patient is male; **(5)** patient is child or young adult; **(6)** additional clinical signs are present (e.g. hoarseness, suspicious lymph nodes, evidence of distant metastases); **(7)** serum calcitonin is elevated (a marker for medullary carcinoma).

Hyperparathyroidism

PRIMARY HYPERPARATHYROIDISM is the condition in which there is excessive secretion of parathyroid hormone by one or more parathyroid glands despite the fact that the plasma ionized calcium is elevated. _Etiology:_ The pathogenesis of the more or less unrestrained secretion of parathormone is unknown. A single benign parathyroid adenoma accounts for 80% cases. The remainder are nearly all due to hyperplasia of all 4 glands. Parathyroid cancer accounts for < 2% cases of primary hyperparathyroidism. _Age and sex prediliction:_ Two thirds or more of patients with primary hyperparathyroidism are women. The condition is rare in children. _Multiple endocrine neoplasia syndrome_ (MEN) is found in some cases of primary hyperparathyroidism. MEN is described in a separate chapter.

Signs/symptoms are those of hypercalcemia (see "Hypercalcemia" chapter). Bone pain may be present. Severe back pain may be due to vertebral compression fracture(s). In addition, primary hyperparathyroidism may be associated with kidney stones, hypertension, gout, or pancreatitis. And so the clinical features of these entities may also be present. Patients are frequently asymptomatic and the diagnosis is suspected because an elevated serum calcium is found on a routine lab screen.

Laboratory: The principal diagnostic findings are: ●Serum calcium is generally > 10.1 mg/100ml. In some cases, serum calcium is only intermittently elevated, or the serum total calcium is in the upper range of normal and yet the ionized fraction is elevated. ●Serum parathyroid hormone as measured by radioimmunoassay will be elevated or inappropriately elevated relative to the hypercalcemia. ●Hypophosphatemia and hyperchloremic acidosis are common. They are the consequence of parathyroid hormone–induced increases in renal excretion of phosphorus and bicarbonate. _Other commonly found laboratory abnormalities_ include elevated serum alkaline phosphatase, normochromic normocytic anemia, elevated 24 hr urinary calcium, elevated serum uric acid, elevated urinary cyclic AMP/creatinine ratio.

X-ray may disclose osteoporosis; subperiosteal resorption of the phalanges; vertebral compression fractures; bone cysts; osteitis of the skull; chondrocalcinosis; soft tissue calcification (e.g. of pancreas, lung, tendons); kidney stones.

Treatment: Hypercalcemia is treated as outlined in "Hypercalcemia" chapter. Single parathyroid adenomas are resected. If all 4 glands are hyperplastic, three and one-half glands are resected. To preclude development of _HYPO_parathyroidism, all 4 glands may be resected and a portion of one parathyroid gland is implanted into the forearm for easy surgical access should hyperparathyroidism recur. Parathyroid cancer is resected. Hypocalcemia may follow parathyroid surgery as calcium is taken up by the bones in the reparative process ("hungry bones"). This is especially likely to occur if there is severe osteitis fibrosa cystica, or if the preoperative serum alkaline phosphatase is elevated. Surgery is not imperative in asymptomatic patients who are not significantly hypercalcemic (serum calcium < 11.0 mg/dl) and who show no evidence of renal stones, renal impairment (e.g. decreased creatinine clearance), or signs of bone disease. In these patients; the serum calcium, alkaline phosphatase, and creatinine clearance should be obtained twice yearly, and x-rays of the hands yearly. In order to preclude renal complications, thiazide diuretics are avoided, excessive calcium ingestion is discouraged, and patients are urged to drink a generous amount of fluid daily. Phosphate ingestion should be increased if there is hypophosphatemia.

ECTOPIC HYPERPARATHYROIDISM may occur when a malignancy (e.g. of lung, kidney, pancreas) secretes a peptide similar to parathyroid hormone. Consequently, the patient may also be subject to the additional clinical consequences ascribed above for primary hyperparathyroidism.

SECONDARY HYPERPARATHYROIDISM (parathyroid hyperplasia in reaction to hypocalcemia) is a normal adaptive response to hypocalcemia. The parathyroid glands sensing a decrease in serum calcium react by increasing parathyroid hormone output. The glands eventually hypertrophy.

Etiology: Disorders provoking hypocalcemia with ensuing secondary hyperparathyroidism include renal failure; GI malabsorption; vitamin D deficiency; renal tubular defects leading to increased calcium loss (e.g. renal tubular acidosis, Fanconi syndrome); drugs interfering with vitamin D metabolism and hence GI calcium absorption (e.g. phenytoin or phenobarbital).

Laboratory: Serum calcium is low or low-normal. Serum parathyroid hormone is elevated. Patients with hyperparathyroidism secondary to chronic renal failure usually have parathyroid hormone levels that are much greater than that observed in primary hyperparathyroidism. Serum phosphorous level is usually decreased unless there is renal insufficiency. Serum alkaline phosphatase may be elevated.

In severe or chronic renal failure, impaired excretion of phosphate leads to elevated plasma phosphate. As a consequence (since the solubility product of calcium x phosphate is a constant), the plasma calcium falls. At saturation levels, calcium phosphate may be precipitated in the soft tissues. Renal osteodystrophy (bone disease resulting from chronic renal failure) develops in most cases. Renal osteodystrophy has 4 manifestations: osteomalacia, osteoporosis, osteitis fibrosa cystica, and osteosclerosis. The latter 3 are due to the influence of the markedly elevated parathyroid hormone levels on bone metabolism. Osteomalacia is largely due to impaired conversion by the kidney of 25-OH-vitamin D to the active metabolite 1,25-OH-vitamin D. Lack of latter leads to decreased intestinal absorption of calcium.

Treatment of secondary hyperparathyroidism: Secondary hyperparathyroidism due to chronic renal failure is treated with aluminum hydroxide antacids to bind phosphate in the GI tract. Once the serum phosphate has decreased, and if hypocalcemia or renal osteodystrophy are worrisome, oral calcium and 1,25-OH-vitamin D may be prescribed. These agents, it is emphasized, must not be used until the serum phosphate level has been controlled with antacids for otherwise precipitation of calcium phosphate may occur intravascularly and in the soft tissues. Partial parathryroidectomy may be required in unremitting cases in which there is soft tissue calcification or osteitis fibrosa cystica. Secondary hyperparathyroidism and osteomalacia resulting from anticonvulsant medication may be corrected with vitamin D.

TERTIARY HYPERPARATHYROIDISM is the *autonomous* production of parathyroid hormone that sometimes results from severe and chronic secondary hyperparathyroidism. The gland(s) are not responsive to fluctuations in serum calcium and thus hypercalcemia may ensue.

Hypoparathyroidism is usually the consequence of excision

of (or damage to) the parathyroid glands at thyroid or parathyroid surgery. Other examples of hypoparathyroidism include DiGeorge syndrome (incomplete development of the 3rd branchial arch with absent parathyroid glands and thymus), idiopathic hypoparathyroidism, hypomagnesemia–induced hypoparathyroidism, pseudhypoparathyroidism.

Signs/symptoms of hypoparathyroidism are in general the manifestations of hypocalcemia. Refer to "Hypocalcemia".

Hypocalcemia following parathyroid/thyroid surgery may be transient. In this case IV calcium gluconate is administered as needed. See "Hypocalcemia" chapter. If hypoparathyroidism lasts more than a week or if it is permanent, vitamin D therapy (refer to drug section) is required to prevent hypocalcemia. Diet plus calcium supplementation should provide 1–2 gram of elemental calcium/day. The serum calcium should be checked twice weekly at first, and then every few months when the serum calcium has been stabilized. The urine calcium should also be measured periodically. If the urine calcium exceeds 250 mg/24hr, the fluid intake should be increased in order to preclude development of renal stones.

Idiopathic hypoparathyroidism is rare. It is most commonly associated with other endocrine abnormalities (e.g. diabetes mellitus, hypothyroidism, adrenal insufficiency, early menopause); pernicious anemia; candidiasis. It appears to be an autoimmune disorder since the glands are infiltrated with lymphocytes and there are antibodies directed against affected tissues. Treatment is as described above for surgically–induced hypoparathyroidism.

Pseudohypoparathyroidism (end–organ resistance to parathyroid hormone in the absence of parathyroid hormone deficiency) is characterized by elevated serum parathyroid hormone, hypocalcemia, and hyperphosphatemia. In most cases, phosphate excretion and urinary cyclic AMP fails to increase following injection of parathyroid hormone. Patients may be of short stature, obese, and have short metacarpals. Treatment is as described above for surgically–induced hypoparathyroidism.

Hypomagnesemia (a common problem in alcoholics) may provoke hypoparathyroidism. Magnesium deficiency appears to impair parathyroid hormone secretion so that hypocalcemia ensues. Magnesium administration corrects the parathyroid hormone deficiency and hence the hypocalcemia.

Hypercalcemia (total serum calcium > 10.5 mg/100ml).

Etiology: Hypercalcemia due primarily to increased bone resorption may be the consequence of prolonged immobilization; hyperthyroidism; osteolytic malignancy (e.g. carcinoma metastatic to bone, leukemia, lymphoma, multiple myeloma). Primary hyperparathyroidism or ectopic hyperparathyroidism (e.g. bronchogenic carcinoma) induces hypercalcemia by 3 mechanisms: increased GI absorption of calcium, increased renal reabsorption of calcium, induction of bone resorption. Enhanced intestinal absorption of calcium with increased resorption of bone may be the consequence of sarcoidosis, hypervitaminosis A or D, Addison's disease. Increased renal calcium reabsorption may be due to thiazide diuretics, Addison's disease. Ingestion of large amounts of calcium carbonate and milk may result in hypercalcemia (milk–alkali syndrome).

Signs/symptoms: renal: polyuria (calcium inhibits binding of ADH to receptor sites in distal convoluted tubules), renal stones (with risk of urinary obstruction), azotemia (due to the effects of calcium precipitation in renal parenchyma); gastrointestinal: anorexia, nausea, vomiting, constipation, ileus, abdominal pain; cardiac: shortening of QT interval; skin: pruritis; muscle weakness due to myopathy; neuropsychiatric: headache, labile emotions, confusion, delirium, lethargy, stupor, coma.

Treatment: Treat underlying disorder. This alone may suffice if the serum calcium is < 11.5. General measures that may mitigate hypercalcemia: dietary calcium restriction, maintain physical activity, generous fluid intake. If the serum calcium exceeds 13.0, administer IV isotonic (0.9%) saline 3–4 liters/24 hour concurrently with furosemide 80–160 mg/day divided. This regimen is of course only suitable for patients with adequate renal function. To preclude hypernatremia, D5W may be substituted for isotonic saline every 4th liter of fluid. In patients with limited cardiac reserve, insertion of a central venous line is advised in order to avoid fluid overload. EKG monitoring is advised. Serum electrolytes including calcium and magnesium are monitored daily (potassium and magnesium depletion is a common consequence of saline and furosemide therapy). ●Calcitonin has low toxicity and may be added to the regimen of saline diuresis and furosemide. It may also be used in conjunction with corticosteroids. Calcitonin is most likely to be effective if hypercalcemia is due to thyrotoxicosis or hyperparathyroidism. Additional measures to be considered in life–threatening hypercalcemia: ●Hemodialysis or peritoneal dialysis with low or calcium–free dialysate. ●Intravenous phosphate therapy for hypercalcemia is effective but dangerous. Patients with hypercalcemia < 13.0, including patients whose serum calcium has been brought down by the foregoing measures may be treated with PO fluids (3–4 liters/day), PO sodium chloride tablets (500 mEq/day), and PO furosemide (40–160 mg/day in divided doses). Other regimens that may be useful depending on the clinical circumstances:
●Oral inorganic phosphates (sodium or potassium phosphate providing 1–2 gram of elemental phosphorus/day) may be given if prolonged therapy is required for mild–moderate hypercalcemia. However, phosphates must not be administered in the presence of severe renal insufficiency or hyperphosphatemia. Serum electrolytes (including calcium and phosphorous) and renal function must be monitored. To forestall metastatic calcification, the serum phosphorous should not be allowed to rise above 5 mg/dl. ●Mithramycin may be used to lower serum calcium if phosphate therapy is ineffective, but it is a toxic drug. ●Corticosteroids (e.g. prednisone 60 mg/day) may help reduce serum calcium but the effect may not be seen for several days. Hypocalcemia due to sarcoidosis, multiple myeloma, or hypervitaminosis D are the conditions most likely to respond to steroids. ●Indomethacin thru its inhibition of prostaglandin synthesis may sometimes help decrease serum calcium in malignancy–associated hypercalcemia. ●Cyclical estrogen administration may benefit

postmenopausal women with chronic hypercalcemia. Women with primary or ectopic hyperparathyroidism are the patients most likely to benefit.

Hypocalcemia (total serum calcium < 8.4 mg/100ml in adult and < 8.8 in child).

Etiology: Hypoparathyroidism (e.g. excision of or damage to the parathyroid gland at thyroid or parathyroid surgery, DiGeorge syndrome, idiopathic hypoparathyroidism, hypomagnesemia–induced hypoparathyroidism, pseudohypoparathyroidism). Subtotal parathyroidectomy for hyperparathyroidism may subsequently lead to hypocalcemia as calcium is taken up by the bones in the reparative process ("hungry bones"). Vitamin D–related abnormalities: Vitamin D deficiency; vitamin D resistance (e.g. familial hypophosphatemic rickets); GI malabsorption of calcium and vitamin D; conditions (e.g. renal osteodystrophy) or drugs (e.g. phenytoin or phenobarbital) impairing vitamin D metabolism and hence GI calcium absorption. Renal disease: Renal failure with hyperphosphatemia and impaired vitamin D metabolism may induce hypocalcemia (see *renal osteodystrophy* in "Hyperparathyroidism" chapter). Renal tubular defects may lead to increased calcium loss (e.g. distal renal tubular acidosis, Fanconi syndrome). Liver disease may result in impaired 25-hydroxylation of vitamin D. Consequently, there is a deficiency of the active metabolite 1,25 hydroxy–vitamin D. In the absence of this metabolite, calcium absorption is impaired and hypocalcemia ensues. Acute pancreatitis sometimes results in hypocalcemia. Multiple transfusions of citrated blood can cause hypocalcemia. Hypoalbuminemia is associated with decreased total serum calcium but since about 60% of serum calcium is protein bound (mainly to albumin), the level of the metabolically active ionized (unbound) fraction may be normal and the patient is therefore asymptomatic. It is possible to measure the ionized fraction but a rough estimate of what the total serum calcium would be if hypoalbuminemia where not present can be made as follows: add 0.8 mg/100ml to the measured total serum calcium for each 1 gram/100ml the serum albumin is below normal.

Signs/symptoms may be absent, especially if hypocalcemia develops slowly. Patients with slowly developing hypocalcemia are sometimes asymptomatic with total serum calcium 5–6 mg/100ml. Tetany is the most striking presentation of hypocalcemia. Carpal, facial and/or pedal spasm are common. Sometimes spasm is so severe that the patient cannot talk, and breathing may be impaired if there is laryngeal spasm. Trousseau's sign: In hypocalcemic patients without overt spasm, carpal spasm may be induced by inflating a blood pressure cuff on the arm and maintaining the pressure above systolic for 3 minutes. Chvostek's sign: Tapping the facial nerve in front of the ear may elicit facial contraction. Parasthesias (e.g. numbness/tingling of the hands, feet, tongue, or lips) are common consequences of hypocalcemia. Alkalosis and hypocalcemia: Because alkalosis reduces the amount of ionized serum calcium (calcium ion binds to albumin sites that would otherwise be occupied by hydrogen ion), the manifestations of hypocalcemia are aggravated by either respiratory or metabolic alkalosis. In fact, hyperventilation can, by reducing the amount of ionized (unbound) calcium, provoke tetany in normocalcemic patients. Chronic hypocalcemia may result in weakness; fatigue; myalgias; psychic disturbances (e.g. irritability, depression, dementia). Prolonged hypocalcemia may be associated with dermatological sequelae—e.g. dry scaling skin, coarse hair, hair loss, longitudinally–ridged fingernails. Neurologic consequences of prolonged hypocalcemia: There may be calcification of the basal ganglia with ensuing extrapyramidal manifestations—possibly including parkinsonism. Secondary hyperparathyroidism may ensue from hypocalcemia (see "Hyperparathyroidism"). Other possible consequences of hypocalcemia: hypotension, prolonged QT interval, cataracts, malabsorption, elevated intracranial pressure with papilledema.

Laboratory: Total serum calcium is < 8.4 mg/100ml in adult and < 8.8 in child. Tetany is usually associated with serum calcium < 7 but tetany occurs at higher levels if alkalosis is present. In renal failure–associated hypocalcemia, the serum phosphate level will be elevated along with elevated BUN and creatinine. In hypoparathyroidism–associated hypocalcemia, the serum phosphate is elevated. This also true of pseudohypoparathyroidism. However, pseudohypoparathyroidism is distinguished by the presence of elevated serum parathyroid hormone. In vitamin D deficiency–associated hypocalcemia (e.g. rickets, osteomalacia); the serum phosphate is decreased, alkaline phosphatate is elevated, urinary calcium decreased. A similar picture is seen if the metabolism of vitamin D is impaired (e.g. phenytoin or barbiturate therapy).

Treatment: Severe hypocalcemia with tetany: 10 ml of 10% calcium gluconate IV over 15 minutes. Repeat as needed. The goal of emergency intravenous therapy is to provide symptomatic relief and/or to bring the serum calcium up to 7.5–8.5 mg/dl. If prolonged therapy is required, add 20–30 ml 10% calcium gluconate to liter of D5W and infuse IV over 12–24 hours. EKG monitoring is required if the patient is on digitalis. PO calcium may be begun while the patient is still on IV therapy. In less urgent cases, therapy consists of vitamin D or an analog (see "Vitamin D" in drug section) together with ingestion of 1–2 gram elemental calcium/day from diet and/or supplements. A gram of calcium carbonate contains 400 mg elemental calcium while a gram calcium gluconate contains 90 mg elemental calcium. Hypocalcemia due to renal failure: see *secondary hyperparathyroism* in "Hyperparathyroism" chapter.

Osteoporosis is a decrease in bone mass arising from a decrease in

both bone matrix and bone mineral. In contrast to other forms of osteopenia (poorly calcified bone), the bone has a normal histologic appearance. For instance, in osteopenia due to osteomalacia, bone is replaced by osteoid, a histologically abnormal bone matrix that is poorly calcified.

Causes:

Involutional osteoporosis (aging–associated osteoporosis) is most prevalent in women, particularly slender caucasian women who are sedentary. As bone loss progresses the bones become increasingly fragile (e.g. the incidence of traumatic distal forearm fractures in women starts to increase at about age 45). Generally, however, osteoporosis is relatively far advanced before becoming clinically apparent, usually within 20 years following menopause. Clinical expression is heralded in most cases by the onset of back pain from vertebral body compression fracture. About a fourth of white women over 60 have osteoporosis–associated spinal compression fractures. Black women (or black men) seldom develop involutional osteoporosis because they have greater bone mass to start with. Women are 5 times more likely than men to develop symptomatic spinal osteoporosis. Premature menopause or castration may hasten bone loss in susceptible women. There may be other concurrent conditions exacerbating involutional osteoporosis (e.g. see the following list).

Other possible causes of osteoporosis include alcoholism, chronic obstructive pulmonary disease, immobilization, malabsorption, malnutrition, alactasia, chronic obstructive jaundice, primary biliary cirrhosis, hypogonadism, hyperparathyroidism, hyperthyroidism (rarely leads to osteoporosis), adrenocortical hormone excess (endogenous or exogenous).

Signs/symptoms: Back pain following a vertebral compression fracture is a common presentation. Often, the fracture ensues from such seemingly innocuous activity as straining to open a window or lifting an object, or even walking. Spinal deformity and loss of height is the consequence of multiple compression fractures of the lumbar and thoracic spine. Multiple thoracic compression fractures leads to thoracic kyphosis ("dowager's hump"). Patients may lose as much as 5 inches in height. Hip fractures are a common cause of morbidity and mortality in elderly women and men with involutional osteoporosis. Although many osteoporosis–associated hip fractures result from a fall, about as many are spontaneous. Other fractures: Patients are also susceptible to other fractures, particularly of the wrist or ribs.

X-ray findings: Osteopenia (decreased bone density/calcification) is not apparent until bone mass has decreased by more than 25%. The central portion of vertebral bodies become relatively radiolucent and eventually become as radiolucent as the surrounding soft–tissue. Until osteoporosis becomes advanced, however, the vertical trabeculae are actually accentuated because the horizontal trabeculae vanish first. The cortex of the vertebral bodies are thinned but are nevertheless highlighted by contrast with the more radiolucent central portion of the bodies. Vertebral body compression fractures are common. While a vertebral body may collapse uniformly, a characteristic finding: (**1**) in the lumbar region is for vertebral body end–plates to buckle centrally thus giving a biconcave profile to an involved vertebral body, (**2**) in the thoracic spine is a anterior wedged–shaped compression fracture(s). The latter leads to thoracic kyphosis.

Laboratory tests are indicated in order to rule out causes for osteopenia other than osteoporosis. Serum calcium, phosphorus, and alkaline phosphatase are characteristically normal in uncomplicated osteoporosis. However, the serum alkaline phosphatase may be mildly elevated after a fracture. All three are abnormal in osteomalacia. Serum albumin is ordered since deviation of the serum albumin level will cause a change in the total serum calcium. About 60% of serum calcium is protein–bound (mainly to albumin) while the remaining fraction (the metabolically active ionized fraction) is unbound. If the serum albumin should decrease for instance, the total serum calcium would also decrease as a consequence of a decrease in albumin–bound calcium. However, the level of the metabolically active ionized fraction would (in uncomplicated osteoporosis) remain the same. It is possible to measure the ionized fraction but a rough estimate of what the total serum calcium would be if hypoalbuminemia were not present can be made as follows: add 0.8mg/100ml to the measured total serum calcium for each 1 gram/100ml the serum albumin is below normal. Serum and urine electrophoresis are indicated to exclude multiple myeloma. Serum creatinine and BUN are obtained to screen for chronic renal disease. Thyroxine level is measured to rule out hyperthyroidism. Other tests are ordered as clinical circumstances suggest.

Treatment: Pain; Acute back pain following a spinal compression fracture may be eased by analgesics and local heat. Bed rest may be necessary for a short time. Stool softeners are advised in order to avoid straining. Chronic back pain may be mitigated by judicious back extension exercises aimed at increasing the tone of paravertebral muscles. Wearing of a correctly fitted surgical corset may be recommended. Diet; In order to slow bone demineralization, calcium intake should be adequate. At least 1000–1500 mg elemental calcium/day is recommended. A calcium supplement is advisable if diet is deficient; a 500 mg calcium carbonate tablet (e.g. Tums) contains 200 mg of elemental calcium. The diet should also be adequate in protein and vitamins. Vitamin D supplementation is generally not indicated unless the diet is deficient (the recommended daily allowance in an adult is 400 IU/day). Activity; The patient should be reasonably active since immobility accelerates bone loss. Estrogens appear to be beneficial in curbing bone loss if they are begun soon after menopause: conjugated estrogens (Premarin) 0.625 mg/day is taken cyclically (e.g. 3 wk on, 1 wk off). To decrease the risk of endometrial hyperplasia/carcinoma, medroxyprogesterone acetate (Provera) 10mg/day is given along with estrogen during the 3rd wk. Neither estrogen nor progesterone is given during the 4th wk. Etidronate appears to curb bone loss to some extent. It reduces bone resorption thru inhibition of osteoclastic activity. There are almost no side effects with this drug.

Multiple Endocrine Neoplasia (MEN)

MEN syndromes are a group of familial syndromes with autosomal dominant inheritance in which neoplasia or hyperplasia arises in more than one endocrine organ. Any patient presenting with evidence of hyperplasia/neoplasia of one endocrine organ should be investigated for the presence of other endocrine disorders and a family history should be obtained.

MEN type I (Wermer syndrome) is associated with neoplasia or hyperplasia of parathyroid glands, pancreatic islet cells, pituitary gland, and/or adrenal cortex in assorted combinations. Parathyroid hyperplasia with ensuing hypercalcemia is present in about 90% of patients. Pituitary adenomas (65% MEN I patients) are usually nonfunctional but they may secrete prolactin, growth hormone, or ACTH. Pancreatic islet tumors are found in 5% MEN I patients. Islet tumor possibilities include: (**1**) insulinoma–induced hypoglycemia; (**2**) gastrinoma–provoked Zollinger-Ellison syndrome (Excessive gastrin causes hypersecretion of hydrochloric acid by gastric parietal cells with ensuing peptic ulcers. Gastrinomas may be single or multiple, and may be malignant and metastasize locally and/or to the liver.); (**3**) glucagonoma–induced hyperglycemia and dermatitis; (**4**) somatostatin–secreting tumor with ensuing hyperglycemia; (**5**) ACTH-secreting tumor; (**6**) vasoactive intestinal peptide–secreting tumor possibly leading to diarrhea, hypokalemia, hyperglycemia;. (**7**) serotonin–secreting tumor leading to carcinoid syndrome; (**8**) prostaglandin E–secreting tumor with consequent diarrhea.

   MEN type II (Sipple syndrome) includes various combinations of parathyroid hyperplasia (also seen in MEN I), medullary thyroid carcinoma, or pheochromocytoma. Parathyroid hyperplasia is present in about 90% patients but only 40% patients with histologic evidence of parathyroid hyperplasia are hypercalcemic. Medullary thyroid carcinoma (90% MEN II patients) arises from the calcitonin–secreting parafollicular cells (C cells). Elevated levels of serum calcitonin may be found basally or following calcium or pentagastrin infusion. Pheochromocytoma (20% MEN II patients) arises from the adrenal medulla or from sympathetic ganglia. The tumors are often multiple, bilateral, and/or malignant. See "Hypertension" chapter for further discussion of pheochromocytoma.

   MEN type III (IIb) is genetically distinct from MEN II. Parathyroid hyperplasia is rare in MEN III. Medullary thyroid carcinoma occurs in 90% patients and pheochromocytoma 50%. MEN III is also distinguished from MEN II by the presence of multiple mucosal neuromas (90% patients) of the eyes, mouth, upper respiratory tract, and GI tract. Furthermore, 90% patients have a Marfanoid habitus.

Hematology

Anemia is defined as a less than normal hemoglobin, hematocrit, or number

of RBC's. The normal range varies according to age, sex, and pregnancy. ●Laboratory investigation of anemia begins with evaluation of the CBC (including RBC indices, reticulocyte count) as well as microscopic exam of the peripheral blood smear, urinalysis, test of stool for occult blood. **Reticulocyte count:** A normally productive bone marrow will respond to anemia by increasing production and release of erythrocytes into the bloodstream. A recently released erythrocyte (reticulocyte) contains remnants of ribosomal RNA. This is indicative of continued hemoglobin synthesis; the RNA disappears in about 24 hours. RNA stains with methylene blue thereby enabling one to count the number of reticulocytes as a percentage of the total number of erythrocytes (reticulocyte count). Since erythrocytes survive about 120 days, the normal reticulocyte count is about 1 % (normal range is 0.5–1.5%). An elevated reticulocyte count indicates that there is blood loss, hemolysis, or recovery from anemia. Examples of the latter include treatment of B–12, folate, or iron deficiency; and remission of aplastic anemia or leukemia. Chronic hemolytic anemia is characterized by a constant hematocrit with a persistently elevated reticulocyte count. In contrast, recovery from an *acute* hemolytic episode or other anemias is associated with an increasing hematocrit and an elevated reticulocyte count. A low or normal reticulocyte count in the face of anemia indicates that the marrow is not adequately increasing erythrocyte production. **Reticulocyte index** (corrected reticulocyte count). The reticulocyte count may be misleading because in the setting of a low hematocrit the release of even a small number of reticulocytes by the bone marrow may substantially increase the reticulocyte count. The reticulocyte index is therefore calculated in order to verify the adequacy of the bone marrow response to anemia: reticulocyte index = reticulocyte count X (observed hematocrit / normal hematocrit). **Mean corpuscular volume (MCV)** is the average volume of a person's erythrocytes—i.e. MCV = (hematocrit / RBC count) X 10. The normal range varies with age (see appendix). **Mean corpuscular hemoglobin (MCH)** is the average amount of hemoglobin contained in an individual's erythrocytes—i.e. MCH = (hemoglobin / RBC count) X 10^6. The normal range varies with age. **Mean corpuscular hemoglobin concentration (MCHC)** is the average percent hemoglobin per erythrocyte—i.e. MCHC = (hemoglobin/ hematocrit) X 0.1. The normal range varies with age (see appendix).

MICROCYTIC ANEMIA (MCV < 80 cu microns) is usually the result of iron deficiency (e.g. blood loss, inadequate dietary iron) or thalassemia. Microcytic anemia may also be seen in chronic renal insufficiency and chronic inflammation (conditions usually associated with normocytic anemia). In sideroblastic anemia, microcytic as well as normocytic erythrocytes are seen but the MCV is usually in the normal range (see below under "Normocytic anemia").
  Iron deficiency anemia is usually described as microcytic and hypochromic (decreased MCV and MCHC respectively). However, iron deficiency anemia in the early stages may be normocytic normochromic; the MCV often remains in the normal range until the hematocrit has fallen to about 35 and the MCHC is often normal until the hematocrit is quite low. Moreover, the peripheral blood smear frequently appears normal until the hematocrit falls below 30. Microscopic appearance: With worsening anemia the RBC's may exhibit central pallor with a rim of hemoglobin, target cells may be seen, and there be variation in shape and size of the RBC's. Reticulocyte count is low to normal. When iron deficiency is suspected, serum iron, TIBC (total iron–binding capacity), and serum ferritin are ordered. Serum iron is usually low in the case of iron deficiency anemia (normal range 60–135mcg/100ml). TIBC (total iron–binding capacity) is an indirect measure of the level of transferrin (an iron transport protein). It is usually elevated in iron deficiency anemia, although it may remain in the normal range (250–350mcg/200ml) until the hematocrit falls below 30 as the microcytic hypochromic picture emerges. Transferrin saturation (serum iron ÷ TIBC) is < 15% (normal 20–40%). Serum ferritin is low (normal > 15 ng/ml). Ferritin is an iron storage protein found in the reticuloendothelial system—mostly in the bone marrow and liver. Small amounts are also found in the bloodstream and this reflects the body's iron stores. Serum ferritin is the first of the laboratory parameters so far described to become abnormal with the onset of iron deficiency. Bone marrow iron stain is sometimes obtained if the diagnosis is uncertain.

A decrease or absence of stainable bone marrow confirms that iron stores are low. Treatment: Ferrous sulfate is the usual therapy (see drug section). Parenteral iron therapy is used in selected cases (see iron dextran in drug section). **Non–anemic iron deficiency** refers to the condition in which the total amount of body iron is low but not deficient to the point of impairing normal RBC production. The serum ferritin is low (< 15–20 ng/ml) and bone marrow stain reveals depleted bone marrow iron stores. However—in the absence of other deficiencies or diseases—the peripheral smear is normal, the RBC indices are normal, the hemoglobin and hematocrit are normal, and the patient is asymptomatic.

Thalassemia may be confused with iron deficiency anemia. It is important to make the distinction because patients with thalassemia are not uncommonly treated inappropriately for iron deficiency and thus risk iron overload. Beta thalassemia minor (trait) is the most common form of thalassemia. The blood smear shows microcytic hypochromic RBC's and this reflected in a decreased MCV and MCH. MCHC is normal. Target cells, tear drop cells, and ovalocytes may be seen on the blood smear. Serum iron and TIBC are generally normal. A transferrin saturation of about 30% with a TIBC of about 350 is suggestive of beta thalassemia minor. In the absence of concurrent iron deficiency, the serum ferritin level is normal. Anemia is either absent or mild because there is a compensatory increase in the number of RBC's. The reticulocyte count is slightly elevated in many cases. Hemoglobin electrophoresis is confirmatory (per cent Hgb A2 is increased). Persons with beta thalassemia minor trait are asymptomatic. Alpha thalassemia minor (trait) is also asymptomatic and has a similar blood profile except that hemoglobin electrophoresis is sometimes normal. Refer to "Thalassemia" chapter for further details.

MACROCYTIC ANEMIA (MCV > 100 cu microns) : Megaloblastic anemia due to B–12 or folate deficiency is the most common cause of macrocytic anemia. Refer to "Megaloblastic Anemia" chapter for details. Macrocytic anemia in absence of megaloblastosis may be seen in liver disease, alcoholism (even in the absence of evidence of liver disease), preleukemia, and sideroblastic anemia. Neonates normally have an MCV > 100. Marked reticulocytosis is associated with an MCV > 100 because reticulocytes are larger than the more mature erythrocytes. Idiopathic cases of macrocytosis occasionally occur. Lab error: A falsely elevated MCV measurement may occur in the setting of immune–mediated RBC agglutination when automated methods of measurement are used.

NORMOCYTIC ANEMIA (MCV 82–98 cu microns):

Chronic diseases such as malignancies or chronic inflammatory conditions (e.g. autoimmune diseases, chronic infection) are probably second only to iron deficiency as the most common cause of anemia. Multiple interrelated factors are postulated to account for chronic disease–associated anemia: iron sequestration by macrophages of the reticuloendothelial system, iron sequestration by hepatocytes and GI mucosal epithelial cells, decreased iron uptake and utilization by marrow normoblasts, decreased erythropoietin, decreased RBC survival. Microscopic appearance: Erythrocyte morphology is typically normal. Anemia is not severe. If the hemoglobin is < 9 or hematocrit < 30, chronic disease alone is probably not causing the anemia. Reticulocyte count is in the "normal" range but low considering the anemia and assuming adequate iron stores. Serum iron and TIBC are decreased. Transferrin saturation is decreased. Serum ferritin (a measure of the body's iron stores) is normal to elevated. Bone marrow iron stain discloses normal to increased iron. Chronic disease–associated anemia is not always normocytic normochromic. Microcytic hypochromic anemia is not uncommon.

Chronic renal failure patients may have multiple reasons for their anemia—e.g. anemia of chronic disease; hemolysis; blood loss (from GI tract, hemodialysis, repeated blood drawing); hemodialysis–induced folate deficiency. Consequently, the peripheral blood smear is unpredictable. Anemia is usually normocytic normochromic or microcytic hypochromic. Schistocytes or burr cells may be seen on the peripheral smear if there is hemolysis. Stool should be tested for occult blood. Bone marrow exam may be needed to establish the presence of iron deficiency. Treatment: Dialysis patients should receive folate supplements. Epoetin (a recombinant human erythropoietin) may be used to correct the anemia. Iron deficiency should be corrected before beginning epoetin. Anemia is sometimes severe enough to require transfusion. Anemia may resolve with successful renal transplantation.

Endocrine insufficiency (e.g. thyroid, adrenal, pituitary) may cause anemia—usually a mild normochromic normocytic anemia. Anemia results from decreased marrow production—the consequence of decreased erythropoietin. Anemia in hypothyroid patients may be compounded by pernicious anemia and/or by iron deficiency secondary to heavy menses. Also be aware that the serum iron is usually decreased in myxedema even if there is no iron deficiency.

Chronic liver disease is frequently associated with normocytic normochromic anemia. However, macrocytic or microcytic anemia may also occur. The hematologic picture is often unclear because anemia may be due multiple factors. For instance, an alcoholic with cirrhosis may have anemia because: (1) ethanol suppresses marrow production; (2) folate deficiency; (3) blood loss (e.g. varices, gastritis, ulcer, coagulation factor deficiency); (4) decreased RBC survival secondary to portal hypertension-induced splenomegaly with hypersplenism.

Aplastic anemia is usually associated with normocytic normochromic anemia, although the MCV is sometimes slightly elevated. Reticulocytes are absent or rare. Pure red cell aplasia is rare and consequently, the peripheral smear usually also discloses thrombocytopenia and neutropenia. The absolute lymphocyte count, however, is typically normal. The bone marrow is acellular or hypocellular. Serum iron is elevated. Etiology: About half the cases are idiopathic. Drugs are the most common known precipitants (e.g. chloramphenicol, phenylbutazone, gold, quinacrine, trimethadione, antineoplastic). Aplastic anemia may be familial (e.g. Fanconi syndrome). Other precipitants include toxins (e.g. benzene); infection (e.g. viral hepatitis, EB virus); ionizing radiation; pregnancy; thymona. Chloramphenicol is an example of a drug that may cause either a dose-independent (idiosyncratic) or a dose-dependent aplastic anemia. The aplasia that results from antineoplastic drugs or ionizing radiation is dose-dependent.

Marrow infiltration (myelophthisis) results in premature release of blood cells into the circulation. Consequently, the peripheral smear may disclose immature cell types—e.g. nucleated red cells, myelocytes, giant platelets. Poikilocytosis is evident (e.g. teardrop shaped RBC's). Extensive marrow displacement may lead to leukopenia and thrombocytopenia in addition to anemia. Bone marrow exam is necessary to confirm the diagnosis. Etiology: Bone marrow infiltration may be the consequence of metastatic carcinoma; leukemia; myelofibrosis (e.g. primary, secondary to leukemia or metastatic cancer); infection (Tb, fungal); osteopetrosis; lipid storage disease (e.g. Gaucher's disease).

Sideroblastic anemias are disorders of globin synthesis (in the case of thalassemia) or heme synthesis that result in decreased production of hemoglobin with ensuing intracellular accumulation of iron. Impaired heme synthesis leading to sideroblastic anemia may be due to: (**1**) drugs/toxins—e.g. alcohol; antituberculous drugs (isoniazid, pyrazinamide, cycloserine); lead; chloramphenicol; (**2**) autoimmune diseases; (**3**) neoplasia—e.g. multiple myeloma, certain leukemias; (**4**) megaloblastic anemia; (**5**) severe hemolysis; (**6**) hereditary sideroblastic anemia—a rare X-linked recessive disorder; (**7**) acquired idiopathic sideroblastic anemia. Bone marrow stain with Prussian blue demonstrates the characteristic ringed sideroblasts. A ringed sideroblast is a normoblast (a nucleated RBC) containing mitochondria that are loaded with non-heme iron (and cosequently stain with Prussian blue) and that partially or completely surround (ring) the nucleus. The mitochondria are the site of heme synthesis. Bone marrow exam also reveals erythroid hyperplasia. Peripheral smear shows both normochromic normocytic RBC's and microcytic hypochromic RBC's. The MCV usually remains in the normal range or may even be slightly increased. Reticulocyte count is decreased. WBC and platelet count are normal. Serum iron is elevated. TIBC is normal. Transferrin saturation is increased. Serum ferritin is elevated. Treatment: Remove possible offending drugs/toxins. Treat underlying disorder if possible. Megaloblastic anemia–associated sideroblastic anemia is treated with folate or B–12 (see "Megaloblastic Anemia"). Alcohol-related cases are treated with folate and abstinence. Chelation therapy in used in cases associated with lead poisoning. Hereditary or idiopathic–acquired sideroblastic anemia sometimes responds to pyridoxine (vitamin B–6) 100–200 mg/day. Some patients who do not improve with pyridoxine may respond to pyridoxal phosphate.

Concurrent iron deficiency and megaloblastic anemia may result in an MCV that is low, normal, or high. The peripheral smear may reveal features of both megaloblastic anemia (e.g. hypersegmented granulocytes, macroovalocytes) or iron deficiency (microcytic hypochromic RBC's). Serum folate, serum B–12, and the laboratory studies outlined above for iron deficiency are obtained.

Hemolysis–provoked anemia is usually normocytic normochromic. However, the MCV may be elevated slightly because more reticulocytes (which are slightly larger than mature RBC's are released into the circulation. Chronic <u>intrav</u>ascular hemolysis results in urinary iron loss which may lead to a microcytic hypochromic anemia. The other laboratory features of hemolytic anemia are discussed in other chapters: "Laboratory Findings in Hemolysis", "Immunoglobulin/Complement-Mediated Hemolysis", and "Hemolysis not Involving Immunoglobulin or Complement".

Acute hemorrhage results in normocytic normochromic anemia. However, a decrease in hematocrit and hemoglobin is not immediately observed. These parameters may not decrease for several hours—until fluid has had time to shift from the tissues into the intravascular space and thereby dilute the remaining RBC's. Reticulocytosis begins in 3–5 days and peaks at 7 days.

Megaloblastic Anemia is usually due to vitamin B–12
and/or folate deficiency; both of which in turn have sundry causes. Megaloblastic anemia may also result from disorders unresponsive to B–12 or folate therapy.
Biochemistry: Megaloblastic anemia results from impaired DNA synthesis. The metabolism of folate and B–12 are closely interrelated. One of the derivatives of folate (N 5,10–methylene tetrahydrofolate) serves in the transfer of one–carbon units. Specifically, in the context of DNA synthesis, the role of this molecule is to transfer a one–carbon methyl group to deoxyuridine to form thymidylate (the methylated pyrimidine nucleotide found in DNA). However, much of the body's THF is in the form of N 5–methyl THF, a form which is unable to transfer its methyl group to deoxyuridine. This methyl group must be removed in a B 12–dependent reaction to form THF (see diagram below). THF in turn accepts a one carbon moiety from serine to form N 5,10–methylene THF.

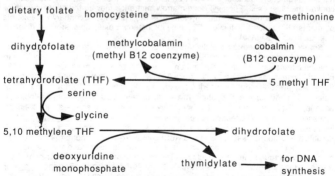

B–12 also serves as a coenzyme in a reaction that converts methylmalonyl Co–A to succinyl Co–A. This defect somehow affects myelin synthesis and leads to the neurologic sequelae associated with B–12 deficiency. Impaired conversion of methylmalonyl Co–A leads to increased urinary excretion of methylmalonic acid. While B–12 deficiency or folate deficiency alone or in combination may cause megaloblastic anemia, neurologic complications are due to B–12 deficiency. Neurologic complications are not associated with folate deficiency alone. **Laboratory findings common to both folate and B–12 deficiency:** It is not possible to distinguish folate deficiency from B–12 deficiency by simply examining the peripheral blood smear or bone marrow. <u>Peripheral blood smear</u> typically shows RBC's that vary in both size and form. Some of the RBC's are large and oval (macro–ovalocytes). In the absence of iron deficiency, the RBC's are normochromic. Reticulocytes are decreased. Nucleated

RBC's may be present in advanced cases. Howell–Jolly bodies and Pappenheimer bodies may be found. The neutrophils tend to be enlarged and some have hypersegmented nuclei (i.e. > 5 lobes)—one of the first indications of megaloblastic anemia. Hypersegmentation is not found in other types of macrocytic anemia. Platelets may be abnormal in size and shape. Bone marrow exam: The term megaloblastic is used to describe the anemia because the erythroblasts seen in the bone marrow are unusually large. Since the other bone marrow cell lines are also affected by the defect in DNA synthesis, one also sees megaloblastic changes in the myeloid line (e.g. giant metamyelocytes) and abnormal megakaryocytes. Iron stain of the marrow reveals abnormal sideroblasts, sometimes including ringed sideroblasts. Erythrocyte indices: As expected the MCV is > 100 and often exceeds 115. The MCH is high and the MCHC is normal in the absence of concomitant iron deficiency. Neutropenia ensues and thrombocytopenia is common in advanced cases. Serum indirect bilirubin is often found to be elevated as a consequence of the hemolysis of abnormal RBC's within the bone marrow. Serum LDH and serum iron may also be elevated because of hemolysis.

FOLATE DEFICIENCY is most often due to inadequate dietary intake. Green leafy vegetables, eggs, milk, liver, yeast are good sources of folate. Alcoholics are prone to megaloblastic anemia because their diet is often poor and because alcohol may interfere with folate metabolism. Normally the body has a sufficient reserve of folate so that the blood smear will not show evidence of megaloblastosis until 3–4 months after curtailing intake. Hypersegmented neutrophils is one of the first signs of folate deficiency. Folate deficiency may also arise because of increased requirements—e.g. pregnancy, infancy, chronic hemolysis (e.g. sickle cell anemia). Other causes of folate deficiency include malabsorption (e.g. sprue), drugs that interfere with folate absorption (e.g. phenytoin, oral contraceptives); hemodialysis. ●Inhibitors of dihydrofolate reductase (e.g. methotrexate) act to purposefully block folate utilization. The block may be circumvented by administering folinic acid (N 5–formyl FH4). **Signs/symptoms:** There may be manifestations of anemia in general (e.g. fatigue, pallor) and/or evidence of poor epithelial cell proliferation secondary to impaired DNA synthesis—e.g. glossitis (sore smooth tongue), diarrhea. **Diagnosis:** Laboratory findings common to both folate and B–12 deficiency; see above. Serum folate level is < 3–5 ng/ml. Be aware, however, that a short–term improvement in diet or a transfusion may bring the serum folate into the normal range. RBC folate level: When the body's store of folate is exhausted, the RBC folate level will fall to < 150 ng/ml. For unknown reasons, about half of folate deficient patients have slightly decreased serum B–12 levels in the absence of B–12 deficiency. Administration of small doses of folate or B–12 may help distinguish folate from B–12 deficiency (see Diagnosis B–12 deficiency below). **Treatment:** Folic acid 1 mg PO once daily is usually adequate therapy. Alcoholics require larger doses. Multivitamin B complex supplementation is a good idea because combined vitamin B complex deficiencies are not uncommon. With adequate therapy, reticulocytosis is noted in 3–5 days and peaks in about 7 days. Anemia usually takes over a month to correct. Neutropenia and thrombocytopenia begin to resolve in about a week. The serum potassium level may fall due to increased intracellular potassium incorporation. Be aware that folate therapy alone (by inducing reticulocytosis) may ameliorate anemia and thereby mask megaloblastic anemia due to B–12 deficiency.

B–12 DEFICIENCY Liver, meat, fish, eggs, milk are good sources of B–12. Usually, the body's store of B–12 is such that deficiency will not develop until years after the onset of an absorptive defect or dietary insufficiency. **Causes:** Pernicious anemia is the most common B–12 deficiency–associated syndrome. The gastric mucosa is atrophic and the gastric parietal cells are incapable of secreting a glycoprotein called intrinsic factor. Intrinsic factor normally combines with ingested B–12. When the combination arrives at the distal ileum, intrinsic factor binds to specific mucosal receptors thereby enabling B–12 absorption. Absence of intrinsic factor, therefore, greatly impairs B–12 absorption. Gastric HCl secretion is also impaired in pernicious anemia since the gastric parietal cells are also the source of hydrogen ion (there is failure to produce acid following administration of histamine). Many patients with pernicious anemia have autoantibodies directed against intrinsic factor and/or gastric parietal cells. Other causes of B–12 deficiency include dietary deficiency (usually in strict vegetarians); total gastrectomy or rarely partial gastrectomy; disease or resection of the ileum; competition for B-12 within the GI tract (e.g. bacterial overgrowth as in blind loop syndrome, fish tapeworm infestation); Imerslund's syndrome. The latter is a rare inherited ileal defect in B-12 absorption associated with normal gastric acid and intrinsic factor secretion and otherwise normal GI absorption. **Signs/symptoms:** B-12 deficiency may provoke the same manifestations as described above for folate deficiency. In addition, however, B-12 deficiency may also have neurologic consequences (sometimes even without megaloblastic anemia) with eventual degeneration of both the dorsal and lateral portions of the spinal cord (i.e. subacute combined degeneration). Neurologic abnormalities may include paresthesias (e.g. numbness/tingling/burning extremities); impaired position and/or vibration sense; ataxia; hyper or hypoactive deep tendon reflexes; positive Babinski; psychologic disturbances (e.g. irritability, depression, confusion, paranoia, dementia). **Diagnosis:** Laboratory findings common to both folate and B-12 deficiency; see above. Serum B-12 level is low: < 150 pg/ml and often < 100 pg/ml. However, radioimmune assay techniques may give falsely normal serum levels in 10% cases of B-12 deficiency. Administration of small doses of folate or B-12 may help distinguish folate from B-12 deficiency. If a person is administered a single 50 µg PO or IM dose of folate, it will induce reticulocytosis if there is folate deficiency but not if there is B-12 deficiency. On the other hand, a single 1 µg IM dose of B-12 will induce reticulocytosis in B-12 deficiency but not in folate deficiency. Larger doses of either vitamin may mask deficiency of the other by causing improvement of the megaloblastic anemia. Schilling test may be used to confirm the diagnosis of pernicious anemia. (see the chapter "Malabsorption" for details). Histamine-induced gastric acid secretion is impaired in pernicious anemia. Urinary levels of methylmalonate are increased in B-12 deficiency. However, this measurement is seldom needed to diagnose B-12 deficiency. **Treatment:** B-12 1000 µg IM daily for 2 wk followed by 1000 µg IM monthly. Injections are continued for life if B-12 deficiency is due to permanently impaired B-12 absorption. If there are neurologic findings, bimonthly shots are recommended for 6 months followed by the monthly regimen. In severe cases of megaloblastic anemia, it is permissible to start therapy with both B-12 and folate before laboratory confirmation can be obtained provided that blood for testing is drawn prior to initiating therapy. Response to treatment: The patient may feel better within 1-2 days. Reticulocytosis is noted in 3-5 days and peaks in about 7 days (and may exceed 30% in severe anemia). Anemia usually takes over a month to correct. Neutropenia and thrombocytopenia begin to resolve in about a week. Serum potassium level may fall because of increased intracellular potassium incorporation. Neurologic abnormalities may take over a year to resolve and some neurologic deficits may be permanent. ●Treatment of B-12 deficient patients with over 400 µg/day doses of folate may partially improve the hematologic picture and thereby mask the B-12 deficiency. Furthermore, yet larger doses of folate alone may precipitate neurologic abnormalities in the B-12 deficient patient.

FOLATE and B-12 UNRESPONSIVE MEGALOBLASTIC ANEMIA: Antineoplastic drugs by impairing DNA, RNA, and/or protein synthesis may provoke megaloblastic anemia (e.g. doxorubicin, daunorubicin, cytosine arabinoside, hydroxyurea, mercaptopurine, azathioprine, 5-fluorouracil). Inhibitors of dihydrofolate reductase (e.g. methotrexate) are used to purposefully block folate utilization. The block may be circumvented by administering folinic acid (N 5-formyl FH4). Rare hereditary disorders of folate metabolism, purine metabolism (e.g. Lesch-Nyhan syndrome), or pyrimidine metabolism (hereditary orotic aciduria) may lead to megaloblastic anemia.

Certain myelodysplastic disorders (e.g. chronic myelomonocytic leukemia, refractory sideroblastic anemia); and pyridoxine and thiamine-responsive megaloblastic anemias may be responsible for megaloblastic anemia.

Laboratory Findings in Hemolysis

Reticulocytosis: When there is depletion of RBC's, the bone marrow (if it is capable) compensates by increasing production and release of RBC's. This manifests on the peripheral blood smear as an increased percentage of immature erythocytes (reticulocytes). Anemia ensues if marrow compensation cannot keep up with hemolysis. Under normal circumstances the reticulocyte count (i.e. % of circulating RBC's that are reticulocytes) is 0.5–1.5 %. Reticulocyte index: The reticulocyte count by itself may be misleading because in the setting of a low hematocrit the reticulocyte count may be substantially increased by the release of even a small number of reticulocytes by the bone marrow. Therefore, as a check on the adequacy of the bone marrow response to anemia, a corrected reticulocyte count (reticulocyte index) is calculated. The reticulocyte index = % reticulocytes X (observed hematocrit ÷ normal hematocrit).

Hyperbilirubinemia: Hemolysis leads to an elevated serum bilirubin because there is an increased load of free plasma hemoglobin from ruptured erythrocytes.

INTRAVASCULAR HEMOLYSIS: Markedly elevated plasma hemoglobin with consequent red–brown discoloration of the serum is characteristic of intravascular hemolysis. Discoloration of the serum may be detected on gross inspection after the lysis of only a few milliliters of RBC's. Haptoglobin (a hemoglobin–binding plasma globulin) binds to the hemoglobin released from the ruptured RBC's, and the hemoglobin–haptoglobin complex is rapidly cleared by the reticuloendothelial system. Haptoglobin is thus consumed and the serum haptoglobin level is nil or markedly decreased. Hemoglobinuria: Hemoglobin is filtered by the glomerulus when haptoglobin is expended. Filtered hemoglobin is taken up by the renal tubular cells. Hemoglobin appears in the urine once the the renal tubular cells have become saturated with hemoglobin. ●Hemoglobinuria may be distinguished from myoglobinuria by gross inspection of urine and plasma. Myoglobin (a smaller molecule than hemoglobin) is rapidly filtered by the kidneys, and so the urine may be discolored by myoglobin but the plasma is not discolored. Hemoglobin, on the other hand, is less easily filtered. Consequently, hemoglobin is present in appreciable amounts in both plasma and urine and so both may be discolored red–brown. Hemosiderinuria appears after a few days. As previously stated, the hemoglobin that is filtered at the glomerulus is taken up by renal tubular cells. Consequently, those renal tubular cells that slough into the urine will stain positive for iron. Serum LDH is usually markedly elevated because LDH is released from the lyzed RBC's.

EXTRAVASCULAR HEMOLYSIS The majority of hemolytic disorders are associated with extravascular hemolysis—i.e. the RBC's are phagocytized by macrophages of the reticuloendothelial system, primarily within the spleen and liver. **Contrast with intravascular hemolysis:** Haptoglobin: Even though hemolysis is extravascular, a small amount of hemoglobin is released into the bloodstream. In contrast to intravascular hemolysis, however, *plasma* hemoglobin is generally normal or only slightly elevated (and consequently red–brown discoloration of the serum is absent) because haptoglobin (a hemoglobin–binding plasma globulin) binds to the free hemoglobin and the hemoglobin–haptoglobin complex is rapidly cleared by the reticuloendothelial system. Haptoglobin is thus consumed and the serum haptoglobin level decreases as with intravascular hemolysis but generally not to as great an extent. Hemoglobinuria and hemosiderinuria are absent (and therefore red–brown discoloration of the urine is absent) because the *plasma* hemoglobin level is not elevated, and consequently little if any hemoglobin is filtered at the glomeruli. Serum LDH is generally elevated because of the release of LDH from ruptured RBC's. However, the serum LDH does not reach the markedly elevated levels observed with intravascular hemolysis. Spherocytes: Sometimes an RBC is not completely phagocytized and only a portion of the RBC membrane is removed; the damaged membrane seals; and the RBC again enters the bloodstream and is seen as a spherocyte on a blood smear. The presence of many spherocytes is associated with an elevated MCHC.

IMMUNOGLOBULIN/COMPLEMENT–MEDIATED HEMOLYSIS may be intravascular or extravascular and so the comments made above regarding intravascular versus extravascular hemolysis are relevant. However, most cases of immunoglobulin/complement–mediated are <u>extra</u>vascular (e.g. warm antibody–mediated hemolysis, cold agglutinin–mediated hemolysis). An acute hemolytic transfusion reaction is an example of an immune–mediated <u>intra</u>vascular reaction. **Direct Coombs' (direct antiglobulin) test** detects antibody, complement, or other plasma proteins bound to the RBC membrane. Serum from animals immunized with human serum is mixed with the patient's RBC's. If the patient's RBC's are coated with certain plasma components (e.g. IgG, complement), antibodies in the animal antisera directed against constituents of human serum will attach to those components coating the RBC's and the RBC's will agglutinate (clump). <u>Identifying the specific serum component responsible for a positive direct Coombs' test:</u> Antisera are available from animals that have been specifically immunized with human immunoglobulin alone (or even classes of immunoglobulin) or human complement alone to permit identification of the specific plasma component(s) coating the RBC's. <u>False–negative direct Coombs' test:</u> Sometimes there is sufficient antibody attached to the RBC membrane to induce hemolysis but not enough to yield a positive direct Coombs' test. **Indirect Coombs' (indirect antiglobulin) test** detects free circulating antibody capable of binding to RBC's. A sample of the patient's serum is mixed with a sample of another person's normal RBC's. In the event that antibody from the patient's serum binds to the normal test RBC's, the subsequent addition of animal antisera directed against human immunoglobulin will result in agglutination of the normal test RBC's. <u>The indirect test may be positive if:</u> **(1)** antibody has been produced by the patient in excess—i.e. all the specific antigen sites on the patient's RBC's are saturated and so immunoglobulin directed against the specific RBC membrane antigen continues to circulate freely. In this case the *direct* Coombs's test will also be positive. **(2)** all the susceptible RBC's have been destroyed (e.g. hemolytic transfusion reaction) but the responsible immunoglobulin continues to circulate. In this case the *direct* Coombs' test is negative. <u>A positive indirect Coombs' test in the absence of hemolysis</u> is not uncommon.

Immunoglobulin and/or Complement–Mediated Hemolysis

PATHOGENESIS: <u>Immunoglobulin/complement–mediated hemolysis may occur by various mechanisms.</u> For example: **(1)** Immunoglobulin binds to a RBC membrane antigen. Complement component C1 then binds to the RBC membrane–bound immunoglobulin. The complement cascade proceeds to completion leading to the *intra*vascular destruction of RBC's. **(2)** Same initial mechanism except that the complement cascade is interrupted before it can be completed. The complement component–coated RBC's undergo *extra*vascular destruction by the reticuloendothelial system (primarily in the liver) where they encounter and are engulfed by macrophages. **(3)** Immunoglobulin binds to RBC membrane antigen. However, complement is not fixed. The immunoglobulin–coated RBC's undergo *extra*vascular destruction by the reticuloendothelial system (chiefly in the liver and spleen) where they encounter and are engulfed by macrophages. **(4)** Rarely, complement alone may bind to RBC's and lead to *intra*vascular hemolysis without involving immunoglobulin (see Paroxysmal Nocturnal Hemoglobinuria below). <u>The antigenic stimulus to immunoglobulin–mediated hemolysis is varied</u>—e.g. **(1)** autoimmune—when the inducing antigen is an integral part of the patient's RBC membrane; **(2)** alloimmune [isoimmune] when foreign incompatible RBC's enter or are introduced into the patient's circulation and are subsequently lyzed (see Alloantibody–Induced Hemolysis below); **(3)** drug–induced by various mechanisms (see below).
LABORATORY INVESTIGATION: Refer to previous chapter "Laboratory Findings in Hemolysis".

ALLOANTIBODY–MEDIATED HEMOLYSIS An alloantibody (isoantibody) is an antibody produced in response to exposure to an alloantigen (antigen from another individual that is foreign to the patient)—e.g. transfusion of incompatible blood, leakage of incompatible fetal blood into maternal circulation. Sometimes, so–called natural alloantibodies are formed in response to an individual's own intestinal bacteria.
Hemolysis following transfusion: Alloantibodies that have been induced by expo-

sure to incompatible blood are directed against antigenic components (e.g. Rh, Lewis) on *foreign* RBC's. Subsequent transfusion of RBC's bearing the same alloantigen(s) may lead to binding of the patient's alloantibodies to and hemolysis of the transfused RBC's. The patient's own RBC's are not hemolyzed. Hemolysis may be intravascular (acute hemolytic transfusion reaction) or extravascular (delayed hemolytic transfusion reaction). Coombs' testing: If the transfused RBC's have not been completely destroyed, the direct Coombs' test may be positive. In the event that hemolysis of the transfused RBC's is complete, the alloantibody can only be detected by the indirect Coombs' test. **Erythroblastosis fetalis:** In the case of a mother who has been previously sensitized by either prior transfusion or prior pregnancy, a subsequent pregnancy with fetal–maternal incompatibility may cause erythroblastosis fetalis. In this condition, maternal alloantibodies leak across the placenta into the fetal circulation and cause hemolysis of the fetal RBC's.

WARM ANTIBODY–MEDIATED HEMOLYSIS is the hemolysis that is provoked by an IgG (occasionally IgM or IgA) that has affinity for a RBC membrane antigen, and that affinity is maximal at body temperature. Hemolysis is usually not intravascular because either the IgG molecule fails to fix complement or the complement cascade is interrupted before completion. Rather, the IgG–coated and possibly complement component–coated RBC's are destroyed in the reticuloendothelial system (mostly in the spleen or liver) by macrophages with receptors for IgG molecule (the Fc portion) or complement component. **Etiology:** idiopathic; infection (usually viral); autoimmune (e.g. systemic lupus, rheumatoid arthritis, scleroderma); lymphoproliferative disorder (e.g. lymphoma, CLL); ovarian teratoma; ulcerative colitis; certain drugs (see below). **Laboratory:** Specific direct Coombs' testing reveals RBC's to be coated with IgG alone, both IgG and C3, or in rare cases C3 alone. Indirect Coombs' test will also be positive if the patient produces excess antibody directed against his own RBC's (i.e. the RBC antigen binding sites are saturated). Other findings consistent with extravascular hemolysis (see "Laboratory Findings in Hemolysis" chapter). **Therapy:** Treat the underlying disorder if possible and discontinue suspect drugs (see below). Specific therapy is not required in mild hemolysis. In more severe cases, prednisone 1–2 mg/kg/day is begun and can usually be tapered after 2–3 weeks as the anemia begins to resolve. Continued low–dose maintenance may be required. Patients not responding to prednisone are candidates for splenectomy, and those patients refractory to both prednisone and splenectomy are treated with immunosuppressants (e.g. azothioprine, cyclophosphamide). Severe hemolytic anemia may necessitate transfusion but crossmatching is difficult, particularly if the indirect Coombs' test is positive. This is because a positive indirect Coombs' test means that the culpable antibodies will bind to RBC's of all possible donors and thus obscure detection of alloantibodies.

COLD AGGLUTININ–MEDIATED HEMOLYSIS Cold agglutinins are antibodies that bind to RBC's at 0 to 4° C with ensuing RBC agglutination (clumping). Cold agglutinins are virtually always IgM, rarely IgA or IgG (see Donath–Landsteimer hemolysis below). Clinically significant cold agglutinins: Only those cold IgM antibodies whose affinity for RBC's extends to physiologically feasible temperatures are capable of causing clinical hemolysis (i.e. to at least 30° C—temperatures that may occur in the extremities, nose, ears). In fact, cold antibodies are commonly produced that have no clinical significance since they only react with RBC's at subphysiologic temperatures. Extravascular hemolysis: The complement cascade is activated when IgM binds to the RBC membrane. However, the cascade is usually interrupted before RBC membrane injury can occur, and consequently intravascular hemolysis is uncommon. However, hemolysis does occur in the reticuloendothelial system (mostly in the liver) where the complement component–coated RBC's encounter and are destroyed by macrophages. **Laboratory:** Tube test: Cold agglutinins can be demonstrated simply by observing the effects of cooling on a sample of the patient's blood in an anticoagulant–containing tube. Cool the tube in ice water for 5 minutes. With cooling, IgM attaches to the RBC membrane antigen and the RBC's agglutinate (clump). Upon rewarming, IgM dissociates and clumping disappears. In some cases clumping is seen without cooling in ice water. Sometimes, in fact, agglutination is so exuberant that clumping is noted in an anticoagulant–containing tube even as the blood is being drawn. Direct Coombs' test is positive using anti–complement sera because the RBC's are coated with complement component (C3). The test is performed after warming the blood in order to dissociate IgM from the RBC's and thereby reveal a pure complement–positive direct Coombs' test. Cold agglutinin titer is elevated to > 1:32. To insure an accurate reading, the serum should be separated promptly after the blood is drawn (before the blood sample cools and IgM binds to the RBC's). Blood smear reveals RBC agglutination. Erroneous measurements of the RBC count, hematocrit, and indices may occur as a consequence of RBC agglutination when automated measurement methods are used. **Causes:** Infection (e.g. mycoplasma, infectious mononucleosis, cytomegalovirus, malaria, trypanosoma) may induce production of cold agglutinins but seldom do the IgM levels become elevated enough for them to cause clinical signs. Furthermore, IgM–mediated hemolysis is self–limited. Lymphoproliferative disease, particularly histiocytic lymphoma, may be associated with chronic cold agglutinin hemolysis. The cold agglutinin is a monoclonal IgM (kappa or lambda). Idiopathic cold agglutinin hemolysis is a rare syndrome occurring in elderly males. It is associated with chronic hemolysis and a monoclonal elevation of IgM. Exposure to cold characteristically precipitates or exacerbates agglutination. The normally cooler areas of the body (extremities, nose, ears) is where agglutination occurs. Upon exposure to cold, the patient may experience ischemic pain in those areas. **Treatment of clinically significant cases:** Treatment is directed at the underlying disorder if possible. Patient should avoid cold exposure. ●Chlorambucil is sometimes used in severe cases of idiopathic cold agglutinin hemolysis. ●Transfusions are dangerous in patients with cold agglutinin hemolysis because the cold agglutinins will agglutinate the transfused RBC's. Furthermore, crossmatching is difficult because the agglutinins bind to RBC's of all possible donors and therefore obscure detection of alloantibodies.

Donath–Landsteimer hemolysis (paroxysmal cold hemoglobinuria) is a rare form of cold agglutinin hemolysis mediated by an IgG antibody with affinity for the P antigen on RBC's. Upon cold exposure classically, the IgG antibody attaches to the RBC's and complement is fixed. Intravascular hemolysis with hemoglobinuria ensues. The condition is idiopathic or may be associated with syphilis or viral infection. In the case of viral infection, hemolysis may be provoked in the absence of cold–exposure. The Donath–Landsteiner antibody test is diagnostic.

DRUG–INDUCED IMMUNE–MEDIATED HEMOLYSIS:

Drugs inducing complement–fixing antibody—e.g. quinidine, quinine, sulfonamides, phenothiazines. The drug binds to a plasma protein forming a drug–protein antigen. The induced antibody forms a complex with the drug–protein and the complex in turn activates complement. Complement components subsequently coat the RBC's. Hemolysis may be intravascular if the complement cascade is not aborted. More often, however, the RBC's are destroyed in the reticuloendothelial system (mostly in the liver) where the complemented–coated RBC's are recognized and destroyed by macrophages. The direct Coombs' test is negative when animal antisera directed against human IgG is added to a sample of the patient's blood because immunoglobulin is not bound to the RBC's. However, the direct test is positive if anti–complement antisera is used. The indirect Coombs' test is usually negative.

Methyldopa (Aldomet) may induce production of an IgG antibody that binds to RBC's. Methyldopa is not itself bound to the RBC's. Complement is not fixed and therefore hemolysis (if it occurs) is extravascular: the IgG–coated RBC's encounter and are destroyed, in the spleen mostly, by macrophages with receptors for the Fc portion of the IgG molecule. Hemolysis develops in about 10% of those with a positive Coombs' test. Methyldopa may be continued in Coombs' postive cases provided that there is no hemolysis. Levodopa and mefenamic acid (Ponstel) may also provoke hemolysis by this mechanism.

Penicillin attaches to RBC's and may act as a hapten upon binding to the RBC membrane. The induced IgG antibody binds to RBC's but complement is not fixed. Consequently, the direct Coombs' test is positive with anti–IgG sera but not with anti-–complement sera. In performing the indirect Coombs test, penicillin must be present on the test RBC's in order to yield a positive test (i.e. normal test RBC's mixed with the patient's serum will not bind the IgG in question without prior addition of penicillin to the normal test RBC's).

PAROXYSMAL NOCTURNAL HEMOGLOBINURIA is a very rare acquired complement–mediated hemolysis. Some of the patient's RBC's fix increased amounts of complement and so they are prone to intravascular lysis. Immunoglobulin is not involved in the hemolytic process. Complement may also affect platelet function (with increased incidence of thrombosis) and granulocyte function. **Laboratory:** Sucrose hemolysis test (in vitro hemolysis of patient's RBC's in a hypotonic sugar solution) and/or Ham's test (in vitro hemolysis of patient's RBC's upon addition of slightly acidified normal human test serum) are diagnostic. Direct Coombs' test is generally negative. Intravascular hemolysis results in hemoglobinuria (most obvious in the concentrated first–voided morning urine), hemosiderinuria, decreased serum haptoglobin, elevated serum LDH. Peripheral smear discloses reticulocytosis. RBC's are hypochromic secondary to urinary iron loss with ensuing anemia. **Treatment:** iron and folate supplements. Therapy may also include androgens, prednisone, and/or blood transfusion.

Hemolysis not Involving Immunoglobulin or Complement

LABORATORY INVESTIGATION: The chapter "Laboratory Findings in Hemolysis" outlines the differences between intravascular and extravascular hemolysis and is relevant here since examples of both are described below.

EXAMPLES of EXTRAVASCULAR HEMOLYSIS:

Hereditary spherocytosis is an autosomal dominant inherited disease. A defect in the RBC membrane causes many of the RBC's to assume a spheroidal shape. The RBC's exhibit increased osmotic fragility (i.e. more susceptible to hemolysis in hypotonic solution). The MCV is normal but the MCHC is increased. The RBC's, because they are unable to alter their shape, have difficulty traversing the spleen. Consequently, there is increased splenic destruction with ensuing anemia. The spleen enlarges. Indirect hyperbilirubinemia is characteristic and there may be jaundice. Infection may precipitate aplastic crisis. Patients are prone to bilirubin gallstones. Treatment: splenectomy, but usually not before the age of 6. Pneumococcal vaccination is advised 1–2 months before surgery and prophylactic penicillin is recommended for at least 2 years following surgery.

Hereditary elliptocytosis is an autosomal inherited disorder of the RBC cell membrane. The blood smear reveals RBC's with an oval profile. Most patients do not exhibit increased osmotic fragility or increased splenic destruction. Splenectomy is therefore not usually necessary.

Hypersplenism refers to the condition in which there is excessive sequestration and destruction of blood cells (RBC's, WBC's, and/or platelets) by the spleen. Since any or all of the blood cell types may be depleted, one may see any combination of anemia, thrombocytopenia, and/or leukopenia. The spleen is enlarged. The bone marrow attempts to compensate for the depletion of blood cells by increasing production. Consequently, the marrow is hypercellular. *Etiology:* Hypersplenism is sometimes idiopathic. Known precipitants include congestive splenomegaly (e.g. cirrhosis, thrombosis or compression of portal or splenic vein); neoplasia (e.g. leukemia, lymphoma, polycythemia vera, myeloid metaplasia); autoimmune (Felty's syndrome, SLE); acute infection (infectious mononucleosis, infectious hepatitis, bacterial endocarditis); chronic infection (e.g. miliary Tb, malaria, trypanosoma, leishmaniasis, brucellosis); hereditary RBC abnormalities (e.g. spherocytosis, elliptocytosis, thalassemias, hemoglobin SC); other (amyloidosis, sarcoidosis, Gaucher's disease, Niemann–Pick disease).

Hemoglobinopathies: thalassemia, sickle cell anemia.

EXAMPLES of INTRAVASCULAR HEMOLYSIS:

Glucose–6–phosphate dehydrogenase (G6PD) deficiency: Pathogenesis: G6PD is the enzyme in the hexose monophophate (HMP) shunt that catalyzes the conversion of G-6-P to glucose. The HMP shunt generates the reducing agent NADPH. Without sufficient NADPH the RBC is susceptible to oxidative injury with hemolysis. Inheritance: G6PD deficiency is an X–linked disorder, and thus most patients are male. However, heterozygous females (in addition to homozygous females) may have G6PD deficiency to a variable degree. In black Americans: 10% males have G6PD deficiency, 20% females are heterozygous, 1% females are homozygous. G6PD deficiency is not uncommon in persons originating from the Mediterranean area (e.g. Greeks, Italians, Arabs, Sephardic Jews); and in Chinese and Thais. In these groups, G6PD deficiency is often more severe than in blacks. In some cases, in fact, hemolysis is chronic and not associated with oxidant stress. In blacks, hemolysis tends to be less severe since only the older RBC's (older RBC's have less G6PD) are subject to hemolysis; and consequently no more than 25% of the RBC's will be hemolyzed. <u>Precipitants:</u> Many oxidative drugs are known to precipitate hemolysis in G6PD–deficient persons (e.g. primaquine, sulfonamides, sulfones, nitrofurantoin, quinine, quinidine, probenecid, large doses of aspirin, some water–soluble vitamin K derivatives). Naphthalene (found in moth balls) is also a precipitant. Fava beans are a precipitant in G6PD–deficient persons of Mediterranean origin.   A febrile illness or severe acidosis may also induce hemolysis. <u>Laboratory</u> findings may include decreased hematocrit, elevated reticulocyte count, hemoglobinuria, elevated *plasma* hemoglobin, and/or hemosiderinuria. The peripheral smear, in addition to disclosing increased numbers of reticulocytes, may show bite cells (bites appear to have been taken out of the periphery of some RBC's). Heinz bodies (denatured hemoglobin deposits within RBC's) are an early and transient finding that may be revealed with special staining methods. Diagnosis is confirmed by measurement of G6PD enzyme activity (i.e. quantitative measurement NADPH production by hemolyzates of patient's RBC's). G6PD enzyme activity may be normal during or soon after an attack (particularly in black patients) because the older RBC's have lower levels of G6PD and are therefore preferentially destroyed. Consequently, confirmation of G6PD deficiency may not be possible until a few weeks following an attack when older RBC's are again present and reticulocytosis has subsided.

Mechanical hemolysis: In this type of intravascular hemolysis, schistocytes are a characteristic finding on blood smear. *Causes include:* <u>external trauma</u>—e.g. march hemoglobinuria (prolonged marching, marathon); repeated hand trauma (e.g. karate); <u>prosthetic heart valve or diseased natural heart valve</u> (particularly aortic); <u>trauma–related AV fistula</u>; <u>thrombosis in small vessels</u> (DIC, TTP, hemolytic uremia); <u>endothelial damage</u> (e.g. vasculitis, malignant hypertension, eclampsia, renal transplant rejection, giant hemangiomas); <u>severe and widespread burns</u>.

Toxins: heavy metals, snake or spider venom, certain mushrooms, amphotericin B, castor beans, certain bacterial toxins (e.g. Clostridrium perfringes sepsis).

RBC parasites: Malaria and babesiosis is associated with hemolysis secondary to RBC invasion. In bartonellosis, bacteria only proliferate on the RBC surface.

Sickle Cell Disorders
An erythrocyte of a normal adult contains 3 types of hemoglobin: 97% Hgb A, 2% Hgb A2, and 1% Hgb F (fetal hemoglobin). Hgb A consists of two α globin chains and two β globin chains ($\alpha2\beta2$), Hgb A2 consists of two α chains and two δ chains ($\alpha2\delta2$), and Hgb F consists of two α chains and two γ chains ($\alpha2\gamma2$). ●Persons with sickle cell disease (SS genotype) or sickle trait (AS genotype) have an abnormal hemoglobin in their erythrocytes—Hgb S. Hgb S consists of two normal α globin chains and two abnormal β globin chains designated β^S. Thus Hgb S in shorthand is $\alpha2\beta^S2$. The abnormal β globin chain β^S is due to a substitution of valine for glutamic acid at the 6 position of the β globin chain. ●Under conditions of low oxygen tension when the hemoglobin molecule is deoxygenated, Hgb S has a tendency to polymerize with other Hgb S molecules to form elongated crystalline structures (tactoids) that distort the RBC and cause it to assume a sickle shape. ●Acidosis (because it favors deoxygenation) and dehydration also promote sickling. ●The presence of substantial amounts of hemoglobin other than Hgb S may decrease the likelihood of sickling. For example, the erythrocytes in sickle trait (genotype AS) do not ordinarily sickle even though they contain 40–45% Hgb S; the substantial presence other hemoglobins (primarily Hgb A 55–60%) prevents sickling. On the other hand, the erythrocyte in sickle cell disease (i.e. genotype SS) is very susceptible to sickling because it contains no Hgb A and 85–95% Hgb S.

SICKLE CELL TRAIT occurs in 8% of American blacks. In certain areas of Africa where malaria is endemic as many as 30% may have the trait. The trait apparently confers resistance to falciparum malaria. The trait is not uncommon in Greeks, Italians, Asian Indians, and Arabians. ●Sickle cell trait is a heterozygous condition (genotype AS) with one gene coding for normal β globin chain and the allele coding for the $β^S$ globin chain. Thus, an erythrocyte contains Hgb S ($α2β^S2$), normal Hgb A ($α2β2$), a hybrid ($αβ$ $αβ^S$), and the other two normal hemoglobins whose composition does not include β globin chain: Hgb A2 ($α2δ2$) and Hgb F ($α2γ2$). Hemoglobin electrophoresis demonstrates the presence of Hgb A (55–60%), Hgb S (40–45%), Hgb A2 (2–3%), and Hgb F (about 1%). The hybrid is not detected by electrophoresis. A routine blood smear does not reveal sickling. However, sickling is revealed when hemoglobin is deoxygenated by the addition of sodium metabisulfite to the blood sample (sickle cell prep). ●Persons with the trait are not anemic. Symptoms are absent unless the patient is subjected to markedly hypoxic conditions. Under normal conditions, however, sickling does occur in the renal medulla where the erythrocytes are subjected to a hypertonic environment and become dehydrated. As a consequence there is local ischemia and infarction. Injury to the renal tubules leads to hyposthenuria (inability to produce a concentrated urine). Episodes of microscopic hematuria are common and gross hematuria may occur.

SICKLE CELL DISEASE occurs in about 1 in 500 U.S. blacks. It is a homozygous condition (genotype SS). Thus there are no genes coding for normal β globin chains, and so Hgb A is absent. Hemoglobin electrophoresis demonstrates 85–95% Hgb S ($α2β^S2$), 2–3% Hgb A2 ($α2δ2$), and 5–15% Hgb F ($α2γ2$). Hgb F is not distributed uniformly amongst the erythrocytes. Those erythrocytes containing more Hgb F survive longer.

Clinical manifestations of sickle cell disease begin in infancy after most of the Hgb F has been supplanted by Hgb S. Vascular occlusive crisis is due to sickling with occlusion of small blood vessels. Microinfarction commonly ensues. Patient usually presents with abrupt onset of severe pain in the back, chest, and/or limbs. There may also be abdominal pain or this may be the only complaint. Fever is common; it may be the consequence of infection (which often provokes a crisis) or tissue infarction. A vascular occlusive crisis is not a hemolytic crisis and so the hemoglobin and hematocrit do not fall. The crisis may be brought on by infection, dehydration, hypoxia, or acidosis. Often, there is no obvious precipitant. Acute vascular occlusion may have a number of consequences depending on the organ(s) affected—e.g. stroke, priapism, pulmonary infarction, abdominal crisis, hepatic crisis, renal complications. These disturbances are discussed below. Splenic sequestration crisis may occur in childhood (usually in children 2–5 yr of age) before autosplenectomy is complete. Sickled erythrocytes become trapped in the spleen in large numbers and the hematocrit falls. There is left upper quadrant pain, fever, chills. Shock and death may ensue. Splenomegaly may be present until about 8 years of age, but the spleen is generally not enlarged thereafter because repeated infarctions lead to autosplenectomy. In fact, the spleen is usually nonfunctional by 1–2 year of age. The absence of a functional spleen predisposes to bacterial infections. Aplastic crisis may be induced when an infection by parvovirus C–19 suppresses bone marrow RBC production. The hemoglobin, hematocrit, and reticulocyte count fall dramatically. Infection with parvovirus C–19 usually confers immunity so that adults are seldom subject to an aplastic crisis. Other infections may suppress marrow function but seldom to the life-threatening degree seen with parvovirus C–19 infection. Toxins, or folic acid deficiency may also suppress marrow function. Abdominal crisis is characterized by diffuse abdominal pain/tenderness with paralytic ileus. There are no localizing signs. Hepatic crisis may result when there is sickling within the hepatic sinusoids. Ensuing bile stasis combined with hemolysis often causes marked elevations of the serum bilirubin and liver enzymes. The liver is enlarged. Right upper quadrant pain may be confused with cholecystitis. Chronic jaundice is common and is due to chronic hemolysis–induced elevation of plasma bilirubin. Bilirubin gallstones are present in about half of adult patients. They are the consequence of chronic hemolysis. Cholecystitis may result. Strokes due to intracerebral sickling with infarction occur in up to 8% patients. Subarachnoid and subdural bleeding are also possible. Retinopathy is common. Sickling with occlusion of the retinal capillaries leads to retinal neovascularization. Vitreous bleeding occurs when and if these fragile neo–vessels rupture. The subsequent scarring may cause retinal detachment and blindness. Pulmonary infarction may ensue from (1) deep venous thrombosis with embolism, (2) fat emboli that originate from sickling–induced infarction of the bone marrow, or (3) sickling with thrombosis within the pulmonary microvasculature itself. Pulmonary infarctions may appear as infiltrates on chest x–ray and be confused with pneumonia. Cor pulmonale may ensue from widespread or repeated episodes of pulmonary thrombosis or embolism. Cardiomyopathy is common. It generally results from repeated sickling–induced occlusion of the cardiac microvasculature with ensuing microinfarction. The anemia–induced high–output state itself stresses the heart. Renal disease: Sickling with microvascular occlusion and ensuing renal ischemia/infarction may manifest in several ways. Papillary necrosis may cause hematuria and possibly result in acute obstructive uropathy. There is interstitial fibrosis. Ischemic renal tubular damage causes permanent hyposthenuria (inability to concentrate urine) to develop in all patients, usually by age 5. An antigen derived from damaged tubular epithelium may induce immune–complex glomerulonephritis. Tubular injury may also manifest as a partial distal renal tubular acidosis. Priapism is common. It occurs when sickling occludes blood vessels of the corpus cavernosum. Hand–foot syndrome (sickle cell dactylitis) is the transient painful swelling of the hands and feet due to sickling–induced ischemia in the marrow of the small bones. Children are most susceptible. Osteomyelitis is not uncommon. It is most often due to S. aureus followed by salmonellae. Avascular necrosis of femoral heads is due to repeated episoces of vascular occlusion with infarction. Avascular necrosis may also occur in the humeral heads, patella, and vertebrae. Hyperplasia of the marrow may lead to the following x–ray findings: widened medullary cavities, thinned cortices, irregular trabeculae, "hair on end" appearance of skull trabeculae, cupped vertebrae. Ischemia–induced skin ulcers are common, particularly about the medial maleolus and shins. Delayed puberty is characteristic. Consequently, patients tend to be tall due to delay in closure of the epiphyses.

Laboratory findings in sickle cell disease: Routine blood smear reveals distorted RBC's some of which may be sickled. Target cells, erythroblasts, and polychromatophilia are also seen on the routine smear. Howell–Jolly bodies and Pappenheimer bodies appear after autosplenectomy has occurred. Sickle cell prep (addition of sodium metabisulfite to deoxygenate the hemoglobin and thereby promote tactoid formation) may be needed to demonstrate sickling on a blood smear. Solubility test (e.g. Sickledex) may also disclose Hgb S by demonstrating the reduced solubility of Hgb S. Hemoglobin range is typically 6–8 gram/100ml and the hematocrit 18–24. Reticulocytosis is chronic (10–25%). Reticulocyte level falls during an aplastic crisis. MCV may be slightly increased because there is an increased percentage of reticulocytes—which are larger than mature erythrocytes. Chronic neutrophilia with WBC count of about 15,000 is common. The WBC count may in the absence of infection reach 30,000–40,000 during a painful crisis. Hemoglobin electrophoresis demonstrates absence of Hgb A. There is 85–95% Hgb S, 2–3% Hgb A2, and 5–15% Hgb F. Serum bilirubin is chronically elevated. Sedimentation rate is low. Serum haptoglobin (a hemoglobin–binding globulin) is decreased. Haptoglobin is consumed because hemoglobin from lyzed RBC's binds to haptoglobin and the complex is rapidly cleared from the circulation.

Treatment of sickle cell disease: Oxygen at 3–4 liter/min via nasal cannulae is administered in any vasoocclusive crisis. However, it is uncertain how helpful this is in the absence of hypoxia. Oral and/or IV fluids are administered in sufficient quantity to maintain high urine output. A hypotonic IV solution such as D5 1/2NS is usually recommended. Correct acidosis because it favors sickling. Narcotic analgesics are usually needed during a painful crisis. Rule out infection: All vasoocclusive crises should be investigated for the presence of infection (urinalysis, blood culture, chest x–ray) and antibiotic administered as needed. However, most sickle crises are not associated with infection. Transfusion: Because of the risk of iron overload, transfusion is not indicated merely to correct anemia unless the hemoglobin is less than 7 gram/dl. ●Neither is transfusion indicated for the usual painful crisis. However, exchange transfusion may be considered if a painful crisis persists for > 6–10 days or if the patient is disabled by frequent painful episodes. ●Transfusions are required for aplastic crisis; the goal is to maintain the hematocrit at about 20%. ●Exchange transfusion is necessary in splenic sequestration crisis.

•Exchange transfusions are indicated for a patient undergoing a stroke. For several years thereafter, monthly prophylactic exchange transfusions are advised. The goal is to maintain hemoglobin S at < 30% of total hemoglobin. •Exchange tranfusion is advised prior to general anesthesia and during the last half of pregnancy. •Other indications for exchange transfusions are retinopathy, persistent priapism, severe skin ulceration, severe dactylitis, selected cases of aseptic necrosis. Priapism: (1) apply ice compresses, (2) give exchange transfusions if priapism persists over 24 hours, (3) an urologist may need to aspirate blood from the penis. Retinopathy: Exchange transfusions are indicated and laser photocoagulation may be needed to control proliferative retinopathy. Folic acid (1mg PO once daily) is administered chronically because the chronic accelerated rate of erythropoeisis imposes an increased demand for this vitamin. Vaccination against pneumococcus is advised because functional asplenism increases the risk of this infection.

OTHER SYNDROMES:

Hemoglobin S–C disease is a double heterozygous condition with one gene coding for production of β^c globin chain and the allele coding for the production of β^S globin chain. Both β^c globin chain and β^S globin chain are the consequence of substitutions for glutamic acid at position 6 of the β globin chain (lysine in the case of Hgb C and valine in the case of Hgb S). Erythrocytes contain approximately equal amounts of Hgb C ($\alpha2\beta^c2$) and Hgb S ($\alpha2\beta^S2$). Hgb A ($\alpha2\beta2$) is absent. Electrophoresis reveals 45–50% Hgb S, 45–50% Hgb C, 2–3% Hgb A2, and about 1% Hgb F. Blood smear shows numerous target cells and some sickle cells. All the erythrocytes are found to sickle with a sickle cell preparation. Anemia (hemoglobin 10–12 gram/100ml) is milder than SS disease. Clinical consequences: SC disease is in most respects clinically milder than SS disease. However, the sundry manifestations of SS disease may also occur in SC disease. •In contrast with SS disease, adults with SC disease often have an enlarged spleen and may therefore undergo splenic sequestration crisis or infarcts. SS disease after childhood is not associated with splenic enlargement or sequestration crisis because repeated splenic infarctions have generally resulted in autosplenectomy by age 8. •Retinopathy (e.g. retinal infarction/hemorrhage/detachment) and pregnancy–related problems are more common in SC disease than SS disease.

Hemoglobin CC disease (homozygous with genotype CC) is NOT a sickling disorder. There is substitution of lysine for glutamic acid at position 6 of the β globin chain. The predominant hemoglobin is Hgb C ($\alpha2\beta^c2$). Hgb A ($\alpha2\beta2$) is absent. The blood smear shows 30–100% target cells but sickling does not occur. There is a normocytic hypochromic (decreased MCHC) anemia with mild reticulocytosis. Electrophoresis is confirmatory. The disorder is less common and clinically milder than hemoglobin SC disease. There is a mild hemolytic anemia with splenomegaly and there may be mild janndice. The trait (i.e. heterozygous with genotype AC) is found in 2–3% American blacks. Target cells are seen on the blood smear but there is neither anemia nor symptoms.

Combined sickle cell–thalassemia is a double heterozygous condition: there is one gene that codes for the abnormal β^S globin chain while another gene (the gene for thalassemia) suppresses production of normal β globin chain. Hgb S ($\alpha2\beta^S2$) accounts for 60–95% of hemoglobin with 0–30% Hgb A ($\alpha2\beta2$), 3–5% Hgb A2 ($\alpha2\delta2$), and 0–30%. Hgb F ($\alpha2\gamma2$). There is a hypochromic microcytic anemia (decreased MCHC and MCV). Splenomegaly is common. The clinical course varies from mild to severe depending on the amount of Hgb A and Hgb F produced relative to Hgb S.

Hemoglobin S–F (hemoglobin S—hereditary persistence fetal hemoglobin) is rare. The electrophoretic prophile is similar to sickle cell anemia (genotype SS) but contrasts in that there is a higher proportion of Hgb F (about 30%). Further testing shows that, in contrast to sickle cell anemia, Hgb F is uniformly distributed amongst the erythrocytes. There is neither anemia nor clinical disease.

Thalassemias

are inherited disorders of hemoglobin synthesis characterized by a decrease or absence of synthesis of one of the globin chains of hemoglobin but without abnormalities in the structure of that chain.

ALPHA THALASSEMIAS are most prevalent in those from Southeast Asia, Mediterranean basin, or blacks. There are defects in the genes that control synthesis of the α globin chains of hemoglobin. Depending on the exact genetic defect, manifestations range from completely adequate hemoglobin synthesis (and abnormalities may even be undetectable by usual laboratory methods) to complete absence of α globin chain synthesis with death in utero.

Alpha thalassemia trait has genotype $\alpha \alpha/- -$ or $\alpha -/\alpha -$. The blood smear shows microcytic hypochromic RBC's and this reflected in the decreased MCV and MCHC. Anemia is mild or absent because there is a compensatory increase in the number of RBC's. Hemoglobin electrophoresis is normal. Persons with this condition are asymptomatic and suffer no ill effects. This condition may possibly confer resistance to malaria.

Silent carrier (genotype $\alpha \alpha/- \alpha$) can only be detected by pedigree analysis or special lab research methods. The blood smear is normal, the blood count and indices are normal, hemoglobin electrophoresis is normal, and the condition is clinically silent.

Hemoglobin H disease ($\alpha -/- -$ genotype). Blood smear shows microcytic hypochromic RBC's which have intracytoplasmic inclusions due to precipitation of hemoglobin H (tetramer of the β chain). Hemoglobin H forms because there are excess β chains over α chains. RBC fragments (secondary to hemolysis) are also seen on the smear. Hemoglobin level is typically 7–10 g/dl but this does not truly reflect the clinical severity of the anemia because the hemoglobin H fraction (30–40% of the total hemoglobin) has such a high affinity for oxygen that it is incapable of releasing oxygen to the tissues and is therefore of no use to the patient. Hgb A constitutes 60–70% of the hemoglobin while Hgb A2 and Hgb F each account for 2–5% of the total. Splenomegaly is common but splenectomy is not indicated unless there is evidence of hypersplenism–induced thrombocytopenia, leukopenia, and increasing anemia. Exchange transfusions are administered as needed. Oxidants (e.g. sulfonamides) are avoided since they may exacerbate hemolysis.

Alpha thalassemia with hydrops fetalis ($- -/- -$ genotype) is not compatible with life. Death in utero or soon after birth is inevitable since no α chains are produced and, except for embryonic hemoglobin, hemoglobin lacking α chains cannot deliver oxygen. The only hemoglobins produced after synthesis of embryonic hemoglobin ceases in the early stages of pregnancy are Hgb H ($\beta 4$ tetramer) and Hgb Barts ($\gamma 4$ tetramer); neither which is capable of delivering oxygen to the tissues. Hydrops fetalis ensues from the severe congestive heart failure engendered as synthesis of embryonic hemoglobin wanes. Antenatal diagnosis may be made by analysis of amniotic fluid DNA.

BETA THALASSEMIAS are most prevalent in peoples of Mediterranean origin (especially Greeks and Italians), blacks, and asiatics. There are defects in the genes that control synthesis of the β globin chains of hemoglobin. Depending on the exact genetic defect, manifestations range from completely adequate hemoglobin synthesis without anemia or symptoms to complete absence of Hgb A ($\alpha 2 \beta 2$) with severe clinical anemia.

Thalassemia major (Cooley's anemia) results from a complete or almost complete lack of β globin chain synthesis due to homozygous defect at the β gene locus. Severe anemia develops in the first year of life when Hgb F ($\alpha 2 \gamma 2$) levels decline as γ globin chain synthesis wanes. Normally, Hgb A ($\alpha 2 \beta 2$) rises at this time. However, this cannot occur in this case because β globin chain synthesis is inadequate. ●Despite the lack of β chains required for Hgb A synthesis, α globin chains continue to be produced in excess of that needed for Hgb F or Hgb A2 synthesis. The α globin chains precipitate in the RBC cytoplasm. This thwarts the development of erythroblasts and decreases the life span of RBC's that do reach maturity. ●The ensuing severe anemia induces erythropoietin synthesis. This in turn accelerates erythroblast production in the bone marrow (which shows a predominance of erythrocyte precursors) and also leads to extramedullary hematopoiesis by the liver and spleen. <u>Hemoglobin electrophoresis:</u> 90–95% Hgb F, 4–10% Hgb A2 ($\alpha 2 \delta 2$), very little or no Hgb A is found. <u>Blood smear</u> shows microcytic hypochromic RBC's, RBC fragments, target cells, many nucleated erythroblasts. <u>MCV and MCHC</u> are decreased. <u>Reticulocyte count</u> is increased. <u>Hemoglobin</u> is 3–6 g/dl. <u>Bone abnormalities:</u> The bone marrow is hyperplastic. Consequently, widening of the marrow space and cortical thinning is seen in the skull and long bone x–rays. The osteoporotic bones are prone to pathologic fracture. Spinal cord compression may ensue from pathologic fractures of the vertebrae. Abnormal development of the facial bones leads to the so–called "hemolytic" or "chipmunk" facies. <u>Treatment:</u> Without blood transfusions, many patients die in infancy and early childhood. Regular transfusions may extend life to early adulthood. Regular transfusions to maintain the hemoglobin at 8–10mg/100ml will allow normal growth and sexual development to about 10–12 years. However, the ameliorative effects of transfusions in this regard are frequently thwarted thereafter. ●With frequent transfusions there is iron overload. The main clinical impact of iron overload falls on the heart (e.g. arrhythmias, pericarditis, congestive heart failure). Hypersplenism–provoked increase in transfusion requirements, leukopenia, or thrombocytopenia is an indication for splenectomy. Liver abnormalities (hepatomegaly, elevated liver enzymes, fibrosis) occur and there may be endocrine dysfunction (e.g. diabetes mellitus, hypothyroidism). ●Deferoxamine IM or preferably via slow subcutaneous infusion pump is used to reduce iron stores. ●Bone marrow transplantation from a normal HLA identical sibling is sometimes curative.

Thalassemia intermedia rmay result from any one of several genetic mutations (inherited from both parents) governing β globin chain synthesis that yet allows the hemoglobin to exceed 6 g/dl. Patients with this condition have increased amounts of Hgb F and Hgb A2, and may have some Hgb A. They may suffer from the same clinical conditions as Thalassemia major but the disease course is less severe and there is less need for transfusion. Growth and sexual development is less impaired than in thalassemia major. Patients often survive childhood.

Beta thalassemia minor (trait) occurs in individuals heterozyqous for a defect in the gene governing β globin chain synthesis. There is anisocytosis with microcytic hypochromic RBC's. MCV and MCHC are decreased. Anemia is either absent or mild (hgb 10–12 g/dl) because there is a compensatory increase in the number of RBC's. Hemoglobin electrophoresis is slightly different from normal in many cases: Hgb A 90–95%, Hgb A2 5–7%, Hgb F 2–10%. Persons with this trait are asymptomatic and suffer no ill effects. They generally should not be treated with iron supplements since serum iron and transferrin levels are typically normal. This condition may possibly confer resistance to malaria.

Erythrocytosis/Polycythemia

Erythrocytosis is defined as an excessive total erythrocyte volume or mass (i.e. excessive number of circulating erythrocytes). The terms erythrocytosis and polycythemia are commonly used interchangeably. Strictly speaking, however, polycythemia refers to conditions in which, not only erythrocytes, but other blood cell line(s) are increased as well.

RELATIVE POLYCYTHEMIA refers to an increase in the hematocrit due to a decrease in the plasma volume. The red cell mass is not elevated.

Dehydration is the most common cause of relative polycythemia.

Gaisbock's syndrome (stress polycythemia) occurs primarily in middle–aged obese hypertensive males. The hematocrit is usually in the 55–60 range. Reduction of elevated blood pressure will often relieve this condition; antihypertensive medication other than diuretics is recommended. Smoking–induced carboxyhemoglobinemia may be a contributing factor; smoking should therefore be discouraged.

SECONDARY ERYTHROCYTOSIS

Impaired tissue oxygenation induces erythropoietin production which in turn stimulates increased RBC production by bone marrow. This mechanism is responsible for erythrocytosis in the following conditions: high altitude residence; chronic lung disease (e.g. COPD, interstitial fibrosis); cyanotic heart disease; smoking–induced carboxyhemoglobin; chronic hypoventilation (e.g. Pickwickian syndrome); hereditary hemoglobins with high–oxygen affinity; congenital 2,3–DPG deficiency. **Autonomous secretion of erythropoietin or erythropoietin–like substances:** hepatoma; cerebellar hemangioblastoma; ovarian carcinoma; large uterine myoma; pheochromocytoma; renal tumor; kidney disease (e.g. renal cysts, hydronephrosis, nephotic syndrome, renal transplant, hemodialysis). **Androgens**, exogenous or endogenous (e.g. adrenal–derived) may induce erythrocytosis.

POLYCYTHEMIA VERA is a myeloproliferative disorder due to neoplastic transformation of a bone marrow stem cell. There is proliferation of all bone marrow cell lines. However, the erythroid cell line is most noticeably affected. The erythrocyte mass is increased. Erythropoietin levels are very low or absent. Proliferation of the myeloid cell line and megakaryocytes leads to increased granulocytes and platelets respectively. **Signs/symptoms:** Some patients are asymptomatic. Common manifestations include fatigue, headache, dizziness, tinnitus, splenomegaly, hepatomegaly, pruritis, skin rubor, cyanosis of the face and mucous membranes, hypertension. Patients are susceptible to peptic ulcers; bleeding (e.g. spontaneous ecchymoses, GI bleeding, nosebleeds); venous thrombosis, pulmonary thromboembolism; and arterial thrombosis. **Laboratory:** RBC mass (using ^{51}Cr–labeled RBC's) is elevated > 36 ml/kg in men and > 32ml/kg in women. When making this determination in obese patients, substitute the patient's actual weight with his ideal weight plus 20% of the excess weight. Hematocrit is generally > 60% in men and > 55% in women. RBC count is elevated (range 6.5–10 million). Blood smear: Erythrocytes may be normocytic normochromic or microcytic hypochromic. The latter occurs if iron stores are insufficient relative to the increased numbers of erythrocytes. In fact, the serum iron level is frequently found to be low, and bone marrow stain often fails to reveal iron stores. With progression, the peripheral smear may reveal erythrocytes of varied size and shape, and there may be nucleated erythrocytes. Leukocytosis is present in approximately 60% cases. The peripheral blood smear shows increased neutrophils and bands, and often there are more immature forms (myelocytes, metamyelocytes). The differential often reveals increased basophils and eosinophils. Platelets are increased to > 400,000 in about half the cases. Counts > 1 million/μl are not unusual. Platelet morphology is often found to be abnormal. The bleeding time may be prolonged. Leukocyte alkaline phosphatase is elevated in most cases. Serum B12 is elevated to > 900 pg/ml in about a third of cases. This is the consequence of increased levels of the B12–binding proteins, transcobalamins I and III. The increased levels of transcobalamins reflect the increased granulocyte mass. Erythropoietin level is very low or absent. Bone marrow is hypercellular with increased numbers of erythrocyte and granulocyte precursors, megakaryocytes, and fibroblasts. In advanced stages ("spent" polycythemia), there is fibrosis of the marrow with evidence of decreased RBC production; anemia ensues. Hyperuricemia is common (a reflection of the increased cell turnover). **Diagnosis:** Polycythemia vera is very probable if all 3 of the following conditions are met: (**1**) elevated RBC cell mass—see above, (**2**) normal arterial oxygen saturation—i.e. > 92%, (**3**) splenomegaly. If the spleen is not enlarged, two of the following may be used to supplant that stipulation: (**1**) leukocytosis > 12,000, (**2**) thrombocytosis > 400,000, (**3**) elevated leukocyte alkaline phosphatase > 100, (**4**) elevated serum B12 > 900 pg/ml or B12–binding capacity > 2200 pg/ml. **Treatment:** Phlebotomy 2–3 times a week until a hematocrit of about 45 is achieved. About 500 ml of blood may usually be removed at a time. Phlebotomy of the aged patient with cardiac disease or arteriosclerosis is more safely carried out with 250 ml aliquots. Once the desired hematocrit is attained, maintenance of that level may only require phlebotomy 2–4 times/year. Myelosuppression: If the patient is over 70, treatment consists of both phlebotomy and myelosuppression (hydroxyurea or radioactive phosphorous). Myelosuppression is not advocated in patients < 50 yr unless there is an increased risk of thrombosis. Whether or not myelosuppressive therapy is indicated in the 50–70 age group is debated. Hydroxyurea is often recommended if the platelet count exceeds 1 million. Excessive iron deficiency anemia with marked microcytosis should be avoided. Judicious iron supplementation while following the hematocrit may be recommended if the MCHC falls below 22 with repeated phlebotomy.

Thrombocytopenia
may be defined as a platelet count less than 150,000. In the absence of platelet dysfunction, spontaneous bleeding is generally not likely until the platelet count falls below 20,000, and a bleeding tendency is not usually observed until the count is below 50,000. <u>Factors influencing bleeding tendency</u>: At comparable platelet counts, patients with decreased platelet production are more likely to bleed than those with increased platelet destruction or sequestration. The explanation is that in thrombocytopenia due to increased destruction or sequestration, young platelets (which are presumably more effective at controlling bleeding) are being released into the circulation. ●At the same platelet level, patients with acute thrombocytopenia are more susceptible to bleeding than those with chronic stable thrombocytopenia. ●Fever and anemia enhance the bleeding tendency in thrombocytopenia. <u>Platelet transfusion</u> may be useful in those with thrombocytopenia resulting from decreased platelet production but are not generally effective in conditions associated with increased destruction or sequestration. <u>Manifestations of thrombocytopenia</u> may include petechiae, ecchymoses, epistaxis, bleeding from the GI or GU tract, vaginal bleeding, CNS bleeding. Hemarthrosis is unusual.

DECREASED PLATELET PRODUCTION may be associated with a decreased or increased number of megakaryocytes (the platelet precursor) in the bone marrow. Thrombocytopenia with decreased megakaryocytes is seen with myelophthisis, radiation, certain drugs or toxins, infections. Thrombocytopenia with increased megakaryocytes indicates ineffective platelet production (see below).

Marrow displacement (myelophthisis) may be due to metastatic carcinoma; acute leukemia; chronic lymphocytic leukemia; myeloma; lymphoma; myelofibrosis; granulomatous disease (e.g. tuberculosis, sarcoidosis).

Radiation/drugs/toxins: Some agents (e.g. radiation, benzene, antineoplastic drugs, gold salts, phenylbutazone, chloramphenicol, quinacrine) may suppress production of all cell lines so that there is leukopenia and anemia in addition to thrombocytopenia. Others (e.g. chronic ethanol abuse, thiazides, estrogens, tolbutamide) may provoke selective inhibition of platelet production.

Infections (e.g. viremia, bacteremia) may temporarily depress production but thrombocytopenia is generally not severe. Infections may also cause thrombocytopenia by other mechanisms—e.g. DIC due to bacterial sepsis, immune–mediated destruction.

Ineffective production: Megakaryocytes may be found in increased numbers in the marrow but maturation is impaired. Folate or B12 deficiency results not only in thrombocytopenia but also in leukopenia and anemia (refer to "Megaloblastic Anemia" chapter). Other conditions which may be associated with ineffective platelet production include preleukemia; sideroblastic anemia; paroxysmal nocturnal hemoglobinuria; congenital abnormalities (e.g. Wiskott–Aldrich syndrome, May–Hegglin anomaly).

INCREASED PLATELET DESTRUCTION: Typically, (1) there are increased numbers of megakaryocytes in the bone marrow, and (2) large and often elongated platelets are seen on the peripheral blood smear (the older smaller platelets having been destroyed).
<u>Immune–mediated platelet destruction:</u>

Idiopathic thrombocytopenic purpura (ITP): Antiplatelet IgG antibody is frequently demonstrated. The spleen is not enlarged. Increased numbers of megakaryocytes are seen in the bone marrow and the blood smear reveals large platelets. ●In acute ITP, there may be eosinophilia and lymphocytosis in addition to findings just mentioned. Acute ITP usually follows a viral infection, usually occurs in childhood, and is usually self–limited. ●Chronic ITP is more common in adults, more often women. <u>Treatment</u> may not be required if the platelet count remains above 30,000 provided that there is no significant bleeding and the patient is followed closely. Prednisone 1mg/kg/day is administered if the platelet count is < 30,000; 2mg/kg/day is recommended if there is serious bleeding or if the platelet count is < 10,000. In most cases, the platelet count will rise within a week. If successful, prednisone is subsequently tapered to a dose that sustains the platelet count above 30,000. ●Splenectomy is advised if the patient does not respond to prednisone

2mg/kg/day after 2 weeks or if prednisone is still necessary after 3 months. ●If the patient is refractory to prednisone and splenectomy, several other measures are available. However, patients with platelet counts in the 10,000–30,000 range are often asymptomatic and do not require chronic therapy. In the short run, the following measures may be helpful: gamma globulin (0.4mg/kg/day IV for 5 days), vincristine (2mg/week for 3 weeks), platelet transfusions. For patients requiring chronic therapy, danazol (200mg PO three times/day) or cyclophosphamide (2mg/kg/day PO) may be used. Colchicine (2mg PO twice daily) may be tried if other therapies fail. ●Prior to surgery, the prednisone–responsive patient should receive prednisone to raise the platelet count to an acceptable level.

Drug–mediated platelet destruction is usually an immune phenomenon whereby the drug acts as a hapten upon binding to a plasma protein. The resulting antigen (i.e. drug–protein combination) stimulates antibody production. An antigen–antibody complex forms which attaches to platelets. These immune complex–coated platelets are subsequently destroyed by the spleen and other elements of the reticuloendothelial system. Commonly implicated drugs include thiazides, quinidine, quinine, sulfonamides, phenytoin, methyldopa, desipramine, rifampin, gold salts, heparin.

Viral infection (e.g. infectious mononucleosis, rubella) may induce production of cold antibodies that in turn attach to platelets. These antibody–coated platelets are susceptible to destruction by the reticuloendothelial system. HIV infection may also be associated with thrombocytopenia.

Post–transfusion purpura is a rare phenomenon that occurs about a week following transfusion of Pl^{A1} (a platelet antigen) positive blood to a patient who is Pl^{A1}negative and who has been previously sensitized to produce anti–Pl antibodies by prior blood transfusion or pregnancy. Other platelet antigens may also cause this syndrome. Thrombocytopenia is severe in many cases and may last for weeks. Treatment consists of prednisone, IV gamma globulin, plasmapheresis, and/or exchange transfusions with appropriate platelet antigen–negative blood.

Neonatal purpura occurs when there is transplacental passage of a specific anti-platelet antibody (usually anti–Pl^{A1}antibody) to a fetus whose platelets do not have the corresponding antigen. Treatment is with exchange transfusion of appropriate platelet antigen–negative blood. Corticosteroids and platelet transfusions have also been used.

Autoimmune disease, particularly systemic lupus, may result in thrombocytopenia. The treatment guidelines set forth under ITP above are applicable. Rheumatoid arthritis and hypothyroidism may be associated with mild thrombocytopenia. Evans' syndrome is characterized by the presence of thrombocytopenia with a Coombs' test--positive hemolytic anemia.

Lymphomas (Hodgkin's and nonHodgkin's) and **chronic lymphocytic leukemia** may be associated with immune–mediated thrombocytopenia. However, thrombocytopenia is usually the consequence of marrow infiltration.

Allergens (e.g. foods, insect stings, vaccines) may provoke formation of antigen–antibody complexes that then bind to platelets. These immune complex–coated platelets are subsequently recognized and destroyed by the reticuloendothelial system.

<u>Non–immune platelet destruction</u> **(increased platelet consumption):**

Thrombotic thrombocytopenic purpura (TTP) is a rare but often lethal disorder in which there is endothelial injury with widespread formation of thrombi that leads to occlusion of arterioles and capillaries. Platelets are consumed and thrombocytopenia ensues. A Coombs' test–negative microangiopathic hemolytic anemia develops. An elevated LDH, and a blood smear showing schistocytes and increased reticulocytes gives evidence of that hemolysis. <u>Signs/symptoms</u>: There is fever. The pathologic process involves multiple organs including the skin (petechia, purpura); CNS (sundry possible neurologic complications); GI tract (bleeding); and kidneys (proteinuria, hematuria, casts, renal failure). <u>Treatment</u> is begun with prednisone (50mg PO qid) and daily plasma exchange transfusions with fresh frozen plasma (40ml/kg) until the platelet count exceeds 100,000 and the serum LDH has dropped significantly. As the patient's condition improves; (**1**) prednisone and exchange tranfusion therapy are tapered; and (**2**) aspirin 300mg tid, dipyridamole 100mg PO qid, and sulfinpyrazone 100mg PO qid are begun and continued for 6 months.

Hemolytic–uremic syndrome occurs in childhood, mainly in infancy. The syndrome begins with GI symptoms (vomiting, diarrhea, abdominal pain) and is followed in a few days by thrombocytopenia, hemolytic anemia, and renal failure (usually with hematuria and proteinuria). There may be hypertension, cardiac failure, and/or hepatomegaly. Renal histology reveals varying degrees of occlusion of the microvasculature and collapsed glomerular capillary loops. Treatment may include peritoneal dialysis and RBC transfusions. Renal function usually improves within a month. Aspirin, dipyridamole, plamapheresis, and/or fresh frozen plasma may have a therapeutic role.

Disseminated intravascular coagulation (DIC) may result in thrombocytopenia as platelets are consumed in the coagulation process. Refer to "Disseminated Intravascular Coagulation" chapter for further information.

Cavernous hemangioma is associated with thrombocytopenia in < 1% cases. DIC and hemolytic anemia are also possible consequences.

Extracorporeal circulation may provoke thrombocytopenia by influencing platelet aggregation and/or by DIC mechanism.

HYPERSPLENISM (splenic platelet sequestration) may occur when the spleen is enlarged from virtually any cause. The spleen normally holds approximately 1/3 of the body's platelet pool. That fraction increases as the spleen enlarges. There may be concurrent thrombocytopenia, leukopenia, and anemia. The bone marrow shows normal or increased numbers of megakaryocytes. The platelet life span is not curtailed in uncomplicated hypersplenism since accelerated splenic destruction of platelets as seen in immune–mediated phenomenon does not occur. Seldom is thrombocytopenia sufficiently severe to cause bleeding or to warrant splenectomy.

PLATELET DILUTION may occur in the setting of massive blood transfusion. In general, there is no bleeding tendency unless the platelet count falls below 50,000. Below this level, platelet transfusion may be needed if clinical circumstances so dictate. In uncomplicated cases, platelet levels recover spontaneously in 3–5 days.

Neutropenia is said to be present when the absolute neutrophil count

(WBC count x per cent neutrophils) is < 1500–2000/μl. However, some normal individuals may have absolute neutrophil counts approaching 1000/μl. In general, the risk of infection is not great if the absolute neutrophil count is 1000–1500/μl. However, a serious infection is very likely to develop within a few weeks if the absolute count drops below 500.

Etiology: Drugs are the most common cause of neutropenia. Most drug–induced neutropenias are due to suppression of bone marrow neutrophil production, and bone marrow exam discloses reduced numbers of neutrophil precursors. With some drugs the pathogenesis of neutropenia is an immune reaction. ●Some drugs consistently produce neutropenia in all exposed individuals if large enough doses are administered—e.g. antineoplastic drugs, ethanol, chloamphenicol, rifampin. ●Some other drugs also produce neutropenia in a dose–dependent manner but only certain persons are affected. The most noteworthy example is chlorpromazine and other phenothiazines. Other examples include phenylbutazone, antithyroid drugs, sulfonamides, semisynthetic penicillins, isoniazid, gold. Acute agranulocytosis is said to be present if marrow production fails and the neutrophil count falls below 200. If the patient does not die from infection, neutropenia corrects spontaneously within a couple of weeks once the offending drug is removed. ●A dose–independent neutropenia may develop in patients hypersensitive to certain drugs (e.g. phenylbutazone, sulfonamides, thiazides, chloamphenicol, penicillin, ampicillin, procainamide, quinidine, gold). Eosinophilia is is common. Aplastic anemia (bone marrow failure resulting in pancytopenia with a hypocellular marrow) may occur with these drugs. Systemic infections may provoke neutropenia by various mechanisms—e.g. bone marrow suppression, immune mechanisms, hypersplenism, margination. Margination refers to the phenomenon in which neutrophils attach to walls of the microvasculature. The marginated neutrophils are in dynamic equillibrium with the circulating neutrophils. At any one time, about half the neutrophils are circulating and the other half are marginated. ●Viremia (e.g. infectious mononucleosis, influenza, measles, yellow fever) may induce neutropenia by margination. ●Protozoa (e.g. malaria) may also cause neutropenia by margination. ●Severe bacterial infections may provoke neutropenia when the neutrophils are used up so quickly that bone marrow production and release cannot keep up. Margination may also play a role here. Leukemia, lymphoma, or metastatic carcinoma may decrease neutrophil production by invading/displacing the marrow. Folate or B-12 deficiency causes megaloblastic anemia with thrombocytopenia and neutropenia. Blood smear reveals decreased numbers of neutrophils. The neutrophils are enlarged and have hypersegmented nuclei (i.e. ≥ 5 lobes). In severe deficiency the RBC's vary in shape (poikilocytosis) and size (anisocytosis). ●Drugs that interfere with folate metabolism (e.g. phenytoin, methotrexate, cytosine arabinoside) may also cause neutropenia. In Felty's syndrome (rheumatoid arthritis with splenomegaly and neutropenia), neutropenia is due to decreased neutrophil survival which is presumably the consequence of production of an antibody directed against neutrophils. Systemic lupus is associated with neutropenia in about half the cases but only a small percentage have severe neutropenia. Isoimmune neutropenia is a temporary neutropenia of infants. It results from the transplacental transfer of maternal IgG antibody that is directed against the fetal neutrophils. Hypersplenism may cause neutropenia as well as anemia and thrombocytopenia. Neutrophils are sequestered in the spleen along with platelets and RBC's. Congenital abnormalities in both bone marrow production or release of neutrophils are known. Some are benign, others lethal (e.g. Kostmann's neutropenia, reticular dysgenesis). ●An interesting autosomal dominant example is cyclic neutropenia: severe neutropenia due to decreased bone marrow production recurs at 3 week intervals. Hemodialysis or cardiopulmonary bypass may induce neutropenia by activating complement which in turn leads to neutrophil aggregation.

Laboratory: CBC and blood smear exam may be diagnostic (e.g. megaloblastic anemia, leukemia). Bone marrow exam is necessary if the cause of neutropenia is uncertain. Bone marrow exam may be delayed and serial blood counts performed if there is a likely cause for the neutropenia (e.g. drug, viral infection). ●A marrow showing decreased numbers of neutrophil precursors (i.e. myeloblasts, promyelocytes, myelocytes, metamyelocytes) is consistent with impaired neutrophil production (e.g. drug-induced neutropenia, marrow infiltration by metastatic carcinoma). ●A marrow revealing increased neutrophil precursors and no neutrophils indicates that there is normal release from the marrow with subsequent peripheral destruction (e.g. Felty's syndrome). ●Neutropenia with a marrow that is cellular and shows 25% of the myeloid cells to be neutrophils (both band and segmented forms) is consistent with impaired release of neutrophils from the marrow or with margination. ●Folate or B-12 deficiency discloses a cellular marrow with abnormal cells in the myeloid line as well as the other cell lines. Other diagnostic tests may be obtained as circumstances suggest: ANA, rheumatoid factor, Coombs test, serum immunoelectrophoresis, serum folate and B12 levels, etc.

Treatment: Stop exposure to all possible offending agents such as drugs or toxins (e.g. solvents, paints). Lithium therapy may stimulate the bone marrow and help neutropenic patients receiving antineoplastic drugs. Glucocorticoid therapy may alleviate neutropenia secondary to systemic lupus or Felty's syndrome. Splenectomy may be helpful in Felty's syndrome. Marrow transplantation may be considered for severe aplastic anemia and selected congenital neutropenias. Androgens may be useful in selected patients with congenital or acquired bone marrow abnormalities. Prevention of infection: If there are no signs of infection, neutropenia by itself is not an indication for hospitalization since the hospital may increase the risk of infection. Anal and oral hygiene is emphasized. Patient should use a soft toothbrush. Stool softeners are prescribed. Invasive procedures should be minimized. Treatment of infection: Patient must be hospitalized if fever or other signs of infection develop. Reverse isolation is required and scrupulous hygiene is imperative. Cultures are obtained of blood, urine, throat, sputum, and any other suspicious sites (e.g. stool, CSF). Chest and sinus x-rays are obtained. Antibiotic therapy may be delayed if the temperature is < 38.3 C (101F) and there is a likely noninfectious cause of fever (e.g. transfusion reaction, drug reaction). If the temperature is > 38.3 C, cultures are obtained and antibiotics are begun without delay—e.g. an extended spectrum penicillin (e.g. carbenicillin, ticarcillin, mezlocillin) plus an aminoglycoside (gentamycin, tobramycin). Amphotericin B may be added to cover fungal infection if fever persists 1-2 days and the infection has not been identified.

Hereditary Coagulation Disorders

LABORATORY INVESTIGATION: **Initial screening** of any patient with a bleeding disorder consists of prothrombin time (PT), activated partial thromboplastin time (aPTT), examination of the peripheral smear, and platelet count. The aPTT measures the performance of the intrinsic pathway: XII → XI → IX → VIII → X + V leading to conversion of II (prothrombin) to thrombin which in turn converts fibrinogen to fibrin. PT measures performance of the extrinsic pathway: VII → X + V leading to conversion of prothrombin to thrombin and so forth. Common pathway: X + V is at the convergent point of both pathways so that abnormalities of the coagulation cascade from this point on will lead to prolongation of both PT and aPTT. Note that the aPTT tests for all the coagulation factors except for factor VII.

```
    XII
      \
       XI
         \
          IX
            \
             VIII    VII
               \    /
                X
                +
                V
                |
          II (prothrombin) ──────→ thrombin

             I (fibrinogen) ──────→ fibrin
```

Coagulation factor deficiency versus inhibitor of coagulation? When a prolonged PT or aPTT is first discovered, the test should be repeated. If the abnormality is confirmed, one can ascertain whether the prolongation is due to a deficiency of a coagulation factor or to the existence of an inhibitor of coagulation. This can be done by mixing equal amounts of a sample of the patient's plasma with control plasma and repeating the test. The test will then be normal if the patient has a coagulation factor deficiency but will remain prolonged if an inhibitor of coagulation is responsible. **Prolonged aPTT, prolonged PT, or both?** Prolonged aPTT with a normal PT is the combination found in von Willebrand's Disease and nearly all cases of hemophilia. This narrows the diagnostic possibilities to a defect in the intrinsic pathway prior to the origin of the common pathway, and the diagnosis is thus focused on factors VIII, IX, XI, XII, prekallikrein, or high molecular weight kininogen. Deficiencies of the latter 3 factors are associated with prolonged aPTT but there is no bleeding tendency. Factor VIII deficiency (Hemophilia A) accounts for 85% cases of hemophilia, factor IX deficiency (Hemophilia B) 12%, and factor XI deficiency about 1 %. Von Willebrand's Disease is about as common as Hemophilia B. Prolonged PT with a normal aPTT suggests a deficiency of factor VII, a rare phenomenon. Prolongation of both the PT and aPTT points to a defect in the common pathway. The inherited possibilities are rare—e.g. deficiency of factors X, V, or II; or inherited fibrinogen disorders (dysfibrinogenemia, afibrinogenemia/hypofibrinogenemia). The fbrinogen abnormalities are associated with a prolonged thrombin time as well. **Determining the specific coagulation deficit:** The usual method of determining the specific coagulation deficit is by specific factor assays. When (as is almost always the case) the aPTT is prolonged with a normal PT, assays of factor VIII and IX are performed first since they account for the majority of hemophilias. Assays are performed by adding various dilutions of the patient's plasma to plasma known to be deficient in a specific coagulation factor. Failure to correct the prolonged aPTT (or PT) of the known deficient plasma identifies the patient's deficit. Another method that will help identify a coagulation deficit is to (**1**) add normal SERUM (which is deficient in factors V and VIII but retains factors IX, X, XI, XII) to a sample of the patient's plasma, and (**2**) add normal PLASMA which has been adsorbed with barium sulfate (deficient in vitamin K–dependent factors II, VII, IX, X but retains factor VIII) to another sample of the patient's plasma. If the patient has factor VIII deficiency, the addition of barium sulfate–adsorbed normal plasma corrects the prolonged aPTT but the addition of normal serum does not. If factor IX deficiency exists, the opposite results are obtained. With factor V deficiency the addition of barium sulfate–adsorbed normal plasma will correct the prolonged PT and aPTT but the addition of normal serum will not. If factor X deficiency exists, the opposite results are obtained. **Von Willebrand's disease:** see below for laboratory parameters.

HEMOPHILIA is characterized by a prolonged aPTT, prolonged PT, or both. However, in the great majority of hemophiliacs, there is a prolonged aPTT with a normal PT. This means that the deficiency is in the intrinsic pathway prior to the origin of the common pathway and thus narrows the possibilities (see Laboratory Investigation above).

Hemophilia A (Classic hemophilia) is the most common inherited coagulation disorder, accounting for about 85% cases or 1 in 10,000 males. Hemophilia A may result from a quantitative deficiency of factor VIII or from a defective factor VIII molecule. Inheritance is X–linked recessive and therefore virtually all patients are male. The rare exception is the homozygous female resulting from the union of a female carrier and an affected male. On the average, half of the female offspring of carrier women will themselves be carriers and half of the male offspring will have hemophilia. The absence of a family history in 30% of Hemophilia A patients reflects the relatively high incidence of spontaneous mutation. Female carriers will on the average have about half the normal factor VIII activity since only one of the X chromosomes in each cell may express itself; the other is permanently inactivated. If the random balance of X chromosome inactivation in each cell results in more of the X chromosomes with the normal gene being inactivated, the carrier female may even show some of the stigmata of hemophilia. Laboratory: aPTT is characteristically prolonged but may be normal if the coagulation deficiency is mild. PT, TT (thrombin time), fibrinogen level, and bleeding time are all normal. Signs/symptoms: Mild hemophiliacs may only have significant bleeding in the setting of surgery, trauma, or dental extraction. More severely affected patients may have repeated episodes of muscular bleeding and hemarthroses, sometimes spontaneous and sometimes exercise–induced. Joint bleeding may eventually lead to joint destruction. Other potential problems include nosebleeds, retroperitoneal bleeding, CNS bleeding (usually trauma–related), oropharyngeal bleeding (sometimes leading to airway obstruction). Treatment/prevention life–threatening bleeding—e.g. severe hemorrhage, major surgery, bleeding in critical regions (e.g. about airway, head trauma): administer sufficient factor VIII concentrate to bring the patient's factor VIII level to 80% of normal. The units of factor VIII initially required = (desired % of normal – observed % of normal) x (patient's weight in kg ÷ 2). For instance, a 70 kg with critical bleeding and a factor VIII level of 10% of normal would require 2450 units of concentrate: (80 – 10) x 70/2. Half this dose is repeated every 8 hours for 3–6 doses, and continued every 12 hours for 3–5 days after bleeding has stopped. Factor VIII level is measured after the initial dose and then daily. Treatment in less critical circumstances (e.g. hemarthrosis, symptomatic noncritical hematoma): Using the foregoing formula, administer sufficient factor VIII concentrate to bring the level of factor VIII activity up to 50% of normal. The initial dose is repeated every 12 hours for 2–4 days. Treatment of mild bleeding: Desmopressin is the preferred treatment. It acts by inducing release of factor VIII and von Willebrand factor from endothelial cells. Options are cryoprecipitate (which contains about 100 units of factor VIII per bag) or heat–treated factor VIII concentrate. Hemarthrosis: Blood is aspirated from joints only if hemarthrosis is large, tense, and painful; and then only after factor VIII levels have been brought up to at least 50% of normal. Aminocaproic acid may be used adjunctively to control bleeding in certain situations (see Hemophilia B).

Hemophilia B (Christmas disease) is also a X–linked recessive disorder. It is usually due to a quantitative deficiency of factor IX and occasionally to functional defects in the factor IX molecule. Hemophilia B accounts for about 12% cases of hemophilia. As in Hemophilia A, (1) the aPTT is prolonged, and (2) the PT, TT (thrombin time), fibrinogen level, and bleeding time are all normal. Clinical findings are the same as Hemophilia A. Treatment: Minor bleeding can be treated with fresh frozen plasma (500ml twice daily in adult). Serious bleeding (e.g. CNS, retroperitoneal, large muscular or joint bleed) is treated with prothrombin complex concentrates

(PCC) which contains factors II, VII, IX, and XI. In life–threatening situations, the goal is to bring the patient's factor IX level to 60% of normal. In less critical circumstances, a level of 40% should suffice and a level of 20% may control mild bleeding. The units of PCC required = (desired % of normal − observed % of normal) x (patient's weight in kg). Repeat doses are given twice daily as needed. To reduce the risk of PCC–associated thromboembolism, 5–10 units heparin is administered for each ml of PCC administered. Aminocaproic acid (an antifibrinolytic) may be used adjunctively to control bleeding in certain situations—e.g. nosebleed, dental surgery. However, this agent is contraindicated in the presence of hematuria or if prothrombin complex concentrates are administered.

Other hemophilias are rare. All are autosomal recessive. Some coagulation deficiencies (e.g. factor XII, prekallikrein) cause prolongation of the PTT but there is no bleeding tendency. The diagnostic approach follows the guidelines set forth above. Identification of the deficiency is by specific factor assays.

VON WILLEBRAND'S DISEASE (VWD) is an inherited disorder of which there are several known variants—some autosomal dominant, others autosomal recessive. It is not known why VWD is more common in females. The disorder is due to a deficiency or functional abnormality of Von Willebrand factor (VWF), a protein that circulates in the blood attached to factor VIII. Infusion of plasma from a patient with Hemophilia A (factor VIII deficiency) corrects the derangements of VWD. <u>Laboratory:</u> ●The abnormal or deficient VWF impairs platelet adhesiveness. Consequently, the bleeding time is prolonged. ●Most patients also have decreased factor VIII activity, and the aPTT may therefore be prolonged. ●In most cases, in vitro platelet aggregation is decreased by addition of ristocetin. Platelet aggregation is normal in other respects. Ristocetin–induced platelet aggregation is actually increased in patients with type II B variant. ●The PT, TT, and platelet count are all normal. <u>Signs/symptoms:</u> Heterozygotes usually only have significant bleeding in the setting of trauma or surgery. Homozygotes often have skin and mucosal bleeding (e.g. epistaxis, ecchymoses); GI bleeding; heavy menses. Joint and muscle bleeding seldom occurs. <u>Treatment</u> of bleeding is usually with cryoprecipitate. The dose is individualized (5–10 bags twice daily is effective in many cases). Fresh frozen plasma is also effective but, because of the large volume required, is impractical in other than mild cases. Intravenous desmopressin may be effective in mild cases but is contraindicated in patients with type II B variant. Women with heavy menses may benefit from hormonal medication (e.g. oral contraceptive).

Acquired Coagulation Disorders are the most
common coagulation disorders encountered.

Vitamin K deficiency results in deficiency of vitamin K–dependent factors II, VII, IX, X. The prothrombin time should correct 24 hours after administering 15 mg vitamin K subcutaneously.

Coumadin anticoagulation also leads to deficiency of vitamin K–dependent factors.

Liver disease is often associated with prolonged aPTT, PT, and/or TT. In many cases, this is due to a deficiency of vitamin K–dependent factors (II, VII, IX, X) and this may be corrected with vitamin K. However, there may also be deficiencies of other clotting factors manufactured in the liver (e.g. fibrinogen, V, XI, XII, plasminogen). Fresh frozen plasma will correct these deficiencies but may be impractical because large volumes may be needed. Prothrombin complex concentrate (PCC) may be used instead but PCC carries the risk of thrombosis/embolism. Mixing FFP with PCC may reduce that risk.

Acquired coagulation factor inhibitor (e.g. systemic lupus, postpartum). To test for the presence of an inhibitor, see Coagulation factor deficiency versus inhibitor of coagulation? in "Hereditary Coagulation Disorders" chapter.

Disseminated Intravascular Coagulation

Pathogenesis: Depending on the nature of the underlying disorder, there is widespread activation of either the intrinsic or extrinsic coagulation pathways, or both. Increased formation of fibrin with depletion of coagulation factors is the consequence. Platelets are also consumed in the coagulation process. Fibrinolysis occurs concurrently with coagulation because, in the coagulation process, substances are formed or released that convert plasminogen to plasmin. Plasmin in turn digests fibrin/fibrinogen yielding fibrin/fibrinogen degradation products (FDP). FDP interfere with formation of the fibrin polymer by binding to the fibrin monomers. FDP therefore interfere with formation of the final clot and thereby contribute to prolongation of the PT and PTT. DIC may lead to thrombosis or, as is usually the case, bleeding. Which occurs is a function of the relative balance of determinants that includes rate of coagulation, concentration of inhibitors of coagulation cascade (e.g. antithrombin III), rate of replenishment of clotting factors, rate of fibrinolysis, platelet levels, and the characteristics of the underlying disorder. Fibrinolysis, depletion of clotting factors, and thrombocytopenia all favor bleeding.

Etiology: Infection is a common precipitant of DIC. Gram–negative or gram–positive bacteremia are the usual culprits although rickettsiae (e.g. Rocky Mountain Spotted Fever), viruses, fungi, or protozoa may also cause DIC. Other causes include shock; malignancy (e.g. carcinoma, leukemia—particularly progranulocytic leukemia); hemolytic transfusion reaction; extracorporeal circulation; crush injury; burns; heat stroke; obstetric complications (abruptio placentae, amniotic fluid embolism, retained dead fetus, retained placenta); snake bite; lupus; giant hemangioma.

Diagnosis: DIC may express itself diversely—both in the severity and spectrum of clinical findings, and in the laboratory profile. Some patients with mild DIC may only have abnormal laboratory parameters. Or there may be thrombosis or, more often, bleeding. Bleeding manifestations may range from mild bruising or a few petechiae to bleeding from multiple sites (gums, nose, vagina) with extensive ecchymoses, hematomas, and severe GI or GU hemorrhage. In acute severe DIC (e.g. DIC–associated hemorrhage), there is prolonged PT, prolonged PTT, prolonged TT; thrombocytopenia; elevated fibrin/fibrinogen degradation products, decreased fibrinogen. With milder degrees of acute DIC the laboratory profile may not be so clear. The PT, PTT, or TT may not be abnormal. Usually, however, there is thrombocytopenia, hypofibrinogenemia, and elevated fibrin/fibrinogen degradation products. Chronic DIC (a common example is the DIC that may accompany disseminated malignancy) also may not be obvious. The PT, PTT, or TT may be normal to moderately prolonged; the platelet count may be normal or decreased; and the fibrinogen level may be elevated to decreased. However, fibrin/fibrinogen degradation products are generally increased. Microangiopathic hemolysis may occur as a consequence of the injury incurred by erythrocytes when fibrin is deposited in the microvasculature. Evidence of this hemolysis may be seen (particularly with chronic DIC) on the peripheral blood smear: schistocytes, burr cells, microspherocytes.

Treatment: Treat underlying disorder if possible. Replacement therapy is advised If there is significant bleeding: (**1**) fresh frozen plasma (2–10 unit/day in adult), (**2**) platelet transfusion (e.g. 10 units initially in adult) if the platelet count falls below 50,000 with a prolonged bleeding time, (**3**) cryoprecipitate if serum fibrinogen level falls below 100mg/dl. ●Mild bleeding (e.g. minor bruising) is not an indication for replacement therapy, especially when it is anticipated that the underlying disorder can be promptly corrected. Heparin therapy is advocated: (1) if replacement therapy fails to increase platelet and coagulation factor levels, and significant bleeding is not curtailed; (2) if there are manifestations of fibrin deposition–e.g. venous thromboembolism, skin necrosis, peripheral ischemia; (3) if significant DIC–associated bleeding is due to giant hemangioma; (4) before inducing labor in the case of intrauterine fetal demise with fibrinogen level < 150mg/dl; (5) before starting chemotherapy in patient with acute promyelocytic leukemia. ●Heparin is administered by continuous IV infusion. In adult, start with 500 unit/hour and increase gradually to therapeutic level. Heparin therapy is not advised in the following circumstances: CNS bleeding, surgery in last few days, major localized bleeding, uncontrolled hypertension with diastolic > 110.

Acute Lymphoblastic Leukemia

ALL incidence is highest in children under 10 (peak 5 yr) but it may occur at any age. ALL is due to the proliferation of a single malignant clone of immature lymphocytes (lymphoblasts). **Risk factors** include history of ionizing radiation, sibling (particularly a twin) with acute leukemia, certain chromosomal abnormalities (e.g. Down's syndrome), prior treatment with alkylating agent, human T–cell leukemia virus (HTLV–1) infection.

Signs/symptoms derive from: (**1**) suppression and displacement of the normal marrow by the leukemic cells. Consequently, there is decreased production of RBC's, platelets, and normal WBC's. This in turn leads respectively to anemia, bleeding, and susceptibility to infections. (**2**) infiltration of leukemic cells into the tissues—e.g. CNS, liver, spleen, lymph nodes. Consequences of anemia: Depending on the severity of anemia; there may be weakness, fatigue, headache, dizziness, tinnitus, heart failure, angina. Consequences of thrombocytopenia: If the platelet count is severely depressed, there may be petechiae, bruising, nosebleed, GI bleeding, menorrhagia, etc. Enlargement of lymph nodes, spleen, and/or liver may result from invasion by leukemic cells. Bone pain is common and there may be painful and swollen joints. Invasion of the thymus with development of a mediastinal mass may occur—usually in patients with T cell type of ALL. In these cases, there may be signs and symptoms due to compression of the airway (e.g. cough, dyspnea, hoarseness, obstruction) or mediastinal vessels (e.g. superior vena caval syndrome). With CNS invasion, there may be evidence of meningitis. Stroke may result when lymphoblasts sludge and block small cerebral vessels. Infarction and then bleeding ensue.

Laboratory: WBC count may range from < 3000 to > 100,000 (about a third cases > 50,000 and about a third < 10,000). Peripheral smear: Blast forms are usually evident on the peripheral blood smear when the WBC count is > 5000. However, the distinction between ALL and AML is not always obvious on a peripheral smear. Moreover, normal lymphoblasts may be "forced" into the peripheral blood when in fact the patient has AML with infiltration of the marrow by myeloblasts. The peripheral smear is occasionally normal. Morphology: ALL is divided into 3 morphological subtypes, L1–L3. In general, L1 has the best prognosis and L3 the worst. L1 is found in 85% of childhood cases of ALL but in less half of adults. The L1 lymphoblast is small with a homogenous staining nucleus surrounded by a thin rim of nongranular cytoplasm. L2 lymphoblasts (14% of childhood ALL) are large with an irregular folded nucleus surrounded by substantial basophilic cytoplasm. L3 cells resemble those seen in Burkitt's lymphoma (i.e. vacuolated strongly basophilic cytoplasm). Auer bodies are absent (see "Acute Myelogenous Leukemia"). Bone marrow must always be examined to confirm the diagnosis of leukemia. Most of the cells will be blasts and the normal cell lines will be diminished (i.e. decreased erythroid cells, megakaryocytes, and granulocytic forms). Terminal deoxynucleotidyl transferase enzyme activity is increased in about 95% ALL patients (absent in patients with B–cell ALL). However, the enzyme is also found in 5–10% of AML patients. Immunological markers are present on ALL cells in most patients. The markers not only identify them as ALL cells but also permit subcategorization: (**1**) About two–thirds of children and about half of adult ALL patients are CALLA (common ALL antigen) positive, a favorable prognostic sign. (**2**) About 20% of ALL patients have the T cell type of ALL and these patients typically present with a mediastinal mass and a high leukocyte count. The leukemic cells in T cell type of ALL have receptors on their surface that bind sheep RBC's to form rosettes. (**3**) B–cell ALL accounts for < 5% ALL patients. B–cells are positive for Ia (immune response antigen) and smIg (surface membrane immunoglobulin). B–cells have L3 morphology. Prognosis is poor. (**4**) In pre–B–cell ALL, intracytoplasmic heavy immunoglobulin chains are detected in the leukemic cells and they are CALLA +. (**5**) Null–cell ALL has no immunological markers. It is uncommon and has a poor prognosis. Serum uric acid level is usually elevated because nucleic acid catabolism is increased as a consequence of the turnover of large numbers of leukemic cells. Hyperuricemia may lead to uric acid nephropathy with renal failure. DIC sometimes occurs but is more common in the promyelocytic form of AML.

Supportive measures: Allopurinol is begun prior to chemotherapy to prevent hyperuricemia, and fluid intake should be generous in order to assure brisk urine ouput. Stool softeners are administered to reduce the risk of rectal bleeding. Platelet transfusion may be needed to control bleeding and/or to bring the platelet count to above 40,000–50,000. RBC transfusion may be required to maintain an acceptable hematocrit, particularly prior to and during chemotherapy. Infection (the most common cause of death in adults) is aggressively treated. Broad spectrum antibiotic coverage is begun pending culture results. Leukophoresis is indicated to reduce markedly elevated leukocyte counts if for some reason chemotherapy must be delayed. Patients with WBC counts > 100,000 are at risk for stroke since the large numbers of lymphoblasts may sludge and block cerebral vessels so that infarction and then bleeding ensue. Large numbers of circulating leukocytes increase blood viscosity which may lead to circulatory compromise with congestive heart failure. For these reasons, chemotherapy is not delayed unnecessarily. Oral contraceptives are administered when appropriate in order to suppress menstruation during chemotherapy. Treat hypokalemia: Urinary potassium loss is common. Potassium supplementation is begun if hypokalemia develops. Treat hyperkalemia (see "Hyperkalemia"): Hyperkalemia frequently occurs with chemotherapy as large numbers of cells die and release potassium. However, diagnose hyperkalemia cautiously (particularly when the WBC is > 100,000) since potassium may be released from the WBC after a blood sample is drawn (pseudohyperkalemia). To verify hyperkalemia, a heparinized sample of blood is drawn and the serum potassium is measured immediately. Transient hyperphosphatemia with ensuing hypocalcemia may occur during chemotherapy as phosphates are released from lyzed cells. Acutely, severe hyperphosphatemia may be treated with glucose and insulin infusion.

Note: The information presented below is extracted from National Cancer Institute PDQ State-of-the-Art Cancer Treatment Information 6/1/90 for children and 9/28/90 for adults. However, since cancer treatment is evolving, this information may not be current. The most up-to-date standard treatment options may be obtained by calling the National Cancer Institute Cancer Information Service at 1–800–4–CANCER. Newly diagnosed patients should be considered for inclusion in clinical trials. Descriptions of these trials are also available.

Chemo and radiation therapy in children: Remission induction is usually with a 3-drug combination—e.g. prednisone + vincristine + asparaginase. Daunorubicin may be substituted for asparaginase. A 4-drug combination is usually reserved for children at high risk (e.g. prednisone + vincristine + asparaginase + daunorubicin). CNS prophylaxis: ●For children with good prognosis, the standard options are: (1) triple intrathecal therapy with methotrexate, cytarabine, and hydrocortisone without cranial irradiation; (2) intrathecal methotrexate (administered during induction and consolidation, and continued periodically during maintenance) without cranial irradiation; (3) five intrathecal doses of methotrexate during induction and consolidation + cranial irradiation. Because of possible long-term neurotoxicity, the latter regimen is not advised unless there is established CNS disease at the time of diagnosis. ●For children with intermediate prognosis, standard options for CNS prophylaxis include the options presented above for those with good prognosis or the following options: (1) intermediate-dose systemic methotrexate + intrathecal methotrexate without cranial irradiation; (2) high-dose systemic methotrexate alone. ●Children with poor prognosis: five intrathecal doses of methotrexate + cranial irradiation. Maintenance: Chemotherapy is necessary for an additional 2–3 yr after remission has been achieved. ●In children with good prognosis, the usual maintenance regimen consists of methotrexate + mercaptopurine. Monthly pulses of vincristine + prednisone may be included in the regimen. ●Children with intermediate to poor prognosis commonly receive methotrexate + mercaptopurine along with pulses of additional drugs (e.g. prednisone, vincristine, cytarabine, cyclophosphamide, doxorubicin, asparaginase, thioguanine, methotrexate).

Chemo and radiation therapy in adult: Remission induction options include: (1) prednisone + vincristine + asparaginase + daunorubicin; (2) prednisone + vincristine + doxorubicin + intrathecal methotrexate. CNS prophylaxis options are: (1) intrathecal methotrexate + cranial irradiation, or (2) intrathecal methotrexate + high-dose systemic methotrexate without cranial irradiation. Maintenance: The best maintenance regimen remains to be clarified. Sundry regimens using combinations of such drugs as methotrexate, mercaptopurine, cyclophosphamide, cytarabine, prednisone, vincristine, carmustine, daunorubicin, doxorubicin have similar outcome.

Acute Myelogenous Leukemia in contrast to ALL,

is more common in adults. However, AML may occur at any age. AML is due to the proliferation of a single malignant clone of immature granulocytes (myeloblasts). **Morphologic subtypes of AML:** acute myelocytic without maturation (M1), acute myelocytic with maturation (M2), acute promyelocytic (M3), acute myelomonocytic (M4), acute monocytic (M5), acute erythroleukemia (M6), acute megakaryoblastic (M7). Except for M5, which may have poorer prognosis, the response to treatment of subtypes is comparable. **Signs/symptoms** are similar to ALL.

   Laboratory: Blood count; WBC count (as in ALL) may range from < 3000 to > 100,000. Patients with WBC count > 20,000 have poorer prognosis. Anemia and thrombocytopenia are common. Sometimes the CBC is normal. Peripheral smear nearly always shows myeloblasts but distinguishing them from lymphoblasts may not be obvious with Wright's stain. In contrast to lymphoblasts, myeloblasts have a granular cytoplasm and typically have more than one nucleolus. Auer bodies (rod-shaped cytoplasmic granular aggregates that stain red with azure–eosin stains) may be found in AML. ●Myeloblasts often contain granules that stain positive for myeloperoxidase. In contrast, the lymphoblasts of ALL are myeloperoxidase negative. ●Other stains that may help identify myeloblasts are nonspecific esterases, and Sudan black. Bone marrow erythroblasts of M6 subtype stain strongly with PAS stain. TdT (terminal deoxyribonucleotidyl transferase) enzyme activity is increased in about 95% of ALL patients but is increased in only 5–10% of AML patients. Identification of cell surface antigens using monoclonal antibodies may support the diagnosis of AML. Bone marrow is crowded with myeloblasts. Lysozyme, an enzyme released from myeloblasts, is elevated in the serum and urine of some AML patients (M4–5 subtypes). Lysozyme is believed to injure the renal tubular cells. This may account for the frequent finding of hypokalemia secondary to urinary potassium loss. Bleeding; Thrombocytopenia is the usual cause of bleeding, However, patients with the promyelocytic form (M3 subtype) of AML are particularly susceptible to DIC-associated bleeding because certain substances are released from granules of the promyelocytes that activate the coagulation cascade. Chromosomal analysis is used in prognosis. Monosomy 7 is an unfavorable sign while inv 16, t(8; 21), and t(15; 17) are more favorable indicators of treatment response.

Note: The following information is largely extracted from National Cancer Institute PDQ State-of-the-Art Cancer Treatment Information 9/28/90 for children and 11/1/90 for adults. However, since cancer treatment is evolving, this information may not be current. The most up-to-date standard treatment options may be obtained by calling the National Cancer Institute Cancer Information Service at 1–800–4–CANCER. All patients should be considered for inclusion in clinical trials. Descriptions of these trials are also available.

   Treatment of children should be supervised by experienced pediatric oncologists at facilities that are able to cope with possible complications of therapy (e.g. severe myelosuppression with bleeding or infection). Remission induction: (1) cytarabine + daunorubicin ± thioguanine, or (2) cytarabine + doxorubicine ± thioguanine. In order to induce remission, chemotherapy must be aggressive enough to produce marrow aplasia. Therefore, until the marrow recovers, supportive measures are often crucial to survival. The general supportive measures described under ALL apply to AML. In particular, transfusion of RBC, platelets, WBC, fresh frozen plasma, and/or cryoprecipitate may be necessary. ●Patients who develop infections during chemotherapy. Broad-spectrum antibiotics are administered if neutropenia is severe. It is common practice to administer a nonabsorbable PO antibiotic (e.g. neomycin) in order to reduce the risk of infection by enteric bacteria. CNS prophylaxis is usually recommended: (1) intrathecal methotrexate and/or cytarabine, or (2) cranial irradiation with intrathecal chemotherapy. Post–remission therapy consists of chemotherapy or (if a suitable donor is available) bone marrow transplantation.

   Treatment of adult: Remission induction commonly consists of cytarabine + daunorubicin ± thioguanine. In order to induce remission, chemotherapy must be aggressive enough to produce marrow aplasia. Therefore, until the marrow recovers, supportive measures are often crucial to survival. The general supportive measures described under ALL apply to AML. In particular, RBC and platelet transfusions are often necessary. ●Patients who develop infections during chemotherapy. Broad-spectrum antibiotics are administered if neutropenia is severe. It is common practice to administer a nonabsorbable PO antibiotic (e.g. neomycin) to reduce the risk of infection by enteric bacteria. CNS prophylaxis/treatment: Prophylaxis is not advocated because < 5% patients develop CNS disease. If there is CNS disease, treatment is intrathecal methotrexate or cytabarine. Post–remission therapy; Bone marrow transplantation may be considered if the patient is < 40 yr and a histocompatible donor sibling is available. Otherwise, chemotherapy is advised. However, the most effective regimen has yet to be determined. Clinical trials are underway.

Chronic Myelogenous Leukemia

CML may occur at any age but it is primarily an adult disease with a peak incidence at 40–45 yr. Persons who have received ionizing radiation or perhaps those that have been exposed to certain chemicals are at increased risk for developing CML.
Cellular characteristics: CML arises from the malignant transformation of a single myeloid stem cell. CML is associated in > 90% of cases with an acquired chromosomal abnormality—the Philadelphia chromosome (reciprocal translocation of a segment of the long arm of chromosome 22, usually to chromosome 9). These malignant monoclonal myeloid stem cells are still able to and do differentiate into mature cells. The evidence for this is that the Philadelphia chromosome is found in precursors of erythrocytes, megakaryocytes, granulocytes, and monocytes. Furthermore, the mature cells of the malignant clone are still able to function in their usual roles. ●Thus, the CML patient has 2 populations of myeloid cells—a normal population derived from normal stem cells, and a population belonging to a malignant clone with precursors containing the Philadelphia chromosome. As the disease progresses, the malignant clone gains ascendancy so that, usually by the time the diagnosis is made, the majority of myeloid cells belong to the malignant clone. ●The fact that the Philadelphia chromosome is not found in cells other than hematopoietic cells and is not present in the unaffected twin of a patient with CML are evidence that the chromosomal aberration is acquired. ●CML tends to be a more aggressive with a shorter life expectancy when the Philadelphia chromosome is absent. ●The Philadelphia chromosome is not pathognomonic for CML. It is sometimes present in patients with AML, ALL, or other myeloproliferative diseases.

CLINICAL & LABORATORY FINDINGS: WBC count usually ranges from 15,000 to 500,000. Occasionally, the WBC count exceeds 1 million. Peripheral blood smear discloses immature granulocytic forms (e.g. myeloblasts, promyelocytes). There are also increased numbers of mature granulocytes—mostly neutrophils, often with increased basophils and eosinophils. The absolute lymphocyte count is usually normal even though the differential count discloses a decreased percentage of lymphocytes. Occasionally, a few nucleated RBC's are seen. Bone marrow is hypercellular with increased numbers of granulocytes at all developmental levels. This contrasts with the acute leukemias which are characteristically associated with impaired maturation leading to a dearth of mature white cells. There are usually normal numbers of erythroblasts, although the myeloid/erythroid ratio is markedly increased. Megakaryocytes may be increased. Philadelphia chromosome is present in over 90% cases and helps confirm the diagnosis. It is found by bone marrow cytologic analysis of dividing myeloid cells. Leukocyte alkaline phosphatase activity is decreased. Serum uric acid is elevated as a consequence of increased nucleic acid catabolism secondary to increased cell turnover. Leukostasis tends to occur when the WBC count is > 100,000. Sludging with occlusion of blood vessels may ensue and have diverse possible consequences—e.g. strokes, priapism. Hyperviscosity (due to large numbers of circulating leukocytes) may stress the heart so that congestive heart failure develops. Hyperviscosity may also be associated with headaches, blurred vision, abdominal pain. Fever in the absence of infection is common and is attributed to hypermetabolism. Fever subsides when the WBC count is reduced.
Three successive phases of CML are recognized:

The first or **chronic phase** usually lasts 3–5 years. Nonspecific complaints are typical during this phase (e.g. fatigue, malaise, weight loss). Splenomegaly is usually present, and may be associated with left upper quadrant discomfort and early satiety. Occasionally, patients are asymptomatic at the time of diagnosis when a routine CBC is obtained and is found to be abnormal. Typically, there is a mild normocytic normochromic anemia. Platelet count is usually normal to mildly elevated. Occasionally, there is thrombocytopenia. During the chronic phase, the peripheral blood and marrow contains < 5% myeloblasts and promyelocytes.

The subsequent **accelerated phase** may begin suddenly or develop gradually over months to a year or so. The peripheral blood and marrow reveal an increased number of immature granulocytes. Between 5–30% blasts are seen on the peripheral smear and bone marrow exam. During this phase, CML becomes more aggressive and less amenable to chemotherapy. There is worsening anemia. Thrombocytopenia or occasionally thrombocytosis develops. Consequently, there may be hemorrhagic or thrombotic complications. There is further splenic enlargement and the liver often enlarges; lymphadenopathy is common; lytic bone lesions develop and bone pain is common; there is increased susceptibility to infection; other organs are invaded (e.g. lungs, kidneys, GI, skin, gonads).

The terminal **blastic phase** has the characteristics of an acute leukemia. There is a rising WBC count with a blood and marrow differential showing > 20–30% blasts. Death usually occurs in < 6 months. The blast phase is due to additional malignant transformation(s) leading to increased proliferation of leukemic cells that are incapable of differentiating past the blast stage of development. Transformation usually results in the proliferation of myeloblasts, but in about a fourth of patients there is transformation leading to proliferation of lymphoblasts. If the latter occurs, markers characteristic of acute lymphoblastic leukemia may be detected in these cells—e.g. terminal deoxynucleotidyl transferase, CALLA (common acute lymphoblastic leukemia antigen). This has practical significance because chemotherapeutic agents employed in ALL may be temporarily ameliorative.

Note: The following information is largely extracted from National Cancer Institute PDQ State-of-the-Art Cancer Treatment Information 12/3/90. However, since cancer treatment is evolving, this information may not be current. The most up-to-date standard treatment options may be obtained by calling the National Cancer Institute Cancer Information Service at 1-800-4-CANCER. All patients should be considered for inclusion in clinical trials of new regimens. Descriptions of these trials are also available.

Treatment: Allopurinol is begun prior to chemotherapy to prevent hyperuricemia. Generous fluid intake is advised to assure brisk urine ouput. Systemic chemotherapy is palliative not curative. Chemotherapy may be withheld in the asymptomatic patient with moderately elevated WBC count because chemotherapy does not on the average appear to prolong life. ●When symptoms appear, busulfan or hydroxyurea are the recommended drugs. The initial adult dose of busulfan is 4–8 mg/day PO. The dose is reduced by half as the WBC count is reduced by half, and discontinued when WBC is reduced to 25,000. The drug is reinstituted when the WBC count again rises. Ongoing therapy is individualized. ●Similarly, hydroxyurea therapy is titrated according to the WBC count. The initial dose is 1–1.5 grams/day or 30 mg/kg/day PO. ●Vincristine + prednisone may be used to treat patients in the blastic phase in whom there has been a transformation to lymphoblastic cells that are terminal deoxynucleotidyl transferase (TdT) positive. Meningeal involvement is an indication for intrathecal methotrexate, intrathecal cytarabine, or cranial irradiation. Splenectomy may be indicated during the chronic phase in patients with hypersplenism–related hematologic complications or in distress because of a massively enlarged spleen. Leukophoresis may be required if the WBC count exceeds 300,000. Plateletphoresis is indicated for very high platelet counts. Transfusions may be needed during the accelerated phase. Radiation of lytic bone lesions may be necessary. Marrow transplantation is being used with some success in patients with an identical twin or HLA identical sibling. Whether long–term survival can be expected is not yet known. Alpha interferon has been shown to reduce the WBC count with a decrease in number and percent of Philadelphia chromosome–positive metaphases. The spleen concurrently returns to normal size.

Chronic Lymphocytic Leukemia

Over 90% cases occur after the age of 50. CLL seldom occurs before age 30. Men outnumber women 2 to 1. **Cellular characteristics:** ●CLL is almost always a proliferation of abnormal B lymphocytes; T cell CLL accounts for < 5% cases. ●In B–cell CLL, the abnormal lymphocytes can be shown to belong to a single clone: (1) a single light chain type is found on the surface of the abnormal lymphocytes, and (2) furthermore, a complete immunoglobulin of a discrete idiotype is also detected on the surface. In a small percentage of cases, these cells secrete sufficient immunoglobulin to be detected as a monoclonal spike on electrophoresis. Other surface characteristics include Ia antigen, receptors for Fc portion of immunoglobulin, receptors for C3 complement, receptors for mouse RBC's. ●The abnormal B lymphocytes are functionally impaired, and their presence frequently appears to impair the function of the normal B lymphocyte population and T lymphocytes. Increased susceptibility to infection and ultimately a reduced serum gammaglobulin level bear witness to the immunologic dysfunction. Furthermore, autoantibody may be produced, and this may lead to a direct Coombs–positive hemolytic anemia or to immune thrombocytopenia. ●The uncommon T–cell CLL is identified by the fact that the T cells characteristically bind sheep erythrocytes to their surface and thereby form rosettes. Moreover, immunoglobulin is not found on the surface of these cells.

Signs/symptoms: CLL usually has an insidious course. About a fourth of patients have no symptoms at the time of diagnosis when an abnormal CBC is noted or enlarged lymph nodes are found. ●Common findings include fatigue, malaise, weight loss, enlarged lymph nodes, enlarged spleen and liver. ●The leukemic cells may invade the skin, GI tract, lungs, heart, and other areas. ●A thrombocytopenia–associated bleeding tendency may develop. ●There is increased susceptibility to infections. Fever may be due to intercurrent infection or to the effects of CLL itself. Infection is ultimately the cause of death in many cases.

Laboratory: Peripheral blood smear discloses lymphocytosis > 15,000. WBC count may exceed 100,000 and occasionally may even surpass 1 million. The abnormal lymphocytes are small, well–differentiated, and often it is not possible by light microscopy to distinguish them from the normal lymphocytes. Bone marrow is hypercellular with > 40% lymphocytes. Anemia, thrombocytopenia, and granulocytopenia eventually develops as a consequence of marrow displacement by the excessive number of lymphocytes. Hypersplenism and/or autoimmune–mediated destruction may also contribute to anemia and thrombocytopenia. Positive direct Coombs' test is found in about a fourth of cases. Hemolysis, however, is uncommon and responds to prednisone. Serum gammaglobulin levels are depressed or eventually become depressed in most cases.

Note: The information presented below is largely extracted from National Cancer Institute PDQ State–of–the–Art Cancer Treatment Information 12/3/90. However, since cancer treatment is evolving, this information may not be current. The most up-to-date standard treatment options may be obtained by calling the National Cancer Institute Cancer Information Service at 1–800–4–CAN-CER. Patients may be considered for inclusion in clinical trials of new regimens. Descriptions of these trials are also available.

Treatment: There is no cure. Asymptomatic patients are not treated as a rule. Chemotherapy: When there is a compelling reason (e.g. thrombocytopenia, anemia, symptomatic lymphadenopathy or splenomegaly); chlorambucil is the usual therapy. A corticosteroid (e.g. prednisone) is often used as an adjunct to chlorambucil. A corticosteroid is especially helpful when there is immune–mediated hemolytic anemia or thrombocytopenia. Because RBC or platelet transfusion (should that become necessary) is difficult in such cases, it is best to curb the immune–mediated phenomena with a corticosteroid before starting chlorambucil. Patients with large nodal masses undergoing chemotherapy should receive allopurinol, and receive a generous amount of fluid to maintain brisk urine output. Local irradiation of enlarged lymph nodes or spleen is sometimes needed. Splenectomy may be considered for hypersplenism, for immune–mediated thrombocytopenia, or for hemolytic anemia that is unresponsive to chemotherapy. Leukopheresis may be employed in certain situations—e.g. markedly elevated lymphocyte counts with severe thrombocytopenia, bone marrow failure due to prior chemotherapy. Leukopheresis must be performed frequently because the response is transient. Other therapeutic approaches under investigation include biologic response modifiers (stages II–IV), splenic irradiation alone (stages II–IV), new chemotherapy regimens (stages III–IV), total body irradiation (stages III–IV).

Prognosis: Absolute lymphocytosis > 15,000 in the absence of anemia, thrombocytopenia, lymphadenopathy, or hepatosplenomegaly: median survival 12+ years. Absolute lymphocytosis + lymphadenopathy in absence of anemia, thrombocytopenia, or hepatosplenomegaly: median survival 8+ years. Absolute lymphocytosis + lymphadenopathy + splenomegaly or hepatomegaly: median survival 6 years. Absolute lymphocytosis with anemia (hemoglobin < 11 gm/dl) and/or thrombocytopenia (<100,000/cu mm): median survival 1+ years.

Leukemoid Reaction is defined as a persistently elevated WBC count > 30,000 not due to a hematologic malignancy.

NEUTROPHILIC LEUKEMOID REACTION: Causes: sundry cancers (e.g. breast, lung, renal, sarcoma); inflammation (e.g. rheumatoid arthritis); chronic infection possibly (e.g. tuberculosis).

Characteristic features of neutrophilic leukemoid reaction: (**1**) Peripheral WBC count seldom > 100,000 and usually < 50,000. (**2**) Peripheral smear discloses mostly mature neutrophils with < 10% bands. Cells of the myeloid line less mature than metamyelocytes are seldom seen. (**3**) Peripheral smear does not show increased numbers of basophils, eosinophils, or monocytes. (**4**) Nucleated RBC's are absent from the peripheral smear. (**5**) Thrombocytopenia is absent. There may be thrombocytosis but not greater than 600,000–700,000. (**6**) Splenomegaly is absent. (**7**) Bone marrow discloses myeloid hyperplasia. (**8**) No chromosomal abnormalities are detected.

Differential diagnosis includes: Chronic myelogenous leukemia; (**1**) WBC count often > 100, 000; (**2**) peripheral smear discloses some cells of the myeloid line that are less mature than metamyelocytes; **(3)** leukocyte alkaline phosphatase usually decreased; **(4)** Philadelphia chromosome present in > 90% cases; **(5)** splenomegaly present. Idiopathic myelofibrosis: **(1)** peripheral smear shows nucleated RBC's, teardrop RBC's, early myeloid forms; **(2)** there is splenomegaly and frequently hepatomegaly; **(3)** "dry" marrow aspiration with subsequent marrow biopsy revealing fibrosis. Polycythemia vera may be associated with markedly elevated neutrophil counts. In contrast to a leukemoid reaction, however, the RBC count is increased and other blood cell types (platelets, basophils, eosinophils) are often increased as well. Splenomegaly is typical. Acute myelogenous leukemia: Myeloblasts are seen on the peripheral smear. Anemia and thrombocytopenia are common. Auer bodies may be found. Bone marrow is crowded with myeloblasts. See "Acute Myelogenous Leukemia" for additional features.

Multiple Myeloma is uncommon before the age of 40. Peak incidence

is in the 60s. ●Multiple myeloma arises from the malignant transformation of a single cell leading to the proliferation of a single clone of plasma cells that secrete a discrete monoclonal immunoglobulin (IgG, IgA, IgD, or IgE) and/or portion thereof (kappa or lambda light chain). ●If the malignant clone secretes the relatively small light chains (either solely or in addition to intact immunoglobulin), they will be filtered at the glomeruli. These light chains (Bence Jones proteins) are detected in the urine if more is filtered than the renal tubular cells can reabsorb and catabolize. ●The malignant plasma cells typically proliferate within the bone. Sometimes a solitary locus is found within the bone (isolated plasmacytoma of bone) or soft tissue (isolated extramedullary plasmacytoma).

Signs/symptoms: Bone pain is characteristic. Pathologic fractures are common. Manifestations of anemia (e.g. pallor, fatigue, weakness) may be apparent. Infections: Compromised immune function leaves patient susceptible to recurrent infections. Pneumococcal respiratory infections are particularly common. Bleeding may occur secondary to thrombocytopenia, platelet dysfunction, or myeloma protein–induced inhibition of coagulation factors. Renal insufficiency may develop. Renal injury may be the consequence of Bence Jones nephropathy, calcium nephropathy, uric acid nephropathy, and/or amyloidosis. Symptoms of hypercalcemia (e.g. polyuria, constipation, confusion) may develop. Lymphadenopathy, splenomegaly, or hepatomegaly may be present. Hyperviscosity and its manifestations: Rarely, the serum immunoglobulin level becomes markedly elevated to the point that hyperviscosity with sludging and impaired circulation develops. Consequences may include congestive heart failure; bleeding of the skin or mucosa; sundry neurologic manifestations (e.g. headache, confusion, tinnitus, vertigo, blurred vision). Nerve or spinal cord compression–induced neurologic abnormalities may develop as a consequence of an enlarging plasmacytoma or a pathologic vertebral fracture.

Laboratory: Serum protein electrophoresis discloses a monoclonal immunoglobulin spike (M protein) in about 75% of multiple myeloma patients. In the remainder: (1) the spike is too small to be detected, (2) the malignant clone does not secrete immunoglobulin, or (3) the malignant plasma clone synthesizes light chains (Bence Jones proteins) only. The latter circumstance, which accounts for most of the serum protein electrophoresis negative cases, characteristically manifests as a hypogammaglobulinemic electrophoretic pattern. Urine protein electrophoresis of concentrate of 24 hr urine collection will reveal an immunoglobulin spike or narrow band in about 75% myeloma patients. Monoclonal light chains (Bence Jones protein) are detected in the urine not only of patients whose malignant plasma cells only synthesize light chain but also in the majority of myeloma patients whose malignant plasma cells synthesize intact monoclonal molecules. The latter patient's malignant cells often synthesize light chains in excess of heavy chains so that excess light chains are detected in the urine. Immunoelectrophoresis of the serum or the urine will identify the specific class of immunoglobulin secreted by the malignant plasma clone. In about 55% patients that monoclonal immunoglobulin is IgG, in about 25% cases it is IgA, and in about 20% only an immunoglobulin light chain (kappa or lambda) is secreted. IgD accounts for 1% cases and IgE multiple myeloma is rare. Immunoelectrophoresis is also useful in that it may detect a monoclonal spike that is too small to be discerned on serum protein electrophoresis. Immunofluorescence or immunoperoxidase stain of bone marrow biopsy specimen may be needed to identify monoclonal protein within the malignant plasma cells of the approximately 1% of multiple myeloma patients whose malignant plasma cells apparently fail to secrete immunoglobulin and who are therefore not detected by other methods. Some of these "nonsecretory" cases may possibly be explained by the presence of a malignant plasma clone that synthesizes free monoclonal light chain only and only in small amounts. In these cases, the light chain (Bence Jone protein) is not detected in the urine since the amount filtered at the glomeruli does not exceed the amount that is reabsorbed and catabolized by the renal tubular cells. Consequently, Bence Jones proteinuria does not occur. Urine dipstick tests detect anionic proteins. Since Bence Jones proteins are cations, they will not be detected by this method. However, other nonspecific protein tests are reliable (e.g. sulfosalicylic acid method). Heat testing of urine is not a dependable means of detecting Bence Jones protein; it is falsely negative in about half the cases. When heat testing is positive, the classical finding is that Bence Jones protein precipitates as the urine is slowly heated to 45–60° C and redissolves on boiling. Bone marrow exam is an essential part of the workup.

Characteristically, over 15–20% of the marrow cells are plasma cells (normal < 5%). Hematologic profile: Usually there is normocytic normochromic anemia. There may be leukopenia. The peripheral blood smear shows RBC rouleaux formation. Sedimentation rate is elevated and may exceed 100 mm/hr. X-rays may simply reveal osteoporosis or osteolytic lesions may be evident. Pathologic fractures may be seen (e.g. vertebral compression fracture). Renal function: Bence Jones proteins appear to damage the renal tubules, and so there may be evidence of renal failure (e.g. elevated BUN and creatinine). The ability to produce a concentrated urine may be impaired (I.e. nephrogenic diabetes insipidus) and/or the patient may be unable to produce an acid urine (i.e. distal renal tubular acidosis). Hypercalcemia is common and may result in renal failure. Hyperuricemia/hyperuricosuria is also common and may contribute to renal injury.

Essential diagnostic criteria: presence of > 10% plasma cells on bone marrow exam (or presence of extraskeletal plasmacytoma) together with clinical evidence of multiple myeloma plus at least one of the following: (1) detection of myeloma protein in the serum or urine, (2) x-ray evidence of osteolytic lesions.

Staging/prognosis: Stage I patients meet all of the following criteria: hemoglobin > 10 g/dl, normal serum calcium, absence of osteolytic lesions, serum IgG < 5 g/dl or serum IgA < 3 g/dl, Bence Jones proteinuria < 4 g/24 hr. The 5 yr survival is 25–40%. Stage II patients do not fulfill the criteria of stage I or stage III. The 5 yr survival is 15–30%. Stage III patients have at least one of the following abnormalities: hemoglobin < 8.5 g/dl, serum calcium > 12, more than 3 osteolytic lesions, serum IgG > 7 g/dl, serum IgA > 5 g/dl, Bence Jones proteinuria > 12 g/24 hr. The 5 yr survival is 10–25%.

Treatment: Treatment is withheld in stage I asymptomatic patients until there is there is evidence of disease progression. Chemotherapy: Symptomatic stage I patients, and stage II and III patients receive chemotherapy. The most common regimen consists of melphalan + prednisone. Other multiple drug regimens may be employed but they have not improved survival. Local radiotherapy may be used to alleviate a painful bone lesion, to preclude a pathologic fracture, or to relieve a vital organ that is being encroached upon by an extraskeletal plasmacytoma. Local radiation therapy is also standard treatment for an isolated plasmacytoma of the bone or soft tissues. Adequate hydration is important to prevent renal failure in patients with Bence Jones proteinuria. Sufficient fluids are taken to maintain urine output at > 1500 ml/day. Hydration is especially important if an IVP is to be performed since this study may precipitate renal failure. Packed red cell transfusion is indicated for severe anemia. Hypercalcemia: refer to "Hypercalcemia" chapter. Allopurinol is administered to prevent hyperuricemia. Infections are treated aggressively. Recurrent infection is common and infection is the most common ultimate cause of death The most frequent sites of infection are the lungs (particularly pneumococcus and gram–negative bacteria) and the urinary tract. Plasmapheresis together with chemotherapy is recommended if symptoms of hyperviscosity develop.

Benign monoclonal gammopathy (monoclonal gammopathy of unknown significance) is more common than multiple myeloma. An M spike is discovered on serum electrophoresis, but the serum myeloma protein level is < 3 g/dl and the other stigmata of multiple myeloma are absent (e.g. anemia or osteolytic lesions are absent, < 5% plasma cells in bone marrow). About 10% of these individuals go on to develop multiple myeloma.

Waldenström's Macroglobulinemia results

from the malignant transformation of a single cell in the B lymphocyte line. There is proliferation of plasmacytoid lymphocytes that secrete a monoclonal IgM. The disease is most often seen in the elderly. In contrast to multiple myeloma, the malignant clone frequently proliferates in the spleen and lymph nodes in addition to the bone marrow.

Signs/symptoms: Hepatomegaly, splenomegaly and lymphadenopathy are common. Sundry neurologic manifestations (e.g. headache, confusion, tinnitus, vertigo, blurred vision, peripheral neuropathy, paresis, paresthesias) may develop as a consequence of the hyperviscosity–induced sludging and impaired circulation that arises as the serum immunoglobulin level becomes elevated. Hyperviscosity–induced retinal abnormalities may be evident: the retinal veins are dilated from congestion and often have a sausage–link appearance. Retinal hemorrhages and exudates may be present. Hyperviscosity–induced congestive heart failure may develop. Bleeding of the skin or mucosa may also ensue from hyperviscosity. Recurrent bacterial infection is common. Cold–induced cyanosis of the digits, nose, ears may occur in those patients who secrete a monoclonal IgM that is a cryoglobulin. In contrast to multiple myeloma, bone pain is not present and renal failure is unusual.

Laboratory: Serum protein electrophoresis reveals a monoclonal immunoglobulin spike (M protein). Immunoelectrophoresis shows that immunoglobulin to be IgM. Bence Jones proteinuria is found in approximately 10% patients. In these cases, the malignant clone synthesizes excess light chains. Hematologic profile: Normocytic normochromic anemia is typical. Peripheral smear reveals plasmacytic lymphocytes and rouleaux formation of RBC's. Sedimentation rate is quite high. Bone marrow typically discloses increased numbers of plasma cells and plasmocytoid lymphocytes. Xrays: The malignant cells proliferate within the bone marrow but the lytic bone lesions seen in multiple myeloma are rare. Cold agglutinins and the direct Coombs' test: In some cases, the malignant clone synthesizes an IgM that is a cold agglutinin and so the direct Coombs' test is positive. In a few of these patients, cold–exposure induces hemolysis (refer to "Immunoglobulin/complement–mediated Hemolysis" chapter).

Treatment: <u>Chemotherapy</u>: Chlorambucil is the preferred chemotherapeutic agent. Melphelan plus prednisone is one alternative. <u>Plasmapheresis</u> is indicated if there is hyperviscosity–associated bleeding or neurologic manifestations. In order to avoid gel formation or erythrocyte agglutination, plasmapheresis must be performed at a warm ambient temperature if the monoclonal IgM is shown to be a cryoglobulin or a cold agglutinin.

Adult Hodgkin's Disease is often curable. This malig-
nancy arises in the reticuloendothelial system (lymph nodes, spleen, liver, marrow). The histologic hallmark is the Reed–Sternberg cell, a large reticular cell with pale-staining eosinophilic cytoplasm and 1–2 large nuclei. Hodgkin's is more common in males. Incidence is binodal with a peak at about age 30 and another at about age 70. **Four histologic types** of Hodgkin's disease are recognized: lymphocyte predominance, nodular sclerosis, mixed cellularity, lymphocyte depletion.

Signs/symptoms: <u>Regional adenopathy</u> is the characteristic finding. The involved nodes are enlarged and nontender. Hodgkin's disease typically spreads in a predictable step–wise fashion to contiguous nodes, <u>Nonspecific complaints</u> are common (e.g. fatigue, fever, night sweats, weight loss). <u>Itching</u> may develop and is sometimes severe. <u>Other possible manifestations</u> include: bone metastases–associated pain, superior vena cava syndrome due to compression by a bulky mediastinal tumor, mediastinal tumor–associated compression of airway, signs of biliary obstruction in an advanced case of liver involvement, metastatic tumor–associated spinal cord compression with neurologic sequelae, susceptibility to infections.

Investigations: <u>Laboratory</u>: ESR, CBC, urinalysis, BUN, creatinine, uric acid, liver function tests, alkaline phosphatase. <u>Chest x–ray</u> and <u>CAT scan of abdomen, pelvis, and chest</u> are obtained. <u>Bilateral lower extremity lymphangiogram</u> is indicated if CAT scan is negative below diaphragm. <u>Bone marrow biopsy</u> is performed if there are systemic symptoms or clinical stage III. <u>Bone scan and local bone x–rays</u> are ordered if there is bone pain. <u>Laparotomy with splenectomy</u> for the purpose of establishing the pathologic stage is indicated only if the findings might change the treatment plan. Staging laparotomy is not necessary if the physician is confident of the extent of disease. Staging laparotomy may be recommended for clinical stages I, II, or IIIA. Staging laparotomy is not done in patients with clinical stages III B or IV, nor must it be done in patients with massive mediastinal involvement. <u>Liver biopsy</u> via peritoneoscope may be recommended in clinical stage III patients who do not undergo staging laparotomy.

Note: The following information is largely extracted from National Cancer Institute PDQ State–of–the–Art Cancer Treatment Information 2/1/91. However, since cancer treatment is evolving, this information may not be current. The most up-to-date standard treatment options may be obtained by calling the National Cancer Institute Cancer Information Service at 1–800–4–CANCER.

Staging: Clinical staging is based on history, physical exam, radiological tests, lab. Pathologic staging is based on biopsies. The stages presented below are also assigned the letter B if the patient has had unexplained fever > 38°, night sweats, or unexplained weight loss > 10% in the 6 months prior to diagnosis. Patients without these findings are assigned the letter A.

<u>Stage I</u>: involvement of a single lymph node region or a single extralymphatic organ or site.

<u>Stage II</u>: involvement of 2 or more lymph node regions on the same side of the diaphragm.

Stage II E: involvement of 1 or more lymph node regions plus an extralymphatic organ or site. Involvement is restricted to one side of the diaphragm.

<u>Stage III</u> indicates involvement of 2 or more lymph node regions on opposite sides of the diaphragm; and may also include an extralymphatic site (stage III E), spleen (stage III S), or both (stage III ES).

<u>Stage IV</u>: diffuse or disseminated involvement of one or more extralymphatic sites or tissues with or without lymph node involvement.

Treatment overview:

<u>Stage I and II patients with supradiaphragmatic presentation</u>: Radiation alone is appropriate in many cases. However, radiation plus combination chemotherapy is: (1) usually advised for patients with massive mediastinal involvement, (2) advised for clinical stage IB and IIB patients who do not undergo staging laparotomy.

<u>Stage I and II patients with infradiaphragmatic presentation</u>: Radiation alone is appropriate in many cases. However, combination chemotherapy plus radiation (1) may be recommended for stage IA and IIA patients with para-aortic nodal involvement, (2) is advised for clinical stage IB patients who do not undergo staging laparotomy. Chemotherapy ± radiation is advised for stage IIB patients.

<u>Stage IIIA treatment</u>: Most patients receive combination chemotherapy ± radiation.

<u>Stage IIIB and stage IV</u> are treated with combination chemotherapy. Patients may also receive radiation to regions of bulky disease or sites of initial involvement.

Commonly employed combination chemotherapy regimens include: MOPP (mechlorethamine + vincristine + procarbazine + prednisone), MOPP/ABV hybrid (MOPP + doxorubicin + bleomycin + vinblastine), MOPP alternating with ABVD (doxorubicin + bleomycin + vinblastine + dacarbazine), MVPP (mechlorethamine + vinblastine + procarbazine + prednisone).

Radiation fields: Mantle field (cervical, supraclavicular, infraclavicular, axillary, mediastinal, and hilar nodes); Para–aortic/splenic field (para–aortic nodes from diaphragm to aortic bifurcation, and spleen or splenic bed if the spleen has been extirpated); Inverted Y field (para–aortic–splenic field + iliac + inguinal–femoral nodes); Subtotal lymphoid field (mantle + para–aortic/splenic field); Total lymphoid field (mantle + inverted Y field).

Prognosis with treatment:

	5 yr disease–free survival	10 yr survival
Stage I	up to 90%	up to 90%
Stage II	75–90%	80–90%
Stage III A–1*	65–85%	80–90%
Stage III A–2*	65–85%	65–80%
Stage III B–1*	50–85%	80–90%
Stage III B–2*	50–85%	50–65%
Stage IV	40–65%	40–65%

*The number 1 indicates that abdominal disease is limited to the upper abdomen while the number 2 indicates involvement of pelvic and/or para–aortic nodes.

Childhood Hodgkin's Disease

See "Adult Hodgkin's Disease" above for general information on Hodgkin's disease including signs, symptoms, histology, diagnostic tests.

Note: The facts presented below are extracted from National Cancer Institute PDQ State-of-the-Art Cancer Treatment Information 12/3/90. However, since cancer treatment is evolving, this information may not be current. The most up-to-date treatment recommendations may be obtained by calling the National Cancer Institute Cancer Information Service at 1–800–4–CANCER. Treatment is best administered as part of a clinical trial at a major medical center proficient in pediatric cancer care. Descriptions of these trials are also available.

STAGING: The stages presented below are also assigned the letter B if the patient has had unexplained fever > 38°, night sweats, or unexplained weight loss > 10% in the 6 months prior to diagnosis. Patients without these findings are assigned the letter A.

Stage I; involvement of a single lymph node region, or a single extralymphatic organ or site.

Stage II; involvement of 2 or more lymph node regions on same side of the diaphragm or (stage II E) localized involvement of a single extralymphatic organ/site and regional nodes ± other node regions. All disease is restricted to same side of diaphragm.

Stage III; involvement of 2 or more lymph node regions on opposite sides of the diaphragm. This may also include an extralymphatic site (stage III E), spleen (stage III S), or both (stage III ES).

Stage IV; diffuse or disseminated (multifocal) involvement of 1 or more extralymphatic organs or sites with or without associated lymph node involvement or involvement of an isolated extralymphatic organ with distant (nonregional) lymph node involvement.

TREATMENT:

Key to radiation fields: Mantle field (cervical, supraclavicular, infraclavicular, axillary, mediastinal, and hilar nodes); Para–aortic/splenic field (para–aortic nodes from diaphragm to aortic bifurcation, and spleen or splenic bed if the spleen has been extirpated); Inverted Y field (para–aortic/splenic field + iliac + inguinal–femoral nodes); Subtotal lymphoid field (mantle + para–aortic/splenic field); Total lymphoid field (mantle + inverted Y field). NOTE: Radiation should be administered at institutions with modern linear accelerators delivering 4–10 MeV energy and treatment planning simulators. Protective blocks tailored to each patient should be used to protect normal tissues.

Chemotherapy regimens: The most experience with combination chemotherapy has been with MOPP (mechlorethamine + vincristine + procarbazine + prednisone). Other regimens that may be employed are: ABVD (doxorubicin + bleomycin + vinblastine + dacarbazine), MOPP alternatiing with ABVD.

Stage I and stage II:

Disease above diaphragm without massive mediastinal involvement; ●Children who are full–grown are usually treated with mantle + para–aortic/splenic field irradiation (the pelvic lymph nodes are spared). Mantle field alone is an option if there is very limited involvement. ●In younger children, it is recommended that only the involved field be irradiated (at a reduced dose) and that combination chemotherapy be employed.

Disease above diaphragm with massive mediastinal involvement (i.e. mediastinal mass > 1/3 chest diameter) or pericardial or chest wall involvement is usually treated with mediastinal or mantle radiation + combination chemotherapy. It is best to shrink the mediastinal mass with at least part of the chemotherapy regimen before commencing irradiation. ●An alternative approach is subtotal lymphoid radiation with boost to mediastinum, and with chemotherapy reserved for relapse. This regimen must not be employed if the mediastinal mass overlaps the heart to such an extent that administration of a full dose of radiation is precluded.

Stage III A may be treated with combination chemotherapy alone. ●Total lymphoid irradiation is an alternative provided that: (1) subdiaphragmatic involvement restricted to the upper abdomen and (2) < 5 nodules visible on cut section of the spleen. Those who do have splenic involvement may also receive low–dose irradiation of the liver. ●Combination chemotherapy plus irradiation of regions of bulky disease is yet another option.

Stage III B is treated with combination chemotherapy. Radiation of regions/sites of bulky disease may be employed in conjunction with combination chemotherapy.

Stage IV is treated similarly to stage III B.

PROGNOSIS:

	5 yr disease–free survival	10 yr survival
Stage I:	75–85%	up to 100%
Stage II:	75–85%	Up to 90%
Stage IIIA	65–90%	65–85%
Stage III B	50–75%	50–75%
Stage IV	40–80%	50–65%

Adult non-Hodgkin's Lymphoma

Identifying cell characteristics: Hodgkin's disease accounts for about a fourth of all lymphomas. The remaining three–fourths—the non–Hodgkin's lymphomas (NHL)—-includes a variety of histologic types (see histologic classification below). Nonlymphoblastic NHL's account for the majority of NHL's. Most nonlymphoblastic NHL's are malignant derivatives of B–lymphocytes. Consequently, in most cases, immunoglobulins (usually IgM) can be demonstrated on the cell surface. Also, other B–cell surface markers can usually be identified. Lymphoblastic NHL's: Most are of T–lymphocyte origin. They are usually positive for the T cell enzyme, terminal deoxynucleotidyl transferase (TdT). They can also usually be identified by the fact that they form rosettes when mixed with sheep erythrocytes.

Etiology: Predisposing conditions: hereditary immunodeficiency (e.g. Wiskott–Aldrich syndrome, ataxia–telangectasia, congenital agammaglobulinemia, Chédiak–Higashi syndrome); acquired immunodeficiency (autoimmune disease, AIDS, renal and cardiac allograft recipients receiving immunosuppressants); radiation exposure, exposure to certain herbicides. Viruses have been associated with some cases of non–Hodgkin's lymphoma. However, a causal relationship has not yet been proven. Ebstein–Barr virus has been linked to Burkitt's lymphoma in African children. HTLV–1 virus has been linked to adult T–cell leukemia/lymphoma. HIV virus may be associated with some types of non–Hodgkin's lymphomas developing in AIDS patients. Certain chromosome translocations and oncogenes may be implicated in pathogenesis of some non–Hodgkin's lymphomas. Burkitt's and follicular NHL are commonly associated with chromosomal translocations.

Signs/symptoms: Painless adenopathy is the most common finding (80% newly diagnosed patients). Patients often discover a painless swelling in an axilla, groin, or neck. It should be noted that NHL's do not spread predictably to contiguous nodes like in Hodgkin's disease. Instead, NHL often disseminates to distant nodes and other organs. This has important therapeutic implications since NHL's are thus less often curable with regional radiotherapy. Waldeyer's ring is involved in as many as 30% of patients (e.g. tonsillar enlargement is common). Nonspecific systemic complaints (fever, night sweats, fatigue, weight loss) may be elicited in some patients. Splenic enlargement is common. Painless abdominal mass may be the initial complaint. Urinary tract complications may occur. For instance, tumor may encroach on an ureter so that obstruction and flank pain ensue. Sometimes, tumor encroaches upon and blocks the renal blood vessels. In other cases, the kidney itself is invaded. Hyperuricemia–provoked renal complications may occur (e.g. uric acid nephropathy, stones). Liver enlargement and/or jaundice may develop. Jaundice may result from encroachment on the biliary tract or from invasion of the liver itself. Gastrointestinal involvement may lead to malabsorption or possibly manifest as GI obstruction, bleeding, or perforation. Bone marrow involvement may result in bone pain/tenderness, and/or anemia. Lymphatic obstruction may lead to chylous ascites or pleural effusion. Neurologic syndromes may arise by various mechanisms—e.g. spinal cord compression from an epidural or paraspinal tumor, meningeal involvement. Anterior mediastinal mass is particularly common in lymphoblastic NHL. The mass may (1) obstruct the superior vena cava leading to swelling of the head and neck; (2) obstruct the airway resulting in dyspnea, wheezing, or stridor; (3) compress the esophagus with ensuing dysphagia.

Routine blood tests: <u>Hematology</u>; Anemia may develop as a consequence of one or a combination of factors—e.g. marrow involvement, marrow suppression from chemo– or radiation therapy, hypersplenism, immune–mediated (Coombs' positive) hemolysis, GI invasion–associated bleeding. There may be thrombocytopenia. The peripheral smear may reveal abnormal lymphocytes, particularly in patients with follicular and diffuse well–differentiated lymphocytic types of NHL. <u>Liver function tests</u> abnormalities suggest liver involvement. <u>Serum LDH</u>; High levels are associated with poorer prognosis. <u>Other</u>; Obtain BUN, creatinine, uric acid, serum calcium.

Radiologic tests: Obtain chest x–ray. Order CT scan of chest, abdomen, and pelvis. Bone pain/tenderness is an indication for plain x–ray of suspect site and for bone scan. Bipedal lymphangiogram (retroperitoneal lymphangiogram) is ordered if additional staging information is needed to decide optimum therapy.

Biopsy of suspicious nodes or other tissue is necessary to establish the diagnosis and the grade of tumor. Bone marrow biopsy (bilateral iliac crest biopsy) is advised only if it is required in making the diagnosis, or if the information so obtained may alter the mode of therapy. Liver biopsy is not advised, except perhaps in the case of an aggressive lymphoma.

Staging laparotomy is seldom necessary since most patients are found to require chemotherapy. Staging laparotomy may be of value if the patient is a possible candidate for radiation therapy alone.

Staging:

<u>Stage I</u>; involvement of a single lymph node region <u>or</u> a single extralymphatic organ or site.

<u>Stage II</u>; involvement of 2 or more lymph node regions on the same side of the diaphragm <u>or</u> involvement of 1 or more lymph node regions with associated localized involvement of an extralymphatic organ or site. In stage II, lymphatic and extralymphatic involvement are restricted to one side of the diaphragm.

<u>Stage III</u>; involvement of lymph node regions on both sides of the diaphragm, with or without associated localized involvement of the spleen and/or extralymphatic organ or site.

<u>Stage IV</u>; involvement of bone marrow or liver <u>or</u> diffuse or disseminated (multifocal) involvement of 1 or more extralymphatic organs or sites with or without associated lymph node involvement <u>or</u> involvement of an isolated extralymphatic organ with distant (nonregional) lymph node involvement.

<u>Note</u>; Each stage is subdivided into either A (without systemic symptoms) or B (with systemic symptoms). Those in the B category have: (1) unexplained fever > 38° C, (2) night sweats, and/or (3) > 10% weight loss in the 6 months prior to diagnosis.

Histologic classification:

WORKING CLASSIFICATION	RAPPAPORT CLASSIFICATION EQUIVALENT
Low grade;	
Small lymphocytic, consistent with CLL (SL)	Diffuse, well–differentiated lymphocytic (DWDL).
Follicular, mainly small cleaved cell (FSC)	Nodular, poorly differentiated lymphocytic (NPDL).
Follicular, mixed small cleaved & large cell (FM)	Nodular, mixed lymphocytic & histiocytic (NM).
Intermediate grade;	
Follicular, mainly large cell (FL)	Nodular histiocytic (NH)
Diffuse, small cleaved cell (DSC)	Diffuse, poorly differentiated lymphocytic (DPDL).
Diffuse, mixed small & large cell (DM)	Diffuse, mixed lymphocytic & histiocytic (DM).
Diffuse, large cell cleaved or noncleaved (DL)	Diffuse, histiocytic (DH).
High grade;	
Immunoblastic, large cell (IBL)	Diffuse, histiocytic (DH)
Lymphoblastic, convoluted or nonconvoluted (LBL)	Lymphoblastic (LBL)
Small noncleaved cell (SNC) Burkitt's or non–Burkitt's	Diffuse, undifferentiated (DU) Burkitt's or non–Burkitt's.

Treatment varies according to such factors as stage and histologic classification. Regional radiotherapy plays a more limited role in the treatment of NHL than Hodgkin's disease. This is because NHL's do not spread predictably to contiguous nodes like in Hodgkin's disease and they more often disseminate to distant nodes and other organs. Consequently, except for low grade stage I and stage II disease which may be treated with regional radiotherapy alone, all patients should generally receive chemotherapy. Combination chemotherapy alone is standard treatment in most cases. Adjunctive radiotherapy may be indicated—e.g. to control a large mass, to control a mass compressing the superior vena cava or airway. Cancer treatment is evolving. The most up-to-date standard treatment options are found in the National Cancer Institute PDQ State–of–the–Art Cancer Treatment Information. This information may be obtained by calling the National Cancer Institute Cancer Information Service at 1–800–4–CANCER. Patients should be considered for inclusion in clinical trials aimed at improving therapy. Descriptions of these trials are also available.

Prognosis: <u>Low grade non–Hodgkin's lymphoma</u>; Low grade stage I and stage II patients may possibly be cured with radiation alone. Stage III and IV is not presently curable. Despite the dearth of cures, 50–75% of patients are alive after 5 yr. <u>Intermediate and high grade non–</u>

<u>Hodgkin's lymphoma</u>; Combination chemotherapy may cure many of these patients (e.g. 30–60% intermediate grade patients are curable). <u>Lymphoblastic lymphoma</u>; Patients have about a 90% chance of cure if the serum LDH is not high and if stage IV disease is not present. Patients with stage IV disease or elevated serum LDH have a 20% chance of 5 year relapse–free survival.

Childhood non-Hodgkin's Lymphoma

Non–Hodgkin's lymphoma (NHL) is responsible for about 10% of the cancers in patients under 20 years of age. About 60% of these patients can be cured. Refer to the previous chapter "Adult non–Hodgkin's Lymphoma" for information on etiology, signs/symptoms, tests, etc. One distinction between childhood and adult NHL is that the nodular histologic types are seldom seen in children. Lymphoblastic NHL accounts for 30% of NHL cases in children with the remainder designated nonlymphoblastic NHL. Lymphoblastic NHL usually arises from the malignant transformation of a T–cell. An anterior mediastinal mass is found in the majority of lymphoblastic NHL's.

Note: The information presented below is extracted from National Cancer Institute PDQ State–of–the–Art Cancer Treatment Information 9/28/90. The most up-to-date standard treatment options may be obtained by calling the National Cancer Institute Cancer Information Service at 1–800–4–CANCER. Cancer treatment is evolving. All patients should be considered for inclusion in clinical trials aimed at improving therapy. Descriptions of these trials are also available.

Staging (slightly modified from system used at St Jude Children's Research Hospital)**:**
<u>Stage I</u>; single tumor or single nodal region involvement outside mediastinum or abdomen.
<u>Stage II</u>; single tumor with regional node involvement <u>or</u> 2 or more tumors or nodal regions on one side of diaphragm <u>or</u> primary GI tract tumor ± regional node involvement.
<u>Stage III</u>; tumors or lymph node involvement on both sides of diaphragm <u>or</u> any primary intrathoracic disease <u>or</u> extensive intraabdominal disease <u>or</u> any paraspinal or epidural tumor.
<u>Stage IV</u>; bone marrow or CNS disease. Those patients with marrow involvement showing > 25% malignant cells of lymphoblastic type are usually treated with regimens used in the treatment of leukemia.

Another staging system (Children's Cancer Study Group) divides patients into those with localized disease and those with nonlocalized disease. Localized disease means that tumor is restricted to a single extranodal site ± positive regional nodes, or is restricted to lymph nodes in 2 adjacent lymphatic regions. Localized disease corresponds to stage I or II above. All others including mediastinal disease are designated nonlocalized.

Treatment: Combination chemotherapy is the cornerstone of therapy. Intrathecal chemotherapy for CNS prophylaxis is part of standard therapy. Radiotherapy may be needed as an adjunct—e.g. to control a mass compressing the superior vena cava, airway, or esophagus, to help control CNS disease. Since optimal treatment requires the efforts of specialists experienced in pediatric oncology, therapy should be administered as part of a clinical trial at a major medical center proficient in pediatric cancer care.

Rheumatoid and Autoimmune Disease

Rheumatoid Arthritis (RA) is a chronic inflammatory disorder of unknown cause associated with inflammation/destruction of synovial joints, and with the potential for causing disease in multiple organs. RA affects about 1–2% of the population. Females outnumber males 2–3 to 1. RA usually begins in the 20–50s but onset may occur at any age.

Pathology: The synovium is infiltrated with inflammatory cells, mostly neutrophils at first then shifting to lymphocytes along with macrophages, and plasma cells. There is hyperplasia/hypertrophy of the synovium. The synovium forms a pannus that extends over the cartilage and erodes it and underlying bone.

Signs/symptoms: Onset and progression of RA is variable. Onset may be abrupt but more often there is a several week prodrome which may include fever, malaise, fatigue, stiffness, generalized aching, poorly defined/localized joint symptoms. RA is a polyarthritis with symmetrical involvement although symmetry may not be seen initially. The first joints involved are usually the PIP and MCP joints of the hands (the DIP joints are seldom involved unless there is severe arthritis) and the joints of the feet (e.g. MTP). The fingers typically take on sausage–like appearance due to swelling of the PIP joints. Eventually, joint destruction, laxity of tendons and ligaments, and muscle contractures combine to produce deformities typical of RA—e.g. "swan neck" deformity (flexed DIP with hyperextended PIP), "boutonniere deformity" (flexed PIP), ulnar deviation of the fingers at the MCP joint. Deformities of the toes also occur (e.g. hammer toe, cock–up toe). Other joints often involved early in the disease are the wrists, elbows, knees, ankles. Knee involvement with effusion sometimes results in a Baker's cyst (popliteal cyst). Any synovial joint may be involved (e.g. temporomandibular joint, intervertebral facet joints, cricoarytenoid). Involvement of the cricoarytenoid joint of the larynx can cause hoarseness or even asphyxia. Rarely, spinal cord compression may occur when there is subluxation of the atlanto–axial joint.

Potential extra–articular complications: Subcutaneous nodules are granulomatous lesions. They are firm, nontender, and usually movable. They are most common over the elbows, dorsal forearm, occiput, ischial tuberosities, anterior tibia, Achilles tendon. They are virtually always associated with the presence of rheumatoid factor and usually with aggressive disease. Cutaneous vasculitis may lead to ischemic ulcers. Many patients bruise easily. Felty's syndrome (RA with splenomegaly and neutropenia, thrombocytopenia, anemia, lymphadenopathy) occasionally occurs. Pulmonary : pleuritis with or without effusion, interstitial fibrosis, pulmonary nodules, Caplan's syndrome (RA with pulmonary nodules and pneumoconiosis). Cardiac: pericarditis (often accompanied by a small effusion, rarely there is a large effusion with tamponade); nodules on heart valves (sometimes leading to valvular incompetence); nodules in myocardium (occasionally causing conduction abnormalities); coronary arteritis (sometimes leading to myocardial infarction). Eyes: scleritis (nodule forms in sclera, sometimes the sclera perforates); episcleritis; uveitis. Neurologic: carpal tunnel syndrome (due to thickening of synovial tendon sheaths of the wrist); mononeuritis multiplex (sensorimotor neuropathy due to vasculitis of vessels supplying a peripheral nerve); rare CNS lesions.

Laboratory: Rheumatoid factor is + in 75% cases. Seronegative patients tend to have milder disease. High titers correlate with more serious disease and are frequently associated with rheumatoid nodules. Rheumatoid factor may also be found in many other disorders (e.g. other autoimmune disorders, bacterial endocarditis, sarcoidosis, leprosy, chronic liver disease) and in 1–4% of normal individuals, especially with advancing age. Rheumatoid factors are immunoglobulins (IgM, IgG, or sometimes IgA) that react with the Fc locus of IgG. They are not the culprits responsible for RA. Antinuclear antigen (ANA) is + in up to half the cases. Normocytic normochromic anemia is a common finding. Eosinophilia sometimes occurs. Sedimentation rate may be increased. Synovial fluid analysis: WBC 5000–20,000 (50–75% neutrophils), decreased viscosity, decreased glucose, decreased complement, poor mucin clot test. The latter test is performed by adding 1% acetic acid to synovial fluid when/if fibrin clot has formed. In RA, hyaluronic acid will be broken down. Consequently, mucin clot formation is impaired: there is a poor mucin precipitate of synovial fluid (i.e. it is cloudy with shreds).

Diagnostic criteria: Definite diagnosis requires 5 of the following criteria while a probable diagnosis requires 3 of these criteria. Inclusion of any of criteria 1–5 requires that it be present for minimum of 6 weeks. (**1**) morning stiffness, (**2**) pain on motion or tenderness of at least 1 joint, (**3**) soft tissue swelling or fluid in at least 1 joint, (**4**) swelling of at least one other joint, (**5**) symmetrical joint swelling with simultaneous involvement of the same joints on both sides of the body (distal interphalangeal joints do not qualify), (**6**) subcutaneous nodules, (**7**) x-ray changes characteristic of RA, (**8**) positive rheumatoid factor, (**9**) poor mucin precipitate of synovial fluid (cloudy with shreds), (**10**) characteristic histologic changes in synovium, (**11**) characteristic histologic changes in nodules.

Treatment: Measures aimed at maintaining joint function; rest, warmth, judicious exercise and/or physical therapy. Aspirin is usually the first drug used and is titrated to achieve serum level of 20–30 mg/dl (refer to drug section for dosage in arthritis). Other nonsteroidal anti–inflammatory drugs (e.g. ibuprofen) are indicated when aspirin is not tolerated or is contraindicated. Sulfasalazine (Asulfidine) 2 grams/day is often effective. Hydroxychloroquine (an antimalarial) may be used in conjunction with aspirin or other nonsteroidal if sufficient relief is not achieved with one of the latter agents. Hydroxychloroquine is discontinued if improvement does not occur after 6 weeks. Eye exam is advised at least every 6 months because corneal and retinal abnormalities occasionally occur with this drug. Gold salts (gold sodium thiomalate) are an alternative to hydroxychloroquine if that drug is ineffective. Because of the potential for marrow and renal toxicity; a CBC, platelet count, and urinalysis are obtained prior to beginning therapy and before each injection. Penicillamine, methotrexate, or azathioprine (Imuran) are other options in refractory cases but they may also have toxic consequences. Corticosteroids may be indicated to control extra–articular manifestations of RA (e.g. Felty's syndrome, pleuritis, pericarditis, vasculitis, neural or ocular complications) but they are generally not recommended for the chronic treatment of joint disease alone. They may sometimes be used to control an acute exacerbation of joint disease. Synovectomy or joint replacement may become necessary.

Juvenile Rheumatoid Arthritis is divided into 3 clinical categories.

Systemic category (Still's disease) may occur in adults as well as children. Signs/symptoms may include high fevers, morbilliform salmon-colored rash, generalized lymphadenopathy, hepatosplenomegaly, pericarditis, pleuritis, anemia. Polyarthritis may be present early in the course of the disease, or onset may be delayed for months or even years. There is leukocytosis and an elevated sedimentation rate, but rheumatoid factor and ANA are usually negative.

Polyarticular category is more common in girls. Fever, malaise, lymphadenopathy, and/or anemia may be present, but the extra–articular manifestations of the systemic category are otherwise absent. Besides the peripheral joints, the apophyseal joints of the cervical spine (particularly C2–3) are frequently involved. Rheumatoid factor is negative in most cases. ANA is positive in many patients.

Pauciarticular category (≤ 5 joints affected). ●In some cases, mostly girls, a positive ANA in the absence of rheumatoid factors is found. These patients have a propensity to develop iridocyclitis and this may lead to blindness. ●Some cases, mostly boys, are associated with histocompatibility antigen HLA–B27 and spinal involvement (see "Ankylosing Spondylitis").

Systemic Lupus Erythematosus (SLE) is an autoimmune inflammatory disease that may involve any organ—one organ alone or multiple organs concurrently. SLE may be recurrent or chronic. It may undergo exacerbations and remissions. Onset may occur at any age but in the majority of cases, SLE begins between 13–45 yr. About 90% patients are female. The incidence in black females is 3 times that of whites females. A genetic predilection is apparent since close relatives of patients with SLE are more likely to have SLE. The association is particularly strong between monozygotic twins (70%).

Pathogenesis: Autoantibody may combine with antigen at the site of inflammatory injury, or the antigen–antibody complex is formed elsewhere and transported to that site. In either case, the antigen–antibody complex activates the complement cascade which in turn mediates the inflammatory response with ensuing tissue injury. Immune complexes are commonly demonstrated at the glomerular basement membrane and at the dermal–epidermal junction. Vasculitis appears to play a major role in the pathogenesis of SLE, and immunoglobulin–complement deposits are also demonstrated in the blood vessels of affected organs. Histologic findings in vessel walls may include presence of inflammatory cells, endothelial hyperplasia, and/or fibrinoid necrosis. **Drug–induced SLE:** Certain drugs (e.g. procainamide, hydralazine, isoniazid) may induce an SLE–like syndrome with a positive ANA. Drug–induced SLE is distinguished by the fact that anti–nDNA antibody and anti–Sm antibody are always absent. Furthermore, renal or CNS involvement is unusual. The syndrome resolves after discontinuing the drug, although a positive ANA may persist for some time.

SIGNS/SYMPTOMS:

General: fever, fatigue, weakness, anorexia, weight loss.

Cutaneous: "Butterfly rash" is an erythematous (usually symmetrical) rash over the malar area and the bridge of the nose that occurs in about 60% cases. ●Photosensitivity is a common problem. Exposure to sunlight often provokes or exacerbates rashes and/or other manifestations of SLE. Sometimes a photosensitive maculopapular eruption resembling a drug eruption develops over the face, neck, and other light–exposed areas. ●*Discoid lupus* is the term used to describe patients with lupus confined to the skin. However, about 10% discoid patients do go on to develop SLE. The lesions of discoid lupus consist of chronic or recurrent erythematous scaling papules or plaques that are associated with plugged follicles. There may be telangiectasias, scarring, and/or hypo– or hyperpigmentation. Discoid rash is most common on the face, ears, scalp, neck, upper torso, and the extensor surfaces of the extremities. ●Other possible cutaneous manifestations of SLE include alopecia, Raynaud's phenomenon, palmar erythema, livedo reticularis, splinter hemorrhages, panniculitis.

Mucous membranes: Ulcers may occur on the oral or nasal mucosa, or in the vagina.

Joints: Migratory arthralgias occur in 90% patients; it is the most common and often the presenting complaint. However, objective evidence of joint inflammation is often absent. There may be a symmetric polyarthritis; most commonly involving the PIP and MCP joints, wrists, elbows, knees, and ankles. Mild joint deformity may occur but destructive lesions like that of rheumatoid arthritis are uncommon.

Muscle: There may be myalgias, with or without muscle tenderness, and with or without elevation of serum CPK.

Kidney disease occurs in about half the cases and is severe in 20% patients. Renal disease accounts for half of SLE fatalities. During active renal disease, there is proteinuria, and urine microscopy reveals RBC, WBC, and red and white cell casts. Renal biopsy findings in lupus glomerulonephritis vary (e.g. mesangial involvement, focal glomerulonephritis, diffuse proliferative glomerulonephritis, or membranous glomerulonephritis). Hypertension may ensue from kidney disease.

Heart: ●Myocarditis (manifesting as tachycardia) occurs in about a third of cases and is occasionally severe enough to cause CHF. ●Pericarditis is common and symptomatic but seldom leads to serious consequences such as effusion with tamponade. ●Libman–Sacks endocarditis (nonbacterial vegetations on the heart valves and chordae) is usually asymptomatic. Valvular malfunction with either systolic or diastolic murmurs sometimes occurs.

Lungs: Pleuritis develops at one time or another in many patients. There may be an associated effusion but it is usually small. Pneumonitis is usually due to infection; noninfectious pneumonitis rarely occurs. Interstitial fibrosis is uncommon.

Gastrointestinal: vomiting; abdominal pain (secondary to mesenteric arteritis or peritonitis); dysphagia (e.g. due to impaired esophageal peristalsis, due to esophageal ulceration secondary to candidal infection or arteritis).

Nervous system: seizures, chorea, depression, psychosis, peripheral neuropathy, cranial nerve deficits, migraine, stroke, aseptic meningitis, transverse myelitis.

Blood: normochromic normocytic anemia, lymphopenia, thrombocytopenia, hemolysis (with + or – Coombs' test), coagulation disorders (due to antibodies directed against coagulation factors). Purpura may result from the individual or combined effects of capillary fragility, vasculitis, thrombocytopenia, coagulation deficits, corticosteroids.

Eyes: conjunctivitis, episcleritis, keratoconjunctivitis sicca. With active CNS disease, cytoid bodies (white lesions adjacent to retinal vessels) may be seen on fundoscopic exam and be confused with exudates.

Gynecologic: irregular menses, spontaneous abortions. Disease may worsen during pregnancy, postpartum, postabortion, or during last half of menstrual cycle.

Other: lymphadenopathy, splenomegaly, hepatomegaly.

LABORATORY: There is no single pathognomonic test for SLE. **ANA (antinuclear antibodies)** is a very sensitive test for SLE. It is positive in almost all cases. The test is performed as follows: (1) the patients serum is incubated with a frozen section of animal tissue; (2) the section is subsequently washed to remove any unbound immunoglobulin, (3) then fluorescein–labeled anti–immunoglobulin is added, (4) section is then examined microscopically under UV light to determine if immunoglobulin from the patients serum has reacted with nuclear constituents of the animal tissue. A diffusely stained nucleus (indicating antibodies in the patients serum directed against DNA–histone complex) or a peripherally (rim) stained nucleus (indicating antibodies in the patients serum directed against DNA) is consistent with SLE. A speckled nuclear staining pattern of the nucleolus is consistent with scleroderma. **Anti-nDNA antibody** (antibodies in the patients serum directed against native DNA—i.e. double–stranded DNA) is one of the most specific tests for SLE. Elevated anti–nDNA antibody is found in 60–70% patients with SLE. Anti–nDNA antibody may also be found in other disorders, but this is very unusual and the titers are usually low. Anti–nDNA antibody titers correlate with disease activity, and can be used to follow the progress of therapy. **Anti–Sm antibody** is an antibody in the patients serum directed against the Sm antigen (a component of extractable nuclear antigen [ENA]). Test is specific for SLE but it is positive in only 20–30% patients. It is more likely to be positive in SLE patients with renal involvement. **LE cell reaction** is positive in 75–90% cases SLE. The test is now less commonly used because it is time–consuming, and because the ANA test is more sensitive and more specific. Furthermore, the LE cell reaction is almost never positive in a patient with SLE who is ANA negative. The basis for the LE cell phenomenon is that certain immunoglobulins in the serum of an SLE patient will react with the DNA–histone complex from nuclei of damaged cells. The resulting immunoglobulin–DNA–histone aggregates will be phagocytized by neutrophils to thus form the characteristic LE cell (a neutrophil whose cytoplasm contains a homogenous eosinophilic material that stains purple with Wright's stain). The LE cell can be demonstrated by incubating a sample of anticoagulated blood from an SLE patient (or by incubating the serum of an SLE patient with heterologous nuclear material and then adding neutrophils). LE cells are also sometimes discovered in pleural and synovial effusions of SLE patients. **Serum immunoglobulins** are elevated. **Serum complement** is decreased during active disease. **Cryoglobulins** (serum proteins that precipitate when cooled) consisting of aggregates of IgG, IgM, and complement are demonstrated during active disease. **Rheumatoid factor** is positive in about 15% cases. **Other tests:** false positive VDRL (about 20% SLE cases), elevated sedimentation rate, + Coombs test, prolonged PT and PTT.

TREATMENT is individualized. Aspirin or some other nonsteroidal anti–inflammatory drug alone may suffice in mild disease without major organ complications. For example, such agents will usually suffice for mild fever, arthralgias/arthritis, myalgia, or uncomplicated pleuritis or pericarditis. To mitigate or reduce the risk of rash patients should avoid sunlight and/or use sunscreens, avoid agents that enhance the effects of ultraviolet light (tetracyclines, psoralens), avoid sulfonamides. Hydroxychloroquine may be added if necessary to help control rash and/or arthritis. Corticosteroids: A patient with moderate disease who is not sufficiently improved with the foregoing measures, may benefit from the addition of low–dose prednisone as a daily morning dose. Once control is achieved, a morning dose on alternate days is tried. Tapering and discontinuation of prednisone may be attempted periodically. ●Major organ complications (e.g. glomerulonephritis, CNS disease, myocarditis, noninfectious pneumonitis, thrombocytopenic purpura, serious hemolytic anemia) are treated with corticosteroids (e.g. 1–2 mg/kg/day prednisone or its equivalent and increased as necessary to achieve control). The clinical response and laboratory parameters (e.g. anti–nDNA antibody, serum complement levels, urinalysis, sedimentation rate) are used to guide therapy. Slow tapering may be tried once control is achieved. Azathioprine (an immunosuppressant) may be used in conjunction with corticosteroids for the treatment of glomerulonephritis if corticosteroids alone are not sufficiently effective.

Polymyositis
is an inflammatory disease of skeletal muscle. About a third of patients also have involvement of the skin (**dermatomyositis**). About 10% of patients with polymyositis have a coexisting malignancy, and the majority of these patients have dermatomyositis. Polymyositis is twice as common in females. Females outnumber males by an even greater margin when polymyositis or dermatomyositis is associated with other connective tissue disorders (see "Mixed Connective Tissue Disease"), but the male to female incidence is roughly equal in cases associated with malignancy.

Signs/symptoms: Symmetrical muscle weakness develops slowly—first the hips and proximal leg muscles (e.g. difficulty walking up stairs) and then the shoulder and proximal arm muscles. With progressive disease; weakness of the distal muscles, abdominal muscles, and neck flexors may develop. Dysphagia may appear with involvement of posterior pharyngeal muscles and striated muscle of upper esophagus. Weakness of facial or extraocular muscles can occur. Muscular atrophy occurs in about half and contractures in about a fourth or cases. Muscle tenderness or pain is present in about half the patients. Rash; Patients with *dermato*myositis have a red scaly rash over the elbows, PIP and MCP joints, knees, medial maleoli, and frequently the face. Sometimes there is the pathognomic lilac rash on the upper eyelids (heliotrope rash). Arthralgias or arthritis is present in about a fourth of patients but is usually not serious. Heart block or heart failure develops in ≤ 5% patients. Pulmonary disease occurs in a few patients (pulmonary fibrosis, interstitial pneumonitis). A coexisting malignancy is present in about 10% patients. Therefore, evidence of neoplasia must be sought, especially in a patient over 40.

Laboratory: Serum CPK is virtually always found to be elevated at some point in the disease course. The CPK rises as disease activity increases. Other enzymes are also released from injured muscle and may be elevated in the serum (e.g. SGOT, SGPT, LDH). Myoglobin is also released from damaged muscle and the serum levels increase during active disease. Sedimentation rate is an unreliable indicator of disease activity. ANA and/or rheumatoid factor are sometimes positive, particularly when polymyositis is associated with mixed connective tissue disease (overlap syndrome). Electromyographic findings; fibrillation, repetitive runs of high frequency action potentials, voluntary muscle contraction–associated low–amplitude short–duration polyphasic potentials. Muscle biopsy reveals inflammatory cells together with degeneration/necrosis of muscle fibers. EKG is sometimes abnormal (e.g. nonspecific ST–T abnormalities, Q waves, bundle branch block, arrhythmias).

Treatment: Prednisone 50–100 mg/day, depending on the clinical severity, is the usual adult regimen. The serum CPK and clinical response is used to guide therapy. As the CPK returns to normal (usually over 1–3 months), prednisone is slowly tapered. When clinical condition permits, prednisone may be tried as a single AM dose (or as a single alternate–day AM dose) in order to reduce corticosteroid side effects. In many cases, chronic therapy will be required (7.5–20 mg/day). Immunosuppression (azathioprine or methotrexate) is indicated in patients who fail to respond to prednisone after 1–2 months. Resection of a tumor may result in a complete remission of polymyositis/dermatomyositis and thereby preempt drug therapy.

Scleroderma
(progressive systemic sclerosis) is a connective tissue disease of unknown cause that may involve multiple organs (e.g. skin, joints, GI tract, lungs, heart, kidneys). The nervous system is seldom involved primarily. Female to male incidence is 4: 1. Onset is usually between 20 and 50 years of age. **CREST syndrome** is a variant of scleroderma (see below). **Overlap syndrome** refers to a syndrome in which scleroderma is associated with manifestations of one or any combination of the following: lupus, rheumatoid arthritis, polymyositis. See "Mixed Connective Tissue Disease" chapter as an example. **Histology** of involved tissues discloses collagen deposition and endothelial hyperplasia in the arteries/arterioles with reduction or obliteration of the vessel lumina. Capillaries are dilated and reduced in number. The vascular changes are accompanied by inflammation with subsequent fibrosis of the skin and other affected organs. **Prognosis** is variable. The disease may follow a relatively benign and protracted course consistent with a long life. Others may suffer rapidly progressive renal failure with malignant hypertension; or have severe complicating pulmonary, cardiac, or GI disease.

Signs/symptoms: Raynaud's phenomenon (cold–induced cyanosis and pallor of the digits) may precede other signs of scleroderma by months or years. Scleroderma; Initially, there is edema—typically of the fingers which may assume a sausage–like appearance. As edema resolves the skin becomes tight and thick (scleroderma) and eventually becomes taut and shiny. Scleroderma of the digits is called sclerodactyly. Skin changes are symmetric and may be restricted to the fingers or to a varying extent involve the rest of the extremities, trunk, face, or entire body. A diffuse melanotic hyperpigmentation may develop, or there may be patchy hypopigmentation. Telangiectasias may eventually appear. Skin ulcers may develop, particularly on the fingertips and over the finger joints. The tight skin contributes to joint immobility. Facial Involvement results in loss of skin folds, pursed lips, and reduced facial expression. The skin becomes progressively atrophied. <u>Subcutaneous calcinosis</u> may develop. Palpable calcifications are most commonly found on the fingertips, or over the knees or elbows. X-ray of the fingers shows the subcutaneous calcifications, and may disclose resorption of the phalangeal tufts. <u>Joint pain/stiffness</u> is a common complaint and may be the initial complaint. There is fibrosis of the synovium and also fibrosis of the tendon sheaths so that a friction rub may be felt over an involved joint and tendon. Tendinous calcinosis may also be present. Joint stiffness/immobility is due to the combined effects of the tight skin overlying the joint, contractures of involved tendons and fascia, and muscle contractures. <u>Myositis</u> resembling polymyositis (elevated CPK and proximal muscle weakness) is a not an uncommon development. Muscle atrophy may ensue. <u>Gastrointestinal</u>: Esophageal dysmotility is present in 90% patients; it is due to atrophy and fibrosis of the smooth muscle (lower 2/3 of esophagus). Inadequate or absent esophageal peristalsis results in dysphagia. Lower esophageal sphincter incompetence leads to reflux esophagitis which in turn may lead to esophageal ulceration and/or stricture. Esophageal hypomotility and dilation of the lower 2/3 of the esophagus is demonstrated on barium swallow. Often, the remainder of the GI tract is also involved. GI series may show intestinal hypomotility; dilated 2nd and 3rd segments of duodenum (loop sign); and/or wide mouthed diverticula (sacculations) of the jejunum, ileum, and/or colon. Atrophy of the muscularis mucosa may allow air to enter the bowel wall (pneumotosis intestinales). Stagnation of intestinal contents from GI hypomotility leads to bacterial overgrowth with ensuing malabsorption and weight loss. Intestinal hypomotility may be severe enough to provoke signs consistent with intestinal obstruction (e.g. vomiting, bloating, abdominal distension). Not surprisingly, constipation is a common complaint. <u>Pulmonary</u> Interstitial and alveolar fibrosis may develop. Chest x-ray will then reveal interstitial fibrosis. Dyspnea on exertion, nonproductive cough, rales are common manifestations. Recurrent episodes of pleuritis (associated with pleural friction rub) and pneumonia are not uncommon. Pulmonary function testing initially shows a reduced diffusing capacity (decreased diffusing capacity carbon monoxide). As pulmonary fibrosis progresses, further testing reveals abnormalities consistent with both obstructive and restrictive lung disease (decreased vital capacity, increased residual lung volume, reduced total lung capacity). <u>Cardiac</u> disease may be the consequence of fibrosis of the myocardium or be due to pulmonary disease. Fibrosis of the conducting system may lead to heart block and arrhythmias. Cardiac failure ensues if there is extensive fibrous replacement of the myocardium. Pericarditis/pericardial effusion is occasionally seen. Pulmonary hypertension with cor pulmonale is a rare development in the diffuse form of scleroderma but is not uncommon with the CREST syndrome (see below). <u>Renal</u> disease occurs in about a fourth of patients with diffuse scleroderma. There is glomerulosclerosis with intimal proliferation and fibrinoid necrosis of the small renal arteries and arterioles. Proteinuria, microscopic hematuria, and hypertension are common. Acute renal failure develops in many cases and is almost always associated with development of malignant hypertension.

Laboratory: <u>ANA</u> (antinuclear antibodies) are found in over two thirds cases (often with a speckled or nucleolar immmunofluorescence pattern). About a third of patients with diffuse form of scleroderma have ANA directed against the scleroderma–70 nuclear antigen but rarely against the centromere (these tests help distinguish the diffuse form of scleroderma from the CREST syndrome, see below). <u>Rheumatoid factor</u> is positive in about a third of patients. <u>Urinalysis</u>: Patients with hypertensive renal involvement typically have proteinuria, microscopic hematuria, and urinary casts. <u>Hematology</u>: Chronic disease–associated normochromic normocytic anemia is common. Malabsorption–induced folate or B–12 deficiency may lean the anemia toward a macrocytic profile. If there is blood loss because of esophageal ulceration, there will be a tendency toward microcytic hypochromic anemia.

Treatment: Avoid cold or other inducers of vasospasm (e.g. nicotine, caffeine). <u>Reflux esophagitis</u>: antacids, H2–antagonist (cimetidine or ranitidine). See "Gastroesophageal Reflux" chapter. <u>Malabsorption</u> due to bacterial overgrowth is treated with broad spectrum antibiotic (e.g. tetracycline). <u>Hypertension</u> is treated with captopril. <u>Corticosteroids</u> are generally not helpful. They are sometimes tried if severe myositis or rapidly worsening interstitial lung disease develops.

CREST SYNDROME (calcinosis, Raynaud's phenomenon, esophageal dysmotility, sclerodactyly, telangectasia) is a variant of scleroderma that usually follows a more benign course. **Distinguishing features:** <u>Skin</u>: Edema with subsequent thickening of the skin is restricted to the fingers. <u>Subcutaneous calcinosis</u> tends to be more prominent. <u>Kidneys</u> are seldom affected. <u>Pulmonary fibrosis</u> is rare. <u>Myositis and arthritis</u> are less common. <u>Myocardium</u> is involved in < 5% cases. <u>Esophagus</u> is as commonly involved (90% cases) as in diffuse scleroderma. <u>Pulmonary hypertension and cor pulmonale</u> develop in about 10% cases as a conseuence of fibrosis of the small pulmonary arteries. <u>A distinguishing laboratory feature</u> is the presence of antinuclear antibody directed against the centromere in 70–90% CREST patients—a finding observed in ≤ 10% of patients with diffuse scleroderma. Furthermore, antibody to the scleroderma 70 antigen is rarely found in CREST patients.

Mixed Connective Tissue Disease

(MCTD) is an autoimmune disorder which shares some of the features of 3 other connective tissue diseases: scleroderma, polymyositis, and systemic lupus. ANA is positive with a speckled immunofluorescence pattern. Corticosteroid therapy is frequently beneficial.

Sjögren's Syndrome is a chronic autoimmune disorder whose

salient feature is the decreased secretion of saliva and tears (sicca complex). These glands and other involved organs are infiltrated with lymphocytes and plasma cells. Women account for over 90% of cases. A genetic predilection to Sjögren's syndrome is suggested by the fact that there is a common association with certain HLA antigens (e.g. B8, DR3). Another autoimmune disease is found in about half the cases (e.g. rheumatoid arthritis, lupus, scleroderma, polymyostis, primary biliary cirrhosis). Lymphoma is a not uncommon development in patients with Sjögren's syndrome.

Signs/symptoms: Dry eyes (xerophthalmia) is due to decreased tear production by the lacrimal glands which are damaged by chronic inflammation. The Schirmer test may be positive (< 5 mm wetting of a piece of filter paper placed on conjunctiva for 5 minutes). Photosensitivity, reddened conjunctiva, a gritty foreign body sensation of the eyes, and decreased visual acuity are typical manifestations. Staphylococcal conjunctivitis is a not uncommon complication. Keratoconjunctivitis sicca refers to the erosive lesions of the cornea and bulbar conjunctiva that result from prolonged xerophthalmia. These superficial erosions are made readily visible by applying rose bengal stain. Sloughing of the corneal epithelium is revealed on slit–lamp exam by the presence of corneal debris and corneal filaments. Dry mouth (xerostomia) is due to decreased salivary gland secretion. The severity of xerostomia is not predictably related to the severity of xerophthalmia. Dysphagia is common. Dysphagia may be aggravated by impaired secretion of the esophageal mucosal glands. The lips, tongue, and buccal mucosa may be dry, cracked, and ulcerated. There is a predilection to dental caries. Parotid glands may enlarge because of lymphocytic infiltration and/or salivatory duct obstruction. This may be a chronic painless phenomemon or there may be recurrent painful episodes. Respiratory: Dryness of the larynx and tracheobronchial tree may lead to hoarseness and to respiratory infections. Dyspnea may occur as a consequence of interstitial pneumonitis and/or obstructive disease (both associated with lymphocytic infiltration). Nasal mucosa may be dry and epistaxis may result. Sense of smell and taste may be impaired. Ears: The eustachian tubes may be blocked by inspissated secretions. Otitis media and hearing loss may ensue. Vaginal dryness with dyspareunia may occur. Gastrointestinal: Decreased gastric acid secretion and pancreatic insufficiency may develop. Other findings may include Raynaud's phenomenon, dependent nonthrombocytopenic purpura (usually associated with polyclonal hypergammaglobulinemia), renal tubular acidosis (associated with renal interstitial lymphocytic infiltration), vasculitis–associated peripheral and cranial neuropathy.

Laboratory: Histology: Biopsy of minor salivary glands of the lower lip confirms the diagnosis by revealing infiltration by lymphocytes and plasma cells. ANA (antinuclear antibodies) are present in 50–80% cases. Antibodies to the nucleoprotein antigens SS–A and SS–B are helpful diagnostically but both may also be positive in systemic lupus. Antibody to SS–B is the more specific for Sjögren'syndrome since it is less often positive in lupus. Rheumatoid factor is positive in about 75% cases. Polyclonal hypergammaglobulinemia is found in over half the cases. Anemia, leukopenia, and elevated sedimentation rate are often found.

Treatment: Dry eyes are treated with 0.5% methylcellulose eye drops. Staphylococcal blepharitis is treated with either topical or parenteral antibiotics according to clinical judgment. Dry mouth may be alleviated by increased fluid intake and sucking sour sugarless candies. Dental hygiene including plaque control is essential since there is a predilection to dental caries. Vaginal dryness may be relieved with topical preparations (e.g. proprionic acid gel). Diuretics are avoided if possible because they may further impair salivary and lacrimal gland secretion. Corticosteroids or other immunosuppressants are reserved for severe pulmonary or renal disease, or for those who are seriously disabled by the disease.

Reiter's Syndrome in many cases follows a sexually acquired

infection (e.g. Chlamydia trachomatis) or an episode of bacterial dysentery (shigella, salmonella, Yersinia enterocolitica). However, a causal relationship has not been established. A genetic predisposition is likely since many patients are found to have the HLA–B27 antigen. Over 90% patients are male, usually young adult males.

Signs/symptoms: Triad of urethritis, conjunctivitis, and arthritis is the classical presentation. Sometimes, however, only 2 of these are present—perhaps because the other symptom was mild or evanescent. Besides the triad, mucocutaneous lesions are common (balanitis, stomatitis, keratodermia blennorrhagicum). Reiter's syndrome may have a gradual or sudden onset. A low–grade fever is common. The disease may be self–limited or the patient have relapses or chronic symptoms. Urethritis often heralds the syndrome. There is dysuria with a (usually clear) mucoid discharge. Cystitis may accompany the urethritis. Conjunctivitis most often manifests as a mild reddening and burning of the conjunctiva. A minority of patients have more severe inflammation progressing to uveitis and/or corneal ulceration that left untreated may lead to visual impairment. Arthritis is asymmetric and can involve any joint but has a predilection for knees, ankles, or metatarsophalangeal joints. The affected joint is swollen and warm. Arthritis tends to persist after conjunctivitis and urethritis have disappeared. About half the patients have recurrent episodes of arthritis, sometimes over a period of several years. Sacroiliitis and spondylitis are common. About 15% of those so affected eventually develop ankylosing spondylitis. Tendinitis with periostitis at the insertion of the Achilles and patellar tendons is common. Periostitis may also develop over the distal tibia, the plantar surface of the heel or other tarsal bones, metatarsals, or toes. Circinate balanitis is a painless condition of the glans penis. Initially there are small vesicles. These may later evolve into larger confluent lesions. Stomatitis may develop. There are small painless vesicles on the tongue and buccal mucosa that progress to painless ulcers. Keratodermia blennorrhagicum, if it occurs, is most likely to manifest on the soles. There are painless hyperkeratotic papules/pustules that subsequently desquamate. Such lesions appear at other sites less frequently (e.g. palms).

Laboratory: Gonorrhea must be excluded—e.g. negative gram stain of urethral discharge. Hematology: There may be leukocytosis, elevated sedimentation rate, normochromic normocytic anemia. HLA-B27 antigen is positive in about 75% whites and about a third of blacks. X-ray findings may include demineralization of bone adjacent to affected joints; fluffy areas of new bone formation (e.g. of calcaneous, tarsal bones); vertebral syndesmophytes.

Treatment: ●Rest. ●Nonsteroidal anti-inflammatory drug (e.g. aspirin, ibuprofen, indomethacin). ●Ophthalmologist should follow the patient.

Ankylosing Spondylitis (AS) is an inflammatory disease

of unknown cause whose primary foci are the sacroiliac joints and the spine. Inflammation of affected joints ultimately leads to fibrosis and ossification with ensuing ankylosis (= joint stiffening or fixation). Onset is usually between 10 and 30 years of age. Predisposing factors: The disorder is most common in whites and in males. A genetic predisposition is likely since over 90% white patients have the HLA-B27 antigen compared to about 10% of the white population in general. About 20% HLA-B27 positive individuals develop AS. AS is less common in blacks. Furthermore, only about half of black AS patients are HLA-B27 positive.

Signs/symptoms: Typically, there is insidious onset of aching low back pain, and morning stiffness that is relieved by exercise. About 10% patients experience pain in the sciatic distribution. Over a period of months to years there is progressive ascending involvement of the lumbar and then thoracic spine, and in some cases the neck is affected. Lumbar spine: The normal lumbar lordotic curve becomes progressively flattened. The loss of lumbar mobility may be demonstrated by having the patient bend forward to touch his toes and observing that the lumbar lordotic curve may not reverse itself as is normally the case but remains flat. Lumbar tenderness and muscle spasm are characteristic. Cervical spine: Decreased mobility of the neck may be noted. Thoracic spine: In severe cases the patient may assume a stooped posture and kyphosis (hump back) may develop. Costovertebral joints are also involved and this may restrict chest expansion. Large peripheral joints are affected in about a third of cases (shoulders, hips, and/or knees). Fatigue and weight loss may occur.

Extra-articular complications: Anterior uveitis occurs in about 25% patients and there may be recurrent episodes. This condition is usually self-limited but topical corticosteroids are occasionally required. Cardiac conduction abnormalities (e.g. 1st degree heart block) develop in 10% patients. Aortic regurgitation (due to medial necrosis of the proximal aorta with ensuing dilation of the aortic ring) occurs in 1–4% cases. Pulmonary fibrosis of the upper lobes occurs in some patients with severe disease and may be associated with cough and dyspnea. Cauda equina syndrome (urinary and rectal incontinence with leg pain) is an unusual complication of advanced disease.

X-ray findings: The spine and sacroiliac joints are symmetrically affected. Sacroiliac joint: The first sign is seen on the iliac side of the sacroiliac joint where there is blurring of the margins of the subchondral bone. Bone erosion with subsequent sclerosis progresses on both sides of the sacroiliac joint so that there is narrowing of the joint space. After several years the joint space is obliterated and the joint is fused. The same process takes place in the vertebral apophyseal joints and costovertebral joints. Vertebrae: Bony erosion of the anteroinferior and anterosuperior corners of the vertebral bodies leads to "squaring" of the vertebral bodies. The anterior and lateral spinal ligaments calcify. Bony bridges linking adjacent vertebrae (syndesmophytes) may develop as a consequence of ossification of the outer layer of the anulus fibrosus and adjacent fibrous tissue. After many years the squaring and calcification process may progress to the point that x-ray reveals the vertebral column to have a profile resembling bamboo ("bamboo spine"). This is unusual however.

Laboratory: Test for HLA–B27 is obtained if one is unsure of the diagnosis. HLA–B27 is found in > 90% of white patients and about half of black American patients. Sedimentation rate is often elevated.

Treatment: ●Aspirin or some other nonsteroidal anti–inflammatory agent for pain. ●Corticosteroids are <u>not</u> indicated. ●Exercises directed toward maintaining flexibility of the back are encouraged. ●Patient should sleep on a firm mattress with a small pillow in order to minimize flexion of the back and neck respectively. ●Surgery may become necessary if there is deformity.

Gout is an arthritis of the peripheral joints that results from the deposition of sodium urate crystals within the joints. Gout is associated with hyperuricemia—a necessary condition for the development of gout. Normally, the serum uric acid is < 7 mg/100ml in women and < 8 mg/100ml in men.

In primary gout, hyperuricemia is due to an inherited error in purine metabolism—either decreased renal clearance of uric acid or overproduction of uric acid, or a combination thereof. <u>Over 99% cases of primary gout are idiopathic:</u> 95% are male, family history of gout is common, onset most common in the 30–40s. <u>In the remaining < 1% cases of primary gout,</u> a specific inherited enzymatic defect leading to overproduction of uric acid is identified—e.g. Lesch–Nyhan sydrome (X–linked absence of hypoxanthine–guanine phosphoribosyl tranferase), von Gierke's glycogen storage disease.

In secondary gout hyperuricemia is the consequence of <u>increased production of uric acid due to increased turnover of nucleic acids</u> (e.g. leukemia, multiple myeloma, polycythemia vera, chronic hemolysis); <u>or decreased renal excretion uric acid</u> (e.g. diuretics, renal failure, lactic acidosis, ketoacidosis, fasting, hypovolemia).

ACUTE GOUTY ARTHRITIS:

Signs/symptoms: In the first few attacks the majority of patients experience sudden onset of pain in a single joint—most often podagra (gouty inflammation of the MT joint of the great toe), less frequently the instep, ankle, knee, wrist, finger, or elbow. As the disease progresses, acute attacks tend to involve 2 or more of these joints. The hip and shoulder are uncommonly involved, and the sacroiliac and spine seldom involved. The attack often begins at night without warning. Sometimes an attack appears to be brought on by overindulgence in food or alcohol, trauma, or infection. An affected joint becomes intensely painful and tender over several minutes to a few hours. The joint is warm, swollen, and the overlying skin is tense and dusky red to purple. Untreated, an attack may depending on the severity last from a few days to a few weeks. The overlying skin may desquamate as the attack resolves. Fever, chills, elevated sedimentation rate, leukocytosis may attend the attack. The course is unpredictable; ranging from a single episode to increasingly frequent attacks.

Diagnosis of acute gout: Gout may be strongly suspected when there is typical presentation (i.e. sudden onset of severe pain in a single joint of the lower extremity, particularly the great toe) together with a serum uric acid > 7–8 mg/100ml. However, the serum uric acid measurement may be misleading because the serum uric acid may paradoxically decrease during a gouty attack; and conversely there are many individuals with hyperuricemia who never experience gout. A family history of gout, history of renal stones, presence of tophi are additional diagnostic clues. <u>Synovial fluid analysis:</u> The diagnosis of gout is confirmed by examining a sample of synovial fluid from an inflamed joint. To make the diagnosis conclusively, one must find negatively birefringent needle–shaped urate crystals *within* leukocytes. During a quiescent phase of gout, urate crystals may be seen but not within leukocytes. Thus, the finding of extraleukocytic urate crystals alone does not prove that the acute attack of joint pain/inflammation is due to gout. Other synovial fluid findings characteristic of gouty arthritis include cloudy appearance, low viscosity, poor mucin clot test, WBC 1000–100,000 (usually 10,000–20,000) with 60–70% neutrophils. Also, the synovial glucose is no more than 25 mg/dl less than a simultaneously obtained serum glucose. Remember to obtain a gram stain of the synovial fluid in order to rule out septic arthritis. Diagnostic aspiration of a joint in a gout patient is not required in succeeding attacks if the presentation is straightforward. A dramatic response to colchicine may help make the diagnosis of gout (if synovial fluid analysis is not confirmatory) because colchicine will not mask septic arthritis–associated signs of periarticular inflammation as might a conventional anti–inflammatory drug such as indomethacin. It should be remembered, however, that a less marked response to colchicine is also observed in pseudogout and sarcoid arthritis.

Treatment of acute gout: see below.

CHRONIC TOPHACEOUS GOUT develops in 50–60% untreated gout patients, and tends to be more extensive the more elevated the serum uric acid. Tophi are uncommon in those with serum uric acid < 8.5 mg/100ml. Tophi consist of deposits of monosodium urate monohydrate. **Tophi are most often found** in and about the joints (particularly of the hands and feet), the bursae (e.g. olecranon bursa), and tendon sheaths (particularly the Achilles and infrapatellar), extensor surface of the forearm, external ear. Rare tophaceous sites include nasal cartilage, tongue, epiglottis, vocal cords, myocardium, aorta. The lungs, spleen, liver, and CNS are spared. **Consequences of tophi:** Tophi are generally painless. Inflammation resulting from tophaceous deposits about articular surfaces leads to erosion of cartilage and subchondral bone. As a consequence, the involved joints become deformed and there is limitation of movement. Subcutaneous tophi may rupture releasing a chalky or pasty white substance. **X–rays** may reveal "punched–out" radiolucent areas representing urate deposits.

NEPHROPATHY is present in most cases of chronic tophaceous gout. Deposits of sodium urate crystals together with inflammatory cells are found in the renal interstitium. There are degenerative changes in the glomeruli, tubules, and arterioles. While a significant percentage of patients with gout eventually develop renal failure, it is not certain what role gout plays. This is because gout is frequently associated with other conditions known to contribute to renal failure (e.g. hypertension, renovascular disease, diabetes mellitus, pyelonephritis, renal stones). **Uric acid nephropathy** refers to the condition in which urate precipitates in and blocks the renal tubules, collecting ducts, and ureters. This condition may occur when there is marked hyperuricemia due to high turnover of nucleic acids (e.g. lymphoproliferative disease, chemotherapy of neoplasia). Renal failure may ensue. **Urate nephrolithiasis:** refer to "Nephrolithiasis".

TREATMENT OF GOUT:

  General measures: Avoid foods high in purines such as organ meats (e.g. liver, kidney, brain); sardines; anchovies. Weight reduction if obese. However, rapid weight loss is discouraged as this may increase the risk of attacks. Intemperate ethanol ingestion is discouraged—particularly beer and wine. Liberal fluid intake is advised in order to lessen the likelihood of uric acid precipitating in the urine, and thereby lessen the risk of uric acid nephropathy and uric acid nephrolithiasis. Allopurinol is used prophylactically in conditions where nucleic acid turnover is high (e.g. myeloproliferative disease, chemotherapy of neoplasia).

  Treatment of an acute gouty attack: Therapy should if possible begin when the patient feels an attack is imminent. By this expedient an attack is often averted. Indomethacin is the drug most commonly used to treat an acute gout attack (see drug section). Other nonsteroidal anti–inflammatory agents such as ibuprofen may also be effective. Colchicine is an alternative to indomethacin, but intolerable GI side effects are often associated with the large doses of PO colchicine required to treat an acute attack. If, however, the diagnosis is is doubt and the possibility of septic arthritis cannot be excluded, colchicine may be preferred to indomethacin for two reasons: (1) colchicine will not mask the signs of septic arthritis–associated periarticular inflammation as might indomethacin or some other nonsteroidal anti–inflammatory drug; (2) a dramatic response to colchicine makes the diagnosis of gout likely. Remember, however, that arthritic flareups due to pseudogout or sarcoid may also show some response to colchicine. It is emphasized that colchicine should be started as soon as possible and certainly no later than 24 hr after the onset of an attack. About 25% patients will fail to respond if therapy is not initiated within 12 hours of onset. <u>Intravenous colchicine</u> brings about a speedier response (4–12 hours) than PO colchicine (24–48 hours). Furthermore, GI side effects are infrequent by the intravenous route.

Once the attack subsides: <u>If the acute attack is being treated with colchicine,</u> the dosage is reduced to a maintenance preventive dose (see drug section). <u>If the acute attack is being treated with indomethacin,</u> the dose is reduced over 2–3 days, and then discontinued when the patient is asymptomatic. At that point, colchicine at a maintenance dose may be initiated to prevent further attacks. Because of side effects, the longterm use of indomethacin to prevent gout attacks is discouraged. However, indomethacin may again be reinstituted at the first sign of an attack. <u>When the patient is no longer symptomatic,</u> attention is turned to reducing serum uric acid levels.

Lowering blood urate levels: <u>Urate–lowering drugs are advised</u> (**1**) if there are recurrent attacks, (**2**) if tophi are present, (**3**) if there is radiographic evidence of urate deposits, (**4**) if there is renal damage, (**5**) if there is severe hyperuricemia—i.e. serum uric acid > 10 mg/100ml. <u>When to begin urate–lowering therapy:</u> ●Urate-lowering drugs are of no use in the treatment of an acute gouty attack and should not be started during an acute episode. If the patient is already on an urate–lowering drug when an acute gout strikes, that drug should be continued at the same dosage. ●Initially, gouty attacks may actually increase with urate–lowering therapy unless maintenance doses of colchicine are given concurrently for 6–18 months. Urate–lowering drugs are begun after the patient has been on maintenance doses of colchicine for a few days. <u>Allopurinol,</u> an inhibitor of uric acid synthesis, is the drug most often used to reduce serum urate levels (see drug section). It is the drug of choice in patients whose gout stems from the overproduction of uric acid (i.e. patients whose urinary uric acid excretion exceeds 800–1000 mg/24 hr) or in patients with renal failure. The uricosuric drugs <u>probenecid</u> or <u>sulfinpyrazone</u> are alternatives to allopurinol but there are drawbacks. They enhance renal excretion of uric acid but there effectiveness diminishes when the GFR is < 80 ml/min and they are not effective if the GFR is < 30 mg/min. Furthermore, they should not be used if the 24 hour urinary excretion of uric acid exceeds 800 mg/day or if high fluid intake cannot be assured. This is because high urinary uric acid concentrations increase the likelihood of uric acid precipitation, and therefore increase the risk of uric acid nephropathy and uric acid stone formation. <u>The goal of therapy</u> is to reduce and maintain the serum uric acid to ≤ 6 mg/100ml. To that end, one should periodically measure the serum uric acid level.

Asymptomatic hyperuricemia: There is debate as to what level the serum uric acid must reach before asymptomatic hyperuricemia is treated. About 50% patients with serum uric acid > 11mg/100ml or with urinary excretion > 1100 mg/24 hr will develop uric acid stones. Thus, it is reasonable to treat these individuals with allopurinol, particularly if there is a strong family history of gout.

Chondrocalcinosis and Pseudogout

<u>Chondrocalcinosis</u> is defined as the deposition of calcium pyrophosphate dihydrate (CPPD) crystals on cartilage. Why CPPD deposition occurs is unknown. <u>Pseudogout</u> is the inflammatory arthritis that results from the presence of CPPD crystals in the synovial fluid. <u>Risk factors:</u> Chondrocalcinosis occurs in males as often as females. However, pseudogout attacks are more common in men. Chondrocalcinosis is common in the elderly and is often associated with osteoarthritis. The incidence of chondrocalcinosis is increased in gout, hyperparathyroidism, myxedema, hypomagnesemia, hypophosphatasia, hemochromatosis, Wilson's disease, ochronosis, acromegaly. Familial cases of chondrocalcinosis have also been identified.

Signs/symptoms: Many patients with chondrocalcinosis are asymptomatic. In an acute attack there is a sudden onset of joint pain with signs of inflammation, usually in a single joint (most often the knee). Besides the knee, any of the large peripheral joints are commonly involved. The joints of the hands and wrists are less often affected. Without treatment an attack may last a few days to weeks. Some patients have chronic inflammation. Flexion contractures may eventually develop.

X-rays: Chondrocalcinosis is recognized on x-rays in about 75% pseudogout patients by the presence of linear or punctate calcifications in the hyaline and fibrocartilage of the knee, hip, shoulder, or other synovial joints. The lateral meniscus of the knee and the fibrocartilage of the distal radioulnar joint are particularly common sites of calcification. Calcifications may also be seen in the intervertebral disks or the symphysis pubis.

Synovial fluid analysis: Diagnosis of chondrocalcinosis is confirmed by finding rhomboid or rod-shaped CPPD crystals (free or within leukocytes) in the synovial fluid. Viewed under polarizing microscope, the crystals are weakly positive birefringent. This contrasts with the negative birefringent urate crystals characteristic of gout. Both CPPD and urate crystals may be seen in patients with coexisting gout. During an inflammatory episode the synovial fluid is cloudy and has a low viscosity. The synovial fluid WBC count is elevated (3000–50,000) with a left shift. Between inflammatory episodes, the synovial fluid is clear with normal WBC count, but CPPD crystals may still be identified.

Treatment: A pseudogout attack is treated with a nonsteroidal anti-inflammatory drug (e.g. indomethacin, ibuprofen). If necessary, aspiration of the joint fluid will provide relief. Colchicine is an alternate therapy for pseudogout but tends to be less effective than in gout. Patients who experience frequent pseudogout attacks may be prescribed chronic maintenance doses of colchicine or a nonsteroidal drug (e.g. ibuprofen).

Osteoarthritis (degenerative joint disease). DJD is a noninflammatory disease that may involve both diarthrodial (synovial) joints and amphiarthrodial joints (e.g. intervertebral disk). DJD is the most common joint disorder and becomes progressively more prevalent with age so that nearly all persons are affected by age 70. Osteoarthritis is particularly likely to develop in joints that have been damaged by trauma, gout, rheumatoid arthritis, ischemia, hemophilia, ochronosis, acromegaly.

Pathogenesis: The progressive deterioration of cartilage is attributed to mechanical stress/trauma and metabolic factors. With time the cartilage degenerates—thins, cracks, and may eventually disappear and thus expose subchondral bone. Then there is remodeling of the subchondral bone and proliferation of bone at the margins of the joint (osteophytes).

Signs/symptoms depend on the joint(s) affected. In general, the patient complains of pain that is aggravated by movement or weight-bearing, and morning stiffness. Overuse of an affected joint may result in effusion. Heberden's nodes are deformities of the DIP joints of hands due to bony protruberances at the base of the distal phalanx. They are more common in women and there is a familial predilection. Bouchard's nodes are similar osteoarthritic deformities of the PIP joints of the hand. Osteoarthritis of the hip (coxarthrosis): Pain is felt mostly in the groin with referred pain along the medial thigh and knee (i.e. the distribution of the obturator nerve). Pain is aggravated by movement or weight-bearing. Coxarthrosis often occurs against a background of prior hip disorder (e.g. slipped capital epiphysis, congenital hip dysplasia, Legg-Calvé-Perthes disease, avascular necrosis femoral head, rheumatoid arthritis). Osteoarthritis of the knees may manifest as crepitus, effusion, reduced range of movement, bowleg or flexion deformity. Chondromalacia patellae is a distinct form of osteoarthritis of the knee. In many cases, it is attributed to trauma. It is most often seen in the young. Effusions are common. Osteoarthritis of the spine is most common in the spinal segments with the most movement—the neck and lumbar spine. Osteophytes (spurs) may cause neurologic abnormalities by encroaching either on the vertebral foramen and compressing the spinal cord, or by encroaching on the intervertebral foramina and impinging on the nerve roots. Neurologic difficulties may also occur when a degenerative intervertebral disk herniates posteriorly into the spinal cord or laterally against a nerve root. In addition to osteophytes, x-rays may reveal narrowing of the intervertebral space and degenerative changes in the interfacetal joints. Encroachment of osteophytes on the intervertebral foramina may be seen on oblique views. Spinal osteoarthritis is often asymptomatic despite x-ray evidence of severe degeneration.

Laboratory: If an joint effusion is tapped, the synovial fluid is found to be clear, yellow, viscous, and the mucin clot test is good. Synovial WBC count is < 3000 with < 30% neutrophils.

Treatment: <u>Conservative measures</u> consist of rest, local heat, and analgesics (e.g. acetaminophen, aspirin, ibuprofen). In the event that a weight–bearing joint is involved, additional measures might include weight reduction, proper shoes, crutches or cane. Patients with cervical osteoarthritis may benefit from wearing a cervical collar. <u>Surgery:</u> Spinal surgery is indicated if there is spinal involvement with neurologic dysfunction. Surgical options for osteoarthritis of the knee or hip may include debridement, osteotomy, arthroplasty, arthrodesis (joint fusion), joint replacement.

Septic Arthritis may be due to bacteria, fungi, or virus.

ACUTE BACTERIAL ARTHRITIS: The infecting organism usually arrives at a joint via the blood; less frequently by contiguous spread from the bone or by direct traumatic introduction. <u>Pathogens:</u> Staphylococcus aureus is the most common culprit. However, in young sexually active persons, gonococcal arthritis is more common (see below). Less common pathogens include streptococci (pneumococcus, S. pyogenes, S. viridans); meningococci; E.coli; pseudomonas; salmonellae; H. influenza (in young children). <u>Risk factors:</u> prior joint trauma, rheumatoid arthritis, sickle cell anemia, diabetes mellitus, chronic alcoholism, IV drug abuse, promiscuous sex (because of the risk of gonococcal infection), immuodeficiency (including immunodeficiency secondary to administration of corticosteroids or other immunosuppressants).

Signs/symptoms: An involved joint is usually painful, tender, warm, swollen. In most cases, a single joint is involved (gonococcal arthritis is often an exception to this generalization, see below). The knee is the most frequently involved joint. Fever and chills are common.

Laboratory: <u>Synovial fluid analysis:</u> Needle aspiration of a joint must always be performed if there is any suspicion of joint infection. Joint aspiration has both diagnostic and therapeutic value. The synovial fluid should be gram stained and cultured (aerobic and anaerobic). Synovial fluid is characteristically opaque; mucin clot test is poor; crystals are generally not present. Synovial WBC count is typically 20,000–100,000 with > 75% neutrophils. <u>Leukocytosis</u> is common. <u>Cultures:</u> Blood cultures are obtained. Cultures are also obtained of any suspicious sites from which bacteria may have originated (e.g. abscess, urine); see also gonococcal arthritis below.

Treatment: <u>Antibiotics</u> are started immediately and continued for 2–4 weeks. While awaiting culture results, the choice of antibiotic is initially guided by the gram stain—e.g. penicillinase–resistant penicillin (e.g. nafcillin) if gram stain reveals staphylococci, an aminoglycoside if gram–negative bacilli are seen. See gonococcal arthritis below for the treatment of that infection. If no organisms are seen on gram stain, an aminoglycoside plus a cephalosporin is a suitable initial choice. <u>Arthrocentesis</u> via a large–bore needle is performed daily or more often if necessary until purulent synovial fluid no longer accumulates. Lavage with sterile saline solution via the aspirating needle may be used to facilitate drainage of the contents of a purulent joint. <u>Surgical drainage</u> is indicated if there is no significant improvement after 5–7 days of antibiotics and repeated arthrocentesis. Surgical drainage is also indicated when arthrocentesis fails to adequately drain a joint, or if there is septic arthritis of the hip joint.

GONOCOCCAL ARTHRITIS is the most common septic arthritis in young sexually active persons. Gonococcal arthritis develops in about 80% of patients with gonococcal septicemia. **Signs/symptoms:** Diagnosis is suggested when a sexually active patient presents with arthritis affecting more than one joint—particulary if there is articular involvement of the wrists and/or hands. Additional clues might include the presence of tenosynovitis or skin lesions (petechial, macular, vesicular, or pustular). **Laboratory:** Gram stain of the synovial fluid is rouinely performed even though this test often fails to reveal the diagnostic gram–negative intracellular diplococci. Culture of the synovial fluid is not uncommonly unproductive also. Blood cultures are more frequently positive. Additional cultures may be obtained from the urethra (and gram stained), cervix, throat, skin lesions (and gram stained), and/or anus as historical or clinical findings suggest. **Treatment:** Joint effusions are drained by needle aspiration. Antibiotic therapy is begun immediately—e.g. ceftriaxone (Rocephin) 1 gram/day IV as a single dose or divided into 2 daily doses. Once there is improvement, treatment may be switched to an oral antibiotic (e.g. cefuroxime axetil) and continued until the patient has received a total of at least 7 days of antibiotics. Penicillin may be chosen during the PO antibiotic phase of treatment if laboratory testing shows the organism to be sensitive to penicillin.

TUBERCULOUS ARTHRITIS is now uncommon. The patient is usually an adult, often without active pulmonary disease. In most cases tuberculous arthritis is due to reactivation of bacilli that have remained dormant in the subchondral bone since blood–borne dissemination of pulmonary tuberculosis during the primary infection years before. Typically, only one joint is involved; the knee, hip, wrist are common sites. Vertebral involvement (Pott's disease) is rare. Joint pain and swelling begins insidiously. Erythema is usually absent. The regional lymph nodes may be mildly enlarged and tender. X–rays may reveal osteoporosis of subchondral bone. **Diagnosis:** Tuberculin skin test is performed. Synovial fluid acid–fast stain seldom reveals the bacteria; however, synovial fluid cultures are positive in the majority of cases. Biopsy may be necessary for diagnosis. Acid–fast stain of synovial biopsy specimens are usually positive as are cultures of biopsy material. Hopefully, biopsy will also show the typical caseating granulomas. **Drug therapy** is discussed under "Tuberculosis".

FUNGAL ARTHRITIS (e.g. coccidioidomycosis, histoplasmosis, sporotrichosis, blastomycosis, cryptococcosis) is unusual. There is a chronic monoarticular arthritis. Blood–borne dissemination to the subchondral bone is the route of joint infection. However, sporotrichosis infects the joint directly (e.g. rose thorn puncture). Skin tests, synovial culture, and biopsy (to detect granuloma) all aid in the diagnosis.

VIRAL ARTHRITIS manifests as a self–limited polyarthritis. One of the more frequent causes is rubella; the virus has been cultured from the synovial fluid. The attenuated rubella virus used for vaccination may also cause polyarthritis. Mumps, infectious mononucleosis (Ebstein–Barr virus), arboviruses, adenoviruses, hepatitis B are examples of other viruses that may be associated with polyarthritis. However, viruses other than rubella have seldom been recovered from the synovial fluid. The polyarthritis associated with hepatitis B appears to be mediated by immune complexes as part of a serum sickness syndrome.

Vasculitides

POLYARTERITIS NODOSA is a vasculitis of the small and medium–sized arteries of multiple organs. Consequently, protean clinical manifestations may follow from involvement of sundry organs. <u>Pathology:</u> There is segmental inflammation and necrosis of the arterial walls starting in the media, and then involving the intima and adventitia. This is particularly likely at bifurcations and branch points. Proliferation of the intimal layer with thrombosis leads to vessel narrowing or occlusion with ensuing infarction of tissues in their distribution. The weakened arterial walls form aneurysms. The walls of necrotic arterial segments are replaced by fibrous tissue and the adventitia is marked by nodular fibrosis. <u>Kidneys</u> are affected in about 80–90% cases. There may be renal infarction as a consequence of the arterial lesions described above and/or there may be evidence of glomerulonephritis. Hypertension and renal failure are common sequelae. <u>Heart</u> is involved in about 1/3 cases. Coronary arteritis, depending on the extent of occlusion, may lead to angina and infarction. Pericarditis also occurs. <u>Gastrointestinal</u> complications arise in 1/3 cases when mesenteric arteritis leads to impaired GI blood flow. Thus, there may be abdominal pain, GI bleeding, bowel infarction/perforation, and/or retroperitoneal bleeding. The liver, pancreas, and/or gallbladder may also be affected. <u>Neurologic</u> deficits vary according to the area of impaired blood flow—e.g. CNS (e.g. seizures, strokes); peripheral nerves (e.g. motor and sensory deficits). <u>Skin</u> involvement may manifest as purpuric lesions, vasculitic ulcers, painful nodules, livedo reticularis. <u>Arthralgias and myalgias</u> are common complaints. <u>Pulmonary</u> arteries are spared. Lesions of the bronchial arteries may sometimes occur. Even in these cases, however, pulmonary involvement is clinically silent. **Tests:** <u>Histology:</u> Diagnosis is confirmed by biopsy of a lesion. <u>Serology:</u> Hepatitis B antigen is present in about 1/3 cases. <u>Urinalysis:</u> If glomerulonephritis is present; there will be hematuria, proteinuria, and hyaline and/or granular casts. <u>Elevated sedimentation rate and/or leukocytosis</u> are common. <u>Radiology:</u> Mesenteric, hepatic, or renal angiography is sometimes performed to detect aneurysms.

ALLERGIC GRANULOMATOUS VASCULITIS (Churg–Strauss syndrome), like polyarteritis nodosa, is a vasculitis of the small and medium sized arteries. Patients are also afflicted with both allergic rhinitis and asthma. Eosinophilia is present. The arteritis, like polyarteritis nodosa, may involve multiple organs with similar consequences. However, unlike polyarteritis nodosa, the disease also involves the pulmonary arteries and pulmonary granuloma are present. High–dose corticosteroids is the treatment of choice.

WEGENER'S GRANULOMATOSIS is an uncommon multisystem disease characterized by necrotizing vasculitis of small arteries and veins in association with development of granuloma. <u>Upper respiratory tract</u> symptoms are usually present (e.g. sinusitis, purulent and/or bloody nasal discharge, nasal mucosal ulcers, septal perforation, saddle nose deformity, purulent otitis media). <u>Pulmonary</u> involvement is evident in most patients (e.g. cough, hemoptysis, dyspnea, pleuritis, pulmonary infiltrates or nodules, cavitation). <u>Glomerulonephritis</u> develops in over 80% cases and without treatment culminates in renal failure. <u>Ocular</u> disease is found in about half the cases (e.g. conjunctivitis and/or lesions of cornea, sclera, or uveal tract). <u>Skin</u> lesions are found in about a third (e.g. nodules, purpuric papules). <u>Constitutional</u> symptoms include fever, malaise, arthralgias, weight loss. <u>Cardiac</u> involvement is evident in < 20% cases (e.g. coronary arteritis, pericarditis). <u>Neurologic</u> impairment occurs in < 20% cases (e.g. peripheral neuropathy, cranial nerve deficits, cerebral vasculitis). **Diagnosis** rests on the constellation of clinical findings and biopsy (e.g. of nasal mucosal lesion, kidney). **Treatment** is with cyclophosphamide. Prednisone is administered concurrently at first. Corticosteroids alone are ineffective.

HYPERSENSITIVITY VASCULITIS (ANGIITIS) encompasses a group of antigen–induced immune complex–mediated disorders associated with a necrotizing vasculitis of the arterioles or venules. **Examples:** The antigenic precipitant may be a drug (e.g. sulfa, penicillin); infectious agent (e.g. virus, streptococcal); endogenous protein (e.g. autoimmune disease). The syndrome may be associated with malignancy. Henoch–Schoenlein purpura, essential mixed cryoglobulinemia, serum sickness, and congenital complement deficits are other examples. **Signs/symptoms:** The principal target of the vasculitis is the vessels of the skin. However, vasculitis may also involve other organs. A variety of cutaneous lesions may occur (e.g. palpable purpura, papules, vesicles, bullae, ulcers, subcutaneous nodules, urticaria).

Henoch–Schoenlein purpura is a type of hypersensitivity angiitis that mostly occurs in children. Patients present with palpable purpura; glomerulonephritis; fever; arthralgias; GI complaints (e.g. nausea, vomiting, diarrhea, GI bleeding, abdominal pain).

Essential mixed cryoglobulinemia is a form of hypersensitivity angiitis characterized by recurrent attacks of palpable purpura along with arthralgias, lymphadenopathy, splenic and liver enlargement, glomerulonephritis. The serum reveals cryoglobulins composed of polyclonal IgG and IgM. Other laboratory findings include IgM rheumatoid factors, decreased serum complement. The syndrome is sometimes associated with autoimmune disease (e.g. rheumatoid arthritis, Sjögren's syndrome) or a malignancy (e.g. lymphoma).

GIANT CELL ARTERITIS (e.g. temporal arteritis, cranial arteritis) is a segmental arteritis of the medium to large arteries (the smaller arterioles are spared). Almost all patients are over 50 and white, and about two thirds are women. **Clinical findings** are in part a function of which artery(s) are involved: <u>Temporal arteritis</u> causes severe headache with swelling/tenderness/nodularity over the temporal artery. <u>Occlusion of ophthalmic artery</u> or its branches may lead to blindness or diplopia. <u>Occlusion in the internal carotid or vertebral</u> artery distribution may result in stroke. <u>Facial artery</u> involvement is associated with masseter muscle pain. <u>Peripheral arteries</u> (e.g. claudication of an extremity) or <u>aorta</u> may be affected. <u>Polymyalgia rheumatica</u> develops in many patients with giant cell arteritis (see below). **Laboratory:** <u>Sedimentation rate</u> is elevated. <u>Histology:</u> An involved segment of artery is infiltrated with lymphocytes, histiocytes, and giant cells; and there is degeneration of the internal elastic lamina. **Treatment** is with prednisone. Many patients with demonstrated giant cell arteritis on temporal artery biopsy have visual disturbances indicating involvement of the ophthalmic artery. Because of the risk of blindness, patients with visual symptoms must begin prednisone therapy promptly (60 mg/day initially) without awaiting confirmation from results of temporal artery biopsy.

Polymyalgia rheumatica complicates the course of giant cell arteritis in many patients. However, polymyalgia rheumatica may and in most instances does occur without evidence of coexisting giant cell arteritis. There is a sudden or insidious onset of muscular pain/tenderness (neck, back, proximal extremities) and stiffness, but without muscle weakness. Fever, malaise, fatigue, weight loss are characteristic. The sedimentation rate is elevated, often markedly so. CPK, SGOT, aldolase are normal. The patient responds quickly to low doses of prednisone

Synovial Fluid Analysis

Laboratory tests of synovial fluid:

<u>Gram stain and culture</u> specimen is introduced into a sterile heparinized tube. Routine cultures suffice unless clinical circumstances dictate additional cultures—e.g. mycobacterial, fungal, gonococcal. If the latter is suspected, a specimen should be immediately introduced onto a chocolate agar or selective chocolate agar medium (e.g. Thayer–Martin, MTM). <u>Specimen for WBC count and differential</u> is introduced into a heparinized tube. <u>Specimen for clarity, color, and viscosity</u> is introduced into a tube without additives. <u>Presence of crystals</u> is determined by polarized light microscopy. <u>Specimen for glucose concentration</u> is introduced into a tube containing preservative. A serum glucose should also be obtained. <u>Mucin clot test</u> is performed by adding one part synovial fluid to 4 parts 2% acetic acid. In the presence of inflammation, hyaluronic acid will be broken down. Consequently, mucin clot formation is impaired and so the mucin precipitate is poor (i.e. cloudy with shreds).

Normal synovial fluid is transparent, clear or pale yellow, viscous, and does not clot. The mucin clot test is normal. The synovial leukocyte count does not exceed 200, and less than 10% are neutrophils. Synovial glucose is about the same as a simultaneously obtained serum glucose.

Osteoarthritis: If an joint effusion is tapped; the synovial fluid is found to be clear or pale yellow in color. It is transparent but may be slightly turbid. The fluid is viscous and does not clot. The mucin clot test is good. Synovial WBC count is usually < 1000 (with < 30% neutrophils) and seldom over 4000.

Rheumatoid Arthritis: Inflammatory synovial fluid is pale yellow, cloudy, and has low viscosity. It contains clots and the mucin clot test is poor. Synovial WBC count is usually 5000–20,000 with 50–75% neutrophils. Synovial glucose level is about 30 mg/dl lower than a simultaneously obtained serum glucose. Synovial fluid complement is decreased.

Gout: Diagnosis of gout is confirmed by examining a sample of synovial fluid from an inflamed joint. To make the diagnosis conclusively, one must find negative birefringent needle–shaped urate crystals *within* leukocytes. During a quiescent phase of gout, urate crystals may be seen—but not within leukocytes. Thus, the finding of extraleukocytic urate crystals alone does not prove that the acute attack of joint pain/inflammation is due to gout. Other synovial fluid findings characteristic of acute gouty arthritis include cloudy appearance, low viscosity, poor mucin clot test. The synovial WBC count during an attack is usually 10.000–20,000 (range 1000–100,000) with 60–70% neutrophils. Synovial glucose is usually about 10 mg/dl less than a simultaneously obtained serum glucose.

Chondrocalcinosis/pseudogout: Chondrocalcinosis is confirmed by finding rhomboid or rod–shaped CPPD crystals (free or within leukocytes) in the synovial fluid. Viewed under polarizing microscope, the crystals are weakly positive birefringent. This contrasts with the negative birefringent urate crystals characteristic of gout. Both CPPD and urate crystals may be seen in patients with coexisting gout. <u>During an inflammatory episode</u>, the synovial fluid is cloudy, has low viscosity, and the mucin clot test is poor. The synovial fluid WBC count is elevated (3000–100,000) with 70–90% neutrophils. <u>Between inflammatory episodes</u>, the synovial fluid is clear with normal WBC count but CPPD crystals may still be identified.

Septic arthritis: Needle aspiration of a joint must always be performed if there is any suspicion of joint infection. Joint aspiration has both diagnostic and therapeutic value. The synovial fluid should be gram stained and cultured (aerobic and anaerobic). Synovial fluid is characteristically opaque and the mucin clot test is poor. Synovial WBC count is 20,000–250,000 with > 75% neutrophils. Synovial glucose is > 30 mg/dl lower than a simultaneously obtained serum glucose.

Skin Disease

Psoriasis
Seborrheic Dermatitis
Atopic Dermatitis
Contact Dermatitis
Diaper Dermatitis
Acne
Rosacea
Erythema Nodosum
Erythema Multiforme
Pityriasis Rosea
Pemphigus Vulgaris
Pemphigoid
Bacterial Skin Infections
Superficial Fungal Infections
Urticaria and Angioedema
Skin Cancer
Scabies
Pediculosis

Psoriasis
is an inflammatory disease associated with increased prolifera-
tion of the cells of the epidermis so that the epidermal turnover time is accelerated
(4–6 days instead of the normal 29–30 days). About 2% of the U.S. population is
affected—males as often as females. Psoriasis is inherited; the pattern is unknown.
However, there is an association with the histocompatibility antigens HLA B17,
Bw27, or Cw6.

Signs/symptoms: Typical lesion is an erythematous papule or plaque with
white-silvery scaling. Removing a scale leaves pinpoint sites of bleeding. Although
psoriasis may appear anywhere on the body, the most common sites are the scalp,
extensor surface of the extremities (particularly the elbows and knees), genitals, umbilicus, intergluteal cleft. Lesions are likely to develop at sites of minor trauma
(Koebner phenomenon). Itching is sometimes present—particularly of lesions of the
scalp or intertriginous folds. Arthritis develops in a minority of patients and seldom
occurs before age 20. Arthritis may be symmetric or asymmetric. In one form of
psoriatic arthritis, there is involvement of the distal interphalangeal joints of the
hands and feet. In another form, the large joints are affected (particularly the hips,
sacroiliac joints) and also the spine (ankylosis sometimes ensues). Psoriatic arthritis is rheumatoid factor negative. Nail involvement occurs in about a fourth of
patients—e.g. pitting, onycholysis, thickening, subungual keratosis or subungual yellow spots. Guttate psoriasis is an unusual presentation characterized by the rapid
appearance of hundreds of nonpruritic erythematous papular lesions in a generalized
distribution. This condition arises in children and young adults, and often follows a
streptococcal infection. Pustular psoriasis is another atypical form. In one type of
pustular psoriasis (Barber type), pustular lesions appear on the palms and soles. In
the other type (von Zumbusch type), the skin over the entire body becomes
erythematous followed by a generalized eruption of coalescing pustules. The patient
is febrile with leukocytosis and requires hospitalization. Pustular psoriasis is accompanied by arthritis in about a fourth of cases.

Treatment is individualized. Sunlight or artificial ultraviolet B alone may control
psoriasis. In severe cases with widespread involvement, aggressive ultraviolet B radiation under carefully supervised conditions is a very effective treatment. Ultraviolet
B is administered daily or 3–5 times per week. Most cases will clear after 18 treatments. Topical corticosteroid creams or ointments (refer to "Corticosteroids–Dermatologic" in drug section for preparations) are usually effective for treatment of patients with moderate involvement of the extremities. Begin with a potent corticosteroid applied 3 times daily and change to a less potent preparation as improvement
occurs. At night, an occlusive covering such as Saran wrap applied over the topical
steroid will enhance absorption. Topical tar therapy is often used in conjunction
with sunlight or artificial ultraviolet B, or in conjunction with topical corticosteroids.
Tars are best avoided in acute psoriasis because they may irritate and cause more
widespread lesions. Tar therapy may be carried out by applying a gel (e.g. Estar) or
1–5% crude tar overnight. The tar is removed in the morning with mineral oil and
then bathing. After cleansing, the patient may apply a corticosteroid cream, and/or
is exposed to sunlight or artificial ultraviolet B (see Goeckerman regimen below).
Combination preparations (e.g. Pragmatar) that contain tar and a keratolytic to break
up the scale are useful. Other tar preparations that may be beneficial include tar
shampoos (e.g. T/Gel, Zetar, Tegrin, Sebutone); soaps (Polytar); bath preparations
(e.g. Alma–Tar, Balnetar, Lavatar, Zetar). Goeckerman regimen is used in serious
cases with widespread involvement. Therapy consists of ultraviolet B radiation in the
morning followed by the application of a gel (e.g. Estar) or 5% crude tar several times
per day and at bedtime. In the morning, prior to the ultraviolet B treatment, the tar
is removed with mineral oil and then bathing. Ultraviolet exposure should be
sufficient to produce a slight reddening of the skin 12 hours later. Regimen is usually continued for 2–3 weeks. PUVA (psoralen + UVA) therapy may be used in patients with severe and refractory psoriasis. In this method a psoralen (methoxsalen)
is taken PO daily. Two hours later, the patient receives ultraviolet A radiation. This
regimen is carried out 2–4 times/week and tapered as improvement occurs.
Methotrexate as a small periodic dose is an option for patients with severe psoriasis. Regimens combining methotrexate with PUVA or UVB have been shown to be
very effective. **Scalp lesions** may be treated with a topical steroid solution (e.g.
Lidex, Halog). Wearing a shower cap will enhance adsorption. If there is thick scal-

ing or plaques, a keratolytic should be used as an adjunct—e.g. Keralyt gel, Pragmatar (the latter contains tar and a keratolytic). Tar shampoos (e.g. T/Gel, Zetar, Tegrin, Sebutone) will also be beneficial. **Psoriatic arthritis** usually responds to a nonsteroidal drug—e.g. ibuprofen. Hydroxychloroquin (Plaquenil) may be of benefit. Gold salts or methotrexate are used as a last resort in severe refractory cases.

Seborrheic Dermatitis is a chronic hyperproliferative in-

flammation of the epidermis of unknown cause. It is more common in males. It may occur at any age. However, it is less common in young children. It often appears at puberty in association with acne. Exacerbations often occur during periods of stress and during the winter months. Seborrheic dermatitis is relatively common in patients with Parkinson's disease.

Signs/symptoms: Sites of involvement; Common sites are areas where sebaceous glands are numerous—i.e. scalp, eyebrows, face (particularly paranasally), ears, behind ears, and in more severe cases the sternal area and body folds. Erythematous macular and/or papular scaling lesions are characteristic. The scales are typically greasy and yellowish. In severe cases there is crusting. Itching may or may not be present. In infants, scale may accumulate on the scalp to such an extent that it is called "cradle cap".

Treatment: Dandruff; For mild dandruff, daily shampooing with a regular shampoo may suffice. In stubborn or more severe cases, a shampoo that contains an agent that will reduce epidermal cell turnover rate is used. This may be a selenium sulfide shampoo (e.g. Selsun Blue, Exsel, Iosel), zinc pyrithione shampoo (e.g. Head and Shoulders, Danex, Zincon), or a tar shampoo (e.g. Zetar, T/Gel, Ionil T, Sebutone). These shampoos may be used 2–3 times/week but once weekly may suffice. A regular shampoo is used on other days. A topical corticosteroid lotion is prescribed if shampooing alone does not control the scalp lesions. For the face or other body areas, a low potency corticosteroid (e.g. 1% hydrocortisone cream) will usually suffice. High potency fluorinated corticosteroids should not be used on the face. A sulfur–containing cream (e.g. Pragmatar) is a good choice for chronic seborrheic dermatitis of the face. Topical application of ketoconazole cream may be effective. Seborrheic blepharitis; An ophthalmic solution containing 10% sulfacetamide and 0.2% prednisolone (e.g. Blephamide, Vasocidin) is applied 3 times a day with the eyes closed. Corticosteroids should not be used on the eyes for extended periods; the intraocular pressure must be checked periodically. Consultation with an ophthalmologist is best. Sulfacetamide ophthalmic alone is an alternative.

Atopic Dermatitis is an acute or chronic inflammation of the epi-

dermis and dermis that affects 2–3% of the population. The tendency toward atopic dermatitis is inherited. A personal or family history of atopic dermatitis, asthma, or hay fever is present in most patients. About a third of patients have or will develop asthma or hay fever. Age of onset and duration; Atopic dermatitis will develop by age 1 in 60% cases, by age 5 in 90% cases, and by age 20 in all cases. As a rule, the disease is chronic with flares and remissions. The disease disappears or subsides after 15–20 years. Impaired resistance to viral or fungal infection may occur because T cell function is depressed. For example, patients may develop widespread herpes simplex infection (Kaposi's varicelliform eruption), or stubborn cases of Molluscum contagiosum or Verruca vulgaris. Laboratory; Serum IgE levels are often elevated. Eosinophilia is common. Abnormal skin reactions to pharmacologic stimuli are characteristic—e.g. injection of acetylcholine into the skin will elcit blanching instead of vasodilation with erythema.

Signs/symptoms: The distribution and type of lesions varies with age. Pruritus is prominent feature of atopic dermatitis. Dry skin, certain irritants (notably soap and wool), emotional stress, or even bathing may precipitate itching. Normal sweating is often impaired so that sweat retention (which induces pruritis) may occur upon heat exposure. In infancy, there are reddened scaling patches with blisters, oozing, and crusting. There is a predilection for the forehead and cheeks (while sparing the area about the eyes and mouth). Lesions may also be present on the scalp, neck, chest, and extensor surfaces of the extremities. In children, dry papules or plaques are found, especially on the flexor surfaces—e.g. antecubital and popliteal fossae, volar aspect of wrists, anterior neck. There is less oozing than in infancy and lesions tend to be dispersed. Lichenified lesions are common. Periorbital reddening and edema is prevalent. Later in childhood and into adulthood, the lesions are chiefly dry and lichenified. Commonly involved sites are the antecubital and popliteal fossae, wrists, flexor surface of neck, eyelids. Chronic facial edema may result in an infraorbital fold (Dennie–Morgan sign). Anterior subcapsular cataracts develop in about 10% patients.

Treatment: Skin must be kept moist; otherwise itching is exacerbated. Excessive bathing is avoided. Use of soaps is minimized or avoided (e.g. Cetaphyl is an effective alternative cleansing agent). Emollients are applied to retain moisture and soften skin, particularly after bathing—e.g. lotions (e.g. Keri, Lubriderm, Lubrex, Neutrogena); Eucerin; Nivea oil, petrolatum. If the skin is particularly dry, the patient may need to bathe or soak an affected part and then apply an emollient. Oozing lesions are treated with Burrow's solution compresses for 20 minutes 4–6 times/day, or the patient soaks in a tub containing oatmeal (Aveeno) or a bath oil (e.g. Oilated Aveeno, Alpha Keri, Lubrex, Domol). Topical corticosteroids are usually needed. It is common practice to start with a moderately potent corticosteroid (e.g. 0.1% triamcinolone cream) and then switch to a less potent agent (e.g. 1% hydrocortisone) as improvement occurs. Remember that fluorinated corticosteroids must not be used on the face; 1% hydrocortisone is a good choice for facial lesions. Systemic corticosteroids may be administered during an acute severe exacerbation but prolonged systemic steroid therapy is discouraged. A single IM injection is administered—e.g. 40–80 mg methylprednisolone (Depo–Medrol). Alternatively, a short course of prednisone may be prescribed (40–60 mg PO initially and then tapered and discontinued within 10–14 days). Oral antihistamines (e.g. hydroxyzine, diphenhydramine—see drug section) are used to relieve itching. Cut fingernails short in order to minimize excoriation.

Contact Dermatitis is of 2 types: primary irritant contact dermatitis (PICD) and the much less common allergic contact dermatitis (ACD). The 2 types differ in their pathogenesis. **Primary irritant contact dermatitis (PICD)** is not immune–mediated but is caused by direct injury to the skin by an offending substance. Furthermore, in contrast to ACD, a substance that causes PICD will cause dermatitis in *all* individuals who come in contact with it provided that it is irritating enough and contact is sufficiently protracted—i.e. all exposed persons will develop PICD on the first exposure if the irritant is sufficiently injurious (e.g. strong acid or alkali) or upon repeated or prolonged contact with a less irritating substance (e.g. excessive exposure of hands to soaps or detergents). **Allergic contact dermatitis (ACD)** Is mediated indirectly via T cells (type IV delayed hypersensitivity reaction). ACD never occurs on first contact with the offending agent; a person must first become sensitized (allergic)—i.e. a clone of T cells specific for the offending antigen must first be generated by previous contact. Once sensitized and upon reexposure, T cells from that clone move to the newly exposed area of skin contact to cause the dermatitis. A person may be exposed to a substance for years before developing an allergy. Examples of substances commonly causing ACD are poison ivy; ragweed; nickel; dichromates; topical antibiotics (e.g. neomycin, sulfonamide); rubber; ethylenediamine preservative; and the list is endless. **Light–influenced contact dermatitis:** For some substances contact dermatitis is not elicited unless the skin is also subsequently exposed to light. This phenomenon may be primary irritant type (phototoxic PICD) or immune–mediated (photoallergic contact dermatitis).

Diagnosis: Patch testing may be required; if the culpable incitant is not identified by the history, location of the lesion(s), and/or relief of dermatitis after stopping exposure to suspected offending agents.

Treatment: Stop exposure to offending substance. This may be all that is required in mild cases. Blistered and oozing lesions are treated with Burrow's solution compresses for 20 minutes 4–6 times/day or the patient soaks in a lukewarm tub containing oatmeal (e.g. Aveeno). Calamine lotion may alleviate discomfort. Antihistamine (e.g. Benadryl) is administered if there is itching. Topical corticosteroid is applied as circumstances suggest. Use 1% hydrocortisone cream or lotion if the face is involved. A stronger corticosteroid (e.g. 0.1% triamcinolone cream or lotion) may be used on other areas. Systemic corticosteroids are administered in severe allergic contact dermatitis (e.g. severe poison ivy contact dermatitis). Administration is advised for for at least 10–14 days and then tapered over 1 week. Curtailing the regimen prematurely may lead to recrudescence. The usual regimen consists of PO prednisone 40–60/day in adult (1–2 mg/kg/day in child) divided into 3 daily doses. An initial dose of parenteral corticosteroid may be administered (e.g. dexamethasone 0.25 mg/kg IV or IM).

Diaper Dermatitis develops in the setting of excessive moisture

as the natural skin oils are lost. Sundry irritants may further promote inflammation— e.g. bacterial enzymes in the feces; diaper detergents; topical medications; superimposed infection (e.g. Candida, S. aureus). Other conditions that may play a part in the inflammation include contact dermatitis, seborrheic dermatitis, atopic dermatitis, or psoriasis. **Laboratory:** If there are pustules, they should be sampled for microscopic exam (gram stain, KOH preparation) and culture. **Prevention:** Keep diaper area dry as possible. Change diaper frequently. Use no diaper at all when possible. Cleansing: Refrain from washing excessively. Use mild soaps (e.g. Neutrogena) or Cetaphil lotion for cleansing. After cleansing, apply Talcum powder or a protective cream (e.g. Diaparene). **Treatment:** 1% hydrocortisone cream applied daily for a week or so will help ease inflammation in mild cases. Burrow's solution compresses may be needed in severe cases with exudation. Fungal infection: If small satellite lesions suggestive of Candidiasis are seen, an antifungal cream is indicated— e.g. miconazole (Micatin), clotrimazole (Lotrimin). Bacterial infection is treated with a combination topical antibacterial—e.g. Neosporin, Polysporin.

Acne is an inflammation of the sebaceous glands and associated hair follicles.

Pathogenesis: The folliclar outlet becomes obstructed with cellular debris and sebum. Sebum contains triglycerides which when acted upon by bacteria (e.g. Propionibacterium acnes) produces fatty acids that mediate the inflammation. If the plug is at the surface, an open comedome (blackhead) results. The black color is due to the presence of melanin–containing keratinocytes in the plug. If the plug is deeper a closed comedome (whitehead) is formed and the melanin is not visible. Sebum accumulates behind the obstruction and eventually the follicle ruptures releasing free fatty acids into the surrounding tissue. The ensuing inflammation leads to the formation of inflammatory papules, pustules, nodules, and/or cysts. Hormonal influence: Acne usually begins at puberty when, under the influence of increased androgens, the sebaceous glands enlarge and sebum production is increased. Acne is generally more severe in males because of the comparatively high levels of testicular–derived androgens. Androgens in females originate from the ovaries and adrenals. Acne may be a manifestation of endocrine disease—e.g. Cushing's syndrome, polycystic ovarian syndrome. Drug causes: Acne may also be due to or be aggravated by iodides, bromides, lithium, systemic corticosteroids, androgens, isoniazid, phenytoin.

Treatment is individualized according to severity. Mild acne may respond to topical therapy alone. Retinoic acid (tretinoin, vitamin A acid) is a topical keratolytic agent that promotes peeling and disrupts comedone plugs. Exposure to sunlight should be minimized when using this agent. It is usually applied nightly. Reddening and peeling is to be expected. However, less frequent application may be necessary if irritation is excessive. Preparations include 0.05% and 0.1% Retin-A cream, 0.01% or 0.025% Retin-A gel, 0.05% Retin-A liquid. Patients with fair complexion and sensitive skin should first try the lowest concentration cream or gel. Benzoyl peroxide is another keratolytic agent that may be used alone or in conjunction with retinoic acid (retinoic acid at night and benzoyl peroxide in the morning). Benzoyl peroxide (Desquam X, Fostex) is available as a 5 or 10% wash or 2.5, 5, or 10% gel. Both retinoic acid and benzoyl peroxide are irritants. Therefore, the use of these agents alone or in combination must be individualized. Antibiotics are needed for more severe acne (i.e. papules, pustules, and/or cysts). Tetracycline is usually the best choice but is contraindicated in pregnancy or patients < 8 years of age. The dose is 1 gram/day PO divided into 2–4 daily doses until there is significant improvement followed by gradual tapering to 250 mg/day. Erythromycin in the same dose is the usual choice when tetracycline is contraindicated. In mild cases (i.e. absence of papules, pustules, or cysts) a topical antibiotic may be effective—e.g. topical clinda-mycin (Cleocin T) lotion or gel applied twice daily. <u>Accutane</u> (13–cis–retinoic acid, isotretinoin) may be used in severe cystic acne refractory to other therapy. This agent is teratogenic. Females of reproductive age must therefore have a pregnancy test before starting the drug, and effective contraception must be assured while ther-apy is in progress. <u>Oral vitamin A</u> (100,000–300,000 units/day) may be an effec-tive treatment. Chronic high dose vitamin A is toxic. However, an adult receiving vi-tamin A will not usually develop signs of toxicity until at least 50,000 unit/day has been ingested for over a year. <u>In females, oral contraceptive pills</u> with relatively high estrogen potency will usually bring about substantial improvement. Conversely, certain oral contraceptives with a relatively high androgen potency (e.g. Lo/Ovral) may cause acne to worsen. Demulen has a relatively low androgen potency and may be tried first. If acne does not improve with Demulen, then Enovid E (which has greater estrogen potency and virtually no androgen potency) may be tried. <u>Spironolactone</u> may ameliorate acne.

Rosacea is more common in women and in persons with fair complexion.

The greatest incidence is from 30 to 50 years of age.

Signs/symptoms: Rosacea is a chronic inflammatory skin condition—primarily of the face—whose main features are flushing, telangectasias, and inflammation of the pilosebacious units. The latter leads to papules, pustules, and cysts. Rosacea may resemble acne but, in contrast, comedones are absent. The cheeks, nose, chin, and forehead are the usual sites affected. Involvement of the neck, trunk, or extremities is unusual.

Complications: With time, men may develop rhinophyma (soft tissue overgrowth of the nose). Eye complications may occur (e.g. blepharitis, conjunctivitis, keratitis).

Treatment: <u>Avoid conditions that cause cutaneous vasodilation</u> (e.g. hot drinks, alcohol, hot showers). Menopause–associated flushing may be treated with estrogens (e.g. Premarin). <u>Tetracycline</u> if often effective. Start with 250 mg PO 4 times/day and then gradually taper to 250 mg once daily as improvement occurs. Rosacea may recur after tetracycline is stopped. Prolonged antibiotic therapy may be required. <u>Erythromyin</u> in the same dosage may be used if tetracycline is contrain-dicated or ineffective. <u>Topical antibiotics</u> may be effective. Try tetracycline; or if tet-racycline is contraindicated, use topical erythromycin or clindamycin. <u>Metronidazole</u> (Flagyl) is often effective in patients with papulo–pustular lesions. Oral (200 mg twice daily) or topical (1% cream or 0.75% gel twice daily) administration may be tried. <u>Topical benzoyl peroxide</u> is sometimes used as an adjunct to tetracycline in those patients with papulo–pustular lesions. <u>Accutane</u> (13–cis–retinoic acid, isotret-inoin) may be used in severe intractable cases. This agent is teratogenic. Therefore, women of childbearing age must have a pregnancy test before starting the drug, and effective contraception must be assured while therapy is in progress. <u>Rhinophyma</u> may be treated by various methods: CO_2 laser, dermabrasion, elec-trodessication. <u>Telangectasias</u> may be treated by electrodessication or with argon laser.

Erythema Nodosum is an immune–mediated inflammatory re-action of the skin and subcutaneous tissue. It is more common in women by 3 to 1.

Incidence is greatest between 15 and 30 yr of age. Erythema nodosum can occur at any age but seldom before age 6 or in the elderly.

Precipitants: Sundry precipitants of erythema nodosum have been identified. In many cases, however, no inciting factor can be found. Known incitants include <u>infections:</u> streptococcus; tuberculosis; leprosy; Yersinia enterocolitica; syphilis; gonorrhea; lymphogranuloma venereum; fungi (e.g. histoplasmosis, coccidioidomyco-sis, other systemic or cutaneous fungal infections); measles and other viral infec-tions); <u>noninfectious conditions:</u> sarcoid; ulcerative colitis; Crohn's disease; Bechet's syndrome; malignancy; <u>drugs:</u> sulfonamides; oral contraceptives; iodides.

Signs/symptoms: <u>Skin lesions:</u> Painful/tender erythematous indurated nodular lesions are found, most often on the shin(s). The lesions measure 3–10 cm in diameter and are slightly elevated with poorly defined borders Less frequent sites are the knees, thighs, extensor surface of arms, neck, or face. Skin lesions usually resolve spontaneously within 4–6 weeks. Fever, malaise, and/or joint pain may precede the appearance of the skin lesions.

Work-up requires clinical discretion taking into account such factors as the patient's age, recent medical history, geography, physical exam. Initial laboratory work-up usually consists of CBC, urinalysis, ESR, throat culture, ASO titer, chest x-ray. Other tests may include tuberculin skin test, coccidioidin skin test, VDRL, test for Yersinia.

Treatment: Bed rest is recommended. Nonsteroidal anti-inflammatory drug (e.g. aspirin, ibuprofen) is administered. Potassium iodide for 3–4 weeks may be used to alleviate disabling pain and swelling: potassium iodide 360–900 mg/day PO or SSKI (saturated solution potassium iodide) 6–15 drops/day PO. Corticosteroid: Intralesional injection of a corticosteroid, or 1–2 weeks of PO prednisone may be needed if no underlying cause can be found and symptoms persist despite foregoing measures.

Erythema Multiforme is an immune–mediated inflammatory

reaction of the skin (specifically, a vasculitis of the dermis) and mucosa. The greatest incidence is between 10 and 30 years of age. Majority of patients are male.

Precipitants: Sundry incitants have been identified including infections (e.g. *herpes simplex*, Mycoplasma, infectious mononucleosis, hepatitis, mumps, adenovirus, coxsackie; drugs (e.g. *sulfonamides*, *penicillin*, *barbiturates*, phenytoin, phenolphthalein, oral contraceptives, phenybutazone, gold); autoimmune disease; malignancy.

Signs/symptoms: Skin lesions may develop over several days. The lesions start as macules or papules that then develop into iris or target lesions (1–2 cm in diameter) with a purpuric center surrounded by a pale ring (due to edema) which is in turn surrounded by a erythematous ring (due to vasodilation). The central purpuric center may subsequently develop into a vesicle or bulla. The lesions are found on the hands and feet (particularly the palms and soles) with progressively fewer lesions proximally. The trunk is spared unless involvement of the extremities is extensive. Facial lesions may also be present. There may be itching. Lesions are painless or there may be stinging sensation. Large blisters may be painful. Mucosal lesions: Erosive lesions are often found on the lips and oral mucosa. The genital mucosa may also be involved. Ocular complications: Conjunctival lesions with conjunctival discharge may be present. Corneal ulcers, and/or anterior uveitis may develop. The cornea may become scarred and vision may be permanently impaired. Pulmonary involvement is not infrequent. Stevens–Johnson syndrome is a severe manifestation of erythema multiforme. The patient is quite ill with high fever, myalgias, arthralgias, nausea, vomiting. There are widespread skin lesions with rapid development of bullae. Erosive lesions appear on the oral, nasal, and/or genital mucosa. Eye lesions are usually present (see above). Nephritis and renal failure may develop. There may be erosive lesions of GI mucosa. Toxic epidermal necrolysis: Rarely, the bullae become confluent and the epidermis desquamates.

Treatment: Most cases require no treatment. As a rule the lesions resolve spontaneously within 3 weeks, although there is sometimes a recurrence. For itching, an antihistamine and/or a topical corticosteroid may be prescribed. An ophthalmologist is consulted if there is eye involvement. Stevens–Johnson syndrome: Hospitalize. IV fluids are usually administered, the amount gauged by the adequacy of urine output. The pain from oral lesions may be mitigated by rinsing the mouth with 2% viscous xylocaine and/or Benadryl elixir. Bacitracin or Polysporin ointment may be applied to lip or skin lesions. The use of systemic corticosteroids is controversial. High doses are advocated (e.g. 80–100 mg/day prednisone or its equivalent) until there is improvement and then tapered over 2–3 weeks. An ophthalmologist must be consulted if there is eye involvement. Toxic epidermal necrolysis is treated as a 2nd degree burn.

Pityriasis Rosea is a maculopapular rash believed to be provoked
by a viral infection. It may occur at any age but is most common from 10 to 35 yr.

Signs/symptoms: In 80% of cases, the rash begins with a solitary red "herald" patch 2–5 cm across, usually on the trunk. The patch resembles tinea corporis in that there is some fine scaling. This is followed, usually in 1–2 weeks, by the appearance of multiple red macules that progress to papules and then to 0.5–2 cm oval slightly scaling plaques (smaller replicas of the herald patch) whose long axes lie parallel to the lines of cleavage of the skin. On the back, this alignment resembles a Christmas tree design. The lesions are found mostly on the trunk and to a lesser extent on the proximal extremities, neck, groin, and axillae. The rash may become confluent in areas. In blacks, the rash may involve the extremities more than the trunk. Children may also develop the lesions on the face, hands, and feet but this is not a characteristic finding in adults. New lesions may continue to develop for a few weeks. Occasionally, there is blistering. The rash usually resolves within 6–8 weeks but may occasionally persist for months. Pruritis occurs in about 20% cases. Recurrences are unusual.

Differential diagnosis: tinea corporis, tinea versicolor, secondary syphilis, drug eruption (e.g. clonidine, captopril, barbiturates, gold).

Laboratory: Serologic test for syphilis is advised. The characteristic absence of lesions on the palms or hands helps differentiate pityriasis rosea from secondary syphilis.

Treatment: An oral antihistamine and/or an antipruritic lotion (e.g. Calamine, Caladryl) may be used if there is itching. Otherwise, treatment is usually unnecessary. Sunbathing or artificial ultraviolet B appears to limit spread of the rash. The rare severely inflamed rash may be treated with topical or systemic corticosteroid.

Pemphigus Vulgaris is a chronic autoimmune disease with greatest
incidence in persons over 40. It is rare in children. Males are affected as often as females. The incidence is greater in Jews and those of Mediterranean descent. A relatively high incidence has been observed in Brazil (Brazilian pemphigus, also known as folgo salvagem). **Signs/symptoms:** Skin lesions: Skin bullae develop in seemingly normal skin. Common sites of involvement are the face, scalp, chest, axillae, groin. Nikolsky's sign is present (the epidermis separates from the underlying skin with stroking or minor trauma). The bullae break easily leaving a raw area that subsequently crusts but fails to heal. Pruritis is unusual. Mucosal lesions: Bullae not infrequently develop in the mouth before skin lesions appear. The bullae break leaving a raw and often painful erosion. Mucosal lesions may not remain confined to the mouth but may also develop in the pharynx, larynx, and esophagus. **Diagnosis** is confirmed by biopsy. Histology discloses adjacent cells within the epidermis separated from one another. This demonstrates that the bullae develop above the basal cell layer. By immunofluorescence method, one discovers that the serum contains IgG directed against intercellular epidermal antigen. The serum levels of indirect immunofluorescent anti–intercellular antibody correlate with disease severity. **Differential diagnosis:** pemphigoid, erythema multiforme, toxic epidermal necrolysis, dermatitis herpetiformis, bullous contact dermatitis, bullous drug eruption. **Treatment:** In severe disease, prednisone 100–150 mg/day is administered initially. Even more may be needed to achieve control. In less severe cases, 60–80 mg/day may suffice. Cyclophosphamide (100 mg/day) or azathioprine (150 mg/day) are often administered concurrently with prednisone so that lower doses of prednisone may be used.

Pemphigus foliaceus is a less severe form of pemphigus which is characterized by scaling with fewer and more superficial blisters. The oral mucosa is seldom involved.

Pemphigoid is a chronic autoimmune disease. Patients are typically over 60.
Pemphigoid is seen as often in men as in women. Immunofluorescence discloses IgG and C3 deposition on the basement membrane at the dermal–epidermal junction.

Signs/symptoms: Skin lesions: Bullae may be localized or generalized. Bullae arise from skin that is erythematous or has a normal appearance. Because the bullae develop from a subepidermal location, they are not as easily ruptured as those of pemphigus and may remain intact for many days. Another contrast to pemphigus is that Nikolsky's sign is absent (see "Pemphigus" above). The lesions heal spontaneously while new bullae arise. Except for occasional itching, the patient is usually otherwise asymptomatic. Mucosal lesions: About a third of patients develop lesions of the oral, vaginal, anal mucosa. Mucosal lesions are small and heal quickly.

Diagnosis: Light microscopy of a skin biopsy specimen reveals subepidermal blister formation. By immunofluorescence method, it is revealed that the patient's serum contains IgG directed against the basement membrane.

Treatment: Pemphigoid is a relatively benign disease that, even without treatment, usually does not significantly impair the health of the patient. Treatment consists of prednisone 40–60 mg every morning for a few weeks and then tapered to a maintenance dose. Azathioprine is an alternative, or azathioprine may be used concurrently with prednisone so that lower doses of prednisone may suffice.

Bacterial Skin Infections

CELLULITIS is an infection of the skin and subcutaneous tissues that is nearly always due to staphylococcus or streptococcus. Rarely, other bacteria are responsible- —e.g. H. influenza, pneumococcus, Clostridium perfringens.

Erysipelas (streptococcal cellulitis) manifests as a reddened, tender, and indurated area of skin whose advancing edge is usually well–delineated and slightly elevated. The face or legs are common sites of involvement; the abdomen is a common site in infants. There is a high fever—often with chills, headache, nausea. Sometimes there is regional adenopathy. There is leukocytosis. The diagnosis is usually obvious, and so treatment should not await laboratory confirmation. Blood, throat, nasal, or eye culture is sometimes positive. Attempts to culture and gram stain the organism from the advancing border are usually fruitless. Treatment: penicillin for 10 days. Alternatives are erythromycin or a cephalosporin–e.g. cephalexin (Keflex).

Staphylococcal cellulitis occasionally has a clinical presentation identical to erysipelas. In most cases however and unlike erysipelas, there is usually not a well–delineated advancing edge and the infection usually spreads more slowly. Like erysipelas, the skin is reddened, tender, and swollen. Red streaks extending from the region of cellulitis, indicating spread via dermal lymphatics, may be seen. Treatment: penicillinase–resistant penicillin (e.g. dicloxacillin). A cephalosporin or erythromycin are alternatives.

PYODERMA (purulent skin infection):

Impetigo is superficial skin infection usually due to group A streptococcus and less often to Staphylococcus aureus. Impetigo may occur at any age but it is most common in children. It starts with transitory vesicles and/or pustules that rupture to form yellow crusts. The face is the most frequently involved site. The lesions are contagious and there is often autoinoculation from one site to another. Treatment: single injection benzathine penicillin (to prevent possible development of poststreptococcal glomerulonephritis) or oral penicillin VK for 10 days. Alternatives are a 10 day course of erythromycin or a cephalosporin–e.g. cephalexin (Keflex).

Ecthyma is an ulcerated form of impetigo, usually due to group A streptococcus and/or staphylococcus. It characteristically arises at a site of minor skin trauma or excoriation. The ulcer is covered with a yellow crust and has a violaceous elevated margin. All skin layers are involved and the lesion heals with a scar. Treatment: penicillin or erythromycin.

Bullous impetigo is due to phage group II Staphylococcus aureus (i.e. staphylococci that produce an extracellular exotoxin). Typically, one finds scattered thin–walled flaccid bullae that break easily leaving red erosive lesions or white to yellow crusted lesions. The lesions are nonpruritic and well–demarcated from the surrouding nonerythematous normal skin. Treatment: dicloxacillin. Alternatives are erythromycin or a cephalosporin–e.g. cephalexin (Keflex).

STAPHYLOCOCCAL SCALDED SKIN SYNDROME (toxic epidermal necrolysis of the Rittner type) is, like bullous impetigo, due to exotoxin–produding phage group II Staphylococcus aureus. The syndrome is seen most often in infants and small children. The skin becomes diffusely reddened and tender and has the feel of sandpaper. Erythema is particularly noticeable in the skin folds of the neck, antecubiti, axillae, and groin. After about 2 days, the superficial epidermis desquamates as in a scald injury. Nikolsky's sign is present (involved epidermis peels when it is stroked). Desquamation continues for about a week. There is no scarring. Treatment: (1) Severely ill patients will require hospitalization for skin care and IV fluid support. (2) Administer antibiotic as for bullous impetigo; use IV antibiotic if patient is toxic. (3) Analgesics as needed.

HAIR FOLLICLE INFECTION and EXTENSION:

Folliculitis is an infection of the superficial part of the hair follicle. It is usually due to Staphylococcus aureus. Superficial pustules are seen about the hairs. Gram-negative bacteria (Pseudomonas, Proteus, Klebsiella, E. coli) may occasionally cause folliculitis. Treatment: warm moist compresses. In stubborn cases, an antibiotic may be prescribed—dicloxacillin, erythromycin, or a cephalosporin (e.g. cephalexin [Keflex]). In the case of gram-negative folliculitis, antibiotic therapy is based on culture results.

Furuncles (boils) are perifollicular tender nodules that develop when the infection of superficial follicultitis extends deep into the follicle. Furuncles are usually due to Staphylococcus aureus. The nodule typically develops into a pustule which subsequently drains. Treatment: A solitary furuncle can usually be managed with moist warm compresses to promote drainage. In some cases, the furuncle is incised to allow drainage. An antibiotic (see folliculitis above) may be needed (e.g. dicloxacillin, erythromycin, cephalexin).

Carbuncle is an abscess of the skin and subcutaneous tissue that results from extension of a furuncle. Typically, multiple sites of purulent drainage develop. The back and nape of neck are common areas of involvement. The patient is often febrile and "sick". Lesions heal with scarring. Treatment: drainage, obtain culture, penicillinase–resistant penicillin (e.g. nafcillin) or cephalosporin.

HIDRADENITIS SUPPURATIVA is a localized infection that develops when apocrine glands become occluded and rupture into the surrounding tissue. This condition usually occurs in the axillae or groin; sometimes about the nipples or anus. There is a tender firm nodular area that subsequently becomes fluctuant and may drain spontaneously. Hydroadenitis suppurativa does not develop until after puberty. It is more common in females, blacks, and the obese. Treatment: (**1**) warm compresses; (**2**) 1–2 month course of antibiotic—e.g. 250 mg PO 4 times/day of penicilliin, erythromycin, or cephalexin. (**3**) Excision may be required in stubborn or recurrent cases.

Superficial Fungal Infections

DERMATOPHYTES are fungi that cause tinea (ringworm). Dermatophytic fungi grow only on nonviable tissue—i.e. stratum corneum of skin, nails, or hair. Tinea may be due to any one of several species of the genera Trichophyton (e.g. Trichophyton rubra), Microsporum (e.g. M. audouini), or Epidermophyton (e.g. E. floccosum).

Diagnosis may be confirmed by microscopic exam of a KOH preparation, or if doubt persits by culture on Sabouraud's agar. Certain dermatophytes (e.g. M. audouini, M. canis, T. schoenleini) will fluoresce under Wood's light (long wave ultraviolet).

Treatment: Most fungal skin infections may be effectively treated with a topical antifungal—e.g. miconazole (Micatin) or clotrimazole (Lotrimin) creams or lotions (see drug section). Other effective topical agents include ketoconazole, econazole, ciclopirox, haloprogin. Tinea pedis ("athlete's foot") may respond to topical agents (e.g. 2% ketoconazole cream is curative in most cases). A keratolytic agent (e.g. Whitfield's ointment, Keralyt gel) may be necessary if the soles are involved and may alone be curative, or may be used in conjunction with one of the aforementioned topical antifungals. Macerated interdigital infection may first need to be treated with applications of 20% aluminum chloride hexahydrate twice daily for 7–10 days. Tinea pedis may also be treated with PO griseofulvin; concurrent application of a topical antifungal may increase the cure rate in those with intertriginous infection. Tinea capitus is treated with griseofulvin. Nail infections (tinea unguium) are treated with griseofulvin (see drug section). However, griseofulvin alone may not be curative. In many cases, consequently, the nail may have to be removed (surgically or with application of 40% urea ointment) and griseofulvin prescribed as well.

TINEA VERSICOLOR (due to Pityrosporum orbiculare) is recognized by the presence of scattered brown or white patches. There is slight scaling but no evidence of inflammation and the patient is asymptomatic. White areas are due to inhibition of melanin synthesis. A faint fluorescence may be seen under Wood's light.

264

<u>Treatment:</u> Selenium sulfide lotion (Selsun) left on the skin for half hour daily for 2 weeks is one of several effective regimens.

CUTANEOUS CANDIDIASIS usually develops where warmth and moisture are conducive to Candidal growth—e.g. in the body folds (axillae, groin, inframammary), on the feet of persons wearing occlusive shoes. Persons whose hands are frequently wet are prone to candidal paronychia (which manifests as erythema and swelling of proximal nail folds) and infection in the web space of the fingers. <u>Risk factors</u> (besides chronically moist skin) include obesity; diabetes mellitus; antibiotic therapy; pregnancy; corticosteroid therapy; impaired immunity (e.g. leukemia, chemotherapy, AIDS); psoriasis; seborrheic dermatitis. <u>Treatment of skin infection:</u> miconazole or clotrimazole cream (see drug section). Other effective topical agents include ketoconazole, econazole and haloprogin. All these drugs are also effective against dermatophytic fungi. The affected areas should be kept dry. <u>Treatment of paronychia:</u> The infection may respond to any of the aforementioned creams. However, topical application of absolute alcohol is more effective. **Mucocutaneous candidiasis:** refer to "Candida" chapter.

Urticaria and Angioedema <u>Urticaria</u> (hives) is

recognized by the presence of wheals (transitory circumscribed edematous areas in the superficial dermis) that are usually accompanied by itching. <u>Angioedema</u> is said to be present if the edema is more diffuse and reaches to the deeper layers of the dermis, subcutaneous tissue, and/or submucosa. <u>Definition acute versus chronic urticaria/angioedema:</u> acute if attacks have been occurring for < 1 month and chronic if > 1 month.

Etiology: <u>Foods</u> (e.g. shellfish, fish, nuts, eggs, milk, tomatoes, strawberries, pork); <u>antibiotics</u> (e.g. penicillins, cephalosporins) that act as haptens; <u>Hymenoptera venom</u> (bees, wasps, fire ants, etc); <u>inhalants</u> (pollen, dander). These inhalants induce urticaria or angioedema via an IgE–mediated mechanism (type I reaction) in persons who have been previously sensitized to the offending allergen (antigen). That antigen induces the production of IgE which subsequently coat the surface of mast cells, and basophils. On reexposure, the antigen bridges adjacent IgE molecules coating the mast cells and thereby induces the mast cells to release histamine and other substances that alter the permeability of capillaries and venules. Urticaria and/or angioedema ensue. <u>Physical agents</u> may induce urticaria/angioedema via IgE–mediated mechanism—e.g. cold, light, prolonged pressure, dermatographism (i.e. wheal elicited by stroking skin firmly). <u>Serum sickness</u> (e.g. due to certain drugs, horse antisera) is immune–mediated but is IgE is not involved. Instead, antigen–antibody complexes (IgG–antigen) are formed which activate complement leading to lysis of platelets with release of histamine. <u>Certain infections</u> (e.g. hepatitis B, infectious mononucleosis, parasites) and <u>autoimmune disease</u> (e.g. lupus) may also induce urticaria via formation of antigen–antibody complexes with ensuing activation of complement. <u>Blood transfusion–induced</u> urticaria or angioedema may be mediated by formation of antigen–antibody complexes with activation of complement, or less often it is mediated by IgE. <u>Certain malignancies</u> (leukemia, lymphoma) may cause urticaria/angioedema—presumably thru immune mechanisms. <u>Aspirin or other nonsteroidal anti–inflammatory drugs (e.g. indomethacin, ibuprofen); certain food additives (tartrazine, benzoate)</u> may induce urticaria/angioedema or anaphylaxis but the phenomenon is not immune–mediated. The reaction may therefore occur on the first exposure to the offending agent. The reaction mechanism is mediated via arachidonic acid metabolism. <u>Agents that directly induce release of histamine from mast cells</u>—e.g. narcotics, radiographic contrast agents, curare, polymyxin B. <u>Cholinergic urticaria</u> is mediated via endogenous release of acetylcholine. Urticaria is provoked by elevation in body temperature (exercise, hot bath, fever) or emotion. Interestingly, injected cholinergic drugs reproduce this phenomenon in only a minority of patients. Cholinergic urticaria has a characteristic appearance (1–2 mm urticarial lesions with surrounding erythema). <u>Hereditary angioedema</u> is an autosomal inherited deficiency of the inhibitor of activated C1 component of complement. As a consequence, the patient is subject to recurrent attacks of angioedema (not urticaria alone) due to the unrestrained activation of the complement system with ensuing release of histamine from mast cells. Pain rather than pruritis is characteristic. Serum C4 is decreased and bioassay or immunodiffusion tests show a deficiency of C1 esterase. An acquired form of the disease sometimes occurs in patients with certain malignancies or SLE. <u>Cutaneous necrotizing vasculitis</u>, a syndrome associated with chronic urticaria, may be due to lupus, Sjögren's syndrome, or be idiopathic. Skin biopsy is diagnostic.

Signs/symptoms: <u>Urticarial lesions</u> (hives) are tense, edematous, and may vary in size from 1–2 mm papules (e.g. cholinergic urticaria) to large plaques over 10 cm across. The larger lesions may show central clearing. The color is a function of the amount of fluid separating the layers of skin (i.e. pink to white). Blanching occurs when finger pressure is applied. The lesions are characteristically pruritic. Individual lesions last < 24 hours but an acute urticarial episode may persist for some time with new crops appearing as others clear. Angiodema: There is more diffuse swelling. This may be noted in the face including the eyelids and lips, the tongue, and/or the extremities (particularly the dorsum of hands and feet). The upper airways may become edematous, and so respiratory distress and stridor may ensue Hypotension may develop. Additional clinical findings may suggest the cause of urticaria/angioedema. For instance the presence of arthralgias might suggest hepatitis, serum sickness, or cutaneous necrotizing venulitis.

Identifying the precipitant: As a rule, tests are not diagnostically fruitful or indicated in cases of acute urticaria/angioedema (i.e. urticaria that has been occurring for < 1 month). The history and/or physical exam usually suggests the cause, and indicates the need for and direction of laboratory testing. Elimination diet may uncover a culpable food. Skin biopsy is indicated if urticaria is associated with petechiae or if *individual* urticarial lesions persist for more than 24 hours because in these instances, urticaria may be due to cutaneous necrotizing vasculitis. CBC and sedimentation rate may be useful as an initial screen: elevated sedimentation rate (? autoimmune disease, ? cutaneous necrotizing vasculitis, ? infection); eosinophilia (? worm infestation). Hepatitis panel may be indicated. ANA is obtained if autoimmune disease is suspected. Serum complement levels (C3, CH50) may be altered in certain diseases (e.g. autoimmune disease, cutaneous necrotizing vasculitis). C1, C4, C1 INH levels are useful for diagnosing deficiency of inhibitor of activated C1 component. If there is a deficiency, the characteristic findings are a normal C1 level with low C4 and C1 INH. Skin testing is seldom helpful. RAST (radioallergoabsorbent test) to detect specific IgE antibody directed against suspected allergens is likewise seldom helpful.

Treatment: Remove/avoid the offending agent if it can be identified. Subcutaneous epinephrine (see drug section for dose) is required if there is respiratory distress from laryngeal/pharyngeal edema or if significant hypotension develops. Antihistamine usually helps relieve symptoms. Diphenhydramine (Benadryl) is recommended for acute urticaria (25–50 mg PO, IV, or IM every 4–6 hours as needed) and is an useful adjunct to epinephrine if there is anaphylaxis. Hydroxyzine (Atarax, Vistaril) may be beneficial in chronic urticaria. H–2 antagonist antihistamine (e.g. cimetidine) may be tried concurrently with a regular antihistamine if the latter does not provide adequate relief. Oral ephedrine or terbutaline may also be combined with an antihistamine if an antihistamine alone is not adequate. A combination drug containing both a sympathomimetic and an antihistamine may be more convenient (e.g. Tedral). Cromolyn sodium (Intal) may be tried in cases of chronic urticaria unresponsive to antihistamines. Oral or parenteral corticosteroids are usually not needed and topical corticosteroids are of no value. Chronic urticaria/angioedema (i.e. recurrent episodes of urticaria lasting over 1 month) for which no cause can be found is sometimes treated empirically. The following drugs may be tried in succession: metronidazole for 5 days, oral ketoconazole for 1–2 weeks, erythromycin for 10 days. An antihelminth (thiabendazole for 3 days) may also be tried. Hereditary angioneurotic edema is treated with an anabolic steroid (e.g. danazol).

Skin Cancer

BASAL CELL CARCINOMA is the most common type of skin cancer. **Risk factors:** Seldom occurs in dark–skinned persons or before the age of 40. Long–standing exposure to sunlight is the most common risk factor. Other risk factors include history of ionizing radiation, history of arsenic exposure, basal cell nevus syndrome. **Appearance:** The tumor grows slowly. Most cases occur on the face or scalp, and less often on other sun–exposed areas—e.g. chest, arms. Typical appearance: In the early stages, one usually sees a small firm shiny translucent papule or nodule. Color varies: pale, red, or (in the case of a pigmented type) brown to black. At the edges, telangiectasias may be seen under a magnifying glass. As the tumor enlarges, the center ulcerates and crusts but the border remains smooth, shiny, and firm. Other presentations sometimes occur—e.g. indurated scar–like plaque on the face or neck, slightly raised plaque resembling eczema on the trunk. **Local invasion** may occur but metastasis does not. **Biopsy** diagnosis is essential. **Treatment:** Excision is the usual therapy. Superficial radiation, electrocautery, or cryotherapy are sometimes used because of cosmetic concerns.

SQUAMOUS CELL CARCINOMA usually develops on sun–exposed areas of the skin in persons over 55 with actinic keratoses. Fair–skinned individuals are most susceptible. Besides excessive sun–exposure, factors that may increase the risk include x–radiation, arsenic, burn scars, skin ulcers, xeroderma pigmentosum, discoid lupus. **Appearance:** The tumor grows slowly. It starts as a reddish papule, or it may commence as a scaling or crusting plaque. Further growth leads to a nodular or wart–like appearance and ultimately there is ulceration. **Metastasis** is most likely to occur in patients with risk factors other than sun–exposure. An exception is an actinic keratoses–associated squamous cell carcinoma of the lip, Left untreated, this lesion has about 10% chance of metastasizing. **Biopsy** confirmation is necessary. **Treatment:** Excision is the safest course.

MELANOMA may arise in any location where melanocytes are found—e.g. skin, mucous membranes, CNS, eye. Cutaneous melanomas may arise from melanocytes in normal skin or a pre–existing nevus. They usually develop on sun–exposed areas. **Three types of cutaneous melanoma** are recognized: <u>Superficial spreading melanoma</u> accounts for about 70% cases. It occurs in women as often as men. It is usually seen in those areas of skin where there has been excessive sun–exposure. It grows relatively slowly over a period of years. It is usually seen as a brown black slightly raised plaque with irregular borders. The more advanced lesions may have blue, red, or white areas; and a papular or nodular surface. <u>Nodular melanoma</u> (15% cases) has the worst prognosis. It is rapidly growing with little radial growth. It is usually darkly pigmented dark brown to black. It presents as a plaque or it may have a papular or nodular contour. There may be erosion of the central area. <u>Lentigo maligna melanoma</u> develops in elderly persons and seldom occurs in other than Caucasians. This type of melanoma develops in sun–exposed areas from a lentigo maligna (Hutchinson's freckle). Lentigo maligna is a 2–20 cm diameter hyperpigmented macular area with different shades of brown and traces of black. Growth is slow and confined to the epidermis for a number of years before finally extending into the dermis. With progression—red, blue, or white areas may develop and the tumor surface may become papular or nodular. **Treatment:** excision.

MYCOSIS FUNGOIDES (cutaneous T–cell lymphoma) is an uncommon malignancy. **Appearance:** Mycosis fungoides is often difficult to diagnose in the early stages when an eczematous condition develops. Patients are often thought to have psoriasis, seborrheic dermatitis, or nummular dermatitis. With time the lesions progressively thicken and become nodular. Patients often present with large superficial erythematous plaques in no particular distribution. The lesions may scale. There may be pruritis and it may be severe. **Metastasis** occurs in about two–thirds of cases—e..g. to lymph nodes, liver, spleen, lung. **Sēzary's syndrome** may develop: there is generalized erythroderma with exfoliation, lymphadenopathy, severe pruritis, lymphocytosis, and the peripheral blood contains Sēzary cells (atypical lymphocytes with large convoluted nucleus and a scanty cytoplasm that is PAS–stain positive). **Diagnosis:** Histologic exam of skin biopsy specimen discloses so–called mycosis cells (hyperchromatic lymphocytes with irregular nuclei), band–like dermal infiltrate of atypical lymphocytes, and Pautrier's abscesses (accumulations of abnormal lymphocytes in the epidermis). **Treatment option**s: total skin electron beam irradiation, topical nitrogen mustard, PUVA (psoralen with ultraviolet A radiation). Cures are uncommon and currently are only possible in the early stage.

Scabies is due to a mite, Sarcoptes scabiei. The mites are usually transmitted by close personal contact, and unusually via the clothes or bedclothes of infested persons. The gravid female burrows into the epidermis and lays eggs as she goes. The larvae emerge and establish residence in the hair follicles, mature, and mate.

Signs/symptoms: <u>Pruritis</u>; A severe allergy–induced itch develops 2–6 weeks after exposure at the sites of the burrows or papules. <u>Areas of involvement</u>; Common sites are the sides and webs of the fingers; volar aspect of the wrists and elbows; axillary folds; the areolae; breast folds of women; male genitalia. The head, palms, soles are generally spared in adults. However, in infants and small children, burrows may be seen on the palms or soles, and papules may be found on the head and neck. Burrows, if they are not obscured by excoriations or secondary infection, may be recognized as slightly elevated dark lines 0.5–1.5 cm long with a tiny papule at the open end. The lines may be straight or tortuous. In many cases, burrows are not found. Papules and/or vesicles also contain the mite and are more frequently observed than burrows. Other lesions: Excoriations are common. There may be secondary bacterial infection—e.g. pustules, impetigo. Slowly resolving reddened and indurated inflammatory nodules up to about a centimeter in diameter may arise. Eczema may develop. Urticaria sometimes occurs. Crusted scabies is a rare, severe, and very contagious form of scabies that is most likely to occur in immunocompromised patients. It is characterized by a widespread scaling dermatitis that frequently involves the hands and feet in association with dystrophic nails.

Diagnosis of scabies is confirmed by finding the adult female in a skin scraping of a burrow or a papule. The specimen is examined microscopically X 50–100. A drop of mineral oil preferably or 20% KOH may be adVded to the specimen prior to viewing. ●With the help of a magnifying glass, the female may sometimes be identified by extricating her from her burrow with a needle.

Treatment: lindane (Kwell, Scabene); refer to drug section. Crotamiton (Eurax) is an alternative which may also relieve itching. Close contacts should be treated as well. Clothing, bedclothes, and towels should be washed in hot water or dry cleaned. Itching may be relieved with antihistamines. If not, a topical corticosteroid or even a short course of PO prednisone may be required to relieve itching. Pruritus may continue for some time following successful treatment; it is not necessarily an indication that treatment has failed.

Pediculosis (lice infestation) may be due to either of 2 obligatory blood-sucking species: (**1**) Phthirus pubis—the cause of lice infestation of the pubic hair principally; (**2**) Pediculus humanus—the cause of lice infestations of the scalp and body. Body lice are vectors for typhus, trench fever, and relapsing fever.

Mode of transmision/signs/symptoms: Body lice are transmitted via infested clothes and bedclothes. Nits (eggs) may be found attached to body hair. The lice are seldom found on the body, but they and their nits may be found along the seams of clothing. The bites of the adult lice may leave reddened papules and there may be itching with excoriation; and possibly secondary bacterial infection. In sensitized persons, the bites may provoke widespread erythema, urticaria, lymphadenopathy. Scalp lice are transmitted by contact with infested clothes, hats, or hairbrushes. Besides the scalp; the eyebrows, eyelashes, and/or beard may sometimes be infested. The eggs (nits) are found attached to the shaft of the scalp hair but the adult lice may not be easy to find. The bites of the adult lice provoke itching with excoriation. There may be dermatitis. Not uncommonly, there is secondary bacterial scalp infection with posterior cervical and posterior auricular adenopathy. Pubic infestation ("crabs"): Transmission is by person–to–person contact, or by contact with infested clothes and bedclothes. Nits are found attached to the pubic hair and perianal hair chiefly; less often on the hair of the thighs, body, axillae, beard, or eyelashes; and seldom on the scalp hair. Adults are not found easily. Dark brown specks (lice excrement) in the infested regions or on undergarments may be seen. The lice bites may leave reddened papules and/or small dark bluish spots on the skin (maculae ceruleae). Itching with excoriation is common.

Treatment: Topical applications of pyrethrins + piperonyl butoxide (e.g. RID, A–200 Pyrinate) or lindane (Kwell, Scabene) are effective. Lindane (see drug section) is also effective against scabies. A repeat application may be required in 7–10 days if living lice are found, or if nits are found at the base of the hair shaft next to the skin (this is indicative of newly–laid eggs). Sexual contacts of patients with pubic lice should be treated as well. Eyelid infestations may be treated by twice daily application of petrolatum for 7–10 days. Suspected fomites (infested clothes, bedclothes, hats, towels) should be washed in hot water or dry cleaned. Infested brushes or combs should be boiled. Removal of the lice and nits after treatment is not necessary unless it reassures the patient. A fine–toothed comb or forceps may be used for this purpose.

Ear, Nose, Throat, and Mouth

Otitis Media
Rhinitis
Sinusitis
Pharyngitis
Peritonsillar Abscess
Retropharyngeal Abscess
Diptheria
Stomatitis
Dental Abscess

Otitis Media (inflammation of the middle ear).

Pathogens: Acute bacterial otitis media: Pneumococcus is the most common pathogen in all age groups. Haemophilus influenza is the 2nd most common in infants and children; incidence declines after 8 yr of age. Less common pathogens include Strep. pyogenes (group A); Branhamella catarrhalis; coliforms (E. coli, proteus, klebsiella); Staph. aureus, mycoplasma, viruses. Infants < 6 wk of age: The most prevalent pathogens after pneumococcus and H. influenza are coliforms (E. coli, Proteus, Klebsiella) and less often Staph. aureus. Chronic otitis media is usually due to a gram–negative aerobe (e.g. klebsiella, proteus, pseudomonas). Serous otitis media: In many cases there is no infection but simply the accumulation of secretions due to obstruction of the eustachian tube. Serous otitis media may follow acute bacterial otitis media. Eustachian tube may be obstructed because of allergic inflammation (in association with allergic rhinitis), adenoid hyperplasia, or tumor.

Signs/symptoms: Acute infectious otitis media often follows an upper respiratory infection. Besides earache, there is often fever and perhaps impaired hearing. Eardrum is reddened (However, this also seen in a child without infection who is crying.). The eardrum may bulge. Bony landmarks (i.e. the underlying maleus) behind the tympanic membrane are obscured. Fluid behind the eardrum may be disclosed by observing decreased movement of the pars flaccida when air is insufflated into the external auditory meatus via a pneumatic otoscope. If the tympanic membrane perforates, there is a serosanguinous to purulent discharge. In small children, otitis media is often associated with vomiting and diarrhea. In chronic otitis media, there is perforation of the eardrum with chronic or recurrent discharge. This condition is due to chronic obstruction of the eustachian tube or to chronic mastoiditis.

Treatment: Antibiotic therapy for acute bacterial otitis media: Amoxicillin or ampicillin for 10 days is usually effective. The most common pathogens are covered (pneumococcus, H. influenza, group A streptococci). Ampicillin–resistant strains of H. influenza are not uncommon. When this is known or suspected, Augmentin (amoxicillin with potassium clavulanate) or cefaclor are options since H. influenza, pneumococcus, and group A streptococci will be covered. In infants < 6 wk of age, cefaclor is a good choice since it will also cover coliforms and Staph. aureus. Trrimethoprim–sulfamethoxazole (Bactrim, Septra); sulfisoxazole–erythromycin (Pediazole) will cover H. influenza and pneumococcus but sulfonamides are contraindicated in infants < 2 months of age, nursing mother, or last 3 months of pregnancy. Infants that do not respond to oral antibiotics in 24 hours should be admited for septic workup and IV antibiotics administered. Tympanocentesis may be needed to relieve severe pain in some cases. Tympanocentesis is also helpful when the response to antibiotics is inadequate, and also affords the opportunity to obtain a sample for gram stain, and culture. Tympanocentesis is also advised in immunosuppressed patients with otitis media. Tympanostomy: Selected patients with persistent middle ear effusions (either serous or infectious) are candidates for placement of tympanostomy tubes. Chronic otitis media which fails to respond to antibiotics may improve with adenoidectomy if the adenoids are blocking the eustachian tube. Mastoidectomy may be required if persistent and antibiotic–unresponsive mastoid infection is the source of otitis media. Allergy–associated serous otitis media: A decongestant/antihistamine combination may be tried (e.g. Sudafed, Actifed).

Complications: Spread of the infection medially may lead to labyrinthitis with vertigo and sensorineural hearing impairment, and/or involve the facial nerve so that facial palsy ensues. Posterior spread leads to mastoiditis, and from here infection may involve the sigmoid sinus where it may provoke thrombosis. Upward extension into the cranial fossa may lead to meningitis, subdural empyema, and/or cerebral abscess. Choleastoma: Chronic otitis media is associated with perforation of the eardrum. A marginal perforation may lead to the development of a choleastoma as follows: Squamous epithelium from the external auditory canal moves in to cover or to attempt to cover the perforation. In the process, the squamous epithelium proliferates and desquamates within the middle ear to form a choleastoma (revealed as an accumulation of white debris in the middle ear). A choleastoma may destroy adjacent bone (possibly seen on otoscopic exam or on x–ray) and predisposes to the other complications just cited.

Rhinitis (inflammation of the nasal mucous membranes) may be due to infection (e.g. common cold), inhaled allergens (allergic rhinitis), inhaled irritants (vasomotor rhinitis), medications.

ALLERGIC RHINITIS is divided into seasonal allergic rhinitis (hay fever) which is due to airborne pollens (tree pollens, weed pollens, grass pollens) and perennial allergic rhinitis which results from inhalation of nonseasonal allergens (e.g. dust, animal dander, molds). **Pathogenesis:** In sensitized individuals, IgE molecules are bound to mast cells in the nasal submucosa. Upon inhalation, the offending antigen attaches to IgE molecules and this induces the mast cell to release substances (e.g. histamine, bradykinin, prostaglandins, ECF–A, etc.) that mediate nasal mucosal inflammation. **Signs/symptoms:** The nasal mucosa is usually bluish–red to normal in color. The mucosa is swollen, often to the point of nasal obstruction so that the patient must breathe thru his mouth. There is a clear nasal discharge which contains many eosinophils. The patient complains of nasal itching and sneezing. Conjunctival involvement is common: conjunctival itching, injection, and tearing. Postnasal "drip" and pharyngitis are common concurrent complaints. Mucosal inflammation may extend to the eustachian tubes so that obstruction with serous otitis media and impaired hearing may ensue. Sinusitis may also complicate allergic rhinitis. **Tests:** Blood differential may be normal or reveal eosinophilia. Smear of nasal discharge typically shows many eosinophils. Skin testing may identify the causative allergen. **Treatment:** Avoid offending allergens Electrostatic air purifiers may help reduce exposure. Antihistamines provide some relief. Chlorpheniramine (Chlor–Trimeton) or brompheniramine (Dimetame), terfenadine (Seldane), astemizole (Hismanal) are among the least sedating antihistamines. Antihistamines are often combined with a sympathomimetic (e.g. phenylpropanolamine, pseudoephedrine) as in certain combination preparations (e.g. Actifed, Sudafed). Cromolyn sodium nasal solution spray (Nasalcrom) may be effective. However, it may take 2–4 weeks before beneficial effects are realized. Initially, concurrent use of an oral antihistamine–sympathomimetic combination (e.g. Actifed, Sudafed) may be helpful. Nasal corticosteroid inhalants such as beclomethasone (Beconase, Vancenase) are effective in the treatment of allergic rhinitis. Systemic corticosteroid side effects do not occur at the recommended doses. Desensitization by subcutaneous injections of a specific known allergen may be tried if the above measures fail or are not feasible. Starting at very low doses, increasing doses are injected at 1–2 week intervals until a maximum dose is reached. Maintenance injections are then continued at monthly intervals. Desensitization is associated with decrease in serum IgE levels, and an increase in serum IgG blocking antibodies directed against the allergen.

INFECTIOUS RHINITIS is usually an acute phenomenon due to infection by a virus (i.e. the common cold). Many viruses have been implicated (e.g. rhinoviruses, coronaviruses, influenza, parainfluenza, respiratory syncytial virus, adenoviruses, coxsackievirus, echoviruses). ●Group A streptococci may also cause acute rhinitis. ●Rhinitis may be the consequence of chronic infections including tuberculosis, leprosy, syphilis, histoplasmosis, blastomycosis, leishmaniasis. **Common cold syndrome** is associated with swollen and reddened nasal mucosa. Neutrophils (not eosinophils as in allergic rhinitis) are found in the nasal discharge. Fever, chills, sore throat, cough, headache, bodyache are common accompanying complaints. **Treatment** of the common cold is symptomatic; many oral decongestant–antihistamine combination "cold" preparations are available. Nasal sprays or drops containing a vasoconstrictor (e.g. phenylephrine) may also provide relief. However, rebound nasal mucosal vasodilation occurs with overuse as the nasal mucosa becomes insensitive to the topical agent. Penicillin (or erythromycin in the penicillin–allergic) is used to treat rhinitis due to group A streptococci.

VASOMOTOR RHINITIS is a nonallergic phenomenon of unknown cause that is associated with engorgement of the nasal mucosal blood vessels. The nasal mucosa is swollen and reddened to bluish in color. Typically, there is a small amount of clear discharge without eosinophils. Dry air or inhaled irritants may worsen the condition. Relief may be obtained with humidified air and oral sympathomimetics (e.g. pseudoephedrine). Topical nasal vasoconstrictors should not be used.

RHINITIS MEDICAMENTOSA is most often due to the overuse of topical nasal vasoconstrictors. Nasal mucosal congestion subsides upon discontinuation of these
agents. Nasal mucosal congestion may also be associated with hydralazine or reserpine therapy. Ovarian hormones may also mediate rhinitis (e.g. oral contraceptives,
pregnancy, premenstrual).

Sinusitis
Acute sinusitis is most often due to H. influenza or pneumococci, and less frequently to Staphyloccocus aureus, S. pyogenes, or anaerobes.
Acute sinusitis is frequently precipitated by a viral upper respiratory infection. Chronic sinusitis is often a mixed anaerobic infection. Predisposing factors; allergic rhinitis, anatomic abnormalities impeding sinus drainage, impaired immunity, cystic fibrosis, Wegener's granulomatosis, Kartagener's syndrome.

Diagnosis: Pain; The frontal sinus is supplied by the superior orbital nerve. Consequently, pain from frontal sinusitis may be felt over the forehead and up to the vertex of the scalp. Maxillary sinusitis is felt over the distribution of the infraorbital
nerve (pain over the cheek and upper teeth). Ethmoid sinusitis typically causes pain
behind or between the eyes. Sphenoid sinusitis causes occipital or frontal pain.
Sinusitis–associated pain may be worsened by straining or bending forward.
Tenderness may be present over the frontal sinus (press upward on medial part of
the superior orbital margin), ethmoid sinus (press against the medial wall of the
orbit), or the maxillary sinus (press on the face below the inferior orbital margin).
Failure to transilluminate; The maxillary sinus may not transilluminate if there is
accumulation of fluid within that sinus (in a dark room shine a light upward into the
roof of the mouth or thru the sinus). Check the frontal sinuses similarly by shining a
penlight upward against the medial margin of the orbit. Associated findings may include septal deviation, congested nasal mucosa, purulent nasal discharge. Maxillary
sinusitis may be associated with or follow dental infection. Sinus x–rays may demonstrate air–fluid levels in or opacification of involved sinuses. These findings
usually indicate the presence of purulent fluid. Congestion of the sinus mucosa also
contributes to radio–opacity. The sinus mucosa may be thickened in chronic sinusitis.

Treatment: Antibiotic; Amoxicillin or ampicillin for at least 10 days is standard
therapy. Alternatives are trimethoprim–sulfamethoxazole (Septra, Bactrim); or
doxycycline. Several weeks of antibiotic therapy may be required in chronic cases.
Decongestant such as PO pseudoephedrine and steam inhalation may promote
drainage. Surgical drainage is indicated when sinusitis is refractory to antibiotics or
when the patient is septic.

Pharyngitis
Causes: Viral infection is the most common cause—e.g. rhinoviruses, coronaviruses, adenoviruses, Coxsackie A (herpangina), respiratory syncytial virus, influenza,
parainfluenza, Ebstein–Barr (infectious mononucleosis), cytomegalovirus, herpes
simplex. Bacterial infection; Group A streptococcus is a common cause of pharyngitis. Other bacterial causes of pharyngitis are relatively uncommon—e.g. gonococcus, Vincent's disease (a symbiotic infection due to spirochetes and fusiform bacteria). Diptheria is rare in the U.S. Other bacteria may be cultured from the pharynx
(e.g. pneumococcus, H. influenza, staphylococcus) but do not cause pharyngitis in
immunocompetent individuals. Fungal infection; Candida may cause pharyngitis.

Signs/symptoms: Sore throat is characteristic. However, mild or asymptomatic pharyngeal infection may occur. A sore throat combined with nasal discharge
and/or conjunctivitis suggests a viral infection. Dysphagia is a common complaint
with streptococcal pharyngitis. Pharyngeal exudate may or may not be present. An
exudate does not differentiate streptococcal pharyngitis from viral pharyngitis. Adenoviruses, herpes simplex, infectious mononucleosis are often associated with a
pharyngeal exudate. Furthermore, an exudate may be absent in streptococcal pharyngitis. Adenopathy: Tender cervical nodes are common in both viral and bacterial
pharyngitis. Infectious mononucleosis is suggested by generalized adenopathy
and/or splenomegaly. Vesicles may be seen with either Coxsackie A (herpangina) or
herpes simplex. Pseudomembrane that bleeds when it is removed is characteristic
of diptheria.

Laboratory: Routine throat culture is obtained to identify group A streptococcus. Monospot test is performed if infectious mononucleosis is suspected. Atypical lymphocytes may be seen on blood smear of patients with mononucleosis. Throat culture specific for gonorrhea (Thayer–Martin) is obtained in homosexuals or when a history of fellatio is elicited.

Treatment: Symptomatic relief of both viral and streptococcal pharyngitis may be obtained with salt–water gargles, and aspirin or acetaminophen. Streptococcal pharyngitis is usually self–limited. However, antibiotic therapy is recommended to prevent spread of the infection and to prevent complications (e.g. rheumatic fever, glomerulonephritis, peritonsilar abscess). Administer a single IM dose of benzathine penicillin G 1.2 million unit (600,000 unit IM for child < 27 kg). An alternative is penicillin VK 250 mg PO tid–qid for 10 days (12.5 mg/kg PO qid x 10 days for child, maximum 1 gram/day). Erythromycin is used in penicillin–allergic patients: 250 mg PO qid for 10 days (10 mg/kg PO qid x 10 days for child, total daily dose not to exceed 1 gram). Gonococcal pharyngitis: refer to "Gonorrhea" chapter for treatment. Diptheria: see "Diptheria" chapter.

Peritonsillar Abscess (Quinsy) is an unilateral abscess between the tonsil and superior constrictor muscle. It is a complication of group A streptococcal pharyngitis. However, streptococci are not isolated from the abscess but other oropharyngeal bacteria are found instead. The tonsillar region bulges medially, the uvula is displaced contralaterally, and the soft palate anteriorly. The neck is swollen on the involved side. Swallowing is very painful and trismus often develops. Initially there is a phlegmon and this is amenable to penicillin therapy alone. Once an abscess forms (revealed by fluctuance on palpation with a gloved finger), incision and drainage is necessary.

Retropharyngeal Abscess (abscess between the prevertebral fascia and superior constrictor muscle) is an uncommon complication of pharyngitis that may result in obstruction with dysphagia and inspiratory stridor. There is fever and the neck is stiff and hyperextended. Bulging and fluctuance of the posterior pharynx may be noted. Lateral x-ray of the neck shows widening of prevertebral soft tissue. Treatment: surgical drainage and IV antibiotic.

Diptheria is a rare disease in the U.S. It is due to Corynebacterium diptheriae—a gram–positive nonmotile aerobic bacillus. The disease is spread person–to–person by nasopharyngeal secretions or by infected skin lesions. Asymptomatic carriers are often the source of infection. **Pathogenesis:** Incubation takes about 2–6 days. The organism typically invades the tonsilar mucosa and destroys the superficial epithelium to produce a grayish pseudomembrane consisting of fibrin, necrotic epithelium, leukocytes, bacteria. A pseudomembrane may also form on the rest of the pharynx, the soft palate, and nasal mucosa; and the process may even extend down to involve the larynx, trachea, and/or bronchi. The proliferating bacteria produce an exotoxin which is systemically absorbed. The major clinical consequence of the exotoxin is myocarditis which may lead to heart failure and arrhythmias.

Signs/symptoms: Sore throat ia present. Dysphagia is common. Mucosal bleeding characteristically results if the adherent pseudomembrane is removed. Dyspnea, stridor, and possibly asphyxia may result if there is pseudomembrane formation and edema in the larynx, trachea, and bronchial mucosa. Heart failure and/or arrhythmias may develop as a consequence of exotoxin production.

Treatment is begun immediately without awaiting laboratory confirmation (e.g. growth on Loeffler's medium). Diptheria antitoxin and an antibiotic (erythromycin or penicillin) are administered. Bed rest with isolation for 10–14 days. Airway management: Intubation or tracheostomy is sometimes required. Bronchoscopy is necessary to remove pseudomembrane if the bronchi are involved. Coronary care: Cardiac monitoring is necessary if there are EKG abnormalities. Arrhythmias or heart failure are treated in the usual manner.

Prevention: diptheria immunization (see "Routine Immunizations" chapter).

Stomatitis (inflammation of the mucous membranes of the mouth)

APTHOUS STOMATITIS (canker sores) is a common and often recurrent disease of unknown cause. Apthous lesions are common in patients with inflammatory bowel disease and are seen as part of Beçhet's syndrome. **Signs/symptoms:** Shallow painful ulcers (usually < 6 mm in diameter but sometimes larger) are found on the oral mucosa—usually the buccal or labial mucosa. The ulcers are typically covered with a pseudomembrane and surrounded by erythema. The number of ulcers varies from 1 to 15, but 2 to 3 are usually found. **Treatment:** Spontaneous healing (without scarring) over 1–2 weeks is the rule, although large lesions may persist longer. Rinsing the mouth with a tablespoon of 2% viscous xylocaine before eating or every 3–4 hours provides pain relief.

VINCENT'S DISEASE (Vincent's angina, acute necrotizing ulcerative gingivitis, trench mouth) is an acute gingivitis caused by normal oropharyngeal anaerobes (fusiform bacteria and spirochetes). Poor dental hygiene and poor nutrition appear to be predisposing conditions. **Diagnosis:** Ulcers are seen on the interdental papillae and marginal gingiva. The ulcers are covered with a purulent exudate and tend to bleed. A foul breath is typical. The buccal mucosa is involved rarely. Gram stain of the lesions shows many spirochetes and fusiform bacteria. **Treatment** is with PO penicillin, or with PO erythromycin if the patient is allergic to penicillin.

THRUSH is a stomatitis due to overgrowth of Candida albicans—a normal intraoral inhabitant. Antibiotic or corticosteroid therapy, impaired immunity, diabetes mellitus, xerostomia are predisposing conditions. **Signs/symptoms:** Thrush is common in otherwise normal infants but should not be confused with milk curds which are easily wiped away. White patches are seen on the tongue and buccal mucosa, and may also be found on the gums, palate, and throat. Removal of a thrush "patch" leaves a reddened oozing area. **Laboratory:** If the diagnosis is in doubt, microscopic exam of a KOH preparation of a sample taken from the lesions may show pseudohyphae and yeast. **Treatment:** nystatin or clotrimazole (see drug section).

OTHER CONDITIONS associated with oral mucosal ulcers include herpes simplex (see "Herpes Simplex" chapter), syphilis (primary chancre or mucous patch), herpangina (small vesicles and ulcers on the soft palate due to Coxsackie A virus), blood dyscrasia, erythema multiforme, lichen planus, pemphigus, pemphigoid, drug eruption, oral cancer.

Dental Abscess usually develops as a consequence of tooth decay

(caries). Cold or sweets may, in the absence of infection, provoke a toothache in a patient with caries alone. ●As tooth decay advances, the pulp is eventually involved and becomes inflamed (pulpitis). With pulpitis, there is often a spontaneous unprovoked throbbing toothache which is aggravated by heat or cold. ●Infection then extends thru the apex of the tooth and a periapical abscess forms. Pain on percussion of the involved tooth suggests the presence of a periapical abscess. A periapical radiolucency is seen on dental x-ray. ●Further extension of the infection may result in facial swelling with fever and regional adenopathy. **Treatment:** penicillin therapy followed by root canal or tooth extraction. Fluctuant abscesses are drained, usually thru an intraoral incision.

LUDWIG'S ANGINA (infection/suppuration of the floor of the mouth) is uncommon. It is usually a complication of an untreated dental abscess. The tongue is upwardly displaced and protrudes. There is indurated cervico-facial swelling. Airway obstruction may ensue.

Eye Disease

Conjunctivitis
Orbital Cellulitis
Cavernous Sinus Thrombosis
Hordeolum
Chalazion
Dacrocystitis
Uveitis
Glaucoma
Central Retinal Artery Occlusion
Cataract
Ultraviolet Keratitis
Strabismus
Corneal Abrasion
Corneal Foreign Body
Traumatic Iritis
Hyphema
Orbital Blow–out Fracture
Chemical Eye Injury

Conjunctivitis (inflammation of the conjunctiva—the mucous membrane covering the posterior surface of the lids and anterior surface of the sclera).

Blepharitis is the term used when only the mucous membrane of the eyelid is involved. **Etiology:** Infection is the most common cause—e.g. viral, bacterial, chlamydial, rickettsial, fungal (rare), parasitic (rare). Allergy or chemicals may be responsible. Other conditions that may be associated with conjunctivitis include psoriasis, Sjögren's syndrome, Reiter's syndrome, gout, rosacea, erythema multiforme, dermatitis herpetiformis, carcinoid, thyroid disease, pemphigoid, Wegener's granulomatosis. **Signs/symptoms:** Conjunctival reddening is characteristic. Itching is a frequent complaint, particularly with allergic conjunctivitis. Gritty foreign body sensation may be present. Tearing is common. Tearing is often profuse in viral conjunctivitis. Photophobia and/or pain may be present If the cornea is also involved. Chemosis (edema of the ocular conjunctiva) is seen as a swelling about the cornea. It is common in hay fever conjunctivitis. It may also occur in bacterial conjunctivitis (N. gonorrhea, N. meningitidis) and in adenovirus keratoconjunctivitis. Discharge: A mucopurulent discharge is typical of bacterial conjunctivitis. A profuse purulent discharge is characteristic of Neisseria gonorrhea or N. meningitidis. A scanty exudate is typical of viral infections. A stringy white mucoid discharge occurs in allergic conditions.

BACTERIAL CONJUNCTIVITIS is most often due to pneumococcus, H. influenza, and staphylococci. Less common causes include streptococci, Neisseria gonorrhea, N. meningitidis, Moraxella, H. aegyptius. **Signs/symptoms:** Usually both eyes are involved. There is a mucopurulent discharge and a foreign body sensation. The lids may be edematous. **Laboratory:** A gram stain and culture of the exudate may be obtained. Giemsa stain of conjunctival scraping will reveal the presence of many neutrophils. However, these tests are not necessary in routine cases. If gonorrhea is suspected, a Thayer–Martin culture is obtained. **Treatment:** Antibiotic drops are prescribed (e.g. gentamycin, Neosporin) although most cases of bacterial conjunctivitis resolve spontaneously in 2 weeks. Gonococcal conjunctivitis must be treated aggressively with saline irrigation and intravenous acqueous penicillin G (neonate: 25,000 unit/kg IV twice daily for 7 days, adult: 10 million units/day IV in divided doses for 5 days). **Prevention neonatal gonococcal conjunctivitis:** At birth, instill 0.5% erythromycin ointment (within 30 minutes of birth), or one drop of 1% silver nitrate solution in the conjunctival sac of both eyes.

ADENOVIRUS KERATOCONJUNCTIVITIS is associated with conjunctival injection, pain, photophobia, and tearing with a scanty secretion. A tender preauricular node may be present. Other findings may include epithelial keratitis, subepithelial opacities, conjunctival pseudomembrane. Giemsa stain of conjunctival scraping discloses many mononuclear cells. With some adenovirus strains there may also be fever, pharyngitis, cervical adenopathy. **Therapy:** Conjunctivitis resolves spontaneously within 3–4 weeks. However, a topical antibiotic is usually prescribed since it may not be clinically possible to distinguish viral from bacterial conjunctivitis.

HERPES SIMPLEX CONJUNCTIVITIS is usually due to herpes simplex type 1 (HSV 1). HSV 2 conjunctivitis is uncommon. The conjunctiva are injected, there is photophobia, and there is tearing with a mucoid discharge. A tender unilateral preauricular node is a common finding. In the initial episode, vesicles may be present on the lid margins or adjacent skin. If the cornea is also involved (i.e. keratoconjunctivitis), the typical finding is dendritic keratitis. Dendritic keratitis is easily recognized with fluorescein stain as a branched ulcer of the corneal epithelium. There may be a foreign body sensation followed by decreased corneal sensation. With recurrences the cornea may scar and vision may be affected. **Therapy** is not indicated if only the conjunctiva is affected. Topical antiviral agents (e.g. vidarabine, acyclovir) are used if there is keratitis.

ACUTE HEMORRHAGIC CONJUNCTIVITIS (due to picornavirus type 70) is characterized by profuse tearing, serous discharge, foreign body sensation, pain, and photophobia. The eyelids are edematous and there may be chemosis. There is conjunctival suffusion with development of subepithelial follicles, and subconjunctival hemorrhages. Other findings may include tender preauricular nodes, fever, myalgias. The condition resolves spontaneously in about a week.

INCLUSION CONJUNCTIVITIS

In the newborn, infection is acquired during passage thru the birth canal from a mother with cervicitis due to C. trachomatis immunotypes D–K. Signs of conjunctivitis become evident 5–14 days after birth: mucopurulent discharge, conjunctival suffusion, chemosis, lid swelling. Hypertrophy of papillae in the conjunctival folds may be apparent. Chlamydia may be isolated from the conjunctiva and also from the neonate's nasopharynx, rectum, vagina, urethra. Not uncommonly, infants go on to develop pneumonitis and occasionally otitis media. Diagnosis is confirmed by: (1) finding epithelial–cell inclusion bodies on Giemsa or immunofluorescent stains of conjunctival scrapings, (2) culture of conjunctival scrapings. Treatment of either inclusion conjunctivitis and pneumonitis is erythromycin 12.5 mg/kg PO 4 times/day for 2–3 weeks. Prevention: Silver nitrate does not prevent inclusion conjunctivitis. Erythromycin ophthalmic ointment is the recommended prophylaxis.

In adults the infection is acquired by contact–spread from infections of the genital mucosa. Conjunctivitis is milder than that seen in newborn. Treatment is with tetracycline 500 mg PO 4 times/day for at least 7 days to eradicate both conjunctival and possible genital infection. Erythromycin is an alternative.

TRACHOMA is a chronic conjunctivitis due to Chlamydia trachomatis immunotypes A-C. It is most prevalent in hot dry climates in the setting of poor sanitation. Trachoma is particularly common in Asia and Africa. Infection is transmitted from the eyes of infected patients by direct contact, fingers, contaminated towels, flies, etc. Many millions are infected and millions of untreated persons go blind. **Signs**: After about a week of incubation, there is conjunctival suffusion with lacrimation and lid edema. Over the next several weeks or months, there is a progressive follicular conjunctivitis that is particularly prominent in the conjunctiva of the upper lids. This folliicular conjunctivitis is associated with enlargement of the subepithelial lymphoid follicles and hypertrophy of surrounding papillae. With chronicity, there is progressive pannus formation. Pannus (corneal vascularization with fibrosis) starts at the limbus of the upper cornea and works down. Continuing invasion of the cornea by blood vessels with fibrosis culminates in corneal opacification. In the eyelids, follicular and papillar hypertrophy eventually gives way to atrophy and scarring with infolding of the lids (entropion). Lacrimal glands and ducts are also involved, and so impaired tearing ensues. **Diagnosis**: Giemsa or immunofluorescent stains of conjunctival scrapings show typical inclusions within conjunctival epithelial cells. Cultures from the conjunctiva may also be diagnostic. **Treatment** is with topical or oral tetracycline or erythromycin.

ALLERGIC CONJUNCTIVITIS:

Hay fever conjunctivitis is associated with allergic rhinitis. Typical findings include bilateral ocular itching, tearing, conjunctival injection, chemosis (in severe attack), and a small amount of stringy white discharge. Treatment consists of cool compresses, and a PO antihistamine concurrent with topical vasoconstrictor drops—e.g. tetrahydrozoline (e.g. Visine, Murine Plus).

Vernal keratoconjunctivitis is a recurrent spring–summer seasonal condition. The patient complains of lacrimation and itching. There is a papillary conjunctivitis of the eyelids, and so the conjunctival surface of the eyelids typically has a "cobblestone" appearance due to the presence of enlarged closely packed papillae. The limbic area of the bulbar conjunctiva may also become hypertrophied. Treatment consists of cool compresses and topical corticosteroids. Refer to ophthalmologist.

Atopic keratoconjunctivitis is characterized by nonseasonal conjunctival itching and/or burning. There is photophobia with tearing and a mucoid discharge. The conjunctiva have a pale milky appearance and fine papillae are noted. Corneal involvement may with time lead to corneal vascularization with impaired vision. This condition is usually associated with other evidence of atopy (e.g. hay fever, atopic dermatitis, asthma). Treatment: topical cromolyn (Opticrom).

Orbital Cellulitis is most often due to staphylococci, streptococci,

or pneumococci. The infection usually spreads to the orbit from infected sinuses (most often the ethmoid or maxillary) either by direct extension or via orbital veins. Infection may also arrive along venous channels from a focus of infection in the skin of an eyelid, or be introduced by eye trauma. **Signs/symptoms:** Typically the eyelids quickly become red, swollen, and tender. The conjunctiva are edematous. There may be proptosis of the affected eye. Fever and leukocytosis often develops. **Laboratory:** Obtain CBC as well as gram stain and culture of conjunctiva, nasopharynx, or other likely sources of infection in the area. **Treatment:** Intravenous antibiotics and warm compresses usually leads to improvement within 2–3 days. Antibiotics are continued for 7–14 days. Surgical drainage may be required (e.g. abscess of eyelid, sinus, or orbit). **Complications** include cavernous sinus thrombosis, meningitis, brain abscess, optic neuritis.

Cavernous Sinus Thrombosis may result when

there is a focus of infection in a region which has venous drainage into the cavernous sinus (e.g. face, ear, sinuses). **Signs/symptoms:** Impaired or absent pupillary reflexes and ocular movement is due to involvement of the cranial nerves (III, IV, and VI) that control these functions and that pass thru the cavernous sinus. Severe eye pain is the consequence of involvement of the ophthalmic division of the trigeminal nerve which also passes thru the cavernous sinus. Additional findings include papilledema, impaired vision, exophthalmos, edema of the lids, fever. Sometimes there is bilateral involvement. **Treatment**: intravenous antibiotics and anticoagulation.

Hordeolum (stye) is a suppurative infection of a gland of the eyelid.

EXTERNAL HORDEOLUM is an abscess of one of the glands of Zeis (a sebaceous gland connected to the follicle of an eyelash) or glands of Moll (modified sweat glands). **Signs/symptoms:** The stye is found at the margin of the eyelid. There is a red swollen tender area at the lid margin. This focus subsequently suppurates, usually points to the skin side of the lid, and then drains spontaneously. **Treatment**: warm compresses, antibiotic drops. Incision is advised if the infection does not improve within 2 days.

INTERNAL HORDEOLUM is an abscess of one of the meibomian glands (sebaceous glands within the tarsal plate). **Signs/symptoms:** There is a localized area of pain, redness, and swelling. The abscess almost always points to the conjunctival surface. Examination of the conjunctival surface of the lid discloses a small (sometimes yellowish) swelling. Spontaneous drainage is unlikely. **Treatment** is as for external hordeolum.

Chalazion (chronic inflammatory granuloma of a meibomian gland of the

eyelid) presents as a firm nontender swelling within an eyelid. Examination of the conjunctival surface reveals a small red or gray lump. Chalazion may follow from a hordeolum. **Treatment**: The lump often resolves spontaneously within a few months. Furthermore, treatment may be unnecessary if the lump is small. The lump is excised by an ophthalmologist if it is causing a problem.

Dacryocystitis (inflammation of the lacrimal sac) is usually associ-

ated with obstruction of the nasolacrimal duct. In infants, Haemophilus influenza is the most common infecting organism. In acute adult cases, the most common pathogens are Staphylococcus aureus or beta-hemolytic streptococcus.

Signs/symptoms: In acute dacryocystitis, the area about the lacrimal sac is red, tender, and swollen; and there is an associated conjunctivitis. Since the normal outlet for tears is usually blocked, tears overflow onto the cheek (epiphora). In chronic cases, there is swelling in the region of the lacrimal duct and epiphora. In many cases, pus can be expressed from the blocked nasolacrimal duct back thru the puncta into the medial conjunctival area. **Treatment:** In acute cases, warm compresses are applied, and oral or parenteral antibiotic is administered (e.g. a cephalosporin pending culture results). Definitive treatment of chronic dacrocystitis is accomplished by unblocking the nasolacrimal duct.

Uveitis is subdivided into anterior uveitis (also called iritis or iridocyclitis) if

there is inflammation of the iris and/or ciliary body, and posterior uveitis if the choroid is inflamed. Posterior uveitis is usually associated with retinitis (i.e. there is chorioretinitis).

ANTERIOR UVEITIS is usually idiopathic. Known associations include inflammatory conditions (e.g. ankylosing spondylitis; juvenile rheumatoid arthritis, sarcoidosis); infections (e.g. syphilis, tuberculosis). **Signs/symptoms**: Vision is slightly blurred and there is moderate to severe pain. The pupil is small and reacts sluggishly to light. The cornea is clear but the conjunctiva, particularly the conjunctiva immediately around the cornea, is injected. Intraocular pressure is normal. Slit lamp examination is diagnostic: there are bright spots in the anterior chamber due to the presence of free-floating cells. **Treatment**: Mydriatic drops and topical corticosteroid is standard therapy. Antibiotics are administered if infection is the suspected cause.

CHORIORETINITIS is often idiopathic. Known causes include congenital toxoplasmosis, cytomegalovirus, herpes, syphilis, tuberculosis, cryptococcus. **Signs/symptoms**: Vision may be impaired. There may be eye pain, photophobia, and/or lacrimation. Fundoscopic exam typically discloses white or yellow retinal lesions.

Glaucoma is the optic nerve damage with ensuing visual field defects

that results from elevated intraocular pressure. The intraocular pressure increases when there is impaired outflow of acqueous humor thru Schlemm's canal of the anterior chamber. Increased intraocular pressure per se does not define glaucoma.

Open-angle glaucoma versus closed-angle glaucoma: In closed-angle glaucoma, the root of the iris abuts on the trabecular absorptive surfaces and/or cornea thereby preventing the outflow of acqueous humor from the anterior chamber. In open-angle glaucoma the trabecular resorptive surfaces in the angle between the iris and the cornea are unobstructed but ouflow is impaired for other reasons.

Primary versus secondary glaucoma: Glaucoma is also classified as primary if the precipitant is unknown and secondary if there is a known cause.

PRIMARY OPEN-ANGLE GLAUCOMA is the most common form of glaucoma (> 90% cases). There is an abnormality of the trabeculae and Schlemm's canal that leads to impaired outflow of acqueous humor. However, mechanical obstruction of outflow due to the abutment of the peripheral iris on the trabeculae as in closed-angle glaucoma is not present. **Diagnosis**: The disease process leading to increased intraocular pressure affects both eyes. The patient is asymptomatic until late in the disease when visual impairment ensues (loss of peripheral field with preservation of central vision). Tonometry discloses the elevated intraocular pressure (usually > 25–30 mm Hg). Fundoscopic exam reveals increased cupping of the optic disc (cup to disc diameter ratio exceeds 0.3–0.6) and pallor of the optic disc may be discerned. Quantitative perimetry testing may reveal scotomas or more extensive peripheral field loss. Crude methods of assessing visual field such as confrontation with moving finger will only reveal large visual field deficits. Gonioscopy is performed to verify that the anterior angle is open. **Treatment** consists of one or a combination of a miotic (e.g. 0.5–4% topical pilocarpine one drop 4 times/day), a topical drug to reduce acqueous humor production (e.g. 0.25% or 0.5% timolol), and acetazolamide. Surgery is employed (e.g. laser trabeculoplasty) if medical therapy fails to control intraocular pressure.

PRIMARY CLOSED-ANGLE GLAUCOMA accounts for < 2% cases of glaucoma. This condition may occur in persons with a narrow angle between the iris and cornea. The shallow anterior chamber may be demonstrated by shining a penlight from the temporal side of the eye and noting that a shadow is cast on the nasal side of the iris. Primary closed–angle glaucoma may sometimes be precipitated by factors that cause the pupil to dilate (e.g. drugs with anticholinergic properties, topically applied mydriatics). **Signs/symptoms**: In acute cases, usually only one eye is affected. There is sudden onset of blurred vision followed by severe eye pain. A halo is seen about lights. The pupil is mid–position and fixed. The cornea has a steamy appearance that may obscure the iris somewhat. The conjunctiva at the corneal–scleral junction is injected. There may be nausea and vomiting. Elevated intraocular pressure (sometimes > 50 mm Hg) is confirmed by tonometry. **Treatment acute case**: intravenous acetazolamide (Diamox), oral glycerin (1ml/kg), topical 4% pilocarpine (2 drops every 15 minutes). Administer intravenous mannitol (see drug section) if the intraocular pressure is still elevated after 30 minutes. Once the acute attack is controlled, laser iridotomy (preferably) or surgical iridectomy is performed on the peripheral iris in order to allow outflow of acqueous humor from the angle of the cornea and iris.

In chronic primary closed–angle glaucoma, the iris starting superiorly gradually extends its arc of contact with the trabeculae until the resorption of acqueous humor is so impaired that the intraocular pressure rises. The patient may experience intermittent episodes of blurred vision with halos about lights and perhaps mild pain. An acute attack of glaucoma may supervene if the remaining open portion of trabecula becomes abruptly occluded.

SECONDARY GLAUCOMAS may be of the open–angle or closed angle type. Examples of secondary glaucoma follow. **Trauma** may lead to increased intraocular pressure with ensuing glaucoma by various mechanisms: (**1**) blood leaking into the anterior chamber as a consequence of injury to the iris or ciliary body may block outflow of acqueous humor outflow via the trabeculae, (**2**) direct injury to the trabeculae may impair acqueous humor resorption, (**3**) an open corneal wound may seal by forming senechiae that obstruct acqueous outflow, (**4**) the lens may be displaced anteriorly thereby obstructing acqueous flow thru the pupil into the anterior chamber. **Cataracts** may lead to glaucoma: (**1**) the lens may swell so that outflow of acqueous into the anterior chamber is blocked, (**2**) the lens may press the iris toward the cornea so that the iris abuts on the cornea and acqueous is unable to pass out thru Schlemm's canal of the anterior chamber, (**3**) the lens may leak proteins that block the trabecular meshwork. **Cataract surgery** may lead to glaucoma: (**1**) The corneal or conjunctival epithelium may grow into the anterior chamber and cover the iris and trabeculae so that acqueous outflow is prevented. (**2**) The surgical wound may leak acqueous so that the anterior chamber is emptied and the iris therefore lies against the cornea. Anterior synechiae with outflow obstruction ensue. **Uveitis (iridocyclitis)** may cause open–angle glaucoma by generating inflammatory cells and protein that occlude the trabecular meshwork. Furthermore, chronic uveitis may lead to anterior synechiae and further compromise outflow. **Rubeosis iridis** (neovascularization of the anterior surface of the iris and trabecular meshwork) with obstruction of the trabecular outflow is a form of secondary open–angle glaucoma most often associated with diabetes mellitus or central retinal vein occlusion.

Central Retinal Artery Occlusion may be due

to an embolus; disease of the vessel itself (e.g. atheromatous plaque, polyarteritis nodosa, giant cell arteritis); or carotid artery obstruction. **Diagnosis**: There is a sudden unilateral loss of vision. There is no pain. Initially, fundoscopy reveals narrowing of the arterioles with segmentation of the venules (due to venous stasis). After a few hours the retina becomes pale except for a "cherry red macula" (the thinner retinal region of the fovea appears red by contrast because blood supply to the underlying choroid is unimpaired). The pupil fails to react to light but the consensual reflex is preserved. **Treatment** must be instituted within the first hour if any vision is to be saved. Initial therapy, before an ophthalmologist is available, consists of massaging the eyeball in an attempt to dislodge an embolus. Rebreathing into a paper bag in order to raise the CO_2 level may also be helpful for its vasodilating effect. The ophthalmologist performs anterior chamber paracentesis.

Cataract (opacification of the crystalline lens or its capsule).

Etiology: Cataracts may be congenital (e.g. secondary to rubella in pregnancy). Most cataracts are associated with advanced age. Other causes or contributing conditions may include diabetes mellitus, eye trauma, glaucoma, hypocalcemia, Paget's disease, certain drugs (e.g. corticosteroids, chlorpromazine). **Signs/symptoms:** Usually, there is a gradual impairment of visual acuity and perhaps color perception. Fixed spots may be seen before the eyes (in contrast to vitreous "floaters" which move). There is no pain. Ophthalmic exam reveals opacification of the lens. Cataracts secondary to diabetes mellitus may develop rapidly. **Treatment:** The lens is removed when vision becomes significantly impaired.

Ultraviolet Keratitis (flash burn) may result from exposure to

light from arc welder or intense exposure to sunlight (e.g. snow blindness). About 12 hours after exposure, the patient experiences severe eye pain with photophobia. There is tearing with reddened conjunctiva. Examination of fluorescein–stained eye under cobalt blue light reveals minute punctate lesions of the cornea. **Treatment**: systemic analgesics. Topical analgesics are not prescribed. Symptoms will resolve spontaneously within 1–2 days.

Strabismus (heterotropia, squint) is said to be present when the visual

axes of the eyes are such that the image of an object falls on the fovea of only one eye. In the other eye (the deviant or squinting eye), the image of an object falls on some other point on the retina. By contrast, when a person with normal binocular vision looks at a point, the image falls simultaneously on the fovea of both eyes.

Strabismus and development of amblyopia: Diplopia would be the logical consequence of strabismus were it not for the fact that the brain, in order to avoid confusion, adapts by suppressing the image from the deviant eye. At first, vision of the squinting eye is normal if the good eye is covered. Ultimately, if the condition is not corrected, the vision of the deviant eye is impaired (strabismic amblyopia).

Types of strabismus: The most common type of strabismus is esotropia (internal convergence or cross–eyed) in which the abnormal eye deviates inward followed in decreasing incidence by exotropia (external deviation or wall eyes), hypertropia (upward deviation of an eye), hypotropia (downward deviation of an eye).

Diagnosis: Strabismus is sometimes subtle and may be intermittent. Two tests are commonly used to diagnose strabismus. In one test, the patient is asked to look at a penlight held 1–2 feet away and directed at one pupil and then the other. Normally, the reflection of the penlight should remain centered at the pupil of each eye. In the cover–uncover test, the patient is asked to look at an object and the examiner observes the left eye as the right eye is covered. Normally, the left eye should not move. If it does, there is a squint. The test is repeated for the opposite eye. The test should be performed while observing near and distant objects.

Treatment: Patching of the good eye is used to restore normal vision in the strabismic eye (i.e. treat amblyopia). To be effective in children, patching must be started before the age of 7. The earlier patching is instituted the better since the later strabismus is diagnosed the longer patching is required. Once normal vision of the strabismic eye is restored, eyeglasses and/or surgery are indicated to straighten the eye for cosmesis.

Corneal Abrasion There is pain with a foreign body sensation.

There may be lacrimation and conjunctival injection. The abrasion may sometimes be visible to the naked eye when a penlight is directed obliquely at the cornea. Application of fluorescein stain and examination with cobalt blue filtered light will delineate the abrasion. Slit lamp exam is best. Thorough exam to rule out foreign body is imperative. **Treatment**: No therapy is necessary for small abrasions. For large abrasions, pain may be mitigated by application of a firm patch over the eye. Before patching, an antibiotic solution is instilled into the eye. If there is evidence of traumatic iritis (e.g. photophobia, small poorly reactive pupil); instilling a cycloplegic (e.g.

0.25% scopolamine) will relieve ciliary spasm and make the patient more comfortable. An oral analgesic may be needed to relieve pain. Topical analgesics or steroids should never be prescribed.

Corneal Foreign Body
There is a foreign body sensation, pain, and lacrimation. The foreign body is usually visible to the naked eye. Application of a topical anesthetic will facilitate further exam and foreign body removal. The eye should be examined under magnification. Slit lamp is best. Exam of fluorescein--stained eye under cobalt blue filtered light will clarify additional lesions. **Treatment:** After applying a topical anesthetic (e.g. proparacaine [Ophthaine]), foreign body removal can usually be accomplished with a sterile needle tip or corneal spud. Following removal, antibiotic drops are instilled and a firm patch is applied over the eye. If there is evidence of traumatic iritis (e.g. photophobia, small poorly reactive pupil); instillation of a cycloplegic (e.g. 0.25% scopolamine) will relieve ciliary spasm and make the patient more comfortable. An oral analgesic is prescribed and the patient is referred to an ophthalmologist. Topical analgesics or steroids should never be prescribed.

Traumatic iritis
Moderate pain, blurred vision, and photophobia are characteristic. The pupil is small and reacts poorly to light. Intraocular pressure is normal. Uncomplicated traumatic iritis may be treated by instilling a mydriatic–cycloplegic (e.g. 0.25% scopolamine) to reduce ciliary spasm, and thereby relieve pain and photophobia.

Hyphema
(hemorrhage into the anterior chamber of the eye) may follow eye trauma. Visual acuity may be impaired. Blood is usually seen in the anterior chamber but may not be seen if bleeding is slight. Glaucoma may develop and there may be blood-staining of the cornea. **Treatment:** Unless the anterior chamber is completely filled with blood, hyphema usually resolves spontaneously with bed rest—which should be continued for at least 5 days. Tonometry is performed daily. If the intraocular pressure is elevated, the patient is treated with acetazolamide and topical timolol. Surgery is indicated if the intraocular pressure persistently exceeds 50 mm Hg, or if there is blood-staining of the cornea

Orbital Blow-out Fracture
results from blunt trauma to the eye. As the eye is struck, there is a sudden increase in intraorbital pressure. The weakest part of the orbit is the medial wall and the floor. If the floor collapses, the eye may appear "sunken in". ●Entrapment of the inferior rectus muscle may impair upward gaze and cause diplopia. However, this finding may be difficult or impossible to elicit if there is substantial periorbital swelling. ●The infraorbital nerve runs along the orbital floor. If it is injured, there may also be unilateral hypesthesia of the cheek, buccal mucosa, or upper gum. ●X–ray (stereo Waters view) may confirm the diagnosis, or tomograms or CT scan may be necessary. **Repair** by an ophthalmologist is necessary if movement of the globe is impaired or if there is enophthalmos.

Chemical Eye Injury
may result from a variety of agents. Acid (e.g. battery acid) and alkali (e.g. lime, Drano) burns are of greatest concern. Alkaline burns have the worst prognosis. Immediate copious irrigation of the eye is the key to preventing/mitigating injury. Medical assistance may be sought after irrigation is in progress. In the case of severe alkali burns, irrigation may have to be prolonged for many hours.

Obstetrics and Gynecology

Diagnosis of Pregnancy

Positive (certain) diagnosis: <u>Ultrasound B–scan</u> can reveal intrauterine gestational sac at 5th week gestation. <u>Doppler ultrasound</u> detects fetal heart tones at 12 week gestation. <u>Stethoscope</u> detects fetal heart at 18 week. <u>Fetal movements</u> may be felt by examiner by 5th month.

Probable diagnosis: <u>Enlarged and softened uterus</u> may be felt on pelvic exam at 4–6 week gestation. <u>Hegar's sign</u> (softening of junction of cervix and corpus) can be felt on bimanual exam at about 4 week gestation. <u>Braxton Hick's contractions</u> are pregnancy–associated irregular painless contractions of the uterus. <u>Positive pregnancy test.</u>

Presumptive diagnosis: <u>Chadwick's sign</u> is the pregnancy–associated bluish discoloration of cervix. <u>Quickening</u> (maternal awareness of fetal movements) occurs at 16–18 weeks gestation. <u>Breast</u> tenderness/swelling and nipple sensitivity may be present at 2 weeks gestation. <u>Fatigue, nausea, urinary frequency</u> may also be noted at about 2 week. <u>Other</u> presumptive symptoms include amenorrhea, darkening of areola, colostrum secretion.

PREGNANCY TESTS: Pregnancy tests are based on the level of human chorionic gonadotropin (HCG)—a hormone secreted by the syncytiotrophoblast that is necessary for the perpetuation of the corpus luteum. The corpus luteum is essential to the survival of pregnancy during the first 10 weeks gestation. Even before uterine implantation begins (about 5–8 days following fertilization) the conceptus secretes HCG. HCG peaks at about 10 weeks gestation and then drops to much lower level by the 16–20th week. ●LH (luteinizing hormone) has a composition similar to HCG. Both consist of an alpha and a beta subunit. The alpha subunits are identical, but the beta subunits differ. Tests, therefore, that are not specific for the beta subunit of HCG may give a false positive pregnancy test when LH levels are elevated (e.g. during midcycle surge of LH at time of ovulation, perimenopausal woman).

Types of pregnancy tests: <u>Serum radioimmunoassay</u> is specific for the beta subunit and therefore does not cross–react with LH. It is also very sensitive (detects ≤ 25–50 mIU HCG/ml) and can detect pregnancy within 7 days of fertilization (i.e. before the next anticipated menses). Besides revealing early normal pregnancy, the test is sensitive enough to detect the low levels of HCG associated with ectopic pregnancy. Serum radioimmunoassay can also be employed to quantitatively evaluate diseases in which HCG levels may be increased (e.g. trophoblastic disease, teratoma, carcinoma testes/ovary/breast/lungs). Moreover, quantitative serial measurements may be used to follow the course of the disease. HCG level is greater than usual in multiple gestation. Sequential quantitative meaurement may be useful in detecting the fall in HCG level that is associated with impending spontaneous abortion. <u>Enzyme–linked immunoassays</u> of serum or urine are also specific for the beta subunit and can detect pregnancy within 12 days after fertilization. <u>Serum radioreceptor assay</u> can detect pregnancy within 14 days of conception. It is not specific for the beta subunit. Thus, an elevated serum LH may give a false positive result. <u>Routine serum or urine immunoassays</u> (latex–inhibition slide test, latex–agglutination slide test, hemagglutination–inhibition tube test) can detect pregnancy in the range of 7–28 days after fertilization (i.e. 3–6 wk after onset of LMP). They are not specific for the beta subnunit. Consequently, an elevated serum LH may give a false positive result. They are not sensitive enough to be reliable in the diagnosis of ectopic pregnancy because the low level of HCG associated with ectopic pregnancy gives false negatives in over 20% cases. <u>Home pregnancy tests</u> are about as reliable as the routine immunoassays provided that the instructions are carefully followed.

Causes of inaccurate pregnancy test results: <u>False–positives</u> may occur in the following circumstances: elevated LH when the test is not beta subunit specific (e.g. LH surge at time of ovulation, elevated LH at peri– or post–menopause); persistent corpus luteum; thyrotoxicosis; trophoblastic disease; HCG–secreting malignancy; tubo–ovarian abscess; drugs (e.g. phenothiazines, antidepressants, anticonvulsants, methadone, aldomet, marijuana, high–dose aspirin); hematuria or proteinuria (when using urine tests); hyperlipidemia (with serum tests); termination of pregnancy within last 1–2 weeks. In regards to the latter circumstance, the pregnancy test will usually turn negative within 7–10 days following termination of pregnancy with the less sensitive tests but may remain positive 2 weeks or longer with more sensitive tests. <u>False–negatives</u> may arise when HCG levels are low (e.g. ectopic pregnancy, missed or threatened abortion, early pregnancy). A false negative urine–based test may result if urine is overly dilute.

Contraception

Failure rates of contraceptive methods among typical couples who initiate use of a method (not necessarily for the first time): The percentage who experience an accidental pregnancy during the first year if they do not stop use for any other reason is as follows: chance—85%, spermicides—21%, periodic abstinence—20%, withdrawal—18%, cervical cap—18%, sponge in parous women—28%, sponge in nulliparous women—18%, diaphragm—18%, condom—12%, IUD—3%, oral contraceptive—3%, injectable DMPA—0.3%, injectable NET—0.4%, implants—0.03–0.04%, female sterilization—0.4%, male sterilization—0.15%. Foregoing data extracted from: James Trussell, Robert A. Hatcher, Willard Cates, Jr., Felicia Hance Stewart, and Kathryn Kost, "Contraceptive Failure in theUnited States: An Update." <u>Studies in Family Planning</u> 21 (1), January/February 1990, pages 51–54.

Sterilization: <u>Vasectomy</u> (division of the vas deferens) is a simple and brief procedure that does not require hospitalization. Patients undergoing vasectomy should anticipate that sterility will be permanent although many vasectomies can be successfully reversed. Sterility is not immediate; as a rule the patient will have to have ejaculated at least 10 times to clear the tubes. To be safe, microscopic exam of the semen should be performed to rule out the presence of sperm. Vasectomy procedure fails to prevent pregnancy in 0.15% cases—usually because the patient has had intercourse before the tubes are cleared of residual sperm. <u>Tubal sterilization</u> is usually done with the aid of a laparoscope, by mini–laparotomy, or by colpotomy. The latter 2 methods do not require special equipment. The tubes may be coagulated, ligated, or interrupted with clips or rings. Depending on the amount of tubal destruction, some tubal sterilizations can be successfully reversed.

Condoms besides being a good method of contraception, protect against venereal disease and may thereby possibly protect against development of cervical cancer. Spermicidal condoms (e.g. Ramses Extra, Trojan Plus, Sheik Extra, Contracept Plus) are available that not only enhance contraception but also reduce the risk of infection (the associated lubricant has spermicidal as well as antibacterial and antiviral properties). Natural membrane condoms (made from lamb cecum) should not be relied upon to prevent sexually transmitted infection. The risk of a condom rupturing during intercourse is about 0.6%. Rubber condoms should not be exposed to heat as the rubber will deteriorate. Petroleum lubricants (e.g. Vaseline) will also cause deterioration. Condoms should not be reused.

Foam, cream, gels must (because of the limited duration of spermicidal effect) be inserted intravaginally no more than 30–60 minutes prior to intercourse. An additional dose is advised if > 30 minutes has elapsed before anticipated intercourse or if intercourse is to be repeated. Douching is avoided for at least 8 hours. Creams and gels may be used alone or, for increased effectiveness, in conjunction with a diaphragm or cervical cap. The antiviral and antibacterial properties of these products may also reduce the risk of sexually transmitted infection.

Suppositories must be allowed to dissolve in the vagina for 10–15 min before intercourse. They must not be inserted more than 30–60 minutes prior to intercourse because maximal spermicidal effect lasts < 1 hour. An additional suppository is advised if intercourse is repeated. Douching is avoided for 8 hour following intercourse.

Vaginal contraceptive sponge serves as a barrier and also contains a spermicide. The sponge is more effective in nulliparous women; parous women are twice as likely to become pregnant using this method as nulliparous women. In nulliparous women, the sponge is about as effective as a diaphragm. The sponge must be left in place for a minimum of 6 hours following intercourse but removed (because of the increased risk of toxic shock syndrome) before 24 hours elapses. Because the sponge continues to confer protection while it remains in the vagina, additional intercourse is possible during the first 18 hours following insertion. Douching is prohibited while the sponge is in place. The sponge should not be used if there is vaginal bleeding or abnormal discharge, or for 6–12 weeks following childbirth.

Diaphragms act as a barrier by covering the cervix. To enhance the contraceptive effect, spermicidal cream or gel is placed in the diaphragm. The diaphragm remains in place a minimum of 6–8 hours following intercourse and douching is avoided during that time. Each time intercourse is repeated, additional cream or gel is inserted into the vagina without disturbing the diaphragm. The diaphragm should not be worn for more than 24 hours. The diaphragm should not be used if there is vaginal bleeding or abnormal discharge, or for 6–12 weeks following childbirth. Diaphragms come in 4 basic types and a variety of sizes. They must be fitted to each patient; the largest fit that is comfortable is recommended. Patients with cystocele, rectocele, prolapse uterus, vaginal abnormalities, or recurrent urinary infections may not be good diaphragm candidates.

Cervical caps (like diaphragms) cover the cervix, are used in conjunction with spermicidal creams or gels, and must be individually fitted. Contraceptive effectiveness is about the same as a diaphragm. The cap remains in place for at least 6–8 hours following intercourse and douching is prohibited during that time. If intercourse is repeated, it is advised that the user insert additional cream or gel into the vagina without moving the cap. The cap should not remain for more than 24 hours. The cap should not be used if there is vaginal bleeding or abnormal discharge, or for 6–12 weeks following childbirth.

Birth control pills are covered in more detail in the drug section under "Oral Contraceptives". Certain antibiotics and anticonvulsants may increase the metabolism of contraceptive hormones and reduce their effectiveness. Combination oral contraceptives: Women are usually started on a combination pill containing 30–35 mcg estrogen (e.g. Ovcon–35, Modicon, Brevicon). Noncontraceptive benefits of combination oral contraceptives include decreased incidence of PID: benign breast disease (fibroadenomas, fibrocystic disease); functional ovarian cysts; and ectopic pregnancy. There is decreased blood loss and decreased incidence of iron–deficiency anemia. There is also a possible decreased incidence of uterine fibroids and rheumatoid arthritis. Progestin–only pill (minipill) is slightly less effective than combination pill. The minipill is often used when estrogens are not advised (e.g. over 35 and smoker; history of hypertension, migraines, or chloasma) or when estrogen–containing pills are not tolerated. A progestin–only pill may be begun immediately postpartum and is the pill of choice in the breast–feeding mother. A disadvantage of progestin–only pills is that spotting, irregular menses, or amenorrhea are relatively common complaints. In contrast to combination pills, progestin–only pills are taken daily without cyclical breaks.

Progestin injections: Medroxyprogesterone (Depo–Provera) 100–150 mg is injected IM every 3 months. An alternative is norethindrone enanthate (Noristerat) 200 mg IM every 7–10 weeks. **Progestin implants:** Norplant is a subcutaneously implanted capsule that slowly releases levonorgestrel.

Post–coital contraception: The risk of becoming pregnant after unprotected midcycle intercourse is estimated, depending on the authority, to be 2–30%. Ovral can prevent pregnancy if given early enough. Administer two Ovral pills (ethinyl estradiol 100mcg/norgestrel 1 mg) within 24–72 hours of unprotected intercourse and another two pills 12 hours after the first dose. Pregnancy testing is advised if menses does not occur within 3 weeks. High–dose estrogens are no longer approved for postcoital contraception. Insertion of a copper–containing IUD within 5 days of unprotected intercourse is also an effective means of post–coital contraception. However, this method should not be used in women who are nulliparous or who have any of the absolute or relative contraindications to IUD use (see below).

Intrauterine device (IUD) does not prevent ovulation and fertilization may occur. The IUD is believed to work by producing an inflammatory reaction in the endometrium and by stimulating prostaglandin production. The environment thereby engendered prevents implantation of the blastocyst and may impair sperm motility. Copper in the copper–containing T380A (Paragard T380A) somehow adds to the contraceptive effect. The copper–containing IUD must be replaced every 4 years. Contraindications to IUD: Absolute contraindications: pregnancy; pelvic infection. Relative contraindications: recent or repeated pelvic infection; multiple sex partners; history of ectopic pregnancy; distortion of uterine cavity; vaginal bleeding of unknown cause; abnormal PAP smear; possible uterine or cervical malignancy; acute cervicitis; significant anemia; valvular heart disease; coagulation disorder; impaired ability to respond to infection (e.g. leukemia, diabetes mellitus, steroid therapy). Caution: Because of the increased risk of pelvic infection, an IUD is not the best contraceptive choice in a nulligravida or any woman considering future pregnancies. Neither is an IUD optimal for a woman with dysmenorrhea or menorrhagia. When to insert IUD: An IUD may be inserted during any part of the menstrual cycle provided that pregnancy is excluded. Some advocate that IUD's be inserted only during the menses when pregnancy is unlikely and the slightly dilated cervix facilitates insertion. However, the risk of infection and expulsion are greater if the IUD is inserted during the menses. Because of the increased risk of expulsion and uterine perforation, an IUD is usually not inserted until 4-8 weeks postpartum. An IUD may be inserted following unprotected intercourse (see "post-coital contraception" above). If pelvic infection occurs, the safest course is to remove the IUD and treat the infection. Another IUD is not inserted for 3 months. If pregnancy occurs, the IUD should be removed because of the risk of infection. Spontaneous abortion will occur in 50% cases if the IUD is left in place, while 25% will spontaneously abort if the IUD is removed. If the patient does not wish to continue the pregnancy, the IUD is removed at the time of induced abortion. Ectopic pregnancy: Even though an IUD appears to reduce the risk, ectopic pregnancy must be considered when pregnancy occurs in a woman with an IUD. IUD string should be felt by the patient after each menses. The expulsion rate is 5-20% during first year of IUD use. If the string cannot be felt and if it is not seen on vaginal exam, the string can often be retrieved from the cervical canal with alligator forceps. If the string is still not located, a pregnancy test is advised before proceeding further (the string may be drawn up by an enlarging gravid uterine cavity). Sometimes an IUD string gradually disappears when the uterus has been perforated at the time of IUD insertion. IUD may be located by x-ray (after pregnancy is ruled out) or by ultrasound. A lenghtening string may indicate partial expulsion. Increased menstrual bleeding is often noted with IUD's. Menses may be longer and there may be intermenstrual spotting. IUD should be removed if the hematocrit is < 32% or falls 5% or more. IUD users should receive iron supplementation.

Abstinence during predicted fertile part of menstrual cycle Three methods are described that predict the interval during which ovulation occurs. Success is most likely if the menstrual cycles are regular. Accuracy may be enhanced by using these methods in conjunction. Calendar method: Subtract 18 days from the shortest of the previous 8-12 cycles and subtract 11 days from the longest cycle and abstain during that interval. For instance, if the shortest cycle is 27 days and the longest 30, then 27-18 = **9** and 30 - 11 = **19** implies that intercourse should be avoided from day 9 to day 19 of each cycle with day 1 being the first day of bleeding. Basal body temperature (BBT) method is based on the fact that body temperature increases after ovulation. The temperature is taken every morning before arising (for convenience, special BBT thermometers are available) and recorded on a BBT chart. In order to gain expertise in predicting the time of ovulation, a chart should be plotted for 3-4 cycles. After ovulation has occurred, the temperature should increase by 0.4-0.7° F. Intercourse is avoided until the temperature has been elevated for 72 hours. To maximize the effectiveness of this method, intercourse is avoided throughout the first part of the cycle (i.e. from the onset of menses, through ovulation, and until the temperature has been elevated for 72 hours). If there is intercourse during the first part of the cycle, it should be restricted to the first 4 days (assuming menstrual cycles are longer than 25 days) because ovulation can occur by day 7. Once proficiency is achieved, the temperature need only be taken from day 3 until the temperature rises and remains elevated for 3 days. Mucus method depends on estrogen-induced changes in the cervical mucus. As ovulation approaches, the cervical mucus becomes progressively more abundant, clear, and less viscous. At the time of ovulation, spinnbarkheit is pronounced (mucus can be stretched between the fingers to ≥ 6 cm). In using the mucus method, it is assumed that no unusual vaginal discharge is present, that semen or other substances have not been introduced into the vagina, and that the patient is not douching.

Induced Abortion

Preliminaries: Confirm pregnancy. See "Diagnosis of Pregnancy" above. Obtain ultrasound if gestational age is uncertain. Obtain history: LMP, pregnancy history and complications, surgery uterus/cervix, uterine abnormalities (e.g. fibroids), allergies, medications. Physical exam is thorough. Note in particular the size of uterus, position of uterus (a retroverted uterus may for instance make procedure more difficult), adnexal masses. Tests: Obtain hemoglobin or hematocrit. Ascertain blood type and Rh. Rh immune globulin will need to be administered at time of abortion if patient is Rh negative. Discuss plans for contraception following the abortion.

First trimester abortion (thru 13 weeks gestation) is usually accomplished by vacuum curettage. This can be done in an outpatient setting. In order to facilitate the procedure, the cervix may be painlessly dilated by placing a laminaria in the cervix 6–24 hours in advance. Before the procedure, a paracervical block is performed with a local anesthetic. If laminaria have not been used, instrument dilation may be needed (e.g. Pratt dilators). To insure complete evacuation, sharp curettage is advised after vacuum curettage Tissue obtained should be examined, under magnification if necessary, to confirm removal of products of conception. Methylergonovine (see drug section) is often prescribed to contract the uterus following the procedure. RU 486 is an orally administered progesterone antagonist recently developed in France but not available in the U.S. that induces early first trimester abortion.

Second trimester abortion (13–20 weeks gestation). D & E (dilation & evacuation) is done in a hospital setting. Cervical dilation is accomplished by placing laminaria in the cervix 6–24 hours before the procedure. Suction curettage is performed after paracervical block (e.g. submucosal injection 5–7 ml 1% lidocaine at 4 and 8 o'clock of cervico–vaginal junction) or under general anesthesia. Crushing instruments may be required to facilitate evacuation. Some clinicians use oxytocin adjunctively, but others do not until the procedure is completed because of concern that contraction of the uterus will make evacuation of the uterus more difficult. Methylergonovine (see drug section) is often prescribed following the procedure in order to contract the uterus. Prostaglandin vaginal suppository–induced abortion: In this method, 20 mg prostaglandin E2 intravaginal suppository every 3 hours is used to stimulate uterine contractions and expel the products of conception. Nausea and vomiting are common side effects, and there may be fever and chills. In order to dilate the cervix, laminaria may be inserted into the cervix 6–24 hours in advance. The prostaglandin will itself soften the cervix. Transabdominal intra–amniotic infusion of abortifacient: Intra–amniotic infusion of prostaglandin F2, hypertonic urea, or hypertonic saline are other methods sometimes used to induce abortion.

Complications of abortion: Infection (e.g. fever, discharge, pelvic pain) must be reported to a physician immediately. Mild infections confined to uterus may sometimes be treated as an outpatient with oral antibiotics and bed rest. Patients with more severe infections that have extended beyond the uterus are admitted and treated with IV antibiotics (see "Pelvic Inflammatory Disease"). To insure that no products of conception remain, D & C is performed once IV antibiotics are on board. Retained products of conception may cause cramping pelvic pain and bleeding. Vacuum curettage or D & C is performed. An oral antibiotic and methylergonovine (see drug section) is subsequently prescribed. Retained blood clots may provoke cramping pelvic pain in the absence of vaginal bleeding. Treatment is by vacuum curettage or D & C. Bleeding is to be expected following an abortion. However, unusually heavy bleeding or bleeding that continues for over 3 weeks mandates investigation to rule out retained products of conception, cervical/uterine trauma, or DIC. Uterine perforation may result in laceration of uterine blood vessels with severe blood loss and shock. Abdomen may be tender and there may be rebound tenderness due to presence of intraperitoneal or retroperitoneal blood. Abdominal x-rays (flat, upright, decubitus) may reveal free–air or intraperitoneal fluid. Laparoscopy may assist in diagnosis. Small uncomplicated uterine perforation in absence of significant bleeding or other trauma can be managed by observation since the uterus will heal without surgical intervention. GI trauma or continuing intra or retroperitoneal bleeding mandates laparotomy. Cervical lacerations: Incidence is reduced by dilating cervix with laminaria beforehand.

Threatened or Spontaneous Abortion

THREATENED ABORTION is defined as uterine bleeding during the first 20 weeks of pregnancy in the absence of cervical dilation or passage of products of conception. About half of threatened abortions will proceed to abortion.

Signs/symptoms: Bleeding and pain: Vaginal bleeding is often accompanied by lower abdominal cramping and sometimes by low back pain. Ectopic pregnancy must be excluded if there is unilateral pain/tenderness. Absence of pregnancy symptoms ? Ask patient if she is still experiencing symptoms of pregnancy (e.g. nausea, breast fullness/tenderness). Vaginal exam: There may be bleeding from the cervical os but the os is closed. Vaginal exam should rule out cervical or vaginal lesions as the source of vaginal bleeding. Assess size of uterus by bimanual exam. Doppler exam may reveal fetal heart tones if the uterus is ≥ 12 weeks size. Hartman's sign (implantation bleeding) refers to the light menses that not uncommonly occurs after becoming pregnant. It occurs about the time of the normally anticipated menses had the woman not become pregnant. Abdominal pain/cramping is absent. The pregnancy is not in jeopardy.

Laboratory: Pregnancy test is obtained unless fetal heart tones are heard. However, the pregnancy test is usually still positive when the patient is first seen even if the fetus is dead. Routine (slide test) urine tests turn negative within 7–10 days while more sensitive tests may remain positive for about 2 weeks after fetal demise. A falling serum HCG level as measured by serial quantitative serum radioimmunoassay may used to detect impending spontaneous abortion. Ultrasound may identify the gestational sac and ascertain fetal viability. CBC is routinely obtained. Urinalysis of catheter–obtained specimen is performed to exclude urinary tract bleeding, especially if no blood is noted on vaginal exam.

Treatment is conservative (bed rest, avoid intercourse), unless fetal demise is confirmed. Close follow–up is recommended and the patient is advised to keep any tissue that passes per vagina.

INEVITABLE ABORTION (uterine bleeding during the first 20 weeks pregnancy that is associated with dilation of the cervix but without passage of products of conception). Vaginal bleeding and lower abdominal cramping are characteristic. Vaginal exam reveals a dilated cervix and there may be bleeding. The cervix may be leaking amniotic fluid and/or the amniotic sac may be visible. **Treatment:** The pregnancy cannot be salvaged. An IV is established and oxytocin may be administered (see oxytocin drug section). The uterus is evacuated by suction curettage. Crushing instruments may be required if the fetus is ≥ 13 weeks gestation. Rh immune globulin is administered to Rh negative patient.

INCOMPLETE ABORTION (passage of only part of the products of conception). Vaginal exam reveals a dilated cervix and the products of conception may be visible in the vagina or cervix. Bleeding may be heavy because a retained placenta prevents uterine contraction. Clots are commonly found in the vagina. Management is as for inevitable abortion.

MISSED ABORTION (fetal demise with prolonged in utero retention of products of conception). Patient may report that she is no longer experiencing pregnancy symptoms. Spotting may occur. The cervical os is closed. Fetal heart tones are absent. **Tests:** Pregnancy test may have turned negative depending on the interval since fetal demise and the sensitivity of the pregnancy test. Ultrasound may confirm fetal demise. Obtain CBC, PT, PTT, and blood type and Rh. **Treatment:** If the uterus is < 14 week size, the uterus is evacuated by vacuum curretage. Laminaria placed in the cervix 4–12 hours beforehand will dilate the cervix and thereby facilitate the procedure. If the uterus is ≥ 14 weeks size, the cervix is first dilated with laminaria. This is followed by suction curettage. Procedure is performed after paracervical block or under general anesthesia. Crushing instruments may be required to enable evacuation. ●An alternative method if the uterus is > 14 weeks is to dilate the cervix with laminaria for 4–12 hours, and then stimulate uterine contractions and delivery with 20 mg prostaglandin E2 intravaginal suppository every 3 hours. Rh negative women receive Rh immune globulin (refer drug section). **Disseminated intravascular coagulation** is a rare complication of missed abortion. Nosebleed, bleeding gums, bruises, etc should arouse suspicion. See "Disseminated Intravascular Coagulation" chapter for further information.

Ectopic Pregnancy (pregnancy at a site other than within the

uterine cavity) is almost always due to a pregnancy within a fallopian tube. About one in 100 pregnancies is a tubal pregnancy. A third to a half of patients with ectopic pregnancy give a history of previous pelvic infection. Ectopic ovarian and abdominal pregnancies are uncommon. They are almost always due to secondary implantation of a ruptured tubal pregnancy. Cervical pregnancy is rare.

Symptoms: Symptoms of pregnancy in general may be present (e.g. anorexia, nausea, vomiting, breast tenderness). Most patients have missed a period. Abdominal pain develops in 95% cases, usually 6–8 weeks after the last normal period. Classically, pain is initially unilateral lower quadrant and crampy (attributed to streching of the involved tube). However, the patient may complain of bilateral lower quadrant, upper quadrant, or diffuse abdominal pain. A sudden sharp abdominal pain may occur when the tube ruptures, and more than one instance of sudden sharp pain may occur over a few days. In many cases, pain is made worse by movement. Paradoxically, one third of those patients who experience unilateral lower quadrant pain actually have pregnancy in the tube opposite from the side of pain. Shoulder pain may result when intraperitoneal blood irritates the diaphragm. Vaginal bleeding occurs in about 75% cases, usually 1–2 weeks after a missed menses. Occasionally, vaginal bleeding occurs at the time of the normally expected menses. Vaginal bleeding typically begins after the onset of pain because endocrine support (HCG is secreted by the trophoblast and progesterone by the corpus luteum) of the endometrium persists until the embryo dies. The amount, number of episodes, and duration of bleeding is variable. Intraperitoneal hemorrhage with hypovolemia may result in faintness and/or syncope. This may occur after an episode of sudden abdominal pain when the tube ruptures.

Physical exam: Temperature; Patient is generally afebrile. Abdominal exam; Abdominal tenderness is nearly always present. It may be unilateral or bilateral lower quadrant, upper quadrant, or diffuse. Intraperitoneal bleeding may provoke peritoneal signs (e.g. rebound tenderness, guarding, rigid abdomen, hypoactive bowel sounds). Bimanual pelvic exam; A tender, usually poorly defined, adnexal mass is a common finding. Movement of the cervix typically elicits adnexal pain. The uterus is often found to be enlarged since the uterus usually grows during the first 6–8 week of ectopic gestation. Blood may accumulate and clot in the cul-de-sac, and the clot is sometimes felt on vaginal or rectovaginal exam. If intraperitoneal hemorrhage has occurred, there may be signs of hypovolemic shock (e.g. tachycardia, postural hypotension, thready pulse, cool clammy pale skin, confusion, tachypnea, flat neck veins, oliguria). Abdominal ectopic pregnancy is rare. Suspicion is aroused in advanced cases when abominal exam reveals the presence of easily-felt fetal parts. Furthermore, the fetus is often oriented abnormally (e.g. transverse lie).

Laboratory tests/diagnostic procedures: If the patient is in shock or has a surgical abdomen, do not delay laparotomy to await the results of diagnostic tests or to perform diagnostic procedures. However, culdocentesis (see below) can usually be rapidly performed without delaying therapy. Pregnancy test; Serum radioimmunoassay (serum beta HCG) is positive in about 99% cases of ectopic pregnancy. Routine (urine) slide tests are not reliable for diagnosing ectopic pregnancy because false–negatives occur in 20–50% cases. CBC; The hemoglobin and hematocrit will (1) be unchanged if intra-abdominal bleeding is acute, or (2) may have decreased if bleeding has been present for sufficient time to allow for dilutional shifts into the intravascular space. The WBC count is usually normal or slightly elevated (< 15,000 in 75% cases, < 10,000 in 50%). Sedimentation rate is normal. Arterial blood gas; There is metabolic acidosis if hypovolemic shock is present. Ultrasound may exclude an ectopic pregnancy by revealing an intrauterine gestational sac (detectable 5–6 weeks after the last menstrual period). A positive serum radioimmunoassay pregnancy test in the absence of an intrauterine gestational sac is consistent with ectopic pregnancy. Culdocentesis; Presence of *non*clotting blood is diagnostic of intraperitoneal bleeding. However, the presence of blood that clots or a negative culdocentesis does not rule out ectopic pregnancy. Laparoscopy is performed if the diagnosis is still in doubt provided that the patient's condition does not demand immediate laparotomy.

Differential diagnosis: ovarian cyst (e.g. ruptured follicular or corpus luteum cyst), pelvic infection, threatened or incomplete intrauterine abortion, adnexal torsion, appendicitis.

Treatment: Large bore IV is established as soon as the diagnosis is suspected. Hypotension is corrected. Type and crossmatch for at least 4 units. Surgery is mandatory. The involved tube is excised or sometimes more conservative measures are undertaken. Abdominal ectopic pregnancy may sometimes go to term. Because of the danger of hemorrhage, however, surgery to remove the fetus is advocated when the diagnosis is made. The placenta is usually left in place because removal may precipitate hemorrhage.

Hyperemesis Gravidarum (severe pregnancy–associated nausea and vomiting resulting in weight loss or dehydration) usually occurs at 2–4 month gestation. Incidence is increased with multiple gestation or molar pregnancy.

Signs/symptoms: Weight loss may have occurred. Signs of dehydration may be present (e.g. dry mouth, poor skin turgor, hypotension, tachycardia). Breath may be ketotic. Abdomen should be nontender and there should be no costovertebral angle tenderness. Urine is concentrated and ketones are characteristic.

Laboratory: Hemoglobin and hematocrit may be elevated as a consequence of hemoconcentration. Electrolyte abnormalities may be found (e.g. hyponatremia, hypokalemia, hypochloremia, metabolic alkalosis). Other tests may be indicated depending on the clinical circumstances (e.g. serum amylase, bilirubin, SGOT).

Differential diagnosis: gastroenteritis, bowel obstruction, appendicitis, hepatitis, cholecystitis, pancreatitis, peptic ulcer, pyelonephritis, diabetic ketoacidosis, intracranial lesion. ●The patient who presents with severe vomiting after 16 weeks gestation should be carefully evaluated to rule out other causes of vomiting besides hyperemesis gravidarum.

Treatment: Establish IV and administer 1–2 liter D5 LR over 1 hour. Administer antiemetic—e.g. promethazine (Phenergan) 25 mg IM or rectal suppository as needed at 4–6 hour intervals. Oral fluids may be tried when vomiting is controlled. Once oral fluids are tolerated, some patients may be sent home provided that dehydration and electrolyte abnormalities have been corrected, urine ketones are no longer present, and there are no other complications. Antiemetic suppositories are prescribed as needed and a bland diet is recommended (while).

Preeclampsia/Eclampsia (toxemia of pregnancy).

Preeclampsia is defined as pregnancy–associated (or recent pregnancy–associated) presence of (1) hypertension and (2) proteinuria and/or edema. **Eclampsia** is said to be present when convulsions and/or coma are present in addition to the signs of preeclampsia.

Risk factors: primigravida, teenager, poor nutrition, preexisting hypertensive vascular disease, family history preeclampsia, diabetes mellitus, multiple gestation, molar pregnancy, fetal hydrops (Rh isoimmunization).

Pathogenesis: The incitant is unknown, perhaps uteroplacental ischemia. Whatever the mechanism, the result is arteriolar spasm with ensuing hypertension and impaired organ perfusion. The renal consequences include sodium retention, proteinuria, and decreased glomerular filtration rate.

Onset: In most cases preeclampsia develops after the 20th week of pregnancy (and the incidence increases thereafter) but it may appear sooner in the presence of trophoblastic growths (e.g. molar pregnancy).

Symptoms: Patient may notice swelling of face or hands (e.g. rings may feel tight). Symptoms suggesting possible development of severe preeclampsia include headache (cerebral edema ?), impaired vision (retinal edema ?), epigastric pain (hepatic edema ?).

Signs: Hypertension (based on BP taken on at least two occasions at least 6 hours apart): (1) ≥ 140/90 or (2) a diastolic ≥ 15mm Hg above usual or systolic ≥ 30mm Hg above usual. Generalized edema, not just dependent edema. Note particularly the face and hands. Rapid weight gain of > 3 lb/wk. Hyperreflexia ±

clonus is characteristic. Fundoscopy sometimes reveals arteriolar spasm. Liver tenderness may be present.

Laboratory: Obtain CBC, urinalysis, serum glucose, serum electrolytes, BUN, creatinine, platelet count, PT, PTT, SGOT. Proteinuria: ≥ 1+ or > 0.3 gram/24 hr. In severe cases, urine protein is 3-4 + or > 5 gram/24 hr. Serum creatinine and BUN are usually normal unless there is preexisting kidney disease. Serum uric acid may be elevated because of decreased renal clearance. In severe cases, additional abnormalities may include: evidence of liver dysfunction (e.g. elevated SGOT, LDH, bilirubin); evidence of disseminated intravascular coagulation (e.g. decreased platelets, presence of schistocytes, prolonged PT and PTT); evidence of decreased plasma volume (e.g. elevated or increasing hematocrit).

Differential diagnosis: (1) Chronic hypertension is suggested by the following: hypertension before 20th week, multiparity, absence of proteinuria. (2) Kidney disease may be associated with proteinuria, hypertension, and edema. (3) Some otherwise normal patients develop proteinuria or generalized edema during pregnancy but BP is not elevated or increased above usual levels. They are therefore not preeclamptic by definition

Complications include placental abruption, acute renal failure, stroke, pulmonary edema, heart failure, hemolysis, DIC, hypofibrinogenemia, retinal detachment, jaundice, liver rupture.

Treatment of mild preeclampsia (blood pressure < 140/90 but diastolic pressure > 15 mm Hg above usual on at least 2 instances 6 hours apart, 1+ proteinuria): ●Patient is placed at bedrest and sodium intake is restricted. ●If signs of mild preeclampsia persist and the L/S ratio is > 2:1, delivery is indicated. ●If signs of mild preeclampsia persist and the fetus is not yet mature and there is no evidence of fetal distress, delivery may be delayed until the lecithin/sphingomyelin (L/S) ratio is > 2:1. ●If signs of mild preeclampsia persist and there is evidence of fetal distress (e.g. abnormal contraction stress test, diminished fetal movement, ultrasound reveals oligohydramnios), delivery is advised even though the fetus may be immature.

Treatment of moderate preeclampsia (blood pressure 140/90 to 160/110 and/or proteinuria > 2+): Hospitalizion, bed rest, and sedation (e.g. phenobarbital 30-60 mg PO/IM every 6 hours) are necessary. Magnesium sulfate (see administration instructions below) is begun when delivery is anticipated within 24 hours. ●Delivery is advised if the L/S ratio is > 2:1. ●If the patient improves and is stable and the fetus is not yet mature and there is no evidence of fetal distress, delivery may possibly be delayed until the lecithin/sphingomyelin (L/S) ratio is > 2:1. Dexamethasone may be indicated to hasten fetal lung maturity. ●Delivery is required irrespective of fetal maturity if the mother fails to improve or if there are signs of fetal distress (e.g. abnormal contraction stress test, diminished fetal movement, ultrasound reveals oligohydramnios).

Treatment of severe preeclampsia: Preeclampsia is considered severe if any one of the following exists: (1) systolic ≥ 160 or diastolic ≥ 110, (2) urine protein 3-4 + or > 5 gram/24 hr, (3) urine output < 500 ml/24 hr, (4) visual or CNS abnormalities, (5) pulmonary edema or cyanosis, (6) epigastric pain/impaired liver function. Bedrest and NPO is required. Intravenous fluids: Start with D5W to run at 100 ml/hr. Make subsequent adjustments according to urine ouput and electrolyte determinations. Closely monitor blood pressure, urine output (preferably with Foley catheter in place), urine protein, IV intake, respirations, reflexes, fetal heart monitor. Magnesium sulfate (see drug section) is administered to prevent seizures. The loading dose is 4 gram which is diluted in D5W to 100 ml and administered IV over 20 minutes. After the loading dose is administered, the usual maintenance infusion is 1 gram/hr. However, the rate of infusion should be titrated to: (1) achieve serum magnesium level of 6-8mEq/liter; (2) the knee jerk, the dose is increased if hyperreflexia or clonus is present, and the dose is decreased or discontinued when areflexia occurs (serum magnesium ≥ 8 mEq/l). Magnesium sulfate is also discontinued if respiratory depression occurs (serum magnesium ≥ 10 mEq/l) or if urine output falls to < 30 ml/hr. If necessary, the antidote for magnesium toxicity is calcium gluconate 10 ml of 10% solution IV over 3 minutes. Intravenous hydralazine: Magnesium sulfate has a mild antihypertensive effect. However, if the blood pressure remains > 110 diastolic or > 170 systolic, intravenous hydralazine (see drug section) is administered. Titrate to diastolic BP of 90-100. Delivery: After the patient has been stabilized, labor is induced with oxytocin or C–section is performed.

Treatment of eclampsia: If the patient is seizing, protect airway and administer diazepam 5–10 mg IV. Follow the guidelines above for severe preeclampsia. Delivery should be accomplished within 24 hours, hopefully within 6 hours.

Treatment after delivery: Seizures may still occur after delivery, particularly the first 2–4 days postpartum. For this reason, the urine protein, urine output, blood pressure, reflexes, hematocrit, BUN, and creatinine should still be monitored. Furthermore, if magnesium sulfate was required, it should be continued for at least 24 hours following delivery. Therapy is then continued with a sedative (e.g. phenobarbital 30–60 mg PO 3 times/day). Proteinuria and edema usually disappear within a few days. Hypertension resolves within 10 days postpartum in about half the patients and within a few weeks in the remainder.

Placenta Previa (implantation of the placenta in the lower segment of the uterus such that the placenta either covers or encroaches upon the internal os). The placenta may cover the internal os completely (total placenta previa), partially (partial placenta previa), or may simply encroach upon the internal os without covering it (marginal placenta previa/low lying placenta).

Risk factors: older or multiparous woman, multiple gestation, prior C–section, prior placenta previa. The incidence of placenta previa is 0.4%.

Signs/symptoms: Time of onset of vaginal bleeding: Bleeding occurs in the 3rd trimester of pregnancy because this is the time that the cervix thins and dilates so that the placental segment covering the internal os separates and bleeds. Vaginal bleeding due to placenta previa seldom occurs before the 7th month. Painless vaginal bleeding is characteristic and is usually sudden in onset. The blood is bright red (by contrast blood may be dark in abruptio placentae). Bleeding may be scant to massive. Bleeding may stop spontaneously, but tends to recur and is usually increasingly severe. If bleeding is severe there may be signs of hypovolemic shock (e.g. tachycardia, postural hypotension, thready pulse, cool clammy pale skin, confusion, tachypnea, flat neck veins, oliguria). Abdominal exam: Typically, the uterus is nontender with normal tone and without contractions. The fetus is not engaged in the pelvis. Breech or other abnormal presentations are common. Fetal heart sounds are normal in most cases. Pelvic exam *must not* be performed until the patient is in the operating room—prepared for emergency C–section if necessary and with blood available for transfusion if needed. This "double setup" precaution is necessary because vaginal or rectal exam may precipitate massive uncontrollable bleeding. Before the bimanual exam, a vaginal speculum is inserted to rule out a nonobstetric lesion as the cause of vaginal bleeding (e.g. laceration, cervical carcinoma, cervical erosion). Ultrasound: If the patient is stable, ultrasound exam may be performed to locate the placenta. If placenta previa is confirmed, vaginal exam is deferred thus sparing the patient the risk of exam–induced hemorrhage. Ultrasound will also reveal fetal age and presentation.

Laboratory: Blood tests: CBC, type and crossmatch blood, PT, PTT. Urinalysis: Urine should be obtained via catheter so that bleeding from the urinary tract can be ruled out. Amniocentesis may be performed if fetal maturity is uncertain in order to determine the lecithin/sphingomyelin (L/S) ratio.

Differential diagnosis: abruptio placenta, bloody show (the blood–stained mucous discharge associated with cervical dilation during the first stage of labor), uterine rupture (rare), vaginal or cervical lesions, vasa previa. Vasa previa (a rare abnormality of the umbilicus in which the umbilical vessels separate in the membranes before reaching the placenta and cross the internal os) may result in bright red painless bleeding if the membranes rupture and the umbilical vessels are disrupted. Fetal heart tones are often absent or abnormal. Since vaginal blood is fetal in origin, testing for fetal blood is diagnostic (e.g. Kleihauer test, Apt test, multinucleated fetal RBC on blood smear).

Treatment of placenta previa: Insert large bore IV as soon as diagnosis is suspected. If hypovolemic shock is present, administer crystalloid (e.g. Ringer's lactate) and transfuse blood.
If massive or continuous bleeding is present or if the patient is in labor, proceed with C–section regardless of whether the fetus is mature or not.

If the fetus is mature and there is either a total or a partial placenta previa, proceed with C-section.

If the fetus is mature and there is a marginal previa, a vaginal delivery may *sometimes* be allowed provided that there is no fetal distress, vaginal bleeding is slight, there is a cephalic presentation, and the patient is a multigravida. In this situation, the membranes are ruptured and labor is induced with oxytocin.

If the fetus is immature and bleeding has abated, it may be possible to delay delivery while observing the patient in the hospital. However, if significant bleeding continues or recurs, C-section is the only recourse.

Abruptio Placentae (premature separation of the placenta, ablatio placentae) is the premature separation of all or part of a normally positioned placenta after the 20th week pregnancy. <u>Risk factors:</u> Abruption occurs in about 1% pregnancies with about 10% chance of recurrence in subsequent pregnancies. Hypertension, multiparity, and/or abdominal trauma may predispose to abruption.

Signs/symptoms: <u>Vaginal bleeding:</u> Blood tends to be darker than with placenta previa. The amount of vaginal bleeding is variable. In some cases, there is no vaginal bleeding because bleeding is concealed (i.e. blood remains confined behind the placenta). The uterus may enlarge if there is concealed hemorrhage. Consequently, if abruption is suspected, it is useful to mark the top of the fundus and note any change in fundal height. <u>Evidence of hypovolemic shock</u> may be present if bleeding is severe. <u>Abdominal pain/tenderness:</u> In severe cases there is constant uterine pain with a tense and tender uterus. Pain and uterine signs are proportionally less remarkable with less serious abruption. <u>Fetal heart tones:</u> Obviously, the more extensive the abruption the more likely it is that fetal heart tones will be absent or abnormal (e.g. bradycardia, late decelerations). <u>Pelvic exam:</u> Unless placentae previa can be ruled out by ultrasound, pelvic exam must be deferred until the patient can be examined in the operating room (prepared for emergency C-section and with blood available for transfusion if needed). <u>Note:</u> In some cases abruption develops after the onset of labor.

Tests: <u>Blood tests:</u> Obtain CBC. Type and crossmatch blood. Since DIC sometimes occurs, a coagulation panel is also obtained (PT, PTT, platelets, fibrinogen, and fibrin split products)—refer to "Disseminated Intravascular Coagulation" chapter. <u>Ultrasound</u> may locate the placenta, delineate the abruption, and also ascertain fetal age.

Differential diagnosis includes placenta previa, bloody show (the blood-stained mucus discharge associated with cervical dilation during the first stage of labor), vasa previa (rare), uterine rupture (rare), abdominal pregnancy-associated hemorrhage, nonobstetric causes of abdominal pain.

Treatment: Insert large bore IV as soon as diagnosis is suspected. <u>Monitor</u> vital signs, urinary ouput, fetal heart tones. <u>If hypovolemic shock is present,</u> administer crystalloid (e.g. Ringer's lactate) and transfuse blood.

<u>If the fetus is immature and abruption is not severe</u> (i.e. patient stable, minimal bleeding, uterine pain/tenderness absent, normal fetal heart tones, normal coagulation tests, relatively unimpressive ultrasound); it may be possible to delay delivery while monitoring patient and fetus in the hospital. Obtain serial hemoglobin and hematocrit. Serial ultrasound may be used to determine if the abruption is enlarging.

<u>All other patients are delivered.</u> Vaginal delivery is permitted provided that: (**1**) the patient is stable and bleeding is not severe, (**2**) there is no evidence of fetal compromise or the fetus is dead, (**3**) conditions for vaginal delivery are favorable (e.g. cervix ripe, cephalic presentation). If these criteria are met, the membranes are ruptured and if necessary labor is induced with oxytocin. Vaginal delivery should be completed in 6-8 hours in order to preclude potential complications of abruption (e.g. DIC, acute renal failure). C-section is indicated for other patients.

Complications: <u>Couvelaire uterus</u> may be a complication of abruption. Blood extravasates into the uterine muscle so that it becomes discolored blue. Hysterectomy is required if the uterus fails to contract with oxytocin administration. <u>Other complications:</u> disseminated intravascular coagulation, renal failure.

Premature Rupture of Membranes is the

spontaneous rupture of membranes more than an hour before the onset of labor irrespective of gestational age.

Diagnosis: Leaking or a gush of fluid from the vagina not accompanied by labor pains is the usual report. Note, however, that it is not unusual for a pregnant woman to complain of vaginal leaking when in fact there is actually urinary incontinence. Vaginal exam with a sterile speculum: That the membranes have ruptured may be obvious (e.g. exposed fetal parts). Testing of vaginal fluid is indicated if the diagnosis is not obvious. Nitrazine paper: Because it is alkaline, amniotic fluid will turn nitrazine paper blue on contact. Remember, however, that blood can also turn nitrazine blue. "Fern" pattern: Vaginal fluid is placed on a glass slide, allowed to dry, and viewed under a microscope. Amniotic fluid is revealed by presence of fern pattern. However, the presence of comingled blood or inflammatory secretions may interfere with ferning.

Infection workup: If infection is likely, samples are obtained during the sterile speculum exam for the following tests: cervical culture (GC, chlamydia, beta strep); gram stain; smear for WBC. If the patient is febrile or shows other evidence of infection, additional tests are ordered: blood cultures, urinalysis, urine gram stain and culture. As clinical circumstances suggest and assuming delivery is not imminent, amniocentesis be perfomed to obtain amniotic fluid samples in order to exclude chorioamnionitis and to assess fetal maturity.

Assessing fetal maturity: L/S ratio: If the pregnancy is not yet at term, a sample of amniotic fluid from the vagina may be tested to determine the lecithin/sphingomyelin (L/S) ratio and thereby assess fetal lung maturity. If necessary, amniocentesis may be performed to determine L/S ratio and to rule out chorioamnionitis. Ultrasound may be indicated to determine fetal age.

Treatment: Avoid bimanual or vaginal speculum exams (except for the initial speculum exam) until labor is in progress in order to not provoke infection. If intrauterine infection is present, expeditious delivery is mandatory regardless of fetal age. If pregnancy is over 34–36 weeks or if the lecithin/sphingomyelin (L/S) ratio > 2:1, delivery is advised within 24 hours. In pregnancies at term, rupture of membranes is followed by spontaneous labor within 12 hours in 70% cases and within 24 hours in 85%. If the fetus is < 34 weeks or the L/S ratio is < 2:1 and there is no evidence of intrauterine infection, it may be possible to delay delivery until the fetus becomes more mature. It is emphasized that vaginal and bimanual exams are avoided so as to not precipitate intrauterine infection. In pregnancies at 26–34 weeks gestation, betamethasone (12 mg IM and repeated in 12–24 hours) is administered to hasten lung maturation and thus hopefully prevent infant respiratory distress syndrome.

Amnionitis (infection of the amniotic sac) is usually due to ascending

vaginal contamination. **Risk factors:** premature rupture of membranes, protracted labor, and multiple vaginal exams are the main risk factors. Other factors are internal fetal monitoring, low socioeconomic status, nulliparity, young age, pre-existing vaginosis. **Pathogens:** More than one pathogen is usually isolated from the amniotic fluid. The most common pathogens are bacteroides species; aerobic gram-negative bacilli (mainly E. coli, Klebsiella pneumoniae, proteus); anaerobic streptococci, group B streptococci, staphylococci. Uncommon pathogens are Listeria Monocytogenes, gonococcus, Chlamydia trachomatis. **Unusual pathogens and routes of infection:** ●Amnionitis may occur when the membranes are intact and the route of infection is either ascending or hematogenous. Organisms that have thus been implicated include rubella, herpes simplex, cytomegalovirus, toxoplasmosis, syphilis. ●Infection may also be introduced by amniocentesis.

Signs/symptoms: There may be fever, and/or uterine pain/tenderness. Tachycardia and tachypnea may be present. If the membranes are ruptured, vaginal exam may reveal foul smelling or purulent amniotic fluid. Fetal heart monitor may reveal tachycardia and/or decreased variability.

Laboratory: CBC; cervical culture (GC, chlamydia, beta strep); cervical gram stain, blood cultures (aerobic and anaerobic). Limulus assay of amniotic fluid may detect presence of endotoxin from aerobic gram-negative bacilli. The latex fixation test may reveal group B streptococci. Uterine culture is obtained if C–section is performed, or the placenta is cultured upon vaginal delivery.

Treatment: Prompt delivery is advised even if the fetus is immature. Vaginal delivery is generally preferable to C–section because maternal morbidity is greater with C–section and neonatal prognosis is generally not improved by C–section. Thus, the decision to perform C–section is customarily based on the usual standard criteria. Dysfunctional labor is common and many patients will require C–section despite oxytocin administration. Broad spectrum antibiotics are begun as soon as amnionitis is suspected, and cervical and blood cultures have been obtained. Intravenous ampicillin plus an aminoglycoside (e.g. gentamycin, tobramycin) is a suitable regimen for patients who will deliver vaginally. A 3rd drug (metronidazole or clindamycin) is added to the regimen if C–section is necessary. Duration of therapy: If blood culture is negative, antibiotic treatment may generally be stopped after the patient has been asymptomatic and afebrile for 24 hours. If blood culture is positive, a 2nd set of cultures is promptly obtained and antibiotic therapy is continued until the patient is asymptomatic and afebrile, and the 2nd set has been shown to be negative for at least 48 hours. If blood culture is positive for staphylococci, antibiotic therapy must be continued for at least 10–14 days.

Labor and Delivery

True labor is characterized by regular contractions that increase in frequency and duration. At first the contractions may occur every 15–30 minutes, and are often first felt in the lower back. True labor contractions become progressively more intense and frequent so that by the latter part of labor, contractions are occurring every 2–3 min and lasting 45–60 seconds.

False labor contractions, in contrast to true labor, are irregular and do not progressively increase in intensity or result in dilation of the cervix.

There are 3 stages of labor:

First stage (from onset of true labor when contractions become regular until the cervix is completely dilated) is itself divided into 2 phases: (1) *latent* phase during which the cervix effaces and dilates to about 2.5 cm, and (2) the *active* phase that follows sees the cervix progress to complete dilation.

	Nullipara	Multipara
First stage usual duration	10–14 hr	6–8 hr
Latent phase		
average duration	8.5 hr	5 hr
max normal duration	20 hr	14 hr
Active phase		
average rate cervical dilation	3 cm/hr	5.7 cm/hr
minimum normal rate dilation	1.2 cm/hr	1.5 cm/hr

Second stage (complete cervical dilation to birth) of normal labor is ≤ 1 hour.

Third stage (birth to delivery of placenta) normally lasts 15–30 minutes.

Initial assessment and preparation of patient in labor: Obtain vital signs and perform brief general physical exam. Is edema present?

Abdominal exam: Assess fetal size and verify presence of fetal heart tones. Are uterine contractions regular? Note their duration.

Vaginal exam: Remember: if there is more vaginal bleeding than the small amount associated with bloody show, vaginal exam is contraindicated unless special precautions are taken (see "Placenta Previa"). Assess for (**1**) rupture of membranes (nitrazine paper and/or fern test if there is doubt); (**2**) presentation (e.g. vertex, breech); (**3**) cervical effacement; (**4**) cervical dilation (0–10 cm); (**5**) station. The station is the level of presenting part with reference to the ischial spines—e.g. – 2 station means the presenting part is 2 cm above the spines, 0 station means the presenting part is even with the spines, and + 2 station means that the presenting part is 2 cm below the spines. Abnormalities in the position of the head, molding of the head, or caput succedaneum may mislead the examiner into judging the station to be lower down than it really is.

Other steps: establish IV (e.g. D5 LR), NPO, enema. Laboratory: CBC, blood type & Rh. Perform urinalysis to rule out proteinuria or glycosuria.

Fetal heart rate (FHR) monitoring may be accomplished directly via a fetal scalp electrode if the membranes have ruptured, or by sensors on the abdomen (e.g. electrode, ultrasound transducer). If electronic monitor is not available, the FHR should be checked with a doppler fetoscope or fetal stethoscope every 15–30 minutes during the first stage of labor and every 5–10 minutes during the second stage.

Baseline FHR: The baseline FHR is the FHR in the absence of fetal stimulation, or between contractions if the patient is in labor. The normal baseline FHR is 120–160. A baseline FHR of 100–120 is common in prolonged pregnancy. In general, a baseline FHR consistently < 100–120 is considered abnormal. Fetal bradycardia (baseline FHR < 120) may be due fetal heart block (e.g. congenital, maternal systemic lupus). Fetal tachycardia (baseline FHR > 160) may be due to fetal hypoxia, maternal fever, maternal hyperthyroidism, sympathomimetic or parasympatholytic drugs.

Variability: The normal fetal heart rate tracing shows both short–term variability (beat–to–beat variability) and long–term variability (the variability seen over the course of a minute). Short–term variability is normally 5–10 bpm. Long–term variability is normally 10–25 bpm and gives the fetal heart tracing its wavy appearance. Diminished variability may be the consequence of fetal hypoxia, indicate that the fetus is asleep, or may be associated with fetal tachycardia. Administration of sedatives or narcotics, or parasympatholytics will also diminish variability.

Early decelerations: As the uterus contracts in the course of normal labor, the fetal head is compressed. This causes a vagally–mediated decrease in the FHR which coincides with the contraction (i.e. the FHR decreases when the contraction begins and returns to baseline when the contraction ends). The FHR tracing of early decelerations are uniform and smooth.

Late decelerations, unlike early decelerations, are consistently late (i.e. begin after the onset of uterine contraction). However, like early decelerations, they have a smooth and uniform contour. Late decelerations are the consequence of fetal hypoxia. Late decelerations are particularly worrisome if they are associated with (**1**) fetal tachycardia, (**2**) diminished or absent baseline variability, or (**3**) less than 45 second delay between onset of uterine contraction and decelerations.

Variable decelerations: Uterine contraction may compress the umbilical cord causing variable decelerations. The onset of a variable deceleration is abrupt, and the onset often varies with respect to the onset of uterine contractions. Furthermore, the shape of the deceleration curve is characteristically variable and irregular. Variable decelerations are worrisome if cord compression leads to progressive hypoxia so that: (1) short–term variability is lost, (2) there is fetal tachycardia, and/or (3) the deceleration ends with a gradual return to baseline. In many cases, cord compression is alleviated by changing position of the patient.

Care of patient with abnormal FHR tracing: Turn patient on her side if she is on her back. Administer oxygen. Stop oxytocin infusion. Cord prolapse should be excluded by vaginal exam. If signs of fetal distress persist, obtain a blood sample from the fetal scalp. A scalp pH < 7.2 is an indication for emergency C–section unless vaginal delivery is imminent.

Analgesia and regional anesthesia: The most common means of providing pain relief during labor and delivery is to administer small doses of narcotics (e.g. 25–50 mg meperidine IV q1–2 hr) after active labor has dilated the cervix to 3–4 cm in the primigravida and 5 cm in the multigravida, and then perform a pudendal block during the 2nd stage. Mild sedation (e.g. hydroxyzine) may be used in the early latent phase of labor, but narcotics are not generally recommended until after cervical dilation is in progress.

Pudendal block: The pudendal nerve carries sensation from the lower vagina, vulva, and perineum. A pudendal block may therefore be used to partially relieve pain when pressure is exerted on this region during the 2nd stage of labor and delivery. The pudendal nerve is blocked with the aid of a needle guide introduced into the vagina and aimed just medial and below the ischial spine. About 8 ml of 1% lidocaine or 2% chloroprocaine are injected and the procedure is repeated on the opposite side.

Lumbar epidural anesthesia interrupts pain sensation from the uterus, cervix, and perineum; and can therefore be used to provide pain relief during both the 1st and 2nd stage of labor.

Subarachnoid saddle block interupts pain sensation from the saddle area and may therefore provide some pain relief after the cervix is completely dilated.

Paracervical block may be used during the 1st stage of labor to interrupt pain associated with uterine contractions and dilation of the cervix. With the aid of a needle guide introduced into the vagina, 5-7 ml of 1% chloroprocaine preferably or 1% lidocaine are injected at the cervicovaginal junction at 3-4 o'clock; the procedure is repeated at 8-9 o'clock. Paracervical block may cause fetal bradycardia. Consequently, this procedure is best avoided in cases of fetal compromise, prematurity, or uteroplacental insufficiency.

Dystocia (difficult labor) may be due to disorders of powers (uterine contractions), passage (pelvis), passenger (fetus), or combination thereof. The stage 1 latent phase is considered prolonged if it is > 20 hr in the primigravida and > 14 hr in the multipara. The stage 1 active phase is said to be protracted if the cervix dilates < 1.2 cm/hr in the nullipara and < 1.5 cm/hr in the multipara.

    Passenger: Fetal abnormalities impeding labor or delivery that may make C-section necessary include large fetus; hydrocephalus; abnormal presentation (e.g. shoulder presentation, transverse lie).

    Passage: The bony pelvis (passage) may make vaginal delivery difficult or impossible if it is too small or if the configuration is abnormal. Pelvic abnormalities may be congenital or be the result of trauma or malnutrition. Diagnosis is based on manual exam and x-ray pelvimetry.

    Powers: Effective uterine contractions (powers) generate pressures of 25-60 mm Hg; pressures ≤ 15mm Hg are inadequate. At the peak of an effective uterine contraction, the uterus does not indent easily with external pressure. Conditions leading to inadequate uterine contractions include uterine overdistension (e.g. multiple gestation), prolonged labor with maternal exhaustion, and administration of narcotics or sedatives before true labor is in progress and the cervix has begun to dilate. If weak uterine contractions are judged to be the cause of impaired labor (and assuming that there are not also abnormalities of either passenger or passage preventing normal progress of labor), it is common practice to (1) perform amniotomy if the membranes are intact and provided that the head is engaged, and (2) augment labor with oxytocin. If labor has not progressed past the latent phase of stage 1 and the patient is tired, an alternative approach is to first rest the patient for several hours (e.g. administer morphine 10-15 mg SC or IM) before proceding as just outlined.

Vaginal delivery with vertex presentation: Just before delivery, as the head is crowning, the mother is told not to bear down but to pant. If it looks as if perineum is going to tear, an episiotomy is performed. When the head emerges, the mouth and nose are suctioned. If the umbilical cord is wrapped around the neck, an attempt is made to remove it (do not place undue tension on the cord that might result in rupture of the cord and fetal blood loss). Failing this, the cord is doubly clamped and cut before delivering the shoulders. After parturition, a sample of cord blood is obtained for neonatal blood type and Rh.

APGAR score of infant is obtained at 1 and 5 min after birth. Point totals are interpreted as follows: severely depressed (0-3), moderately depressed (4-6), good (≥ 7)

SIGN	0	1	2
Appearance (color)	blue, pale	body pink, blue limbs	all pink
Pulse (heart rate)	absent	< 100	> 100
Grimace (reflex response to nasal catheter)	none	some motion, grimace	cough, sneeze
Activity (muscle tone)	limp	some flexion limbs	active
Respirations	absent	slow, irregular	good cry

Note: Administration of narcotics to the mother during labor may be the cause of neonatal depression. The infant will respond to naloxone if this is the case.

Delivery of the placenta and after: The placenta is normally delivered within 15-30 minutes after parturition. Once the placenta is delivered, oxytocin (Pitocin) is administered (e.g. add 10 unit to 500 ml IV solution) to augment contraction of the uterus. Alternatively, 10 unit oxytocin may be given IM. Methylergonovine 0.2 mg IM or 0.2 mg PO q4h x 6 is yet another option. Placenta should be examined to verify that it is complete and the uterine cavity must be manually explored if it is not. The umbilical cord is assessed for the presence of 2 umbilical arteries (a single artery may be associated with congenital anomalies). The cervix, vagina, and perineum are inspected for lacerations. <u>Rh immune prophylaxis:</u> The unsensitized Rh-negative mother who delivers an Rh-postive infant should receive Rh immune globulin (e.g. RhoGAM). <u>Lactation suppressant</u> may be administered if the mother will not be breast feeding (e.g. bromocriptine 2.5 mg PO twice daily for 14 days).

Postpartum bleeding: In the patient that does not require episiotomy, blood loss normally averages about 300 ml. Postpartum hemorrhage (> 500 ml blood loss in the 24 hours following delivery) is most frequently caused (75-90% cases) by uterine atony followed by injury to the genital tract (vagina, cervix, or uterus) or retained placental fragments. Uterine atony is most likely to be due to prolonged labor;

multiparity; general anesthesia, uterine overdistension (e.g. twins, polyhydramnios); uterine fibroid; placenta previa, abruption. <u>Treatment:</u> IV fluids (e.g. Ringers lactate) are administered, and blood is typed and crossmatched. A CBC and coagulation panel are obtained. Uterine atony is managed by uterine massage and oxytocin infusion. If bleeding continues and inspection of the vagina and cervix does not reveal a bleeding site, the uterine cavity is manually explored for retained placental tissue and to exclude uterine rupture.

Isoimmunization

Persons with the D antigen on the surface of their erythrocytes are said to be Rh–positive. During pregnancy or delivery some fetal RBC's may pass thru defects in the placenta into the maternal circulation. If the fetus is Rh–positive and the mother is Rh–negative, the fetal RBC's that gain access to the maternal circulation will provoke her immune system to produce anti-Rh (anti-D) antibodies. These maternal anti-Rh antibodies then pass across the placenta into the fetal circulation where they cause lysis of the fetal RBC's. The fetus is seldom affected during the first pregnancy, but the risk of serious fetal hemolysis is increased with each successive pregnancy in which the maternal immune system is challenged by a Rh–positive fetus. **Maternal injections of Rh immune globulin** are given to prevent sensitization of an Rh–negative mother by Rh–positive fetal RBC's. The injected Rh immune globulin contains anti-Rh antibody that "coats" the fetal Rh–positive RBC's that have gained access to the maternal circulation, and so the maternal immune system is not induced to produce anti-Rh (anti-D) antibodies.

Rh genotype: All the children resulting from the union of a Rh–negative (i.e. dd genotype) female and a homozygous Rh–positive (i.e. DD genotype) male will be Rh–positive, while half of the offspring on the average will be Rh–positive if the father is heterozygous (Dd genotype).

D^u antigen refers to weak antigenic forms of the D antigen. About 1% of whites and 8% of blacks are D negative but D^u positive. Immune prophylaxis of these patients is the same as for patients who are simply D-negative (Rh-negative).

Other Rh antigens (e.g. c/C, e/E) derived from the Rh gene locus may be implicated in Rh isoimmunization.

Erythroblastosis fetalis and antigens other than Rh antigens: Antibody directed against the antigenic products of the Rh locus is not the only possible cause of erythroblastosis fetalis. Other maternal antibodies either natural, or induced by transplacental passage of fetal erythrocytes or by incompatible blood transfusion are capable of causing fetal hemolysis. Notable examples include antibodies directed against the ABO blood group antigens, anti-Kell antibody, and anti-Duffy antibody. Maternal-fetal ABO incompatibility may actually prevent maternal Rh sensitization. For instance, when the RBC's of a blood type A Rh-positive fetus enter the circulation of a blood type O Rh–negative mother; the mother's anti-A antibodies bind to and hemolyze the fetal RBC's before antibody against the D antigen can be induced.

Clinical consequences of fetal and neonatal hemolysis: <u>Fetal hydrops:</u> Fetal hemolysis causes fetal anemia. Anemia in turn induces the fetal bone marrow to release immature RBC's or erythroblasts into the fetal circulation (hence the term erythroblastosis fetalis). The severely anemic fetus may develop hydrops fetalis (e.g. generalized edema, ascites, pleural effusions) with congestive heart failure. Fetal death may ensue. Polyhydramnios and a large placenta in the setting of Rh sensitization should arouse suspicion of hydrops fetalis. <u>Kernicterus:</u> The bilirubin derived from the breakdown of fetal hemoglobin crosses the placenta, and is metabolized and excreted by the mother. After delivery, however, the immature neonatal liver may not be able to cope with the large amount of bilirubin generated by hemolysis. Bilirubin therefore accumulates and jaundice ensues. Serious neurologic consequences may result if sufficient bilirubin is deposited in the brainstem nuclei and basal ganglia (hence the term kernicterus). Initial signs may include poor feeding, vomiting, lethargy. Flaccidity, convulsions, opisthotonus, and/or apnea may follow. Neurologic sequelae may include mental retardation, choreoathetosis, cerebral palsy, deafness, upward gaze palsy. The treatment/prevention of kernicterus consists of exchange transfusions with the goal of maintaining the serum bilirubin below 20 mg/dl in the fullterm neonate and below 15 mg/dl in the premature neonate.

Rh immune prophylaxis:

Antepartum: On the first prenatal visit, blood is drawn fo ascertain blood type and Rh, and to screen for antibodies (including anti-Rh antibodies if the patient is found to be Rh-negative) known to cause erythroblastosis fetalis.

If the woman is Rh-positive and the antibody screen is negative, further antibody screening is unnecessary and Rho(D) immune globulin is contraindicated.

If the woman is Rh-negative and the antibody screen is negative, antibody screening is repeated at 28 weeks gestation. If the repeat screen is negative, a 300 mcg dose of Rho(D) immune globulin is administered. The same approach is used in the woman with a negative antibody screen who is Rh-negative but D^u positive.

Note: Rh-immune globulin is *not* given to a Rh–negative woman who *has* been Rh-sensitized (i.e. has developed anti–Rh antibodies either during the course of this pregnancy or a previous pregnancy). Administering Rh-immune globulin (which contains anti–Rh antibodies) to a sensitized woman who already has anti–Rh antibodies is futile.

Postpartum: Upon delivery, the Rh-negative mother's blood is once again tested for the presence of anti–Rh antibody, and the cord blood is tested to determine if the neonate is Rh–positive or D^u positive. A direct Coombs' test is also performed on the cord blood to detect whether antibodies other than anti–Rh antibody have been induced in the mother and are present on fetal RBC's. The mother receives Rh-immune globulin prophylaxis if all 4 of the following are true: (**1**) mother is Rh–negative (D-negative) and D^u negative, (**2**) anti–Rh antibody is not present in maternal serum, (**3**) neonate is Rh–positive or D^u positive, (**4**) direct Coombs' test of cord blood is negative (or is positive because of the presence of antibodies other than anti–Rh antibody). Note: Rh-immune globulin is *not* given to a Rh–negative woman who *has* been Rh–sensitized (i.e. already has anti–Rh antibodies). Neonates should not receive Rh-immune globulin.

Other circumstances requiring Rh immune prophylaxis: Rh-immune globulin is also administered to an Rh–negative woman following antepartum hemorrhage, induced or spontaneous abortion, ectopic pregnancy, amniocentesis, or transfusion of Rh-positive blood.

Prevention/treatment of erythroblastosis fetalis if maternal sensitization has occurred:

Antepartum: Steps may be needed to prevent fetal morbidity and mortality.

If the maternal indirect Coombs' test is positive at < 1:8 dilution, the test is repeated monthly. As long as the titer remains < 1:8 (and in the absence of symptoms), the pregnancy is allowed to progress to 36–38 weeks gestation, at which time delivery is advised.

If the maternal indirect Coombs' titer reaches ≥ 1:8 dilution, amniocentesis is indicated. Amniocentesis is usually delayed until after 26 weeks gestation, but may be performed earlier if titers are high or if there is prior history of erythroblastosis fetalis. The results of spectrophotometric analysis of the amniotic fluid for bilirubin concentration is plotted against gestational age on a special semilogarithmic graph (see Management of Rh disease, *AGOG Technical Bulletin* July 1972). Specific recommendations depend on position on the graph and on gestational age. At slightly to moderately elevated amniotic fluid bilirubin concentrations, amniocentesis is repeated periodically (at 1–4 week intervals depending on position on the graph and whether or not amniotic bilirubin is rising or falling) and delivery is advised as soon as the L/S ratio is mature. If the amniotic fluid bilirubin concentration is high and the gestational age is 26–32 weeks, transabdominal intrauterine transfusions into the fetal abdominal cavity are recommended at 10–21 day intervals until 34–35 weeks gestation, at which time delivery is advised. Intrauterine transfusions are restricted to tertiary centers experienced in the procedure. If the amniotic fluid bilirubin concentration is high and the patient does not receive intrauterine transfusion, immediate delivery is advised if ≥ 34 wk gestation or upon reaching 32–34 weeks gestation. For further information refer to: *AGOG Technical Bulletin*, No. 79: *Management of Isoimmunization in Pregnancy*. Chicago; Aug. 1984.

Postpartum: A sample of cord blood is sent to the lab to ascertain the newborn's blood type and also to perform a direct Coombs test. A positive direct Coombs test indicates that maternal antibodies are present on the neonates RBC's. In this case, the newborn's hematocrit, reticulocyte count, and serum bilirubin should be determined; and a blood smear should be examined for the presence of nucleated RBC's (erythroblasts). Exchange transfusion is indicated if the hematocrit is < 40%, if reticulocytes are > 15%, and/or if unconjugated bilirubin is > 5 mg/dl. If by these criteria an exchange transfusion is not immediately required, serial hematocrit and bilirubin levels are obtained over a period of weeks in case neonatal exchange transfusion becomes necessary.

Pelvic Inflammatory Disease (PID) refers to

infection of the fallopian tubes (salpingitis) which may be accompanied by infection of the ovaries (oophoritis), cervix, endometrium, broad ligament, or pelvic peritoneum.

Pathogens: The most common pathogens are gonococcus and Chlamydia trachomatis. Others possibilities include Mycoplasma hominis; Ureaplasma urealyticum; anaerobes (e.g. bacteroides, gram–positive cocci, clostridia); aerobic gram-negative rods (e.g. E. coli, enterobacter, klebsiella, proteus, pseudomonas); Actinomyces israeli, tuberculosis (rare).

Risk factors include promiscuity, prior episode of PID, presence of intrauterine device, cervical instrumentation.

Signs/symptoms: Pain and possibly menorrhagia; Pain often starts during menses (and flow may be heavier than normal) or within a few days following menses. There may have been bleeding between periods. Pain is usually bilateral lower quadrant, although at first the pain may be unilateral or suprapubic. Generalized abdominal pain may develop. Movement is painful and the patient often walks bent forward so as to minimize the pain. Fever and chills may be present. GI complaints are sometimes present (e.g. nausea, vomiting, proctitis symptoms). GU complaints (dysuria, frequency, urgency) may be present if there is urethral involvement. With gonorrheal infection there may also be a purulent discharge from the urethra, Skene's glands, or Bartholin's glands. Abdominal exam typically reveals bilateral lower quadrant tenderness. If the peritoneum is involved, there will also be rebound tenderness with guarding, and there may be abdominal rigidity or distension, and diminished bowel sounds. Right upper quadrant tenderness and/or shoulder pain may be present if gonorrheal infection has spread up the paracolic gutter so that perihepatitis develops (Fitz–Hugh–Curtis syndrome). Vaginal exam; Often, there is a purulent cervical discharge. Bimanual exam; Pain is elicited or aggravated by movement of the cervix and palpation of the adnexa. Culdocentesis is sometimes performed: (**1**) to ascertain if there is blood in the cul–de–sac (? ectopic pregnancy), and (**2**) to obtain fluid from the cul–de–sac for diagnostic aerobic and anaerobic culture, and gram stain. Laparoscopy to directly inspect the tubes may be necessary if the diagnosis is uncertain.

Laboratory: Leukocytosis with neutrophilia is characteristic. Sedimentation rate is usually elevated. Gram stain of the urethral or cervical discharge disclosing gram–negative diplococci *within* neutrophils is diagnostic of gonococcal infection. However, gram stain taken from the endocervix is falsely negative in about half the women shown to have gonococcal infection by cervical culture. Furthermore, because of the presence of nonpathogenic species of neisseria, gram stain of cervical discharge is falsely positive in as many as 20% patients. Thayer–Martin cultures of the cervix and the rectum should be obtained. Chlamydial testing of the cervix is also appropriate. Blood cultures (aerobic and anaerobic) are obtained if there is a fever. Serologic test for syphilis (e.g. RPR, VDRL) is ordered. If negative, the test is repeated in several weeks. Serum radioimmunoassay pregnancy test is obtained to rule out ectopic pregnancy. Urinalysis is generally negative. Ultrasound may be useful if a pelvic abscess is suspected.

Differential diagnosis includes appendicitis, ectopic pregnancy, diverticulitis, ovarian cyst, endometriosis, uterine fibroids, Crohn's disease.

Complications: Pyosalpinx (distension of the fallopian tube with pus) may occur when a tube becomes blocked at both ends. The tube(s) may feel enlarged on bimanual exam. A hydrosalpinx may develop as the pus is reabsorbed. Tubo–ovarian abscess may develop when the tubal infection spreads to the adjacent ovary and the two organs adhere. On bimanual exam, an adnexal mass may be palpated and sometimes a mass can be felt in the posterior cul–de–sac. Ultrasound may identify the abscess. If a mass is suddenly not palpable, and peritoneal signs and/or septic shock rapidly develop; it is likely that rupture of a tubo–ovarian abscess has occurred. Intravenous antibiotics are begun immediately and emergency laparatomy is required. Other complications include infertility, septic thrombophlebitis, lymphangitis.

TREATMENT of PID is begun immediately. Initiation of antibiotic therapy should not await culture results. Criteria for hospitalization; pregnant, not responding to or unable to take oral antibiotics, suspected or known pelvic abscess, diagnosis uncertain and surgical emergencies cannot be ruled out, severely ill patient, adolescent

Inpatient treatment of nonpregnant adult consists of intravenous doxycycline in conjunction with cefoxitin, ceftizoxime, or cefotetan. ●For example, administer doxycycline 100 mg IV q12h plus cefoxitin 2 gram IV q6h for at least 4 days and until the patient is clinically improved and afebrile for at least 48 hours. Treatment is then continued with oral doxycycline (100 mg PO bid) until a total of 10–14 days of antibiotic therapy has been completed. ●An alternative consists of clindamycin 600 mg IV q6h plus (assuming normal renal function) gentamycin or tobramycin (2 mg/kg as initial dose followed by 1.5 mg/kg IV q8h) for at least 4 days and until the patient is afebrile for at least 48 hr. Treatment is then continued with oral clindamycin (450 mg PO qid) until a total of 10–14 days of antibiotic therapy has been completed.

Outpatient treatment: Single dose of ceftriaxone 250 mg IM followed by doxycycline 100 mg PO bid for 10–14 days. If there is a history of severe penicillin allergy, the preferred regimen is spectinomycin 2 gram IM followed by doxycycline 100 mg PO bid for 10–14 days. A single dose of ceftriaxone 250 mg IM followed by erythromycin 500 mg PO qid for 10–14 days is recommended if doxycycline/tetracyclines are not tolerated or contraindicated (e.g. pregnancy).

Vaginitis and Cervicitis

TRICHOMONAS VAGINITIS is due to a flagellated protozoan, Trichomonas vaginalis. It is sexually transmitted and both sexes may be asymptomatic carriers. The urethra and endocervix may be infected as well. **Signs/symptoms:** <u>Vaginal discharge</u> may vary in amount and character. It may be thin or frothy, malodorous, grey to yellow–green. <u>Vaginal pruritis/soreness</u> is common. <u>Other manifestations may include:</u> painful Intercourse, postcoital spotting (endocervix bleeds on contact), sore and reddened vaginal mucosa and vulva. **Laboratory:** Diagnosis is confirmed by placing a sample of the discharge with a drop of saline on a glass slide and identifying the motile flagellated trichomonads on microscopic exam. **Treatment:** <u>Metronidazole</u> (Flagyl) is the treatment of choice, either 2 gram PO as a single dose or 250 mg PO 3 times/day for 7 days. Both the patient and sexual partner should be treated at the same time. <u>Pregnant women</u> may be treated with povidone–iodine douche. Should this treatment fail, metronidazole may be used in the 2nd or 3rd trimester but it is contraindicated in the 1st trimester (refer to drug section for contraindications/cautions).

MONILIAL (candidal) VAGINITIS is due to a yeast, Candida albicans. It is not transmitted sexually. Predisposing factors: diabetes mellitus, pregnancy, oral contraceptives, corticosteroid therapy, antibiotic therapy, obesity, heat/moisture-retaining underwear. **Signs/symptoms:** <u>White vaginal discharge</u>, is the characteristic finding. The discharge often has a "cottage cheese" appearance. <u>Other common associated manifestations include:</u> reddened and swollen labia, vaginal/vulvar burning and pruritis, dysuria and dyspareunia. **Laboratory:** The diagnosis is often made on gross exam of the discharge. If there is uncertainty, microscopic exam of a KOH preparation of the discharge usually discloses candidal hyphae and spores. False–negative microscopic exam may occur. **Treatment:** miconazole (Monistat), nystatin (Mycostatin), or clotrimazole (Mycelex, Gyne–Lotrimin). Refer to drug section. In stubborn cases oral ketoconazole for 7–10 days beginning on day 16–18 of the menstrual cycle may be effective.

GARDNERELLA VAGINITIS is due to a gram–negative facultative anaerobic bacillus, Gardnerella vaginalis (formerly Haemophilus vaginalis). It may possibly be a sexually transmitted infection. **Signs/symptoms:** <u>Vaginal discharge</u> is gray or white, and has a characteristic fishy odor. <u>Pruritis and burning</u> may be present. **Laboratory:** Diagnosis is usually based on exclusion of Candida or Trichomonas. <u>A positive sniff test</u> is characteristic: add 10% KOH to discharge specimen and note a significant worsening of the odor. <u>Clue cells</u> (epithelial cells whose cytoplasm contains bacilli) are diagnostic if they can be found on microscopic exam of a saline preparation. **Treatment:** metronidazole 500 mg PO twice daily for 5–7 days, or 250 mg PO 3 times/day for 5–7 days. Amoxicillin/clavulanate 500 mg PO 3 times/day for 10 days may be effective in resistant cases.

ATROPHIC VAGINITIS occurs almost exclusively in postmenopausal women and results from estrogen deficiency. **Signs/symptoms:** The vaginal epithelium appears thin, pale, and dry. Symptoms may include pruritis, burning, soreness, painful intercourse. **Treatment:** An atrophic vagina is common in the postmenopausal woman but treatment is not required unless the patient is symptomatic with signs of vaginal inflammation. Symptomatic atrophic vaginitis may be treated with oral medications as described under "Menopause/Climacteric" chapter or with topical intravaginal estrogen creams (e.g. Premarin). Treatment is usually continued for 3 months, and then tapered and discontinued if possible. Topical creams, it should be noted, are readily absorbed systemically, and so the contraindications to oral estrogens apply to topical estrogens as well.

CERVICITIS is often the cause of vaginal discharge. Many women are diagnosed as having a vaginitis when in fact an endocervicitis is the cause of the discharge. Known pathogens include gonorrhea, trichomonas, herpes simplex, Chlamydia. **Signs/symptoms:** A yellow discharge is common. Vaginal symptoms, aside from the discharge, are usually absent. The cervix is inflamed and may bleed on contact. **Laboratory:** GC culture, wet smear to rule out trichomonas. Herpes culture is obtained as clinical circumstances suggest. Chlamydial testing may also be done.

Dysfunctional Uterine Bleeding

Definition: abnormal uterine bleeding that is not associated with an anatomic or organic abnormality. That is to say, dysfunctional uterine bleeding (DUB) is bleeding that is _not_ associated with systemic disease, pelvic infection/inflammation, neoplasia (malignant or benign), nor any of the causes of abnormal uterine bleeding listed below under differential diagnosis. **Incidence:** Overall, 75% cases of abnormal vaginal bleeding are DUB. In adolescents DUB accounts for 90% cases of abnormal vaginal bleeding.

Anovulatory DUB: Most cases of DUB are the consequence of anovulation and this most often occurs (**1**) soon after menarche when anovulation is attributed to hypothalamic immaturity with the consequent absence of the midcycle surge of estradiol and LH necessary for ovulation, or (**2**) before menopause as ovarian function declines. When anovulation occurs between these age groups, it is often associated with stress, chronic strenuous exercise, obesity, or rapid weight gain/loss, or polycystic ovarian syndrome (Stein–Leventhal syndrome). Mechanism: When ovulation fails to occur, the corpus luteum does not form and therefore ovarian progesterone is not secreted. As a consequence, there is persistent secretion of estrogen unopposed by progesterone. This results in a hyperplastic proliferative endometrium that is fragile and tends to bleed easily and randomly (estrogen breakthrough bleeding). Should estrogen secretion wane, estrogen withdrawal bleeding will ensue. Bleeding may be irregular and frequent, or there may be heavy persistent bleeding following an interval of amenorrhea.

Ovulatory DUB is usually due to malfunction of the corpus luteum (e.g. persistent corpus luteum with prolonged secretion of progesterone, corpus luteum secreting insufficient progesterone, early progesterone withdrawal). Ovulatory DUB is suspected when a patient with DUB presents with any of the signs characteristic of ovulatory cycles: e.g. dysmenorrhea, breast tenderness/swelling, fluid retention, mid–cycle pain (mittelschmerz).

Tests: The following tests are routinely recommended: serum pregnancy test, CBC, urinalysis, rectal exam for occult blood, PAP smear, endometrial biopsy. The latter two may be deferred in adolescent. If blood dyscrasia is suspected, obtain PT, PTT. If the CBC indicates insufficient platelets, also obtain platelet count. If thyroid malfunction is suspected, obtain thyroid panel. FSH and LH level may be ordered in an adult with persistent DUB but is seldom useful in perimenarchal female. Pelvic ultrasound indicated if a pelvic mass is suspected or felt on physical exam.

Differential diagnosis (i.e. abnormal vaginal bleeding other than DUB): complications of pregnancy (e.g. ectopic pregnancy, abortion, trophoblastic disease); uterine lesions (e.g. endometriosis, adenomyosis, leiomyomas, polyps, neoplasia, infections including Tb and sexually transmitted diseases, intrauterine device); cervical lesions (e.g. infection, neoplasia, trauma); vaginal lesions (e.g. infection, trauma, foreign body, atrophic vaginitis); ovarian lesions (e.g. estrogen–secreting granulosa cell tumor); endocrine disease (e.g. hypo or hyperthyroidism, adrenal hyperplasia); abnormal estrogen metabolism (e.g. hepatitis, cirrhosis); blood dyscrasias (e.g. thrombocytopenia, coagulation factor deficiencies); exogenous hormones (e.g. birth control pills, corticosteroids).

Treatment: Preliminaries: Adults should first have a pelvic exam, PAP smear, and endometrial biopsy before undergoing therapy. Adolescents should have a pelvic exam (or rectal exam if a vaginal exam is likely to be traumatic) before proceding with therapy, but may forego PAP smear and endometrial biopsy unless there is a compelling reason. Standard treatment: Administer any combination progestin–estrogen birth control pill (1 PO 4 times a day continued for 5–7 days even if bleeding ceases). Bleeding should subside within 24 hours of starting pills. D & C is indicated if it does not. Withdrawal bleeding will begin 2–4 days after completing the pills. On the 5th day of withdrawal bleeding, begin a *low–dose* combination progestin–estrogen birth control pill in the usual prescribed manner and continue for 3 months, or longer if contraception is desired. If contraception is not desired, the pill is discontinued after 3 months and the patient is allowed to cycle spontaneously. However, if she does not spontaneously menstruate, administer Provera 10 mg PO once daily for 5 days every 2 months to insure periodic withdrawal bleeding. <u>High-dose estrogen therapy</u> is indicated initially in the following circumstances: (**1**) bleeding has been heavy and prolonged over many days leaving a denuded endometrium, (**2**) the patient has been receiving progestins (e.g. oral contraceptives, progestin shots) so that there is a shallow atrophic endometrium, (**3**) endometrial biopsy yields minimal tissue. In these circumstances, the endometrium must first be built up with high–dose estrogen (e.g. Premarin 25 mg IV q4h until bleeding stops or maximum 6 doses have been given). Once bleeding stops, follow the standard treatment outlined above starting with a combination birth control pill (1 PO 4 times/day for 5–7 days). D & C is indicated if high–dose estrogen therapy does not stop bleeding within 24 hours. <u>An alternate method of treating DUB (especially in women over 35 or others in whom estrogen therapy is not ideal)</u> is to administer a progestin alone (Provera 10 mg PO once daily for 5 days or one dose of progesterone in oil 100 mg IM). Progestin treatment may be repeated at two month intervals if necessary to insure withdrawal bleeding. This method may not be effective if bleeding has been heavy and prolonged over many days. In this case, high–dose estrogen therapy is needed or D & C is considered.

Dysmenorrhea (painful menstruation)

Primary dysmenorrhea (dysmenorrhea in the absence of a specific pelvic abnormality) usually begins within 2 yr following menarche. It is associated with ovulatory cycles and is probably due to prostaglandin–induced contractions of the myometrium. Pelvic exam is normal. Many patients will benefit from a prostaglandin inhibiting analgesic (e.g. aspirin, ibuprofen, naproxen) or from birth control pills (ovulation is suppressed and so prostaglandin levels are reduced).

Seconday dysmenorrhea (dysmenorrhea in the presence of a specific pelvic abnormality) may be due to acute or chronic pelvic inflammatory disease, endometriosis, adenomyosis, intrauterine or intracervical tumor (e.g. submucous leiomyoma), intrauterine device, cervical or vaginal stenosis, congenital uterine abnormalities.

Endometriosis (endometrial tissue at locations other than within the

uterine cavity) is most commonly found on the ovary followed in decreasing order by the posterior cul de sac, uterosacral ligaments, rectovaginal septum, fallopian tubes, rectosigmoid colon, bladder. Rarely, endometriosis is found in such remote locations as the pleura, lymph nodes, extremities. **Pathogenesis:** One theory is that endometriosis results when there is retrograde menstruation thru the Fallopian tubes. Hematogenous or lymphatic spread of endometrial tissue is another possibility. The endometrial tissue implants are cyclically stimulated just as the normal endometrium. They appear grossly as "powder burns" on the peritoneum or serosa. The ensuing scarring and adhesions may compromise function of the fallopian tubes with and thus cause infertility, or it may possibly lead to bowel or ureteral obstruction. Endometrioma ("chocolate cysts") may develop. They are hemorrhagic cysts lined with endometrial tissue and are usually located on the ovaries. Endometrioma may rupture causing pain and intraperitoneal bleeding. **Predisposing factors:** Endometriosis does not occur before puberty or after menopause. Pregnancy may ameliorate the condition. The risk appears to be reduced in women who have had an early pregnancy, who have short menstrual periods, who have long menstrual cycles (> 35 days), or who engage in regular strenuous exercise. Nulliparous women between 30 and 40 have the greatest risk. The risk seems to be increased in patients with menstrual periods longer than 8 days or cycle lengths < 27 days.

Signs/symptoms: <u>Pelvic pain</u> is worst during menses. It tends to begin a few days before menses, continue thru menses, and persist for a few days afterward. Sometimes pain persists the entire month. Low back pain is also common. In some cases, endometriosis is asymptomatic. Menorrhagia: Menses are commonly irregular and heavy. Dyspareunia (painful intercourse) may be due to endometriosis of the posterior cul-de-sac, uterosacral ligaments, or vaginal fornix. Tenesmus may be the consequence of endometriosis of the rectum or rectovaginal septum. Urinary complaints: Bladder involvement may manifest as dysuria, suprapubic pain, urgency, frequency, and/or cyclic hematuria. Pelvic exam may be normal. In advanced cases, adhesions may result in a fixed and retroverted uterus. The ovaries are often found to be enlarged by endometrioma and may adhere to the uterus. Tender nodules are sometimes seen in the posterior vaginal fornix, or felt (best on rectovaginal exam) on the uterosacral ligaments and rectovaginal septum. Laparoscopy with biopsy: Laparoscopy discloses the characteristic "powder burns" and "chocolate cysts". Biopsy is required to confirm the diagnosis.

Treatment: Mildly symptomatic patients with minimal disease can often be treated with mild analgesics. Hormonal therapy may be tried in the following circumstances: (**1**) infertile woman with periovarian or peritubal adhesions who desires future pregnancy, (**2**) fertility is not a concern, (**3**) surgery is contraindicated or patient refuses surgery, (**4**) recurrent endometriosis following surgery. Acceptable hormonal medications include: (**1**) nafarelin, a gonadotropin–releasing hormone (GnRH) analog administered via intranasal spray 200 mcg twice daily; (**2**) danazol 400 mg twice daily for 3–9 months. Conservative surgery for infertile women desiring future pregnancy: When laparoscopy discloses endometrioma and/or tubal or periovarian adhesions, fertility may sometimes be restored with conservative surgery consisting of lysis of adhesions and excision or cauterization of endometrioma while preserving reproductive organs. If the ovaries are significantly enlarged, noncyclical administration of an oral contraceptive for 6–8 weeks is recommended prior to surgery. However, surgery should not be delayed if ovaries are > 6 cm diameter. Radical surgery for women not desiring further pregnancies who have intractable and recurrent pain despite hormonal therapy: Hysterectomy with or without oophorectomy often cures the patient even when all endometriotic lesions are not removed. Ideally, the ovaries, an ovary, or part of an ovary is preserved in younger women. Depending on the circumstances, more conservative surgical measures may suffice. Additional surgical indications: (1) adhesions and/or scarring causing bowel or ureteral obstruction, (2) rupture of endometrioma ("chocolate cysts") with hemorrhage. Also, surgery is not delayed for hormonal therapy if an ovary is enlarged to > 6 cm diameter or if an undiagnosed adnexal mass is present.

Premenstrual Tension Syndrome is the month-

ly syndrome that many women undergo during the luteal phase of the cycle in the days prior to the onset of menses. **Pathogenesis** is uncertain but fluid retention due to cyclical changes in estrogen and progesterone levels is probably implicated.

Symptoms may include nervousness, irritability, depression, headache, edema, breast tenderness/fullness, abdominal bloating.

Treatment: Sundry regimens have been advocated. However, none are consistently effective. Diuretics occasionally help women with evidence of fluid retention (weight gain, headache, swelling) when administered in the days prior to onset menses (e.g. spironolactone 25 mg 3–4 times/day or a thiazide diuretic). Oral contraception is sometimes helpful. Select a combinatiion pill with low estrogen and low progestin potency (e.g. LoEstrin 1/20, Ortho–Novum 1/50, Norinyl 1/50) or a progestin–only pill. Up to 30% improve and up to 30% get worse with birth control pills. Other remedies yet unproven include vitamin B6, regular vigorous exercise, well balanced nutrition, vitamin A, vitamin E, magnesium.

Amenorrhea

Primary amenorrhea is the absence of menstruation by the age of 18. Investigation is warranted if menarche has not occurred by age 16, or at age 14 if signs of puberty are absent. **Secondary amenorrhea** is the absence of menses for at least 3 months in a female who has had menarche. Amenorrhea may be normal for up to 6 months following pregnancy, especially when breastfeeding.

Workup of amenorrhea: Pregnancy should be excluded. Menopause is the usual expectation in the 48–55 yr old; the serum FSH will be > 40 mIU/ml (see "Menopause/Climacteric" chapter). History or physical exam may suggest the diagnosis. Following protocol may be used if the cause of amenorrhea is not obvious:

● Challenge patient with progesterone (Provera 10 mg PO once daily for 5 days or single IM injection 200 mg progesterone in oil). If bleeding occurs (usually 2–7 days after the injection or after taking the last pill), then the ovaries are secreting sufficient estrogen to prime the endometrium but ovulation is not occurring. The presence of bleeding indicates an intact endometrium and a patent outflow tract as well as a functioning (although not normally functioning) hypothalamic–pituitary–ovarian axis.

● On the initial visit, also obtain serum prolactin. If the serum prolactin is elevated (i.e. > 20 ng/ml) or if there is galactorrhea, CAT scan the pituitary to rule out a pituitary tumor.

● If serum prolactin is normal and bleeding does not occur following progesterone challenge, administer estrogen for 25 days (e.g. Premarin 1.25 mg PO once daily) and add progesterone (Provera 10 mg PO once daily) during the last 10 days of estrogen administration. If bleeding does not ensue, the abnormality lies in the endometrium or outflow tract. Bleeding demonstrates patency of the outflow tract and an endometrium which responds normally with appropriate hormonal influence.

● If bleeding occurs following the combined challenge of estrogen and progesterone, wait 2 weeks and then obtain serum FSH. An elevated FSH (> 40mIU/ml) indicates ovarian failure. A normal or low FSH indicates malfunction of the pituitary and/or hypothalamus. In the latter case, obtain a CAT scan, and a thyroid panel that includes TSH.

● If ovarian failure is present and the patient is over 35, the conclusion is that premature menopause has occurred and further evaluation is generally not required. Younger patients with ovarian failure require chromosome karyotyping to exclude a Y chromosome. There is an increased risk of gonadal malignancy if the Y chromosome is present.

Differential diagnosis: Endometrial destruction (Asherman's syndrome) is almost always due to curettage and rarely to infection (e.g. Tb, schistosomiasis). Other outflow tract abnormalities include cervical stenosis; congenital anomalies such as imperforate hymen, absence of uterus/cervix/vagina. See also 'Testicular Feminization' below. Ovarian abnormalities; ovarian destruction (radiation, autoimmmune, toxins); resistant ovary (i.e. ovarian insensitivity to FSH and LH); persistent corpus luteum; androgen or estrogen–secreting ovarian tumor; premature menopause. See also 'Turner's Syndrome' below. Pituitary abnormalities: **(1)** pituitary tumors—either nonfunctioning or functioning. Prolactin–secreting tumor is the most common functional tumor and it is often associated with galactorrhea. Less common are ACTH–secreting tumors (Is there evidence of Cushing's syndrome ?) and growth hormone–secreting tumors (Is there evidence of acromegaly?). Other functional pituitary tumors (e.g. TSH, LH, FSH) are very rare. **(2)** empty sella syndrome—subarachnoid space extends below the diaphragma sella compressing the pituitary gland and thereby compromising production of FSH, LH, and growth hormone. **(3)** other pituitary lesions leading to pituitary insufficiency: Sheehan's syndrome (postpartum pituitary infarction), granulomatous disease, gummas, trauma, hemachromatosis, cerebral aneurysm. Hypothalamic dysfunction (e.g. from anorexia, stress, hypogonadotropic hypogonadism). Stein–Leventhal syndrome (polycystic ovary syndrome) is possibly the consequence of hypothalamic dysfunction. Typical signs include hirsutism, obesity, infertility, enlarged white polycystic ovaries, elevated LH with decreased FSH, elevated estradiol and 17–ketosteroids. Other endocrine abnormalities: hyper or hypothyroidism, adrenal insufficiency (Addison's disease), adrenal androgen excess (adrenal hyperplasia or tumor ?), diabetes mellitus. Certain drugs (e.g. phenothiazines, methyldopa, reserpine) inhibit dopamine secretion by the hypothalamus. Dopamine is thought to inhibit prolactin release from the pituitary. Consequently, drugs that inhibit dopanine secretion may lead to elevated prolactin level with ensuing galactorrhea and amenorrhea. Chromosomal abnormalities: Turner's syndrome (XO karyotype, streak gonads, absence of secondary sex characteristics, short stature, web neck, shield chest, decreased estrogen levels and elevated FSH); mosaicism (patient with cells varying in chromosome composition—e.g. XX/XO or XX/XY karyotype); testicular feminization (XY karyotype but cells are insensitive to androgens so that patients are phenotypic females with following structural findings: blind vagina; absent uterus; intra–abdominal, inguinal, or vulvar testes); hermaphroditism. Other: chronic disease, renal or hepatic dysfunction.

Menopause/Climacteric

Menopause is the permanent cessation of menstruation. Menses will have been absent for over 6–12 months. Menopause usually occurs between 48 and 55 years of age (mean age 51.4). The climacteric encompasses the menopause and refers to the entire period of declining ovarian function which may span 15–20 years. The climacteric typically starts at about age 40 when ovulation becomes less frequent and fertility diminishes. Gradually, ovulation becomes less predictable, period(s) may be skipped. Eventually, ovulation ceases and, in the absence of corpus luteum, progesterone is no longer produced. For a time, ovarian follicles still produce estrogen (estradiol) which continues to stimulate the endometrium. However, without the cyclical influence of progesterone on the endometrium, menses are often irregular in both timing and flow. Menopause ensues when the ovarian follicles are exhausted and cease to produce estrogen. Low levels of estrogen are still maintained, owing chiefly to the conversion of androstenedione (derived from the adrenals) to estrone by the fat, skin, and liver. The level of estrogen thus derived may in some postmenopausal women be sufficient to sustain estrogen–dependent tissues and prevent vasomotor symptoms. However, the majority will experience the effects of estrogen withdrawal. As ovarian estrogen secretion decreases, estrogen inhibition of pituitary FSH (follicle stimulating hormone) and LH (luteinizing hormone) secretion is removed. Consequently, serum FSH and LH levels become elevated, and thus confirm that ovarian (follicular) failure has occurred.

Signs/symptoms of estrogen deficiency: Vasomotor instability: hot flashes, sweats. Nonspecific complaints: anxiety, depression, irritability, insomnia, headaches. Atrophy of estrogen–dependent tissues: (**1**) atrophy of the vaginal epithelium may result in dyspareunia and pruritis; (**2**) thinning of the urethral epithelium may manifest as dysuria, urgency, incontinence; (**3**) atrophy of the breasts and skin may be evident. Osteoporosis is most likely to develop in white, fair–skinned women of slight build who are sedentary. Other risk factors include menopause before age 40, smoker, excessive alcohol consumption, corticosteroid treatment, family history of osteoporosis. See "Osteoporosis" chapter for further information.

Treatment of menopausal complaints: Before starting therapy, progestin (e.g. Provera 10 mg PO once daily for 5 days) is administered to confirm that withdrawal bleeding does not occur. Absence of withdrawal bleeding indicates that the endometrium is no longer being primed by estrogen. A standard therapeutic regimen is to administer conjugated estrogens (Premarin) cyclically, 3 wk on and 1 wk off. Use the smallest effective dose that relieves symptoms and yet does not provoke vaginal bleeding (usual range Premarin is 0.625 to 1.25 mg PO once daily). Refer to drug section for estrogen contraindications and cautions. In order to protect against some of the possible adverse consequences of unopposed estrogen administration, it is common recommended practice to administer medroxyprogesterone acetate (Provera) 5–10 mg PO once daily along with the estrogen during the 3rd week of estrogen administration. Duration of treatment depends on the patient's specific climacteric problem. For instance, hot flushes usually last 1–2 years. After that interval, hormone administration can often be tapered over 3–6 months and then discontinued. Some postmenopausal women, however, may have persistent vasomotor symptoms for over 5 yr. Patients at risk for developing osteoporosis require prolonged hormonal therapy along with calcium supplements. Alternate treatment of vasomotor symptoms if estrogens are contraindicated: progestin (e.g. Depo–Provera 150 mg IM every 3 months). Atrophic vaginitis may be treated either with oral estrogen medications as described above or with topical intravaginal estrogen creams (e.g. Premarin cream). Treatment is usually continued for 3 months and then tapered and discontinued if possible. The patient may be able to judge for herself the frequency of application needed to maintain remission during the tapering stage. Topical creams, it should be noted, are readily absorbed systemically, and so the contraindications to oral estrogens apply to topical estrogens as well.

Galactorrhea is defined as inappropriate milk secretion; (i.e. milk secretion not resulting from pregnancy and nursing). Milk secretion normally ends within 6–8 weeks after nursing is diccontinued.

Workup: The patient complaining of both galactorrhea and amenorrhea is evaluated according to the guidelines set forth under "Amenorrhea" chapter. Obtain serum prolactin. A normal level (< 30 ng/ml) in a patient with normal menstrual cycles usually indicates that galactorrhea is benign. A prolactin level > 300 ng/ml indicates a prolactin–secreting pituitary tumor. If prolactin is elevated but < 300 ng/ml, administration of TRH (thyrotropin releasing hormone) 500 mcg IV may help differentiate between a prolactin–secreting tumor and other causes of elevated prolactin. If a tumor is present, TRH will fail to increase the prolactin level significantly. CAT scan of the pituitary can detect a pituitary tumor as small as 10 mm or possibly less. Other tests may be obtained as clinical circumstances suggest (e.g. thyroid panel).

Etiology: Idiopathic with menstrual cycles accounts for about a third of cases of galactorrhea. About 85% of these patients will have normal prolactin level. Idiopathic with amenorrhea accounts for about 10% cases of galactorrhea. Prolactin–secreting pituitary tumor is responsible for about 20% cases of galactorrhea. Growth hormone–secreting pituitary tumor: Acromegaly may be associated with galactorrhea. Cushing's syndrome or Addison's disease is sometimes associated with galactorrhea. Empty sella syndrome is occasionally associated with galactorrhea. Hypothalamic or pituitary stalk lesions may compromise delivery of prolactin inhibiting factor (dopamine) to the pituitary, and thus allow prolactin secretion to increase. Neurally–mediated increase in prolactin secretion: suckling; chest wall lesion (e.g. herpes zoster, thoracotamy scar); cervical cord lesion. Hypothyroidism: In the absence of negative feedback inhibition by thyroid hormone, there is an increase in TRH which is in turn thought to induce prolactin release. Renal failure or liver failure may lead to decrease metabolism and clearance of prolactin. Certain drugs: Prolactin–inhibiting factor (dopamine) is normally secreted by the hypothalamus. Drugs that deplete dopamine (e.g. benzodiazepines, tricyclic antidepressants, methyldopa, reserpine, cimetidine) or block dopamine receptors (e.g. phenothiazines) may lead to an increase in prolactin with ensuing galactorrhea. Prolactin levels also rise with administration of estrogens (e.g. combination oral contraceptives) or drugs that increase estrogen levels (e.g. opiates, marijuana, digitalis) because estrogen suppresses hypothalamic synthesis and secretion of dopamine.

Treatment: ●Discontinue drugs known to cause galactorrhea. ●Treat underlying disorder if possible. ●Bromocryptine may be used to suppress idiopathic galactorrhea if the amount of breast discharge is disturbing. Patients with idiopathic galactorrhea and amenorrhea will often resume menses. Bromocryptine acts as a dopamine (prolactin inhibiting factor) agonist and thus inhibits prolactin secretion. ●Galactorrhea secondary to a prolactin–secreting pituitary tumor will also respond to bromocryptine and the tumor may actually shrink. Large tumors and tumors with suprasellar extension are resected via transphenoidal approach.

Hirsutism

is defined as excessive hair growth in a woman, particularly the androgen-sensitive areas (face, chest, upper back, shoulders, lower abdomen, anterior thighs). Hirsutism is due to the influence of endogenous androgens on hair follicles. Hypertrichosis refers to an increase in soft vellous hair (not the terminal hair—the coarse pigmented hair resulting from androgen stimulation). Hypertrichosis may be the consequence of drugs (e.g. phenytoin, minoxidil, diazoxide); anorexia nervosa; acromegaly; CNS disease (e.g. multiple sclerosis, head trauma, encephalitis). Source of endogenous androgens: In women, endogenous androgens are derived from either the ovaries or the adrenals. In a normal female, the 17-hydroxysteroids (e.g. testosterone, dihydrotestosterone, androstenediol, androstanediol) account for nearly all of the androgenic activity. They are derived from the 17-ketosteroids—e.g. dehydroepiandrosterone (DHEA), dehydroepiandrosterone sulfate (DHEA-S), androstenedione, androsterone. Differentiating excess androgens of adrenal origin from those of ovarian origin: In virtually all cases in which the adrenal gland secretes excessive testosterone, the levels of 17-ketosteroids will be elevated. In contrast, the ovaries secrete testosterone more efficiently and markedly elevated levels of testosterone are possible with little or no elevation of 17-ketosteroids. Of the 17-ketosteroids, the serum DHEA-S is the most useful assay of adrenal androgen secretion because about 95% of the DHEA-S secreted is derived from the adrenals.

INVESTIGATION: Family history of hirsutism and ethnic background. Women of Mediterranean origin are often normally hirsute. Drug history (e.g. phenytoin, minoxidil, steroids, diazoxide). Age of onset and rate of development of hirsutism. Hirsutism that slowly progresses from the time of puberty is most often associated with Stein-Leventhal syndrome, idiopathic hirsutism, or ethnic/familial hirsutism. Rapidly progressing hirsutism with masculinization arouses suspicion of an ovarian or adrenal tumor. Menstrual history: Women with idiopathic or ethnic/familial hirsutism generally have normal menstrual cycles. Physical exam should be comprehensive. In particular, be alert to any of the following: short stature (? congenital adrenal hyperplasia); hypertension (? adrenal lesion); masculinization (male hair pattern, enlarged clitoris, deep voice, unusual muscle development); presence of acne; signs of Cushing's syndrome; abdominal or pelvic masses. **Tests:** Measurement of the serum total testosterone and serum dehydroepiandrosterone sulfate (DHEA-S) is basic to the work-up of hirsutism. If the serum total testosterone is > 2.0 ng/ml (normal < 0.2-0.8 ng/ml), an ovarian tumor is likely. Patients with Stein-Leventhal syndrome (polycystic ovaries) or idiopathic hirsutism often have elevated testosterone levels but seldom is it > 2.0 ng/ml. An elevated serum DHEA-S suggests an adrenal lesion (benign or malignant adrenal tumor, or congenital adrenal hyperplasia). A normal serum DHEA-S (i.e. < 2.5 mcg/ml) almost always rules out adrenal disease as the source of excessive androgens and shifts attention to the ovaries. Elevated DHEA-S levels will be suppressed by administration of dexamethasone (0.5 mg PO 4 times/day for 3 days) if congenital adrenal hyperplasia is present. However, DHEA-S will not be suppressed if an adrenal tumor is responsible for the elevated DHEA-S. If Cushing's syndrome is suspected, refer to "Adrenocortical Excess" chapter for laboratory evaluation. CAT scan may be used to search for an adrenal tumor. However, because of the risks of radiation, it is best to visualize the ovaries with ultrasound.

EXAMPLES of ANDROGEN-MEDIATED HIRSUTISM:

Cushing's syndrome: refer to "Adrenocortical Excess" chapter.

Stein-Leventhal syndrome (polycystic ovary syndrome) is typically associated with enlarged white polycystic ovaries. Anovulation is common and manifests as amenorrhea or irregular bleeding, and infertility. Hirsutism and obesity are also common. LH is elevated and FSH is low or normal. In many cases, the serum FREE testosterone and serum androstenedione are moderately increased. Hirsutism is treated with cyclical administration of estrogen-progesterone birth control pills (serum free testosterone levels will fall over 1-3 months but an improvement in hirsutism may take 6 months or more). If oral birth control pills are contraindicated, Depo-Provera (150 mg IM every 3 months) may also be effective. Nafarelin, a gonadotropin-releasing hormone (GnRH) analog administered via intranasal spray will also reduce serum androgen level and hopefully lead to improvement of hirsutism. Spironolactone 100–200 mg/day is yet another therapy that may be effective.

Idiopathic hirsutism is in many cases associated with mild elevation of androgens, particularly if the free 17–hydroxysteroids are measured. Assay of the serum free testosterone, for instance, will often be found to be elevated even though the serum total testosterone is normal. This is because elevated androgens lead to a reduction in sex hormone–binding globulin and hence a reduction in bound testosterone. These patients may ovulate normally. The source of the increased androgens may be ovarian, adrenal, or both. A serum free testosterone and serum DHEA–S are obtained and guide the need for further evaluation. Treatment of idiopathic hirsutism is hormonal as described under Stein–Leventhal syndrome.

Ovarian tumor–associated hirsutism typically presents with rapidly progressing hirsutism and virilization. The serum total testosterone is > 2.0–2.5 ng/ml. An ovarian mass may be felt in about half of cases. Pelvic ultrasound, CAT scan, and/or laparoscopy may be used to locate the tumor.

Adrenal tumor–associated hirsutism: Rapidly progressive hirsutism and virilization are characteristic. Cushing's syndrome secondary to excessive glucocorticoid production is present in many cases. The 17–ketosteroids are elevated: serum DHEA–S > 9 mcg/ml (normal < 2.5 mcg/ml), urinary 17–ketosteroids > 20 mg/24hr (normal 7–13 mg/24hr). Sometimes the serum total testosterone is also elevated: > 2 ng/ml (normal < 0.2–0.8 ng/ml). When Cushing's syndrome is present, the serum cortisol will be elevated and ACTH will be decreased. In the case of an adrenal carcinoma, high–dose dexamethasone (2 mg PO q6h for 2–5 days) will not significantly suppress excessive hormone production, while high–dose dexamethasone may occasionally suppress an adrenal adenoma. Ultrasound, CAT scan, and sometimes arteriography may be used to locate the tumor.

Congenital adrenal hyperplasia (CAH) is due to inherited enzymatic defects in the production of cortisol. Inheritance is autosomal recessive. Cortisol (which normally exerts a negative feedback inhibition on ACTH release) is decreased and so the ACTH level rises. Elevated ACTH stimulates the adrenals so that hyperplasia and increased production of androgens ensues. 21–hydroxylase deficiency is the most common type of CAH. Diagnosis is based upon elevation of serum 17–hydoxyprogesterone (usually > 1000 ng/dl) with marked increase of this metabolite (usually ≥ 3000 ng/dl) 30 minutes after IV administration of ACTH 250 mcg. Furthermore, serum 17–hydoxyprogesterone should be suppressed to normal following administration of dexamethasone 0.5 mg PO 4 times/day for 3 days. Aldosterone deficiency occurs in about half the cases and this may lead to salt–losing crises and hyperkalemia. Two other rare examples of CAH leading to hirsutism and virilization are 11–hydroxylase and 3–hydroxylase deficiency. Treatment of CAH is with glucocorticoids to suppress ACTH production. A mineralocorticoid may also be needed.

Breast Cancer

follows lung cancer as the most common cause of cancer death in women. Breast cancer seldom occurs before the age of 30. The incidence rises sharply after menopause.

Risk factors include positive family history (2–3 fold increase in risk), cystic mastitis (4–fold increase in risk), early menarche or late menopause (slight increase in risk). Full term pregnancy before age 18 reduces the risk. There is diminishing protection with age so that a woman who first delivers after age 35 or remains nulliparous has a 3–fold risk over a woman who first delivers before age 18. Pregnancies after the initial term pregnancy confer slight if any additional protection. Lactation does not reducce the risk, except perhaps when ovulation is suppressed by prolonged breast feeding.

Screening: Women should regularly perform self breast exam. Physicians should make breast exam a routine part of the physical exam. Ideally, mammography is first performed at age 35, every 2 years between 40 and 50, and every year thereafter. Mammography is especially important in those with a prior history of breast cancer, or those over 40 whose mother or sister have had breast cancer.

Signs, symptoms, diagnosis, detection of metastases: Breast mass is the most common manifestation. The mass is usually painless. A breast lump < 1 cm in diameter may not be palpable by the examiner but is sometimes detected by the patient. Other breast findings may include retraction or dimpling of skin or areola, bloody or serous nipple discharge, skin edema with peau d'orange (i.e. like an orange skin). Axillary or supraclavicular nodes may be felt. However, 1–2 movable axillary nodes ≤ 5 mm in size is not an abnormal finding. On the other hand, nodes are not usually felt in the infra- or supraclavicular area; firm or hard nodes in this region is very suspicious. In Paget's disease of the nipple there may be burning or itching of the nipple with crusting or ulceration. In inflammatory breast cancer (an aggressive form of breast cancer that metastasizes early and has a poor prognosis), anaplastic cells invade the subdermal lymphatics resulting in what looks like a skin infection (i.e. warm, red, indurated, and painful skin). Histology confirms this type of breast cancer. Mammography may reveal breast cancer even before there is a palpable lump. Mammography is advised if there is a poorly defined or equivocal breast mass, or if there are other worrisome breast findings. Cystic mass: If the breast mass feels cystic, needle aspiration for cytology may be attempted to confirm the diagnosis. Otherwise—needle, excisional, or incisional biopsy is indicated. Metastasis: Once breast cancer is confirmed, one should carefully search for metastases before considering surgery. To this end, perform a careful physical exam (e.g. ? palpable lymph nodes, ? liver involvement, ? mass in other breast) and obtain CBC, liver function tests; serum calcium; chest x–ray, and perhaps a bone scan. The most susceptible sites of metastases are the regional lymph nodes, the bones, and the viscera. Estrogen/progesterone receptors: A portion of the tumor at the time of biopsy or definitive surgery is either assayed immediately for estrogen and progesterone receptors or frozen at – 70° C until such time as assay can be performed.

Note: The following information is extracted from National Cancer Institute PDQ State-of-the-Art Cancer Treatment Information 12/3/90. Breast cancer treatment is complex and is evolving. The most up-to-date standard treatment options may be obtained by calling the National Cancer Institute Cancer Information Service at 1–800–4–CANCER. All newly diagnosed breast cancer patients may be considered for inclusion in ongoing clinical trials of regimens aimed at improving survival and decreasing morbidity. Descriptions of these trials are also available.

   TNM classification: Primary tumor: **TX**—minimum requirements to assess primary tumor cannot be met; **T0**—no detectable primary tumor; **Tis**—carcinoma in situ (e.g. intraductal in situ, lobular in situ, Paget's disease of nipple with no tumor); **T1**—tumor ≤ 2 cm in greatest dimension; **T2**—tumor 2–5cm in greatest dimension; **T3**—tumor > 5 cm in greatest dimension; **T4**—tumor of any size with direct extension to skin or chest wall, or inflammatory carcinoma. NOTE: Skin involvement is identified by skin edema with peau d'orange, ulceration, or satellite skin nodules; but not merely dimpling or skin retraction. The latter two signs may be seen in T1, T2, or T3 without changing tumor classification. Chest wall involvement is defined as involvement of the ribs, intercostal muscles, or serratus anterior—not just the pectoral muscle or fascia. Regional nodes: **NX**––regional nodes cannot be assessed (e.g. because of prior removal), **N0**—negative nodes, **N1**—positive ipsilateral axillary nodes, **N2**—positive ipsilateral axillary nodes with fixation to one another or to adjacent structures, **N3**—positive ipsilateral internal mammary lymph nodes. Distant metastasis: **MX**—minimum requirements to assess for distant metastasis cannot be met, **M0**—no known distant metastasis, **M1**—distant metastasis.

   Staging: Stage 0 (Tis, N0, M0)—carcinoma in situ; Stage I (T1, N0, M0); Stage IIA (T0–T1, N1, M0 or T2, N0, M0); Stage IIB (T2, N1, M0 or T3, N0, M0); Stage IIIA (T0–T2, N2, M0 or T3, N1–N2, M0); Stage IIIB (any T, N3, M0 or T4, any N, M0); Stage IV (any T, any N, M1). Inflammatory breast cancer is an aggressive form of breast cancer with poor prognosis. The tumor is classified as T4d. Anaplastic cells invade the subdermal lymphatics resulting in what looks like a skin infection (i.e. warm, red, indurated, and painful). Histology confirms this type of breast cancer. Inflammatory breast cancer is not to be confused with other types of breast cancer in which there is inflammation or secondary infection.

   Treatment: Surgery is standard treatment for stages 0 thru stage IIIA. The surgical procedure employed is individualized. Factors that may enter into which surgical option to use include cancer stage, tumor location and size, breast size, regional nodal involvement, patient concern about breast preservation. Surgery is only recommended in certain circumstances for stage IIIB (mastectomy for patient who responds poorly to radiation) or stage IV (hygienic mastectomy to control local disease). Radiotherapy: Radiation is used as an adjunct to surgery in stage I and stage II when there is less than complete resection of breast tissue or there is residual tumor. Radiation is part of the standard treatment of stage III disease. Radiation may be recommended to control local disease in stage IV. Chemotherapy and/or the anti-estrogen tamoxifen are used in the treatment of stages I thru IV. Which or whether both modalities are used depends on such factors as whether or not the tumor is estrogen receptor-positive, disease stage, whether the patient is pre or postmenopausal, whether or not there is visceral disease. If chemotherapy is employed, several combination chemotherapy options are available—e.g. CMF (cyclophosphamide + methotrexate + fluorouracil), CMFP (= CMF + prednisone), CMFVP (= CMF + vincristine + prednisone). Hormonal options other than tamoxifen may be considered for the adjunctive treatment of stage IIIB or stage IV disease. In the premenopausal patient, oophorectomy or androgen may be considered. In the postmenopausal: estrogen, progesterone, or androgen.

Prognosis (5 year survival with treatment): <u>Stage 0</u>: > 95%, <u>Stage I</u>; 85%, <u>Stage II</u>; 66%, <u>Stage III</u>; 41%, <u>Stage IV</u>; 10%.

Cervical Cancer is responsible for 6% of cases of cancer in

women. **Types:** About 90% of the cases are squamous cell carcinoma, about 10% are adenocarcinoma. Adenosquamous carcinoma, small cell carcinoma, sarcomas, and lymphomas of the cervix are rare. **Risk factors:** inception of intercourse at an early age, multiple sex partners, low socioeconomic status, history or serologic evidence of herpes simplex type 2 infection, genital warts. **Invasion:** There is probably a delay of several years between the time the cancer first arises in the cervical epithelium until it becomes invasive. This supported by the observation that carcinoma in situ is diagnosed most commonly in the 30s whereas invasive cancer is most frequently discovered in the 50s. **Metastasis:** Cervical cancer spreads by direct extension to the vagina and parametrium and thence by the lymphatics to regional pelvic nodes and to periaortic nodes. Metastases to the bone, liver, lung, brain may occur. **SIGNS/SYMPTOMS/DIAGNOSIS: Disease course:** Blood–tinged vaginal disharge or postcoital spotting is the initial complaint in many cases. The bleeding progressively increases both in volume and frequency. As the tumor spreads the patient may develop (**1**) lumbar, hip, and leg pain due to invasion of the lumbosacral plexus; (**2**) suprapubic pain, dysuria or hematuria secondary to bladder involvement; (**3**) flank pain (? involvement of ureter); (**4**) rectal pain or bleeding; (**5**) lower extremity edema due to lymphatic obstruction. Fistulas may develop between the vagina and bladder, or vagina and rectum. Eventually the ureters may become obstructed so that hydronephrosis and uremia ensue. **Pap smear** is obtained from the external cervical os (with a wood spatula or cotton–tipped applicator) and the posterior vaginal fornix (by aspiration with a glass pipette). The smear must be fixed at once. Pap smears are designated class I (no abnormal cells), class II (atypical yet benign cells present), class III (cells suspicious for malignancy), class IV and V (malignant cells present). The incidence of false–negative Pap smears is 20–45%. **Endocervical curretage and cervical punch biopsies** are performed (**1**) if there is a clinically suspicious lesion even if the Pap smear is negative, (**2**) if the Pap smear reveals malignant cells, (**3**) if the Pap smear is suspicious and there is no evidence of infection, (**4**) if the Pap smear is suspicious and there is an infection but atypical cells are still seen on Pap smear after the infection has been treated. Selection of punch biopsy sites may be guided by colposcopy or Schiller's test (the latter is based on fact that abnormal cervical epithelium does not take up iodine/potassium iodide stain). **Cone biopsy** is performed if punch biopsy reveals cancer that appears to be noninvasive. This is done to exclude invasive cancer that may be present at other cervical sites. Cone biopsy is also performed if endocervical curretage is positive, or if punch biopsy is negative with suspicious or positive Pap smear. Cone biopsy is not necessary if punch biopsy shows invasive cancer. **Additional tests** to assess the extent of disease may include IVP, cytoscopy, proctoscopy, chest x–ray, CAT scan pelvis.

Note: The following information is extracted from National Cancer Institute PDQ State–of–the–Art Cancer Treatment Information 11/1/90. However, since cancer treatment is evolving, this information may not be current. The most up-to-date standard treatment options may be obtained by calling the National Cancer Institute Cancer Information Service at 1–800–4–CANCER. Patients may also be candidates for clinical trials of new therapeutic regimens. Descriptions of these trials are also available.

STAGING: Stage 0: carcinoma in situ, intraepithelial carcinoma. **Stage I A:** Carcinoma confined to cervix, or may extend to corpus without advancing the stage. Stage IA is not clinically evident. It can only be detected by microscopy. <u>Stage IA1</u> designates minimal stromal invasion. <u>Stage IA2</u> means that lesions can be measured microscopically but that (1) the depth of invasion from the base of either the surface epithelium or the glandular epithelium is ≤ 5 mm, and (2) horizontal spread is ≤ 7 mm. **Stage I B** like stage IA is confined to cervix, or may extend to the corpus without advancing the stage. In contrast, (1) the lesions may or may not be clinically apparent, and (2) the dimension of the lesions exceeds limits of stage IA2. **Stage II A** is carcinoma that has spread beyond the cervix to involve the upper 1/3 of the vagina but has not spread to the lower 1/3 of the vagina. Carcinoma has not extended to pelvic wall, and there is no obvious parametrical involvement. **Stage II B** is defined like stage II A except that there is obvious parametrical involvement. **Stage III A:** Tumor has spread to lower 1/3 of the vagina but not to the pelvic wall. **Stage III B:** Tumor has (1) spread to pelvic wall, and/or (2) there is hydronephrosis or nonfunctioning kidney not attributable to other causes. **Stage IV A** means that tumor has invaded adjacent organs. Specifically, there is involvement of mucosa of bladder or rectum. Biopsy of the bladder and/or rectum is positive. **Stage IV B** means that there has been spread beyond true pelvis to distant organs.

TREATMENT: Stage 0 is commonly treated by simple abdominal or vaginal hysterectomy if fertility is not a consideration. Cervical conization is an alternative in those wishing to preserve fertility or avoid hysterectomy. Other options are laser cauterization or cryotherapy. **Stage I A** standard treatment is hysterectomy. Lymph node dissection is not necessary if depth of invasion is < 3 mm and there is no evidence of vascular/lymphatic invasion. The ovaries may be retained in younger women. If surgery is contraindicated, the treatment is intracavitary radiation. **Stage I B** standard treatment is either (1) radical hysterectomy with pelvic node resection ± postoperative external beam radiation or (2) combined intracavitary and external beam radiation. **Stage II A** standard treatment is as for stage I B. **Stage II B** standard treatment is radiation. Patients who are surgically staged as part of a clinical trial who are to undergo postoperative external beam radiation: (1) are less likely to have radiation–provoked complications if node sampling is done by the extraperitoneal approach rather than the transperitoneal approach, (2) are more likely to realize local control from radiation if macroscopically involved nodes are removed, (3) may be cured by pelvic and para–aortic radiotherapy if there is small volume para–aortic nodal disease and controllable pelvic disease. **Stage III** is generally treated similarly to stage II B, and the comments concerning postoperative radiation are applicable. Anterior, posterior, or total pelvic exenteration is sometimes recommended in certain cases in which the tumor has not spread to the parametrial regions nor outside the pelvis. **Stage IV A** standard treatment is radiation. Pelvic and para–aortic radiotherapy may cure some surgically–staged patients with small volume para–aortic disease and controllable pelvic disease. Anterior or posterior pelvic exenteration is sometimes recommended in certain cases in which the tumor has not spread to the parametrial regions nor outside the pelvis. **Stage IV B** treatment is palliative radiation. Investigational chemotherapeutic regimens may be tried.

PROGNOSIS (5 yr survival with treatment): **stage 0:** 100%, **stage I:** 80–90% (adenocarcinoma: 70–75%), **stage II:** 45–80% (adenocarcinoma: 30–40%), **stage III:** up to 61% (adenocarcinoma: 20–30%), **stage IV:** < 15%.

Endometrial Cancer is responsible for 13% of cases of

cancer in women. It is postmenopausal in about three–fourths the cases. The median age at diagnosis is 61. **Risk** appears to be increased by unopposed estrogen stimulation. Thus, women who are frequently anovulatory, obese, nulliparous, or who begin menopause late (i.e. menopause after 52 yr) are at increased risk. Diabetics are also at increased risk. **Five histologic types:** adenocarcinoma (75% cases) consists of malignant glandular epithelial components and is often accompanied by squamous metaplasia; adenosquamous (18% cases) consists of both malignant glandular epithelial cells and malignant squamous cells; papillary serous carcinoma (6% cases) has proclivity for vascular and myometrial invasion; clear cell carcinoma (1% cases) is a mullerian derivative with histologic similarity to clear clear cell carcinomas of vagina, fallopian tube, and ovary. ●The latter two types have the poorest prognosis. Mucinous carcinoma is rare.

   Signs/symptoms: Vaginal bleeding: Postmenopausal bleeding is due to cancer of the endometrium in about 40% of cases. Metrorrhagia is the most common presentation in premenopausal women. Pain does not usually accompany the bleeding. Cervical stenosis and pyometra may ensue if there is invasion of the cervix. An enlarged uterus on bimanual exam is consistent with myometrial invasion.

   Diagnosis: Outpatient endometrial biopsy with histology will frequently confirm the diagnosis. Fractional curretage under anesthesia is necessary if the foregoing method is negative. Fractional curretage consists in sequence of: (**1**) curretage of the endocervix for histologic assessment of involvement of the cervix, (**2**) dilation of the cervix, (**3**) curretage of the endometrium for histologic confirmation and grading of the tumor. PAP smear and vaginal cytology are not reliable methods for diagnosing endometrial carcinoma.

NOTE: The following information is extracted from National Cancer Institute PDQ State-of-the-Art Cancer Treatment Information 9/28/90. However, since cancer treatment is evolving, this information may not be current. The most up-to-date standard treatment options may be obtained by calling the National Cancer Institute Cancer Information Service at 1–800–4–CANCER. Some patients may be candidates for clinical trials of new therapeutic regimens. Descriptions of these trials are also available

Staging: NOTE: Hysterectomy is necessary to ascertain the degree of myometrial invasion.
Stage 0 is defined as atypical hyperplasia or carcinoma in situ.

Stage I refers to carcinoma restricted to the corpus uteri.
  Stage IA means that tumor is restricted to the endometrium.
  Stage IB stands for depth of invasion to < half of myometrium.
  Stage IC stands for depth of invasion to > half of myometrium.
Stage II indicates tumor involvement of corpus and cervix, without extending outside the corpus.
  Stage IIA means that the cervical disease only involves the endocervical glandular tissue.
  Stage IIB means the cervical stroma is invaded.
Stage III means the that the tumor has spread outside the uterus but not outside the true pelvis.
  Stage IIIA: invasion of serosa and/or adnexae and/or positve peritoneal cytology.
  Stage IIIB: metastases to pelvic and/or para-aortic nodes.
Stage IV indicates spread to bladder or bowel mucosa, or distant metastasis.
  Stage IVA: tumor spread to bladder or bowel mucosa.
  Stage IVB: distant metastasis. Involvement of inguinal or intra-abdominal nodes is included in category of distant metastasis.

Treatment:
Stage 0 treatment is abdominal or vaginal hysterectomy if infertility is not of concern or if patient requires estrogen treatment for another medical condition. Treatment of patients wishing to remain fertile is meticulous dilation and curretage (with high-dose progestin therapy for recurrence) and avoidance of estrogens.
Stage I:
  ●Patients who meet all the following criteria undergo TAHBSO (total abdominal hysterectomy with bilateral salpingo-oophorectomy) with removal of any target nodes: (1) well to moderately differentiated tumor involving upper 2/3 corpus, (2) myometrium invaded to < 1/3, (3) absence of vascular space invasion, (4) peritoneal cytology negative. Postoperative treatment is unnecessary unless target nodes prove to be positive.
  ●All other stage I patients undergo (in addition to TAHBSO) selective sampling of pelvic and periaortic nodes. If the samplings are negative, the pelvis is irradiated. If the pelvic nodes are positive and the periaortic nodes are negative, the patient receives total pelvic irradiation that includes the common nodes. If the periaortic nodes are positive, the patient may enter clinical trials that include radiation and/or chemotherapy.
  ●If surgery cannot be performed, the treatment is radiation alone.
Stage II treatment options are: (1) preoperative intracavitary and external irradiation followed by TAHBSO with biopsy of para-aortic nodes, (2) TAHBSO with node biopsy and postoperative radiotherapy, (3) radical surgery in selected patients—i.e. TAHBSO with resection of parametria and pelvic lymph nodes.
Stage III treatment is individualized. Those with operable tumors also receive radiation. If surgery is not feasible (e.g. tumor reaches pelvic wall), the treatment of choice is combined external beam and intracavitary irradiation. If neither surgery nor radiation is possible, progestins are indicated—e.g. medroxyprogesterone (Provera).
Stage IV treatment is individualized. Large pelvic tumors are treated with combined external beam and intracavitary irradiation. Those with distant metastases are treated with a progestin—e.g. medroxyprogesterone (Provera). Investigational chemotherapy protocols are an option.

Prognosis (5 yr survival with treatment): stage 0; 100%, stage I; 75-100%, stage II; up to 60%, stage III; up to 30%, stage IV; up to 5%.
NOTE: In stage I and II patients, it is important to assay the tumor for progesterone receptor level since this is a significant predictor of disease-free survival in these patients: 93% of those with progesterone receptor level > 300 are disease-free at 3 yr, while only 36% with level < 100 are disease-free at 3 yr.

Ovarian Cancer
ranks as the 4th most common cause of death from cancer in women. **Risk factors:** family history of ovarian cancer, personal history of breast or uterine cancer, history of ovarian irradiation, low fertility. Use of oral contraceptives may be protective.
  Signs/symptoms are usually absent until late. Furthermore, ovarian cancer is seldom discovered by pelvic exam of asymptomatic patient (once per 10,000 pelvic exams). Common initial manifestations are pelvic/abdominal mass, abdominal enlargement, lower abdominal pain. Often, there is a pressure sensation in the pelvis and there may be low back pain. Weight loss is common. Dysuria or constipation often ensues from tumor compressing the bladder and rectum respectively. Intestinal obstruction may develop when the tumor invades the colon. Ascites (usually secondary to peritoneal implants) develops in about a third of cases. Meig's syndrome (ovarian tumor with ascites and hydrothorax) may develop. Meig's syndrome is most commonly due to ovarian fibroma, Krukenberg tumor (metastatic carcinoma to the ovary), or Brenner tumor. Abnormal vaginal bleeding occurs in about a fifth of cases. This may be due to estrogen production by a hormonally active tumor or to tumor invading the uterus. Acute abdomen may be the initial pre-

sentation if there is torsion of the tumor. Pseudotumor peritonei results when a mucinous cystadenoma or a mucinous cystadenocarcinoma ruptures and releases a gelatinous material. There is a gradual increase in abdominal girth. Intestinal obstruction and fistulas may develop. Pelvic exam may provide a clue as to whether a tumor is benign or malignant. Benign tumors are generally smooth, unilateral, cystic, moveable, and < 8 cm across. Malignant tumors often have an irregular contour, may be fixed, and often have a solid consistency or have both solid and cystic areas. Nodular implants may sometimes be felt in the cul-de-sac. An enlarged ovary in a menopausal or postmenopausal women is due to a malignancy until proven contrary.

Diagnostic tests: Plain x-ray may sometimes show a soft tissue mass. Occasionally, a dermoid cyst is revealed by the presence of teeth or bone. Occasionally, a serous cytadenocarcinoma is suspected from the presence of calcifications (psammoma bodies). Ultrasound may delineate a cystic tumor. CAT scan may clarify the lesion. Other tests that may shed further light are barium enema, IVP, lymphangiography. Laparoscopy or culdoscopy may be used to confirm the diagnosis. Paracentesis for cytology is performed if there is ascites.

Differential diagnosis: functional ovarian cyst, endometriosis, uterine myoma, pelvic kidney, tubal pregnancy, tuboovarian abscess, hydrosalpinx, diverticulitis, colon tumor, retroperitoneal tumor, peritoneal cyst, feces in the colon or full bladder.

CLASSIFICATION of OVARIAN NEOPLASMS:

Benign versus malignant: About 80% of all ovarian neoplasms are benign. Benign tumors in decreasing order of frequency are fibroma (30%), mucinous cystadenoma (25%), serous cystadenoma (20%), cystic teratoma [dermoid cyst] (15%), granulosa cell tumor (4-10%), Brenner tumor (1%), theca cell (< 1%), arrhenoblastoma (< 1%), lipoid cell (1%). Malignant tumors in decreasing order of frequency are serous cystadenocarcinoma (45%), mucinous cystadenocarcinoma (10-15%), endometroid carcinoma (15%), unclassified carcinomas (5-10%), granulosa cell tumor (5%), Krukenberg tumor (< 2%), solid teratoma (1%), dysgerminoma (< 1%), Brenner tumor (< 1%), clear cell carcinoma (< 1%), theca cell tumor (< 1%), arrhenoblastoma (< 1%), lipoid cell (< 1%), hilus cell (< 1%), fibrosarcoma (< 1%).

Cystic versus solid neoplasm: Cystic tumors include serous or mucinous cystadenoma, serous or mucinous cystadenocarcinoma, and benign cystic teratoma (dermoid cyst).

Neoplasms derived from the surface epithelium: Serous cystic tumors are typically loculated and contain a transudate. About 50% are benign (serous cystadenoma) and the remainder malignant (serous cystadenocarcinoma). Serous tumors are uncommon before age 20. Serous cystadenomas tend to be pedunculated and are therefore prone to torsion. Serous cystadenocarcinomas are bilateral in 50% cases. Mucinous tumors contain a viscid material and are often loculated. About 90% are benign (mucinous cystadenoma) and the remainder malignant (mucinous cystadenocarcinoma). Mucinous tumors are uncommon before age 20. Mucinous cystadenomas are bilateral in 5% cases; they may become very large; they may undergo torsion, hemorrhage, or infarction. Mucinous cystadenocarcinoma are bilateral in 20% cases. Pseudomyxoma peritoneii may result if a benign or malignant mucinous tumor ruptures. This may be fatal ultimately. Endometroid carcinoma is bilateral in 30% cases. There is a histologic resemblance to endometrial carcinoma. Clear cell carcinomas are usually solid but may be cystic. About 5% are bilateral. Brenner tumors are small solid tumors that are most common after age 40 and rare before 20. About 5% are bilateral. Malignant degeneration is rare.

Neoplasms derived from germ cells are most common in children and young women. Teratomas: 97% are benign cystic teratomas (dermoid cyst) of which 12% are bilateral. Many types of tissue may be found within a dermoid cyst (e.g. skin, sebaceous glands, teeth, hair, bone). Rarely, functional thyroid gland tissue is found (struma ovarii). About 3% of teratomas are solid malignant teratomas; most commonly a squamous cell carcinoma but there are many other possibilities (e.g. malignant melanoma, basal cell carcinoma, osteosarcoma, choriocarcinoma). The latter may secrete chorionic gonadotropin. Malignant teratoma is more common in the young and is more common in blacks than whites. Dysgerminomas have the same histologic appearance as seminomas in males. They occur principally in young women. They are all malignant and 15% are bilateral. They may secrete chorionic gonadotropin or androgens. Gonadoblastoma is derived from both stromal and germ cell elements. The tumor most commonly develops in dysgenetic gonads or in intersexes. About half are malignant, about half are associated with a dysgerminoma, about 40% are bilateral. Hormone (androgens principally) production sometimes occurs. Other germ cell tumors are endodermal sinus tumor, embryonal carcinoma, polyembryoma.

Neoplasms derived for ovarian sex cord stroma: Granulosa cell tumor is the most common hormone-secreting ovarian neoplasm. It is most common in young girls. Estrogens are the principal hormones produced. Sufficient may be secreted to cause pseudopuberty in children, menstrual abnormalities during reproductive years, or postmenopausal bleeding. About 5% are bilateral and about 5-20% are malignant. Theca cell tumor secretes estrogens principally. Less than 1% are malignant. Gonadoblastoma (see above). Arrhenoblastoma (Sertoli-Leydig cell tumor) secrete androgens mainly. About 20% are malignant. Rarely are they bilateral. Lipoid cell tumor; androgen secreting, about 20% are malignant, rarely bilateral. Hilus cell tumor; androgen secreting, rarely malignant.

Other: Fibromas are solid tumors composed of connective tissue elements, probably derived from ovarian stroma. Meig's syndrome (ascites with hydrothorax) sometimes develops and resolves when the fibroma is resected. Malignant degeneration to a fibrosarcoma is rare. Most patients are in their 30–50s. Krukenberg tumors are tumors metastatic from the GI tract, breast, or GU tract. Over 80% are bilateral.

Note: The following information is extracted from National Cancer Institute PDQ State–of–the–Art Cancer Treatment Information 12/3/90 for epithelial carcinoma and 11/1/90 for ovarian germ cell tumors. However, because ovarian cancer treatment is evolving, this information may not be current. The most up-to-date standard treatment options may be obtained by calling the National Cancer Institute Cancer Information Service at 1–800–4–CANCER. Patients should be considered for inclusion in clinical trials. Descriptions of these trials are also available.

STAGING: Stage I (growth confined to ovaries) is divided into stage IA (growth confined to one ovary, no ascites, absence of tumor on external surface, capsule intact); stage I B (same criteria as IA except that both ovaries involved); and stage I C; one or both ovaries involved with (1) growth on external surface, (2) capsule ruptured, or (3) malignant cells in ascites fluid or peritoneal washing. **Stage II** (involvement of one or both ovaries with spread to other pelvic sites) is divided into stage II A (spread to uterus and/or tubes); stage II B (spread to other pelvic tissues); and stage II C. Stage II C includes the criteria of either IIA or II B and also includes any or all of the following: (1) there is growth on external surface, (2) capsule is ruptured, or (3) malignant cells are found in ascites fluid or peritoneal washings. **Stage III:** involvement of one or both ovaries with (1) peritoneal implants outside the pelvis, (2) positive retroperitoneal or inguinal nodes, and/or (3) superficial liver metastases. Stage IIIA designates tumor grossly confined to true pelvis but with proven microscopic seeding of abdominal peritoneum. Nodes are negative. In stage III B abdominal peritoneal implants are up to 2 cm in diameter. Nodes are negative. In stage III C abdominal peritoneal implants exceed 2 cm, and/or retroperitoneal or inguinal nodes are positive. **Stage IV** = distant metastases. Pleural effusion does not mean stage IV unless proven by cytology. Parenchymal liver metastasis counts as stage IV.

TREATMENT of EPITHELIAL CARCINOMAS (e.g. serous cystadenocarcinoma, mucinous cystadenocarcinoma, endometroid cystadenocarcinoma, clear cell cystadenocarcinoma).

Stage IA and I B, well–moderately well differentiated (grade I–II): Standard treatment is TAHBSO (total abdominal hysterectomy with bilateral salpingo–oophorectomy) + omentectomy. Procedure should include biopsy of pelvic & periaortic nodes or pelvic & abdominal peritoneum, peritoneal washings, visualization and biopsy of undersurface of diaphragm. Unilateral salpingo–oophorectomy is permitted in certain cases when the patient wishes to remain fertile.

Stage IA–1B with grade III differentiation, or stage I C, or large volume ascites: TAHBSO (total abdominal hysterectomy with bilateral salpingo–oophorectomy) + omentectomy. Procedure should include biopsy of pelvic & periaortic nodes or pelvic & abdominal peritoneum, peritoneal washings, visualization and biopsy of undersurface of diaphragm. Surgery is followed by one of the following options: intraperitoneal P–32 radiation, total abdominal–pelvic radiation, or systemic chemotherapy (e.g. cyclophosphamide + cisplatin).

Stage II: Standard treatment is TAHBSO + omentectomy with excision of all or as much tumor as possible. If clinically evident residual disease is absent, the procedure should include sampling of abdominal peritoneum and selected pelvic & periaortic nodes, and visualization & biopsy of undersurface of diaphragm. If after surgery there is < 2 cm residual tumor, the postsurgical treatment options are systemic chemotherapy (e.g. cyclophosphamide + cisplatin), total abdominal–pelvic radiation (only if residual tumor is < 0.5 cm), or intraperitoneal P–32 radiation (only if residual tumor is < 1mm). If there is > 2 cm residual pelvic tumor, postsurgical treatment is systemic chemotherapy (e.g. cyclophosphamide + cisplatin).

Stage III: Standard treatment is TAHBSO + omentectomy with excision of as much gross tumor as is safe. If after surgery there is < 2 cm residual tumor, the postsurgical treatment alternative is either systemic chemotherapy (e.g. cyclophosphamide + cisplatin) or total abdominal–pelvic radiation (only if there is < 0.5 cm residual tumor). If there is > 2 cm residual pelvic tumor, postsurgical treatment is systemic chemotherapy (e.g. cyclophosphamide + cisplatin).

Stage IV treatment consists of chemotherapy (e.g. cyclophosphamide + cisplatin).

TREATMENT of DYSGERMINOMA: Surgery; Total abdominal hysterectomy + salpingo–oophorectomy (TAHBSO) is the standard for all stages. (Unilateral salpingo–oophorectomy may be considered in the younger patient who wishes to remain fertile.) In more advanced stages, surgery includes removal of as much gross tumor as is safely possible but without resecting kidney or large segments of small or large bowel. Postoperative therapy is indicated in all but stage IA patients. Stages IB thru stage III may be treated with radiation or chemotherapy (e.g. bleomycin + etoposide + cisplatin). Chemotherapy may be preferred in stage III patients with bulky residual disease. Stage IV patients receive chemotherapy. Chemotherapy is preferred in the patient who has undergone unilateral salpingo–oophorectomy in order to preserve fertility.

TREATMENT of GERM CELL TUMORS OTHER THAN PURE DYSGERMINOMA (e.g. endodermal sinus tumor, embryonal carcinoma, polyembryona, choriocarcinoma, teratoma): Surgery as for dysgerminoma. Postoperative chemotherapy (e.g. bleomycin + etoposide + cisplatin) is required in all but low–grade immature teratoma. Preoperative chemotherapy may also be used in order to shrink extensive intra-abdominal tumor in a patient who might not tolerate debulking surgery.

Trauma

Initial Care, Airway, Hemorrhage

INITIAL CARE: Maintain and protect airway; stop obvious life–threatening bleeding; and if indicated perform CPR (cardiopulmonary resuscitation). Protect and immobilize spine, especially if there is any question of cervical spine trauma. Establish intravenous lines and administer fluids as outlined under hemorrhage below.

AIRWAY AND VENTILATION: Clear the mouth of blood, false teeth, or other debris. In the unconscious patient, the tongue may fall back and obstruct the airway. This is remedied by placing one's fingers behind the lower incisors and lifting the jaw anteriorly (chin lift). Subsequently maintain the tongue in proper position with an oropharyngeal airway. If the patient is not breathing, initiate mouth–to–mouth or bag–valve mask ventilation pending tracheal intubation. Nasotracheal intubation is preferred if there is significant oral trauma and vice versa. **Warning:** If cervical spine trauma is suspected, tracheal intubation should if possible be delayed until x–rays can be obtained. Furthermore, cervical spine injury is to be assumed (until x–rays prove otherwise) in any unconscious patient with head trauma. When cervical spine injury is present or suspected, great care must be exercised to avoid flexing or hyperextending the neck during tracheal intubation or in any other maneuver. An assistant should apply gentle traction to the head in the line of the long axis of the spine while the most skilled intubationist available intubates. If endotracheal intubation cannot be performed without undue cervical motion, the wisest course is to perform a cricothyroidotomy or insert an esophageal obturator airway (EOA)—both of which can be accomplished without moving the cervical spine.

HEMORRHAGIC SHOCK: In order to preserve cerebral and coronary blood flow, shock evokes compensatory mechanisms that oppose a fall in blood pressure and cardiac output: (**1**) Venoconstriction increases venous return thereby opposing a drop in stroke volume and hence cardiac output. (**2**) Tachycardia maintains cardiac output in the face of decreased stroke volume. (**3**) Arteriolar constriction supports the diastolic pressure although the pulse pressure may be reduced (decrease in pulse pressure reflects the drop in stroke volume secondary to decreased venous return). (**4**) Also vasoconstriction, while sparing the heart and brain, reduces blood flow to other organs (e.g. skin cool pale, reduced kidney perfusion with decreased urine output).

Assessing severity of shock: Tachycardia is not always a reliable gauge of hypovolemia since apprehension and pain increase the pulse rate. Nor is the blood pressure the most sensitive indicator of hypovolemia (a young otherwise healthy patient may have a normal blood pressure with a 25% blood loss). Pulse pressure (systolic–diastolic difference) is more sensitive; it may be reduced when the systolic or diastolic pressures are in the normal range. Postural signs are an early indicator of shock (the pulse rate increases by > 15 and/or the systolic pressure decreases > 15 mm Hg in going from supine to sitting position). Pale, cool, and moist skin also appear in the early stages of shock as a reflection of the increased sympathetic activity associated with shock. Capillary refill is delayed if blood loss is over 15%. Arterial blood gas can detect early shock. As the adequacy of perfusion decreases the cells rely more on anaerobic metabolism. Consequently, lactic acid accumulates and so metabolic acidosis ensues. Tachypnea may reflect shock–induced hypoxia and metabolic acidosis. The increased respiratory rate serves to generate a compensatory respiratory alkalosis. Remember that pain and anxiety may also increase the respiratory rate. Thirst increases with worsening shock. Urine output progressively falls as perfusion of the kidney decreases. Mental status ranges from anxiety in mild shock to agitation, confusion, and finally coma in severe shock.

	mild shock	moderate shock	severe shock †
percent blood loss*	< 15%	15–30%	> 30%
decreased blood pressure	no	±	yes
decreased pulse pressure	no	yes	yes
tachycardia	slight	> 100	> 120
tachypnea	no	20–30	> 30
delayed capillary refill	no	yes	yes
cool pale skin	no	±	yes
urine output	30–35ml/hr	20–30ml/hr	< 15 ml/hr
CNS signs	± anxious	anxious	anxious, confused → lethargy → coma

*Normal total blood volume in adult is 70ml/kg (i.e. 5 liters in 70kg adult).
†Patients in severe shock require blood transfusion in addition to crystalloid.

Treatment of hemorrhagic shock: Lay patient flat (if this does not impair respiratory function) and elevate legs 10°. Establish 2 large bore IV's and administer Ringer's lactate or normal saline. Adjust rate to clinical status: (**1**) If the patient is in severe shock, administer 1–2 liters rapidly (20 ml/kg in child) over 5 minutes and assess response. The goal is to restore a strong pulse (i.e. normal pulse pressure), and eliminate orthostatic changes in pulse rate and systolic blood pressure. (**2**) In less urgent cases, adjust the rate according to clinical judgment while monitoring pulse, blood pressure, urine output, etc. Run IV at TKO (to keep open) rate when signs of hypovolemia resolve. MAST suit is used if the situation is critical. Central venous pressure (CVP) line may be inserted to follow the effectiveness of fluid replacement and to preclude fluid overload. CVP monitoring is especially useful in the elderly or patients with cardiac compromise. The normal CVP range is 5–15 mm H20. The CVP may help clarify situations in which shock persists in spite of fluid administration: (**1**) CVP > 15 mm H20 with jugular venous distention suggests other complications such as: cardiac failure secondary to cardiac contusion/infarction, cardiac tamponade, tension pneumothorax, etc.; (**2**) CVP that remains low (< 5 mm H20), falls, or does not increase with fluid challenge may indicate persistent blood loss or inadequate fluid administration. CVP may to some extent be a misleading indicator of volume status because shock induces vasoconstriction which by itself elevates the CVP. Consequently, the CVP is not a substitute for monitoring of the other usual paramaters (i.e. pulse rate, blood pressure, urine output, etc). Blood transfusion is required in those patients, who in the absence of continued blood loss, continue to deteriorate even with ostensibly adequate crystalloid administration, or who have lost sufficient blood to develop frank uncompensated shock. Generally, these patients have lost over 25% of their blood volume. Depending on the urgency, 3 choices are available: (**1**) uncrossmatched type O negative is administered when blood must be given immediately (uncrossmatched type O positive is the second choice in this situation); (**2**) type specific blood (i.e. blood of the same type and Rh as the patient's but not crossmatched) when the usual delay of 5--10 minutes for blood typing can be tolerated; (**3**) typed and crossmatched blood (delay of 45–60 minutes). The normal total blood volume is estimated to be about 70 ml/kg in an adult and 80 ml/kg in a child.

Head Trauma

GLASGOW COMA SCALE estimates the severity of impaired brain function based on the best response in three categories added together. The highest and best score is 15 and the worst is 3.

Eye opening		Verbal response		Motor response	
spontaneous	4	oriented	5	obeys commands	6
to command	3	confused speech	4	to painful stimuli:	
to pain	2	inappropriate words	3	localizes pain	5
no response	1	incomprehensible sounds	2	flexion–withdrawal	4
		none	1	decorticate posturing	3
				decerebrate posturing	2
				no response	1

CONCUSSION is an immediate and transient neural deficit following head trauma that is without a demonstrable neuropathologic lesion.

Signs/symptoms concussion: Altered consciousness is attributed to impairment of the reticular activating system as a consequence of mechanical stress on the brain stem. The patient loses consciousness or is temporarily dazed. When there is loss of consciousness, it is instantaneous. The patient is briefly flaccid, apneic, and bradycardic; and the pupils are dilated and unreactive to light. Consciousness is regained rapidly, usually within seconds or a few minutes and seldom more than an hour. ●To diagnose concussion the patient must consistently improve after the traumatic incident. A patient who is initially conscious or regains consciousness, and then loses consciousness or later develops focal neural deficits cannot have those manifestations attributed to concussion alone. Barring metabolic or drug–related causes, the patient must have undergone (1) some other brain trauma, or (2) concussion in addition to other brain trauma. <u>Amnesia:</u> Upon regaining consciousness, the patient seldom remembers the traumatic incident itself and is frequently unable to remember events that occured several minutes after the incident (anterograde amnesia). Commonly, there is permanent amnesia for events just prior to the incident and occasionally there is a temporary retrograde amnesia that may extend to more remote events. <u>Other manifestations</u> may include dizziness, loss of equilibrium, altered vision, headache, nausea, vomiting, convulsions. These complaints frequently last for hours. <u>Focal neurologic signs are absent:</u> The presence of aphasia, unequal pupils, abnormal respirations, or focal motor or sensory impairment cannot be attributed to concussion alone. <u>Postconcussion syndrome:</u> In many cases, there are persistent complaints for weeks or months—e.g. headache, dizziness, anxiety, irritability, insomnia, poor memory.

CAT scan is not required if the patient rapidly regains consciousness and remains alert with full neurologic function. A CAT scan is obtained if there is vomiting, seizures, or some other neurologic abnormality.

Treatment concussion: none indicated. Patient should be admitted for 24 hour observation if the patient was unconscious for more than 5 minutes, or if there are convulsions or persistent vomiting. Otherwise, the stable patient can be discharged after a few hours of observation provided that there is a reliable observer at home.

BRAIN STEM CONTUSION: **Signs/symptoms:** <u>Loss of consciousness</u> is immediate and (in contrast to a concussion) prolonged. <u>Pupils</u> are generally small, equal, and react to light. However, they may be unequal if the area in the midbrain from which the third cranial nerves emanate is contused unilaterally. <u>Focal motor abnormalities</u> may be present if there is involvement of the corticospinal tracts. Findings will be unilateral if the contusion is unilateral. <u>Decorticate or decerebrate posturing</u> may develop. <u>Respiratory aberrations</u> may be evident and may identify the region of brainstem involvement: (**1**) central neurogenic hyperventilation (rapid regular breathing) if the midbrain is contused, (**2**) apneustic breathing (inspiratory gasping) with upper pons contusion, (**3**) cluster (periodic) breathing with lower pons contusion, and (**4**) ataxic breathing with a contused medulla. **CAT scan** is obtained. **Treatment** is supportive. Intubate and provide artificial ventilation and oxygen as needed. Insert nasogastric tube and empty the stomach. Insert Foley catheter. Establish IV and, in the absence of hypotension, administer D5 1/2 NS with 20 mEq KCl per liter at a maintenance rate. Osmotic diuretics are not indicated.

CEREBRAL CONTUSION, INTRACEREBRAL BLEEDING, and SUBARACHNOID BLEEDING: The region of the cerebrum contused may be beneath the impact site or opposite from the impact site (contrecoup). Contrecoup contusions commonly occur along the inferior surfaces of the frontal and temporal lobes. The region surrounding the contusion is edematous. Often, there is bleeding at the contusion site, and there may be bleeding into the subarachnoid space.

Signs/symptoms: <u>Consciousness is preserved if injury is restricted to the cerebrum.</u> A *cerebral* contusion does not by itself result in loss of consciousness; for this to occur there must also be injury to the brain stem (e.g. concussion, brain stem contusion, expanding intracranial hematoma leading to temporal lobe herniation against the brainstem). <u>Clinical presentation is variable and depends on the area contused or bleeding:</u> e.g. unilateral weakness/paralysis (precentral gyrus of contralateral frontal lobe), unilateral focal sensory impairment (contralateral parietal lobe), expressive aphasia (Broca's area of frontal lobe of dominant hemisphere), receptive aphasia (Wernicke's area of temporal lobe of dominant hemisphere), impaired memory or behavorial abnormalities (temporal lobe). <u>If there has been subarachnoid bleeding</u>, there may be photophobia and nuchal rigidity. <u>Intracerebral bleeding</u> may result in an expanding hematoma with herniation (see Subdural Hematoma).

CAT scan is obtained and repeated if the neurologic status deteriorates.

Treatment of cerebral contusion alone is supportive as for brainstem contusion. Surgical intervention is necessary if there is an expanding intracerebral hematoma with a midline shift or herniation. While awaiting surgery, the treatment outlined below under Subdural Hematoma is applicable with the exception that a burr hole is not a consideration unless there is a concurrent subdural or epidural hematoma.

SUBDURAL HEMATOMA (accumulation of blood between the dura and the arachnoid) usually results from rupture of veins that bridge from the dural venous sinuses to the brain. Subdural bleeding is occasionally arterial. Morbidity is high even with prompt surgical intervention because in many cases there is substantial concomitant brain trauma. Cerebral atrophy (e.g. elderly, alcoholics) predisposes to subdural hematoma because the delicate bridging veins traverse a greater distance and are therefore more vulnerable to rupture.

Signs/symptoms: Neurologic signs due to the hematoma itself do not appear immediately; they evolve as the expanding subdural hematoma exerts increasing pressure. Immediate neural effects suggests that the patient has undergone additional brain injury (e.g. concussion, cerebral or brain stem contusion). Increased intracranial pressure due to an expanding hematoma and exacerbated by cerebral edema manifest as lethargy, vomiting, papilledema, increased systolic blood pressure, bradycardia, bradypnea. Herniation: A subdural hematoma may exert sufficient pressure against the cerebral hemisphere to herniate the medial portion of the ipsilateral temporal lobe thru the tentorial opening and thus force it against the brain stem. If this occurs: (**1**) the third cranial nerve is compressed and so there is dilation of the ipsilateral pupil, (**2**) contralateral hemiparesis may result from injury to the corticospinal tract, (**3**) decreased level of consciousness may ensue from impairment of the reticular activating system. Bilateral subdural hematomas are not uncommon. If this is the case and herniation ensues, neurologic signs may not be lateralized since herniation may not be directed from just one side. Diffuse cerebral swelling may also lead to herniation in the absence of lateralized neurologic signs. Hypotension? The presence of hypotension should prompt a search for bleeding from an extracranial site because isolated head trauma does not result in hypotension except when (**1**) patient is near death, (**2**) there has been massive bleeding from a scalp wound, or (**3**) there is epidural or subgaleal bleeding in patient < 2 years old.

Tests: Obtain CAT scan, arterial blood gas, CBC, UA, PT, PTT, fibrinogen, electrolytes, type and cross. As circumstances suggest, also obtain blood alcohol and toxic screen.

Treatment subdural hematoma while awaiting surgical evacuation: Intubate those patients whose level of consciousness has deteriorated sufficiently to tolerate an endotracheal tube and who are unable to speak or obey commands. Insert a nasogastric tube and empty stomach. Insert Foley catheter and monitor urine output. Establish IV and, unless the patient is hypotensive, initially administer D5W at a TKO rate. Consult a neurosurgeon immediately. Ask for advice in instituting the following measures to reduce intracranial pressure: (**1**) hyperventilation of the intubated patient. Maintaining the pCO2 at 26–28 induces cerebral vasoconstriction and thus reduces cerebral blood flow. Caution must be exercised, however, since excessive hyperventilation may cause cerebral ischemia. (**2**) intravenous mannitol (see drug section) to shrink the brain. Mannitol induces intracellular dehydration by osmotic effect. Be aware, however, that shrinking the brain may allow increased intracranial blood flow and thus increase intracranial bleeding. (**3**) dexamethasone (10 mg IV every 6 hours) may be administered but is of unproven value in reducing cerebral edema in this situation. (**4**) burr hole may be necessary if surgery is delayed and neurologic status is rapidly worsening. Intravenous phenytoin (see drug section) is routinely administered to prevent seizures.

EPIDURAL HEMATOMA (blood accumulates between the dura and the skull) tends to extend less widely than a subdural hematoma because it must first dissect the dura from the bone; it is also less common. It most frequently results from a blow to the squamous region of the temporal bone where the middle meningeal artery lies in a groove on the inner table of the skull. ●Owing to the fact that the bleeding is usually arterial, clinical signs develop more rapidly than with subdural hematoma. However, the clinical consequences are the same—i.e. expanding intracranial hematoma leads to increasing intracranial pressure which in turn may lead to herniation. ●Although epidural hematonas can be rapidly fatal, early surgical intervention usually results in lower morbidity than a subdural hematoma because in most cases there is less concomitant brain trauma. Occasionally an epidural hematoma results from *venous* hemorrhage from dural sinuses or diploic veins. **Tests and treatment:** as for subdural hematoma.

SKULL FRACTURE: A **linear** skull fracture (seen as a radiolucent line on x–ray) per se requires no specific treatment. However, one should be particularly alert for an epidural hematoma if there is a fracture in the temporo–parietal region extending across the groove of the middle meningeal artery. A **depressed** skull fracture requires surgical elevation if it is depressed more than 5 mm or the thickness of the skull. A depressed fracture may not be recognized as depressed unless tangential x–ray views of the fracture site are ordered or a CAT scan is obtained.

A **basilar** skull fracture (fracture of the base of the skull) is not usually seen on skull x–rays, although the diagnosis is suggested if intracranial air is discerned or if blood is seen in the paranasal sinuses. A Towne's view may disclose an occipital fracture. CAT scan is more sensitive than skull x–rays in identifying basilar skull fracture. A basilar skull fracture may be associated with the following clinical signs: (**1**) Battle's sign (ecchymosis of mastoid area) is associated with fractures across the middle fossa; (**2**) "raccoon eyes" are the periorbital ecchymoses (not attributable to direct eye trauma) that may develop when there is a fracture of the floor of the anterior fossa and blood leaks into the periorbital space; (**3**) hemotympanum or blood in external auditory canal; (**4**) otorrhea or rhinorrhea. **Bedside tests for detecting CSF leakage:** There may be uncertainty regarding CSF leakage if concurrent bleeding obscures the CSF. Two tests may help clarify the situation: (**1**) Uristix (used in detection of urine sugar) will turn blue in presence of blood and CSF but there is usually no color change in presence of blood alone; (**2**) A drop of the suspected CSF–blood mixture placed on a piece of filter paper will form clear CSF rings about a central area of blood if there is in fact a CSF–blood mixture. For comparison, a drop of known uncontaminated blood may be placed on the same paper at a separate location. **Antibiotic prophylaxis** (e.g. ampicillin) against meningitis is advocated for basilar skull fractures even though this is of unproven value.

Spine Trauma

X–RAY EXAMINATION OF THE SPINE:

Cervical spine x–ray exam begins with a cross table lateral view. This view alone will disclose 80–90% of cervical spine fractures or dislocations, and can be obtained without moving the patient. The lateral film should show all 7 cervical vertebrae and the C7–T1 interspace. To this end, gentle in–line traction of the arms may be needed to visualize the lower segments. A swimmer's view is ordered if a complete view of the lower segments is still not possible. Normally, a lateral view of the cervical spine should show a smooth lordotic curve with the anterior and posterior margins of the vertebral bodies as well as the posterior spinal elements arranged in parallel lines. Soft tissue swelling in front of the upper cervical vertebrae is a clue to cervical trauma. In particular, the soft–tissue density in front of C3 should not normally exceed 4 mm in adults. In children, however, considerable prevertebral soft tissue is not necessarily an abnormal finding, especially if the film happens to be taken during forced expiration as when the child is crying. Next obtain the AP and the odontoid (open–mouth) views, both of which can also be obtained without moving the patient. The odontoid view ascertains the integrity/alignment of the odontoid and the lateral masses of C1 and C2. If the foregoing views are judged to be normal or indicate a stable fracture, oblique films may then be taken by "log rolling" the patient so as to not move the neck. Oblique views reveal the condition of the pedicles and laminae, and may further clarify the degree of dislocation or subluxation. Lastly, if the previous films are negative and if history (e.g. whiplash) and physical exam still suggest C–spine injury, then carefully supervised lateral flexion and extension films are taken to rule out subluxation. Tomograms may be obtained if uncertainty remains.

Thoracic spine x–ray: AP and lateral views are obtained. However, because the shoulders obscure the upper thoracic vertebrae on the routine lateral view, a swimmer's view or a slightly oblique lateral projection (Fletcher view) is needed to confirm the integrity of the upper thoracic segment.

Lumbar spine x–ray: A cross table lateral and AP views can be obtained without moving the patient and are the only films needed in the initial investigation of lumbar trauma.

ASSESSING THE LEVEL OF SPINAL CORD INJURY:

Sensory landmarks: top of shoulder (C4), thumb (C6), middle finger (C7), little finger (C8), nipples (T4), xyphoid (T7), umbilicus (T10), pubis (L1), great toe (L5), little toe (S1).

Motor landmarks: Transection above C3–5 cord level: The diaphragm is innervated by the phrenic nerve thru cervical levels C3–5. Therefore, transection above this level results in respiratory paralysis since innervation of the intercostal muscles is also interrupted. However, the patient may still be able to breathe for a while without ventilatory support by using the trapezius, sternomastoid, and platysma muscles. Transection of the lower cervical or upper thoracic cord, as seen in quadriplegics, causes paralysis of the intercostal muscles and makes the patient dependent on diaphragmatic breathing. Complete transection at C4 cord level or above causes complete quadriplegia. Lesions at C4 will allow some neck movement and some diaphragmatic contraction. C5–T1 cord level trauma spares some upper limb function, depending on level and extent of injury: the biceps is innervated by C56, triceps by C678, extension wrist/fingers by C6–8, flexion fingers by C78–T1, abduction/adduction fingers by C8–T1. Cord trauma below T1 entirely spares upper limb function, but complete transection at any level down to T12 results in paraplegia. Lumbar cord segments L1–5 lie behind vertebral bodies T11–L1. Injury in this region results in varying degrees of lower limb paralysis/weakness: hip flexion is mediated by L2–3, the quadriceps is innervated by L2–4 (knee extension and knee jerk reflex), gastrocnemius by L5–S12 (plantar flexion of ankle and ankle jerk reflex), tibialis anterior by L45–S1 (dorsiflexion ankle). The cremasteric reflex (L1) may be absent. Cauda equina injury: The spinal cord ends at the lower border of vertebra L1 and perforce vertebral injury below this level may result in injury to nerves of the cauda equina (L2--S5). Since the cauda equina consists of lower motor neurons, nerve transection here (just like any peripheral nerve) results in immediate *flaccid* paralysis with absence of reflex in the distribution of the affected muscle(s). In contrast, a spinal cord lesion with transection of upper motor neurons results in (after spinal shock resolves) *spastic* paralysis and hyperactive reflexes.

Sacral sparing (preservation of anal and scrotal sensation as well as voluntary contraction of the anal sphincter) is a hopeful prognostic sign. It indicates that transection of the spinal cord is not complete, and that at least some recovery of neurologic function is possible.

Reflexes: Recall that the spinal cord levels of the most commonly assessed reflexes conveniently number from 1 to 8: gastrocnemius or ankle jerk (S1), quadriceps or knee jerk (L2–4), biceps (C5–6), triceps (C7–8).

SPINAL SHOCK (absence of all reflexes below the level of spinal cord injury) immediately follows spinal cord trauma and may last hours to up to 2–6 weeks. In some cases, spinal shock does not occur. **Signs/symptoms:** Depending on the severity of the spinal cord trauma, there will be flaccid paralysis and absent reflexes below the level of the spinal cord lesion. Rectal sphincter tone is lost. Priapism may be present. Urinary retention occurs if there is loss of sensation in the saddle area. Hypotension may ensue in quadriplegic cases. In contrast to hypovolemic shock, the typical patient: (**1**) is not tachycardic and may in fact be bradycardic, and (**2**) the skin is warm and dry. In any hypotension–associated traumatic spine incident, it is mandatory that other causes of shock be ruled out before concluding that hypotension is neurogenic. As spinal shock resolves the patient develops spastic paralysis with hyperactive reflexes below the level of the cord lesion. This is because, although the upper motor neurons are damaged, the lower motor neurons and reflex arc are intact. The bladder is then able to fill and reflexively empty if the cord trauma is above S2–4 (the level where the parasympathetic outflow governing bladder contraction is located). **Treatment:** Hypotension is managed by administration of IV fluids (Ringer's or normal saline) titrated to systolic pressure of about 100. Take care to avoid overhydration with pulmonary edema. Insert Foley catheter and monitor urine output.

CERVICAL TRAUMA:

Fracture of C1 (atlas) most often results from an axial force that drives the occipital condyles inferiorly and ruptures the ring of the atlas (Jefferson bursting fracture). AP film shows the inferior articular surfaces of C1 dislocated laterally from their normal position over the superior articular surfaces of C2. Often, there is an associated C2 fracture.

Fracture of the odontoid (dens) is usually due to a flexion injury and the base of the dens is the most common fracture site. The fracture is usually identified on an AP open mouth film. However, improper positioning may sometimes cause the space between the upper central incisors to overlie the dens and thus give the false impression of a vertical fracture. Cord damage occurs if the dens is sufficiently displaced posteriorly.

Hangman's fracture (bilateral pedicle fracture of C2 with C2–3 dislocation) is an extension injury combined with either distraction or compression. Cervical traction should not be applied if distraction is the cause of the fracture.

Hyperextension injury of cervical spine and cord: Severe hyperextension buckles the ligamemtum flavum. In so doing, there may be narrowing of the anteroposterior diameter of the spinal canal with ensuing compression of the spinal cord. In many cases, the spinal cord escapes injury because the spinal canal at the cervical level has a relatively large diameter. <u>Central cord syndrome:</u> If the spinal cord is injured, it is often mainly the central part of the spinal cord that is contused. Characteristic consequences are: (**1**) weak and hyporeflexic upper extremities possibly with sensory impairment (e.g. loss of pain/temperature sensation in the hands), (**2**) spasticity of legs with weakness of the legs that is less pronounced than the arms. <u>X–ray</u> may be normal or there may be (as a result of tension on the anterior longitudinal ligament) a small avulsion fracture of the anterosuperior aspect of a vertebral body (extension tear drop fracture).

Hyperflexion injury of cervical spine and cord: Hyperflexion may result in a anterior wedged–shaped compression fracture of a vertebral body. This is a stable fracture (though not necessarily benign neurologically) unless the the posterior ligaments or elements are also disrupted. Lateral x–ray view may disclose a fragment broken off the anterior–inferior part of the vertebral body (flexion tear drop fracture). Spinal cord injury may occur without x–ray evidence of fracture or dislocation, and conversely there may be fracture/dislocation without neurologic sequelae. However, cervical spinal cord injury occurring by either a pure flexion or pure extension mechanism usually means that there has been a complete unilateral or bilateral facet dislocation. Hyperflexion–provoked spinal cord injury results when an intervertebral disc or posterior portion of a vertebral body is driven backward into the spinal cord. <u>Anterior cord syndrome</u> is one possible consequence of hyperflexion with incomplete spinal cord injury. Below the level of the lesion there is loss or impairment of motor function and pain/temperature sensation. Posterior column function (i.e. touch, vibration, position sense) is preserved. The anterior cord syndrome may be attributed to compression of the anterior spinal cord and/or compression of the anterior spinal artery.

Cervical spine dislocation, unlike the lumbar or thoracic spine dislocations, can occur without fracture because the orientation of the interarticular facets allows the inferior articular facet of one vertebra to slip forward over the superior articular facet of the vertebra below. Dislocations are most likely at the 4th–5th and the 5th–6th cervical vertebrae. Bilateral facet dislocation is suspected if lateral x–ray shows a vertebral body to be displaced anteriorly by > 50% on the vertebral body below while < 50% displacement implies an unilateral facet dislocation. Oblique x–ray view may be needed to reveal unilateral dislocation (the outline of the intervertebral foramen will be altered if there is a dislocation). The spinal cord usually escapes injury with unilateral dislocation. However, pain may ensue if the nerve is pinched in the ipsilateral intervertebral foramen. Bilateral dislocations are associated with disruption of the anulus and posterior intervertebral ligaments; cervical cord injury is likely.

Cervical dislocation–fracture may or may not result in cord damage depending on the degree of vertebral displacement. However, a fracture–dislocation is an unstable fracture unless the dislocated intervertebral facets are locked. Consequently, careful cervical spine immobilization is mandatory to preclude (or prevent further) cord injury.

Cervical subluxation (incomplete dislocation in which the joint surfaces still retain some contact) implies damage to the joint capsule and the posterior ligaments. On lateral view, one vertebral body may sometimes be seen to have moved slightly anteriorly with reference to the vertebral body below and the interspinous space may be widened if the interspinous ligament is torn. A lateral film with the neck flexed (with careful supervision by a knowlegeable clinician) may be needed to demonstrate subluxation.

Compression fracture of the vertebral body without disruption/dislocation of posterior elements may result in cord damage if the posterior portion of the body is driven back against the spinal cord.

THORACIC SPINE TRAUMA: In contrast to the cervical canal, the thoracic segment of the spinal canal is narrow relative to the spinal cord. Consequently, if thoracic cord damage does occur, it is likely to be severe. Moreover, complete transection is not uncommon. The rib cage bolsters the thoracic spine so that (**1**) considerable force is necessary to alter the alignment of the thoracic spine, (**2**) thoracic spine fractures tend to be stable (although not necessarily benign). **Simple compression** of the vertebral body, the most common fracture of the thoracic spine, is due to flexion–compression of the spine (e.g. fall, heavy object falling on shoulders). The fracture, depending on the force, may be limited to wedge deformity of the anterior aspect of the body or the whole body may be compressed. **Comminuted compression** fractures of the body may result from compression–flexion. The adjacent discs are injured, the interarticular facet joints may be fractured or dislocated, the pedicles may be fractured, and the posterior ligaments may be torn. Cord injury will result if vertebral body fragments are pushed posteriorly. A **shear** fracture is a fracture–dislocation occurring in the transverse plane at or near the intervertebral disc. It is associated with fracture of the pedicle or articular process. Paraplegia is likely.

THORACOLUMBAR FRACTURE (i.e. fracture of T11, T12, or upper lumbar vertebrae). A flexion–rotary force exerted at this level may result in fracture–dislocation. In many cases, this is an unstable fracture because the vertebral body may be fractured transversely, the articular facet joints are fractured and/or dislocated, and the posterior ligaments may be torn. Neurologic impairment is probable. Whether the spinal cord and/or cauda equina are involved depends on the vertebral level traumatized.

LUMBAR SPINE FRACTURES are in principle the same as outlined above for thoracic spine trauma. However, thoracic fractures tend to be more stable by virtue of the supporting rib cage. Also, lumbar fracture results in neurologic deficits that are due to injury to the cauda equina rather than to the spinal cord. The most common fracture is a hyperflexion–provoked compression fracture of the vertebral body. An unstable fracture results if the rotational force also disrupts the posterior elements.

INTERVERTEBRAL DISC RUPTURE AND HERNIATION: refer to neurology section.

Thoracic Trauma

RIB FRACTURE **Signs/symptoms:** There is pain at the fracture site that is made worse by inspiration. Gentle pressure on the sternum or simultaneous pressure on the lateral chest walls may provoke pain in the region of the fracture. Besides tenderness there may be crepitus at the fracture site. **Chest x–ray** (preferably upright PA) is obtained to rule out pneumothorax, hemothorax, lung contusion, etc. An expiratory PA view may be needed to detect a pneumothorax. Additional views solely to identify rib fractures are unnecessary; and furthermore, fractures thru the anterior rib cartilage may not be visualized. **Complications/associated injuries:** Respiratory complications: In order to lessen pain, the patient voluntarily minimizes respiratory effort on the affected side. Consequently, elderly or debilitated patients (especially those with emphysema) are prone to atelectasis, accumulation of bronchial secretions, and pneumonia. Fractures of ribs 1–2 are often associated with severe trauma to the head, neck, spine, large vessels, heart, and/or lungs. Fractures of the lower ribs are often associated with intra-abdominal trauma, particularly of the spleen or liver. **Treatment:** Analgesics: Narcotic analgesics are generally needed to ease pain. Intercostal nerve blocks are especiailly useful for relieving intense pain that compromises ventilation. Intercostal nerve blocks with 0.5% bupivacaine (Marcaine) are performed at the level of the fractured ribs as well as two ribs above and two ribs below. Rib belts or taping the chest wall may ease pain but may also compromise ventilation. Consequently, they are contraindicated except in robust individuals.

LUNG CONTUSION is seen as an infiltrate on chest x-ray. The infiltrate may not appear until several hours after the injury. Hemoptysis may be present. Dyspnea, which may be minimal or absent at first, tends to become worse as the contused lung becomes progressively edematous and therefore progressively noncompliant. **Treatment:** Patients should be admitted and observed for signs of respiratory failure. Intercostal nerve blocks (see Rib Fracture above) are indicated if pain is significantly compromising ventilation. Clearing of respiratory secretions by coughing or nasotracheal suction is important. Intubation and assisted ventilation (IMV + PEEP) may become necessary if the patient is unable to maintain pCO_2 at < 45, or a pO_2 > 50 while on room air or a pO_2 > 80 while on supplemental oxygen.

FLAIL CHEST may result if 3 or more adjacent ribs are fractured with the individual ribs fractured at 2 or more sites. There is paradoxical movement of the flail segment (i.e. it moves in on inspiration and out on expiration). This may not be readily apparent with shallow breathing but is obvious if the patient takes a deep breath. The paradoxical motion may further injure the underlying contused lung (see Lung Contusion above). Paradoxical motion and the noncompliant contused lung combine to increase the work of breathing. **Treatment:** Gentle pressure over the flail segment will improve ventilation. A sandbag may be used for this purpose. Otherwise, the treatment is as for lung contusion (see above).

SUBCUTANEOUS EMPHYSEMA (air in the subcutaneous tissue) may be traumatic or nontraumatic. Depending on the nature of the chest trauma, air may gain access to the subcutaneous tissue by various routes: **(1)** The most common route is for air to pass via a rent in the tracheal, bronchial, and/or alveolar structures; traverse a breach in the visceral and parietal pleura; and thence to dissect thru the chest wall to the subcutaneous tissue. Blunt chest trauma–associated rib fracture with laceration of underlying tissue or penetrating chest trauma may lead to subcutaneous emphysema by this mechanism. Since the air must traverse the visceral and parietal pleura, there is almost always an associated pneumothorax unless prior disease has caused adhesions to form between the parietal and visceral pleura. **(2)** If there is a breach of the tracheal, bronchial, and/or alveolar structures but the pleura remains intact, air may dissect thru the peribronchial connective tissue to the hilum and into the mediastinum (mediastinal emphysema). Mediastinal air may then pass into the neck to dissect into the subcutaneous tissue of the neck, face, chest, and/or abdomen. **(3)** Uncommonly, air may dissect into the subcutaneous tissue via a skin wound. **Diagnosis:** Subcutaneous emphysema is recognized by the swelling, and by crepitus on palpating the skin. Furthermore, subcutaneous air is visible on x-ray. **Treatment** of subcutaneous emphysema per se is rarely required since the condition resolves spontaneously. However, there is usually a concomitant pneumothorax. Consequently, a chest tube must be inserted beforehand if the patient requires a ventilator or general anesthesia even if a chest x-ray fails to disclose a pneumothorax

MEDIASTINAL EMPHYSEMA (air in the mediastinum, pneumomediastinum). Air may enter the mediastinum directly (e.g. penetrating chest trauma, ruptured esophagus), or indirectly by dissecting thru the peribronchial connective tissue to the hilum and into the mediastinum. In the latter case, as a consequence of either blunt or penetrating chest trauma, air gains access to the peribronchial tissue thru a breach in the tracheobronchial tree or lung parenchyma, or pleura. Mediastinal emphysema may lead to subcutaneous emphysema if the mediastinal air passes into the neck to dissect into the subcutaneous tissue of the neck, face, chest, and/or abdomen. **Diagnosis:** Hamman's sign (a crunching sound synchronous with the heart beat) is common. A chest x-ray revealing mediastinal air confirms the diagnosis. **Treatment** of mediastinal emphysema per se is seldom required since the condition resolves spontaneously. Rarely, mediastinal air may compress mediastinal structures and require mediastinotomy via cervical approach.

PNEUMOTHORAX (air in the pleural space) can result from blunt or penetrating trauma. It may be iatrogenic (e.g. subclavian vein catheterization, assisted ventilation). Pneumothorax may also occur spontaneously by the following mechanism: spontaneous rupture of alveoli leads to formation of a bleb of the visceral pleura; and the bleb subsequently ruptures allowing air into the pleural space. **Signs/symptoms:** There is dyspnea, and there is ipsilateral chest pain that is aggravated by inspiration. If the pneumothorax is large enough, there will be decreased breath sounds and hypertympany of the ipsilateral chest. **Chest x-ray** confirms the diagnosis. An expiratory film may reveal a pneumothorax that is not disclosed on an inspiratory film. **Treatment:** Observation: Depending on the clinical circumstances, it may be possible to leave a small pneumothorax (< 1 cm wide or < 20% of hemithorax) alone, observe the patient, repeat a chest x-ray in 6 hours to confirm that the pneumothorax is not expanding, and wait for the pleural air to resorb spontaneously (about 1–2% of the pleural air will resorb per 24 hour). Insertion of a chest tube in the 5th intercostal space (the nipple line) anterior to the midaxillary line is the standard treatment. In the absence of concurrent hemothorax or hydrothorax, a 24 to 28 French chest tube is suitable in an adult. To verify proper placement, an upright PA and lateral chest x-ray should be obtained after the procedure. Generally, the tube may be removed when there has been < 100 ml drainage and air has not leaked for a 24 hour period. However, if the patient is being mechanically ventilated, it is safer to leave the tube in place in case pneumothorax recurs. Needle aspiration is an acceptable alternative to chest tube insertion in patients with spontaneous pneumothorax who are stable and who are not in respiratory distress—provided that there is neither hemothorax nor hydrothorax, and there is no underlying lung disease. Needle aspiration is accomplished by inserting a 16 gauge needle (attached to a 3-way stopcock) into the 2nd intercostal space midclavicular line. As the lung reexpands, there is a risk that the visceral pleura will be lacerated when it contacts the needle. A chest x-ray is obtained immediately after the procedure, and again at 6 hours and 24 hours to confirm that pleural air is not reaccumulating.

TENSION PNEUMOTHORAX develops if a break in the lung-visceral pleura or the chest wall acts as a one-way valve so that air enters the pleural space during inspiration but is not allowed to escape during exhalation. **Diagnosis:** Accumulating air in the pleural space first collapses the lung (absent breath sounds and hypertympanitic chest wall on the injured side) and then exerts increasing pressure on the mediastinum so that the mediastinum and trachea are shifted toward the opposite side. Tracheal shift is usually obvious on physical exam. Pressure on mediastinal vessels blocks venous return which in turn leads to distended neck veins, decreased cardiac output, decreased pulse pressure, tachycardia, hypotension, and finally vascular collapse. The mediastinal shift also compromises ventilation of the normal lung. The patient is severely dyspneic and may be cyanotic. If the diagnosis is in doubt, insert a 14 gauge over-the-needle catheter into the 2nd intercostal space midclavicular line with an attached 35 ml syringe half filled with saline but without the plunger. Air will bubble actively thru the saline throughout the respiratory cycle if a tension pneumothorax is present (the water acts as a seal if a pneumothorax is not present). Tension pneumothorax is an emergency. Treatment should not be delayed in order to obtain a chest x-ray. **Treatment:** Immediately insert a 14 gauge over-the-needle catheter attached to a 35 ml syringe into the 2nd intercostal space midclavicular line to quickly relieve the pressure. After the air has been aspirated, remove the syringe but leave the catheter in place attached to a finger cot—the closed end of which has been cut so that air can escape. Remove the catheter after a chest tube has been inserted in the 5th intercostal space anterior to the midclavicular line.

OPEN PNEUMOTHORAX (open sucking chest wound) refers to a hole in the chest wall that allows air to move in and out of the pleural space with each breath and thus creates a sucking sound. Dyspnea occurs with large holes (> 2/3 tracheal diameter) because air moves preferentially through the hole into the pleural space thereby "stealing" a volume of air that would otherwise enter the trachea to ventilate the lungs. Small holes may be tolerated with little respiratory distress. **Treatment:** Cover the wound immediately with an occlusive dressing if there is severe respiratory compromise. Then apply a dressing that covers the wound completely and tape it in place leaving one edge untaped to act as a one-way valve so that the hole will be completely occluded during inspiration but will allow air to escape during exhalation. This one-way valve device will prevent development of a tension pneumothorax. Applying a rubber glove with a hole in one finger over the wound will have the same effect. Subsequently, insert a chest tube remote from the wound. Evaluation of the wound for surgical repair can then be made.

HEMOTHORAX (blood in the pleural space) may be due to blunt or penetrating trauma. Air may also be present in the pleural space (i.e. hemopneumothorax), especially in penetrating chest trauma. Common sources of hemothorax include bleeding from intercostal vessels, internal mammary artery, or vessels closely associated with lung parenchyma. Lacerations of the heart or major intrathoracic vessels may also result in hemothorax. Laceration of the liver or spleen that includes penetration of the diaphragm is yet another possible source of hemothorax. Laceration of the lung does not usually cause profuse bleeding because: (1) pressure in the pulmonary vessels is low, and (2) collapse of the lung in the region of the injury helps stanch the bleeding. **Clinical signs** may include: (**1**) dyspnea, (**2**) decreased or absent breath sounds on the affected side, (**3**) dullness to percussion or a hypertympanic percussion note depending on the relative amount of pleural blood or air respectively, (**4**) shock. Shock is usually due to frank blood loss but impaired venous return may be a contributing factor if accumulated blood and/or air in the pleural space shifts the mediastinum to the opposite side so that the inferior vena cava becomes kinked. **Chest x–ray** confirms the diagnosis. An upright or a lateral decubitus view are best at revealing hemothorax. **Treatment:** Patients in shock and exsanguinating require prompt fluid resuscitation: establish 2 large bore IV's and administer Ringer's lactate; type and cross for 8 units of blood; apply MAST trousers. If the situation is critical, administer 0–negative or type specific blood while awaiting cross-matched blood. Autotransfusion is also recommended. An emergency thoracotomy is necessary if these measures fail to restore an adequate blood pressure. Chest tube (32–40 French in adult) is inserted in the 5th intercostal space anterior to the midclavicular line. The amount of blood initially evacuated and the hourly yield should be noted. Thoracotomy is indicated if ≥ 1000 ml is removed initially, if there is continued blood loss > 200 ml/hr for 4 hours, if > 1500 ml is evacuated during the first 12–24 hours, or if chest x-ray shows that the involved hemithorax remains more than half filled with blood despite the chest tube. The chest tube should be clamped if there is worsening of vital signs concurrent with rapid and voluminous blood drainage because the hemothorax may have been tamponading the bleeding site thus preventing exsanguination. Such a patient requires emergency surgery. ●Chest tube drainage alone may not be completely effective in removing pleural blood. However, in most such cases the blood resorbs spontaneously within 4 weeks. Thoracotomy is indicated if it does not. A very small hemothorax may not require chest tube drainage. It may be observed to see if there is spontaneous resolution.

CARDIAC CONTUSION is a common consequence of severe blunt chest trauma. **Diagnosis:** EKG may show abnormalities secondary to myocardial ischemia or infarction. Since the contusion is usually anterior; T wave inversion (the most sensitive EKG sign), ST segment elevation/depression**,** and Q wave are most often seen in the anterior chest leads V1–4. Arrhythmias (e.g. premature ventricular contractions, atrial or ventricular fibrillation) and bundle branch block may also occur. Cardiac isoenzyme CPK–MB is measured. If EKG and CPK–MB are normal in the setting of severe chest trauma, it is prudent to obtain serial EKG's and CPK–MB, and also obtain an echocardiogram or perform radionucleotide angiography. This approach is advised because it is not unusual for the EKG and CPK–MB to be normal despite the presence of a myocardial contusion. **Treatment:** Cardiac monitoring is essential because there is a risk of sudden death from arrhythmias. The patient is placed at bed rest. Treatment is generally the same as for a myocardial infarction.

STERNAL FRACTURE: Besides bruising and tenderness, there may be a depression and movement of the sternum. Breathing is shallow to minimize the pain. Sternal x--ray views will confirm the diagnosis. Surgery to stabilize the sternum is often required. Associated mediastinal or pulmonary injuries should be sought.

AORTIC RUPTURE is most likely to occur at the ligamentum arteriosum just distal to the origin of the left subclavian artery. **Signs/symptoms:** Since aortic rupture is often the result of deceleration, signs of chest trauma may be absent. A systolic murmur may be heard over the precordium and/or medial to the left scapula. Blood flow to the descending aorta may be impaired. Consequently, there may be a weak pulse in the lower limbs, and/or there may be a strong pulse with elevated pressure in the upper limbs. Hoarseness may ensue from compression of the left recurrent laryngeal nerve (this nerve is vulnerable because it hooks around the ligamentum arteriosum and aortic arch). **Chest x–ray** often reveals widening of the mediastinum. If possible an inspiratory upright PA view should be obtained because a flat, AP, or poor inspiratory view may give the false impression that the mediastinum is widened. False–positive widening of the mediastinum may also be seen if the x-ray machine is less than a meter from the patient. Be alert to the possibility of aortic rupture if there is a fracture of ribs 1 or 2. Other possible x-ray signs include: indistinct aortic knob, obliteration of clear space between aorta and pulmonary artery, shift of trachea to right, shift of left mainstem bronchus up or down, and/or shift of esophagus to the right as seen with a nasogastric tube in place. **Aortography** confirms the diagnosis. **CAT scan with contrast** has also been used to identify aortic rupture. **Treatment:** Surgery is mandatory since only the intact aortic adventitia is preventing fatal exsanguination.

TRACHEOBRONCHIAL INJURY may be the consequence of blunt or penetrating trauma, or be due to deceleration shear stress. **Signs/symptoms** may include dyspnea, subcutaneous emphysema, hemoptysis. Tracheal deviation may be due to concomitant tension pneumothorax. Tracheal obstruction may manifest as noisy respirations, inspiratory stridor, and/or hoarseness. **Chest x–ray:** Pneumothorax or pneumomediastinum may be seen. **Endoscopy** may identify the site of injury and decide the need for surgery. **Esophagoscopy** is indicated to exclude concomitant esophageal trauma. **Treatment:** Intubation: Airway patency is best assured by intubation. However, intubation may not always be possible if there is airway distortion. Patients with ruptured bronchus and a large air leak should if possible be intubated with an endotracheal tube of sufficient length to enter a mainstem bronchus. In some cases, maintenance of an open airway with an endotracheal tube until healing occurs is the only specific treatment required (see surgical indications below). Tracheostomy may be necessary to bypass tracheal obstruction in the upper neck. Chest tube is inserted if there is a pneumothorax. However, a single chest tube may not suffice if there is a large air leak (air is seen to bubble out of the tube with each breath). Therefore, an additional chest tube may be needed to reexpand the lung and relieve respiratory distress. Surgery: Indications for surgery include persistent air leak and/or respiratory distress, hematoma compressing trachea, laceration > 1/3 circumference of trachea. Emergency surgery may be required in seriously compromised patients. Bronchoscopy is performed prior to surgery if clinical condition allows the delay.

TRAUMATIC PERICARDIAL TAMPONADE is usually due to penetrating chest or abdominal trauma, and less often to blunt chest trauma. **Clinical signs** may include hypotension, tachycardia, narrowed pulse pressure with thready pulse (due to decreased stroke volume), pulsus paradoxus (systolic pressure falls > 10 mm Hg on inspiration), distended neck veins (due to elevated central venous pressure), distant heart sounds. **Differential diagnosis:** Hemorrhagic shock has some of the same signs as tamponade. In contrast to tamponade, however, central venous pressure is decreased (and consequently the neck veins are flat) and pulsus paradoxus is not characteristic. Left tension pneumothorax may be confused with tamponade. However; breath sounds will be absent on the left, dyspnea is marked, and there may be tracheal shift. **Treatment:** EKG monitoring is essential. Intravenous fluid: Establish 2 large bore IV lines. Intravenous volume infusion is recommended to increase stroke volume. Pericardiocentesis is a temporizing measure until surgery can be performed. Use a 16–18 gauge plastic over–the–needle catheter (6 inch or longer) with a metal needle hub, a 3–way stopcock, and a 30 ml syringe. Attach the V lead of EKG machine to the metal hub of the needle via alligator clip leads. Using sterile precautions, the needle is inserted at a 45 degree angle to the skin just to the left of the xyphoid and aimed toward the tip of the left scapula while applying constant suction on the syringe (aiming toward the right scapula is also advocated). Contact with the ventricular epicardium characteristically causes ST segment elevation while contact with the atrial epicardium causes PR segment elevation. Simultaneous elevation of both ST and PR segments is evidence that the pericardium has been contacted but there is no fluid interposed between pericardium and epicardium. Other EKG signs of epicardial contact may include atrial or ventricular arrhythmias, or widened

QRS. If the epicardium is contacted, the needle is withdrawn slightly while aspirating until the injury current disappears. The catheter is left in place (with the stopcock in the closed position) after blood has been removed in case additional aspiration is required. Pericardial blood may clot and prevent pericardiocentesis. This makes thoracotomy all the more urgent. <u>Emergency thoracotomy</u> is performed if the patient is in shock and not improved with pericardiocentesis.

ESOPHAGEAL PERFORATION is not common. It is usually due to penetrating trauma. Rarely, perforation may follow blunt trauma to the chest or upper abdomen. **Signs/symptoms:** Esophageal pain may be felt in the chest. epigastrum, or neck depending on the level of esophageal perforation. Hamman's sign may be present (pneumomediastinum–associated precordial crunching sound that is synchronous with the heart beat). Other possible findings include dysphagia, hematemesis, hoarseness, dyspnea, subcutaneous emphysema. The patient may go on to develop mediastinitis with fever and leukocytosis, and shock. **Chest x–ray** may reveal widening of the mediastinum, pneumomediastinum, and/or pneumothorax (usually left-sided pneumothorax), hydrothorax, or hydropneumothorax. **Esophagoscopy and/or gastrografin swallow** confirm the diagnosis. **Treatment:** NPO, nasogastric tube to continuous suction, IV fluids, broad spectrum IV antibiotics, surgery.

DIAPHRAGMATIC LACERATION/RUPTURE:

Diaphragmatic laceration due to penetrating trauma: That the diaphragm has been perforated may be obvious from cursory exam (e.g. bullet wound in thorax with exit wound in abdomen). When considering whether the diaphragm has been perforated, remember that the dome of the diaphragm reaches as high as the level of the nipples.

Diaphragmatic rupture due to blunt abdominal trauma is secondary to a sudden increase in intra–abdominal pressure. The membranous area of the left hemidiaphragm is the most vulnerable site for rupture. Rupture of the right hemidiaphragm is unusual because the liver buttresses the diaphragm on the right. <u>Left diaphragm rupture:</u> The rupture may allow herniation of abdominal viscera into the left thorax, and so there is a risk of bowel obstruction and strangulation. Bowel sounds may be heard over the left chest, and obviously breath sounds may be decreased or absent in the same region. The patient may be dyspneic and/or complain of pain in the left shoulder that is aggravated by inspiration or Trendelenberg position. Chest x–ray may reveal a left pleural effusion, an "elevated" or indistinct left hemidiaphragm, loops of bowel or gastric fundus (and/or nasogastric tube) in the left thorax, shift of mediastinum to right. Contrast barium or gastrograffin x–rays, or CAT scan may assist in the diagnosis. Sometimes the diagnosis is made when diagnostic peritoneal lavage is performed and the lavage fluid emerges thru a chest tube which has been inserted for pneumo– or hemothorax. <u>Right diaphragm rupture:</u> A right pleural effusion may be the only hint. When there is a large tear, the liver together with loops of bowel may be seen in the right thorax.

Treatment of diaphragm rupture/laceration: Follow the usual protocols for management of abdominal/thoracic trauma. A nasogastric tube should be inserted and connected to continuous suction in order to decompress the bowel and thereby minimize the risk of strangulation. Surgical repair is indicated even for small defects since viscera may herniate thru the tear even years later.

Abdominal Trauma

PERITONEAL LAVAGE:

Indications: ●physical exam supports possibility of intra–abdominal trauma; ●likelihood of significant intra–abdominal injury suggested by history even if physical exam is unremarkable; ●unexplained hypotension or other signs of significant blood loss in trauma patient; ●level of consciousness of traumatized patient makes abdominal exam difficult to evaluate (e.g. head trauma, drug/alcohol ingestion); ●serious combined chest and lower extremity trauma. **Contraindications:** ●need for abdominal surgery is obvious, ●multiple previous abdominal operations (consider CAT scan instead), ●Pregnancy is a relative contraindication. Consider culdocentesis instead. **Limitations:** Lavage may not detect bleeding from extraperitoneal organs (e.g. kidney, ureter, bladder, pancreas, duodenum, aorta, vena cava, rectum, uterus, vagina).

Method: Prior to procedure, insert a nasogastric tube to decompress the stomach and insert a Foley catheter to empty the bladder. Sterile technique is required. The incision is usually made in the midline a third of the distance from the umbilicus to pubis. Anesthetize the incision site with liddocaine with epinephrine. Insert the lavage catheter using the closed Seldinger method, or the open method with direct visualization and incision of the fascia and peritoneum. Attach a syringe to the catheter and aspirate (return of > 10 ml gross blood indicates a positive test). If no blood is aspirated, Ringer's lactate (10–20 ml/kg up to 1 liter) is infused into the peritoneum via the lavage catheter and allowed to remain for 5–10 minutes. Gentle massage of the abdomen and changes of the patient's position will help distribute the lavage fluid throughout the peritoneal space. The fluid is then withdrawn from the peritoneal cavity by placing the Ringers' lactate container at floor level. If fluid does not return, try moving the catheter and check that the Ringers' container is vented.

Interpretation:
A positive lavage is established by one or more of the following findings:
(1) return of gross blood or the inability to read newsprint through the lavage tubing. A blood-tinged lavage that yet allows one to read newsprint thru the tubing is considered weakly positive and the lavage fluid is sent to the lab for cell count and analysis.
(2) RBC count of unspun lavage fluid over 100,000/ml for blunt trauma, over 10,000/ml for stab wound, over 1000/ml for gunshot wound.
(3) over 500 WBC/ml in unspun lavage fluid.
(4) amylase level of lavage fluid > 200 IU/dl.
(5) lab exam of lavage fluid reveals bile, bacteria, vegetable fiber, or feces.

A negative lavage is crystal clear. In blunt trauma there will be < 20,000 RBC/ml in the unspun lavage fluid.

An equivocal lavage in the setting of blunt trauma is an RBC count of the unspun lavage fluid of 20,000–100,000/ml.

INVESTIGATION/MANAGEMENT of BLUNT ABDOMINAL TRAUMA:

Overview: Any patient who is hypotensive or shows any other signs of shock that has been subjected to blunt abdominal trauma who (1) has a normal chest x-ray, and (2) improves following an IV fluid challenge has intra-abdominal bleeding until proven otherwise. Assessment of the comatose patient for blunt intra-abdominal trauma is often difficult because the abdominal exam is frequently unremarkable in spite of severe intra-abdominal bleeding. Be especially wary for possible intra-abdominal bleeding if a head-traumatized comatose patient presents with hypotension. Remember that intracranial bleeding by itself is not associated with hypotension until the patient is terminal. In fact, isolated intracranial bleeding with ensuing elevation of intracranial pressure characteristically leads to systolic hypertension with an increased pulse pressure. On the other hand, severe blood loss from a scalp wound may lead to hypotension.

First considerations: Follow the guidelines set forth above in the chapter "Initial Care, Airway, Hemorrhage".

Rapid but thorough physical exam: Note areas of tenderness and of rebound tenderness. Are there bowel sounds? Is the abdomen distended? Laparotomy is indicated if there are signs of peritoneal irritation. Do not ignore small contusions; they may signal serious underlying trauma. Also, do not forget to examine the back. Perform rectal exam (check for displacement or bogginess of the prostate, sphincter tone, and for blood). Perform pelvic exam unless pelvic injury is not a consideration.

Nasogastric tube is inserted to ascertain presence of blood in GI tract, to prevent gastric distension, and to remove stomach contents and thus reduce risk of aspiration. Suspected cribiform plate fracture is a contraindication to NG tube placement.

Foley catheter is inserted if serious injury is known or suspected unless (1) pelvic injury is likely, (2) there is blood at the urethral meatus, or (3) rectal exam reveals a displaced or boggy prostate. If any of these conditions prevail, an urethrogram must be performed to rule out urethral trauma before inserting a Foley.

Consult a surgeon as soon as possible if patient is unstable or if serious injury is obvious.

Initial x-rays: Free air under the diaphragm on an upright chest x-ray (or the right flank on a left lateral decubitus film) confirms that a hollow viscus has been perforated. A pelvic film is ordered if there is possibility of pelvic trauma.

Further diagnostic testing: The selection of further tests is guided by the history and physical findings, and whether or not the patient is stable. Do not delay treatment in order to perform radiologic tests if the patient is hypotensive or otherwise unstable. Further diagnostic testing may not be necessary if the need for laparotomy is obvious (e.g. persistent hypotension, peritonitis, x-ray reveals free intra-abdominal air), or if the patient is stable and has an unremarkable physical exam. Peritoneal lavage is the next diagnostic step in many cases. This is particularly true if the situation is urgent. CAT scan with contrast may be used instead of peritoneal lavage if the patient is hemodynamically stable and can tolerate the delay, and CAT scan may be indicated if peritoneal lavage findings are equivocal. In addition to IV contrast, the study may be further enhanced by PO administration of water soluble contrast (gastrografin). CAT scan has two diagnostic advantages over peritoneal lavage: (**1**) CAT may identify the specific site of injury, (**2**) peritoneal lavage generally fails to disclose bleeding from extraperitoneal organs (e.g. kidney, ureter, bladder, pancreas, duodenum, aorta, vena cava). Also, CAT scan with contrast is an acceptable alternative to cystogram and IVP for evaluating a patient with hematuria provided that the patient is hemodynamically stable and can tolerate the delay. Urethrogram must be performed prior to inserting a Foley catheter if pelvic injury is suspected, if there is blood at the urethral meatus, or if rectal exam reveals a displaced or boggy prostate. Cystogram and/or IVP are used to rapidly evaluate a patient with hematuria. See *Steps in X-ray Evaluation of Urinary Tract Trauma* in "Urinary Tract" chapter that follows.

Indications for laparotomy include: (**1**) persistent unexplained hypotension; (**2**) signs of peritoneal irritation; (**3**) free intra-abdominal air detected on x-ray; (**4**) positive abdominal CAT scan with compelling findings; (**5**) positive peritoneal lavage.

INVESTIGATION/MANAGEMENT of ABDOMINAL STAB WOUND: Remember that the dome of the diaphragm reaches as high as the level of the nipples so that a wound that penetrates the thorax often penetrates into the abdominal cavity as well.

First considerations: Follow the guidelines set forth above in the chapter "Initial Care, Airway, Hemorrhage".

Rapid but thorough physical exam: Note areas of tenderness and whether or not there is rebound. Are there bowel sounds? Is there abdominal distension? Laparotomy is indicated if there are peritoneal signs or if there is evisceration. Perform rectal exam and check for blood. In female, perform vaginal exam if penetration into the pelvis is likely. Do not remove the impaling instrument if it is still in place since removal may result in fatal exsanguination. Removal is almost always deferred until the patient is in the operating room. **Nasogastric tube** is inserted to ascertain presence of blood, and to remove stomach contents and thus reduce risk of aspiration. **Foley catheter** is inserted and any blood return noted.

Consult a surgeon as soon as possible if it is obvious or likely that the abdominal cavity has been penetrated.

X-rays: An upright chest x-ray or a left lateral decubitus film of the abdomen are obtained. The presence of free air under the diaphragm on chest film (or in the region of the right flank on a left lateral decubitus film) confirms that the peritoneal cavity has been entered.

Exploration and possibly extension of the wound under local anesthesia is indicated if there is uncertainty as to whether the peritoneal cavity has been penetrated.

Peritoneal lavage is indicated in stab wounds of the anterior abdomen unless (1) wound exploration demonstrates that the abdominal fascia has been penetrated, or (2) there is already an indication for laparotomy (e.g. persistent hypotension, peritoneal signs, evisceration).

Other tests may be advisable as clinical circumstances suggest provided that the patient is stable and can tolerate the delay. CAT scan, for instance, is preferred over peritoneal lavage if there is a stab wound of the back or flank and wound exploration demonstrates that (1) the abdominal fascia has been penetrated or (2) there is uncertainty on this point. CAT scan is *generally* preferred for investigation of back or flank wounds because negative peritoneal lavage does not exclude trauma to retroperitoneal organs. CAT scan is enhanced by the administration of IV contrast, and if necessary by PO administration of water–soluble contrast (gastrografin). IVP and/or cystogram may be ordered if there is hematuria and is quicker than CAT scan. See *Steps in X-ray Evvaluation of Urinary Tract Trauma* in "Urinary Tract" chapter that follows. Upper GI with water–soluble contrast (gastrografin) may be ordered in selected cases to rule out stomach or duodenal perforation.

   Indications for laparotomy include persistent hypotension, peritoneal signs, abdominal evisceration, positive peritoneal lavage, compelling radiologic findings. Note that an abdominal stab wound does not necessarily mandate exploratory laparotomy even if the peritoneum has been penetrated provided that the vital signs remain stable and none of the foregoing indications for laparotomy are present. However, careful observation with monitoring of vital signs is imperative.

INVESTIGATION/MANAGEMENT of MISSILE WOUNDS to ABDOMEN: First considerations: Follow the guidelines set forth above in the chapter "Initial Care, Airway, Hemorrhage". **Rapid but thorough physical exam:** Note areas of abdominal tenderness and whether or not there is rebound. Are there bowel sounds? Is there abdominal distension? Perform rectal exam to check for blood, sphincter tone, and displaced or boggy prostate. In female, perform vaginal exam unless pelvic trauma is not a consideration. **Nasogastric tube** is inserted to check for blood, to decompress stomach, and to remove stomach contents in order to reduce risk of aspiration. **Foley catheter** is inserted unless there is blood at the urethral meatus or rectal exam reveals a displaced or boggy prostate. An urethrogram is performed if any of these conditions prevail. **Consult a surgeon** as soon as possible to report patients's status and ongoing investigation. **X-rays:** Obtain chest x-ray (upright if tolerated) and flat plate of abdomen. A left lateral decubitus film may be obtained if the patient cannot tolerate an upright chest x-ray. Identify the position of the missile or fragments. Also look for free air under the diaphragm on an upright chest film, or in the region of the right flank on a left lateral decubitus film. **Other radiographic tests** (e.g. CAT scan, IVP, cystogram, arteriogram) may be justified depending on the circumstances. **Peritoneal lavage** may be indicated if peritoneal penetration is uncertain. However, peritoneal lavage may not be necessary with *high–velocity* gunshot wounds since exploratory laparotomy may have to be performed regardless of whether or not the peritoneum has been penetrated (see indications below). Refer to "Peritoneal Lavage" above for interpretation of peritoneal lavage. **Indications for laparotomy:** known or uncertain peritoneal penetration. In the case of high–velocity gunshot wounds to the abdomen, exploratory laparotomy is often recommended even when peritoneal penetration has been excluded. This is because the impact alone often results in intra–abdominal trauma.

SPLEEN: The spleen is the organ most commonly injured by blunt abdominal trauma and it is a common site of penetrating trauma as well. Sometimes, following blunt trauma, there is delayed rupture of the spleen: a subcapsular hematoma develops which may rupture days or even weeks later. **Abdominal exam** is often deceptively unalarming or negative. Be suspicious if there are contusions about left flank and ribs overlying the spleen, or if there is a history of significant trauma to this region. Signs of peritoneal irritation (e.g. left upper quadrant rebound tenderness, guarding) or diaphragmatic irritation (e.g. dyspnea, referred pain left shoulder) may be absent since intraperitoneal blood may not be irritating at first. Signs of shock can develop before significant abdominal signs appear. Shifting dullness or abdominal distension reflect an alarming amount of intraperitoneal blood loss. **Diagnostic tests:** Do not delay treatment in order to perform radiologic tests in a patient who is hypotensive or otherwise unstable. Moreover, further diagnostic testing may not be necessary if the need for laparotomy is obvious (e.g. persistent hypotension, peritoneal signs). Plain x-rays may be helpful but negative x-rays do not exclude splenic rupture. Suspicious radiographic signs include: fractured left lower ribs, elevation of left hemidiaphragm, small left pleural effusion, left basilar atelectasis, enlarged or blurred splenic outline, medial displacement of gastric bubble, depression of splenic flexure or left kidney, blurred left psoas. Peritoneal lavage is almost always positive with splenic trauma. CAT scan is also diagnostic of splenic trauma and may be used instead of peritoneal lavage if the patient is stable and can tolerate the delay.

LIVER TRAUMA: In the setting of blunt abdominal trauma, the liver is the 2nd most commonly injured organ after the spleen. The liver is also very vulnerable to penetrating trauma. Like the spleen, the liver is a very vascular solid organ and is therefore quite susceptible to blunt traumatic rupture with severe hemorrhage. **Abdominal exam:** Look for contusions/tenderness over the right upper quadrant and flank. Are there signs of diaphragmatic irritation (referred pain right shoulder)? Signs of peritoneal irritation may be the consequence of blood or bile escaping into the peritoneal space. **Diagnostic tests:** Do not delay treatment to perform radiologic tests if the patient is unstable, especially if the need for laparotomy is obvious. Plain x-rays are generally not helpful. An enlarged liver with a blurred outline is suspicious as is a depressed hepatic flexure. Look for fractures of ribs overlying the liver. Peritoneal lavage is frequently positive. CAT scan with contrast may be used instead of peritoneal lavage if the patient is stable and can tolerate the delay.

PANCREAS and DUODENUM: Because they are contiguous, blunt or penetrating injury to one of these organs is often associated with injury to the other. In crush injuries for instance, the pancreas and duodenum are injured together as they are compressed against the spine. **Signs/symptoms:** Because these organs are retroperitoneal; peritoneal signs (e.g. rebound tenderness, guarding) are typically absent or delayed. The patient may initially complain of mid or upper back pain. **Diagnostic tests:** Plain x-ray may show blunting of the psoas shadow if there is retroperitoneal bleeding. A flat plate may reveal retroperitoneal air if the duodenum is ruptured. Peritoneal lavage: The pancreas and duodenum are retroperitoneal. Therefore, isolated blunt trauma to these organs is characteristically associated with a negative or a weakly positive peritoneal lavage. CAT scan with contrast may be diagnostic. Water–soluble contrast upper GI (gastrografin) can reveal duodenal rupture. Serum or urine amylase may be elevated.

STOMACH and INTESTINES: These organs are most frequently injured by penetrating trauma. With regards to blunt trauma, the small intestine is more frequently ruptured from blunt trauma than is the large intestine or stomach, but all are uncommon. The stomach is most susceptible to blunt trauma and rupture when it is filled with fluid. Compression of a portion of the intestine against the spine is one mechanism for blunt intestinal trauma. Compression of the intestines against the spine may result in intramural hematoma with ensuing GI obstruction and vomiting. **Abdominal exam:** Findings may include diffuse tenderness, rebound tenderness, guarding, distension, decreased/absent bowel sounds, vomiting. Nasogastric tube or rectal exam may reveal blood. **Diagnostic tests:** Plain x-ray: If the stomach or bowel has been perforated/ruptured, there may be free-air under the diaphragm on an upright chest x-ray (or the right flank on a left lateral decubitus film). Air–fluid levels may indicate obstruction. Peritoneal lavage and/or abdominal CAT scan may be indicated. Water–soluble contrast (gastrografin) swallow can be used to determine the integrity of the stomach. Water–soluble contrast enema is sometimes used to look for colon injury.

Urinary Tract Trauma

STEPS in X–RAY EVALUATION of URINARY TRACT TRAUMA:
In males, an **urethrogram** is necessary prior to inserting a Foley catheter if (**1**) pelvic injury is suspected, (**2**) there is blood at the urethral meatus, or (**3**) rectal exam reveals a displaced or boggy prostate. Inserting a catheter in the presence of a torn urethra may cause further injury. **Cystogram and/or IVP** are used to rapidly evaluate a patient with hematuria. The findings may mandate surgery and thus may make diagnostic peritoneal lavage unnecessary. Cystogram is performed first unless historical and/or clinical circumstances make lower urinary tract trauma improbable. The contrast solution (400 ml in adult, 5 ml/kg in child) is infused into the bladder via a Foley catheter with the contrast-containing bottle elevated about 2 ft above the level of the patient. An AP x-ray is obtained, the bladder is then washed out with saline, and an AP x-ray is again taken. An IVP is then obtained (the upper

urinary tract will usually be seen on an x-ray obtained 5 minutes after intravenous injection of contrast material). **CAT scan with contrast** may further clarify the lesion if the cystogram or IVP is abnormal. CAT scan may be used (instead of cystogram and IVP) to evaluate traumatic hematuria provided that the patient is hemodynamically stable and can tolerate the delay. **Arteriography** may be needed to investigate suspected arterial bleeding.

URETHRAL injuries are uncommon in females. In males, the clinical signs depend in part on whether the urethra is injured above or below the urogenital diaphram (see below). With complete urethral transection, the patient is unable to void and dye fails to enter the bladder on retrograde urethrogram. With partial transection, some dye may enter the bladder and the rest will extravasate. A Foley catheter should not be inserted into a male with known or suspected pelvic trauma until a retrograde urethrogram verifies the integrity of the urethra. **Posterior urethral trauma** refers to urethral trauma above the urogenital diaphragm (i.e. urethral trauma anywhere along prostatic urethra to just distal to the prostate). Posterior urethral trauma is common with pelvic fractures. With complete transection, the prostate (which is normally attached to the bladder above) may be displaced superiorly and may not even be palpable. The traumatized prostate may have a boggy consistency. Since the disruption is above the urogenital diaphragm, blood and urine accumulate within the pelvis and examination of the external genitalia may be unremarkable. A pelvic hematoma is sometimes palpated. **Anterior urethral injuries** (i.e. injury below the urogenital diaphragm) are often the result of direct blows to the perineum (e.g. straddle injury). Blood may be seen dripping from the urethral meatus. Blood and urine may extravasate into the scrotum, penis, and even the anterior abdominal wall. As a consequence, these structures may become swollen.

BLADDER is easily injured by penetrating trauma. However, it is seldom injured by blunt trauma when it is empty, unless there is an associated pelvic fracture. When the bladder is full, it rides higher and is therefore more susceptible to both blunt and penetrating trauma. Intraperitoneal extravasation of urine and blood will result if the area of the bladder covered by peritoneum is perforated. Signs of peritoneal irritation may ensue (e.g. rebound tenderness). With extraperitoneal rupture, blood and urine may accumulate in the pelvis so that a pelvic mass may sometimes be palpated rectally and on suprapubic exam. With either intra- or extraperitoneal rupture, there may be suprapubic tenderness, dysuria, hematuria. **Urethrogram:** In males, an urethrogram is obtained first to exclude urethral trauma. A Foley catheter may then be inserted if the urethrogram is normal. **Retrograde cystogram** is then performed. If rupture is intraperitoneal: extravasated dye may be seen along the paracolic gutters and outlining the surfaces of small and large bowel, and the ileal loops may be displaced superiorly. If rupture is extraperitoneal, dye may be seen in the perivesicular space. Occasionally, a pelvic hematoma compresses the bladder so that extravasation is prevented and the bladder has an elongated radiologic profile.

KIDNEY injury should be suspected whenever there is significant trauma to the lower ribs, flank, or upper abdomen. Concomitant liver and/or spleen trauma is common. Renal trauma nearly always results in hematuria but it may only be microscopic. Moreover, significant renal injury can occur in the absence of hematuria. **Plain x-ray:** Certain signs should alert the clinician to the likelihood of renal trauma: fractured lower ribs, fractured tranverse processes, blurring of the psoas or renal shadows due to retroperitoneal blood, lumbar scoliosis. **IVP** is indicated if renal injury is suspected. If the kidney is only contused, there will be no extravasation of dye but there may be distortion of the renal outline and collecting system, and puddling of dye in the contused area. Lacerations through the capsule, cortex, and collecting system will result in extravasation of dye and distortion of the renal outline. The kidney will not be visualized if the renal artery is avulsed or thrombosed. A retroperitoneal hematoma may displace the ureter medially. **CAT scan** is obtained for further clarification if the IVP is abnormal. **Arteriography** is indicated if the kidney is poorly visualized, if there is retroperitoneal hemorrhage, or if there is unremitting hematuria.

Burns

CATEGORIES and CHARACTERISTICS of BURNS:

First degree burns are restricted to the most superficial layers of the epidermis. The basal layer, which contains the germinal cells, remains intact. The skin is red and painful but there is minimal edema. Pain subsides in 48-72 hours. Healing is complete and without scarring in 5-10 days as the damaged epithelium peels to be replaced by the evolving deeper cells. Sunburn or brief scalding are typical first degree burns.

Second degree burn (partial thickness burn) involves both the epidermis and dermis. The skin is red, edematous, moist, painful, and blisters. Superficial 2nd degree burns heal in 2 to 3 weeks. There is usually little scarring although there may be depigmentation. Deep dermal 2nd degree burns must heal from the epithelium of the hair follicles and sweat glands; healing takes about a month and scarring occurs.

Third degree burn (full thickness burn) destroys all layers of the skin including the epidermis and dermis (corium) and involves the subcutaneous tissue. Third degree burn frequently resembles a 2nd degree burn (e.g. blisters may be present). However, the skin often has a tough leathery appearance that ranges from white to brown or black. Furthermore, the skin does not blanch on contact because blood vessels of the dermis have been destroyed. Pain is absent because dermal nerve receptors are also destroyed. All epithelial regenerative elements are gone. Consequently, skin grafting is mandatory unless the burn is quite small.

Fourth degree burn refers to burns that destroy not only the skin but also the underlying tissue such as muscle, bone, etc.

ESTIMATING EXTENT of BURN (%):

	adult	15 yr	10 yr	5 yr	1 yr	0 yr
head*	7	9	11	13	17	19
neck*	2	2	2	2	2	2
one upper arm*	4	4	4	4	4	4
one forearm*	3	3	3	3	3	3
one hand*	3	3	3	3	3	3
anterior trunk	13	13	13	13	13	13
posterior trunk	13	13	13	13	13	13
genitalia	1	1	1	1	1	1
one buttock	2.5	2.5	2.5	2.5	2.5	2.5
one thigh*	9.5	9	8.5	8	6.5	5.5
one lower leg*	7	6.5	6	5.5	5	5
one foot*	3.5	3.5	3.5	3.5	3.5	3.5

*The percentage shown represents entire circumference of structure.
Note: One method of estimating the extent of a burn is to remember that one side of the patient's hand equals about 1% of body surface. In an adult, the "rule of nines" is applicable; entire head 9%, an entire upper extremity 9%, an entire lower extremity 18%, anterior trunk 18%, posterior trunk 18%.

CRITERIA for HOSPITALIZATION:

●2nd plus 3rd degree burns involving ≥ 15-20% of body area in an adult or involving ≥ 10% of body area in a child.
●3rd degree burn involving 2 to 5% or more of body area.
●2nd or 3rd degree burns of face, perineum, hands, feet, or large joints.
●high-voltage electrical burn.
●inhalation injury.
●other significant concomitant trauma.
Note: Criteria should be even more liberal if patient is under 2 years, over 60 years, or is otherwise compromised (e.g. diabetes mellitus, immunosupressed, renal or cardiovascular condition).

SUPPORTIVE MEASURES:

Intravenous fluid is required if the burn exceeds 20% body surface. Ringer's lactate is administered. In an adult, administer 2 to 4 ml/kg/% burn over first 24 hours. In a child, administer 3 to 4 ml/kg/% burn over first 24 hours. For instance, a 70 kg patient with 40% burn would require 5,600 to 11,200 ml (2–4 ml X 70 kg X 40%) over the first 24 hours. Administer half the calculated amount over the first 8 hr and the remaining half over the following 16 hours. Remember to give the usual daily maintenance requirement in addition to that calculated by the above formula. This is especially important in children, for otherwise the patient may be receiving little more than the usual maintenance requirement. The above formula is only an approximate guide to fluid requirements; the urine output is used to gauge the adequacy of fluid administration. A Foley catheter is inserted and the IV rate is adjusted to maintain urine output at 30–50 ml/hr in adult and 1 ml/kg/hr in child < 30 kg.

Analgesia: For severe burns, narcotics are administered intravenously (e.g. morphine, meperidine) in small increments titrated to effect. Even 1st degree burns may be extremely painful; parenteral or PO narcotics may be justified. Third degree burns are painless.

Nasogastric suction is indicated if there is abdominal distension, if the patient is vomiting, or if the combined 2nd and 3rd degree burn exceeds 25% body surface.

Tetanus toxoid and tetanus immune globulin is indicated for 2nd thru 4th degree burns. Both tetanus toxoid and tetanus immune globulin may be required. See "Tetanus" chapter for recommendations.

ELECTRICAL BURNS are often deceptive in that the extent of injury is not always immediately obvious. In its path the current may cause significant damage to muscle, nerve, blood vessels, etc; and yet leave a relatively unimpressive skin lesion. Perform urinalysis. The presence of dark urine (due to myoglobinuria and/or hemoglobinuria) is evidence of deep injury. If this is the case, sufficient fluid must be administered to maintain a high urine output and thus preclude development of obstructive uropathy and acute tubular necrosis. The goal is to maintain, the urine output at 100 ml/hr in adult (1.5–2.0 ml/kg/hr in child) until the urine clears. Addition of mannitol is indicated if increased fluids alone do not induce adequate diuresis. Cardiac monitoring is advisable.

CHEMICAL BURNS: Immediately flush copiously with water and continue for at least 15 minutes. Alkali burns are especially dangerous and generally require longer irrigation than acid burns. See "Chemical Eye Injury" chapter for treatment of that condition.

TREATMENT MINOR BURN: (1) Immersion in cool water (not ice water) will provide pain relief and may limit injury. Immersion of the burn is begun immediately after the burn and continued for up to 30 minutes. **(2)** Gently cleanse with mild soap and water. Remove broken blisters but leave intact blisters. Carefully shave hair about margins of wound. **(3)** An antibiotic ointment or cream (e.g. Silvadene) is not needed but is often applied to 2nd degree burns. **(4)** Apply a nonadherent fine mesh gauze directly to the burn; place a layer of gauze on top of this to act as an absorbent of wound exudate; and finally wrap gently with a bulky immobilizing cotton bandage. A splint may be needed to immobilize and prevent contracture of a joint. **(5)** Remove dressing down to fine mesh gauze to inspect for infection on 2nd or 3rd day and then weekly thereafter (remove dressing daily if Silvadene is applied). **(6)** Provide tetanus prophylaxis and analgesics as needed. Even 1st degree burns may be extremely painful; parenteral or PO narcotics are justified.

Smoke Inhalation and Thermal Respiratory Injury

Dry heat seldom causes damage below the vocal cords because the upper airway exerts a cooling effect and because the vocal cords close reflexively upon heat-exposure. However, the upper airway is susceptible to thermal injury, and so edema with airway obstruction may ensue. Therefore, early intubation may be indicated before edema develops and makes this procedure impossible. **Smoke inhalation** may injure the mucosa of both the upper and lower airway. Both mucosal and interstitial edema may result. The edema fluid mixed with the mucopurulent material that sloughs from the injured mucosa may together block the bronchioles. Bronchopneumonia often develops.

Signs/symptoms arousing suspicion that significant respiratory tract injury may have occurred include: facial burn, singed nasal hair, burned or edematous oral/pharyngeal mucosa, cough, hoarseness, dyspnea, dysphagia. The presence of carbonaceous material on the oral/pharyngeal mucosa or in the sputum is a common finding in patients with smoke inhalation,

Tests: Obtain chest x-ray and arterial blood gas. Carboxyhemoglobin is measured if smoke inhalation is suspected. Carboxyhemoglobin levels below 5% in non-smoker or below 10% in smoker are generally not clinically significant. Chest x-ray or arterial blood gas evidence of smoke inhalation injury may take 12–24 hours or more to develop.

Treatment: Maintain airway: Intubate if there is severe respiratory compromise. In other patients, anticipate that respiratory function may deteriorate and that intubation may become necessary. Encourage coughing. Suction the intubated patient as necessary. Oxygen is administered as needed. Administer humidified 100% oxygen (via nonrebreather mask if patient is not intubated) if the carboxyhemoglobin is over 20% and continue until the level falls below 20%. See chapter entitled "Poisoning" for further information on carbon monoxide poisoning. Bronchoscopy may help establish the presence/extent of respiratory tract injury and may be needed to remove accumulated debris. Bronchodilator (e.g. IV aminophylline, beta–adrenergic inhalant) is administered if there is significant bronchospasm.

Miscellany

Miscellany

Poisoning

GUIDE to MANAGEMENT of TOXIC INGESTION: In general, gastric emptying is indicated if the toxic ingestion has occurred within the last 6 hours, or even after 6 hours if bowel sounds are absent.

Induction of emesis: Emetics; Gastric emptying in an alert patient can usually be accomplished with syrup of ipecac. Anionic or nonionic dishwashing detergents taken with water are an alternative if syrup of ipecac is not available. Induction of vomiting is contraindicated if the patient: (**1**) is comatose or stuporous, (**2**) is seizing, (**3**) is in shock, (**4**) has ingested a strong acid or strong alkali, (**5**) has ingested petroleum distillate [see "specific poisonings" below], (**6**) is < 9 months old.

Gastric lavage: Indications: (**1**) patient is comatose or stuporous, (**2**) syrup of ipecac fails to induce vomiting, (**3**) patient < 9 months old. Furthermore, gastric lavage is preferred to inducing emesis if the patient has ingested a highly toxic substance (e.g. tricyclic antidepressant) that urgently requires administration of activated charcoal immediately after gastric emptying. Intubate the comatose or stuporous patient before lavaging in order to prevent aspiration. Use an uncuffed endotracheal tube if the patient is < 6 years of age. Lavage instructions: Insert orally the largest tube possible (e.g. in adult an Ewald tube or 36–40 French) and suction before starting lavage. Save the aspirate in case toxicologic analysis becomes necessary. In the conscious patient not requiring intubation, the risk of aspiration may be minimized by placing the patient on his left side with the body inclined so that the legs are elevated. Tap water may be used for lavage (isotonic or half–normal saline is preferred in infants). In the adult, 250–300 ml boluses (10 ml/kg boluses in infant) are instilled, left in for a minute, and then drained by gravity. Lavage until there is a clear return, and then with an additional amount (3 liters in adult and proportionally less in child).

Activated charcoal (see drug section) is administered (**1**) via the lavage tube after gastric lavage, or (**2**) PO when the patient is no longer vomiting. Activated charcoal may also be administered 20–30 minutes prior to lavage and then again after lavage. Additional doses may be given at 2–4 hour intervals. The dose in an adult is 50–100 gram in 8 oz of water; in a child 30–50 gram in 4 oz water. Activated charcoal does not adsorb mineral acids, alkalis, lithium. Charcoal adsorbs ferrous sulfate and cyanide poorly.

Cathartics are commonly administered but are of unproven value. The following cathartics are suggested: magnesium citrate (150–300 ml in adult and 10 ml/kg in child), magnesium sulfate (15–20 gram of 10% solution in adult, 250 mg/kg of 10% solution in child), or sorbitol (100 ml of 70% solution in adult). Oil cathartics (e.g. castor oil, mineral oil) must not be used.

Alkalinizing the urine by administering intravenous sodium bicarbonate may hasten urinary excretion of phenobarbital, primidone, salicylates, lithium.

Acid diuresis may speed urinary excretion of amphetamines, PCP, strychnine. Acid diuresis may be most safely accomplished with ascorbic acid (vitamin C). When oral administration is feasible, administer 2 gram PO every 4 hours. When the intravenous route must be used, the initial adult dose is 4 gram ascorbic acid to 1 liter of normal saline infused over 1 hour. Repeat doses are administered as needed to maintain an acid urine. Ammonium chloride is an alternative agent if ascorbic acid fails to promote acid diuresis.

Dialysis is indicated for methanol or ethylene glycol poisoning. Dialysis may be indicated in other severe poisonings if the poison is excreted by the kidney. Dialysis is not effective for the following ingestions: tricyclic antidepressants, antihistamines, benzodiazepines, digitalis, glutethimide, ethchlorvynol, methaqualone.

SPECIFIC POISONINGS:

SPECIFIC DRUGS: Recommendations for certain drugs may be found in the drug section—e.g. acetaminophen, aspirin, iron, narcotics, phenothiazines, tricyclic antidepressant, etc.

PETROLEUM DISTILLATES: The principal danger with petroleum distillate ingestion is aspiration with ensuing pneumonitis. The risk of aspiration is greatest when the substance is of low viscosity. The very low viscosity petroleum distillates (e.g. mineral seal oil in furniture polishes) are particularly dangerous in this regard. The more viscous oils (e.g. tar, fuel oil, diesel oil, motor oil, mineral oil, baby oil, suntan oil) are seldom aspirated. **Treatment:** High–viscosity petroleum distillates: Gastric emptying is *not* recommended for the more viscous oils *unless* it contains a toxic additive such as benzene; halogenated hydrocarbon (e.g. trichloroethylene, carbon tetrachloride); pesticide. Low–viscosity petroleum distillates include mineral seal oil; gasoline; kerosene; turpentine; naphtha; benzin; aromatics (e.g. benzene, toluene, xylene); halogenated hydrocarbon; mineral spirits. Gastric emptying is advised if > 2 ml/kg of a low viscosity distillate has been ingested. Patients who are comatose, stuporous, or in respiratory distress should be intubated in order to prevent aspiration and then lavaged.

CAUSTIC INGESTION (strong acid or alkali): Emesis or lavage is contraindicated. Nasogastric or orogastric tube must *not* be inserted. Diluents: A diluent (milk or water) may be administered if the patient has ingested a *solid* lye but otherwise the patient should be kept NPO. Diluents are contraindicated in liquid lye ingestions. A diluent may be used immediately after an acid ingestion but is probably of no use by the time medical assistance is available. In any case, nothing should be given by mouth if there is respiratory distress, shock, or evidence of esophageal or gastric perforation. Patients in respiratory distress should be intubated if this can be performed without causing further injury. If not, cricothyrotomy or tracheostomy will be necessary. Tests: Obtain chest x-ray. Obtain CBC and type & cross. Tetanus prophylaxis according to immunization status (see "Tetanus" chapter for recommendations). Perform endoscopy to identify esophageal burns. Parenteral analgesics are administered as needed. Corticosteroids are advocated for esophageal burns.

METHANOL is metabolized to the toxic metabolite formic acid by the enzyme alcohol dehydrogenase. Ethanol competes for this enzyme and thereby slows the metabolism of methanol. **Treatment:** Empty stomach and administer charcoal. Ethanol is administered intravenously: 600 mg/kg loading followed by 0.66 mg/kg/hr or sufficient to maintain the blood ethanol level at 100 mg/dl. Sodium bicarbonate is administered IV if there is acidosis. Hemodialysis is indicated for severe poisoning (methanol level > 50 mg/dl, ingestion of > 30 ml, visual or CNS manifestations, unremitting acidosis). If hemodialysis is used, the ethanol infusion will have to be increased to maintain the blood alcohol at 100 mg/dl.

ETHYLENE GLYCOL, like methanol, is metabolized by alcohol dehydrogenase to toxic metabolites. Treatment consists of gastric lavage, activated charcoal, IV ethanol infusion as for methanol, hemodialysis, and IV sodium bicarbonate for acidosis.

ORGANOPHOSPHATES bind to the enzyme cholinesterase and thus inhibit the metabolism of acetylcholine. Consequently, excessive acetylcholine accumulates in the synapses of the autonomic and central nervous system, and is responsible for the toxic effects of organophophosphates. **Signs/symptoms:** Excessive stimulation by acetylcholine at muscarinic receptors leads to heightened parasympathetic effects (e.g. excessive salivation, rhinorrhea, excessive bronchial secretions with difficulty breathing and frothing at mouth, nausea, vomiting, diarrhea, abdominal cramping, urinary/fecal incontinence, blurred vision). Excessive stimulation by acetylcholine at nicotinic receptors of the sympathetic ganglia may cause muscle fasciculations, muscle weakness, paralysis, tachycardia, hypertension. Excessive stimulation by acetylcholine at CNS receptors may manifest as confusion, convulsions, ataxia, dysarthria, coma. **Treatment:** If poisoning occurs by PO route, the stomach is emptied, activated charcoal is administered, and this is followed by a cathartic (e.g. magnesium citrate). If poisoning is transdermal, the clothing is removed and the patient is washed thoroughly with soap and water. IV atropine (see drug section for dosing) is administered until anticholinergic effects are noted (dilated pupils, dry mouth, dry skin). Pralidoxime is administered to reverse the nicotinic effects (e.g. muscle weakness, fasciculations, cramping) and to restore function of the cholinesterase enzyme.

CYANIDE is poisonous because it inhibits the cell's cytochrome oxidase system. Clinical findings may include headache, tachycardia, hypotension, convulsions, coma. The patient must be treated immediately. Administer 100% oxygen. If the poisoning is via PO route, perform gastric lavage until cyanide odor is gone. If clothing is contaminated, remove clothing and wash skin. Cyanide poison kits are available: administer amyl nitrite by inhalation (capsule a minute) followed by intravenous sodium nitrite; and then intravenous sodium thiosulfate.

COCAINE ("coke", "crack", "rock", "snow", "flake","girl", "lady", "she", "her", "nose candy", etc) is a sympathomimetic which, while not physically addicting, may cause severe psychologic addiction. **Routes of administration and preparations:** When ocaine is snuffed, stimulation begins to be felt in minutes and the blood level peaks in about 1 hour. ●Free base ("crack", "rock") is alkaloidal cocaine. It is a purified preparation (derived from cocaine hydrochloride) with more intense effects. It is usually smoked in a cigarette or in a "free base" pipe. ●Cocaine may be injected intravenously for a more intense experience that is maximal in about 5 minutes. ●Cocaine may be orally ingested. However, gastric hydrolysis decreases the amount absorbed. **Signs/symptoms:** CNS stimulation may manifest as increased alertness, euphoria, talkativeness, irritability, anxiety, hallucinations, paranoia. Fatigue is relieved and appetite is suppressed. The pupils are dilated. There is tachycardia, tachypnea, increased blood pressure. An itching or crawling senssation of skin ("cocaine bugs") may occur and provoke excoriation. The chronic user is usually depressed and tired following discontinuation of the drug and this serves as an impetus for continued use. **Complications:** hyperthermia, seizures, cardiac arrhythmias, myocardial infarction, aortic dissection, spontaneous pneumothorax. A psychosis resembling schizophrenia may develop in addicted individuals but it is reversible upon discontinuing use of the drug. **Treatment:** Valium is usually used to treat the anxious excited patient and is the drug of choice for cocaine–induced seizures. Valium will also help relieve tachycardia and hypertension. Intravenous propranolol is usually reserved for life–threatening arrhythmias.

PHENCYCLIDINE (PCP, "angel dust", "crystal", "hog", "Sherman", "PeaCe Pill", "gorilla biscuits", etc) is usually smoked or snuffed. It may also be orally ingested. When smoked, the effects begin to be felt in 2–5 minutes and peak in 15–30 min. The patient remains intoxicated for 4–6 hours. **Signs/symptoms** may include confusion, anxiety, agitation, depersonalization, illusions, delusions, paranoia, megalomania, blank stare, drooling, ataxia, muscle rigidity, increased deep tendon reflexes, grimacing, writhing, bizarre posturing, coma. <u>Activity level</u> of conscious patient is variable (e.g. withdrawn with a blank stare, agitated and violent). <u>Pupils</u> are mid–range or constricted and react to light; they may be fixed and dilated if the patient is comatose. There may be nystagmus (horizontal, vertical, or rotary). <u>Pulse, blood pressure, and/or temperature</u> may be elevated. <u>Loss of pain sensation</u> makes the patient vulnerable to injury and may allow the patient to perform acts of great strength (e.g. break handcuffs). <u>Rhabdomyolysis</u> may result from intense muscular exertion. **Treatment:** <u>Observation in a quiet environment and if necessary sedation with diazepam</u> will suffice in many patients. <u>Ascorbic acid</u> will acidify the urine and thereby hasten urinary excretion of PCP (PCP is ionized in acid urine so that renal tubular reabsorption is reduced). Ascorbic acid may be administered IV (e.g. initially 4 gram in 1 liter of normal saline administered over 1 hr) or PO (1–4 grams). Additional doses may be needed at 4–6 hour intervals to maintain urine pH < 5.5. <u>Forced diuresis</u> with furosemide (in conjunction with urinary acidification) will further hasten urinary excretion. <u>If the patient is comatose</u>, continuous nasogastric suction is indicated because the PCP that is absorbed is in part secreted into the stomach. Repeat doses of activated charcoal every 2–4 hours is also an effective means of preventing PCP reabsorption. <u>Seizures</u> are treated with IV diazepam. <u>Rhabdomyolysis</u> with myoglobinuria is treated with IV fluids, mannitol, sodium bicarbonate. Avoid urinary acidification if there is rhabdomyolysis.

LSD (lysergic acid diethylamide) is a nonaddicting psychedelic drug that is usually taken PO. Effects are noted within 30 minutes of ingestion; the psychic effects peak in 1–3 hours and last 6–12 hours. **Signs/symptoms** may include visual illusions, distortions of colors or sounds, time distortion, depersonalization. Mood runs the gamut from euphoria to depression to panic. Sympathomimetic effects may include mydriasis; elevation of pulse and blood pressure, hyperthermia (rare), piloerection, trembling. There may be lacrimation, salivation, anorexia, vomiting, ataxia. Flashbacks (recurrent psychic effects after discontinuing LSD) may occur for up to 18 months. **Treatment** of the panicky patient consists of providing a quiet supportive environment and if necessary sedation with a benzodiazepine (e.g. diazepam).

CARBON MONOXIDE is toxic by virtue of the fact that its affinity for hemoglobin is about 250 times that of oxygen. Thus, there is diminished delivery of oxygen to the tissues. Smokers may have 5–20% carboxyhemoglobin (COHb). **Signs/symptoms:** At 10% COHb the patient may complain of headache. At 20–40% COHb there may be a throbbing headache, decreased visual acuity, exertional dyspnea, nausea, vomiting, dim vision, dizziness, confusion, ataxia. When COHb exceeds 40%, tachycardia and tachypnea are characteristic. When the COHb is > 50–60%, there may be seizures, coma, respiratory failure, and/or cardiovascular collapse. A variety of EKG abnormalities are possible (e.g. PVC's, atrial or ventricular tachycardia, atrial or ventricular fibrillation, heart block). **Blood gases:** If ventilation is not impaired, the arterial blood gas typically reveals a decreased pH with a normal or decreased pO_2 and a normal or decreased pCO_2. The oxygen saturation is typically decreased but, because it is often derived from a nomogram and not measured directly, the value reported is often higher than the actual value. **Treatment:** On room air, the half-life of carbon monoxide is about 6 hours. The half-life is about 1.5 hours if 100% oxygen is administered via a tight-fitting mask. Hyperbaric oxygen at 2.5 times sea-level atmospheric pressure reduces the half-life to < 30 minutes. **Complications** may include myocardial infarction; pulmonary edema; rhabdomyolysis, myoglobinuria–induced renal failure; DIC. There may be visual disturbances (e.g. scotoma, retrobulbar neuritis, cortical blindness). A variety of neuropsychiatric disturbances may ensue—e.g. impaired hearing; seizures; ataxia; parkinsonism; peripheral neuropathy; impaired mentation, memory, or concentration; personality/behavior disorders.

Snakebite

In the U.S., venomous snake bite is due to pit vipers (Crotalidae) or coral snakes.

PIT VIPERS (Crotalidae) includes the copperhead; cottonmouth (water mocassin); rattlesnakes (e.g. timber, sidewinder, E. and W. diamondback); genus Sistrusus (pygmy, massasauga). Pit vipers can be recognized by the presence of a pit between the nostril and the eye, the presence of vertical pupils, and usually by the triangular shape of the head. Envonomation fails to occur in about a fourth of pit viper bites. Thus, the presence of fang wounds does not necessarily mean that poison has been injected.
  Signs/symptoms pit viper envenomation: Local and regional effects: One or two fang wounds may be present. Local pain is characteristic although pain is sometimes minimal or absent. Local edema and swelling usually develop within 10 minutes. With mild envenomation, swelling remains confined to the area about the bite and systemic effects are absent. Swelling spreads in more severe envenomation, so that without treatment an entire limb may be involved in several hours. Regional lymph nodes may become enlarged and tender. Except in mild envenomation, ecchymoses characteristically develop in the region of the bite in a few hours. The skin becomes tense and blisters, and the blisters often fill with blood. Later, the skin about the bite may necrose. Systemic effects may include nausea, vomiting, sweating, hypothermia, tachypnea, tachycardia, hypotension, shock. Neurologic manifestations may include muscle weakness, muscle fasciculations, dysphagia, paresthesias, paralysis, seizures. There may be bleeding—e.g. bleeding gums, hematuria, GI bleeding, ecchymoses, increased vaginal bleeding (if bite occurs during menses). DIC may develop. Pulmonary edema or renal failure may occur in severe cases.
  Laboratory: Obtain CBC, platelet count, PT, PTT, bleeding time, urinalysis, serum electrolytes, BUN, creatinine, blood type and cross–match. An arterial blood gas and an EKG are also ordered in severe cases. Laboratory findings may include prolonged PT and PTT, thrombocytopenia, elevated fibrinogen, decreased fibrin degradation products, decreased hematocrit and hemoglobin.
  Treatment of pit viper envenomation: Keep patient at rest. Patient should be lying down with extremity immobilized and in dependent position if possible A broad constricting band should be placed proximal and near the bite, sufficiently tight to

prevent superficial venous flow while not interrupting arterial or deep venous flow. Tighter constriction may be necessary in cases of *severe* envenomation when there is to be a delay before antivenom can be administered. Incision and suction should be performed only if the bite has occurred within the last 15 minutes. An incision no longer than 1 cm or deeper than 0.3 cm is made directly over each fang puncture. There is no danger from the venom itself to a person applying mouth suction since inadvertently swallowed venom is innocuous. However, bacterial contamination of the wound by oral flora may result. Antivenom is administered except in cases of mild envenomation without systemic manifestations. To be most effective, antivenom should be administered within 4 hours of the bite; antivenom is of questionable benefit if more than 12 hours have elapsed since the bite. The dose varies according to the severity of envenomation. For moderate envenomation 5–10 vials of Crotalidae antivenom are administered while 10–15 vials are given in severe envenomation. Contents of the vials are diluted in isotonic saline (e.g. 500 ml in adult) and administered intravenously. Swelling and other manifestations should not progress if an adequate dose has been given. Additional antivenom is given if there is evidence of further deterioration. Since the antivenom is derived from horses that have been immunized with snake venom, the patient must be tested for horse serum sensitivity: dilute horse serum 1:10 and inject 0.2 ml intradermally (use 0.2 ml at 1:100 dilution if there is a likely history of horse serum sensitivity). A positive reaction consists of erythema, wheal, and itching within half an hour. Antivenom may still have to be administered despite evidence of horse serum sensitivity if there has been severe envenomation. In this case, diphenhydramine (Benadryl) 50 mg IV is administered prior to slow infusion of the antivenom and the clinician must be prepared to treat anaphylaxis. Tetanus prophylaxis: Tetanus immune globulin and/or tetanus toxoid are administered according to immunization status (refer to "Tetanus" chapter for recommendations). Broad spectrum antibiotic is advised—e.g. cephalosporin. Fasciotomy is necessary if swelling leads to compartment syndrome. Blood transfusion is indicated for severe bleeding. Other supportive measures are instituted as needed.

CORAL SNAKE ENVENOMATION: Coral snakes are small with red, yellow, and black bands such that the interposed yellow bands are narrower than the red and black bands. Coral snake venom acts by blocking acetylcholine receptor sites.
   Signs/symptoms: Local effects: Pain is mild and often transient, or is absent in some cases. Swelling in the region of the bite is either slight or absent. Paresthesias may develop about the bite site. Systemic efects may include nausea, vomiting, salivation, weakness, incoordination, dysphagia, dysphonia, ptosis, dilated pupils, diplopia, sleepiness, confusion, euphoria, respiratory failure, shock.
   Treatment: Tourniquet and incision with suction are of no benefit. Antivenom is available for treatment of eastern coral snake bite. If symptoms develop, 3–5 vials of antivenom are diluted in isotonic saline and administered intravenously. Since the antivenom consists of horse serum, the patient must be tested for horse serum sensitivity prior to administration (see above). ●Unfortunately there is no antivenom available for treatment of western coral snake bite but fortunately it is quite rare.

Spider Bite

Nearly all species of spiders produce venom. However, not many species have bites that can penetrate the skin to introduce the venom. There are only two spiders of medical significance in the U.S.: black widow and the brown recluse.
   BLACK WIDOW (Lactrodectus mactans) is identified by the presence of a red hourglass design on the underside of her abdomen. The body is shiny black and about 1 cm in diameter. The male is smaller and is innocuous. **Signs/symptoms:** Local effects: A sharp burning sensation may be felt or the bite may go unnoticed. The bite site may be reddened and slightly swollen. Systemic effects begin 2–12 hours following the bite. There is muscle pain and spasm with rigidity. These muscular phenomena characteristically involve the abdomen if the bite was on the legs or genitalia. Bites on the arm are often associated with pain and spasm of the chest. Other manifestations may include headache, dizziness, nausea, vomiting, sweating, salivation, respiratory distress, paresthesias, hyperreflexia, impaired speech, abnormal vision. **Treatment:** Muscle pain/spasm may be alleviated with in-

travenous calcium gluconate (10 ml of 10% solution in adult) and repeated at 4 hour intervals as needed. Diazepam may also be helpful. Antivenom is available but seldom necessary. Testing for horse serum sensitivity is required before using this product (see "Snakebite").

BROWN RECLUSE (Loxosceles reclusa) is identified by the presence of a violin design on the back of the thorax. It is small (about 0.1 cm long) and may be brown, tan, or gray-colored. **Signs/symptoms:** Local effects: There may be slight immediate pain or the bite may go unnoticed. A few hours later, the bite site becomes reddened. The central area then blanches and later develops into a small bleb surrounded by an ischemic ring which is in turn surrounded by an erythematous ring—all of which resembles a bullseye. Over the next 1–2 days, the central area develops into a necrotic ulcer and a crust forms. The necrotic lesion may enlarge for a few days or weeks and may even extend into the muscle. Systemic effects may appear within the first 2 days and may include fever, chills, nausea, vomiting, muscle and joint pain, measles–like rash, thrombocytopenia, petechiae, intravascular hemolysis. Hemolysis may lead to hemoglobinuria with renal failure. **Treatment:** The lesion may not heal for several weeks. Debridement and perhaps grafting may be necessary.

Hypothermia (core temperature < 35° C [95° F]).

Causes/contributing factors include: cold–exposure; myxedema; Addison's disease; hypopituitarism; hypothalamic or other CNS disorder (e.g. stroke, head trauma); hypoglycemia; sepsis; uremia; drugs (ethanol, phenothiazines, barbiturates); paralysis/immobilization; liver failure, Wernicke's disease (i.e. thiamine deficiency), burns, erythrodermas.

Signs/symptoms: Note: Be aware that standard thermometers do not measure temperatures < 34.4° C (94° F). Shivering is usually present until the core temperature falls to < 33.3° C (92° F). Patients receiving phenothiazines may not shiver. With core temperatures 32°–35° C (90°–95° F), dysarthria and ataxia occur. With core temperature < 32° C, the following are characteristic: stupor or coma, muscle rigidity, shallow irregular breathing, decreased heart rate, decreased blood pressure. With core temperatures < 28° C; findings may include coma, fixed and dilated pupils, stiffness, apnea, ventricular fibrillation, undetectable pulse or blood pressure. Profoundly hypothermic patients may have undetectable vital signs and yet may recover upon rewarming; thus the addage: "the patient is not dead until warm and dead". **Complications:** thromboembolic consequences, disseminated intravascular coagulation, rhabdomyolysis with risk of ensuing acute tubular necrosis.

Laboratory: EKG abnormalities develop with core temperatures < 30° C: e.g. supraventricular arrhythmias; PVC's, T wave inversion, widened PR, widened QRS, widened QT, Osborn wave (J point elevation). Hemoconcentration (e.g. elevated hematocrit) may occur as a consequence of (1) hypothermia–induced diuresis with hypovolemia and/or (2) fluid shifts from the intra– to extra–vascular space. Acid–base abnormalities; Initially, the patient hyperventilates, and so there is respiratory alkalosis and increased potassium excretion. Respiratory acidosis supervenes when the core temperature falls below 32° C and the patient hypoventilates. Hypoventilation also leads to metabolic acidosis as a consequence of lactic acid accumulation (hypoventilation forces the body to rely increasingly on anaerobic metabolism). In less profound hypothermia, violent shivering (like vigorous exercise in general) may possibly lead to increased anaerobic metabolism with lactic acidemia.

Treatment: Monitor vital signs, EKG, urine output. Treat specific underlying conditions if possible (e.g. hypothyroidism, hypoglycemia). Patients with rectal temperature > 32° C (90° F) and normal cardiovascular status usually respond to passive rewarming (e.g. warm room, blankets). Active rewarming (e.g. warming blankets, warm fluids orally, heated humidified air) may also be used. Warming should proceed slowly so that the core temperature increases by about 1° C/hour. Rectal temperature 29.7°–32° C (85–90° F) and normal cardiovascular status: warming blankets, breathing heated humidified air, warm IV fluids. Warming should proceed slowly so that the core temperature increases by about 1° C/hour. Rectal temperature < 29.7° C (85° F) or unstable cardiovascular status: warm peritoneal lavage (lavage fluid at about 40° C) in addition to active rewarming measures stated above.

Partial cardiopulmonary bypass in conjunction with a heat exchanger is an alternative to warm peritoneal lavage. The patient is warmed rapidly to 30° C. Further rewarming should then proceed slowly at about 1° C/hour. ●Severely hypothermic patients are particularly susceptible to ventricular fibrillation and asystole. Seemingly trivial stimuli may be the precipitants. Handle gently. Avoid all but essential procedures and move patient as little as possible. Ventricular fibrillation and asystole are often refractory to countershock and antiarrhythmic agents until the patient is partially rewarmed.

Heat Stroke is the syndrome that results from high body temperature.

This may occur when the body is: (**1**) subjected to excessive heat (environmental or generated metabolically) and/or (**2**) unable to dissipate heat adequately.

Risk factors: Hot (especially hot humid) weather is the most common precipitant—particularly in elderly, debilitated, or obese individuals; or in those compromised by cardiac or pulmonary disease. Other conditions that increase the risk include: thyroid storm; delirium tremens; CNS disorders (head trauma, inflammation); impaired function of sweat glands (e.g. cystic fibrosis, scleroderma). Strenuous exercise is a common precipitant in otherwise healthy persons. Certain drugs may make one more vulnerable to heat stroke: (**1**) drugs that impair sweating—e.g. beta blockers; diuretics; drugs with anticholinergic properties (e.g. atropine, scopolamine, antihistamines, phenothiazines, tricyclic antidepressants); (**2**) drugs that increase heat generation—e.g. amphetamines, salicylate overdose, LSD, inhalation anesthetics, monoamine oxidase inhibitors.

Signs/symptoms: Rectal temperature is > 39.1° C (102.4° F) and may surpass 43.3° C (110° F). Hot dry skin is the classic finding; although many patients with strenuous exercise–provoked heat stroke may continue to perspire. CNS effects may be evident (e.g. headache, dizziness, confusion, irritability, hallucinations, lethargy, coma). Hypotension is common and shock may ensue.

Complications: brain damage, acute renal failure, adult respiratory distress syndrome, pancreatitis, liver damage with jaundice, cardiac injury and arrhythmias. ●Hemorrhage may result from DIC, fibrinolysis, thrombocytopenia (due to bone marrow injury), clotting factor deficiency (due to liver injury). ●Strenuous exercise–provoked heat stroke is often associated with rhabdomyolysis. As a consequence, there is myoglobinuria, markedly elevated CPK, hyperkalemia, hyperphosphatemia, hypocalcemia, hyperuricemia, hypoalbuminemia, and usually lactic acidosis. Myoglobinuria may cause acute tubular necrosis with renal failure.

Treatment: Rapidly cool the patient down to 39° C (102.2° F). Rectal temperature is monitored. Remove clothing and sponge entire body with ice water while fanning the patient to increase evaporative heat loss. Ice packs may be placed in the axillae and groin. A cooling blanket is an option. Immersion in water at about 11° C (51.8° F) with skin massage will also achieve rapid cooling. In order to not overshoot and cause hypothermia, aggressive cooling is curtailed at 39° C in favor of less intensive therapy. Ice water immersion is *not* recommended because it causes shivering (which generates heat), cutaneous vasoconstriction (which impairs heat loss), and/or seizures. Parenteral diazepam or chlorpromazine may be administered if shivering is a problem. Hypotension may be present and usually resolves with cooling. If not, an IV fluid challenge of normal saline may be required. Vasopressors are used as a last resort.

Heat Exhaustion is the condition that results from heat exposure

in an individual who fails to ingest sufficient water and/or salt.

Signs/symptoms are variable and depend in part on whether or not the patient has ingested some fluid and/or salt. Temperature ranges from normal to 38.9° C (102° F). Skin is cool and clammy. Perspiration may be profuse. With dehydration and hyperosmolality comes thirst and there may be decreased skin turgor, hypotension, tachycardia, weakness, confusion, irritability, incoordination, paresthesias, delirium. If salt depletion is proportionally greater than water depletion; there may be lightheadedness, headache, weakness, lethargy, muscle cramps, nausea, vomiting, confusion, convulsions. Heat stroke may ensue.

Laboratory evidence of dehydration includes hemoconcentration (elevated sodium, osmolality, BUN, hematocrit, etc) and concentrated urine (elevated specific gravity and osmolality).

Treatment: Mild to moderate heat exhaustion can usually be managed with PO fluids and salt supplementation. In severe cases, administer IV fluids. The fluid selected depends on the serum electrolyte findings and hemodynamic status. Normal saline is usually administered if there is hypotension or hyponatremia. If there is hypernatremia; administer D5W and (in order to avoid cerebral edema) adjust the infusion rate so that the serum sodium concentration falls no faster than 2 mEq/hr.

Heat Cramps is the condition that results from strenuous exercise in

hot environments in individuals who drink sufficient water but who fail to ingest sufficient salt to compensate for losses in sweat.

Signs/symptoms: There is an abrupt onset of severe palpable muscle cramps—most often in the muscles being exercised and often following cessation of exercise. Cramps of the abdominal muscles may be mistaken for a perforated viscus.

Laboratory: There is hyponatremia. In severe cases, there may be muscle injury with serum CPK elevation.

Treatment consists of intravenous normal saliine or oral salt–containing solutions.

Bacterial & Viral Diseases

Note: Bacterial or viral disease primarily involving a specific organ system may be presented elsewhere in appropriate sections.

Gonorrhea
Syphilis
Chlamydia Trachomatis
Chancroid
Granuloma Inguinale
Condyloma Acuminata
AIDS
Herpes Simplex Virus
Infectious Mononucleosis
Septic Shock
Toxic Shock Syndrome
Meningococcal Disease
Rickettsial Infections
Lyme Disease
Typhoid Fever
Brucellosis
Leptospirosis
Plague
Tularemia
Nocardiosis
Actinomycosis
Leprosy
Osteomyelitis
Rabies
Botulism
Tetanus
Routine Immunizations
Recommendations for Travelers

Gonorrhea (infection by the gram–negative diplococcus Neisseria gonor-
rhoeae). The likelihood of a woman becoming infected from an infected male is
greater (≥ 50%) than the converse (20–30%). About 60% of female infections and
about 20–50% male infections are asymptomatic. The site(s) of infection rests significantly upon sexual practices (e.g. fellatio, rectal intercourse, vaginal intercourse).
However, women with cervical infection frequently also have anorectal infection (seldom symptomatic) even though rectal intercourse has not occurred.

CLINICAL MANIFESTATIONS:

Urethritis in males usually has an incubation period of 2–7 days. Typically,
there is dysuria and a purulent discharge. Nongonococcal urethritis (e.g. Chlamydia,
Ureaplasma) is associated with similar symptoms but the discharge tends to be thinner and gonococci are not seen on gram stain of the discharge.

Urethritis in females: The diagnosis is complicated by the fact that dysuria and
frequency also accompany cystitis due to coliform bacteria (see laboratory below).

Epididymitis may sometimes complicate gonococcal (and chlamydial) urethritis.
The infection is usually unilateral with swelling, warmth, and tenderness. Bilateral involvement may lead to sterility. The testicle may also be involved (epididymo–orchitis). It is most important to differentiate epididymitis from torsion of the spermatic
cord since the latter is a surgical emergency. See the chapters "Torsion of Spermatic Cord" and "Epididymitis" for further details. Epididymitis after middle age is most
often due to coliforms (e.g. E. coli, enterobacter, proteus, Pseudomonas aerugenosa).

Cervicitis: The endocervix is the most common site of gonococcal infection in females. Symptoms are frequently absent or minimal. Examination typically reveals a
reddened cervix with a purulent discharge. About 15–20% patients with cervicitis go
on to develop pelvic inflammatory disease.

Pelvic inflammatory disease: refer to "Pelvic Inflammatory Disease" chapter.

Anorectal infection is common in both homosexual men and heterosexual
women. However, females are seldom symptomatic even though 40% of females with gonococcal cervicitis also have anorectal infection without having engaged in rectal intercourse. Anorectal infection in males is frequently symptomatic
(mucopurulent and/or bloody discharge, tenesmus, pain). Similar symptoms may
occur with inflammatory bowel disease, shigellosis, amebiasis.

Pharyngeal infection is common in homosexual males and occurs in about 20%
of females with gonococcal infection. Pharyngeal infection is usually asymptomatic
and is usually associated with concurrent infection at other sites. Symptomatic
gonococcal pharyngitis is clinically indistinguishable from other causes of pharyngitis
(i.e. an exudate may be present and there may be cervical adenopathy).

Disseminated gonococcal infection: Gonococcal septicemia may result in the
arthritis–dermatitis syndrome. Characteristic manifestations include <u>fever; migratory arthralgias</u> (particularly of the knees, wrists, and/or hands); <u>tenosynovitis</u> (frequently of the flexor aspect of the wrists and Achille's tendon); and <u>skin lesions</u> of
the distal extremities. Skin lesions begin as petechiae or papules that then
frequently become pustular and then necrotic. Gram stain and/or culture of
specimens from skin lesions are sometimes positive. Blood cultures are usually
positive. As the skin lesions heal (and as blood culture typically turns negative), the
patient may develop <u>septic arthritis</u>—usually in a single joint. Synovial fluid WBC
count ranges from 20,000 to 100,000 with > 90% neutrophils. Synovial fluid culture
is more likely to be positive the more elevated the synovial fluid WBC count. Treatment of septic arthritis is outlined below. <u>Meningitis and endocarditis</u> are unusual
complications of gonococcal septicemia.

Other consequences of gonococcal infection include Bartholin gland abscess,
prostatitis, conjunctivitis, perihepatitis (Fitz–Hugh–Curtis syndrome).

LABORATORY:

Male with urethral discharge: Microscopic exam of gram stain of the discharge
is all that is usually needed to diagnose symptomatic gonococcal urethritis since the
test is both quite sensitive and specific. Diagnosis is based on finding gram–negative diplococci within leukocytes. The diagnosis is uncertain if diplococci are extracellular while the absence of diplococci in the discharge excludes the diagnosis of

gonorrhea.

Asymptomatic male suspected of having gonococcal infection: Only about 60% of asymptomatic males with gonococcal infection have a positive urethral gram stain. Negative or equivocal gram stain is therefore an indication for urethral culture. The anterior urethra is sampled using noninhibitory swab (e.g. calcium alginate swab) and promptly streaked on chocolate agar or a more selective chocolate agar medium (e.g. Thayer–Martin), and incubated with carbon dioxide. The sediment of a sample of spun urine may also be cultured. Other sites may be cultured as sexual practices suggest.

Women suspected of having gonococcal infection: <u>Culture;</u> Endocervical culture is obtained using medium just described. Chlamydial testing of the endocervix is also appropriate. Gonococcal culture may also be taken from the urethra if an urethral discharge is present. Pressing the urethra against the symphysis pubis to express pus will enhance the yield of urethral gonococcal culture. <u>Gram stain</u> of the urethral discharge or endocervix may also be examined. However, gram stain is generally unreliable because the picture is confused by the presence of nonpathogenic neisseria species normally found in the vagina. Nonpathogenic neisseria are responsible for a false–positive test in as many as 20% of those sampled. Furthermore, sensitiviy of gram stain is such that ≤ 60% of patients proven to have gonococcal infection by cervical culture are positive by gram stain. If a gram stain is used, the exam should not be read as positive unless several leukocytes are found to have multiple intracellular gram–negative diplococci. <u>Differentiating gonorrhea from common cystitis;</u> The diagnosis of gonococcal or chlamydial urethritis in females is complicated by the fact that dysuria and frequency also accompany the common bladder infection. When—in a sexually active female—there is uncertainty, the best course is to obtain urethral and cervical cultures specific for gonorrhea as well as routine urine culture (which will not grow gonococci). Bacterial cystitis is diagnosed when there are > 100,000 colony forming units/ml urine. As in males, the urethral discharge may fail to grow gonococci and again Chlamydia may be the culprit.

Culture of the urethra in females, pharynx, or rectum is not routinely indicated unless the patient is symptomatic at that/those sites or unless sexual practices (fellatio, rectal intercourse) suggest a likely site of infection. The rationale for not routinely culturing these sites for gonococcus is that it is unusual in conventional cases for these sites to be infected in the absence of infection of the urethra in males or the cervix in females.

When disseminated gonococcal infection is suspected, the gamut of cultures (cervix, urethra, rectum, pharynx, skin lesion, blood, joint) may need to be obtained as clinical circumstances suggest unless the diagnosis can be made quickly (e.g. gram stain of the urethra in males). <u>Septic arthritis;</u> Needle aspiration of a joint must be performed if there is any suspicion of joint infection. Joint aspiration has both diagnostic and therapeutic value. Obtain a gram stain of the synovial fluid. Also culture the fluid: (1) routine aerobic and anaerobic, and (2) immediately introduce a specimen of synovial fluid onto a chocolate agar or selective chocolate agar medium (e.g. Thayer–Martin, MTM). <u>Blood culture</u> is obtained but should not be done on selective media that contain agents that inhibit the growth of nongonococcal organisms.

Serologic test for syphilis (e.g. RPR, VDRL) is ordered if gonorrhea is suspected or diagnosed. If negative, the test is repeated in several weeks.

AIDS testing may also be advisable.

TREATMENT:

Uncomplicated urethritis, cervicitis, proctitis: Single dose of ceftriaxone 250 mg IM. This is followed by doxycycline (100 mg PO twice daily for 7 days) or tetracycline (500 mg PO 4 times/days for 7 days) to cover possible concurrent chlamydial infection. In homosexual males, anti–chlamydial therapy is optional since chlamydial infection is uncommon in this group. If there is a history of severe penicillin allergy, the preferred regimen is spectinomycin 2 gram IM followed by doxycycline or tetracycline as just cited. However, spectinomycin does not cover gonococcal pharyngitis. <u>Pregnant patients, children, and patients with tetracycline sensitivity</u> are treated with single dose of ceftriaxone 250 mg IM followed by erythromycin (500 mg PO 4 times/day in adult) for 7 days with cervical and rectal culture 4–7 days after finishing treatment.

Pharyngitis: Single dose of ceftriaxone 250 mg IM. If ceftriaxone is contraindicated, a single dose of ciprofloxacin 500 mg is recommended followed by repeat culture 4–7 days later.

Pelvic inflammatory disease: refer to "Pelvic Inflammatory Disease" chapter.

Disseminated gonococcal infection (arthritis–dermatitis syndrome): Hospitalization is usually advised, especially if patient appears severely ill, and is mandatory in following cases: purulent joint effusion, meningitis, or endocarditis. Antibiotic options: ceftriaxone 1000 mg IV or IM q24h, cefotaxime 1000 mg IV q8h, or ceftizoxime 1000 mg IV q8h. Therapy may be switched to ampicillin 1000 mg IV q6h if the organism later proves to be sensitive to penicillin. Patient may be discharged 24–48 hours after becoming asymptomatic, and continued on oral antibiotic therapy until a total of 7 days of parenteral and oral antibiotic has been given. Oral antibiotic options are: (**1**) cefuroxime axetil 500 mg PO bid, (**2**) the combination preparation amoxicillin/clavulanic acid 500mg/125mg (Augmentin '500') PO tid, or (**3**) provided the patient is not pregnant—ciprofloxacin 500 mg PO bid. To cover possible concurrent chlamydial infection, patients are also treated with doxycycline (100 mg bid) or tetracycline (500 mg PO qid) for 7 days. In pregnant patients, children, and patients with tetracycline sensitivity, erythromycin (500 mg PO qid in adult) for 7 days is substituted for doxycycline or tetracycline. In homosexual males, anti–chlamydial therapy is optional since chlamydial infection is uncommon in this group. Purulent joint effusions are aspirated and repeated as needed, but open drainage is not advised except if the hip joint is involved. Gonococcal endocarditis or meningitis requires high–dose IV therapy (e.g. cetriaxone 1–2 gram/24hr IV). Antibiotic therapy must be continued for 10–14 days for meningitis and at least 4 wks for endocarditis.

Epididymitis/orchitis: single dose of ceftriaxone 250 mg IM followed by at least 10 days treatment with either doxycycline 100 mg bid or tetracycline 500 mg PO qid.

Ophthalmia in adult or child > 20 kg: ceftriaxone 1 gram once. Irrigate eyes with saline or ophthalmic solution to flush out the discharge and consult ophthalmologist.

Routine prophylaxis against gonococcal ophthalmia in neonates: Single topical application of 0.5% erythromycin ointment, 1% tetracycline ointment, or 1% silver nitrate solution.

Prophylaxis in newborn of mother with gonococcal infection: ceftriaxone 50 mg/kg (maximum 125 mg) IV or IM. Use with caution in neonates with hyperbiluremia, especially if they are premature.

Infant infection: ceftriaxone 25–50 mg/kg IV or IM once every 24 hours, or cefotaxime 25 mg/kg q12h. Antibiotic therapy is continued for 7 days. Thorough workup is mandatory and should include blood and CSF culture. Antibiotic therapy is continued for 14 days if meningitis is discovered. If the organism proves to be penicillin sensitive, antibiotic therapy may be switched to crystalline penicillin G 100,000 units/kg/day divided bid for infants < 1 week of age and divided qid for those > 1wk. The dose of penicillin is 150,000 units/kg/day if there is gonococcal meningitis. If there is gonococcal ophthalmia, the patient should be treated with parenteral antibiotic and the eyes should also be irrigated with buffered saline solutions to flush out the discharge. Topical ophthalmic antibiotic therapy alone is not acceptable.

Gonococcal infection in child: Children ≥ 45 kg are treated as adults. Children < 45 kg with uncomplicated urethritis, cervicitis, vulvovaginitis, proctitis, or pharyngitis are treated with a single dose of ceftriaxone 125 mg IM. The alternative if ceftriaxone is contraindicated is a single dose of spectinomycin 40 mg/kg IM. Bacteremia or arthritis in child ≤ 45 kg; ceftriaxone 50 mg/kg (max 1 gram) once a day for 7 days. Meningitis in child ≤ 45 kg; ceftriaxone 50 mg/kg (max 2 gram) once a day for 10–14 days. Children ≥ 8 yr of age should also be treated with doxycycline 100 mg bid for 7 days.

TREATMENT FOLLOW–UP: Follow–up cultures are not necessary in patients with uncomplicated urethral, cervical, rectal, or throat infections treated with the ceftriaxone/doxycycline combination. Apparent treatment failures are usually due to reinfection and not gonococcal resistance. Patients treated with other regimens should be cultured 4–7 days after finishing therapy. Follow–up includes evaluation and treatment of sex partners.

Syphilis is due to the spirochete Treponema pallidum. The organism cannot be grown on artificial media.

PRIMARY SYPHILIS: During sexual intercourse (and sometimes by kissing or other direct contact with infectious lesions) spirochetes are introduced via the mucous membranes or skin breaks, and then disseminate. The incubation period, a function of the number of spirochetes inoculated, is usually about 3 weeks (range, 10–90 days). The first clinical sign is the **chancre:** a papule that typically develops into a painless ulcer. There may be more than one chancre but the chancre is usually a solitary lesion. The chancre is most often found on the penis or vulva but many sites are possible (e.g. anus, cervix, mouth, tongue, lips, finger, nipple, etc). A "rubbery" nontender adenopathy is usually present in the region of the chancre. The chancre heals spontaneously after about 3–6 weeks. Spirochetes may be recovered from the chancre.

SECONDARY SYPHILIS begins about the time the chancre is resolving (i.e. 4–8 weeks after chancre first appears). The patient continues to be contagious during secondary syphilis. Secondary syphilis may be brief or last for months. **Constitutional complaints:** There may be fever, headache, arthralgias, sore throat, malaise, anorexia. **Generalized "rubbery" nontender adenopathy** is common. **Generalized, usually nonpruritic, rash** appears in most cases. It may be macular, papular, and/or pustular; and there may be some superficial scaling. A helpful diagnostic clue is the presence of the rash on the palms or soles. After healing, the patient may be left with areas of hyper- or hypo-pigmentation. **Condyloma lata** are flat-topped coalescing papules that may be found in moist areas of the skin such as the perineum, axillae, and at mucocutaneous junctions. These lesions contain many spirochetes and are therefore infectious. **Mucous patches** (superficial erosions of the mucous membranes) appear as gray–white oval patches with a pink border. Patches may be seen in the mouth, or on the anus, vulva, or glans penis. They contain spirochetes and are therefore infectious. **Meningitis,** an uncommon complication, usually occurs during the first year of infection. It is often coincident with the mucocutaneous manifestations of secondary syphilis, or with relapses of mucocutaneous disease during the latent stage. The usual signs and symptoms of bacterial meningitis may be present. And seizures, cranial nerve deficits, and/or hydrocephalus are potential complications. Characteristic CSF findings include leukocytosis with mononuclear predominance, normal CSF glucose, elevated CSF total protein with elevated gamma globulin fraction, and a positive CSF VDRL. Serum VDRL and FTA–ABS are usually positive. **Other potential manifestations** include patchy hair loss, hepatitis (rarely with jaundice), uveitis.

LATENT SYPHILIS is the stage that follows secondary syphilis. The patient is asymptomatic and clinical signs of syphilis are absent. The CSF is normal. Syphilitic infection may still be detected by serologic tests however. The patient may be contagious during the first 4 years of infection (but usually not after the first year). There may be recurrences of mucocutaneous disease during "latent" syphilis and it is during these relapses that the patient is most contagious. The patient is not infectious thereafter except perhaps by blood transfusion or by transplacental transmission to the fetus. The untreated patient may never again develop clinical disease and serologic tests may eventually turn negative.

TERTIARY (LATE) SYPHILIS occurs in about a third of untreated cases. It may manifest as gummatous syphilis, cardiovascular syphilis, and/or neurosyphilis.

   Gummas (a granulomatous reaction characterized by central necrosis surrounded by epithelioid cells, fibroblasts, and giant cells) are destructive lesions that may arise 1–10 years following infection, and may involve the skin and virtually any other tissue (e.g. bone, CNS, liver, lung, heart, GI tract, testicle, nasal septum, palate, pharynx, larynx, eye). Skin gummas form nodules, ulcers, or papulosquamous lesions. Subcutaneous gummas characteristically leave punched–out ulcers. Gummas respond well to antibiotics.

   Cardiovascular syphilis is due to an obliterative endarteritis of the vasa vasorum that leads to injury of the intima and media of the large arteries, particularly the aorta. Most cases of cardiovascular syphilis are clinically silent and the diagnosis is made at autopsy. The diagnosis is suspected if x–rays show linear calcifications of the ascending aorta. Patients that do develop clinically evident cardiovascular syphilis do so after 10–25 years of infection. The most frequent complication is dilation of the aortic root with aortic insufficiency. Aortic aneurysm may develop, usually of the ascending aorta and usually saccular. Rarely, there is scarring and stenosis at the coronary ostia with ensuing angina.

Neurosyphilis may be asymptomatic (i.e. + VDRL of the CSF without neurologic stigmata) or may manifest as meningitis (see Secondary Syphilis above), meningovascular syphilis, tabes dorsalis, and/or general paresis. ●<u>Meningovascular syphilis</u> may develop after the primary stage, but most cases occur 2–10 years after the infection is acquired. There is an obliterative endarteritis leading to CNS infarction with sundry possible neurologic abnormalities according to the region of brain or spinal cord affected. CSF VDRL and serum VDRL are virtually always positive; CSF leukocytes and gamma globulin are typically increased. ●<u>Tabes dorsalis</u> (chronic progressive degeneration of the posterior columns and posterior spinal roots) may develop in untreated cases 10–30 years after acquiring the infection. The pathogenesis of tabes is unknown since spirochetes are not found in the dorsal columns or dorsal roots. Both the serum VDRL and CSF VDRL are not uncommonly negative, but the serum FTA–ABS is virtually always positive. Typically, there is ataxia, areflexia, loss of vibration and position sense (the latter deficit results in a + Romberg sign). Babinski reflex is usually normal. The patient characteristically walks with an unsteady broad–based slapping gait. Impaired position sense may make walking in the dark without the benefit of visual cues particularly difficult. Impaired pain sensation leads to destruction of weight–bearing joints (Charcot joints) and ulcers of the soles of the feet (both are late manifestations of tabes). Lancinating ("lightning") pains in the absence muscle spasm are common, particularly in the lower extremities. Episodes of pain affecting the stomach, bladder, rectum, vagina, larynx, and other organs may occur. Argyll Robertson pupils (pupils that constrict with accomodation but not to light) is a common finding. Optic atrophy is uncommon complication that, without treatment, frequently leads to blindness. Impaired bladder sensation causes urinary retention with incontinence. Constipation, orthostatic hypotension, and impotence are common complications. Tabes dorsalis is not associated with mental impairment unless general paresis is also present. Antibiotic therapy stops progression of the disease and partial neurologic recovery may occur. Carbamazepine may help relieve tabetic pain. ●<u>General paresis</u> usually occurs after 10–20 years (range 2–30 yr) in untreated cases. Spirochetes are present in the brain parenchyma. Neurons are lost, and so cerebral atrophy is typical. Headache, fatigue, nervousness, insomnia, depression are common complaints. Emotional lability (e.g. irritability, tantrums, crying spells, elation) is chararacteristic. Mentation is affected (e.g. confusion, poor judgment and insight, impaired concentration, impaired memory). The patient may neglect personal appearance, be paranoid, or have delusions. Tremor of the tongue and facial muscles is characteristic; the entire body may be affected. Hyperreflexia and sometimes an abnormal Babinski are present. Dysarthria and abnormally reactive pupils are common. Seizures may occur. The CSF VDRL is virtually always positive, CSF total protein and gamma globulin fraction are elevated, and the CSF WBC count is elevated. Serum VDRL and FTA–ABS are usually positive. Early antibiotic therapy usually arrests progression of the disease but the degree of recovery varies.

CONGENITAL SYPHILIS: Blood–borne transplacental infection of the fetus may occur from 9–10 weeks gestation up to term. For this reason it is advisable to perform a serum VDRL (or RPR) early in pregnancy and near term. Fetal infection is most likely early in the course of maternal syphilis but an untreated woman has the potential to infect a fetus for at least 5 years. The clinical consequences of fetal syphilis can usually be avoided in the newborn if the mother is treated prior to 16 weeks gestation.

Early congenital syphilis: In many cases, there is a rash. Like acquired secondary syphilis, it often involves the palms and soles; but unlike secondary syphilis there may be blistering. Other findings may include leukocytosis, thrombocytopenia, hemolytic anemia, jaundice, hepatosplenomegaly, and rhinitis. Rhinitis may lead to snuffles (obstructed nasal breathing). There may be osteochondritis and it may be painful enough to cause immobility of an extremity (pseudoparalysis). Meningitis may occur and may lead to cranial nerve deficits, seizures, and/or hydrocephalus.

Late congenital syphilis (congenital syphilis after 2 yr of age). Findings may include abnormal teeth (Hutchinson's incisors [notched and widely–spaced upper central incisors], mulberry molars); eye abnormalities (interstitial keratitis, chorioretinitis, optic atrophy); evidence of periostitis and abnormal bone development (saber shins [anteriorly bowed tibia], frontal bossing, saddle nose, inadequate development of the maxilla with "bulldog" facies); Clutton's joints (arthritis of the knees); gumma on the nasal septum or palate; 8th nerve deafness. There may be early CSF evidence of neurosyphilis but clinically evident neurosyphilis (due to meningovascular syphilis and/or general paresis) does not appear until after a latent interval, usually later in childhood or in adolescence. Tabes dorsalis is very rare and cardiovascular complications are not seen.

LABORATORY: **Screening tests:** The basis for these tests is that patients with syphilis develop antibody against a normal tissue component called cardiolipin. The most common tests that detect anticardiolipin antibody are the rapid plasma reagin (RPR) test and the serum Venereal Disease Research Laboratory (VDRL). The chancre develops 1–2 weeks before the serum VDRL becomes positive. The VDRL is positive in 77% of primary syphilis, 98–99% cases of secondary syphilis, 95% cases of early latent syphilis, and 73% cases of late latent or tertiary syphilis. The 1--2% false–negative results seen in secondary syphilis is due to the prozone phenomenon (serum antibody levels are in excess but the VDRL becomes positive if the serum is diluted). A false–positive VDRL (usually with a titer of < 1: 8) may occur with autoimmune disease, sundry bacterial or viral infections, malaria, opiate addiction, lymphoma, or in the elderly.

Serial quantitative VDRL's are obtained to confirm treatment adequacy. With successful therapy, the serum VDRL usually turns negative after 12 months in primary syphilis and after 24 months in secondary syphilis. However, persistent low–titer positivity is not unusual in adequately treated late syphilis.

FTA–ABS (fluorescent treponemal antibody absorption) is used primarily to confirm the diagnosis of syphilis. It is both more specific and more sensitive than the VDRL. False positive FTA–ABS is unusual (< 1% of the normal population); but there is an increased frequency in autoimmune disorders. The FTA–ABS becomes positive about 2 weeks earlier than the VDRL. It is positive in 86% cases of primary syphilis, virtually 100% cases secondary syphilis, 99% cases of early latent syphilis, and 96% cases of late latent or tertiary syphilis.

Laboratory testing in the newborn: Because IgG crosses the placenta, the VDRL and FTA–ABS will be positive in infants born to seropositive mothers. However, IgM does not cross the placenta and therefore the IgM FTA–ABS is used to help diagnose congenital syphilis in the newborn. Because the IgM FTA–ABS is not entirely reliable (false–positive about 10% and false–negative about 35%), it is best to also obtain standard serial serum quantitative VDRL's on a newborn of a serologic positive mother. The infant is treated if the titers do not fall. It is also common practice not to rely on serologic tests but to go ahead and treat infants born of serologic positive mothers.

TREATMENT:

Primary syphilis, secondary syphilis, early latent (< 1 yr) syphilis, or syphilis exposure in last 3 months: Standard therapy; single dose of *benzathine* penicillin G 2.4 million units IM. Penicillin allergy: Nonpregnant adult is treated with doxycycline 100 mg twice daily for 2 weeks, or tetracycline 500 mg PO 4 times/day for 2 weeks. If doxycycline/tetracycline are contraindicated (e.g. child < 8 yr, allergy, pregnancy); the treatment is oral erythromycin (500 mg PO qid in adult) for 2 weeks. Post-treatment: Physical exam and quantitative serum VDRL should be performed at 3 and 6 months after treatment. HIV–infected patients should be tested 1,2,3,6,9,12 months post treatment. The VDRL titer should drop fourfold by 3 months in primary or secondary syphilis and by 6 months in early latent syphilis. If the VDRL does not turn negative or decline sufficiently and reinfection has been excluded, the patient is retreated after performing lumbar puncture to exclude asymptomatic neurosyphilis (order CSF VDRL, CSF cell count, CSF total protein and IgG level).

Late latent (>1 yr) syphilis, cardiovascular syphilis, gummas: CSF is obtained prior to treatment to exclude asymptomatic neurosyphilis (order CSF VDRL,

CSF cell count, CSF total protein and IgG level). <u>Standard therapy:</u> *Benzathine* penicillin G 2.4 million units IM once a week for 3 consecutive weeks. <u>Penicillin allergy:</u> Nonpregnant adult is treated with doxycycline 100 mg PO bid for 4 weeks or tetracycline 500 mg PO qid for 4 weeks. If doxycycline/tetracycline is contraindicated (e.g. child < 8 yr, pregnancy, allergy) and there is a history of penicillin allergy, confirm penicillin allergy by skin testing. <u>Post–treatment</u> quantitative serum VDRL should be obtained at 6 and 12 months. If the serum VDRL titer rises fourfold, if the pretreatment serum VDRL titer was ≥ 1:32 and subsequent titers do not decline, or if there is clinical evidence of neurosyphilis; then a thorough investigation for neurosyphilis is carried out and the patient is retreated with a suitable antibiotic regimen.

Neurosyphilis (including asymptomatic neurosyphilis): Aqueous crystalline penicillin G 2–4 million units IV q4h for 10–14 days followed by benzathine penicillin G 2.4 million units IM once a week for 3 consecutive weeks. An alternative is aqueous procaine penicillin G 2–4 million units IM once daily for 10–14 days (concurrently with probenecid 500 mg PO qid) followed by benzathine penicillin G 2.4 million units IM once a week for 3 consecutive weeks. Patients with a history of penicillin allergy should be skin tested to verify the alllergy. If positive, penicillin desensitization is recommended or proceed with the advice of an expert. <u>Post–treatment follow–up neurosyphilis</u> consists of (**1**) physical exam at 6 month intervals; (**2**) serum quantitative VDRL at 3, 6, 12, 24, and 36 months; (**3**) CSF analysis [quantitative CSF VDRL, leukocyte count, total protein, IgG level] every 6 months until the CSF leukocyte count is normal. <u>Retreatment</u> is recommended if the CSF leukocyte count has not fallen after 6 months or has not returned to normal at 2 years. Even with adequate treatment, the CSF leukocyte count may not return to normal for 1–2 years, the CSF protein may remain elevated even longer, and the CSF VDRL may remain positive for years.

Syphilis in pregnancy is treated with penicillin as in the nonpregnant patient. For the duration of the pregnancy, monthly quantitative serum VDRL are obtained to document treatment adequacy. Continuing follow–up after the pregnancy is also necessary as recommended above according to the stage of syphilis. If there is a history of penicillin allergy, skin testing is performed to verify the allergy. If positive, penicillin desensitization is carried out. Doxycycline and tetracycline are contraindicated in pregnancy.

Congenital syphilis: <u>Criteria mandating investigation:</u> An infant born to a mother who tests positive for syphilis (positive serum VDRL or RPR verified by serum FTA–ABS) should be investigated for syphilis if the mother (**1**) was not treated during pregnancy or treatment cannot be verified, (**2**) was treated less than a month prior to delivery, (**3**) was treated with nonpenicillin antibiotic (erythromycin), or (**4**) her serum VDRL titer following treatment did not decrease as anticipated or post–treatment serologic testing was inadequate. <u>The investigation:</u> Signs of congenital syphilis should be diligently sought on physical exam. CSF is obtained (order CSF VDRL, CSF cell count, CSF total protein and IgG level). Also order quantitative serum VDRL and if available a serum 19S–IgM FTA–ABS. Long bone x–rays are obtained. Chest x–ray or other tests may also be ordered as clinical findings suggest. <u>Criteria for treatment:</u> A full 10–14 day course of penicillin therapy (see below) is necessary if any of the following are present: (**1**) clinical or x–ray signs of active disease; (**2**) positive CSF VDRL; (**3**) CSF WBC count ≥ 5; (**4**) CSF protein > 50 mg/dl; (**5**) positive serum 19S–IgM FTA–ABS; (**6**) quantitative serum VDRL titer ≥ 4 times that of mother; (**7**) untreated syphilis in mother; (**8**) mother treated appropriately but she subsequently shows clinical or laboratory signs of recrudescence or reinfection, (**9**) investigation of infant was indicated but was not thorough. Furthermore, single-dose benzathine penicillin therapy (see below) is indicated if the infant required investigation, which was thorough and revealed no abnormalities, but: (**1**) the mother was treated with erythromycin rather than penicillin during pregnancy and/or (**2**) close follow–up of the infant cannot be guaranteed. <u>Anitbiotic regimen in newborns:</u> (**1**) aqueous crystalline penicillin G 100,000–150,000/kg/day (50,000 units q8–12 hr) IV for 10-14 days or (**2**) aqueous procaine penicillin G 50,000 units/kg IM once a day for 10-14 days. Newborns who only require a single–dose of penicillin (see *criteria for treatment* above) receive a single IM dose of benzathine penicillin 50,000 units/kg. <u>Antibiotic regimen in older infants and children:</u> acqueous penicillin G 200,000–300,000 units/kg/day (50,000 units/kg q4–6 h) IV for 10–14 days. <u>Follow–up of</u>

seropositive infants not requiring treatment is advised at 1, 2, 3, 6, and 12 months. As the maternally–derived antibodies are cleared, the infant's serum VDRL titer should have decreased by 3 months and vanished by 6 months. Re–evaluation and a 10–14 day course of penicillin are necessary if the titers are not falling. Treatment is also necessary if the infant's serum FTA–ABS remains positive after a year.
Follow–up of treated infants: By 6 months of age the serum–VDRL titer should have vanished and the CSF–VDRL should also be negative with successful treatment. Re–evaluation and retreatment are indicated if this is not the case. ●CSF leukocyte count (assuming that it is initiallly elevated) should be checked every 6 months until it returns to normal. Retreatment is required if the CSF leukocyte count is not consistently decreasing or if it still has not returned to normal by 2 yr of age. ●FTA–ABS is not an useful follow–up test because it may remain positive even with successful treatment.

Acquired syphilis in older children with normal neurologic exam is treated with a single IM dose of benzathine penicillin G 50,000 units/kg (max 2.4 million units). Post–treatment follow–up is as for adults according to the stage of syphilis.

Chlamydia Trachomatis is an obligate intracellular bacte-
rium. There are 15 immunotypes. Types A–C are responsible for endemic trachoma. Types D–K are (**1**) sexually transmitted and may cause urethritis, epididymitis, cervicitis, PID or (**2**) are transmitted during childbirth from a mother with cervical infection to a neonate in whom it may cause neonatal inclusion conjunctivitis. L types cause lymphogranuloma venereum (LGV).
Trachoma and **inclusion conjuctivitis** are discussed in the "Conjunctivitis" chapter in the eye section.

Urethritis, epididymitis, proctitis, cervicitis, and salpingitis arising from sexual transmission of Chlamydia trachomatis immunotypes D–K.

In males about half the cases of nongonococcal urethritis are due to chlamydial infection. The discharge is mucopurulent but tends to be thinner than in gonococcal urethritis. Some patients develop epididymitis as a complication. Chlamydia proctitis may occur in homosexual males. Laboratory: Chlamydial infection may be diagnosed by immunofluorescence testing of urethral discharge. Treatment of choice for urethritis or proctitis is tetracycline 500 mg PO 4 times/day for 7 days, or doxycycline 100 mg PO twice daily for 7 days. Epididymitis is treated with the same drugs and doses for at least 10 days. If tetracyclines are contraindicated, the alternative is erythromycin 500 mg PO 4 times/day continued for the same duration. Sexual contacts are treated as well.

Females: About a fourth of women with urethritis are infected with Chlamydia. Chlamydial cervicitis is also common, accounting for about 2/3 cases of mucopurulent cervicitis. Ascending infection often results in salpingitis. Chlamydial salpingitis may in fact be more common than gonococcal salpingitis. Occasionally, there is spread from the fallopian tubes into the abdominal cavity, and then along the paracolic gutters to the liver so that perihepatitis (Fitz–Hugh–Curtis syndrome) ensues. Laboratory: Chlamydial infection is usually diagnosed by immunofluorescence testing of cervical secretion. This method is quite specific but sensitivity varies according to specimen adequacy (a vigorous endocervical swab should be obtained). Culture is accurate but is is expensive, requires 4–5 days, and the sample must be properly obtained and transported. Using a dacron or rayon–tipped swab or calcium alginate swab, obtain a vigorous swab that is as free of purulent exudate as possible. Sample should be kept refrigerated and delivered to lab within 24 hours. Treatment: Female urethritis, cervicitis, and proctitis is treated with the same drug regimens as male urethritis (see above). Refer to "Pelvic Inflammatory Disease" chapter for the treatment of chlamydial salpingitis.

LYMPHOGRANULOMA VENEREUM (LGV) is due to the L immunotypes of Chlamydia trachomatis. LGV is a venereal disease that occurs primarily in subtropical–tropical areas, and is rare in the U.S. **Signs/symptoms:** One–three weeks following sexual exposure; about a third of patients develop a small painless papule, vesicle, or ulcer in the genital area. The lesion lasts 2–3 days. Regional adenopathy (usually inguinal) develops within a few weeks of exposure. Involved nodes are firm and tender. They are moveable at first, and then become fluctuant and adherent to deeper tissues. The overlying skin is reddened. The nodes may necrose forming fistulas and sinuses with purulent discharge. Node involvement is bilateral in a third of cases. If nodes above and below the inguinal ligament are affected and if there is fibrosis, "grooves" may form parallel to the inguinal line. Homoxexual males may have involvement of perirectal lymphatics, and go on to develop ulcerative proctitis with blood–tinged mucopurulent rectal discharge. Women may have the same sequelae and may also have involvement of pelvic lymphatics. **Complications:** Lymphatic obstruction may eventually develop in untreated cases so that genital elephantiasis ensues. Rectal stricture is another potential complication of chronic infection. Other possible complications include arthritis, keratoconjunctivitis, pericarditis, erythema nodosum. **Laboratory:** Complement fixation test is diagnostic if the titer is > 1: 16. This is true in over 80% of patients. **Treatment:** doxycycline 100 mg PO bid for 21 days. Options are tetracycline 500 mg PO qid for 21 days, erythromycin 500 mg PO qid for 21 days, or sulfisoxazole 500 mg PO qid for 21 days. To prevent fistula formation, fluctuant nodes are aspirated (thru adjacent normal skin); incision and drainage is contraindicated. Dilation or surgery may be required for rectal stricture.

Chancroid
is a venereal infection due to Hemophilus ducreyi, a gram–negative rod. Infection is uncommon in the U.S., but prevalent in S.E. Asia and Africa. **Signs/symptoms:** After an incubation period of 4–10 days, a papule or small blister forms on the penis or perianus of men, or on the vulva. The lesion then develops into a pustule, and subsequently into a painful shallow ulcer of variable size with irregular undermined borders. There may be multiple ulcers and the ulcers may coalesce. Lesions may be seen in the vagina or on the cervix. Fluctuant, usually unilateral, inguinal nodes (buboes) are found in about half the cases. Buboes may erupt thru the skin to form sinuses. **Laboratory:** Gram stain of material obtained from the ulcer edge reveals the gram–negative bacillus in over half the cases. Culture sample is transported on Amies medium if it cannot be promptly streaked on a chocolate agar plate containing vancomycin. Gram stain and culture material may also be obtained by needle aspiration of involved inguinal node (thru normal adjacent skin so that a fistula does not form). Also screen for syphilis (e.g. RPR, VDRL). **Treatment** is with either erythromycin 500 mg PO 4 times/day for 7 days, or a single dose of ceftriaxone 250 mg IM. Options include (**1**) trimethoprim/sulfametnoxasole 160mg/800mg (Bactrim DS, Septra DS) PO twice daily for 7 days; (**2**) the combination preparation amoxicillin/clavulanic acid 500mg/125mg (Augmentin) PO 3 times/day for 7 days.

Granuloma Inguinale
is due to a gram–negative bacillus, Calymmatobacterium granulomatis. The disease is most common in subtropical–tropical areas; it is uncommon in the U.S (about 50 reported cases/yr). The disease is acquired sexually and perhaps nonsexually. **Signs/symptoms:** After an incubation period of 1 to 12 weeks, a subcutaneous papule forms that erupts thru the skin to form a beefy–red painless nodule (a granulomatous lesion). The lesion may appear on the genitalia, thighs, or (in male homosexuals) about the anus. Vaginal lesions may also be found. With time the nodule may ulcerate to form large irregular friable beefy–red ulcers with thickened borders. New nodules form at the ulcer border. Areas of scarring with depigmentation may be present. Adenopathy is not characteristic but spread of the disease thru the subcutaneous tissue of the inguinal region or groin produces subcutaneous swellings (pseudobuboes). Metastatic spread to the bones or internal organs sometimes occurs. **Laboratory:** Giemsa or Wright's stain of scrapings or biopsy specimens reveal bacilli within macrophages (Donovan bodies). **Treatment** is with tetracycline 500 mg PO 4 times/day for 2 weeks. Trimethoprim–sulfamethoxazole is an alternative.

Condyloma Acuminata
(genital warts) are caused by the human papillomaviruses, the same viruses that causes warts on other areas of the body. Specific types of human papillomavirus have been identified as responsible for genital warts. Spread is by sexual contact. There is concern about the association of genital warts with abnormal PAP smears and cervical carcinoma. **Signs/symptoms:** The incubation period is usually 1–2 months but in some cases the lesions may not appear for up to 9 months. Lesions may be found on the external genitalia, perineum, anus, vaginal introitus, and occasionally the cervix. Genital warts may be flat (condyloma planum) or exophytic. Typically, there is a progression from single to multiple papillomas which subsequently coalesce to form cauliflower–like lesions. Genital warts may be confused with condyloma lata (due to syphilis) or

molluscum contagiosum. Women with lesions about the vulvar or vaginal regions often complain of itching and/or vaginal discharge. Left alone the lesions usually regress spontaneously although recurrences are not uncommon. In some cases the lesions ulcerate and may bleed, or become secondarily infected. **Laboratory:** Diagnosis is usually based on physical exam. If the diagnosis is uncertain, however, a PAP smear or histologic exam of biopsy specimen may disclose the pathognomonic koilocyte ("balloon cells"). Other sexually transmitted infections often coexist. It is therefore prudent to screen for syphilis (e.g. RPR or VDRL), gonorrhea, and possibly HIV. **Treatment:** Cryotherapy is the usual treatment of choice. Topical podophyllin is an alternative for small lesions. Electrocautery is yet another option. Extensive lesions not responding adequately to cryotherapy may require laser therapy or surgical excision.

AIDS (acquired immunodeficiency syndrome) is associated with infection by the

human immunodeficiency virus (HIV). HIV is a retrovirus (specifically HTLV–III), one of the human T lymphotrophic viruses. HTLV–III selectively infects T lymphocyte helper cells. The number of T helper cells declines markedly so that the ratio of T helper to T suppressor cells is decreased. T cell deficiency/dysfunction leads to impaired cell–mediated immunity with increased susceptibility to certain infections and malignancies (see below).

Persons at risk: Homosexual or bisexual men constitute about 70% of all AIDS patients followed by IV drug abusers (17%). Other groups at risk include Haitian immigrants, transfusion recipients (particularly hemophiliacs who have received multiple transfusions of blood products), female sexual contacts of the foregoing high risk groups, infants born to women at risk. ●The risk of contracting AIDS from nonsexual/nonparenteral exposure appears to be small. There is no risk from the usual nonsexual contact with family, schoolmates, etc. However, health workers should take care to avoid needle exposure or splashing of the patient's blood or other body fluids onto the face, eyes, or skin wounds.

Testing for HIV infection: Antibody to HTLV–III is present in almost all patients. A convenient 5 minute latex agglutination test is available as a screening test for the presence of HTLV–III antibody. Enzyme–linked immunoassay (ELISA) is a specific test (false–negatives are quite uncommon). However, since false–positives do occur, the test should be repeated in patients who test positive. ELISA–positive patients require verification with the Western blot assay. **Other laboratory findings:** Serum total globulin is commonly increased due to polyclonal increase in the immunoglobulin fraction. Sedimentation rate may be elevated. Hematology: There may be anemia, thrombocytopenia, leukopenia, and/or lymphopenia. The ratio of T lymphocyte suppressor cells to helper cells is increased.

Clinical expression and treatment: There is no cure for AIDS. However, drug therapy is available that may mitigate the disease and perhaps prolong life. Zidovudine (ZDV also known as AZT) is approved for that purpose. Patients are prone to recurrent infections by opportunistic organisms and are susceptible to certain malignancies (Kaposi's sarcoma, CNS lymphoma). Prodromal febrile illness: In some patients, the disease begins with several weeks to months of recurrent fever and night sweats. Generalized lymphadenopathy is characteristic, and the patient may complain of weight loss and/or diarrhea. Pneumocystis carinii pneumonia is diagnosed by bronchial brushings or lung biopsy. Treatment is with trimethoprim–sulfamethoxazole or pentamidine. Candidiasis may manifest as oral thrush (which may respond to nystatin) or esophagitis (which is treated with ketoconazole or amphotericin B). Cryptococcus neoformans meningitis and/or fungemia is treated with amphotericin B. Disseminated tuberculosis: see "Tuberculosis" chapter for treatment. Disseminated Mycobacterium avium–intracellulare may be mitigated by certain antimycobacterial drugs. Diagnosis rests on blood or bone marrow cultures. Acid–fast bacteria are sometimes identified in the stool. Disseminated cytomegalovirus (CMV): no treatment available. Herpes simplex (disseminated mucocutaneous) is treated with acyclovir. Toxoplasmosis (chorioretinitis, brain abscess) is treated with sulfadiazine plus pyrimethamine. Cryptosporium is a protozoan that causes a diarrheal illness.

Herpes Simplex Virus (HSV) comes in two antigenically related types, HSV 1 and HSV 2. Herpetic lesions of the oral mucosa, lips and adjacent skin, and eyes are usually due to HSV 1. Genital herpes, in contrast, is due in about 90% cases to HSV 2. **Transmission:** Man is the only reservoir of HSV. The viruses are transmitted via oral or genital secretions of active or sometimes inactive cases. The virus is usually introduced via the oral or genital mucosa. Other possible routes of infection include the rectal mucosa (with rectal interourse); the eyes; susceptible skin sites (e.g. fingers of dentists, exposed skin surfaces of wrestlers). A patient with active lesions may autoinoculate (e.g. by finger contact) and cause disease at other locations. **Recurrence:** HSV infection tends to cause recurrent disease. This is because viral DNA (but not complete virus) remains within the neurons of sensory ganglia in the intervals between active disease. The trigeminal ganglion is the reservoir of HSV DNA for recurrent herpetic disease of the eyes and perioral area, and the lumbosacral ganglia are the reservoir for recurrent genital herpes. At the time of a recurrence, HSV are produced within the neuron bodies and travel down the nerve fiber to the skin where the active lesions are produced. The nerves themselves are not damaged.

ORAL/CIRCUMORAL HERPES: Initial infection usually occurs in childhood and is usually asymptomatic. Those that are symptomatic commonly present with gingivostomatitis, and less often with a pharyngitis or a combination of the two. After an incubation period of 2–12 days, there is a 1–3 day prodrome (fever, malaise, cervical adenopathy) before the appearance of lesions. With gingivostomatitis, vesicles which subsequently ulcerate may be found anywhere in the mouth (gums, tongue, buccal mucosa). Healing occurs over 1–2 weeks. The breath may be foul and children may refuse to feed because of the pain. **Recurrent episodes** present as herpes labialis ("fever blisters", "cold sores"). Local itching or burning may warn of an impending attack. Vesicles that subsequently ulcerate and crust over are found on the lips and adjacent skin about the vermilion border. The lower lip is most common site of recurrence, and recurrences usually occur at the same site. Intraoral recurrences are unusual except in the immunocompromised. Recurring *intra*oral lesions are most often due to aphthous stomatitis, not HSV. **Laboratory:** see Genital Herpes below. **Treatment:** Acyclovir is sometimes used in the treatment of primary oral herpes but it is not advised for the treatment of the usual patient with recurrent attacks. During the initial infection with intraoral lesions, the patient may benefit from topical application of viscous xylocaine to lessen the pain and allow feeding.

OCULAR HERPES (herpes simplex keratitis) is usually due to HSV 1. The typical finding is dendritic keratitis—a branched ulcer of the corneal epithelium which is easily recognized with fluorescein stain. In the initial episode, vesicles may be present on the lid margins or adjacent skin. The conjunctiva are injected, and there is photophobia and tearing. There may be a foreign body sensation followed by decreased corneal sensation. Recurrences may lead to corneal ulceration and scarring that may ultimately impair vision. Ocular infections are treated by an ophthalmologist.

GENITAL HERPES: First episode begins 2–7 days following sexual exposure. Besides local pain, there is fever and malaise with bilateral tender inguinal lymph nodes. A cluster of small vesicles is the typical finding. The vesicles quickly rupture to form shallow painful ulcers which subsequently crust and heal over 1–2 weeks or so. In males, lesions are typically found on the glans or shaft of the penis. Homosexual males are at increased risk for perianal and rectal lesions with ensuing rectal discharge and tenesmus. In females, lesions may be found on the clitoris, labia, perineum, buttocks, vagina, cervix; and there may be severe dysuria and possibly urinary retention if the urethra is involved. **Recurrent attacks** occur in over half the patients but subsequent episodes tend to be less severe. Genital itching, tingling, burning, or soreness for about 24 hours may warn the patient of an impending episode. **Complications:** aseptic meningitis, sacral radicular myelitis. Cervical cancer is often associated with history or serologic evidence of HSV 2 infection but a causal link is not established. **Laboratory:** <u>Microscopy:</u> Wright's stain (Tzanck smear), Giemsa stain, or Pap stain of scrapings from the ulcer base reveals multinucleated giant cells (transformed epithelial cells) with intranuclear inclusions. <u>Cultures</u> of vesicular fluid or ulcer base may be obtained, and are more sensitive than stains, However, culture is usually unecessary, especially if there is a typical clinical presentation. Special handling is required unless cell culture medium is immediately available. Serology is not useful, except perhaps in the first episode, because the patient with recurrences already has serum HSV antibodies. **Treatment:** Acyclovir (see drug section) is not a cure but it does shorten the duration of an episode of genital herpes. It may be used (**1**) for the initial episode, (**2**) intermittently for recurrent episodes, or (**3**) as chronic suppressive therapy for up to 12 months (followed by re-evaluation) in patient with frequent recurrent episodes.

NEONATAL HERPES infection occurs as the fetus passes thru the mother's infected birth canal, or by ascending infection if there has been prior rupture of the membranes. The risk of neonatal infection is greatest if the mother has active genital lesions. Therefore, mothers with active genital herpes are delivered by C-section unless the membranes have been ruptured for over 4 hours. The severity and extent of neonatal infection varies (e.g. self-limited localized skin lesions, encephalitis, severe disseminated visceral disease).

IMMUNOCOMPROMISED PATIENTS may develop chronic and widespread mucocutaneous lesions, and are susceptible to visceral disease. These patients may benefit from either chronic or intermittent suppressive treatment with acyclovir.

Infectious Mononucleosis is due to the Ebstein–Barr

virus (EBV), a DNA virus belonging to the herpes group. EBV is excreted in body fluids. Transmission is usually by close person-to-person contact (e.g. kissing) or via contaminated eating utensils. EBV may also be acquired by blood transfusion.

SIGNS/SYMPTOMS:

Typical illness: Prodrome: After an incubation period of 5–7 weeks; there is onset of malaise, lethargy, and headache. Subsequent developments are: fever that lasts about a week and may exceed 39.5° C; sore throat/pharyngitis—an exudate is often seen on the tonsils, there may be palatal petechiae; tender cervical adenopathy is characteristic; generalized adenopathy is common. Recovery: Most patients are improved by 3 weeks and well within 6 weeks, although fatigue may persist for months. **Other manifestations:** Splenomegaly occurs in about half the patients. Hepatomegaly in 10–20% cases with jaundice in 5–10% . Rash occurs in 5–10% cases. Maculopapular lesions are found on trunk and limbs. However, sometimes there are petechial or urticarial lesions. Rash may be precipitated by antibiotics, especially ampicillin. Periorbital edema occurs in about a fourth of cases. Pneumonitis occasionally develops. **Uncommon complications:** neurologic (meningoencephalitis, Bell's palsy, Guillain–Barré syndrome, transverse myelitis); hematologic (hemolytic anemia, thrombocytopenia, agranulocytosis, aplastic anemia); cardiac (myocarditis, pericarditis); splenic rupture occurs rarely in patients who develop an enlarged spleen; airway obstruction may occur secondary to severe pharyngitis.

Atypical illness occurs in about 10% patients, particularly the very young or the aged. There is fever and malaise but pharyngitis is mild or absent. Hematologic or serologic evidence of EBV infection may be delayed.

Chronic or recurrent illness occurs in some patients. Manifestations may include fever, adenopathy, headache, fatigue, pharyngitis, myalgias, arthralgias, splenomegaly, hepatomegaly, weight loss. Serologic evidence of persistent illness is present (see lab below).

LABORATORY:

Heterophile antibodies are agglutinating antibodies (mostly IgM) that react with horse, sheep, and bovine erythrocytes. They are usually detected within the first 1–2 week of clinical illness and peak by the 3rd week. Heterophile antibodies usually disappear in 3–6 months. Monospot test is a rapidly performed heterophile antibody slide test that uses horse erythrocytes. The test is quite specific with only rare false positives (e.g. certain cases hepatitis or lymphoma). Heterophile antibody tests are limited to the extent that about 10% adults with infectious mononucleosis do not develop heterophile antibodies and the percentage is even greater in adolescents and children. Most children < 3 yr do not produce heterophile antibodies.

Tests for specific anti–EBV antibodies: A patient with negative monospot or other heterophile antibody test who is still suspected of having infectious mononucleosis should be tested for specific anti–EBV antibodies. Anti–VCA IgM antibody (IgM antibody directed against the viral capsid antigen [VCA]) is present during the acute illness and then decreases. Anti–VCA IgG antibodies are usually present by the time symptoms appear. By itself, anti–VCA IgG may not be diagnostic of acute disease because IgG persists after the illness is over. However, anti–VCA IgG is diagnostic if the titers are very high, if there is a 4–fold increase in titers (< 20% cases), or if titers later decrease. Anti–EA antibody (antibody directed against the early antigen) with diffuse immunofluorescence staining of both cytoplasm and nucleus is diagnostic and is found in about 3/4 cases. Anti–EA antibody with staining restricted to the cytoplasm is seen in persistent or recurrent cases. Antibody to the Ebstein–Barr nuclear antigen (EBNA) is detected weeks to months after the onset of disease. Anti–VCA positivity with anti–EBNA negativity is diagnostic, especially if the anti–EBNA later becomes positive. In chronic infection; anti–VCA IgG is present, anti–EA antibody is present, and anti–EBNA antibody is borderline or absent.

Other lab findings: WBC count may be low to normal in the 1st week of illness, but usually rises to 10,000–20,000 or sometimes higher by the 2nd–3rd week. In some cases there is neutropenia with neutrophil count sometimes ≤ 500. Lymphocytes are typically increased (> 5000) and over 10% are atypical. Liver function tests: Mild increases in liver enzymes are common. Serum bilirubin is increased (usually slightly) in over half the cases. Sometimes there is jaundice.

DIFFERENTIAL DIAGNOSIS: streptococcal pharyngitis, miscellaneous viruses that cause pharyngitis with adenopathy, cytomegalovirus, viral hepatitis, toxoplasmosis, lymphoma.
TREATMENT is generally symptomatic. Corticosteroids are justified if there are unusual complications (see Uncommon Complications above).

Septic Shock (vascular collapse resulting from the blood–borne dissemination of bacteria or their toxins) is fatal in about half the cases.

Etiology: Most cases are due to a gram–negative organism (E. coli, klebsiella, pseudomonas, enterobacter, serratia, proteus, bacteroides). Staphylococcus aureus is the most common gram–positive bacterium provoking septic shock; other culprits include pneumococcus, streptococcus, clostridia.
Pathogenesis is complex. Bacterial toxins or bacterial cell wall constituents activate the complement cascade. Complement components induce histamine release which in turn causes vasodilation. ●Vasodilation is also due to bradykinin. Bradykinin is produced when bacterial toxin activates Hageman factor (factor XII of the clotting cascade). This leads to formation of kallikrein which in turn cleaves kininogen to form bradykinin. ●Complement components also activate neutrophils, and so there is release of lysosomal enzymes and other factors that result in capillary leakage.
Signs/symptoms: Two stages are recognized in the progression of septic shock, warm stage and cold stage. In the warm stage there is vasodilation. The heart, in order to prevent a fall in blood pressure, compensates by increasing cardiac output (rate and stroke volume increase). The patient is warm, flushed, apprehensive. There is fever and tachycardia with a strong pulse. Cold stage ensues when continued capillary leakage depletes the intravascular volume to the point that cardiac compensation is inadequate, and so the blood pressure drops. Vasoconstriction ensues in response to the falling blood pressure. Urine output is negligible. The patient is cool, clammy, confused, and restless or lethargic. The temperature is subnormal and there is tachycardia with a weak pulse. Adult respiratory distress syndrome is a not an uncommon complication of septic shock.
Laboratory: Gram stain and cultures: Obtain 3 sets of blood cultures (aerobic and anaerobic) from different sites. The urine is gram–stained and cultured. Sputum is cultured. Abscesses are gram–stained and cultured. Gram or Wright's stain of the buffy coat fraction of the blood may reveal the bacteria. Blood gases: As tissue perfusion becomes progressively inadequate, there is proportionately more

anaerobic metabolism, and lactic acid accumulates. Consequently, the arterial blood gas reveals metabolic acidosis. At first, however, the arterial pH may be normal or alkalotic because the patient compensates by hyperventilating. There may be hypoxemia. WBC count is unpredictable. It may be elevated with an increased percentage of neutrophils, or the WBC count may be decreased as neutrophils are consumed in the pathologic process. Thrombocytopenia may also occur. PT and PTT may be prolonged.

Treatment: Intravenous fluid (normal saline or Ringer's lactate) is infused at a rate sufficient to maintain normal blood pressure. In order to better guide fluid therapy, a central venous line may be inserted and fluid administered to achieve CVP of 4–10 cm H_2O. Better yet, a Swan–Ganz catheter is inserted with fluid administration titrated to a wedge pressure of 6–12 mm Hg. An urine output > 50 ml/hr provides assurance of adequate circulatory perfusion. Intravenous dopamine (see drug section) may be given if an adequate blood pressure is not maintained with fluids alone. Obvious sources of sepsis are removed (e.g. abscesses drained, Foley catheter or suspicious IV catheter removed). IV antibiotics are begun promptly as soon as culture specimens have been obtained. Choice of antibiotics depends on the likely source of sepsis and clinical circumstances: e.g. abdominal/pelvic infection (gentamycin or tobramycin + metronidazole + ampicillin), immunocompromised patient or burn patient (tobramycin + nafcillin + ticarcillin). The latter combination may also be used when a likely source of infection cannot be identified. Corticosteroids may be of possible value (e.g. methylprednisolone 30 mg/kg IV administered over 20 minutes, and repeated as needed every 8–12 hours for up to two days).

Toxic Shock Syndrome (TSS) results from the production

of an exotoxin by certain strains of Staphylococcus aureus. Most cases have resulted from tampon–associated vaginal infections. Other settings include prolonged wearing of diaphragm, septic abortion, vaginal or caesarian delivery, mastitis, abscess, fascitis, osteomyelitis, nasal surgery/packing. The site of the S. aureus infection may be inconspicuous or inapparent.

Signs/symptoms: Nonspecific manifestations: Typically, there is an abrupt onset of high fever > 38.9 C (102 F), chills, headache, myalgias, nausea, vomiting, diarrhea (usually watery). There may be sore throat, cough, and/or abdominal pain. Mucocutaneous findings: Skin and mucous membranes are erythematous. There may be edema of face and extremities. About a fourth of patients develop a pruritic diffuse macular erythematous rash 5–10 days after onset of illness. All patients experience diffuse desquamation of the skin during the 2nd week following onset of TSS. This is most pronounced on the palms and soles. Loss of hair and nails may occur in 2–3 months. Postural hypotension may be evident on presentation and shock may ensue. Renal failure and/or adult respiratory distress syndrome may supervene.

Laboratory findings may include decreased total serum protein with hypoalbuminemia (due to capillary leakage of albumin); elevated CPK; hypocalcemia; abnormal liver function tests (e.g. elevated total bilirubin, SGOT); prolonged prothrombin time; leukocytosis with left shift; thrombocytopenia; elevated BUN; proteinuria; pyuria. Obtain cultures of cervix, vagina, tampon, blood, or any other suspicious site. Blood cultures are usually negative.

Differential diagnosis: Rocky Mountain Spotted Fever, tick typhus, meningococcemia, viral illness (e.g. measles), gastroenteritis, septic shock, pelvic inflammatory disease, scarlet fever, scalded skin syndrome, leptospirosis, Kawasaki disease, Legionnaires disease, Reye's syndrome.

Treatment: Treat hypotension with intravenous isotonic electrolyte solution (Ringer's lactate, normal saline) and fresh frozen plasma. Add dopamine if fluid therapy alone does not suffice. Monitor vital signs, urine output, CVP, and wedge pressure. Monitor electrolytes, BUN, creatinine, blood gases. Anti–staphylococcal therapy (cephalosporin or penicillinase–resistant penicillin such as nafcillin) is required. Antibiotic therapy does not change the course of TSS. However, the source of exotoxin must be eliminated because otherwise TSS recurrence is common. Treat ARDS should this complication arise. See "Adult Respiratory Distress Syndrome".

Meningococcal Disease is due to Neisseria meningitidis,

a gram–negative coccus. Serogroups A, B, C, or Y are the most common culprits. Most infections are asymptomatic nasopharyngeal infections. Infection is usually acquired by direct contact with or via infected airborne droplets from an asymptomatic carrier. The asymptomatic carrier state is common and increases when there is crowding, especially during epidemics. Asymptomatic nasopharyngeal infection is sufficient stimulus for the production of protective antibodies. Most people have antimeningococcal antibodies by adulthood.

SIGNS/SYMPTOMS: Meningococcal disease varies in severity, speed of onset, and organs involved. The most common clinical entities are meningitis, meningococcemia, or a combination thereof.

Meningococcal meningitis, after the neonatal period, is the 2nd most common cause of bacterial meningitis (2nd to H. influenza in childhood and 2nd to pneumococcus in adulthood). Meningitis is usually associated with meningococcemia. Meningitis may begin abruptly without warning or onset may be gradual. There may be an antecedent or concurrent URI. Refer to "Meningitis" chapter for signs and symptoms of meningitis in general and for standard laboratory evaluation of meningitis.

Meningococcemia: In mild cases, there is a viral–like illness: fever, chills, muscle and joint pains with spontaneous recovery within a few days. In some cases, this syndrome follows an unremarkable URI. In more serious cases, the preceding symptoms are the prelude to the development over 1–2 days of red macular and/or petechial lesions. Purpura may develop as the lesions coalesce. Meningitis may ensue. Hypotension may occur and further deterioration may lead to shock. Fulminant meningococcemia; Meningococcemia may manifest as an illness of sudden onset with rapid deterioration over a matter of hours. There is high fever, chills, prostration. Numerous coalescing petechiae appear (first on the limbs) followed by purpura. Septic shock ensues. Common complications are DIC, adult respiratory distress syndrome, myocarditis, hemorrhagic infarction adrenal gland (Waterhouse–Friderichsen syndrome). Protracted illness: Meningococcemia sometimes follows a chronic course with recurrent bouts of fever, chills, headache, arthralgias, and maculopapular rash. Meningitis is not an uncommon sequel in untreated cases.

Uncommon manifestations of meningococcic infection: pneumonia, arthritis, pericarditis, conjunctivitis, cervicitis, salpingitis, urethritis

LABORATORY: Gram stain of buffy coat may reveal gram–negative cocci if there is fulminant meningococcemia. Latex agglutination or counterimmunoelectrophoresis (CIE) test of CSF is positive in about 2/3 of those with meningococcal meningitis. A blood specimen will test positive in a fourth or less of those with meningococococcemia. Blood cultures are positive in about 2/3 of patients clinical ill with meningococcemia (with or without meningitis) and about 1/3 of those with clinical evidence of meningitis alone. Blood isolates are usually grown on a blood agar medium with 10% CO_2 at 3 atmospheres. Meningococcus, like other Neisseria, is oxidase positive. It is distinguished by metabolizing glucose and usually maltose, but not lactose. Gram stain and culture of sites of clinically apparent disease may be diagnostic (e.g. skin lesion scraping, CSF, sputum, joint, conjunctiva, cervix, anus). Laboratory evaluation of CSF: See "Meningitis" chapter for the characteristic laboratory findings of bacterial meningitis. If DIC is present, the prothrombin time is prolonged, platelets are decreased, and fibrinogen levels are low.

TREATMENT: Intravenous aqueous penicillin G is begun as soon as the diagnosis is suspected, and continued until the patient has been afebrile for 5–7 days. In an adult, the dose is 2 million units every 2 hours (refer to drug section for pediatric dose). Chloramphenicol is the alternative in the penicillin–allergic patient. Treatment of shock and ARDS are discussed in chapters entitled "Septic Shock" and "Adult Respiratory Distress Syndrome" respectively.

PROPHYLAXIS: Rifampin: A 2 day course is advised for close contacts (adult: 600 mg PO bid, 5–12 year: 10 mg/kg bid, 3–12 month: 5 mg/kg bid). Meningococcal vaccine may be advised to control epidemics, for travelers to epidemic region, or in certain cases for close contacts of meningococcal patient. The vaccine comes as monovalent or combined preparations of groups A, C, Y, and W–135.

Rickettsial Infections (infections by obligate intracellular

bacteria of the order Rickettsiales) include epidemic typhus, murine typhus, scrub typhus, Rocky Mountain spotted fever, Queensland tick typhus, African tick typhus, rickettsialpox, Q fever, trench fever. With the exception of Q fever, rickettsial infections are transmitted to man via an arthropod vector. Ricketsiae, with the exception of Q fever and rickettsialpox, have antigens in common with strains of proteus and this may be of diagnostic value (Weil–Felix reaction).

ROCKY MOUNTAIN SPOTTED FEVER is due to Rickettsia rickettsii. It is transmitted to man by a tick bite. The organism is perpetuated in ticks by transovarial transmission from one tick generation to the next. Mammals, especially rabbits and rodents, are bitten by ticks and are therefore also a reservoir. ●Despite the name, Rocky Mountain spotted fever is actually most common on the Atlantic seabord. Infections are restricted to the western hemisphere and occur from Canada to S. America. ●The clinical consequences are explained in part by the infection and injury to blood vessels that leads to formation of thrombi and occlusion. **Signs/symptoms:** Initial manifestations: 3–12 days after a tick bite; the typical patient experiences abrupt onset of an intense headache, photophobia, myalgias, chills, and fever. The temperature rises to 39–40° C within 2 days. Fever persists for 2–3 weeks. Rash appears within the first week—beginning on the wrists, ankles, palms, soles, and then spreading to the rest of the body. The rash is initially pink, macular, and blanches with pressure. It then darkens to form maculopapular lesions which subsequently become petechial. Petechiae may coalesce to form hemorrhagic lesions that may then ulcerate. Neurologic repercussions may include cranial nerve deficits, restlessness, delirium, seizures, coma. Complications include hypotension and shock; gangrene (e.g. fingers, nose, genitals); and bleeding (GI, renal, nose); pneumonia, DIC, brain damage. About 20% untreated patients die. **Laboratory:** Do not rely on serologic tests to make treatment decisions because it is crucial to begin antibiotic therapy early. Furthermore, the following diagnostic tests (based as they are on the body's antibody response) may not become positive until after the patient has been sick for about a week. Proteus OX 2 and OX 19 agglutinins appear in about a week but are also found in other rickettsial diseases. Indirect fluorescent antibody test may confirm the diagnosis. **Treatment** is begun as soon as the diagnosis is suspected. Delaying treatment to await diagnostic laboratory confirmation may be fatal. Treatment of choice is doxycycline or other tetracycline for 6 days. Chloramphenicol is the second best choice.

EPIDEMIC TYPHUS is due to Rickettsia prowasekii. The reservoir of infection is man. The body louse acquires the organism by biting an infected patient and then passes the infection on to a new human host. It is not the louse bite iiself that results in infection but the contamination of bite or other wound with louse feces or crushed louse. Human infection may also occur when airborne lice feces are inhaled. Lice are not the reservoir of infection. In fact, the louse dies soon after biting an infected patient. **Signs/symptoms:** Initial manifestations: 6–15 days following infection; the typical patient experiences rapid development of fever, malaise, myalgias, intense headache, and photophobia. The conjunctiva are injected. The patient becomes severely debilitated. Hot dry skin is characteristic. Temperature may reach 41° C. Without treatment, high fever persists for about 2 weeks and then declines. Pink macular rash that blanches on contact appears on the upper trunk after 4–7 days of fever. The rash subsequently spreads to the rest of the body—except for the face, palms, and soles which are only involved if there is exceptionally severe disease. The rash may then fade, or as a function of worsening disease progress thru additional stages: maculopapular → petechial → hemorrhagic. Bacterial pneumonia often ensues in untreated cases. Thrombosis–induced gangrene (e.g. fingers, nose) may develop. Neurologic repercussions may include cranial nerve deficits, tremor, delirium, stupor, coma. Hypotension with shock may occur. **Laboratory:** Proteus OX 19 agglutinins are present but the test is also positive in other rickettsial diseases. Other more specific serologic diagnostic tests are available. **Treatment** is with doxycycline (one–time dose of 200 mg PO) or other tetracycline.

Brill–Zinsser disease refers to the recrudescent disease that develops months to years following an untreated primary attack of epidemic typhus. Organisms apparently remain dormant within the host but may cause recurrent disease if immune defenses weaken. Brill–Zinsser disease is similar to epidemic typhus but is less severe and is of shorter duration. Rash is absent or fleeting. Treatment is the same.

ENDEMIC (MURINE) TYPHUS is due to R. mooseri (R. typhi). The organism is commonly found in rats and mice worldwide. The vector to man is the rat flea. Man acquires the infection, not from a flea bite, but from the flea's feces thru breaks in the skin. Infection may also occur by inhalation of flea feces. **Signs/symptoms:** After an incubation period of 6–14 days, the patient develops an illness similar to but less severe than epidemic typhus. **Laboratory:** Proteus OX 19 agglutinins are present but not specific. Other more specific serologic tests are available. **Treatment** is with doxycycline or other tetracycline until the patient is afebrile for 2–3 days.

SCRUB TYPHUS is due to Rickettsia tsutsugamushi. The disease occurs in south and east Asia, and in the west and south Pacific. The organism is perpetuated by transovarial passage from one mite generation to the next. Wild rodents bitten by chiggers (mite larva) also serve as a reservoir of infection. **Signs/symptoms:** <u>Local lesion at chigger bite site;</u> A painless papule frequently arises at the bite site. The papule subsequently blisters, breaks, and forms a scab. The lesion is accompanied by regional adenopathy. <u>Initial systemic manifestations</u> develop 6–21 days after the chigger bite with fever, intense headache, myalgias, malaise, conjunctival suffusion. The temperature may reach 40.5° C; fever persists for 2 weeks or longer in untreated cases. <u>Macular rash</u> often develops on the trunk 5–8 days after the start of fever and may spread to the extremities. The rash may then fade or progress to become maculopapular. <u>Respiratory involvement;</u> Cough is characteristic and pneumonia is common. <u>Splenomegaly and less often hepatomegaly</u> may occur. <u>Neurologic repercussions</u> may include restlessness, cranial nerve deficits, tremor, muscle twitching, delirium, stupor, seizures, coma. <u>Myocarditis</u> may develop. **Laboratory:** Proteus OX–K agglutinins are often detected. Indirect fluorescent antibody test is also diagnostic. **Treatment** is with doxycycline or tetracycline continued until the patient is afebrile for 1–2 days. Chloramphenicol is the second best choice.

Q FEVER is due to Coxiella Burnetii. Domestic animals (especially cattle, sheep, and goats) harbor the organism but are not ill. In these animals, C. burnetii is found in the milk, feces, urine, amniotic fluid, and in tissues—particularly the placenta. C. burnetii may also survive on soil, wool, clothing, or other fomites. Man is infected by inhaling the organism. Wild animals are also infected and the tick is the vector. Domestic animals perpetuate the organism amongst themselves without the tick vector or it may be acquired from the wild animal reservoir by a tick bite. **Signs/symptoms:** After an incubation period of 9–28 days there is a sudden onset of fever, intense headache, myalgias, malaise. Fever persists 1–3 weeks and may reach 40° C (104 F). The absence of rash distinguishes Q fever from other rickettsial diseases. In many cases, the liver is enlarged and tender. Serum liver enzymes may be elevated but jaundice is rare. Pneumonitis with a nonproductive cough develops in many cases. **Laboratory:** Diagnosis is usually confirmed by complement fixation test. In contrast to other rickettsial infections, Proteus agglutinins are not present. **Treatment** is with doxycycline or other tetracycline for 1 week. Chloramphenicol is the second best choice.

Lyme Disease is due to a spirochete, Borrelia burgdorferi. Species

of Ixodes ticks are the vector. The disease usually presents with a characteristic expanding skin lesion, erythema chronicum migrans (ECM). The immune response to the infection may subsequently provoke disease of the heart, nervous system, and/or joints. Disease of these organs is most likely to occur in those cases in which: (1) the total serum IgM is elevated, and (2) there are elevated levels of IgM–containing immune complexes and cryoglobulins.

Signs/symptoms: <u>Initial phase;</u> Starting three days to a month following a tick bite (of which the patient may be unaware), most patients will develop an expanding erythematous circular skin lesion (erythema chronicum migrans) in the area of the tick bite. The culpable spirochete can sometimes be cultured from the ECM lesion. Starting as a papule or macule, there is an enlarging erythematous patch (often with central clearing) that may reach several centimeters across before finally disappearing in about 4 weeks or so. In some cases, multiple red rings are seen within the periphery of the ECM lesion. Smaller secondary lesions may also develop. The regional lymph nodes are often found to be enlarged. Other manifestations may include fever, chills, malaise, fatigue, headache, stiff neck, myalgias, arthralgias, conjunctivitis, periorbital edema, malar rash, diffuse erythema. <u>Weeks to months following onset of the disease,</u> neurologic and/or cardiac complications develop in a minority of patients. Cardiac involvement might manifest as AV block or there may be evidence of myocarditis/pericarditis and possibly cardiomegaly. The cardiac valves are spared however. Possible neurologic consequences include meningitis (with CSF showing lymphocytic predominance), cranial neuropathy (e.g. Bell's palsy), peripheral neuropathy. <u>Rheumatic disease</u> develops in many patients. Migratory polyarthritis and tendinitis are the incipient manifestations. Weeks to many months later, a chronic episodic mono– or pauci–articular arthritis of the large joints (particularly the knees) may supervene.

Laboratory: <u>Serologic testing</u> for presence of anti–spirochete antibody with enzyme–linked immunosorbent assay (ELISA) or indirect immunofluorescent assay (IFA) may be diagnostic. However, the patient may not become seropositive for up to 6 months following exposure. Blood culture is sometimes positive early in the course of the disease. Culture of ECM lesion biopsy specimen is occasionally positive. CSF analysis of those with meningitis discloses about 100 lymphocytes/μl. The spirochete is occasionally cultured from the CSF. Synovial fluid from a swollen joint contains about 25,000 cells/μl, mostly neutrophils. Synovial fluid culture is unproductive.

Treatment: Early uncomplicated disease: ●Nonpregnant adults and children ≥ 8 yr may be treated with doxycycline 100 mg PO twice daily for 10–21 days, or tetracycline 250–500 mg PO 4 times/day for 10–21 days. ●Amoxicillin 250–500 mg PO 3 times/day for 10–21 days (20–40mg/kg/day divided tid in child) is an effective alternative and is the choice in pregnant or nursing mothers, or chidren < 8 yr. ●Erythromycin 250 mg PO 4 times/day for 10–21 days (30 mg/kg/day divided qid in child) may be used if the foregoing antibiotics are contraindicated or not tolerated. Patients with mild cardiac disease (e.g. 1st degree block with PR interval not exceeding 0.30 sec in absence of significant symptoms) are treated with with doxycycline, tetracycline, or amoxicillin as above. Patients with mild neurologic disease (e.g. Bell's palsy) are treated with doxycycline, tetracycline, or amoxicillin as above except that therapy is continued for 1 month. Patients with more than mild neurologic disease: IV penicillin G 20–24 million units/day (250,000–400,000 units/kg/day in child) for 10–14 days. Ceftriaxone (Rocephin) 2 grams/day IV (50–80mg/kg/day in child) for 14 days is alternative. Patients with more than mild cardiac disease are treated with IV penicillin G or IV ceftriaxone in the same dose as above for 10–21 days. High-dose prednisone is administered in conjunction with antibiotic if there is complete heart block with heart failure. Established arthritis is treated with one of following regimens: (1) doxycycline 100 mg PO twice daily for 1 month, (2) amoxicillin 500 mg PO 3 times/day for 1 month, (40 mg/kg/day in child), (3) IV penicillin G 20–24 million units/day (250,000–400,000 units/kg/day in child) for 14–21 days, (4) ceftriaxone (Rocephin) 2 grams/day IV (50–80mg/kg/day in child) for 14–21 days.

Typhoid Fever is usually due to Salmonella typhi. Salmonella paratyphi strains may also sometimes cause typhoid fever. The only source of infection is man: feces of asymptomatic carriers, or the feces or urine of a patient with active disease. Infection occurs when a person ingests contaminated food or water. The small bowel mucosa is invaded. Bacteria then disseminate via the lymphatics and thence via the bloodstream to reach and proliferate within the reticuloendothelial system (liver, spleen, bone marrow).

Signs/symptoms: After an incubation period (which varies inversely with the number of organisms ingested) of 1–3 weeks, bacteria are again released into the bloodstream. When this happens there is gradual onset of fever along with chills, headache, malaise, myalgias. Abdominal pain is common, frequently right lower quadrant. Constipation may be present. The temperature continues to rise for about 7–10 days, remains elevated for another 7–10 days, and then subsides over another week or so. Splenomegaly is often evident by the end of the 1st week. "Rose spots" (diagnostic red macular spots that blanch on pressure) frequently appear at the end of the 1st–beginning 2nd week. They are usually found on the abdomen and chest, and fade after 3–5 days. Delirium, obtundation, and coma may occur in severe cases. Cough and possibly pneumonia may develop. Diarrhea may develop during the 3rd week following fever–onset, and it is at this time that GI bleeding or perforation may occur. These GI complications result from the inflammation with ulceration that begins within the lymphoid follicles of the bowel wall. Recovery and possible relapse: The illness usually spends itself in about 4 weeks but relapse sometimes occurs, usually about 2 weeks following cessation of antibiotics. Relapse is less likely if the patient has not been treated with antibiotics.

Laboratory: Blood cultures will be positive in ≥ 90% cases during the 1st week of illness, but only 30–50% of untreated patients will be culture–positive by the 3rd and 4th week. Stool cultures are usually positive from the 2nd week of illness on (especially during 3rd–5th week) and 50% will continue to have positive stool cultures at 6 weeks even though the illness has resolved. Urine cultures will be positive by the third week in about a third of patients. Bone marrow cultures are positive in 90%, but are only obtained if blood or other cultures are negative and typhoid fever is still suspected. Tissue culture obtained from the rose spots is positive in 2/3 cases. Widal agglutination test becomes positive after the 2nd week but laboratory diagnosis should not rely on this alone because other nontyphoidal salmonella may cross–react.

Differential diagnosis: enteric fever due to other salmonellae, shigellosis, malaria, leptospirosis, brucellosis, rickettsial disease, tuberculosis, infectious hepatitis, mononucleosis, tularemia.

Treatment: Chloramphenicol is the drug of choice. Adult dose is 500 mg IV or PO every 4–6 hours. Dose is decreased as the patient improves. Treatment is continued for 14–21 days. Options if chloramphenicol is contraindicated or in the event of chloramphenicol resistance; ampicillin (adult dose is 1–2 gram IV q6h initially), amoxicillin (adults—500mg PO q6h for 14–21 days), sulfamethoxazole–trimethoprim (adults—800mg/160mg IV or PO bid for 14–21 days). Relapses are retreated with the same antibiotic unless there is drug resistance.

   Chronic carriers (i.e. positive stool cultures for ≥ 1 yr) usually have persistent infection of the gallbladder that seeds the gut. Sometimes, the gallbladder is sterile but there is persistent colonic infection. The carrier state is more common in women, persons over 50 yr, and those with gallbladder disease (e.g. gallstones, chronic cholecystitis). Chronic carriers are treated for 6 weeks with PO amoxicillin, ampicillin, or sulfamethoxazole–trimethoprim. If stool cultures are still positive after 6 weeks of antibiotics, chronic carriers with gallbladder disease should undergo cholecystectomy if continued shedding poses a health risk to the community (e.g. health or food workers).

Brucellosis is an infection that occurs worldwide but is uncommon in the U.S.

Brucella (a small gram–negative rod) mainly infects cattle, hogs, sheep, goats, dogs, caribou. Man acquires the organism: (**1**) by ingestion of unpasteurized milk or cheese, or infected meat; (**2**) thru breaks in the skin upon contact with the secretions/excretions of infected animals or their products; or (**3**) rarely by inhalation or conjunctival contact. **Signs/symptoms:** After an incubation period of usually about 2 weeks (range 1week–3 months), there is a sudden or insidious onset of fever which may reach 40° C, and is accompanied by chills, sweats, malaise. There may also be headache, cough, myalgias, arthralgias, diarrhea or constipation, lymphadenopathy, splenomegaly, hepatomegaly. Intermittent or remittent fevers and other manifestations continue for weeks or months, and there is usually weight loss. **Potential complications** are many and varied and include meningitis, encephalitis, neuritis, pneumonitis, lung abscess, pleural effusion, empyema, endocarditis, myocarditis, orchitis, epididymitis, pyelonephritis, cystitis, osteomyelitis, arthritis, blood dyscrasias, thrombophlebitis, cholecystitis. **Laboratory:** Diagnosis is usually confirmed with the brucella agglutination test. Cultures (e.g. blood, urine) may also be diagnostic but places lab workers at risk; precautions must be taken. WBC count is usually low to normal with absolute or relative lymphocytosis. **Treatment:** Adults are treated with tetracycline 500 mg PO 4 times/day for 4-6 weeks. In severe cases, streptomycin (1 gram IM once daily in adult) is given concurrently with tetracycline for the first 2 weeks. Rifampin may be added in resistant cases. Treatment is repeated if relapse occurs. Consider trimethoprim–sulfamethoxazole if tetracycline is contraindicated.

Leptospirosis is an uncommon disease in man. It is due to an obligate aero-

bic spirochete, Leptospira interrogans. Many animals, domestic and wild, may be infected, but in many cases they are not sick. They may excrete the organism in their urine for extended periods. Man is infected by ingesting contaminated water, or by skin or mucous membrane contact with the tissues or excretions of an infected animal.

   Signs/symptoms: After an incubation period of 1–2 weeks (range 2–20 days), the patient develops a fever which may reach 40°C (104°F) along with chills, headache, myalgias, conjunctival injection. Nausea, vomiting, and abdominal pain are common; diarrhea or GI bleeding are uncommon. There may be cough, pharyngitis, and /or lymphadenopathy. Sometimes there is a rash. Occasionally, the liver is enlarged and there may be jaundice. Splenomegaly is uncommon. The patient is usually well in 4–9 days. Aseptic meningitis: Most patients have CSF evidence of aseptic meningitis, and not uncommonly there is also clinical evidence of meningitis. CSF pleocytosis develops at the time serum antibodies to leptospirosis appear. Immune phase: After improving, some patients actually become sicker for 2–4 days (coincident with the appearance of serum antibodies) and then go on to recover. Weil's syndrome refers to a severe case of leptospirosis. Manifestations (in addition to those described above) may include severe jaundice; hematologic complications (e.g. thrombocytopenia, petechiae, purpura, hemorrhage); azotemia; altered consciousness. Leptospirosis may be fatal; the elderly or those with severe jaundice are the most susceptible.

   Laboratory: Indirect hemagglutination; a four-fold rise in titer is diagnostic. Culture (Fletcher's medium) of blood, urine, or CSF may be obtained but is usually of academic interest since growth may take weeks. Hematology; WBC count usually ranges from normal to up to 15,000 with neutrophils predominating. Leukocytosis sometimes reaches 50,000. Anemia and/or thrombocytopenia may occur. Sedimentation rate is elevated in about half the patients. Renal abnormalities: Proteinuria is common. Microscopy often reveals RBC's and WBC's. BUN may be elevated. Liver function: Serum direct bilirubin is elevated in the sicker patients but usually remains < 20 mg/dl. Moderate elevations of the SGOT and SGPT may also occur. CSF analysis: WBC count ranges from 10 to 1000 (usually < 500) with mononuclear predominance. The CSF glucose is normal and the protein is < 100 mg/dl. Chest x–ray may disclose infiltrates and/or an effusion.

   Treatment: Most cases are self–limited. However, recovery may be more rapid if an antibiotic is started within 4 days of the onset of illness. Doxycycline or tetracycline are the drugs of choice. Penicillin is a possibly effective alternative.

Plague

is due to Yersinia pestis, a gram–negative bacillus. Rodents are the reservoir of infection (e.g. rats, mice, and in the U.S. squirrels, prairie dogs). Infection is usually transmitted to man by a flea bite. Rarely, infection is acquired by eating infected tissue, or by inhalation of organisms from a coughing patient.

Bubonic plague begins suddenly 2–8 days after a flea bite with fever (rising to 38–41° C), chills, headache. Coincidentally or after a period of hours; enlarged, firm, and very tender lymph nodes called buboes appear—most frequently in the groin and less often in axillary, cervical, or multiple regions. Sometimes; a small skin lesion (e.g. papule, vesicle, eschar) is seen at the site of the flea bite in the region drained by the involved nodes. Vasculitis with ensuing thrombosis and vascular occlusion may lead to purpuric and then necrotic skin lesions. Spleen and liver may be enlarged and tender. Patient is usually debilitated, lethargic and may be restless or delirious. Untreated, over half of the patients die from septic shock in 3–5 days.

Pneumonic plague may be secondary to bubonic plague (due to hematogenous spread to the lungs) or rarely primary (due to inhalation of organisms). In either case there is high fever, dyspnea, purulent cough, hemoptysis. Serial x-rays confirm a rapidly worsening pneumonia. Untreated plague pneumonia is usually fatal within 48 hours.

Laboratory: Samples are obtained cautiously using aseptic technique with gloves. A blood–tinged needle aspirate of a bubo is obtained using a 10 ml syringe containing 1 ml of sterile saline to be injected and then withdrawn. The specimen is gram and Wayson stained; and cultured on blood agar, MacConkey's agar, and infusion broth. Blood and, if appropriate, sputum and CSF are also stained and cultured. With Wayson's stain, Yersinia pestis has a characteristic bipolar staining pattern (resembling a safety pin). WBC count ranges from 10,000–20,000 with neutrophils predominating.

Treatment: Antibiotic must be begun as soon as the diagnosis is suspected. Treatment must not be delayed for laboratory confirmation. Streptomycin 15 mg/kg IM twice daily for 10 days is the preferred therapy. Tetracycline or chloramphenicol are options. Chloramphenicol is the drug of choice if there is complicating meningitis. Patients with cough or pneumonia are isolated; routine aseptic precautions suffice in patients with uncomplicated bubonic plague.

Prophylaxis: A killed plague vaccine is recommended for travelers to endemic areas or for persons heavily exposed to wild rodents.

Tularemia

is due to Francisella tularensis, a small gram–negative pleomorphic aerobic bacillus. The reservoir of infection is wild animals, particularly rabbits. Infection is most commonly acquired by skin contact (thru a break in the skin or via hair follicle) with an infected animal, or from the bite of infected ticks or deer flies. Infection may also occur by eating contaminated food or water, or rarely by inhalation.

Ulceroglandular tularemia accounts for most cases. Incubation period is usually 2–4 days (range 1–10 days). A small papule, pustule, and then ulcer develops at the site of skin inoculation. The organism spreads to regional nodes which become enlarged and tender, and rarely may then suppurate and drain. Fever and chills usually develop. Untreated; fever continues for 3–4 weeks, the ulcer heals over several weeks, and nodes subside over a period of months. With antibiotic treatment, virtually all patients survive. Untreated ulceroglandular tularemia is fatal in about 5% cases. Secondary pneumonia sometimes occurs in untreated patients and markedly increases mortality.

Other tularemia syndromes: <u>Oculoglandular tularemia:</u> The eye becomes infected by contact (e.g. contaminated finger). Corneal perforation may ensue if untreated. <u>Primary pneumonia</u> follows inhalation of organisms. <u>Typhoidal tularemia</u> follows ingestion of organisms. There is cervical and mesenteric adenopathy with abdominal pain and ileus.

Laboratory: <u>Serology:</u> Four-fold rise in serum agglutinins is diagnostic (titers begin to climb in 7–10 days, peak 3–4 weeks). <u>Cultures:</u> Because of the risk to lab workers; cultures of blood, ulcer, or other sites is not advised unless special protective facilities are available. <u>Special stains</u> are needed to reveal the bacteria on microscopy. <u>WBC count</u> is usually normal. <u>ESR</u> is elevated.

Treatment: Gentamycin is begun as soon as the diagnosis is suspected and continued for 10 days. Patients need not be isolated since man–to–man transmission does not occur.

Prophylaxis: A live attenuated vaccine is available for individuals at high risk for infection. Infection confers immunity.

Nocardiosis

is due to Nocardia asteroides, a gram–positive and weakly acid–fast aerobic bacterium. The organism is found in soil and vegetation. Infection occurs by inhalation or sometimes by contamination of a skin wound. The disease occurs worldwide. About 3/4 patients are male. About half the patients are immunodeficient. When the immune system is impaired, nocardiosis progresses more rapidly and is more likely to disseminate. Nocardiosis is a suppurative disease that often leads to abscesses in involved organs.

Pulmonary infection is subclinical or transient in about a fourth the cases. Symptomatic patients typically develop fever and cough. Chest x-ray may disclose infiltrates, cavitation, lung abscess, empyema, fibrosis. Even the chest wall may be invaded.

Extrapulmonary infection usually occurs by bloodborne dissemination from the lung. Sometimes, hematogenous dissemination emanates from a primary focus of infection in the skin.

Dissemination may occur to any organ; particularly to the CNS but also not uncommonly to the skin, subcutaneous tissues, kidney, liver, lymph nodes. Dissemination to the CNS results in brain abscess, sometimes meningitis. About half the patients have no evidence of extrapulmonary involvement.

Laboratory: <u>Microscopic exam;</u> Nocardia are gram-positive and weakly acid-fast. Microscopic exam may reveal the bacteria as single coccobacilli or joined to form slender interlacing branching filaments. <u>Specimen sites;</u> Gram stain, acid-fast stain, and cultures are obtained of sputum and other involved sites. If necessary, stain and culture specimens may be obtained by trantracheal aspiration, bronchial brushing, or transbronchial biopsy. Blood, urine, CSF cultures may be obtained but the yield is low. <u>Culture media;</u> Because nocardial growth may not become evident for up to a week, standard bacterial cultures may be overgrown by contaminating bacteria by the time nocardial growth emerges. Therefore, fungal or mycobacterial culture media may be required to identify the organism.

Treatment: Sulfadiazine or sulfisoxazole are the drugs of choice. To hopefully prevent recrudescence, sulfonamide therapy is not stopped until at least 6 weeks after clinical cure is achieved. Antibiotic therapy is continued for 1 year in immunodeficient patients. Alternatives to sulfonamides are amikacin, chloramphenicol, minocycline. Abscesses, especially brain abscesses, often require surgical drainage.

Actinomycosis is due to species of actinomyces (e.g. Actinomyces israeli),

gram-positive anaerobes that normally inhabit the mouth, gut, and vagina. Actinomyces infection is not transmitted person-to-person. Actinomycosis is a chronic suppurative disease that in many cases occurs when tissue integrity is impaired. In the suppurative disease process, abscesses form and there is a surrounding granulomatous reaction with fibrosis. Infection spreads mainly by direct extension to adjacent tissues; hematogenous spread in unusual. Purulent draining sinuses form, The purulent material contains the diagnostic "sulfur granules" (see lab below).

Signs/symptoms: 4 clinical forms of actinomycosis are recognized. <u>Cervicofacial form</u> accounts for over half the cases. Gum disease, dental caries, or some other oral lesion is usually present. Disease is first noted when a hard, sometimes painless, swelling develops beneath the oral mucosa or under the skin (frequently near the jaw). The swelling subsequently softens in areas, and fistulas and purulent draining sinuses typically develop. The bacteria may invade the tongue, cheek, salivary glands, pharynx, larynx. Direct extension to and consequent osteomyelitis of the facial or cranial bones may occur. Further extension may involve the meninges and brain. <u>Thoracic form</u> is the consequence of aspiration, bacteremic spread, or direct extension from the cervicofacial or abdominal form. Mediastinal structures may be involved by contiguous spread from the lungs. Draining sinuses may perforate the chest wall. <u>Abdominal form</u> with involvement of the intestines and peritoneum typically develops weeks–months after GI perforation (e.g. ruptured appendix). Ensuing manifestations may include abdominal mass, GI obstruction, fistulas, sinuses draining thru abdominal wall. Extension to other intra-abdominal organs or lungs may occur, and there may be invasion of the pelvis or spine. Actinomycosis may arise in the pelvis from contamination of the endocervix; IUD's may favor this development. <u>Generalized form</u> is unusual and results from hematogenous spread with multiple organ involvement.

Laboratory: <u>Gram stain</u> of pus or infected tissue, or of crushed "sulfur granules" from these specimens reveals actinomyces as gram-positive branching filaments. <u>On H & E stain</u> the "sulfur granules" have basophilic centers from which radiate eosin-staining filaments with club-shaped ends. The granules range up to 1 mm in diameter. <u>Anaerobic cultures</u> may demonstrate the organism but overgrowth of other associated anaerobes may cause confusion.

Treatment: Penicillin is the preferred treatment. The response is slow and recurrences are not uncommon because penicillin penetrates the abscessed–fibrotic lesions poorly. Aqueous penicillin G (12–20 million units/day divided q4–6h in adult) is administered for 2–6 weeks. The patient is then switched to oral penicillin VK (1 gram PO qid in adult) which is continued for 12–18 months. Penicillin–allergic patients are treated with tetracycline, erythromycin, or clindamycin. Surgical drainage may also be required in selected patients.

Leprosy (Hansen's disease) is due to Mycobacterium leprae, an acid-fast bacillus.

The disease affects 11–20 million worldwide, mostly in the tropics. The mode of transmission is uncertain but it is probably the respiratory route via infected nasal secretions, and less often by skin contact. The incubation period is usually 3–5 years (range 6 months – many years). ●Progression of the disease depends on the hosts immunologic resistance. Most people are completely or partially resistant. The least resistant go on to develop lepromatous leprosy while the more resistant patients develop one of the less active forms of leprosy.

Clinical and histopathologic signs: <u>Indeterminate leprosy</u> represents an early stage of leprosy which may advance to one of the other forms of leprosy, but usually resolves spontaneously. Typically, one to four 1–5 cm reddened or hypopigmented macules are seen. Histology reveals a nonspecific inflammatory reaction. Acid–fast bacilli are seldom found. <u>Tuberculoid leprosy;</u> Characteristic finding is 1–3 well–defined reddened anesthetic dry hairless plaques or macules. Histology reveals a granulomatous reaction with epitheloid and Langhans giant cells and many lymphocytes. Acid–fast stain seldom reveals M. leprae. This form of leprosy sometimes resolves spontaneously. <u>Dimorphous (borderline) leprosy</u> forms are described with a spectrum of histologic and

382

dermatologic signs intermediate between tuberculoid and lepromatous leprosy. The disease may advance to the lepromatous type if the patient's immune defense is poor, or less commonly assume the tuberculoid form if there is more adequate immunity. Lepromatous leprosy: There are numerous widespread macules, papules, plaques, and/or nodules. Histology reveals so-called "foamy" histiocytes with a honeycomb–appearing cytoplasm containing many bacilli. There are few lymphocytes. With progressive disease there may be loss of eyebrows; enlarged earlobes, leonine facies (due to thickening of the skin), saddle–nose deformity (due to destruction of nasal cartilage). Lymph nodes may be enlarged and/or abscessed. Testicular involvement may lead to impaired spermatogenesis and gynecomastia. Eye disease may manifest as conjunctivitis, keratitis, and/or iritis. In advanced disease, the fingers and/or toes may destroyed as a consequence of the infection and the repeated inadvertent trauma to anesthetic digits.

Neurologic impairment: Involvement of the peripheral nerves reflects M. leprae's predilection for the cooler body areas. There may be sensory and/or sensorimotor loss. Examples include foot–drop, wrist–drop, claw hand, claw toes, lagophthalmos, glove and stocking anesthesia. ●Paradoxically, the most rapidly developing and often most severe neurologic deficits tend to occur in those patients with the greatest resistance (i.e. tuberculoid leprosy or the less active dimorphous cases). This is because these patients mount a more formidable inflammatory response that may lead to necrosis of involved nerves. For instance, a patient with tuberculoid leprosy may rapidly develop a foot drop due to destruction of the peroneal nerve. Pain characteristically accompanies the acute inflammatory process. ●By contrast, lepromatous cases undergo more widespread peripheral nerve disease with insidious progression over a period of years while suffering little pain and usually less functional impairment.

Diagnosis is confirmed by skin biopsy. The presence of an anesthetic skin lesion should arouse suspicion. Acid–fast stain of nasal mucosal scraping or acid-fast stain of the blood buffy coat may reveal the bacillus.

Treatment: Lepromatous leprosy and the more active dimorphous forms are treated with a combined triple drug regimen that is continued for at least 2 years. Regimen consists of dapsone (adult 100mg/day) plus rifampin (adult 600mg/day) plus clofazimine (adult 100mg/day). In order to reduce the cost of prolonged therapy, 600 mg rifampin may be administered just once a month. Indeterminate or tuberculoid forms are treated with a 2 drug combination consisting of dapsone plus rifampin. Dapsone (adult 100mg/day) is administered for at least 2 years and rifampin (adult 600mg/day) is administered for the first 6 months. In order to reduce the cost of therapy, a 600 mg dose of rifampin administered just once a month for 6 months is permissible.

Treatment reactions are of 2 types: erythema nodosum leprosum and reversal reactions. Erythema nodosum leprosum (ENL) occurs in the first year of therapy in over half the patients with lepromatous leprosy or the more active dimorphous cases. Multiple widespread painful papules or nodules develop over 1–2 days and this is accompanied by a fever. Other findings may include leukocytosis, neuritis, iritis, arthritis, orchitis, lymphadenitis, glomerulonephritis. Reversal reactions may develop in the tuberculoid and dimorphous forms of leprosy after months into the treatment course. The reaction is the consequence of the improved cell–mediated immune status that sets off an enhanced inflammatory reaction. Pre–existing skin lesions become reddened and edematous, and involved nerves may be severely and irreversibly injured by the inflammatory reaction. Treatment of treatment reactions: Mild cases of ENL or reversal reaction are treated with aspirin while severe cases are treated with corticosteroids (e.g. prednisone 60 mg once daily). ●Thalidomide (contraindicated in pregnancy or when contraception cannot be assured) is effective in severe cases of ENL but is not effective in reversal reactions. In severe cases, thalidomide may be combined with a corticosteroid initially and continued when the corticosteroid is discontinued. Thalidomide is then tapered over 2 weeks from the initial 200 mg twice daily dose to 50–100 mg/day maintenance with later attempts to discontinue the drug. ●Both ENL and reversal reaction respond to clofazimine (300 mg/day in adult) which in severe cases may also be initially combined with a corticosteroid.

Osteomyelitis may be initiated locally (e.g. wound, fracture, surgery, bite) or less commonly by hematogenous spread.

ACUTE HEMATOGENOUS OSTEOMYELITIS (AHO) is more common in children and the metaphysis of the long bones (most often the tibia or femur) is the most likely site of infection. In children, the epiphysis is generally spared because the growth plate acts as a vascular barrier. In infants < 18 months, arteries cross the growth plate so that the epiphyseal region and/or adjacent joint may be involved. In adults, blood vessels cross the area formerly occupied by the growth plate so that contiguous involvement of the metaphysis, epiphysis, and joint may occur. In adults, however, the vertebrae or pelvis are the most susceptible sites of hematogenous infection. **Pathogens:** Staph. aureus accounts for most cases of AHO. IV drug abusers are also susceptible to Pseudomonas aeruginosa. Sickle cell patients are also prone to infection by salmonella. In the aged, vertebral AHO is often due to gram–negative enteric bacteria. **Signs/symptoms:** Typically, there is abrupt onset of pain and tenderness of the involved bone, and the pain is aggravated by movement.

The region over the involved bone becomes swollen and reddened. There are fever and chills. <u>Vertebral AHO</u> typically develops in a more indolent and less obvious manner—e.g. days to weeks of dull back pain as the only complaint. Suspicion should be aroused if a patient presents with back pain and fever. There may be tenderness and calor over an involved vertebra and/or paravertebral spasm. Progression of the disease may lead to a paraspinous abscess with neurologic sequelae, and so a thorough neurologic exam is crucial. **Laboratory:** Leukocytosis and an elevated ESR are characteristic. Blood cultures are obtained and are positive in about half the patients. A technetium bone scan will help verify the diagnosis. X–rays will not reveal bone abnormalities for 2 weeks or more. Specimens for smears and culture are obtained by needle aspiration or open biopsy of the bone. Adjacent joints with evidence of effusion should also be aspirated for culture and smears. **Treatment:** Antibiotics are begun as soon as the diagnosis is suspected and continued for at least 6 weeks. Unless there is evidence to suggest otherwise, antibiotic therapy is directed against Staph. aureus while awaiting culture results—e.g. a penicillinase–resistant penicillin (methicillin, nafcillin, dicloxacillin) or a cephalosporin.

OSTEOMYELITIS SECONDARY to LOCAL INFECTION arises in a variety of circumstances including open fracture; local surgical contamination; cellulitis; overlying ulcer (e.g. due to vascular insufficiency, diabetes, decubitus ulcer); penetrating wound (e.g. human or animal bite); dental abscess. **Laboratory:** Cultures and gram stain are obtained from the adjacent infected site or by aspiration directly from the infected bone. An open biopsy specimen for culture may be needed to make the diagnosis. Blood cultures may also be useful. **Treatment:** <u>Antibiotic</u> choice depends on the clinical circumstances and gram stain findings, and may be modified later according to culture results. ●Antibiotic treatment of surgical and most trauma–related cases of osteomyelitis is initiated with antibiotics that cover S. aureus and gram-negative aerobic bacilli (e.g. E. coli, klebsiella, pseudomonas, proteus, enterobacter). ●Osteomyelitis resulting from decubitus ulcers is often due to anaerobes and gram–negative aerobic bacilli. ●Diabetic ulcer–associated osteomyelitis may also be due to anaerobes and gram–negative bacilli; or staphylococci or streptococci may be implicated. ●Osteomyelitis due to human or animal bites is treated with penicillin to cover oral flora. ●Similarly, an oral lesion–associated osteomyelitis (e.g. dental abscess–associated) is also treated with penicillin to cover anaerobes. <u>Debridement:</u> Antibiotics alone may be effective but debridement of dead tissue and abscess drainage are often required to effect a cure.

CHRONIC OSTEOMYELITIS may manifest insidiously, or it may follow untreated or unresponsive acute osteomyelitis infection. **Signs/symptoms:** There is a variable degree of pain, tenderness, and swelling at the site of infection. The overlying skin may be reddened. A draining sinus may open to the skin. Signs and symptoms may fluctuate in severity, or may be recurrent with intervening quiescent intervals sometimes lasting years. **Laboratory:** <u>X–rays</u> may reveal lucent areas (representing bone destruction) and/or areas of increased density (disclosing regions of bone undergoing necrosis). Rarely, a walled–off region of bone infection (Brodie's abscess) occurs and is seen as a lucent area. Tomograms, sinograms, and/or bone scans may further clarify the extent of disease. <u>Hematology:</u> Leukocytosis and an elevated ESR are inconsistent findings that reflect disease activity. As witness to the chronic disease, there may be normochromic normocytic anemia. <u>Culture and gram stain</u> specimens are obtained by needle biopsy or open biopsy. Cultures and gram stains of draining sinuses may be obtained but should be cautiously interpreted because skin contaminants may be included. **Treatment:** While awaiting laboratory confirmation, initial antibiotic treatment is directed against the most common pathogen—Staph. aureus. However, antibiotic therapy alone does not usually suffice. Abscesses must be drained; sequestra (areas of necrotic bone) must be removed. Surgery is followed by at least 6 weeks of antibiotic. When surgery is not successful or is not possible, a 3–6 month course of antibiotic may effect a remission and occasionally a cure.

TUBERCULOUS OSTEOMYELITIS is a chronic infection. The spine is the most commonly involved site (Pott's disease), usually the thoracic or lumbar spine. The infection usually arises in adults from reactivation of dormant bacilli which arrived at the vertebra by hematogenous or lymphatic dissemination earlier in life. Pott's disease (tuberculous spondylitis): The granulomatous inflammatory process destroys both the intervertebral disc (seen as narrowing of disc space on x-ray) and the adjacent vertebral bodies. Involvement of the thoracic spine may result in a hunchback deformity. Neurologic deficits may ensue from compression of the spinal cord and roots. The inflammatory process may extend to the paravertebral tissues and sometimes an abscess forms beneath the psoas fascia. Pus may then track down the length of the psoas muscle to point as a mass below the inguinal ligament. **Laboratory:** A needle biopsy or sometimes open biopsy is performed to obtain specimens for acid-fast stain, culture, and histology. **Treatment** is with antibiotics as outlined under "Tuberculosis". The advisability of surgical drainage is assessed individually.

Rabies is a lethal neurotropic viral disease of warm-blooded animals, princi-

pally carnivores (e.g. skunks, bats, raccoons, fox, dog, cats). The infection is usually acquired from a bite of an infected animal. Nonbite infection is also possible as when infected saliva or brain comes in contact with mucous membrane or an open wound. On rare occassions, rabies has resulted from inhalation of the virus in bat caves and from infected corneal transplant. **Pathogenesis:** Rabies virus initially replicate in the muscle in the region of inoculation. Virus then spread up peripheral nerves to the spinal cord and brain. Virus subsequently disseminate from the CNS along nerves. The virus is then frequently found in the saliva and sometimes in the urine and CSF. Microscopic exam of infected brain discloses perivasular infiltration by lymphocytes with edema and vascular engorgement. However, there is little apparent damage to the nerve cells. The pathognomic Negri bodies (intracytoplasmic eosinophilic inclusions) are seen within the neurons of infected animals and man at autopsy.

Signs/symptoms: The incubation period is 10 days to over a year (average 30-60 days). The duration of incubation in part reflects the time required for the virus to propagate and move along peripheral nerves before reaching the CNS. Consequently, a bite on the face will generally have a shorter incubation period than a bite on the foot. After the incubation, the patient typically develops malaise, headache, and fever. Paresthesias may occur in the region of the bite. There is progressive neuropsychiatric deterioration (e.g. restlessness, irritability, anxiety, confusion, agitation, neck stiffness, aberrant behavior, convulsions, paralysis, coma). Many patients develop painful spasms of the pharyngeal muscles so that they drool and are unable to swallow liquids (hydrophobia). In some patients, progressive paralysis is the salient feature. The infected animal may be well intially even though the saliva may contain the virus. A rabid animal may present with "furious" rabies (agitated aggressive behavior) or "dumb" rabies (progressive paralysis as the most conspicuous feature).

Laboratory confirmation of rabies in the patient is sometimes possible by detecting rabies antibody in the serum or CSF, or by fluorescent antibody stain of a skin biopsy specimen. Fluorescent antibody stain of the brain is the method used to diagnosis rabies in a suspected animal.

Indications for postexposure rabies prophylaxis: Exposure implies bites as well as nonbites in which the mucous membranes or wounds (e.g. cuts, abrasions) are exposed to potentially infectious material (e.g. saliva, brain rabid animal).

●If the suspected animal is apprehended but remains healthy after 10 days observation: If the animal appears healthy and its behavior is appropriate, it should be confined and observed for 10 days. Immune prophylaxis is not indicated if the animal is still asymptomatic after 10 days. This approach would, for instance, apply in the case of a bite by an apparently healthy but unvaccinated domestic dog or cat.

●If the suspected animal is apprehended and initially appears ill and/or is acting inappropriately, or becomes ill during 10 day observation period, it is sacrificed and sent to a laboratory for testing. Rabies immune prophylaxis is indicated if fluorescent antibody stain of the animal's brain confirms the diagnosis.

●Bite or non-bite exposure to domestic dog or cat who is rabid, suspected rabid, or whose condition is unknown (escaped): Rabies immune prophylaxis is advised.

●Bite or non-bite exposure to a bat, coyote, skunk, fox, raccoon, bobcat, or other wild carnivore: Rabies immune prophylaxis is advised.

●Rabbits and rodents (e.g. rats, mice, gerbils, guinea pigs, hamsters, chipmunks, squirrels) are rarely infected with rabies and have not been known to cause rabies in U.S.

●Other: Cattle, swine, horses, mules, goats, sheep are occasionally infected. Proceed as circumstances suggest.

Postexposure prophylaxis: Clean wounds thoroughly. Washing with soap and water inactivates the virus. Apply antiseptic (iodine, alcohol) after cleansing. Rabies immune globulin (RIG) is administered on day 0: 20 IU/kg (1/2 IM and 1/2 infiltrated about wound). Human diploid cell vaccine (HDCV) is also administered. The regimen in adults or children is 1 ml by intramuscular injection on days 0, 3, 7, 14, 21, and 28. The series may be discontinued if the suspected rabid animal remains healthy after 10 days observation or if fluorescent antibody testing of the animal's brain is negative. Patients who have received pre-exposure immunization and are up to date need only have HDCV injections on days 0 and 3. Tetanus prophylaxis as needed. Immunosuppressed patients should have blood drawn on day 28 of HDCV series to verify that an adequate level of rabies antibody (≥ 0.5 IU/ml) has been attained.

Pre-exposure immunization for persons at high risk of rabies exposure (e.g. veterinarian, animal handlers, animal control officer, certain lab workers, persons in countries where rabies is constant threat): rabies vaccine (HDCV) 1 ml IM on days 0, 7, 21. Persons at continued risk should receive a booster every 2 years.

Botulism
is due to one of 4 protein exotoxins (A, B, E, seldom F) each elaborated by a specific strain of Clostridium botulinum (a gram-positive anaerobic spore-forming bacterium). The exotoxin causes flaccid paralysis by preventing acetylcholine release at peripheral nerve endings.

Sources: Ingestion of preformed exotoxin: Exotoxin is produced by C. botulinum in improperly preserved foods—particularly homemade preserves of fruits, vegetables, mushrooms. Improperly prepared commercially canned foods is another possible source of exotoxin (e.g. mushrooms, vegetables, fish, beef, pork). In many cases the food does not appear spoiled and tastes normal. The exotoxin is a protein that resists digestion by GI enzymes and is absorbed. Infant botulism: In infants < 9 months of age, exotoxin may be produced by C. botulinum bacteria that have colonized the gut. Many of these cases arise from ingestion of raw honey contaminated with C. botulinum spores. Wound botulism resulting from production of exotoxin within a C. botulinum-contaminated wound is rare.

Signs/symptoms usually begin 24–48 hours following exotoxin ingestion. However, the interval between ingestion and onset of neurologic symptoms ranges between 2 hours and 8 days. The initial neurologic manifestations are due to involvement of the cranial nerves: dry mouth/throat; visual disturbances (e.g. diplopia, oculomotor weakness, difficulty focusing, sluggish or absent pupillary light reflexes); difficulty swallowing or talking. There may be nausea, vomiting, diarrhea, and abdominal pain. In severe poisoning, there is bilateral descending motor weakness with ensuing flaccid paralysis that quickly spreads to the limbs and trunk. Muscles of respiration are involved, and the patient may become dyspneic and require ventilatory support. In some cases, innervation of the smooth muscle of the bladder and intestines is compromised so that urinary retention and ileus ensue. There are no sensory deficits. Consciousness is not impaired until the terminal stage. Patients are afebrile. Patients who have ingested smaller amounts of botulinum toxin may only be mildly symptomatic. Signs of Infant botulism may include "floppiness", weak cry, poor suck, failure to thrive.

Laboratory: Diagnosis is confirmed by intraperitoneal injection of patient's serum, extract of patient's stool, or extract of suspected food into mice to observe the effect. As a control, the test is also performed in mice who are given antitoxin. ●The stool or suspicious food is also cultured for C. botulinum.

Treatment: Supportive measures are instituted as clinical circumstances dictate. Assisted ventilation may be necessary. Gastric lavage and cathartics are recommended in order to clear the gut of any unabsorbed toxin. Trivalent antitoxin (A, B, E) is usually administered. Adult dose is one vial IV and one vial IM. An additional vial IV is given in 4 hours if there is further deterioration and may be repeated in 12–24 hours if necessary. The antitoxin is a serum from immunized horses. Consequently, equine sensitivity testing is advised prior to administration. If the patient proves to be hypersensitive and the antitoxin is deemed essential, a desensitization injection protocol is followed starting with dilute subcutaneous injections. The clinician must be prepared to treat anaphylaxis.

Tetanus ("lockjaw") is due to an exotoxin produced by Clostridium tetani—
a gram–positive motile sporulating anaerobic bacillus. The bacteria are found in soil, and in animal or human feces. Spores may remain viable for years. **Pathogenesis:** When the spores are introduced into a wound with favorable anaerobic conditions, they germinate into vegetative bacteria that produce the exotoxin (tetanospasmin). Tetanospasmin is carried by the bloodstream to the peripheral motor nerves where it travels up the axons to the motor cell bodies. Tetanospasmin is subsequently released into the synaptic gap and then enters the presynaptic endings of inhibitory interneurons where it binds to gangliosides. This serves to block release of an inhibitory transmitter. Without the inhibitory transmitter, there is unrestrained firing of the motor neurons with consequent muscle spasms.

Signs/symptoms: The first complaint is generalized or localized stiffness. Jaw stiffness is a particularly common initial symptom. The more severely affected patients typically go on to develop trismus ("lockjaw"), risus sardonicus (characteristic fixed sneering grin due to facial spasm), and dysphagia. Spasm of the neck, back, abdomen, and limbs may be observed. Spasm of the neck and back muscles may be severe enough to cause opisthotonus. Spasm of the larynx, intercostals, and/or diaphragm may interfere with ventilation. In severe cases, tetanospasmin affects the autonomic nerves (e.g. hypertension, perspiration, elevated temperature, tachycardia, arrhythmias).

Treatment: In mild cases, diazepam 10 mg q3–4h IV or PO may suffice to relax stiff muscles and relieve spasm. Protect the airway. If there is dysphagia or respiratory difficulty, the patient should be intubated under general anesthesia in conjunction with a paralyzing agent. If after intubation, spasm of the respiratory muscles prevents adequate ventilation, the patient should be paralyzed with a curariform drug (e.g. pancuronium) and mechanically ventilated. IV diazepam is administered to relieve anxiety. Alpha or beta blocking drugs may be needed to control autonomic–induced aberrations in blood pressure and heart rate. Human tetanus immune globulin (1000 units IV and 2000 units IM) is administered to neutralize the tetanospasmin that has not yet entered the nerves. Tetanus toxoid (0.5 ml IM) is administered since clinical disease does not confer immunity. The injection should be given in a limb other than the one in which the immune globulin is injected. The patient should then go on to receive 2 additional injections (the first 4–6 weeks after the initial injection and the last a year later) and a booster every ten year thereafter. Possible sites of Clostridium tetani infection should be treated (e.g. clean wounds) after tetanus immune globulin has been given. Antibiotic (e.g. penicillin, erythromycin) is administered to eradicate C. tetani.

Tetanus prophylaxis in wound management:

Minor superficial wound that is clean:
- 0–2 prior tetanus toxoid doses or uncertainty: tetanus toxoid 0.5 ml IM.
- 3 or more prior tetanus toxoid doses: tetanus toxoid required only if last injection was over 10 years ago.

All other wounds:
- 0–1 prior tetanus toxoid doses or uncertainty: tetanus toxoid (0.5 ml IM) in one limb and tetanus immune globulin (250 units IM) in another limb.
- 2 prior tetanus toxoid doses: tetanus toxoid is administered. Tetanus immune globulin (250 units IM in another limb) is also required if the last tetanus toxoid injection was over 2 years ago.
- 3 or more prior tetanus toxoid doses: tetanus toxoid required only if last injection was over 5 years ago.

Routine prophylaxis: see "Routine Immunizations".

Routine Immunizations

Key to abbreviations: DPT (diptheria toxoid, killed pertussis, tetanus toxoid); Td (tetanus toxoid, reduced dose diptheria toxoid); OPV (oral polio vaccine); MMR (measles, mumps, rubella); HbCV (Haemophilus b conjugate vaccine).

Primary Immunization Schedule:
- 2 months of age: DPT–1, OPV–1
- 4 months of age: DPT–2, OPV–2
- 6 months of age: DPT–3, (OPV optional; it is given in areas where polio is endemic)
- 12 months of age: tuberculin skin test at this time or at 15 months of age.
- 15 months of age: DPT–4, OPV–3
- 18 months of age: HbCV
- between 4 yr & 7th birthday: DPT–5, OPV–4 preferably at or before entering school.
- between 14 & 16 years of age: Td (tetanus toxoid with reduced diptheria toxoid).
- every 10 years thereafter: Td (tetanus toxoid with reduced diptheria toxoid).

Interval between OPV doses: In order to avoid interference, the dose interval should not ordinarily be less than 6–8 weeks.

Comments regarding 15 month visit: If at least 6 months has not elapsed since DPT–3, give OPV and MMR now and wait until the recommended 6 months has elapsed before giving DPT–4. If the patient has received < 3 DPT's and < 6 weeks have elapsed since the last DPT or OPV, give MMR now and administer DPT–4 and OPV–3 at 18 months of age or at least wait until the recommended 6 weeks have elapsed.

HbCV (Haemophilus b conjugate vaccine) is administered at 18 months even if there is history of invasive Haemophilus b disease because infection prior to 24 months of age does not usually induce an immune response.

Child less than 7 year of age not immunized at recommended times:
- First visit:
  - patient 2–14 months of age: DPT–1, OPV–1
  - patient ≥ 15 months of age: DPT–1, OPV–1, MMR
  - patient ≥ 18 months of age: DPT–1, OPV–1, MMR, HbCV*.
- 2 months later: DPT–2 and OPV–2
- 2 months later: DTP–3
- 6–12 months after DPT–3: DPT–4 and OPV–3
- between 4 yr & 7th birthday: (preferably at or before entering school): DPT–5 and OPV–4. This visit is not necessary if DTP–4 and OPV–3 have been given after the 4th birthday.
- between 14 & 16 years of age: Td (tetanus toxoid with reduced diptheria toxoid).
- every 10 years thereafter: Td (tetanus toxoid with reduced diptheria toxoid).

If immunization is begun before reaching first birthday, give DPT–1, 2, and 3; and OPV–1 and 2 according to the above schedule. Give MMR when the child reaches 15 months and HbCV at 18 months. Tuberculin skin test is performed at 12 months or earliest opportunity thereafter.

* HbCV (Haemophilus b conjugate vaccine) is administered at 18 months (or as soon as possible thereafter) even if there is history of invasive Haemophilus b disease because infection prior to 24 months of age does not usually induce an immune response. However, HbCV is not indicated if there is a documented history of invasive Haemophilus influenza infection after 24 months of age; nor is it indicated in children ≥ 5 year of age.

Child ≥ 7 year of age not immunized at recommended times:
- First visit: Td–1, OPV–1, MMR, tuberculin skin test.
- 2 months later: Td–2, OPV–2
- 6–12 months after Td–2: Td–3, OPV–3
- between 14 & 16 years of age, and booster every 10 years thereafter: Td.

Routine immunization of person ≥ 18 yr of age never immunized: Give Td according to the schedule immediately above. OPV is not routinely given but is advised if traveling to endemic area. Persons born before 1957 are considered immune to measles and mumps. Rubella vaccination may be considered in unimmunized persons, especially unimmunized women of childbearing age. Either the individual rubella vaccine or MMR may be used. Remember that rubella vaccination is contraindicated during pregnancy and should be avoided for 3 months post vaccination.

NOTES ON IMMUNIZATION PREPARATIONS:

DPT (diptheria toxoid, killed pertussis vaccine, tetanus toxoid) should only be used up to the 7th birthday because pertussis immunization is not recommended after the 7th birthday. Older children and adults should receive Td (tetanus toxoid with reduced diphtheria toxoid for adults). Other DPT contraindications are: active infection, history of serious adverse reaction, evolving neurologic disorder, concurrent immunosuppressive therapy (irradiation, corticosteroids, cytotoxic agents). Side effects: fever; malaise; injection site effects (tenderness, erythema, induration); rare reactions to pertussis component (severe fever, convulsions, encephalopathy, uncontrollable screaming, shock, thrombocytopenia, hemolytic anemia).

DT (diptheria toxoid, tetanus toxoid) is indicated for active immunization up to 7th birthday when pertussis vaccine is contraindicated (e.g. history of pertussis or severe reaction to DPT).

Td (tetanus toxoid with reduced diphtheria toxoid for adults) contains a fraction of diptheria toxoid found in the pediatric preparations (DPT, DT) and does not contain pertussis vaccine. Td is indicated for immunization of individuals 7 yr and older. A person who has not been previously immunized should receive 3 injections (the 2nd 4–6 wks after the 1st and the 3rd 6–12 months later) and a booster every ten year thereafter. Contraindication: history of serious side effects. Side effects: fever; malaise; injection site effects (tenderness, erythema, induration).

MMR (measles, mumps, rubella) vaccine (M–M–R II) contains live attenuated viruses that provide active immunity by producing a mild or subclinical infection. The vaccine is given to persons 15 months or older as a one time injection. A booster is not necessary. Infants < 15 months may be vaccinated if the risk of measles infection is increased, or if it is anticipated that vaccination may be logistically impossible in the future. However, it must be realized that residual maternal antibodies may prevent immunization. Therefore, children vaccinated prior to 1 yr of age should be revaccinated at 15 months if possible. Contraindications: pregnancy (and avoid pregnancy for 3 months post vaccination), any active febrile infection; active untreated Tb; blood dyscrasias; leukemia; lymphoma; malignant neoplasia affecting bone marrow or lymphatic system; history of hypersensitivity reaction to eggs or neomycin. Patients with primary immunodeficiency or patients receiving immnunosuppressants (e.g. antineoplastics, corticosteroids) should not ordinarily receive MMR. However, MMR is not contraindicated if a corticosteroid is for replacement therapy (e.g. Addison's disease). Comments: ●Warn woman of potential risk to fetus if pregnancy should occur within 3 months of vaccination. ●Delay vaccination for 3 months following administration of blood or blood products containing immunoglobulin. ●Vaccine may temporarily suppress tuberculin skin sensitivity. If tuberculin testing is anticipated, it should be done prior to or simultaneously with vaccination. Side effects include injection site effects (pain, erythema, induration, wheal and flare); rash; urticaria; malaise; fever; sore throat; headache; nausea; vomiting; regional adenopathy; arthralgias; arthritis; parotitis; orchitis; nerve deafness; polyneuritis; optic neuritis; thrombocytopenia; purpura.

Polio vaccine, live oral trivalent [Sabin strains 1,2,3] (Orimune) is a mixture of three live attenuated polio virus strains that induce active immunity by simulating natural polio infection. Infection is communicable and may confer immunity in nonvaccinated contacts. Indications: infants starting at 6–12 wks of age, unimmunized persons thru 18 yr of age. Contraindications: pregnancy (unless immediate protection is essential); during acute illness; advanced debilitated condition; persistent vomiting/diarrhea; immune deficiency disease; altered immune status (e.g. thymic abnormality, leukemia, lymphoma, generalized malignancy, corticosteroid therapy, radiation therapy, antineoplastic drugs); person being considered for immunization has household contacts who are immunodeficient. Comments: ●Inactivated polio vaccine (see below) is the preferred polio vaccine for immunocompromised patients and their contacts. Patients with altered immune status should avoid close contact with recipients of live oral polio vaccine for at least 6–8 weeks. ●Polio vaccine is ineffectual against incubating or existing polio infection. ●During an epidemic, live oral polio vaccine should be administered to all persons over 6 wks of age (with exception of immunocompromised patients who may be given the inactivated vaccine). ●Polio vaccine may be administered at birth in certain endemic tropical regions. However, since a dose of polio vaccine given before 6 weeks of age does not count toward the standard 3-dose primary immunization schedule, the infant should go on to receive the usual full immunization schedule starting 6–8 wks after the neonatal dose. ●Persons ≥ 18 yr of age do not require routine polio immunization. If an unimmunized adult is at increased risk (e.g. travel to endemic area), then inactivated polio vaccine is preferred. If protection is required in less than 4 weeks, then live oral polio vaccine may be administered and the series completed if increased risk continues. ●Even though immune serum globulin does not seem to interfere with oral polio vaccine, it is best to revaccinate in 3 months if immune serum globulin has been administered at about the same time as oral polio vaccine. Side effects: paralysis rarely.

Polio vaccine, inactivated trivalent (Salk) is an inactivated (killed) virus preparation that provides active immunity to recipient. Indications: (1) unimmunized person ≥ 18 yr of age at risk (e.g. travel to endemic area), (2) immunocompromised patient and their household contacts. Schedule: Primary series consist of 3 IM injections: the 2nd 4–8 weeks after the first, the 3rd 6–12 months after the 2nd. A booster is given to children 4–6 yr of age but is not routinely necessary thereafter. Persons traveling to developing countries receive an additional dose. See "Recommendations for Travelers for more information on administration.

Recommendations for Travelers

Travelers's diarrhea is most often due to enterotoxigenic E. coli. Other causes include salmonellae, shigellae, Campylobacter jejuni, Vibrio parahaemolyticus, Rotavirus, Norwalk virus, Giardia, Entamoeba histolytica. Measures recommended to avoid traveler's diarrhea include avoidance of undercooked meats and fish, raw vegetables and fruit (unless peeled by the traveler), unpasteurized milk or milk products, unboiled water (except water treated with tincture of iodine). Canned or bottled carbonated beverages pose no risk. Ice is not risk–free. Antibiotic prophylaxis is not generally recommended although trimethoprim/sulfamethoxazole, trimethoprim alone, or doxycycline are effective. These agents are also effective in reducing the duration of diarrheal illness. Antimotility drugs (e.g. Lomotil) may be used to relieve diarrhea but must not be used if there is bloody stools or high fever, and must not be used for more than 48 hours.

Prevention of insect–borne infections: Risk may be reduced by wearing protective clothing and applying insect repellent. The best insect repellents contain deet (N, N diethylmetatoluamide) and those with the highest concentrations of deet provide the longest protection. Additional measures include screened living quarters, mosquito nets while sleeping, pyrethrum–containing insect spray.

Diptheria, tetanus, and pertussis immunization: Unimmunized or partially immunized persons < 7 yr of age should receive DPT while those ≥ 7 yr should receive Td. See "Routine Immunizations" chapter.

Polio is prevalent in developing countries. Individuals < 18 yr should if possible complete the standard 3-dose primary series of oral polio vaccine (see "Routine Immunizations" above) prior to arrival in an endemic area. Those who have completed the 3-dose primary series should receive (assuming that at least 6 weeks has elapsed since the last dose) a single OPV booster prior to departure. If never immunized and time allows, the 3 doses should be given at least 6–8 week intervals. If the 3 doses cannot be given in time, administer 2 doses if possible (or at the very least give a single dose prior to departure) and complete the series at the earliest opportunity. Those who have been partially immunized should complete the 3-dose series. Infants < 6 weeks of age: Ordinarily OPV is not recommended prior to 6 weeks of age although a dose may be given prior to 6 weeks of age or even at birth if the risk of exposure is increased. However, a dose of OPV given prior to 6 weeks of age does not count toward the standard 3-dose primary OPV series. Infants who have received OPV prior to 6 weeks of age and who remain in an area of increased risk are given the first dose of the standard 3-dose primary series no sooner than 4 wks after the neonatal dose followed at 4 week intervals by the 2nd and 3rd doses. Infants who have received OPV prior to 6 weeks of age and who have left an area of increased risk are given the first dose of the standard 3-dose primary series 6 wks after the neonatal dose followed by the 2nd dose 6 weeks later and the 3rd dose 8–12 months after the 2nd. Individuals ≥ 18 yr: Those who have never been immunized should receive 3 doses of inactivated polio vaccine (IPV): 4–8 week interval between IPV-1 and IPV-2, and 6–12 months between IPV-2 and IPV-3. If < 8 weeks but > 4 weeks is left before departure, give 2 doses of IPV separated by at least 4 weeks. If < 4 weeks is left before departure, give a single dose of IPV. Incompleted series should be completed as scheduled if increased risk persists. Those who have previously completed either an OPV or IPV primary immunization series should receive a single booster dose of either OPV or IPV. Those who have only received part of the OPV or IPV primary immunization series should receive the remaining OPV or IPV doses irrespective of when the last dose was given. Immunocompromised children and adults should receive IPV as just outlined.

Measles, mumps, and rubella: see "Routine Immunizations" chapter.

Malaria prophylaxis is advised when traveling to endemic regions of Africa, Middle East, Indian subcontinent, S.E. Asia, Oceania, Central and S. America. See "Malaria" chapter for drug prophylaxis recommendations.

Yellow fever vaccination is advised for persons traveling to endemic regions of Africa and S. America. A certificate of vaccination is required of persons entering an endemic country from another endemic country. Some African countries require proof of vaccination from all entering persons regardless of origin.

Hepatitis A is prevalent in developing countries. Prophylaxis consists of immune globulin 0.02 mg/kg IM for persons whose stay is < 3 months. The dose is 0.06

mg/kg every 5 months for prolonged visits. Serology to determine if hepatitis A antibodies are present may make repeated injections unnecessary.

Hepatitis B is also prevalent in developing countries. Vaccination is advised for health care workers, and for persons whose visit will exceed 6 months or who will have close contact with local population. Two equally effective types of vaccine are available (hepatitis B carrier plasma–derived and recombinant DNA). The complete vaccination series consists of 3 IM doses as follows: 1st dose, 2nd dose a month later, 3rd dose 6 months after 1st. Some immunity will develop even if there is only sufficient time to give 1 or 2 injections.

Other vaccines (e..g. cholera, typhoid, typhus, plague, rabies, meningococcus) may be advised when traveling to certain high risk regions.

Fungi

Candidiasis
Histoplasmosis
Coccidioidomycosis
Cryptococcosis
Aspergillosis
Blastomycosis
Paracoccidioidomycosis
Mucormycosis

Note: "Superficial Fungal Infections" are presented in Skin Disease section.

Candidiasis (fungal disease resulting from various species of Candida). C. albicans, the most common candidal pathogen, is a normal and common commensal of the mouth, gut, and vagina. Candida species are also normally found on the skin. ●Settings favoring overgrowth of Candida include diabetes mellitus; systemic antibiotic therapy; and impaired immunity (e.g. corticosteroid or other immunosuppressant therapy including chemotherapy, lymphoreticular neoplasia, AIDS). Pregnancy or oral contraceptives predisposes to candidal vaginitis.

Cutaneous candidiasis has a predilection for warm moist intertriginous areas (axillae, under the breast folds, groin, gluteal folds, between toes). Typically, there are moist or dry scaling red patches with well-defined borders surrounded by red papular or pustular lesions (satellite lesions). Disclosure of single-budding yeast on microscopic exam of KOH preparation taken from a skin scraping is diagnostic. Treatment: topical agents—e.g. miconazole, nystatin, clotrimazole (see drug section).

Chronic mucocutaneous candidiasis is a rare and usually familial form of candidiasis that is associated with impaired cell–mediated (T cell) immunity and is frequently associated with endocrine disease (e.g. diabetes mellitus, hypoparathyroidism, hypothyroidism, adrenal insufficiency). The Candida skin test is negative in most cases. Patients may develop candida granuloma (thick crusted pustular lesions) of the skin, esophagitis (possibly leading to stricture), oral and nasal mucosal lesions (which may cause difficulty with eating or speech). Concurrent skin infection with dermatophytes is common. The disease also often involves the conjunctiva and cornea. Topical and/or systemic (amphotericin B) therapy gives only partial or temporary improvement.

Thrush: refer to "Stomatitis" chapter.

Esophagitis is usually the result of spread of mucosal infection from the mouth in a patient who is immunosuppressed or receiving systemic antibiotics. Typically, there is retrosternal pain that is aggravated by swallowing. Treatment: nystatin oral suspension 5 ml PO 4 times/day.

Vaginitis: refer to "Vaginitis" chapter.

Candida cystitis: If cystitis is the consequence of an indwelling Foley catheter, just removing the catheter may be curative. If a catheter is imperative or if cystitis is not catheter–related, treatment consists of amphotericin B bladder irrigation or IV amphotericin B. Oral flucytosine is an alternative in patients without an indwelling catheter.

Systemic Infection may be associated with endocarditis (see below); renal involvement (e.g. pyelonephritis, papillary necrosis, obstruction), skin involvement (nodular skin lesions); eye involvement (endophthalmitis); meningitis; osteomyelitis; arthritis; pneumonitis (rare). Abscesses may form in the brain, liver, spleen, myocardium, thyroid. Diagnosis of systemic candidiasis is confirmed by cultures (blood, CSF). Urine culture may be obtained but does not differentiate cystitis from kidney involvement. Stains of biopsy specimens from involved organs may also establish the diagnosis.

Candida endocarditis is usually seen in the setting of chronic indwelling IV catheter, IV drug abuse, or prosthetic cardiac valve. The valvular vegetations tend to be large (which is revealed on echocardiogram) and friable (and therefore often embolize to major vessels). Strokes commonly ensue from embolization. Treatment includes valve replacement as well as drug therapy (IV amphotericin B in conjunction with oral flucytosine).

Histoplasmosis is due to the fungus, Histoplasma capsulatum. In the US; infection is very common in the Mississippi, Missouri, and Ohio River valleys. The organism is found as a saprophyte in the soil. The fungus may also be found in bird excrement and on the feathers, but birds are not actually infected. Bats, however, may be infected and shed the organism from GI ulcers. Infection occurs when the spores are inhaled. Histoplasmosis is not contagious. Reinfection can occur.

Primary infection is usually either asymptomatic or causes a self–limited respiratory illness with fever, headache, malaise, myalgias, cough, pleuritic chest pain. Auscultation of the chest is generally normal although the chest x-ray may show an infiltrate and hilar adenopathy. Healing may be associated with the formation of a Ghon complex (pulmonary and hilar calcification). Additional possible manifestations include pericarditis, joint pain, widespread rash, erythema nodosum, erythema multiforme.

Disseminated infection may follow the primary infection or be due to reactivation of a dormant infection in an immunocompromised patient. Characteristic findings include fever, weight loss, lymphadenopathy, hepatomegaly, splenomegaly. Sometimes there is ulceration of the nasal, oral, and/or pharyngeal mucosa. GI ulceration may also occur and result in bleeding, perforation, obstruction. Other possibilities include endocarditis, meningitis, adrenal insufficiency.

Chronic pulmonary infection is most common in patients with COPD. The infection may resolve spontaneously with residual scarring or may progress with further necrosis and cavity formation as in tuberculosis.

Laboratory: In pulmonary disease; obtain sputum cultures and sputum stain (e.g. PAS, Giemsa, methenamine silver). In disseminated infection; cultures may be obtained from various sites as clinical circumstances suggest—e.g. of the blood, urine, oral ulcer, lymph node, CSF, bone marrow, liver. Stains of the sputum, ulcer, buffy coat of the blood, etc. may also disclose the organism. Histoplasmin skin test is not diagnostic because the test is so often positive in the population of endemic regions. Serologic tests are not ideal because both false-positives and false-negatives are not uncommon. The complement fixation test with titer ≥ 1:32 or a fourfold rise in titer, or the latex agglutination test with titer ≥ 1:16 may help in the diagnosis.

Treatment: Most primary infections are self–limited and require no treatment. Chronic pulmonary cavitary disease or disseminated infection is treated with IV amphotericin B (refer to drug section).

Coccidioidomycosis (valley fever) is due to the fungus Coccidioides

immitis. Infection is endemic in the southwestern U.S. (particularly California's San Jaoquin Valley) and contiguous Mexico. Infection also occurs in certain regions of Central and S. America (e.g. Chaco area of Argentina). The organism is a soil saprophyte and infection is acquired by inhaling arthrospore–containing dust. Animals may also become infected and become ill. The disease is not contagious. Infection confers immunity; a positive skin test gives almost complete assurance of protection against reinfection.

Primary pulmonary infection is subclinical in over half the cases. Most symptomatic patients develop a flu–like self–limited respiratory illness with fever, chills, cough (which may be productive), and pleuritc pain. Auscultation of the chest is often unremarkable although there may be scattered rales. There is leukocytosis, often with eosinophilia. Skin/joint manifestations: Joint pains with erythema nodusum or erythema multiforme sometimes occurs. Occasionally, there is a measles–like exanthem. Pneumonia may develop and infiltrates with hilar adenopathy are seen on x–ray. Occasionally there is a pleural effusion. Pneumonia is sometimes prolonged and may heal leaving x–ray evidence of scarring (fibrosis, calcification, bronchiectasis). Pulmonary cavitation is seen in some cases. The cavities (usually one) may remain after clinical illness resolves. However, they are usually asymptomatic and often close within 4 years without therapy. Chronic tuberculosis–like pulmonary infection may develop (e.g. formation of nodules, cavitation with hemoptysis).

Disseminated infection is most likely in blacks, Filipinos, pregnancy, and immunocompromised patients. Dissemination may occur to the skin, bones, joints, meninges, brain, kidneys, liver, spleen, lymph nodes, adrenals, prostate, thyroid.

Laboratory: Coccidioidin skin test usually becomes positive 10–21 days after infection, but will usually be negative in disseminated disease or chronic progressive pulmonary infection. Microscopic exam of a KOH preparation: Diagnosis is confirmed by finding the characteristic spherules that contain many endospores. Any of the following may be examined as clinical findings suggest: sputum, gastric washing, CSF, pleural fluid, abscesses, skin lesions, or biopsy specimen. Standard fungal cultures of these sites may also be obtained. However, caution is advised since the mycelial growths are highly infectious. Culture of urine (first void morning specimen) or bone marrow may also identify the organism. Blood cultures are seldom positive except when the patient is near death. Serologic testing: IgM antibody levels rise first and peak 2–3 weeks after the onset of symptoms. IgG levels subsequently rise. IgM may be detected by latex agglutination, precipitin, or immunodiffusion methods. Complement fixation (CF) detects IgG. In the usual uncomplicated primary infection, CF titers > 1:16 are unusual. A persistent CF titer ≥ 1:16 suggests dissemination, especially if the skin test is negative. However, the serum CF titer may not be elevated when dissemination is limited to one site such as the meninges. CSF testing in meningitis: Microscopic exam of a KOH preparation of the CSF may reveal the characteristic spherules. Fungal culture of CSF is positive in less than half the cases. Complement fixation test of the CSF will be positive in most cases of meningitis. Other CSF findings in meningitis include decreased glucose, elevated protein, elevated WBC sometimes with increased eosinophils.

Treatment: Most primary infections are self–limited and require no treatment. Chronic progressive pulmonary disease or disseminated infection is treated with IV amphotericin B (refer to drug section). A repeat course is indicated if there is relapse. IV miconazole is a less reliable alternative to amphotericin B when amphotericin B is not tolerated. Oral ketonazole may also have some utility. Meningitis is treated with intrathecal amphotericin B.

Cryptococcosis is due to the fungus, Cryptococcus neoformans. Distribu-

tion is worldwide. Infection is thought to be acquired by inhalation. Both man and animals may be infected but the disease is not contagious. The organism is commonly present in the GI tract and excrement of birds (particularly pigeons) and on their exterior but the birds are not infected. Patients with compromised cell–mediated immunity (e.g. AIDS, lymphoma, corticosteroid treatment) are particularly susceptible to cryptococcosis.

Pulmonary infection is inapparent in many cases. Patients with preexisting lung disease are most likely to be symptomatic. The illness is usually self–limited. There is fever and cough (minimally productive). Other possible manifestations include hemoptysis, hilar adenopathy, pleural effusion, pulmonary nodules or masses, cavitation. Some patients develop indolent progressive lung disease spanning many years.

Hematogenous dissemination: Meningitis is by far the most frequent reason that cryptococcosis comes to medical attention. Common manifestations include headache; stiff neck; visual disturbances (photophobia, blurred vision, diplopia); confusion and other mental aberrations; cranial nerve deficits; seizures. Symptoms sometimes develop slowly over a period of weeks or months. Other organs: Cryptococcus may also disseminate to the kidneys (usually inapparent but may cause pyelonephritis or papillary necrosis); skin (e.g. papules, pustules, ulcers, abscess, nodules, cellulitis); bones (osteomyelitis); lymph nodes; liver (hepatitis, necrosis); spleen; prostate;

testes; adrenals.

Laboratory: Lumbar puncture should be part of the workup even in cases without obvious manifestations of meningitis. India ink preparation of the spun CSF reveals the characteristic budding yeast with a clear capsule in about half the cases of meningitis. CSF culture, with repeat taps if necessary will identity the organism in over 90% cases meningitis. Nonspecific CSF findings may include glucose < half of simultaneous blood level, elevated protein, elevated WBC (but usually < 500) with lymphocytes usually predominating, elevated CSF pressure. India ink preparation and culture of other likely sites is also obtained (e.g. sputum, pleural effusion, abscess). Blood and urine culture is also part of the workup. Latex cryptococcal agglutination test of the CSF is positive in most cases of meningitis. This test may also be performed on the blood and pleural fluid.

Treatment: Meningitis is treated with a 6 week regimen consisting of amphotericin B (0.3 mg/kg/day IV) combined with flucytosine (150 mg/kg/day PO). Pulmonary infections are usually self-limited. Progressive pulmonary infection is treated with IV amphotericin B (e.g. adult: 50 mg/day every other day for 5–6 weeks).

Aspergillosis refers to a number of different clinical entities resulting from various species of Aspergillus fungi.

ASPERGILLOMA (fungus ball, mycetoma) is a tangled ball of aspergillus hyphae and associated material (e.g. fibrin, exudate, few inflammatory cells) lying freely within a pulmonary cavity which has usually been created by preexisting lung disease (e.g. cavitary tuberculosis). A fungus ball is identified on chest x-ray as a round intracavitary mass with a thin crescent of air on the superior aspect. The ball usually changes position on lateral decubitus view. Surgical resection is advised if there is severe hemoptysis. Otherwise, in the absence of evidence of invasive infection, no therapy is required.

INVASIVE ASPERGILLOSIS

Acute bronchopneumonia is an opportunistic infection occurring mostly in immunocompromised patients, particularly those receiving systemic antibiotics. Patients develop a necrotizing bronchopneumonia with ulceration and abscess formation. Encroachment on pulmonary vessels may lead to hemorrhagic infarction, thrombosis, or embolization. Hematogenous dissemination to sundry organs is common. Sputum culture is obtained but is usually negative. Therefore, specimens are also obtained by transtracheal aspiration, bronchoscopy, etc. Microscopic exam of stained specimens (e.g. PAS, methenamine silver, H & E) discloses the hyphae. Treatment is with amphotericin B.

Chronic necrotizing pulmonary aspergillosis is a less aggresive form of invasive pulmonary aspergillosis that occurs in patients with preexisting lung disease. There is cavitation and aspergilloma may form within the cavities. A productive cough is characteristic and there may be hemoptysis. Treatment is with amphotericin B.

ALLERGIC ASPERGILLOSIS

Allergic bronchopulmonary aspergillosis is a type I, type III, and possibly type IV–mediated syndrome that results from allergy to Aspergillus spores. Signs/symptoms: The type I (IgE mediated) reaction results in a typical asthmatic response with bronchospasm–induced dyspnea and wheezing. The type III and IV reactions mediate a inflammatory reaction with recurrent bouts of fever, cough, and pulmonary infiltrates that is unresponsive to antibiotics. Bronchiectasis and pulmonary fibrosis may develop in chronic cases. Aspergillus skin test is positive as demonstrated by an immediate wheal and flare (the type I reaction) which may be followed in 4–6 hours by redness, swelling, and tenderness (the type III Arthus reaction). Lab findings; eosinophilia; sputum containing eosinophils with Charcot–Leyden crystals and Curschmann spirals; elevated serum IgE; serum precipitating antibodies to Aspergillus. Treatment: prednisone.

Hypersensitivity pneumonitis (extrinsic allergic alveolitis) may follow inhalation of Aspergillus spores in persons who have been previously sensitized to Aspergillus. Signs/symptoms usually begin 4–8 hours following exposure: there is fever, cough, dyspnea, malaise, rales. Wheezing is usually absent. Pulmonary function tests are abnormal (e.g. decreased lung volume, impaired CO diffusion, restrictive air–flow pattern, ventilation/perfusion mismatch). Aspergillus skin test shows a positive type III Arthus reaction (redness, swelling, tenderness in 4–6 hours) but the immediate type I reaction (wheal and flare) may be absent. Laboratory: Precipitating antibodies to Aspergillus are detected in the serum. Eosinophilia is not present. Infiltrates are seen on chest x-ray. Treatment: If exposure to aspergillosis stops, the condition is self–limited and usually resolves spontaneously over several hours. A short course of prednisone may be needed in severe cases. Chronic or repetitive aspergillus exposure may lead to interstitial lung disease with progressive dyspnea. Aspergillus has been identified as one of the agents causing farmer's lung, malt worker's lung, cheese worker's lung.

Blastomycosis <small>(North American blastomycosis) occurs not only in North</small>

America (principally in the Mississippi and Ohio River valleys and about the Great Lakes) but also occurs in the rest of the Americas and in Africa. Blastomyces dermatitidis may be recovered from the soil. Infection is acquired by inhalation. Blastomycocis is not contagious.

Pulmonary infection is usually inapparent or a self-limited respiratory illness which may present with fever, chills, cough (sometimes productive), pleuritic pain, joint pains, and occasionally erythema nodosum. Chest x-ray may reveal hilar adenopathy. With progressive disease one may see bronchopneumonia (sometimes giving the appearance of malignant mass), cavities, fibrosis.

Hematogenous dissemination sometimes occurs; most often to the skin (producing papules or pustules which progress slowly to wart–like lesions) and next most often to bone (sometimes with sinuses draining to and thru the skin). Other sites of involvement may include prostate, epididymis, testes, kidneys, liver, spleen, adrenal, CNS. Hematogenous dissemination to the lungs may be revealed by a miliary pattern on chest x-ray.

Laboratory: Microscopic exam of a KOH preparation (e.g. sputum, pus, prostatic secretion) may disclose the characteristic single–budding thick–walled yeast. Tissue stains (e.g. H & E, PAS) may also demonstrate the yeast. Cultures from suspicious sites are obtained but growth may not become apparent for 3–4 weeks. Skin testing is not helpful.

Treatment: IV amphotericin B is the preferred treatment if there is dissemination or progressive pulmonary disease. Hydroxystilbamidine is the alternative.

Paracoccidioidomycosis <small>(S. American blastomycosis) is due</small>

to the fungus, Paracoccidioides brasiliensis. The disease is restricted to Mexico, and Central and S. America. The majority of cases occur in Brazil (particularly in coffee-growers). Infection is acquired by inhalation. The disease is not contagious.

Pulmonary infection is usually asymptomatic and most symptomatic cases are mild and self-limited. With progressive disease the chest x-ray may disclose infiltrates, nodules, masses. There is hilar adenopathy and there may be cavitation and/or fibrosis.

Disseminated disease (hematogenous and lymphatic spread) is most likely to occur when immunity is impaired. Dissemination may not occur until years after the primary respiratory infection. There may be ulceration of the nasal, oral, and/or pharyngeal mucosa or even of the larynx and epiglottis. There may be skin ulcers (frequently on the face, commonly at the mucocutaneous borders) and wart–like lesions. Other manifestations may include lymphadenopathy (nodes may abscess and drain), splenic and/or hepatic enlargement, GI ulcers. The bones, kidneys, adrenals, prostate, testes, pancreas, heart, or CNS may be involved.

Laboratory: Microscopic exam of a KOH preparation or a wet mount of sputum or pus from lesions often demonstrates the characteristic yeast with multiple buds. Biopsy specimens stained with methenamine silver or PAS may also identify the yeast. Cultures of other sites (e.g. blood, urine, CSF, or biopsy material) as clinical circumstances suggest may also be diagnostic.

Treatment: Severe infections are treated with IV amphotericin B. Oral ketonazole may be used in milder infections. Sulfadiazine is a less effective option that must be continued for 3–5 yr.

Mucormycosis <small>is a noncontagious infection due to fungi of the order</small>

Mucoraceae (e.g. Mucor, Rhizopus, Mortierella, Absidia). The fungi are ordinarily saprophytes (e.g. decaying vegetation, molding bread, etc.).

Syndromes: Rhinocerebral mucormycosis is most often seen in the setting of diabetic ketoacidosis or impaired immunity. Untreated, it is a rapidly fatal. Inhaled fungal spores infect the nasopharyngeal mucosa and infection extends to the sinuses. A purulent blood–streaked nasal discharge develops with blackened necrotic turbinates and destruction/perforation of the nasal septum. There is invasion and destruction of the sinus bones and the same process destroys the palate. Contiguous spread leads to facial cellulitis and/or orbital cellulitis. The latter commonly results in cranial nerve dysfunction, proptosis, blindness. Unchecked, the disease may encroach on the internal carotids, cranial bones, brain. Pulmonary infection follows inhalation of fungal spores. Immunodeficient patients are the most susceptible. Skin infections are associated with contamination of burns or other wounds. GI infection may follow ingestion of fungal spores in patients with GI disorders. Hematogenous dissemination may occur in immunocompromised patients or those with contaminated burns or other wounds. Virtually any organ may be involved.

Laboratory: ●The diagnosis is best made by microscopic exam of a KOH preparation of a crushed biopsy specimen revealing the characteristic broad nonseptate hyphae. The fungi stain well with methenamine silver or H & E. ●Microscopic exam of the sputum or exudates is not usually helpful. ●Cultures from involved sites do not usually grow the organism. Furthermore, false-positive cultures due to fungal contamination may occur if superficial tissues are sampled.

Treatment: amphotericin B, correction of acidosis (essential in those with rhinocerebral mucormycosis), wound debridement.

Protozoa

Malaria
Chagas' Disease
Sleeping Sickness
Toxoplasmosis
Visceral Leishmaniasis
Cutaneous and Mucocutaneous Leishmaniasis

<u>Note</u>: Giardiasis and amebiasis are presented in gastrointestinal section. Refer to "Vaginitis" for discussion of trichomoniasis.

Malaria

Malaria is due to infection by one or any combination of 4 protozoans: Plasmodium falciparum, P. vivax, P. ovale, P. malariae. **Life cycle** of plasmodium starts when a female anopheles mosquito ingests blood infected with gametocytes. The sexual phase of the cycle occurs within the mosquito and sporozoites are ultimately produced. When the mosquito again bites a person, sporozoites are released from the mosquito's salivary glands into the host's blood. The sporozoites reach the liver where asexual proliferation leads to the production of merozoites which are released into the circulation and infect erythrocytes. Merozoites develop within erythrocytes passing thru stages: ring form → trophozoite → schizont. Schizonts contain, depending on the species of malaria, 6–24 merozoites. Lysis of the erythrocytes releases merozoites which are then free to infect other erythrocytes and thus the erythrocytic stage continues to repeat itself. The periodic fever and chills characteristic of malaria occurs when the erythrocytes are lyzed. In some of the infected erythrocytes, gametocytes are produced instead of schizonts. Gametocytes do not replicate; they eventually die if they are not ingested by an anopheles mosquito, the obligatory site of sexual reproduction. **Resistance:** The sickle trait (HB AS) confers resistance to malarial illness. Other hemoglobin variants, thalassemia, or G6PD deficiency may also provide some protection. The RBC's of persons with elliptocytosis are to some extent resistant to malarial infection. Blacks who are Duffy blood group homozygous negative have specific resistance to P. vivax infection. **Immunity:** Patients with chronic malarial infection develop some immunity which renders the illness less severe. Some may even be asymptomatic. Immunity to one species of malaria does not confer immunity to other species. In the case of P. falciparum, immunity is even more restricted; infection by one strain of P. falciparum does not protect against other P. falciparum strains. Immunity is diminished after several years unless reinfection occurs.

SIGNS/SYMPTOMS begin, depending on the species of malaria, 10–35 days after a mosquito bite. Initially, there is a remittent fever. After 1–2 weeks there is usually synchronous production and release of merozoites from ruptured erythrocytes and the paroxysms of fever, chills, and sweats then occur at regular intervals. In P. vivax and P. ovale, the febrile episodes last 1–8 hours and tend to recur at 48 hour intervals. In P. malaria, episodes tend to recur every 72 hours. In a typical paroxysm, there is a sudden onset of shaking chills and fever. There is headache. There may be nausea and vomiting. Over the next 1–2 hours, the temperature continues to rise and may reach 40.5° C (104.9° F). Subsequently, there is profuse sweating and the temperature falls. After the attack has subsided, the patient feels weak and tired. Hepatosplenomaly is a common finding in malarial infections. Mild jaundice may be present.

P. falciparum is unpredictable; cyclic paroxysms may not occur. There may be a persistent fever. Overwhelming P. falciparum parasitemia may cause severe hemolytic anemia. Blackwater fever (hemoglobinuria resulting from severe hemolysis) is an uncommon complication of P. falciparum parasitemia that may lead to acute renal failure. Severe hemolysis may also be precipitated by quinine in sensitive individuals, or by oxidant drugs (e.g. primaquine, sulfonamides) in patients with G6PD deficiency. Cerebral malaria: High P. falciparum parasitemia may cause sludging of erythrocytes in the cerebral capillaries so that encephalopathy ensues. Manifestations may include confusion, stupor, convulsions, coma, and frequently death.

Untreated outcome: Malarial attacks gradually become milder and irregular over a period of weeks and eventually stop. With the exception of P. malariae, which may persist as a lifelong asymptomatic infection, malarial infection is eventually spontaneously eliminated. Assuming the patient survives, untreated P. falciparum illness may recur for about a year to about 3–4 years at the most. Untreated P. vivax and P. ovale infection may last 3–4 years with the potential to produce recurrent illness during that period.

LABORATORY: Giemsa stain of both a thick and a thin blood film are obtained. The thick film is useful for detecting light infection while the thin film is best for identifying the particular species of malaria. **P. falciparum** is identified by high parasitemia with preponderance of small ring forms of the parasite, and parasites with double nuclei. Erythrocytes containing more than one parasite is a characteristic finding. Crescent–shaped gametocytes are also characteristic. **P. vivax** is recognized by its presence within enlarged erythrocytes with Schuffner's dots (pink stippling of the erythrocyte membrane). The trophozoites are large and ameboid. The mature schizont contains 12–24 merozoites. **P. ovale** is distinguished by its presence within oval–shaped erythrocytes with Schuffner's dots. The mature schizont contains 6–16 merozoites. **P. malariae** is notable in that infected erythrocytes are unaltered in shape or size and Schuffner's dots are not present. The mature schizont contains 6–12 merozoites. **Other hematologic findings** may include anemia, thrombocytopenia,and/or leukopenia.

TREATMENT of CHLOROQUINE–RESISTANT P. FALCIPARUM:
Adult males, nonpregnant adult females, and children over 8 yr of age may be treated with a combination of doxocycline (or tetracycline) plus quinine:
 Doxycycline (100 mg PO twice daily in adult) for 7 days. Tetracycline (250 mg PO 4 times/day in adult) for 7 days is the alternative to doxycycline.
 Oral quinine sulfate: Adult dose is 650 mg PO q8h for 3 to 7 days depending on severity of infection. In renal failure, the adult dose is 650 mg once daily.
 ●Pediatric dose is 25mg/kg/day PO divided q8h.
 Intravenous quinine dihydrochloride should be administered initially if the patient is severely ill or is vomiting. Adult dose is 600 mg in 250 ml of glucose or saline solution infused over at least an hour while monitoring the BP. Dose is repeated q8h (maximum 1800 mg/day). Oral quinine therapy is substituted as soon as is feasible. ●Pediatric dose of intravenous quinine dihydrochloride is 25 mg/kg/day (max 1800 mg/day). Half of this amount is given initially (diluted and infused over at least 1hr) and the remainder is given in 6–8 hours if oral therapy is still not tolerated. Oral quinine therapy is substituted as soon as is feasible.
An alternative regimen consists of a 3 drug combination: quinine plus Fansidar (pyrimethamine with sulfadoxine):
 Quinine as above.
 Fansidar (pyrimethamine and sulfadoxine) is given as a single dose at the initiation of quinine therapy: adult: 2–3 tablets, 9–14 yr: 2 tablets, 4–8 yr: 1 tablet, under 4 yr: 1/2 tablet.
Mefloquine alone is yet another option in patients with mild to moderate illness.

TREATMENT of CHLOROQUINE–SENSITIVE P. FALCIPARUM:
Chloroquine (see below) alone is curative since it eliminates the erythrocytic form and there is no persistent hepatic form of P. falciparum. Intravenous quinine (see above) may be used if the patient is severely ill or vomiting (see regimen above). Chloroquine resistance should be suspected when parasitemia fails to decrease after 1–2 days of chloroquine therapy. With successful therapy, no asexual forms should be seen 5 days after finishing a course of chloroquine. Gametocytes may, however, still be seen in the blood for several weeks until they die. The presence of gametocytes does not indicate treatment failure.

TREATMENT of P. VIVAX and P. OVALE
is with combinatiion of chloroquine and primaquine.
 Chloroquine phosphate: In adults, the regimen is 600 mg base PO initial dose followed by 300 mg base PO at 6, 24, and 48 hours. ●In children, 10 mg/kg base (max 600 mg) PO initial dose followed by half of the initial dose PO at 6, 24, and 48 hr. Chloroquine hydrochloride IM is an alternative when the oral route is not feasible. In adults, the dose is 160–200 mg base IM q6h. PO administration is substituted as soon as feasible. Total dose IM + PO over 3 days is 1500 mg base. ●In children, the dose is 5 mg/kg base IM q12h (maximum 800 mg/24hr). PO administration is substituted as soon as feasible. Total dose IM + PO over 3 days is 25 mg/kg base up to maximum 1500 mg total.
 Primaquine must be administered to achieve a radical cure since chloroquine eliminates the erythrocytic but not the hepatic parasites. Primaquine may be administered concurrently with or after chloroquine therapy. Dose in adults is 15 mg base PO once daily for 14 days. In children, 0.3 mg/kg base PO once daily for 14 days. Patients with G6PD deficiency may have to forego primaquine therapy because of the risk of hemolysis and continue on chloroquine for 3 years. The alternative is to use

a modified primaquine regimen while monitoring (especially during the first 2 weeks of therapy) CBC, serum bilirubin, retic count, and the urine. The primaquine dose in-African variant G6PD deficiency is 45 mg once a week for 8 weeks; and in caucasian or oriental variant the dose is 30 mg once a week for 15 weeks.

TREATMENT of P. MALARIAE: Chloroquine alone (see above) is curative since most experts agree that P. malariae does not persist as a hepatic form, but that relapses are due to persistent erythrocytic parasites.

PROPHYLAXIS:

Mefloquine is recommended for travelers to regions where malaria is endemic, especially those regions where P. falciparum strains resistant to other anti-malarial drugs are known to exist. The drug is taken once a week for 4 weeks beginning one week before arrival in an endemic area. It is then taken once every other week and continued until 4 weeks after departing endemic area. Doses are as follows: adult or child > 45 kg: 1tablet (250mg), child > 31–45kg: 3/4 tablet, child 20–30kg: 1/2 tablet, child 15–19kg: 1/4 tablet. Mefloquine is contraindicated in children < 15 kg, pregnancy, and patients taking beta blockers or other drugs that prolong/alter cardiac conduction (see product insert for further restrictions).

Doxycycline is an alternative to mefloquine. The drug is taken once a day beginning 1–2 days before arrival in an endemic area, continued during the stay, and not discontinued until 4 weeks after departure from the malarial area. Doses are as follows: adult: 100mg/day, child > 8 years of age: 2mg/kg/day (max 100mg/day). Doxycline is contraindicated in children < 8 years of age and in pregnancy.

Chloroquine phosphate is an option if mefloquine or doxycycline are contraindicated. However, most malarial regions have chloroquine–resistant malarial organisms. The drug may be taken in pregnancy. It is administered weekly starting 1–2 weeks prior to arrival, continued weekly during the stay, and then weekly for 6–8 weeks after departure. Dose (of base): adult: 300 mg once a week, pediatric: 5 mg/kg once a week not to exceed adult dose.

*Persons travelling to malarial areas who are using chloroquine prophylaxis may carry a single treatment dose of Fansidar (pyrimethamine and sulfadoxine) in case a febrile illness develops and medical care is not readily available. Adult dose: 3 tablets, child > 45 kg: 3 tablets, child 31–45 kg: 2 tablets, child 21–30 kg: 1 1/2 tablets, child 11–20 kg: 1 tablet, infant 5–10 kg: 1/2 tablet.

Sleeping Sickness (African Trypanosomiasis) is due to the protozoan,

Trypanasoma brucei. There are two subspecies, T. brucei rhodesiense (Rhodesian or East African sleeping sickness) and T. brucei gambiense (Gambian or West African sleeping sickness). The vector is the tse tse fly. The principal host of T. brucei gambiense is man whereas wild animals are the main reservoir of infection for T. brucei rhodesiense.

Signs/symptoms: Rhodesian sleeping sickness is generally a more severe and more often deadly illness than the Gambian form. In Gambian disease, the systemic phase is usually distinct from the CNS phase (the CNS phase typically surfaces months to years after inception of the systemic phase). On the other hand, Rhodesian disease usually advances more quickly, and so it is not always possible to discern when the systemic phase has ended and the CNS phase has begun. Furthermore, the patient not infrequently dies before CNS manifestations can emerge. A chancre (a small node/ulcer from which trypanasomes may be recovered) may form at the bite site 1–2 weeks after the bite and remain for up to 3 weeks. Infection may resolve spontaneously before systemic illness occurs. Systemic illness appears months to years later. Manifestations may include recurrent fever; enlarged and typically nontender lymph nodes (almost always including posterior cervical nodes, often generalized lymphadenopathy); splenomegaly; rash; localized edema, jaundice, heart failure. The latter two occur more often in Rhodesian sleeping sickness. Uncommonly, Gambian infection is eliminated without treatment before there is CNS involvement. CNS involvement: Manifestations may include headache, progressive sleepiness, apathy, tremor, chorea, athetosis, seizures, psychic disturbances ranging from mildly altered behavior to frank psychosis. Without treatment, the disease is uniformly lethal once there is CNS involvement.

Laboratory: Diagnosis is confirmed by finding trypanosomes on microscopic exam of a thick blood smear or of a needle aspirate from an enlarged lymph node. ●With CNS invasion, trypanasomes may be found in the CSF and the CSF IgM will be elevated.

Treatment: Suranim or pentamidine are used before there is CNS involvement. Melarsoprol (Mel B) is required once there is CNS invasion. The CSF should be examined periodically for a minimum of 1 year following treatment. Infection does not confer immunity.

Chagas' Disease (South American Trypanosomiasis) is due to the proto-

zoan, Trypanosoma cruzi. T. cruzi infects both man and animals. The organism is transmitted by species of Reduviid bugs which defecate as they suck blood. The T. cruzi-containing feces contaminates the bite wound or other skin breaks. Congenital infection is possible and the infection may be acquired by blood transfusion. The disease occurs exclusively in the Americas, almost entirely in latin America—particularly Argentina, Uruguay, Chile, Brazil, Venezuela; and rarely Mexico. Both the severity of disease and organ involvement may vary from region to region.

Signs/symptoms: Most infected individuals are asymptomatic. Acute Chagas' disease: Of those that do become symptomatic, a minority (and these are almost exclusively children) first experience an acute illness which starts 4–12 days after being bitten and lasts 2–4 months. Manifestations may include a chagoma (redness and swelling at the bite site), fever, weakness, lymphadenopathy, enlarged liver and spleen, Romañas sign (unilateral edema and purplish discoloration of the eyelids) ± conjunctivitis, facial edema, edema of the legs, rash (rare). Acute myocarditis is common in acute Chagas' disease. It manifests as tachycardia and EKG abnormalities. Acute myocarditis is occasionally fatal. Meningoencephalitis is a rare occurrence. Chronic Chagas' disease may remain latent for years, even for life. Manifest illness may be mild. Some patients develop cardiomyopathy. Most cases are subclinical and are detected by an abnormal EKG. Cardiomyopathic findings may include conduction abnormalities (e.g. PVC's, AV block, bundle branch block); biventricular dilatation with mitral and/or tricuspid regurgitation and heart failure (mainly right-sided). The other major potential complications are gastrointestinal (megaesophagus and/or megacolon).

Laboratory: During the acute infection, the organism may be seen on a blood smear. T. cruzi may also be demonstrated by culture; inoculation of mice; or xenodiagnosis. In the latter, uninfected Reduviid bugs are allowed to bite a patient suspected of having Chagas' disease. After an incubation period, the insects' intestinal contents are examined for the organism. During chronic disease, the diagnosis may be made by xenodiagnosis or by serology (hemagglutination, complement fixation, immunofluorescence).

Treatment: nifurtimox or benznidazole

Toxoplasmosis is due to infection by the obligate intracellular protozoan,

Toxoplasma gondii. Infection occurs worldwide but tends to be more common in tropical areas or in regions where undercooked meats are consumed. Depending on the area surveyed, 7–94% population will have serologic evidence of infection and the great majority will have had asymptomatic infection. The organism can infect any mammal or bird. Cats, however, are the only known host where the sexual phase of the life cycle occurs. **Life cycle:** Oocysts: Sexual reproduction within the intestinal mucosal cells of cats results in the production of oocysts which are excreted in the feces. The mature oocyst may cause infection in any warm-blooded animal (including man) that happens to ingest it. Cysts contain thousands of organisms that have resulted from asexual multiplication within infected cells. They can be found in any tissue. Cysts cause infection when man or other warm-blooded animals eat the raw or undercooked flesh of an infected animal. Trophozoites: After ingestion of either the oocyst or cyst, the organism first proliferates in the form of trophozoites within the intestinal mucosal cells of the host. Trophozoites are then spread via the blood or lymphatics and can infect any tissue. Trophozoites are obligate intracellular forms that undergo asexual replication within the host's nucleated cells. After repeated divisions, the host cell ruptures. The released trophozoites then infect other host cells.

Signs/symptoms of acquired toxoplasmosis: Acquired toxoplasmosis is usually asymptomatic. In symptomatic cases; common manifestations include nontender adenopathy, fever, malaise, fatigue, myalgias, splenomegaly. Some patients have a sore throat (but without exudate) and there may be a maculopapular rash. Therapy is seldom required in immunocompetent patients since the illness is almost always self-limited. After recovery, however, cysts do persist in the tissues for life with the potential to cause recurrent disease should the immune system fail. Immunocompromised patients are vulnerable to a fulminant illness that is fatal in many cases. Manifestations may include high fever, chills, adenopathy, pneumonitis, maculopapular rash, meningoencephalitis, myocarditis, hepatitis.

Signs/symptoms of congenital toxoplasmosis: Congenital infection occurs by transplacental transmission. For this to occur, the mother must become infected shortly before or during the pregnancy. The mother is usually asymptomatic. Approximately 40% of recently infected mothers will have an infected fetus. Fetal infection may result in abortion, miscarriage, or stillbirth. Those that survive may be born with or develop a variety of afflictions (e.g. hydrocephalus, convulsions, microcephaly, microophthalmia, intracerebral calcification, hepatosplenomegaly, jaundice, pneumonitis, chorioretinitis, maculopapular rash, thrombocytopenic purpura). Some congenitally infected infants appear normal at birth. Clinical manifestations that may later emerge include seizures, mental retardation, chorioretinitis. Chorioretinitis characteristically makes its appearance later in childhood or in young adults.

Laboratory: Indirect fluorescent antibody (IFA) is the most common diagnostic test. Sabin–Feldman test is the most sensitive and specific serologic test available but is cumbersome. With either test, antitoxoplasma antibodies are detected 1–2 weeks following infection and peak within 2 months. Titers slowly decrease thereafter but low titers persist for life. Recent infection is demonstrated by conversion from negative to positive, or a 4–fold rise in titer (usually to a dilution of ≥ 1:1000). An infant who registers a positive test does not necessarily have congenital toxoplasmosis because a mother who has been previously infected will pass antitoxoplasma antibodies transplacentally to the fetus. A rising titer is significant however. IgM indirect fluorescent antibody test or IgM–ELISA test are are useful in detecting recent infection (e.g. congenital infection in infant) because IgM levels rise within a few days of infection and vanish within months. Complement fixation test turns positive later than other tests (3–6 weeks following infection) and continues to rise for up to 8 months. A rising titer therefore helps confirm a recent infection in the 2–4 to 6–8 months interval following infection when the IgM titers are falling and the Sabin–Feldman or IFA titers have peaked.

Treatment is not necessary in most cases since the disease is usually self-limited. Adult regimen: pyrimethamine (75 mg PO initial dose followed by 25 mg PO daily for 3–4 weeks) plus sulfadiazine (2–4 gram PO initial dose followed by 1 gram PO q6h for 3–4 weeks). Pyrimethamine is contraindicated in pregnancy because of teratogenicity. Sulfadiazine alone may be of benefit in pregnant patients. Pediatric regimen; pyrimethamine (1mg/kg/day PO for 3 days followed by 0.5mg/kg/day for 3–4 weeks, daily dose not to exceed 25 mg) plus sulfadiazine (100mg/kg/day in divided doses for 3–4 weeks). Note: Both pyrimethamine and sulfadiazine are folic acid antagonists, and may thus provoke bone marrow depression. For this reason, concurrent administration of folinic acid (Leucovorin) is recommended—e.g. 5 mg PO three times a week.

Visceral Leishmaniasis (Kala Azar) is due to the intracellular

protozoan, Leishmania donovani. The vectors are various species of phlebotomine sandflies. Reservoir of infection may be dogs, wild canines, rodents, and in some instances man. Geographic distribution: The disease occurs primarily in northeast India, northeast China, countries bordering the Mediterranean, east Africa, Iran, along the Caspian sea, northeast Brazil, and less often in other parts of Brazil and various other countries of central and south America. Reticuloendothelial system involvement; The organism invades macrophages (i.e. cells of the reticuloendothelial system). Amistodotes (nonflagellated nonmotile form) may therefore be found in the spleen, Kupffer cells of the liver, bone marrow, connective tissue histiocytes, etc. Leishmania multiply within macrophages by binary fission as the amastigote form. The macrophages rupture and amastigotes then infect other macrophages. Promastigotes (flagellated motile form) are found in the sandfly or may be produced in cultures.

Signs/symptoms: Weeks to months following a sandfly bite, there is a gradual onset of illness with intermittent fever, weight loss, splenomegaly (often massive), hepatomegaly, generalized lymphadenopathy. Untreated, the patient becomes progressively debilitated and cachectic and dies, usually from another superimposed infection.

Laboratory: Giemsa stain of an aspirate of the bone marrow or spleen, and less often of lymph node, liver, or blood (buffy coat) may reveal the amastigote. Cultures (NNN medium) of these sites may also be diagnostic. A needle aspirate of the spleen can be obtained (using a 21 gauge needle) but only if the spleen can be felt below the costal margin, and the prothrombin time and bleeding time are normal. Serologic tests (e.g. ELISA, IFA) may also aid in the diagnosis. Leishmanin skin test is negative during active disease and becomes positive only after cure. Other lab findings may include normochromic normocytic anemia, leukopenia (absolute neutropenia with relative lymphocytosis), thrombocytopenia, elevated sedimentation rate, elevated total serum protein (due to increased serum IgG), sometimes hypoalbuminemia.

Treatment: sodium stibogluconate (Pentostam) or meglumine antimoniate (Glucantime).

Cutaneous & Mucocutaneous Leishmaniasis

Cutaneous leishmaniasis (oriental sore) is due to various species of leishmania: Old World cutaneous leishmaniasis (L. tropica); New World cutaneous leishmaniasis (e.g. L. brasiliensis, L. mexicana). Geography: The disease occurs in the Middle East, Africa, India, China, Texas, Mexico, Central and S. America (Chile excepted). Reservoir of infection: usually rodent, sometimes dog or man. Vector: phlebotomine sandflies. Cutaneous lesion; A papule develops at the sandfly bite site after 2–10 weeks. A large ulcer subsequently forms and may crust. There may be more than one lesion. The ulcer usually heals spontaneously over 2–18 months leaving a depigmented scar.

Mucocutaneous leishmamiasis (espundia) is virtually restricted to latin America—particularly Brazil, Bolivia, Peru, Ecuador. The disease develops in patients with cutaneous leishmaniasis when there is hematogenous metastasis of L. brasiliensis or L. mexicana to the mucosa of the nose, mouth, and/or pharynx. Mucosal ulcers usually appear after the skin ulcer has healed. Destruction of the nasal cartilage results in disfigurement.

Laboratory: Leishmanin skin test is positive. Serologic tests are diagnostic (e.g. ELISA). Microscopic exam of scrapings or biopsy specimens may disclose the organism. Culture of the ulcers on NNN medium confirms the diagnosis.

Treatment: Mucocutaneous disease is treated with sodium stibogluconate (Pentostam) or meglumine antimoniate (Glucantime). Cutaneous leishmaniasis is usually self-limited. Drug treatment is advocated in regions where mucocutaneous leishmaniasis occurs.

Metazoa

Pinworm
Whipworm
Ascariasis
Toxocariasis
Hookworm
Strongyloidiasis
Cutaneous Larva Migrans
Trichinosis
Schistosomiasis
Lung Fluke
Liver Flukes
Intestinal Fluke
Filariasis
Beef Tapeworm
Pork Tapeworm
Dwarf Tapeworm
Fish Tapeworm
Hydatid Disease

Pinworm
(Enterobius vermicularis) is a nematode. Infestation is common worldwide, especially in children and institutionalized persons. The eggs are transmitted from the perianal area to the mouth by finger contact, fomites (e.g. bedclothes), or transmission may even be airborne. The ingested eggs hatch in the small intestine releasing larvae that develop into adults in the colon in 2–6 weeks. The females migrate out of the anus at night and lay their eggs on the perianal skin.

Signs/symptoms: Most cases are asymptomatic. The chief complaint is perianal itching due to the presence of eggs on the skin. Sometimes the worms migrate into the bladder of female children bringing with them coliform bacteria; bacterial cystitis may ensue. Vaginitis may result if the worms enter the vagina. Bedwetting sometimes seems to be due to pinworm infestation. Rare consequences of infestation are appendicitis, salpingitis, GI perforation.

Diagnosis is made by seeing the 1 cm long females on the perianal skin. The worms are most likely to be seen 1–2 hours after the child goes to sleep. If the adult females are not seen, the diagnosis can be made by applying the sticky side of Scotch tape to the perianal skin, sticking the tape to a glass slide, and examining for eggs under a microscope.

Treatment of adults and children is a single 100 mg dose of mebendazole (see drug section). The single dose is administered to the entire household (except pregnant woman) and again in 2 weeks. Clothing and bedclothes should be washed but no other extraordinary measures are helpful. Children are often reinfested.

Whipworm
(Trichirus trichiura) is a nematode. Infestation is common worldwide, particularly in warm moist climates with poor sanitation. Simultaneous infection with Ascaris is common. Man acquires the infection by ingesting the eggs (often on raw vegetables) which have incubated in fecally contaminated soil. The eggs hatch in the small intestine. Upon reaching the terminal ileum or cecum, the larvae partially imbed in the mucosa where they develop over 2–3 months into egg–producing adults with a potential life span of 3–10 years. In heavy infestations, the adults are found throughout the colon.

Signs/symptoms are absent in light infestations. In heavier infestations there may be abdominal pain or diarrhea. Rectal prolapse may occur in children with heavy infestations. Rarely, the worms may obstruct the appendix and provoke appendicitis.

Diagnosis is usually confirmed by identifying the characteristic ova in the stool, or occasionally by the passage of the adult worm (2.5–3.0 cm long). Eosinophilia is found in up to 15% cases.

Treatment (adults and children): mebendazole 100 mg PO twice daily for 3 days. Mebendazole (see drug section) is contraindicated in pregnancy.

Ascariasis
is due to the nematode (roundworm) Ascaris lumbricoides. It is a common infestation worldwide, particularly in warm areas with poor sanitation. Man is infested by ingesting the eggs which have incubated in fecally contaminated soil. The ova hatch in the duodenum. The larvae penetrate the intestine and are transported by the lymphatics and venous circulation. They reach the lung capillaries about 4 days following infection. Over the following 10 days, the larvae penetrate into the alveoli, ascend the tracheobronchial tree, and are swallowed. The larvae, upon reaching the gut for the 2nd time, establish residence in the small intestine and develop into egg–producing adults (about 60–75 days from the time of initial infection) with a life span of about 18 months.

Signs/symptoms: Pulmonary: If enough eggs are ingested and depending on the patient's sensitivity, an eosinophilic pneumonitis with patchy infiltrates (Löffler's syndrome) may result from the migration of larvae thru the lungs. Manifestations may include fever, cough, wheezing, dyspnea, or even hemoptysis or respiratory failure. Intestinal infestation by the adult worms may cause abdominal pain, vomiting, diarrhea, and perhaps malnutrition. Complications: Sometimes, heavy infestation results in GI obstruction. Rarely, the worms obstruct the appendix causing appendicitis, the pancreatic duct causing pancreatitis, or the bile ducts causing cholangitis. Other unusual consequences include GI perforation, intussusception, liver abscess, aspiration.

Diagnosis is sometimes confirmed by passage of adult worms (15–45 cm long) in the stool. Occasionally, the adult worms are present in emesis. The ova can be identified on microscopic exam of the feces. ●During the larval migratory phase, larvae may sometimes be seen in the sputum. ●Eosinophilia may occur during the larval stage and occasionally with intestinal infestation by the adult worms.

Treatment is with a single PO dose of pyrantel pamoate (see drug section). Mebendazole (see drug section) or piperazine citrate are alternatives.

Toxocariasis
(Visceral Larva Migrans) is due to infection by the larval stage of the dog or cat Ascarid (Toxocara canis or T. cati respectively). The infection is more common in children. Infection follows ingestion of the eggs which have incubated in the soil following excretion by dogs or cats. The eggs hatch in the small intestine. The larvae burrow thru the intestinal wall and then spread via the bloodstream to virtually any organ or tissue. In humans, the infection does not progress past the larval stage.

Signs/symptoms are absent in most infections. Following an incubation period of weeks to months, the patient may develop various combinations of fever, cough, wheezing, hepatomegaly, splenomegaly, pneumonitis. ●Chorioretinitis may occur and be confused with a retinoblastoma. ●Unusually, the CNS is invaded and neurologic abnormalities result.

Laboratory: ●ELISA (enzyme linked immunosorbent assay) test is useful but both false-positives and false-negatives do occur. ●There is eosinophilia. ●Serum immunoglobulins are elevated.

Treatment is not necessary since the condition is usually mild and resolves spontaneously in 6–18 months. Severe infections are treated with prednisone and possibly thiabendazole.

Hookworm is due to either one of two nematodes, Necator americanus or
Ancyclostoma duodenale. The infection occurs worldwide in warm moist climates where there is poor sanitation.

Life cycle: Larvae that have incubated in the soil penetrate the skin. (Ingestion of Ancyclostoma duodenale larvae is an alternative route of infection.) After penetrating the skin, the larvae proceed via the lymphatics and bloodstream to the lung capillaries where they penetrate into the alveoli and then ascend the tracheobronchial tree. The larvae are then swallowed and attach to the mucosa of the upper third of the small intestine and commence sucking blood. As the worms move from mucosal site to site they leave small ulcers that bleed. Adults may live up to 6 years. The females produce thousands of eggs/day which are passed in the stool and hatch in the soil after 1–2 days releasing rhabditiform larvae. Over the next several days these larvae develop into filariform larvae, the infective stage.

Signs/symptoms: Pruritic rash ("ground itch") commonly occurs where the larvae have entered the skin. Pulmonary: With heavy infections, migration thru the lungs may be associated with cough, wheezing, dyspnea. Gastrointestinal: Light intestinal infestations by the adult worms causes no symptoms. Heavier infestations may cause a gnawing epigastric discomfort and/or diarrhea. Anemia: Continued blood loss may lead to the signs and symptoms of iron deficiency anemia.

Laboratory: Diagnosis is confirmed by finding the characteristic eggs in the feces. There may be eosinophilia, anemia, and/or hypoalbuminemia.

Treatment: pyrantel pamoate (see drug section). Mebendazole (see drug section) is an alternative.

Prophylaxis is accomplished by improved sanitation and the wearing of shoes.

Strongyloidiasis is due to the nematode Strongyloides stercoralis (thread-
worm). Infection almost always occurs in warm moist climates where there is poor sanitation.

Life cycle from skin penetration by the larvae, to migration thru blood and lungs, to residence in the gut is similar to that of hookworm. Strongyloides differs in that: (**1**) The host is only infected by females; there are neither male larvae nor male adults in the host. In the intestine the adult females produce eggs by parthenogenesis and therefore only female larvae result from intestinal reproduction. (**2**) Eggs are not passed in the stool. Instead, the eggs hatch in the intestine releasing rhabditiform larvae which are found in the stool. (**3**) The rhabditiform larvae, instead of passing in the stool, may autoinfect the host by maturing within the intestine into infective filariform larvae that penetrate the intestine, pass via the blood to the lungs, and return to the intestine to develop into adult females. Autoinfection may also occur when mature larvae pass with the stool and then penetrate the perianal skin. As a consequence of autoinfection, a person may without reexposure remain infected for many years. (**4**) The immature (rhabditiform) larvae that pass in the stool may either develop in the soil into infective filariform larvae or they may develop into adult females and mate with adult males. The offspring thus continue to perpetuate themselves in a bisexual cycle outside a host with the potential to produce infective larvae

Signs/symptoms: "Ground itch" as in hookworm may occur when larvae penetrate the skin. Pulmonary: Migration of the larvae thru the lungs may (like hookworm or Ascariasis) cause pulmonary manifestations (e.g. cough, dyspnea, wheezing, infiltrates). Gastrointestinal: Light intestinal infestation by the female adults causes no symptoms. Heavier infestations may cause epigastric pain, vomiting, diarrhea, and sometimes manifestations of malabsorption (e.g. abdominal bloating, bulky greasy foul stools) and malnutrition (peripheral edema due to hypoalbuminemia, weight loss). Immunocompromised patients are susceptible to overwhelming autoinfection with massive larval migration. Enterocolitis leading to gram–negative sepsis is very likely to supervene.

Laboratory: Stool exam disclosing characteristic larvae is diagnostic. Ova are rarely found. Duodenal aspirate may reveal the larvae if the stool is negative. Duodenal samples may be obtained by swallowing and then withdrawing a string (string test). Eosinophilia is common.

Treatment: thiabendazole 25 mg/kg (maximum 1.5 gram) PO twice daily for 2–5 days.

Prophylaxis is accomplished by improved sanitation and the wearing of shoes.

Cutaneous Larva Migrans

Cutaneous Larva Migrans is a skin infection by the larval stage of various species of nematodes whose definitive hosts are other than man. The most frequent culprit is Ancyclostoma braziliense, a hookworm whose definitive host is the dog or cat. Other species of hookworm or strongyloid species may be responsible. The infection is most common in tropical–subtropical climates and is frequently acquired while lying on beaches contaminated by dog feces. **Signs/symptoms:** The filariform larvae invade the skin and may leave a red papular lesion or inflamed area at the entrance site. Subsequently, the larvae tunnel in the subcutaneous tissues so that pruritic erythematous serpiginous lesions are seen on the skin. In humans, the infection does not progress past the larval stage. **Treatment** is with either oral thiabendazole 25 mg/kg (maximum 1.5 gram) twice daily for 2 days, or topical thiabendazole.

Trichinosis

Trichinosis is due to Trichinella spiralis, a nematode that infects omnivorous and carnivorous mammals. Infection occurs worldwide but is uncommon in the U.S. Man becomes infected by ingesting raw or inadequately cooked pork containing the encysted larvae. Bear or walrus meat is a rare source of infection. The first stage larvae excyst in the duodenum, imbed in the duodenal and jejunal mucosa where they mature within 2–3 days, and then mate. Starting 1–6 weeks following infection and continuing for about 4 weeks, the gravid females release larvae. The adult worms are eliminated from the GI tract, usually within a month. The released 2nd stage larvae penetrate the small intestinal mucosa and are spread by the lymphatics and bloodstream; they invade many organs and tissues but only those that arrive at striated muscle survive. The larvae grow and encyst in the muscle over a period of 4–16 weeks and the cyst itself calcifies over 6–18 months. Viable larvae may persist for years within the cysts.

Signs/symptoms are usually absent. <u>Gastrointestinal</u> symptoms (diarrhea, abdominal pain, vomiting) due to mucosal invasion develop only in a minority of symptomatic cases. GI symptoms occur 1–2 days after ingesting flesh that contains the encysted larvae. <u>Systemic manifestations</u> resulting from the spread and invasion of the 2nd stage larvae usually begin 1–3 weeks following ingestion. There may be fever, photophobia, edema of the eyelids, facial edema, myalgias, subconjunctival or retinal petechiae/hemorrhage, pruritis, urticaria, maculopapular rash, subungual hemorrhage, pneumonitis, pleurisy, myocarditis, encephalitis, meningitis.

Laboratory: <u>Bentonite flocculation test</u> is usually positive by the 3rd week following infection. <u>Other confirmatory tests</u> include ELISA, hemagglutination, indirect immunofluorescence, counterimmunoelectrophoresis (CIE). <u>Eosinophilia</u> occurs coincident with the appearance of systemic manifestations. <u>Muscle enzymes</u> (e.g. CPK, LDH) become elevated as a consequence of muscle invasion with myositis.

Treatment: Mebendazole is the drug of choice (100 mg PO twice daily for 4 days) but is contraindicated in pregnancy. ●Severely symptomatic patients are also treated with prednisone 60 mg/day divided for 3–4 days. Prednisone is then tapered and discontinued over 7–10 days.

Schistosomiasis

Schistosomiasis is the disease that results from infection by Schistosoma (**blood flukes**). The most important species infecting man are S. haematobium, S. mansoni, and S. japonicum. **Life cycle:** Infection is acquired when free–swimming larvae (cerceriae) penetrate the skin of a person bathing or wading in a contaminated water. The larvae (male and female) migrate via venous channels to the lungs and eventually reach the liver where, within the intrahepatic portal circulation, they develop into adult worms. The mature worms then migrate to their final residence: S. haematobium—the venules of the bladder and lower ureters, S. mansoni—the inferior mesenteric veins, S. japonicum—the superior mesenteric veins. It is at these sites that the worms copulate and where the females deposit their eggs. Adult worms usually survive within the host for 3–10 years (rarely up to 20–30 years) and during that time are capable of mating and producing eggs. Some of the eggs penetrate the venules and are released into the bladder lumen in the case of S. haematobium and into the GI lumen in the case of S. mansoni and S. japonicum. Eggs begin to be excreted in the urine (S. haematobium) or the feces (S. mansoni and S. japonicum) 5–9 weeks from the time the cerceriae penetrate the skin. The excreted eggs hatch in fresh water releasing miracidia which then infect certain species of fresh–water snails. Asexual reproduction occurs within the snails and numerous cerceriae are released. The cycle repeats.

S. HAEMOTOBIUM infection occurs in the Middle East and Africa, and is particularly common along the Nile valley. **Clinical consequences** of infection are due to the granulomatous inflammatory reaction that occurs around the eggs in the wall of the bladder and lower ureters. Symptoms of cystitis are characteristic (dysuria, hematuria, frequency). Varying degrees of urinary obstruction may develop so that hydroureter or hydronephrosis sometimes ensues. **Diagnosis** is confirmed by finding the characteristic eggs in the urine. On cystoscopy, the bladder appears hyperemic and one may see ulcers, tubercles, or polyps. X–rays frequently disclose bladder calcification. **Treatment** is with a one day regimen of praziquantel consisting of three 20 mg/kg doses.

S. MANSONI infection occurs in the Middle East and Africa (often in the same areas where S. haematobium is found), and in S. America and the Caribbean. **Pathoclinical consequences:** <u>An acute febrile illness</u> may occur 3–7 weeks after cerceriae penetrate the skin. This represents an immune–mediated reaction to the presence of S. mansoni eggs. In addition to fever; there may be headache, abdominal pain, hepatosplenomegaly, lymphadenopathy. Serum immunoglobulins are elevated and there is eosinophilia. <u>Gastrointestinal and hepatic consequences:</u> Eggs deposited in the venules draining the colon may (**1**) penetrate the capillaries and be released into the GI lumen and excreted in the feces; (**2**) remain in the wall of the colon where they provoke a granulomatous reaction; (On colonoscopy, the mucosa has a reddened granular appearance, sometimes with ulceration and bleeding. There may be abdominal pain and bloody stools.) (**3**) be transported via the portal veins to the intrahepatic portal venules and cause portal inflammation. In severe cases, there is intrahepatic portal fibrosis leading to portal obstruction with portal hypertension. The liver and spleen are congested and enlarge. Varices form and the esophageal varices may bleed. Normal liver function is preserved until the later stages. Pulmonary complications: With portal hypertension there is portocaval shunting so that eggs may reach the pulmonary arterioles. As a consequence, there may be pulmonary arteriolar inflammation leading to fibrosis, and this may culminate in pulmonary hypertension with cor pulmonale. **Diagnosis** is confirmed by finding the characteristic eggs in the stool. **Treatment** is with a one day regimen of praziquantel consisting of three 20 mg/kg doses.

S. JAPONICUM infection occurs in the Philippines, Celebes, Japan, Taiwan, central and south China, Laos, Cambodia, Thailand, Cambodia, Malaysia. Domestic animals (e.g. cattle, dogs, cats) are also infected. **Pathoclinical consequences:** Dermatitis ("swimmer's itch") occasionally develops at the time cerceriae penetrate the skin. Immune–mediated acute febrile illness (Katayama fever) similar to the one seen with S. mansoni may develop 5–7 weeks after cercerial skin penetration. Pathoclinical consequences of egg deposition in the intestines, liver, and/or lungs is similar to S. mansoni. In addition, neurologic complications occur in 2–4% of cases as a consequence of egg deposition in the cerebral veins. **Diagnosis** is confirmed by finding the eggs in the stool, or by rectal biopsy if eggs are not seen in the stool. **Treatment** is with a one day regimen of praziquantel consisting of three 20 mg/kg doses.

Lung fluke
infection may be due to one of several species of Paragonimus. Paragonimus westermani is the most common culprit in man. Paragonimus also infect other mammals (e.g. cats, dogs, swine, cattle). Infection occurs in the Far East, India, W. Africa, and S. and Central America. **Life cycle:** Man becomes infected by eating freshwater crustacea (crab, crayfish) infected with metacercariae, a larval stage. The metacercaria penetrates the intestinal wall, enters and migrates thru the peritoneal cavity, penetrates the diaphragm, and finally lodges in the lung parenchyma where it develops into an adult with a life span of 5–6 years. Although more than one adult may inhabit the lung, this is not necessary for completion of the life cycle since the worms are hermaphroditic. The adult worm releases operculated eggs that are coughed up and are found in the sputum or subsequently swallowed and found in the feces. The eggs hatch in freshwater releasing miracidia which invade snails, multiply, and develop into cercariae. Cercariae subsequently leave the snail to infect fresh water crustacea which may be eaten by man to complete the cycle.

Signs/symptoms: Pulmonary: There is a gradual onset of productive cough. The sputum may be blood–tinged or there may be more flagrant hemoptysis. Chest pain and/or dyspnea may be present. A lung absess may develop. X–rays may reveal an infiltrate, cyst, pleural effusion, lung abscess. Abdominal: If a fluke implants in the abdominal cavity; there may be abdominal pain, GI ulceration with bleeding, abscess, or adhesions. Unusual sites of implantation include the brain, spinal cord, muscle, skin, genitals.

Diagnosis is confirmed by finding the characteristic eggs in the sputum or stool.

Treatment: praziquantel 25 mg/kg PO 3 times/day for 2 days.

Liver Flukes

CLONORCHIS SINENSIS infection is most prevalent in the Far East (e.g. China, Korea, Japan) where raw fish is regularly consumed. **Life cycle:** The metacercariae (encysted larval stage) are found in the muscle of a variety of freshwater fish. Upon ingestion by man, the larvae excyst in the duodenum and migrate up the biliary ducts where they develop into adults with a potential life span > 40 years. The worms are hermaphroditic and, about 3 weeks following ingestion, start to produce ova which are discharged with the bile and thence into the feces. The eggs hatch in fresh water releasing miracidia. The subsequent life cycle is similar to the lung fluke except that the last intermediate host is freshwater fish. **Signs/symptoms:** Most infected persons have no symptoms. Acute febrile illness may occur 1–3 weeks after exposure. Manifestations may include diarrhea; abdominal pain; tender and enlarged liver; jaundice; elevated bilirubin and liver enzymes (e.g. SGOT, alkaline phosphatase); eosinophilia. Recurrent pyogenic cholangitis may develop as a consequence of the formation of pigment stones in the bile ducts. There are recurrent episodes of fever with chills, biliary colic, and/or jaundice (Charcot's triad). Chronicity may lead to cirrhosis. Multiple hepatic abscesses may form. Suppurative cholangitis is a life-threatening E. coli infection of the bile ducts with ensuing septicemia that sometimes occurs when the bile ducts become obstructed by flukes. **Diagnosis:** Operculated eggs may be found on microscopic exam of feces or duodenal aspirate. **Treatment** of uncomplicated cases is with a one day regimen of three 25 mg/kg doses of praziquantel PO.

OPISTHORCHIS (O. viverrini, O. Felineus) infection also results from the consumption of raw freshwater fish. It is prevalent in Thailand, Vietnam, Laos, Japan, Philippines, India, Eastern Europe, Russia. The life cycle, clinical presentation, and treatment are the same as for Clonorchis.

FASCIOLA HEPATICA infects mammals worldwide, most notably sheep. **Life cycle:** Infection is acquired by eating aquatic plants (e.g. watercress) which are contaminated with metacercariae (encysted larval stage). The larvae excyst in the duodenum, penetrate the intestinal wall, migrate thru the peritoneal cavity, invade the liver, and eventually reach the biliary tree where they develop into adults. Infection to adulthood takes about 3 months. The worms are hermaphroditic. The ova are discharged with the bile and thence into the feces. The eggs hatch in freshwater releasing miracidia which invade snails, multiply, and develop into cercariae. The cycle is completed when cercariae subsequently leave the snail to infect freshwater aquatic plants which are eaten by man. **Signs/symptoms:** Acute illness: Infection during the migratory and development stage prior to the production of ova may result in a febrile illness with jaundice, hepatomegaly, abdominal pain, eosinophilia. Consequences of chronic biliary tract infection: The continued presence of adult flukes in the biliary tract causes inflammation. This may eventually lead to biliary tract obstruction and biliary cirrhosis. The liver may be enlarged. Urticaria or jaundice may occur. Gallstones are common. Patients may present with acute cholangitis (fever, jaundice, and/or abdominal pain). Extrabiliary implantation: On rare occasions, the flukes implant and develop at other sites—e.g. peritoneum, skin, muscle, lung, brain, eye). Halzoun is an unusual occurrence that may follow ingestion of raw sheep or goat liver infected with flukes. The flukes implant in the upper GI and respiratory tract causing inflammatory edema which in turn may lead to difficulty swallowing and/or breathing. Asphyxia may ensue. **Laboratory:** The characteristic operculated ova may be found in the feces. Complement fixation test may assist in the diagnosis. Other findings may include eosinophilia, elevated bilirubin and liver enzymes. **Treatment** of uncomplicated infection is with praziquantel 25 mg/kg PO 3 times/day for 2 days. Patients who fail to respond are treated with bithionol or possibly albendazole.

Intestinal Fluke
Fasciolopsis buski is medically the most important intestinal fluke. Infection is prevalent in S.E. Asia, S. China, India. **Life cycle:** Pigs are the usual host for the adult worms. Man acquires the infection by eating aquatic plants (e.g. water chestnuts) contaminated with metacercariae (encysted larval stage). Following ingestion; the larvae excyst, attach to the duodenum and jejunum, and develop into adults in about a month. The worm is hermaphroditic. The ova pass in the feces and hatch in freshwater. The remainder of the life cycle is similar to Fasciola hepatica (see above). **Signs/symptoms:** Most patients are asymptomatic. With heavy infections there may be abdominal pain, diarrhea, GI bleed, and/or GI obstruction. Severely affected patients may develop edema and ascites. **Laboratory:** Ova may be found in the stool. Eosinophilia is common. **Treatment:** praziquantel 25 mg/kg PO 3 times/day for 1–2 days.

Filariasis
refers to an infection by species of nematodes that are tissue parasites and are spread by arthropod vectors. The most important medical examples are covered below.

WUCHERERIA BANCROFTI infection occurs worldwide in tropical–subtropical regions. **Life cycle:** W. bancrofti is transmitted from man to man by various species of mosquitoes. The adult male and female roundworms live for years or decades in the lymph nodes and afferent lymphatics where they copulate and the females produce microfilariae. The latter are found in the bloodstream and may be ingested by a mosquito. In the mosquito, the microfilariae develop into infective larvae over a period of 2 weeks. The cycle is completed when an infected mosquito bites the only known definitive host, man. In man, development into the adult worms takes place over a period of months. **Signs/symptoms:** Those with light infections are often asymptomatic. Clinical expression stems mainly from the inflammation that results from the presence of adult worms in the lymphatics. Recurrent febrile illness: Typically, several times per year the patient will experience fever, chills, headache, tender lymphadenopathy, lymphangitis. There is spontaneous remission within several days. Chronic lymphatic injury leads first to lymphedema (due to damage to the lymphatic valves) and eventually to lymphatic obstruction with ensuing elephantiasis. In addition to the limbs, there may be lymphatic involvement of the breasts or genitals (scrotal edema). Chyluria may occur if there is obstruction with ensuing engorgement and rupture of the retroperitoneal lymphatics. Tropical eosinophilia syndrome may occur. Manifestations include fever, cough, wheezing, lymphadenopathy. Blood eosinophils and serum IgE are markedly elevated. Chest x-ray is frequently abnormal (e.g. miliary lesions, opacities). **Diagnosis:** Microfilariae may be found on microscopic exam of blood (Giemsa stain), lymph fluid, or chylous urine. In most regions, blood samples are best obtained at night because the microfilariae are nocturnal. To enhance the yield, the specimen may be filtered (3–5 μm Nuclepore) or concentrated (e.g. mix 1 ml sample blood with 9 ml of 2% formalin, centrifuge, and examine sediment). ●Other lab findings are eosinophilia and elevated serum IgE. **Treatment:** diethylcarbamazine is administered PO after meals for 3 weeks. On day 1, administer 50 mg PO once (25–50 mg in child). On day 2, administer 50mg x 3 (25–50mg x 3 in child). On day 3, administer 100mg x 3 (50–100mg x 3 in child). On days 4–21, administer 2 mg/kg 3 times/day. This regimen kills the microfilariae but additional courses are often needed to eliminate the adults.

BRUGIA MALAYI infection occurs in Malaysia, Indonesia, Philippines, China, Korea, Japan, India. B. malayi differs from W. bancrofti in that the cat is also a definitive host and is therefore a reservoir of infection. Furthermore, involvement of the genital lymphatics is unusual. Otherwise the life cycle, clinical expression, diagnosis, and treatment discussed above for W. bancrofti apply to B. malayi.

ONCHOCERCIASIS (River Blindness) is due to Onchocerca volvulus. It is most prevalent in subsaharan tropical Africa. It also occurs in Yemen, Mexico, Guatemala, Colombia, Venezuela, Ecuador, Brazil. Species of biting black flies spread the microfilariae from man to man. Severe disease occurs in those who have the heaviest worm loads because of repeated bites by infected black flies. The adult worms live together and mate in the subcutaneous tissues, next to long bones and joints, and in fascial planes between the muscles. The offspring microfilariae live in various organs but express themselves clinically by there presence in the skin, lymph nodes, and eyes. Microfilariae live up to 2 years while the adult worms survive up to 15 years. **Signs/symptoms:** Subcutaneous nodules may sometimes be felt and are due to the presence of adult worms. Aside from cosmetic considerations, the presence of the adult worms themselves rarely causes any other manifestations. The main clinical consequences stem from the presence of their offspring, the microfilariae. Skin lesions: Microfilariae migrate locally to produce a pruritic red papular rash. In chronic heavy infections, the skin subsequently becomes thickened, lichenified, and then atrophied. Pigmentary changes accompany. Lymphadenopathy: Regional lymph nodes may be enlarged. Impaired vision or blindness may result when microfilariae invade the eyes and provoke inflammation with the following possible consequences: keratitis with corneal opacities, iridocyclitis culminating in glaucoma, chorioretinal lesions, optic neuritis/atrophy. **Diagnosis** is confirmed by one fo the following: (1) recovering adult worms from a subcutaneous nodule, (2) finding microfilariae on microscopic exam of a bloodless skin-snip of an involved region, (3) observing microfilariae in the anterior chamber or cornea on slit-lamp exam. ●In mild infections, when the diagnosis is suspected but the adult worms or microfilariae cannot be found; a helpful diagnostic maneuver is to challenge the patient with diethylcarbamazine (adult 50 mg PO) and observe for worsening of rash or pruritis over the next 24 hours. **Treatment:** ivermectin 150 mg/kg PO once. For prophylaxis the dose may be repeated every 6–12 months.

LOIASIS (infection by the filarial worm Loa Loa) is restricted to rain forests of west and central Africa. The infection is spread by biting deer flies (Chrysops). The adult worms (5–7 cm long) live in the subcutaneous tissues where they mate and produce microfilariae. **Signs/symptoms:** Many cases are asymptomatic. Sometimes, an adult worm can be seen traversing the eye beneath the conjunctiva, felt moving beneath the skin, or seen by its impression beneath the skin. Calabar swellings (painful pruritic erythematous localized patches of subcutaneous edema) may appear as a consequence of an allergic reaction to the presence of adult worm in the subcutaneous tissue. Unusual complications include peripheral nerve involvement, cardiomyopathy, nephropathy, encephalopathy. **Laboratory:** Microfilariae may be found on microscopic exam of the blood. However, microfilariae are not consistently found, especially in patients who are travelers to endemic areas. The presence of eosinophilia and elevated filarial antibody supports the diagnosis. **Treatment:** diethylcarbamazine as for W. Bancrofti above.

Beef tapeworm (Taenia saginata) infestation is very common in Africa; and

occurs in the Middle East, Asia, and Latin America. It is less common in the U.S.
   Life cycle: Man is infested by eating raw or inadequately cooked beef infected with encysted larvae (cysticerci). In the gut, the larva excysts and attaches by its scolex to the jejunal mucosa. The worm matures into an adult in 1–3 months with a potential lifespan of 25 years. The tapeworm consists of the scolex and a neck from which is produced a succession of proglottids attached in ribbon–like chain that may attain a length of 10 meters with thousands of proglottids. Fertilized eggs are produced within the hermaphroditic proglottids. The egg–containing distal proglottids successively break–off. The eggs are passed in the stool within the proglottid or free. Cattle ingest the eggs which then hatch within the cattle's gut to release oncospheres (embryos). The cycle is completed when the encospheres penetrate the cattle's intestinal mucosa and pass via the bloodstream to the skeletal muscle where they form cysticerci.
   Signs/symptoms: Most cases are asymptomatic. There may be diarrhea, cramping, flatulence, weight loss.
   Laboratory: Gross inspection of stools often reveals the diagnostically characteristic proglottids. Microscopic exam: Eggs that have ruptured from a proglottid may be detected by applying cellophane tape to the anal area and then sticking the tape to a glass slide. However, the eggs cannot be distinguised from those of T. solium. Mild eosinophilia is a common finding.
   Treatment: A single dose of niclosamide (Niclocide) is the treatment of choice (adult——2 gram, child over 34 kg——1.5 gram, child 11–34 kg——1 gram). The tablets are chewed and swallowed with a small amount of water on empty stomach. ●A single dose of praziquantel 10–20 mg/kg is also effective.

Pork tapeworm (Taenia solium) causes 2 types of infection in man: (1) **Intestinal infestation** by the adult tapeworm, and (2) **cysticercosis**—infection of the tissues with cysticerci (encysted larvae).

INTESTINAL INFESTATION is acquired by ingesting raw or undercooked flesh of pigs with cysticerci. The cysticercus (encysted larva) is released within the gut and upon reaching the jejunum fixes by its scolex to the intestinal wall. It matures in 5–12 weeks into an adult tapeworm. The events that follow are similar to that described for human intestinal infestation by beef tapeworm (see above). Intestinal infestation by the adult tapeworm is generally asymptomatic. **Diagnosis** rests on finding characteristic proglottids or eggs in the stool. There may be a mild eosinophilia. **Treatment** is as above for beef tapeworm infestation.

CYSTICERCOSIS develops in man or pigs when they ingest food or water contaminated with human feces containing the eggs. Humans with intestinal infestation may also develop cysticercosis (1) by transferring the eggs from anus to mouth or (2) rarely by regurgitating proglottids into the stomach with the subsequent release of eggs from ruptured proglottids. Whatever the mechanism of infection, the eggs hatch within the gut lumen releasing oncospheres (embryos). These penetrate the intestinal mucosa and pass via the bloodstream to the tissues where they form cysticerci (encysted larvae). Fever and myalgias may result. The encysted larvae die after a number of years and calcify. Serious consequences may occur when cysticerci form in the CNS (e.g. increased intracranial pressure, hydrocephalus, seizures and other neurologic abnormalities). The onset of CNS manifestations may be delayed for years. **Diagnosis** of cysticercosis is established by finding cysticerci within subcutaneous nodules. Skull x-rays may reveal calcified cysticerci. CAT scan may also identify the CNS lesions. Indirect hemagglutination test may be positive. A CSF complement fixation test may also be helpful. There may be eosinophilia.

Dwarf tapeworm (Hymenolepis nana) infestation is acquired by ingesting feces contaminated with the eggs. The definitive host is man, rat, or mouse.

Life cycle: The dwarf tapeworm, unlike other tapeworm infestations, is able to complete its life cycle without an intermediate host stage. Following ingestion, the eggs hatch in the gut lumen releasing an oncosphere (embryo). The embryo invades the small intestinal mucosa and subsequently forms a cysticercus (encysted larva). In a few days, the larva is released from the mucosa into the gut lumen and, upon reaching the ileum, fixes by its scolex to the mucosa. It matures into an adult tapeworm within 2 weeks. A succession of proglottids are produced. Fertilized eggs are produced within the hermaphroditic proglottids. The mature distal proglottids break down releasing their eggs. The cycle is completed when the eggs either: (1) pass with the stool and are subsequently ingested by the same or other host, or (2) hatch within the small intestine.

Signs/symptoms: Infection may be asymptomatic. With heavy infestations, there may be diarrhea or cramping.

Laboratory: Diagnosis rests upon finding the characteristic eggs in the feces. Proglottids are not found. Mild eosinophilia may occur.

Treatment: praziquantel 25 mg/kg once. Niclosamide is alternative.

Fish tapeworm (Diphyllobothrium latum) infestation has a wide distribution. Regions with the greatest incidence include Scandinavia, Canada, Alaska, Minnesota, Michigan.

Life cycle: Humans are infected by ingesting raw or undercooked freshwater fish whose flesh contains sparganum (plerocercoid larvae). A sparganum attaches to the small intestine and develops into an adult tapeworm over 3–6 weeks. The adult, with a potential lifespan of 20 years, consists of the scolex and a neck from which is produced a succession of proglottids attached in a chain sometimes attaining 10 meters in length with thousands of proglottids. Fertilized eggs are produced within the hermaphroditic proglottids. The proglottids do not detach but the distal mature proglottids break down releasing eggs that pass with the stool. In fresh water, the eggs hatch and the embryo is ingested by a copepod (a small crustacea) where the 1st larval stage takes place. The copepod may be eaten by a freshwater fish, the site of the 2nd larval stage. The cycle is completed when man eats contaminated raw or undercooked fish.

Signs/symptoms: There are no symptoms in most cases. There may be mild GI complaints. In rare instances, vitamin B–12 deficiency with megaloblastic anemia develops because the vitamin is taken up by the tapeworm.

Diagnosis is made by finding the characteristic operculated eggs in the stool. The proglottids also have a characteristic appearance.

Treatment is as for beef tapeworm (see above).

Hydatid disease is due to infection by the intermediate larval stage of the

tapeworm Echinococcus granulosus, or much less frequently E. multilocularis. E. granulosus infection occurs worldwide, primarily wherever sheep are raised. Sheep serve as the usual intermediate host and dogs are the usual definitive host for the adult tapeworm. E. multilocularis cycle is perpetuated in the northern hemisphere by the fox (definitive host) and rodents (intermediate host). **Life cycle:** The intermediate host (sheep most commonly, sometimes rodents or man) becomes infected upon ingesting the eggs that have been excreted in the feces of the definitive host (usually dogs, sometimes coyote, fox, cat) where the adult tapeworm resides. ●The eggs hatch in the duodenum of man (or sheep or rodents) releasing the embryo which traverse the intestinal mucosa and are carried via the portal veins to the liver. Implantation and development of the cyst may take place in the liver (> 70% cases), or the embryo may pass through the liver and implant in the lung (20% cases) or other organs. ●A hydatid cyst is composed of an outer fibrous layer derived from the host and an inner germinal layer from which daughter cysts form. The daughter cysts contain embryonic tapeworms which develop into adult tapeworms if they are ingested by a definitive host. The hydatid cyst stage is a dead–end in man. ●The cycle is perpetuated, however, if an infected intermediate host (e.g. sheep, rodent) is eaten by a definitive host (e.g dog). In the definitive host, the larva attaches to the intestinal wall and develops into the adult tapeworm.

Signs/symptoms depend on the site of the cyst. Many cases are asymptomatic. Some cysts eventually calcify and cause no further disease. Liver cyst accounts for over 70% cases of hydatid disease. Symptoms seldom emerge until the cyst is > 10 cm in diameter. Cysts grow about 1cm/yr so that it usually takes many years before symptoms appear. There may be right upper quadrant pain with an enlarged liver. Jaundice sometimes occurs. Ballotment over the liver may elicit a thrill. A cyst may rupture into the peritoneum, gut, bile ducts, or lungs leading to implantation of daughter cysts at other sites. Lung cyst is the 2nd most common cyst site. The patient may have no complaints; or there may be cough, chest pain, and/or hemoptysis. Brain cyst may lead to increased intracranial pressure, convulsions, etc. Allergic complications; Rupture of a cyst may also cause anaphylaxis while gradual leakage may cause recurrent urticaria.

Laboratory: Ultrasound or CAT scan are best for verifying the presence of a cyst. Plain x–ray may identify a calcified cyst. Casoni skin test turns positive if the cyst has leaked. Serology may likewise be positive if the cyst has leaked (e.g. indirect hemagglutination, complement fixation, immunoelectrophoresis). Eosinophilia occurs with leakage. Alkaline phosphatase may be elevated with a liver cyst. Never perform diagnostic needle aspiration of a hydatid cyst since anaphylaxis may result and/or the organism may be disseminated.

Treatment: excision. Mebendazole (see drug section) may be administered preoperatively in order to shrink a cyst or may be used postoperatively if there is leakage.

Clinical Index

Clinical Index

Clinical Index

Clinical Index

Clinical Index

Clinical Index

Clinical Index

Clinical Index

Clinical Index

Clinical Index

Clinical Index

Clinical Index

Clinical Index

Clinical Index

Drug
Section

Notice: The author has made every effort to verify the accuracy of information in this book, particularly in regards to drug use and dosage. However, because of the possibility of human error and because medical therapy including drug recommendations may change, the author cannot categorically guarantee the accuracy or currency of information contained in this book. The author and publisher disclaim responsibility for any adverse effects resulting from inadvertent errors in the text or from misunderstandings of the text. Therefore, readers are urged to consult the most recent reliable references in order to confirm that treatment recommendations are correct and consistent with current sound medical practice. In particular, readers should consult the product information included with each drug they plan to administer in order to verify drug indications, contraindications, and proper dosage. This is especially important with new or infrequently used drugs, and with dosages in elderly or pediatric patients. In short, it is the responsibility of the medical practitioner to ascertain the optimal therapy for each patient depending on the clinical setting and in accordance with the latest authoritative information. That this book is intended as a reference for trained health professionals is inherent in the foregoing comments.

ACETAMINOPHEN (Datril, Liquiprin, Panadol, Phenaphen, Tempra, Tylenol, etc)

Indications: fever, mild to moderate pain. Does not have anti–inflammatory effect.
Contraindication: acetaminophen hypersensitivity.
Caution: Do not exceed 3000 mg/day. Overdose may cause fatal hepatic toxicity.
Side effects are rare: hypersensitivity (rash, uticaria, laryngeal edema, drug fever); hematologic (anemia, leukopenia, thrombocytopenia, pancytopenia).
Overdose: Ingestion of over 140 mg/kg may be hepatotoxic. A post ingestion serum acetaminophen level of 140 mcg/ml at 4 hr, 70 mcg/ml at 8 hr, 35 mcg/ml at 12 hr may be hepatotoxic. Low serum acetaminophen levels obtained before 4 hr have elapsed may not reflect degree of poisoning since GI absorption may not yet be complete. However, a serum level greater than 300 mcg/ml at any time following ingestion is hepatotoxic. Lavage or induce emesis. Start acetylcysteine (refer to "Acetylcysteine" for dose) as soon as possible after serum levels are found to be in the toxic range. Cathartics and charcoal interfere with acetylcysteine absorption and should be withheld. If charcoal has been given, lavage until clear and then administer acetylcysteine.
Supplied as: tablets (80, 120, 325, 500, 650 mg);   elixir (160 mg/5ml);
        drops (80 mg/0.8 ml);   suppository (120, 300, 600 mg).

Dose:	0–3 month:	30 mg q4–6h	3–12 month:	60 mg q4–6h
	1–3 year:	60–120 mg q4–6h	3–6 year:	120–180 mg q4–6h
	6–12 year:	240 mg q4–6h	adult/child > 12 yr:	325–650 mg q4–6h

ACETYLCYSTEINE (Mucomyst)

Action/indications: Inhalant: Acetylcysteine lowers the viscosity of mucus by acting upon the disulfide linkages of mucoprotein. It is useful as a mucolytic when there is inspissated or viscid mucus in such conditions as asthma, bronchitis, emphysema.
Antidote to acetaminophen overdose; Acetylcysteine replenishes body's store of glutathione. Glutathione conjugates with and thereby inactivates hepatotoxic metabolites of acetaminophen.
Comments: ●Bronchospasm may occur with acetylcysteine inhalation therapy. A nebulized bronchodilator will usually provide relief but acetylcysteine must be discontinued if bronchospasm progresses. ●Increased bronchial secretions may occur with acetylcysteine inhalation. Mechanical suction must be available if cough is inadequate. ●After 3/4 of the initial inhalation solution has been nebulized, a volume of sterile water for injection USP equal to the volume of remaining solution is added to the nebulizer to prevent overconcentration of the solution.
Side effects: stomatitis, nausea, vomiting, rhinorrhea, bronchospasm, acquired sensitivity.
Supplied as: 10% solution (100 mg/ml) in 4, 10, and 30 ml vials;
        20% solution (200 mg/ml) in 4, 10, and 30 ml vials.
Dose for inhalation (adult or child):
Nebulization (via face mask, mouth piece, tracheostomy):
  20% solution: 1–10 ml q2–6h. For most patients: 3–5 ml tid–qid.
  10% solution: 2–20 ml q2–6h. For most patients: 6–10 ml tid–qid.
Direct instillation: 1–2 ml of 10 or 20% solution as often as every hour if needed.
Dose as acetaminophen overdose antidote (after emptying stomach):
140 mg/kg PO initial dose followed by 70 mg/kg PO q4h for 17 additional doses.

ACYCLOVIR (Zovirax)

Action: Acyclovir is a purine mucleoside analog which is converted by virus–coded thymidine kinase into acyclovir monophosphate (a nucleotide analog) which is in turn converted by host cell enzymes to acyclovir triphosphate. The latter interferes with viral DNA polymerase thereby inhibiting viral DNA replication. Acyclovir is active against herpes simplex 1 and 2, varicella–zoster, Ebstein–Barr, cytomegalovirus. Acyclovir does not eliminate latent viruses.
Indications:
Oral; ●Initial genital herpes infection. ●To reduce frequency and/or severity of genital herpes episodes in patient with frequent recurrences (6 or more episodes/yr). Treat for up to 6 months only. Do not use acyclovir if recurrences are mild. Patient with infrequent episodes may be treated as needed. ●Immunocompromised patients with recurrent herpes episodes may be treated intermittently as needed or may receive chronic suppressive therapy. ●Herpes Zoster.
Intravenous; ●Initial and recurrent herpes simplex 1 or 2 involvement of skin and mucosa in immunocompromised patient. ●Severe initial genital herpes infection in patient with normal immune function. ●Herpes simplex encephalitis. ●Herpes Zoster in immunocompromised patient.
Topical ointment; ●Initial genital herpes infection (not of clinical benefit in recurrent episodes). ●Limited non–life–threatening mucocutaneous herpes infection in immunocompromised patient.
Contraindications: hypersensitivity to any of components. Product is not for eye application.
Caution: Consider risk/benefit in pregnancy or nursing mother.
Comments: ●If the diagnosis of herpes simples is in doubt, viral cultures of lesions should be used to confirm diagnosis. Presumptive diagnosis is made by finding multinucleated giant cells on Wright or Giemsa stains. ●Avoid intercourse if there are active genital herpes lesions.

●Concurrent probenecid administration prolongs half–life of acyclovir.

Side effects: With PO use: (1) Short–term effects: nausea, vomiting, headache, anorexia, diarrhea, dizziness, fatigue, rash, edema, leg pain, inguinal adenopathy, sore throat, medication taste. (2) Long–term effects: nausea, vomiting, headache, vertigo, arthralgia, rash, insomnia, fatigue, fever, palpitations, sore throat, superficial thrombophlebitis, muscle cramps, pars planitis, menstrual abnormalities, acne, lymphadenopathy, irritability, depression, accelerated hair loss. With IV use: transiently elevated serum creatinine, injection site phlebitis, rash, hives, sweating, hypotension, headache, nausea, hematuria, thrombocytosis, jitters, lethargy, obtundation, tremors, confusion, hallucinations, agitation, convulsions, coma. With topical use, local effects include mild pain, pruritis, rash, or vulvitis.

Supplied as: ●200 mg capsule, ●200 mg/5ml suspension, ●5% ointment in 15 gram tubes, ●10ml vial containing 500 mg for IV injection.

Oral dose:
●Initial genital herpes infection: 200 mg q4h 5 times/day for 10 days.
●Chronic suppressive therapy of recurrent disease: 400 mg twice daily for up to 12 months. Then re–evaluate.
●Intermittent therapy: 200 mg q4h 5 times/day for 5 days. Begin therapy at first sign of recurrence.
●Acute treatment Herpes Zoster: 800 mg q4h 5 times/day for 7–10 days.
●Dosage adjustment in renal failure: Refer to product information.

Intravenous dose (dilute in standard IV solution and infuse dose over 1 hour):
●Herpes simplex 1 & 2 infections of skin & mucosa in immunodeficient patient:
   adult: 5 mg/kg q8h for 7 days,
   child under 12 yr: 250 mg/square meter q8h for 7 days.
●Severe initial genital herpes: same dosage as just described for 5 days.
●Herpes simplex encephalitis:
   adult: 10mg/kg q8h for 10 days.
   child 6 months–12 yr: 500 mg/square meter q8h for 10 days.
●Herpes zoster in immunocompromised patient:
   adult: 10mg/kg q8h for 7 days. Dose obese patient according to ideal body
    weight. Maximum dose for any patient is 500mg/square meter q8h.
   child < 12 yr: 500 mg/square meter q8h for 7 days.
NOTE: (a) Refer to product information for dose adjustment in renal failure.
      (b) Avoid SC or IM injection.

Topical Ointment: apply to affected area q3h six times/day for 7 days using a rubber glove or finger cot so as to prevent autoinnoculation of other body sites or transmission to other persons.

ADRENERGIC BRONCHODILATORS:

albuterol (Proventil, Ventolin)
bitolterol (Tornalate)
isoetharine (Bronkometer, Bronkosol)
metaproterenol (Alupent, Metaprel)
pirbuterol (Maxair)
terbutaline (Brethine, Brethaire, Bricanyl)
   *Find **epinephrine** and **isoproterenol** (Isuprel) under individual headings.

Action: The six drugs presented here selectively stimulate beta–2 receptors in bronchial smooth muscle. The consequent bronchial smooth muscle relaxation results in bronchodilation. Albuterol and terbutaline show greater beta–2 selectivity than metaproterenol or isoetharine. The beta–1 effect that does occur results in cardiac stimulation (tachycardia, increased contractility).

Indications: bronchial asthma, emphysema–associated or bronchitis–associated reversible bronchospasm.

Contraindications: hypersensitivity to any of components.

Caution: hypertension, cardiovascular disease, diabetes mellitus, hyperthyroidism, pregnancy, seizure disorder, patient receiving MAO inhibitor or tricyclic antidepressant. ●Adrenergic aerosols may lose their effectiveness if they are used too frequently. Furthermore, paradoxical bronchospasm may sometimes occur.

Side effects include tremor, headache, anxiety, restlessness, insomnia, nausea, vomiting, dizziness, vertigo, tinnitus, weakness, palpitations, tachycardia, hypertension, angina, heartburn, urinary retention, muscle cramps, dry/irritated oropharynx. ●Because of their beta–2 receptor selectivity, the incidence of side effects is less than with other adrenergic drugs (e.g. epinephrine, isoproterenol).

albuterol (Proventil, Ventolin)
Supplied as: ●2 or 4 mg tablet, ●4 mg extended–release tablet (Proventil Rep-etabs), ●syrup (2mg/5ml), ●inhaler (0.5% or 0.83%) solution for inhalation via nebulizer, ●200 mcg capsule for inhalation (Ventolin Rotacaps), ●Inhalation aerosol (Ventolin).
Dose tablets:
●Adults/child over 12 yr: start with 2–4 mg tid–qid (max 8 mg qid).
●Child 6–12 yr: start with 2 mg tid–qid (maximum 24 mg/day).
Dose extended–release tablet (Proventil Repetab): start with 4–8 mg (1–2 tablets) q12h. Maximum: 16 mg q12 h.
Dose syrup:
●Adult/child > 14 yr: Initially, 2–4 mg (1–2 tsp) tid–qid. maximum. 8 mg qid.
●Child 6–14 yr: start with 2 mg (1 tsp) tid–qid. Maximum 24 mg/day.
●Child 2–6 yr: start with 0.1mg/kg tid (not to exceed 2 mg tid). Maximum dose in child 2–6 yr is 0.2 mg/kg tid or 4 mg tid whichever is less.
Dose Ventolin inhalation aerosol (adult/child over 12 yr): 1–2 inhalations q4–6h.
Dose with nebulizer (adult/child over 12 yr): 2.5 mg tid–qid.
Dose Ventolin Rotacaps (adult/child over 12 yr): inhale contents of 1 capsule q8h.

bitolterol (Tornalate)
Supplied as: metered dose inhaler.
Dose (adult/child over 12 yr): Bronchospasm: one inhalation, wait 1–3 minutes, 2nd inhalation, 3rd inhalation as needed.
Prevent bronchospasm: 2 inhalations q8h.

isoetharine (Bronkometer, Bronkosol)
Supplied as: aerosol inhaler (Bronkometer), 1% solution for nebulization (Bronkosol).
Dose (adult):
●Aerosol inhaler (Bronkometer): 1–2 inhalations; wait 1 minute and give a repeat inhalation if needed. Repeat treatments may be given q4h as needed.
●Inhalation solution (Bronkosol):
  (1) hand nebulizer: 3–7 inhalations (usually 4 inhalations) q4h of undiluted 1% so-lution;
  (2) oxygen aerosolization: 0.25–0.5 ml 1% solution (diluted 1: 3 in normal saline) q4h;
  (3) IPPB: 0.25–1.0 ml of 1% solution (diluted 1: 3 in normal saline) q4h.

metaproterenol (Alupent, Metaprel)
Supplied as: 10 or 20 mg tablet, 10mg/5ml syrup, aerosol inhaler, 5% inhalant solution, inhalant solution in unit dose vials (0.4 and 0.6%).
Dose tablets: ●Adult: 20 mg tid–qid. ●Child > 9 yr or > 27 kg: same as adult. ●Child 6–9 yr or < 27 kg: 10 mg tid–qid. ●Child < 6 yr: not recommended.
Dose syrup: dose is as for tablets.
Syrup has been used in children < 6 yr : 1.3–2.6 mg/kg/24hr divided.
Aerosol inhaler (adult/child > 12 yr): 2–3 inhalations q3–4h. Maximum 12 inhala-tions/24hr.
Hand–bulb nebulizer (adult/child > 12 yr): 5–15 inhalations (usually 10) of undiluted 5% solution.
IPPB (adult/child > 12 yr): contents of 0.4% or 0.6% unit dose vial, or 0.2–0.3 ml of 5% solution diluted in 2.5 ml normal saline. IPPB treatment may be repeated in 4 hours. May give 3–4 treatments/day as needed.

pirbuterol (Maxair)   Supplied as: aerosol inhaler.
Dose (adults/child over 12 yr): one inhalation q4–6h.

terbutaline (Brethine, Brethaire, Bricanyl)
Supplied as: 2.5 or 5 mg tablet, solution for SC injection (1mg/ml), aerosol inhaler (Brethaire).
Dose (adult/child over 12 yr):
●Inhaler: one inhalation, wait 1 minute, 2nd inhalation. Repeat q4–6h as needed.
●Oral: 2.5–5 mg tid (usually 5 mg tid). Maximum 15 mg/24hr.
●SC injection: 0.25 mg (0.25 ml), repeat as needed in 15–30 minutes.
Dose child 12–15 yr: 2.5 mg PO tid. Maximum 7.5 mg/24hr.

ALLOPURINOL (Zyloprim, Lopurin)

Action: Decreases serum uric acid by inhibiting xanthine oxidase (the enzyme catalyzing conversion hypoxanthine to xanthine and xanthine to uric acid).

Indications: ●Hyperuricemia that is associated with gout, uric acid nephropathy, or recurrent renal uric acid stones. ●Prevention of hyperuricemia and its consequences (gout, uric acid nephropathy/nephrolithiasis) in patients susceptible to hyperuricemia—e.g. certain malignancies (e.g. lymphoma, leukemia); during cytotoxic therapy for malignancy. ●Recurrent calcium oxalate nephrolithiasis that is associated with urinary uric acid excretion > 800 mg/24 hr in male and > 750 nmg/24 hr in female.

Contraindications: allopurinol hypersensitivity.

Caution: pregnancy (consider risk vs benefit), nursing mother.

Comments: ●Sufficient fluid intake to maintain urine output of at least 2 liter/day is recommended. ●Allopurinol will not alleviate acute gout attack. Use indomethacin or colchicine to quell the attack and start allopurinol 1–2 weeks after attack subsides. If patient is already on allopurinol when attack occurs, continue allopurinol at same dose. ●Allopurinol by mobilizing uric acid may itself precipitate a gout attack. Consequently, continue prophylactic indomethacin or colchicine for a few months after last gouty attack. ●Patient with infrequent gout attacks may not need allopurinol unless serum uric acid is chronically greater than 9 mg/100 ml (or urinary uric acid excretion greater than 1000 mg/day) or uric acid nephropathy is present. ●Discontinue allopurinol if rash occurs. ●Allopurinol by inhibiting xanthine oxidase inhibits the metabolism of mercaptopurine (Purinethol) and azathioprine (Imuran). Consequently, give 1/4 – 1/3 usual dosage of mercaptopurin or azathioprine when initiating concurrent therapy with allopurinol and make subsequent dose adjustments of mercaptopurin or azathioprine contingent on toxic and/or therapeutic response. ●Obtain CBC, liver function tests, BUN, and creatinine when initiating therapy and periodically. ●Allopurinol prolongs half-life of dicumarol but not warfarin.

Side effects include: <u>skin</u> (maculopapular rash, exfoliation, urticaria, purpura, Stevens–Johnson syndrome, toxic epidermal necrolysis, alopecia); <u>gastrointestinal</u> (occasional nausea, vomiting, diarrhea, abdominal pain, impaired taste); <u>hepatic</u> (elevated alkaline phosphatase, transaminases, bilirubin); <u>drowsiness</u> occasionally (use drug with caution if patient engages in activities requiring alertness); <u>idiosyncratic</u> (fever, chills, rash, pruritis, eosinophilia, leukopenia or leukocytosis, nausea, vomiting, arthralgias); <u>rare side effects</u> (peripheral neuritis, renal failure with concurrent use of thiazide, cholestatic jaundice, hepatitis, hepatic necrosis, vasculitis, necrotizing angitis).

Supplied as: 100, 300 mg tablets.

Adult dose: Dose is individualized and is best tolerated if given after meals. Start with 100 mg PO once daily. Increase daily dose by 100 mg at weekly intervals to achieve serum uric acid 6 mg/100ml or less. Maximum 800 mg/day.
●Usual requirements; mild gout: 200–300 mg/day; moderately severe tophaceous gout: 400–600 mg/day. ●Up to 300 mg may be given as a single daily dose. Dose should be divided if the patient requires > 300 mg/day.

<u>Prevention uric acid nephropathy during aggressive chemotherapy for neoplasia</u>: Start with 600–800mg/day. After 2–3 days, adjust dosage according to clinical judgment. Remember to give a generous amount of fluid in order to assure a high urine output.

<u>Dose adjustment renal failure</u>:	creatinine clearance	dose
	10–20 ml/min	200 mg/day,
	less than 10 ml/min	100 mg/day,
	less than 3 ml/min	100 mg/q 36–48 hr.

Pediatric dose (hyperuricemia secondary to neoplasia):
<u>6–10 yr of age</u>: 300 mg PO once daily, <u>less than 6 yr</u>: 150 mg PO once daily. Adjust dose as needed after 48 hours.

AMINOGLYCOSIDES: amikacin (Amikin), gentamycin (Garamycin), tobramycin (Nebcin)

Find **streptomycin** under separate heading.

Action/Spectrum: Bactericidal by binding to the bacterial 30S ribosomal subunit. <u>Sensitive bacteria include</u>: aerobic gram negative bacilli (Pseudomonas aerugenosa, E. coli, proteus, klebsiella, enterobacter, serratia, citrobacter, acinetobacter, providencia, salmonella, shigella, haemophilus); gram–negative cocci (Neisseria gonorrhea, Neisseria meningitidis); gram–positive rods (corynebacterium, listeria, Bacillus anthracis); staphylococci. <u>Gentamycin or tobramycin–resistant strains of aerobic gram–negaitve bacilli</u> (e.g. some Pseudomonas aeruginosa strains) may be sensitive to amikacin. Bacteria resistant to amikacin are often resistant to the other aminoglycosides. <u>Mycobacterium tuberculosis</u> is sensitive to gentamycin and amikacin. <u>Atypical mycobacteria</u> may be sensitive to amikacin.
<u>Resistant bacteria include</u>; gram–positive cocci (staphylococci excepted); anaerobes (e.g. bacteroides, clostridia); rickettsia.

Indications: Serious infections (not amenable to less toxic antiobiotics) caused by aerobic gram-negative bacilli (Pseudomonas aerugenosa, E. coli, proteus, klebsiella, enterobacter, serratia, citrobacter, providencia). ●Aminoglycosides enter the CSF poorly and, except for intrathecal gentamycin, are not useful in CNS infections. **Aminoglycoside is often combined with:** (l) carbenecillin or ticarcillin in treatment of pseudomonas infection, (2) nafcillin or oxacillin in treatment of acute bacterial endocarditis pending culture results, (3) penicillin G or ampicillin in treatment of enterococcal endocarditis, (4) ampicillin in treatment of neonatal meningitis of unknown etiology, (5) ampicillin in treatment of biliary tract infections unknown etiology, (6) carbenicillin, ticarcillin, or cephalosporin in treatment of immunocompromised patient with severe infection of unknown etiology, (7) cephalosporin in treatment of serious klebsiella infection or nosocomial pneumonia of unknown etiology, (8) doxycycline, chloramphenicol, carbenecillin, ticarcillin, cefoxitin, clindamycin, or metronidazole in treatment of pelvic/abdominal sepsis of unknown etiology.

Contraindications: aminoglycoside hypersensitivity, pregnancy (except in life–threatening infections unresponsive to other antibiotics), nursing mother.

Caution: ●Avoid concurrent or sequential use of other potentially nephrotoxic and/or neurotoxic drugs (e.g. furosemide, ethacrynic acid, other aminoglycosides, vancomycin, cephaloridine, polymyxin B, colistin). ●Use aminoglycosides caution in presence of neuromuscular disorders (e.g. Parkinsonism, myasthenia gravis) or in patient receiving neuromuscular blocking drugs or anesthetics.

Side effects include: nephrotoxicity (albuminuria, casts, elevated BUN and creatinine, oliguria); ototoxicity (tinnitus, feeling of fullness or roaring in ears, deafness, dizziness, vertigo, loss of balance); hypersensitivity (fever, rash, pruritis, urticaria, stomatitis, eosinophilia, anaphylaxis, exfoliative dermatitis); neurologic (headache, lethargy, paresthesias, peripheral neuritis, tremor, neuromuscular blockade which may result in paralysis or apnea); blood (anemia, granulocytopenia, leukopenia, thrombocytopenia); gastrointestinal (nausea, vomiting, diarrhea, stomatitis, enterocolitis); liver (elevated transaminases and bilirubin, transient hepatosplenomegaly).

Dose based on ideal body weight and assuming normal renal function:

amikacin (Amikin)   Supplied as: 50 or 250 mg/ml for IV or IM administration.
Adult/child: 5 mg/kg q8h or 7.5 mg/kg q12h IM or IV (maximum 15 mg/kg/24hr).
Neonate: loading: 10 mg/kg IM or IV, maintenance: 7.5 mg/kg q12h IM or IV.

gentamycin (Garamycin)
Supplied as: IV or IM injection (10 or 40 mg/ml), Intrathecal (2 mg/ml).
Adult: 1 mg/kg q8h IM or IV.
In life–threatening infection: 1.7 mg/kg q8h; reduce to 1 mg/kg q8h when improved.
Child: 2.0–2.5 mg/kg q8h IM or IV.
Infant/neonate > 1 wk age: 2.5 mg/kg q8h IM or IV.
Neonate < 1 wk of age or premature neonate:: 2.5 mg/kg q12h IM or IV.
Intrathecal (adjunct in treatment CNS infection)
    Adult: 4–8 mg once daily.   Pediatric (> 3 months of age): 1–2 mg once daily.

tobramycin (Nebcin)   Supplied as: 10 or 40 mg/ml for IV or IM injection.
Adult: 1 mg/kg q8h IM or IV.
Life–threatening infection: 1.66 mg/kg q8h; reduce to 1 mg/kg q8h when improved.
Child: 2.0–2.5 mg/kg q8h IM or IV (or 1.5–1.89 mg/kg q6h).
Neonate < 1 wk of age or premature neonate: up to 2 mg/kg ql2h IM or IV.

Dose adjustments and administration recommendations:

Intravenous administration: Dilute and infuse IV over 30–60 min in adult; over 1–2 hours in infant. Do not mix aminoglycosides in the same IV line with other drugs.

Dose adjustment in obese patient: Use the following adjusted weight in determining dose: (ideal body weight) + (0.4 x excess body weight).

Adjusting dose according to peak and trough levels: Young patients with normal renal function who are treated 7-l0 days or less are exempted from peak and trough monitoring. In other patients, after 2–3 days of therapy and at 3–4 day intervals; obtain peak level (30 min after completing IV infusion, l hr after IM) and trough level (within 15 min next dose).

Adjust dose to avoid	trough greater than:	peak greater than:
amikacin	10 mcg/ml	30–35 mcg/ml
gentamycin	2 mcg/ml	12 mcg/ml
tobramycin	2 mcg/ml	12 mcg/ml

Duration of therapy: usually 7-l0 days. Longer therapy requires monitoring of renal function and audiometry as well as peak and trough level monitoring as discussed above.

Dose adjustment in renal failure (IM or IV): use guideline below and then adjust dose according to peak and trough levels as discussed above.

	loading dose:	maintenance dose (rough estimate):
amikacin	7.5mg/kg	(7.5mg/kg + serum creatinine) q12h
gentamycin	1.0mg/kg	(1.0mg/kg + serum creatinine) q8h
tobramycin	1.0mg/kg	(1.0mg/kg + serum creatinine) q8h

AMINOPHYLLINE (Aminophyllin)

Aminophylline is the ethylenediamine salt of theophylline. Refer to "Theophylline" for action, indications, contraindications, comments, side effects.
Supplied as: tablet (100, 200mg); oral solution (105mg/5ml); intravenous (25mg/ml).

Dose based on ideal body weight:
Intravenous loading dose for patient who has NOT received theophylline medication in last 24 hours: 6 mg/kg. ●Administer IV loading dose no faster than 25 mg/min. Loading dose is usually diluted in 50–250 ml D5W or normal saline and administered over 15–20 minutes, but the dose may also be given undiluted slowly via syringe.
Intravenous loading dose in patient who IS currently receiving or has received theophylline medication in last 24 hours: 3 mg/kg. ●If a stat serum theophylline level can be obtained, give a sufficient loading dose to raise serum theophylline to therapeutic level (10–20mcg/ml). A 3.1 mg/kg dose will raise serum theophylline by 5 mcg/ml.
Intravenous maintenance dose must be individualized because the rate of theophylline metabolism varies with a number of factors. Young patients and patients who smoke metabolize theophylline more rapidly. Theophylline metabolism is prolonged in patients with cardiac or liver insufficiency, and by certain drugs (e.g. erythromycin, cimetidine, propranolol). Suggested infusions rates are modified according to therapeutic response, signs of toxicity, and if possible the serum theophylline level. The therapeutic level is 10–20 mcg/ml.
Suggested maintenance infusion rate:

6 month–9 yr: 1.0 mg/kg/hr	9–16 yr: 0.8 mg/kg/hr
adult smoker < 50 yr : 0.8 mg/kg/hr	adult nonsmoker: 0.5 mg/kg/hr
elderly: 0.3 mg/kg/hr	cor pulmonale: 0.3 mg/kg/hr
cardiac or liver insufficiency: 0.1–0.2 mg/kg/hr.	

●Example of IV maintenance infusion:
Dilute 1:1 with D5W or normal saline (e.g. 250 mg aminophylline in 250 ml D5W). Then, the infusion rate in ml/hr = (desired mg/kg/hr) x (ideal body weight in kg).
Oral dose:
Adult: 3 mg/kg ideal body weight q6h initially. May increase up to 6mg/kg q6h according to therapeutic response and serum theophylline level (therapeutic level is 10–20 mcg/ml).
Pediatric: 5 mg/kg q6h initially. May increase up to 8 mg/kg q6h according to therapeutic response and serum theophylline level (therapeutic level is 10–20 mcg/ml).

AMOXICILLIN (Amoxil, Polymox, Trimox, Wymox)

Amoxicillin is an analog of ampicillin. It is for oral administration only. In contrast to ampicillin, amoxicillin is better absorbed orally (food does not interfere with absorption) and it is less likely to cause diarrhea. Amoxicillin is less active than ampicillin against shigella; otherwise their spectra are identical.
Indications: Refer to ampicillin. In the absence of inflammation, amoxicillin may not reach therapeutic levels in the CSF or synovial fluid. Therefore amoxicillin is not used to treat meningitis or septic arthritis.
Contraindications/side effects: as for ampicillin.
Supplied as: chewable tablet (125, 250mg); capsule (250, 500mg); oral suspension (125mg/5ml, 250mg/5ml); pediatric drops (50mg/ml).
Dose, adult or child > 20 kg: 250–500 mg PO q8h.
Dose, child < 20 kg: 6.7–13.3 mg/kg PO q8h.
Comments: ●Upper dose range is for severe infections and respiratory infections. ●Continue treatment for at least 48–72 hours after patient is asymptomatic and bac-

terial eradication is assured. ●In order to preclude development rheumatic fever or glomerulonephritis, treat beta–hemolytic strep infection for at least 10 days. ●Refer to "Gonorrhea" in clinical section for dosage of amoxicillin in treatment of gonorrhea. ●Dose interval in patient with renal failure (creatinine clearance——dose interval): 50--80 ml/min——8 hr, 10–50 ml/min——12 hr, less than 10 ml/min——16 hr.

AMOXICILLIN plus CLAVULANATE (Augmentin)

Action: Amoxicillin is an analog of ampicillin. Clavulanate is a beta–lactam that structurally resembles the penicillins. Its usefulness stems from the fact that it is able to inhibit the beta–lactamase enzymes produced by many bacteria.

Indications: ●sinusitis, otitis media, and lower respiratory infections due to beta–lactamase-producing strains of Hemophilus influenza and Branhamella catarrhalis; ●urinary tract infection due to beta–lactamase–producing strains of E. coli, klebsiellae, and enterobacter; ●skin and skin structure infections due to beta–lactamase–producing strains of Staph aureus, E. coli, and klebsiellae.

Contraindications/side effects: as for ampicillin.

Supplied as (amoxicillin/clavulanate)**:** '500' tablet (500mg/125 mg), '250' tablet (250mg/125mg); '250' chewable tablet (250mg/62.5mg), '125' chewable tablet (125mg/31.25mg), '250' oral suspension (250mg/62.5mg per 5 ml), '125' oral suspension (125mg/31.25mg per 5ml).

Dose:
Adult/child over 40 kg: '250' tablet q8h is the usual dose. In more serious infections or in respiratory infections, give '500' tablet q8h.
Note: two '250' tablets should not be substituted for one '500' tablet because both tablets contain 125 mg clavulanate.
Children under 40 kg: In terms of amoxicillin, the usual dose is 6.7 mg/kg q8h. Double the dose if treating more severe infection, sinusitis, otitis media, or lower respiratory infection.

AMPHOTERICIN B (Fungizone)

Action: Fungistatic or fungicidal—depending on fungal susceptibility and drug concentration in body fluids. The drug binds to sterols in fungal cell membrane thereby altering cell membrane permeability with ensuing leakage of small molecules.

Indications:
Intravenous and intrathecal administration reserved for progressive and potentially fatal fungal infections: cryptococcosis, North American blastomycosis, mucormycosis, sporotrichosis, aspergillosis; as well as disseminated forms of coccidioidomycosis, histoplasmosis, and candidiasis. ●Also may be used in American mucocutaneous leishmaniasis but is not drug of first choice.
Topical forms indicated for treatment of cutaneous or mucocutaneous candidiasis.

Contraindications: amphotericin B hypersensitivity (unless there is life–threatening disease untreatable by other means). In pregnancy, consider risk versus benefit.

Comments: ●Before treatment is begun, the diagnosis must be confirmed by microscopy or culture. ●Monitor weekly: (1) BUN, serum creatinine (discontinue or sharply reduce dosage if BUN exceeds 40 mg/100ml or creatinine exceeds 3 mg/100ml); (2) liver function (discontinue if bilirubin or alkaline phosphatase is elevated); (3) CBC, potassium. ●Avoid concurrent administration of other nephrotoxic drugs.

Side effects: Most frequent side effects include: fever; chills; headache; malaise; GI (anorexia, nausea, vomiting, indigestion, epigastric pain, diarrhea); renal (hypokalemia, azotemia, hyposthenuria, renal tubular acidosis, nephrocalcinosis); normochromic normocytic anemia; injection site effects (phlebitis,thrombophlebitis); arthralgias; myalgia. Uncommon or rare side effects: renal (anuria, oliguria); cardiovascular (arrhythmias, cardiac arrest, hyper or hypotension); blood (coagulation abnormalities, thrombocytopenia, leukopenia, agranulocytosis, eosinophilia, leukocytosis, GI bleeding); neurologic (deafness, tinnitus, vertigo, blurred vision, diplopia, peripheral neuropathy, seizures); other (rash, pruritis, anaphylactoid reaction, flushing, liver failure).

Supplied as: ●intravenous (vial containing 50mg);
●topical (3% cream, ointment, or lotion).

Intravenous dose (adult or child): First day: Give test dose (1 mg diluted in D5W and infused over 20–30 minutes). Patients with normal cardiopulmonary status who tolerate the test dose well or who have only a mild reaction are then given 0.2 mg/kg IV infused over 2–6 hours. Patient with cardiopulmonary insufficiency or patient with severe reaction to the test dose may subsequently be given 5–10 mg by slow IV infusion. Subsequent days: In the absence of renal insufficiency, increase the daily dose as tolerated by 0.1–0.2 mg/kg/day increments (or 5–10 mg/day increments) until administering 0.5–1.0 mg/kg/day in adult and 1.0–1.5 mg/kg/day in child. Daily dose is tailored according to the patient's tolerance and the dose necessary to achieve a therapeutic response. ●A double dose administered as a single IV infusion on alternate days may lessen phlebitis, anorexia, and renal toxicity. However, no more than 1.5 mg/kg can be administered on a given day. Method of administration: In preparing the intravenous solution, 50 mg amphotericin B is diluted in 10 ml sterile non–bacteriostatic water which is further diluted in D5W to a concentration of < 0.1 mg/ml. The infusion runs over 4–6 hours while vital signs are monitored. ●Adding 1000 unit heparin to the IV infusion reduces incidence of thrombophlebitis. ●Fever (sometimes with shaking chills) may be mitigated by giving 25–50 mg hydrocortisone IV just before the infusion. Diphenhydramine 25–50 mg IV prior to the infusion will help control nausea and vomiting while aspirin or acetaminophen will help relieve headache and fever. Duration of therapy: Therapy is usually continued for 2–4 months or longer.

Intrathecal injection (via lumbar, cisterna magna, or lateral ventricle) may be necessary for meningitis, particularly coccidioidomycosis meningitis or unresponsive cryptococcal meningitis.

●Adult: Intrathecal injection is 2–3 times/week. Initial dose is 0.1mg. The dose is subsequently increased by 0.1 mg increments until the patient is receiving 0.5–1.0 mg depending on the patients tolerance and the severity of infection. In preparing the injection solution, 50 mg amphotericin B is diluted in 10 ml sterile non–bacteriostatic water which is then diluted in 250 ml of D5W. Then, 0.5 ml (0.1 mg) to 5.0 ml (1.0 mg) of this dilution is withdrawn into a 10 ml syringe and further diluted to 10 ml with CSF from the patient, and finally this mixture is injected into the patient. Hydrocortisone sodium succinate 10 mg may be added to the injection solution to lessen chemical arachnoiditis. When administered via the lumbar route, the patient is placed in 30° Trendelenberg for 30–45 minutes to allow distribution of the solution.

●Pediatric: 1/3 to 1/2 the adult dose.

Topical (treatment of cutaneous candidiasis): Apply cream, lotion, or ointment to affected lesion bid—qid.

AMPICILLIN (Omnipen, Polycillin)

Action: Ampicillin is a broad spectrum penicillin which like penicillin is bactericidal by interfering with bacterial cell wall synthesis.
Spectrum: streptococci (S. pneumoniae, S. pyogenes, S. viridans, S. faecalis); nonpenicillinase–producing staphylococci; Listeria monocytogenes; gram–negative cocci (N. gonorrhoeae—with exception of penicillinase–producing strains, N. meningitidis); gram–negative aerobic bacilli (H. influenzae, E coli, salmonellae, shigellae, Proteus mirabilis).
Resistant bacteria include many gram–negative aerobic bacilli (enterobacter, indole + proteus, klebsiella, serratia, acinetobacter, pseudomonas).
Indications: gonorrhea (except pharyngeal or male anorectal infection); urinary tract infection (e.g. E. coli, Proteus mirabilis, streptococci including enterococci); sinusitis or otitis media (e.g. pneumococcus, susceptible H. influenza); pneumonia (e.g. pneumococcus, H. influenza); biliary infection (e.g. E. coli, enterococci); salmonellae (chloramphenicol–resistant S. Typhii or enteric fevers but not uncomplicated gastroenteritis due to other salmonellae). Pediatric meningitis is often treated with combination of ampicillin and chloramphenicol while awaiting culture and sensitivity results. Listeria monocytogenes is responsive to ampicillin.
Contraindication: hypersensitivity to penicillins.
Comments: ●Continue treatment for at least 48–72 hours after patient is asymptomatic or bacterial eradication assured. ●To preclude development of rheumatic fever or glomerulonephritis, treat beta–hemolytic streptococci for at least 10 days. ●Rashes occur more frequently with ampicillin than with penicillin. 80–90% of patients with mononucleosis develop a rash when given ampicillin. Most rashes are not allergic reactions.
Side effects: ●overgrowth resistant organisms; ●gastrointestinal: glossitis, stomatitis, black "hairy" tongue, nausea, vomiting, diarrhea, colitis, pseudomembranous colitis (latter is due to overgrowth of Clostridium difficile); ●Rash may be allergic or nonallergic. Nonallergic rash is particularly common in the patient with infectious mononucleosis who is being treated for presumed streptococcal infection. ●Hypersensitivity: fever, pruritis, rash, urticaria, angioedema, anaphylaxis, eosinophilia. Hypersensitivity may also be responsible for rare cases of anemia, thrombocytopenia, leukopenia, and agranulocytosis.
Supplied as: capsule (250, 500 mg); oral suspension (125, 250, or 500mg/5ml); pediatric drops (100 mg/ml); IM or IV injection preparation.

Dose, gonorrhea: refer to "Gonorrhea" in clinical section.
Dose, adult or child > 20 kg: Usual dose is 250–500 mg q6h IV, IM, or PO.
●Administer up to 2 gram q6h IV in more severe infection.
●In septicemia or bacterial meningitis, administer 150–250 mg/kg/day (8–14 gram/day) intravenously in equally divided doses q3–4h.
<u>Dose interval in renal failure:</u> creatnine clearance 10–80 ml/min——use 8 hr interval, creatinine clearance < 10 ml/min——use 12 interval.
Dose, child < 20 kg: PO : 50–100 mg/kg/day in equally divided doses q6h.
  IV or IM : 100–200 mg/kg/day in equally divided doses q6h.
  Meningitis : 150–400 mg/kg/day IV equally divided q4–6h.
Neonate > 7 days age: 75 mg/kg/day equally divided q8h IV or IM.
  Meningitis: 200 mg/kg/day equally divided q6–8h IV.
Neonate < 7 days age: 50 mg/kg/day equally divided q12h IV or IM.
  Meningitis: 100 mg/kg/day equally divided q12h IV.

AMPICILLIN plus SULBACTAM (Unasyn)

Action: Ampicillin is a broad spectrum penicillin which like penicillin is bactericidal by interfering with bacterial wall synthesis. Sulbactam extends the spectrum of ampicillin by inhibiting the beta-lactamases produced by otherwise resistant bacteria. Except against Neisseria species, sulbactam by itself has little antibacterial effectiveness. Furthermore, sulbactam does not influence the activity of ampicillin against bacteria sensitive to ampicillin alone.
Spectrum: In vitro studies have shown ampicillin/sulbactam to be active against: <u>gram-positive bacteria;</u> streptococci (S. pneumoniae, S. pyogenes, S. viridans, S. faecalis); staphylococci (S. aureus*, S. epidermidis*, S. saprophyticus*); <u>gram-negative bacteria;</u> H. influenzae*, Branhamella catarrhalis*, E coli*, Klebsiella*, Proteus mirabilis*, Proteus vulgaris, Providencia rettgeri, Providencia stuartii, Morganella morganii, gonococcus*. <u>Anaerobes;</u> Clostridia, Peptococcus, Peptostreptococcus, Bacteroides (including B. fragilis).
*Indicates bacteria with strains capable of producing beta-lactamase.
 <u>Resistant bacteria</u> include Enterobacter, Serratia, Pseudomonas aerugenosa, methicillin–resistant staphylococci.
Indications: <u>Skin and skin structure</u> infections by beta-lactamase–producing strains of Staph. aureus, E. coli, Klebsiella (including K. pneumoniae), Proteus mirabilis, Bacteroides fragilis, Enterobacter, Acinetobacter calcoaceticus; <u>intra-abdominal infections</u> due to beta-lactamase–producing strains of E. coli, Klebsiella (including K. pneumoniae), Bacteroides (including B. fragilis), Enterobacter; <u>gynecologic infections</u> due to beta-lactamase–producing strains of E. coli, Bacteroides (including B. fragilis). <u>Note:</u> This drug combination should not be used to treat meningitis since CSF penetration is not reliable.
Contraindication: hypersensitivity to penicillins.
Comments: ●Rashes occur more frequently with ampicillin than with penicillin. 80–90% of patients with mononucleosis develop a rash when given ampicillin. Most rashes are not allergic reactions. ●Rashes are more common in patients concurrently receiving allopurinol.
Side effects include: <u>overgrowth resistant organisms;</u> <u>gastrointestinal</u> (glossitis, stomatitis, black "hairy" tongue, nausea, vomiting, diarrhea, flatulence, abdominal distension, colitis, pseudomembranous colitis due to overgrowth of Clostridium difficile); <u>rash</u> may be allergic or non-allergic. Nonallergic rash is particularly common in the patient with infectious mononucleosis. <u>hypersensitivity</u> (fever, pruritis, rash, urticaria, angioedema, anaphylaxis, eosinophilia). Hypersensitivity may also be responsible for rare cases of anemia, thrombocytopenia, leukopenia, and agranulocytosis. <u>GU;</u> urinary retention, dysuria; <u>other</u> (fatigue, malaise, headache, chills, edema, facial swelling, substernal pain, epistaxis, submucosal bleeding).
Supplied as preparation for IV or IM administration. The preparation contains ampicillin to sulbactam ratio of 2 to 1 (e.g. 3 grams of the preparation contains 2 grams ampicillin plus 1 gram sulbactam).
Dose (adult): 1.5–3 grams every 6 hours IV or IM.

ANTACIDS

Action: neutralize gastric acid. **Indications:** peptic ulcer, gastritis, esophagitis, hiatal hernia, stress ulcer prolaphylaxis. ●Aluminum hydroxide binds phosphate in the GI tract and is therefore useful as a single–agent preparation (e.g. Amphogel) in the treatment/prevention of hyperphosphatemia due to renal failure. The GI phosphate–binding property of aluminum hydroxide also finds utility in the treatment of patients with phosphate–containing renal stones. **Contraindication:** severe renal failure contraindicates the use of magnesium–containing antacids because of the risk of inducing hypermagnesemia. **Caution:** ●By preventing GI absorption of phosphate, prolonged high doses of aluminum hydroxide–containing antacids may induce hypophosphatemia and osteomalacia. ●Antacids may inhibit the oral absorption of some drugs—e.g. tetracyclines, digoxin, phenothiazines, cimetidine, sulfonamides, nitrofurantoin, nalidixic acid, isoniazid, thyroxine. If antacids must be administered concurrently with these drugs, give them at least 1 hr before or 2

hr after the antacid. ●Excessive calcium carbonate antacid (e.g. Tums) may cause hypercalcemia and hypercalciuria. The milk–alkali syndrome may be induced by prolonged ingestion of calcium carbonate with large amounts of homogenized vitamin D–containing milk or sodium bicarbonate.
Comments: ●Magnesium–containing antacids cause diarrhea; aluminum–containing acids are constipating. A balance is achieved with combination preparations. ●Magnesium hydroxide is a more effective antacid than aluminum hydroxide. A liquid antacid is more effective than a tablet with the same constituents. ●Simethicone is added to many antacids as an antiflatulent but is of dubious value.

Amphogel (aluminum hydroxide):
Acid neutralizing capacity; 20mEq/2 tsp suspension, 16mEq/600mg tablet.
Supplied as: 320mg suspension, 300 mg tablet, 600 mg tablet.
Dose (adult): 2 tsp (or two 300 mg tab or one 600 mg tab) 5–6 time/day between meals and at bedtime. Usual maximum: 12 tsp or twelve 300 mg tablets (six 600 mg tabs) per 24 hr. The 24 hr maximum should not usually be continued for more than 2 weeks.

Maalox (magnesium hydroxide plus aluminum hydroxide)

Supplied as:	magnesium hydroxide + aluminum hydroxide	acid neutralizing capacity
Maalox Suspension	200mg + 225mg	13.3mEq/5ml
Maalox tablets	200mg + 200mg	9.7mEq/tablet
Extra Strength Maalox tablets	400mg + 400mg	23.4mEq/tablet
Extra Strength Maalox Plus Suspension*	450mg + 500mg	29mEq per 5ml
Maalox Plus Tablets*	200mg + 200mg	11.4 mEq/tablet
Maalox TC Suspension	300mg + 600mg	27.2mEq/5ml
Maalox TC tablets	300mg + 600mg	28mEq/tablet

*Contains simethicone.
Dose (usual dose/maximum per 24 hr): The following Maalox recommended doses are to be taken four times a day, 20–60 minutes after meals and before bedtime. Tablets are to be chewed. The 24 hr maximum should not usually be continued for more than 2 weeks.
●Maalox Suspension: 2–4 tsp (maximum 16 tsp per 24 hr),
●Maalox tablets: 2–4 tablets (maximum 16 tablets per 24 hr),
●Extra Strength Maalox tablets: 1–2 tablet (maximum 8 tablets per 24 hr),
●Extra Strength Maalox Plus Suspension: 2–4 tsp (maximum 16 tsp per 24 hr),
●Maalox Plus Tablets: 1–4 tablet (maximum 16 tablets per 24 hr).
●Maalox TC Suspension: 1–2 tsp (maximum 8 tsp per 24 hr),
●Maalox TC tablets: 1–2 tablet (maximum 8 tablets per 24 hr).

Mylanta (magnesium hydroxide plus aluminum hydroxide plus simethicone)

Supplied as:	Acid neutralizing capacity
Mylanta liquid	25.4 mEq/2 tsp
Mylanta II liquid	50.8 mEq/2 tsp
Mylanta tablet	23 mEq/2 tab
Mylanta II tablet	46 mEq/2 tab

Dose (adult):
●Mylanta: 2–4 tsp (2–4 tablets chewed) between meals and at bedtime. Max 24 tsp or 24 tablets per 24 hr. The 24 hr maximum should not usually be continued for more than 2 weeks.
●Mylanta II: 2 tsp (2 tablets chewed) between meal and at bedtime. Maximum 12 tsp or 12 tabs per 24 hr. The 24 hr maximum should not usually be continued for more than 2 weeks.

Riopan (hydrated magnesium aluminate [magaldrate])

Supplied as	Acid neutralizing capacity
Riopan liquid	15mEq/5ml
Riopan swallow tablet	13.5mEq/tab
Riopan chewable tablet	13.5mEq/tab
Riopan Plus liquid*	15mEq/5ml
Riopan Plus chewable tablet*	13.5mEq/tab
Riopan Plus 2 liquid*	30mEq/5ml
Riopan Plus 2 chewable tablet*	30mEq/tab

* contains simethicone
Dose (adult): 1–2 tsp (1–2 tablets) between meals and at bedtime.
Usual maximum: 18 tsp or 20 tablets per 24hr of Riopan or Riopan Plus;
9 tsp or 9 tablets per 24 hr of Riopan Plus 2.
The 24 hr maximum should not usually be continued for more than 2 weeks.

Tums (calcium carbonate)
Acid neutralizing capacity: 10mEq/500mg tablet, 20mEq/5ml.
Sodium content: ≤ 2 mg/tablet, ≤ 5 mg/5ml.
Supplied as: Tums tablet (500mg), Tums E–X tablet (750mg),
Tums Liquid Extra–Strength (1000mg/5ml) with or without simethicone.
Dose: Chew 1–2 tablets. If needed, take repeat dose hourly up to maximum 12 500mg tablets or ten 750mg tablets per 24 hr.
Liquid: 1–2 tsp. Repeat hourly if needed up to maximum 8 tsp per 24 hr.

ANTICHOLINESTERASES:
edrophonium (Tensilon)   physostigmine (Antilirium)
neostigmine (Prostigmin)   pyridostigmine (Mestinon)

Action: Anticholinesterases exert a cholinergic effect. They do so by inhibiting the cholinesterase enzyme thus increasing the level of acetylcholine.

Contraindications: anticholinesterase hypersensitivity, mechanical obstruction of urinary or intestinal tract, peritonitis, bromide hypersensitivity (oral pyridostigmine or neostigmine).

Caution: asthma, cardiac arrhythmias, epilepsy, hyperthyroidism, diabetes mellitus.

Comments: ●Atropine should be available to counteract severe cholinergic reactions. ●Severe muscle weakness may be due to worsening myasthenia or due to cholinergic crisis secondary to anticholinesterase overdose. See edrophonium.

Side effects: nausea, vomiting, diarrhea, abdominal cramps, salivation, sweating, miosis, lacrimation, bradycardia with possible hypotension, urinary urgency, increased bronchial secretions, cardiac arrhythmias, cardiac arrest, muscle cramps, fasciculations, weakness, dizziness, drowsiness, convulsions, respiratory arrest.

edrophonium (Tensilon)   Supplied as: 10mg/ml (1 ml ampul or 10 ml vial).
<u>Diagnosis myasthemia gravis:</u>
●Adult: 0.2ml (2mg) IV initially. Discontinue test if cholinergic reaction occurs (e.g. muscle fasciculations, increased muscle weakness, sweating, salivation, bradycardia, hypotension). If nothing occurs after 45 seconds, inject 0.8 ml (8 mg) IV. Alternative: 10 mg IM.
●Child > 75 lbs: 0.2 ml (2 mg) IV test dose to observe for cholinergic reaction. If nothing accurs after 45 seconds, titrate as follows: 0.1ml (1mg) IV q30-45 sec up to a total of 1 ml (10 mg). Alternative: 0.5 ml (5 mg) IM.
●Child ≤ 75 lbs: 0.1ml (1mg) IV test dose to observe for cholinergic reaction. If nothing occurs after 45 seconds, titrate as follows: 0.1ml (1mg) IV q30-45 seconds up to total 5 ml (5 mg). Alternative: 0.2 ml (2 mg) IM.
●Infant: 0.05 ml (0.5 mg).
<u>Evaluation of treatment requirements myasthenia gravis:</u> In adult, give 0.1-0.2 ml (1-2mg) IV one hr after last PO dose of anti-myasthenic medication. The undertreated patient will show increased muscle strength, the overtreated may exhibit cholinergic reaction.
<u>To distinguish cholinergic crisis due to overtreatment from worsening myasthenia</u> in patient in respiratory distress: In adult, give 0.1ml (1mg) IV and observe for 1 minute. If patient is not further compromised, another 0.1ml (1mg) IV is given. Give no more than 0.2 ml (2 mg). If no improvement occurs, discontinue all anticholinesterase drugs. This test must not be performed until adequate airway and ventilation can be assured.
<u>Curare antagonist</u> (for reversal of curare, tubocurarine, gallamine, etc.): 1ml (10 mg) IV over 30-45 seconds. Observe for cholinergic reaction. Repeat as needed (maximum 40mg).

physostigmine (Antilirium)   Supplied as: 2 ml ampul (1mg/ml).
<u>Indication:</u> antidote to overdose by drugs causing anticholinergic effects—e.g. atropine, scopolamine, tricyclic antidepressants, phenothiazines, antihistamines.
<u>Adult dose:</u> 2 mg IV (no faster than 1mg/min) or 2 mg IM. Give repeat doses as necessary if there are life-threatening signs (e.g. arrhythmia, coma, convulsion).
<u>Pediatric dose:</u> 0.02 mg/kg IM or IV (no faster than 0.5 mg/min). Give repeat dose q5-10 minutes if necessary (assuming no cholinergic reaction occurs), but do not exceed maximum cumulative total dose of 2 mg.

neostigmine (Prostigmin)
<u>Supplied as:</u>   15 mg tablet   injection (0.25mg/ml, 0.5mg/ml, or 1.0mg/ml)
<u>Adult dose:</u>
   <u>Myasthenia gravis:</u> 15-375 mg/24hr PO divided (usually: 150mg/24hr divided). If there is difficulty breathing or swallowing, administer 0.5mg SC or IM. Adjust subsequent doses as needed. Switch to PO when feasible.
   <u>Postoperative distension/urinary retention:</u> 0.25 mg SC or IM.
   <u>Reversal of nondepolarizing neuromuscular blocking agents</u> (e.g. tubocurarine): 0.5-2mg slow IV. Repeat as needed (max 5mg). Give 0.6-1.2 mg atropine IV prior to or concurrently with IV neostigmine. If bradycardia is present, titrate with atropine to pulse rate of 80/min before giving neostigmine. Do not use neostigmine in presence of high levels of halothane or cyclopropane.
<u>Pediatric dose (myasthenia gravis):</u> 2 mg/kg/day divided q3-4h.

pyridostigmine (Mestinon)
<u>Supplied as:</u>   60 mg tablet,   180 mg sustain release tablet,   60mg/5ml syrup,
   2ml ampule (5mg/ml).
<u>Myasthenia gravis</u>
   ●Adult: 600 mg/24 hr spaced to provide optimum relief (range: 60-1500mg/day).
       Dose of sustained release tablet: 1-3 tablets qd-bid
       if oral route is not practical, give 1/30th of oral dose IV (preferred) or IM.
   ●Pediatric: individualize. Average dose is 7 mg/kg/day PO divided into 6 equal doses.

Neonates of myasthenia mothers who have difficulty swallowing, sucking, or breathing: 0.05–0.15 mg/kg IM q4–6h. When feasible, switch to 5 mg PO q4–6h..

Reversal of nondepolarizing muscle relaxants (e.g. tubocurarine): 10–20 mg IV. Give 0.6–1.2 mg atropine IV just before giving pyridostigmine.

ANTI-DIARRHEA DRUGS

loperamide (Imodium)

Action: Inhibits GI motility by direct effect on GI muscle, and possibly decreases GI secretions. The daily fecal volume, and loss of water and electrolytes is decreased. Stool viscosity and bulk is increased.

Indications: nonspecific diarrhea, inflammatory bowel disease–associated chronic diarrhea, to reduce volume of discharge from ileostomies.

Contraindications: loperamide hypersensitivity; conditions in which constipation must be avoided (e.g. hepatic insufficiency), infectious diarrhea with bloody stools, diarrhea due to poisons.

Caution: pregnancy, nursing mother, liver dysfunction, young child, antibiotic–induced diarrhea.
●Toxic megacolon may be induced in patient with acute ulcerative colitis or pseudomembranous colitis; discontinue loperamide if abdominal distension or other untoward symptoms occur.
●Discontinue if clinical improvement of acute diarrhea does not occur in 48 hours.

Side effects: abdominal pain/discomfort/distension, nausea, vomiting, constipation, tiredness, drowsiness, dizziness, dry mouth, hypersensitivity (including skin rash).

Supplied as: 2 mg capsule, liquid (1mg/5ml).

Adult dose: 2 capsules (4 tsp) initally, followed by one capsule (2 tsp) after each unformed stool. Maximum 8 capsules/day or 16 tsp/day.

Dose, child 8–12 yr (> 30 kg): On first day, give 2 mg PO 3 times. On subsequent days: give dose as needed after unformed stool. Maximum 6 mg/day.

Dose, child 5–8 yr (20–30 kg): On first day, give 2 mg PO twice.
On subsequent days: give dose as needed after unformed stool. Max. 4 mg/day.

Dose, child 2–5 yr (13–20 kg): On first day, give 1 mg PO 3 times. On subsequent days: give dose as needed after unformed stool. Maximum 3 mg/day.

diphenoxylate with atropine (Lomotil)

Action: diphenoxylate (an opioid related to meperidine) inhibits GI motility. Atropine is present in subtherapeutic amounts to discourage deliberate overdose.

Indication: diarrhea.

Contraindications: under 2 years of age, hypersensitivity to components, obstructive jaundice, pseudomembranous enterocolitis; diarrhea due bacterial infection (e.g. salmonellae, shigellae, toxigenic E. coli) or poisons.

Caution: young children, pregnancy, nursing mother, liver disease (hepatic coma may result), active ulcerative colitis (toxic megacolon may result), concurrent use CNS depressants (barbiturates, alcohol, or tranquilizers may potentiate effects)

Side effects: anorexia, nausea, vomiting, paralytic ileus, toxic megacolon, dizziness, sedation, headache, malaise, restlessness, euphoria, depression, coma, flushing, tachycardia, pruritis, urticaria, angioedema, hyperthermia, urinary retention, dry skin, dry mouth, respiratory depression. Addiction does not occur at recommended doses even with chronic use but may occur at high dosages.

Supplied as: tablet containing 2.5mg diphenoxylate + 0.025mg atropine per tablet, liquid containing 2.5mg diphenoxylate + 0.025mg atropine per 5 ml.

Adult dose: 2 tablets (10 ml) PO qid until diarrhea controlled.
Then, reduce dosage (1 tablet or 5 ml twice daily may suffice).

Pediatric dose (reduce dose after initial control):
9–12 yr (23–55 kg): 3.5–5.0 ml qid initially;
6–8 yr (17–32 kg): 2.5–5.0 ml qid initially;
5 yr (16–23 kg): 2.5–4.5 ml qid initially;   4 yr (14–20 kg): 2–4 ml qid initially;
3 yr (2–3 kg): 2–3 ml qid initially;   2 yr (11–14 kg): 1.5–3.0 ml qid initially.

opium tincture
camphorated tincture of opium [paregoric]

Action: inhibits peristalsis. Indication: nonspecific diarrhea.

Contraindications: diarrhea secondary to infections (e.g. salmonellae, shigellae, toxigenic E. coli); pseudomembranous enterocolitis; severe liver disease, acute poisoning.

Comments: ●Opium may cause toxic megacolon in patient with active ulcerative colitis or acute colitis due to amebae, schistosomes, or ischemia. ●At the usual therapeutic doses neither analgesia nor euphoria is induced, and for short–term use there is little risk of dependence.

Side effects: nausea, vomiting, constipation, confusion.

Supplied as: ●opium tincture (10 mg morphine/ml).
●paregoric (0.4 mg morphine/ml).

<u>Adult dose:</u>   ●opium tincture: 0.6 ml PO qid (range 0.3–1.0 ml qid).
            ●paregoric: 5–10 ml PO qd–qid.
<u>Children dose, paregoric;</u> 0.25–0.5 ml/kg PO qd–qid.

kaolin & pectin (Kaopectate)

<u>Action:</u> Kaolin (hydrated aluminum silicate) and pectin are adsorbents. Stools are bulkier but total water loss is unchanged. <u>Indication:</u> nonspecific diarrhea.
<u>Contraindication:</u> bowel obstruction.
<u>Comments:</u> ●Kaolin and pectin may interfere with absorption of other PO drugs. Allow 2–3 hours to elapse after taking kaolin and pectin before taking another PO drug. ●Constipation may occur with chronic use.
<u>Supplied as:</u> suspension (200mg kaolin + 4.3mg pectin/ml), concentrate, tablet.
<u>Dose of suspension:</u>
    <u>adult:</u> 60–120 ml (4–8 tbsp) after each bowel movement or as needed;
    <u>over 12 yr:</u> 60 ml (4 tbsp) after each bowel movement or as needed;
    <u>6–12 yr:</u> 30–60 ml (2–4 tbsp) after each bowel movement or as needed;
    <u>3–6 yr:</u> 15–30 ml (1–2 tbsp) after each bowel movement or as needed.

atropine + hyoscyamine + hyoscine hydrobromide (Donnagel)

<u>Action:</u> Kaolin and pectin (see above). Atropine, hyoscyamine, and hyoscine are belladonna alkaloids which decrease intestinal motility and cramping.
<u>Indications:</u> nonspecific diarrhea, gastroenteritis.
<u>Contraindications:</u> hypersenstivity to components, glaucoma, obstructive GI or GU disease, severe ulcerative colitis, toxic megacolon, myasthenia gravis, reflux esophagitis secondary to hiatal hernia, acute hemorrhage with cardiovascular instability. <u>Side effects:</u> blurred vision, mydriasis, cycloplegia, increase intraocular pressure, dry mouth, flushing, difficult urination, impotence, lactation suppression, tachycardia, palpitations, nausea, vomiting, constipation, bloated sensation, headache, weakness, dizziness, drowsiness, insomnia, nervousness, excitement, agitation, allergic reactions.
<u>Supplied as:</u> oral suspension, capsule, tablet
<u>Dose:</u>   <u>adult:</u> 1–2 tablets/capsulesx PO tid–qid, or 1–2 tsp PO tid–qid.
<u>child 45.4 kg:</u> 1tsp q4h or 1.5 tsp q6h;   <u>child 34 kg:</u> 3/4 tsp q4h or 1 tsp q6h;
<u>child 22.7 kg:</u> 1/2 tsp q4h or 3/4 tsp q6h; <u>child 13.6 kg:</u> 1.5 ml q4h or 2.0 ml q6h;
<u>child 9.1 kg:</u> 1 ml q4h or 1.5 ml q6h;   <u>child 4.5 kg:</u> 0.5 ml q4h or 0.75 ml q6h.

ANTIHISTAMINES: astemizole (Hismanal), azatadine (Optimine), brompheniramine (Dimetane), chlorpheniramine (Chlor–Trimeton), clemastine (Tavist), cyclizine (Marezine), cyproheptadine (Periactin), dexchlorpheniramine (Polaramine), dimenhydrinate (Dramamine), diphenhydramine (Benadryl), hydroxyzine (Atarax, Vistaril), meclizine (Antivert, Bonine), methdilazine (Tacaryl), promethazine (Phenergan), terfenadine (Seldane), trimeprazine (Temaril), tripelennamine (PBZ), triprolidine (Actidil).

Actions: Block action of histamine by competing with histamine for cell receptor site. Other actions may include anticholinergic effects, sedation, antivertigo/antimotion sickness effects.
Indications: <u>sedation</u> (e.g. hydroxyzine, diphenhydramine, promethazine); <u>vertigo/motion sickness</u> (e.g. meclizine, dimenhydrinate, cyclizine); <u>nausea/vomiting</u> (e.g. hydroxyzine, promethazine); <u>adjunct in treatment of anaphylaxis</u> (diphenhydramine); <u>acute allergic pruritis/urticaria</u> (e.g. diphendydramine); <u>allergic rhinitis or conjunctivitis</u> (e.g. carbinoxamine, chlorpheniramine, and brompheniramine are among the least sedating); <u>chronic urticaria/allergic dermatoses</u> (e.g. hydroxyzine).
Contraindications: acute asthma attack, narrow angle glaucoma, urinary obstruction, prostatic hypertrophy. ●Phenothiazine antihistamines (methdilazine, promothazine, trimeprazine) are also contraindicated in peptic ulcer disease, GI obstruction, epilepsy, CNS depression, pregnancy, nursing mother, neonate, bone marrow depression.
Comments: ●Use antihistamines with caution in the following circumstances: asthma, increased intraocular pressure, hyperthyroidism, elderly, debilitated, cardiac or renal disease, hypertension. ●Use phenothiazine–type antihistamine cautiously in patient with liver disease. ●Warn patient that drowsiness may interfere with performance of hazardous activities. Coffee or tea can be used to counteract sedation. Alcohol or other CNS depressants will aggravate sedation. ●Hard candy or chewing gum will alleviate dry mouth. ●Antihistamines should be stopped evening prior to skin tests for allergy as they interfere with histamine skin response.
Side effects include: <u>CNS</u> (sedation, incoordination, dizziness, vertigo, tremor, irritability, headache, insomnia); <u>gastrointestinal</u> (anorexia, nausea, vomiting, dry mouth, constipation, diarrhea, cholestatic jaundice); <u>urinary</u> (urinary retention, urinary frequency, dysuria); <u>cardiovascular</u> (palpitations, tachycardia, hypotension, premature ventricular contractions), <u>skin</u> (rash, urticaria); <u>blood</u> (leukopenia, agranulocytosis, thrombocytopenia); <u>other</u> (thickening of bronchial secretions). <u>See also</u> "Phenothiazines" for side effects that may be associated with the phenothiazine antihista-

mines (methdilazine, promethazine, trimeprazine).
Overdose: ●Empty stomach, administer activated charcoal and cathartic. ●Treat seizures with phenytoin. ●Physostigmine may useful for treating coma, seizures, and arrhythmias. ●Propranolol and phenytoin may be effective for refractory ventricular arrhythmias. ●Charcoal hemoperfusion may be considered in severe intoxications. ●Exchange transfusions have been effective in children with severe intoxication. ●Isotonic fluids IV and if necessary dopamine may be admininistered if hypotension develops.

astemizole (Hismanal)   Supplied as: 10 mg tablet.
Dose (adult): 10 mg once/day for seasonal allergic rhinitis or chronic idiopathic urticaria. Astemizole is nonsedating.
azatadine (Optimine)   Supplied as: 1mg tablet.
Dose (adult): 1–2 mg PO twice daily (maximum 4 mg/day). Azatadine is sedating.
brompheniramine (Dimetane)
Supplied as: 4 mg tablet;   elixir (2mg/5ml);   time release tablet (8, 12 ml).
Adult: ●4 mg PO q4–6h. ●time release tablet: 8–12 mg PO bid–tid.
●IM/IV/SC: 5–20 mg q6–12h (maximum 40 mg/day).
Child 6–12 yr: ●4 mg PO tid–qid
●IM/IV/SC: 0.5 mg/kg/day divided into 3–4 daily doses.
Child 2–6 yr: ●1mg PO q4–6h.
●IM/IV/SC: 0.5 mg/kg/day divided divided into 3–4 daily doses.
chlorpheniramine (Chlor–Trimeton)
Supplied as: 4mg tablet;   time–release tablet (8, 12ml);
2mg/5ml syrup;   10mg/ml preparation for IM, IV, or SC.
Adult: ●2–4 mg PO tid–qid ●time-release tablet: 8–12 mg PO qd–tid
●IM/IV/SC: 5–40 mg. IV dose is given over one minute.
Child < 12 yr: 0.35 mg/kg/day divided into 4 daily doses PO or SC.
clemastine (Tavist)   Supplied as: tablet (1.34, 2.68 mg);   syrup (0.5mg/5ml).
Adult: ●tablet: 1.34–2.68 mg twice daily. Maximum daily dose is 6 x 1.34 mg.
●syrup: 2 tsp twice daily. Maximum 12 tsp/day.
Child 6–12 yr: 1–2 tsp twice daily. Maximum 6 tsp/day.
cyclizine (Marezine)   Supplied as: 50 mg tablet, 50 mg/ml injection.
Dose (vertigo/motion sickness):
Adult: 50 mg q4–6h PO/IM (initial dose 1–2 hr before travel). Max 200 mg/24 hr.
Child 6–12 yr: 25 mg q4–6h PO, or 1 mg/kg q8h IM.
cyproheptadine (Periactin)   Supplied as: 4 mg tablet, syrup (2mg/5ml).
Adult: 4 mg tid–qid PO. Maximum 0.5 mg/kg/day.
Child 7–14 yr: 4 mg bid–tid PO. Maximum 16 mg/day.
Child 2–6 yr: 2 mg bid–tid PO. Maximum 12 mg/day.
dexchlorpheniramine (Polaramine)
Supplied as: 2mg tablet;   time–release tablets (4, 6 ml);   syrup (2mg/5ml).
Adult: ●2 mg q4–6h PO.
●time release tablet: 4 or 6 mg at bedtime or q8–10h during day.
Child 6–11 yr: 1 mg q4–6h PO.   ●time release tablet: 4 mg at bedtime.
Child 2–5 yr: 0.5 mg q4–6h PO.
dimenhydrinate (Dramamine)
Supplied as: 50 mg tablet,   15.62 mg/5ml liquid,   50mg/ml injection.
Dose (vertigo/motion sickness/nausea/vomiting):
Adult: ●PO: 50–100 mg q4–6h (maximum 400mg/24 hr) ●IM: 50 mg q3–4h.
●IV: 50 mg (dilute in 10 ml NaCl injection & administer over 2 minutes).
Child: 1.0–1.5 mg/kg q6h PO or IM.
diphenhydramine (Benadryl)
Supplied as: capsule (25, 50 mg);   elixir (12.5mg/5ml), injection (10, 50 mg/ml).
Adult: ●25–50 mg PO tid–qid.
●IV or deep IM: 10–50 mg (maximum 400mg/day).
Child < 12 yr (PO/deepIM/IV): 5 mg/kg/day divided into 4 daily doses (maximum 300 mg/day).
Comments: ●When the drug is given parenterally, IV is preferred over IM. ●Contraindicated in premature and newborns. ●Sedating. ●Useful as adjunct to epinephrine in treatment of anaphylaxis.
hydroxyzine (Atarax, Vistaril)
Supplied as: tablet (10, 25, 50, 100 mg);   capsule (25, 50,100 mg);
oral suspension (25mg/5ml); syrup (10mg/5ml); IM injection (25, 50 mg/ml).

Adult: ●Anxiety: 50–100 mg qid IM or PO; ●Sedation: 25–100mg tid–qid PO or IM.
●Vomiting: 25–100 mg IM. ●Pruritis: 25–100 mg tid–qid PO or IM. ●Pre– and post–operative: 25–100 mg IM.
Child: ●Oral: 0.5 mg/kg q6h. ●IM: 0.25–1.0 mg/kg q4–6h.
Comments: ●Maximum 600 mg/day. ●Contraindicated in early pregnancy.
meclizine (Antivert, Bonine)   Supplied as: 12.5, 25, 50 mg tablets.
Dose (adult): ●Vertigo: 25–100 mg/day in divided doses.
●Motion sickness: 25–50 mg PO qd (initial dose at least 1 hour prior to travel).
methdilazine (Tacaryl) is a phenothiazine.
Supplied as: ●Methdilazine HCl (8 mg tablet, 4mg/5ml syrup)
●Methdilazine chewable tablet (3.6 mg equivalent to 4 mg methdilazine HCl).
Adult: 8 mg PO bid–qid.   **Child > 3 yr:** 4 mg PO bid–qid.
promethazine (Phenergan) is a phenothiazine.
Supplied as: tablet or suppository (12.5, 25, 50 mg);
        syrup (6.25/5ml, 25mg/5ml);   injection (25, 50mg/ml).
Adult: ●Sedation: 25–50 mg PO or IM. ●Vertigo/motion sickness: 25 mg PO bid.
●Nausea/vomiting: 12.5–25 mg q4–6h PO, IM, or PR.
●Allergy (PO or PR): 12.5 mg bid–qid or 25mg at bedtime.
Child: ●Sedation: 0.5–1.0 mg/kg IM q6h, or 12.5–25 mg PO or PR.
●Vertigo/motion sickness: 0.5mg/kg PO q12h.
●Nausea/vomiting: 0.25–0.5 mg/kg q4–6h IM, PO, or PR.
●Allergy: 0.1 mg/kg PO as needed q6h during day and 0.5mg PO at bedtime.
Comments: Subcutaneous injection contraindicated. In children, promethazine is not recommended for uncomplicated vomiting or vomiting of unknown etiology.
terfenadine (Seldane)   Supplied as: 60 mg tablet.
Dose (adult or child > 12 yr): 1 tablet twice daily for seasonal allergic rhinitis.
Note: Terfenadine is nonsedating.
trimeprazine (Temaril) is a phenothiazine.
Supplied as: 2.5 mg tablet,   5 mg sustain–release capsule,   2.5mg/5ml syrup.
Adult: 2.5 mg PO qid.   Sustain–release capsule: 5 mg PO twice daily.
Child > 3 years of age: 2.5 mg PO at bedtime or tid.
Child 6 month–3 years: 1.25 mg PO at bedtime or tid.
tripelennamine (PBZ)
Supplied as: 25, 50 mg tablet; 100 mg extend–release tablet; 25mg/5ml elixir.
Adult: 25–50 mg PO q4–6h.   Extend–release tablet: 100 mg PO bid–tid.
Child: 5 mg/kg/24 hr (maximum 300 mg/24hr).
triprolidine (Actidil)   Supplied as: 2.5 mg tablet, syrup (1.25mg/5ml).
Adult: 2.5 mg PO tid–qid.
Child > 6 yr: 1.25 mg PO tid–qid. **Child < 6 years of age:** 0.3–0.6 mg PO tid–qid.

ASPIRIN = acetylsalicylic acid = A.S.A.

Action: Inhibits prostaglandin synthesis. Exerts analgesic, antipyretic, & antiinflammatory effects.
Indications: Aspirin is used to treat fever; mild pain; or inflammation (e.g. osteoarthritis, rheumatoid arthritis, ankylosing spondylitis, bursitis).
Contraindications: salicylate hypersensitivity, coagulation abnormality (e.g. hemophilia), active GI ulcer, hemorrhage, final 3 months pregnancy. ●The concurrent use of certain drugs is contraindicated—e.g. other nonsteroidal anti-inflammatory drugs (including other salicylates), probenecid, sulfinpyrazone, anticoagulants, methotrexate.
Caution: renal insufficiency, liver disease, pregnancy (avoid high doses and avoid altogether in last 3 months of pregnancy), nursing (salicylates are secreted in milk), hyperuricemia, erosive gastritis ●Administer with caution to patient with history of asthma, nasal polyps, hay fever, or peptic ulcer. ●Use caution if any of the following drugs are administered concurrently with aspirin: corticosteroid, phenytoin, oral hypoglycemic.
Comments: ●Administer with food or milk to minimize GI irritation. ●Suppositories irritate mucosa and absorption is erratic. ●Therapeutic blood level in arthritis is 20–30mg/100ml (blood sample drawn 3 hours after last dose). Levels above 30mg/100ml may be toxic. ●Aspirin causes more GI irritation than other salicylates. ●Aspirin interferes with platelet aggregation which results in increased bleeding time. Consequently, aspirin should be discontinued prior to surgery.
Side effects: GI (nausea, vomiting, anorexia, heartburn, GI bleeding); hypersensitivity (bronchospasm, urticaria, angioedema, rhinitis, anaphylaxis); abnormal liver function (e.g. elevated SGOT, SGPT, alkaline phosphatase, prolonged prothrombin time); renal (decreased creatinine clearance, nephritis). ●With high doses there may be headache, tinnitus, decreased hearing, dizziness, vertigo. Signs of more severe toxicity include fever, sweating, diarrhea, hyperventilation with respiratory alkalosis, metabolic acidosis, tachycardia, vasomotor depression, confusion, drowsiness, excite-

ment, convulsions, coma.

Overdose: ●Patients initially hyperventilate and so there is respiratory alkalosis. Metabolic acidosis rapidly ensues in infants and young children. ●Ingestion of > 200–300 mg/kg of aspirin may be toxic. Toxicity is associated with a 6 hr post–ingestion serum salicylate level > 50 mg/ml. ●Empty the stomach. ●Administer activated charcoal. ●Administer cathartic PO—e.g. magnesium citrate. ●Alkalinize the urine by administering intravenous sodium bicarbonate. This traps the salicylate ion in the urine thereby enhancing urinary excretion. The dose of sodium bicarbonate is 2–3 mEq/kg IV initially. Additional doses (e.g. 2 mEq/kg at 6–8 hr intervals) may be necessary to maintain an alkaline urine. ●Dialysis may be necessary if the serum salicylate level exceeds 160mg/dl. ●Fever is controlled with cooling blanket or sponge bath. ●Treat seizures with intravenous diazepam or phenytoin. ●Administer plasma or whole blood if there is shock.

Supplied as:

> tablets: 65mg (1gr), 75mg, 81mg (1.25gr), 325mg (5gr), 500mg, 650mg;
> suppository: 65mg (1gr),130mg (2gr), 300mg, 325mg (5gr), 650mg (10gr).

Adult dose:

Pain/fever: 325–650 mg q4–6h PO or PR. Maximum 4000 mg per day.
Arthritis: 650 mg PO q4–6h. Maximum 5400mg/24hr in divided doses.

Pediatric dose:

Pain/fever: 10 mg/kg q4–6h (60 mg/kg/24hr divided q4–6h) PO or PR.
     Do not excceed 3600 mg/24hr.
Arthritis: Initially 60 mg/kg/24hr divided q4–6h.
     Increase as needed up to 100 mg/kg/24hr.

OTHER SALICYLATES or DERIVATIVES

Action: Like aspirin, these agents have analgesic, antipyretic, and anti–inflammatory properties. Unlike aspirin, (with exception of diflunisal) they do not interfere with platelet aggregation and thus do not increase the bleeding time. The prothrombin time may be prolonged with high doses.

Indications: The main indication is for inflammatory conditions when aspirin cannot be tolerated because of GI irritation.

Contraindications & cautions are in general as for aspirin.

Side effects are in general as for aspirin. See below for diflunisal side effects in particular.

choline magnesium trisalicylate (Trilisate)

Indications: analgesia, antipyretic, arthritis.
Supplied as: tablets (500, 750, 1000 mg); liquid (500mg/5ml).
Dose: Adult: 2000–3000 mg/day divided bid–tid.
     Child < 37 kg: 25 mg/kg PO twice daily.
     Child > 37 kg: 2250 mg/day PO divided bid–tid.

magnesium salicylate (Magan)   Supplied as 545 mg tablet.
Dose (adult): 1–2 tablets PO tid as needed for inflammation.

salsalate = salcyisalicylic acid (Disalcid, Mono–Gesic, Salsitab, Salflex)
Supplied as: 500, 750 mg tablet.
Dose (adult): 1000 mg PO tid (or 1500 mg PO twice daily) as needed for inflammation.

diflunisal (Dolobid)
Supplied as: 250, 500 mg tablets.
Dose (adult/child ≥ 12 yr):
   Pain: 1000 mg initially followed by 500 mg q12h. Some patients require 500 mg
   q8h. Others may require only 250 mg q8–12h.
   Arthritis: 250–500 mg q12h (maximum maintenance 1500 mg/day).
Note: ●500 mg diflusinal has about the same analgesic effect as 650 mg aspirin or acetaminophen. ●At the higher therapeutic doses (500–1000 mg twice daily) there is some interference with platelet aggregation with a slight increase in bleeding time.
Most common diflunisal side effects: gastrointestinal (nausea, vomiting, diarrhea, dyspepsia, abdominal pain, constipation, flatulence); neurologic (headache, fatigue, somnolence, insomnia, dizziness, tinnitus); rash.

ATROPINE

Action: Parasympatholytic. Blocks action of acetylcholine by binding to acatylcholine receptor sites with following consequences: ●reduces vagal tone thus accelerating the sinus node and facilitating AV conduction; ●mydriasis, cycloplegia; ●Inhibits sweating, salivation, bronchial secretions; ●decreases gastric secretion and GI motility; ●increases bladder sphincter tone.

Indications: ●sinus bradycardia in setting of hemodynamically compromising hypotension; ●sinus bradycardia that is associated with frequent PVC's; ●2nd and 3rd degree heart block; ●asystole; ●prior to anesthesia to reduce salivary/airway secretions; ●anticholinesterase insecticide poisoning.

Contraindications: atrial fibrillation or flutter, glaucoma, GI obstruction, bladder neck obstruction, asthma.

Caution: ●Do not use atropine simply to treat bradycardia. Reserve atropine for bradycardia accompanied by hypotension or frequent PVC's. ●Atropine may precipitate glaucoma in susceptible patients.

Side effects: ventricular fibrillation, ventricular tachycardia, dry mouth, blurred vision, skin flushing, urinary retention.

Supplied as: for IV or IM injection (0.1, 0.4, 0.5, 1.0, and 1.2 mg/ml).

Adult dose:

Asystole, symptomatic bradycardia, high degree AV block; 0.5 mg IV. If necessary, give repeat doses at 5 minute intervals up to maximum cumulative total of 2 mg (may also be given via endotracheal tube). If necessary, give repeat doses at 1–2 hour intervals.

Preanesthesia; 0.4–0.6 mg IM.

Anticholinesterase poisoning (in conjunction with pralidoxime); 2–4 mg every 5–10 minutes until bronchial secretions abate or until atropine side effects occur (mydriasis, tachycardia, dry mouth, dry/flushed skin). Additional 1–3 mg doses at 1/2 to 4 hour intervals may be required for 48 hours.

Pediatric dose:

Asystole, symptomatic bradycardia, high degree AV block; 0.01–0.03 mg/kg (minimum dose 0.1 mg, maximum dose 1.0 mg). If necessary, the dose may be repeated twice at 5 minute intervals. However, do not exceed maximum cumulative total of 1 mg in infants and children, and 2 mg in adolescents.

Preanesthesia (IM): Infant: 0.1mg,   4–12 months age: 0.2 mg,
                     1–3 yr age: 0.3 mg,   3–14 yr age: 0.4 mg.

In anticholinesterase poisoning (in conjunction with pralidoxime); 0.05 mg/kg every 5–10 minutes until bronchial secretions abate or atropine side effects occur. Repeat doses may be required periodically for 48 hours.

AZTREONAM (Azactam)

Action: Aztreonam is a monobactam (i.e. a monocyclic beta–lactam) antibiotic that is bactericidal by interfering with bacterial wall synthesis.

Spectrum is virtually restricted to gram–negative bacilli. Anaerobes and gram–positve cocci are resistant. Clinical spectrum includes E. coli, Enterobacter, Klebsiella pneumoniae and K. oxytoca, Proteus mirabilis, Pseudomonas aerugenosa, Serratia marcescens, Haemophilus influenzae (including ampicillin–resistant strains and other penicillinase–producing strains), Citrobacter. Activity against many other gram–negative organisms has been shown in vitro but not proven clinically.

Indications: Infections due to susceptible gram–negative bacteria: septicemia, lower respiratory tract, urinary tract, gynecologic structures, or skin and skin structures.

Contraindications: allergy to this antibiotic.

Comments: ●Use aztreonam in pregnancy only if clearly needed. ●A small fraction (< 1%) of aztreonam is excreted in human milk. Consider suspending nursing while on drug. ●Safety and efficacy in infants and children unknown.

Side effects: Local effects: phlebitis/thrombophlebitis with IV administration, injection site pain/swelling with IM administration. Systemic reactions occurring in 1–1.3% patients: nausea, vomiting, diarrhea, or rash. Refer to manufacturer information for systemic reactions occurring in < 1% of patients.

Supplied as preparation for IV or IM administration.

Dose: Urinary tract infection; 500–1000mg q8–12h.
        Moderately severe systemic infection; 1–2 gram q8–12h.
        Severe systemic or life–threatening infection; 2 gram q6–8h.

Note: ●The IV route is advised if the patient requires single doses > 1 gram. ●The IV route is also advised in the following circumstances: bacterial septicemia, localized parenchymal abscess, peritonitis, or other severe or life–threatening infection. ●Systemic infections by Pseudomonas aerugenosa should be treated with 2 gram q6–8h, at least initially.

BENZODIAZEPINES:

alprazolam (Xanax) **chlordiazepoxide** (Librium),
clorazepate (Tranxene) **flurazepam** (Dalmane)
lorazepam (Ativan) **oxazepam** (Serax)
prazepam (Centrax) **temazepam** (Restoril) **triazolam** (Halcion)

Find **Diazepam** (Valium) and **midazolam** (Versed) under seperate headings.

Contraindications: benzodiazepine hypersensitivity, acute alcohol intoxication, treatment of psychosis, first trimester pregnancy, acute narrow-angle glaucoma.
Caution: ●Because benzodiazepines are sedating, caution patients about using these drugs in dangerous settings that require alertness. Sedation is enhanced by alcohol and other CNS depressants. ●Benzodiazepines are metabolized in the liver and should be used cautiously in presence of liver disease and in the elderly. ●Chronic therapy may lead to physical dependence. To preclude withdrawal reaction (tremor, sweating, vomiting, convulsions, etc.) benzodiazepines should be withdrawn gradually over 1–2 weeks. ●Benzodiazepines can cause depression. Do not prescribe large amounts to patients with suicidal tendencies.
Side effects: CNS: drowsiness, confusion, amnesia, headache, depression, dizziness, vertigo, ataxia, slurred speech, tremor, blurred vision, diplopia, nystagmus, paradoxical effects (anxiety, hyperexcitability, rage, insomnia, vivid dreams, spasticity); cardiovascular: syncope, hypotension, palpitations; gastrointestinal: nausea, dry mouth, constipation; liver: abnormal liver function tests, jaundice; GU: urinary retention, incontinence; skin: rash, urticaria; other: altered libido, edema, joint pains.

alprazolam (Xanax)   Supplied as: 0.25, 0.5, 1 mg tablets.
Adult (anxiety): 0.25–0.5 mg PO tid (maximum 4mg/day).
                Start with 0.25 mg bid–tid in aged or debilitated.
NOTE: Peak serum level is achieved in 1–2 hours. Elimination half-life is 11–19 hr.

chlordiazepoxide (Librium. Libritabs)
Supplied as: ●5, 10, 25mg capsule ●5, 10mg tablet (Libritabs) ●Injection IV or IM.
Dose, adult:
●Anxiety: 5–10 mg PO tid–qid (5 mg bid–qid in aged or debilitated).
●Severe anxiety: 20–25 mg PO tid–qid (or 50–100 mg IV or IM) initially. If necessary, increase up to 25–50 mg tid–qid. Use oral route when possible. ●Acute alcohol withdrawal: 50–100 mg IV or IM, repeat in 2–4 hr as needed. Alternative, 50–100mg PO; repeat as needed, If necessary, administer up to 300mg/day.
Dose, child > 6 years of age: 5 mg PO bid–qid. Increase as needed up to 10 mg bid–tid.
Comments: ●IM absorption is erratic. ●Elimination half-life of the primary active metabolite desmethylchlordiazepoxide is 1–4 days.

clorazepate (Tranxene)
Supplied as: 3.75, 7.5, 15 mg tablet.
●Preparations for single dose administration every 24 hr (but not for initial therapy): 22.5 mg tablet (Tranxene SD), 11.25mg tablet (Tranxene SD half–strength).
Dose (adult):
●Anxiety: 15–60 mg/24hr divided bid–qid (usually 30 mg/24hr).
  May also be given as single bedtime dose. Try 15 mg at bedtime initially.
  Start with 7.5–15mg/24hr in elderly or debilitated.
●Alcohol withdrawal: day 1: 30 mg initial dose followed by 30–60 mg divided; day 2: 45–90 mg divided; day 3: 22.5–45 mg divided ; day 4: 15–30 mg divided; then, gradually decrease dose as condition improves and discontinue.
Elimination half-life of primary active metabolite, desmethyldiazepam, is 50–100 hr.

flurazepam (Dalmane)   Supplied as: 15, 30 mg capsule.
Dose (adult—to induce sleep): 15–30 mg PO at bedtime.
Elimination half-life primary active metabolite N–desalkylflurazepam is 47–100 hr.

lorazepam (Ativan)
Supplied as: tablet (0.5, 1, 2 mg); IM or IV injection (2 or 4 mg/ml).
Oral dose (adult):
●Anxiety: 1–2 mg PO bid–tid (range: 1–10 mg/day).
                Start with 1–2 mg/day in aged or debilitated.

●Insomnia: 2–4 mg at bedtime.
<u>Intravenous dose (adult)</u>: 0.44 mg/kg or 2 mg whichever is less.
Note: Elimination half–life is 8–25 hr. There are no active metabolites.

oxazepam (Serax)　　　　　Supplied as: 10, 15, 30 mg capsule; 15 mg tablet.
Dose (adult):●Anxiety:　10–15 mg PO tid–qid.
　　　　　　　　　　　　Up to 15–30 mg tid–qid if symptoms severe.
　　　　　　　●Acute alcohol withdrawal: 15–30 mg PO tid–qid.
Note: Elimination half–life is 5–15 hr. There are no active metabolites.

prazepam (Centrax)　　　　Supplied as: 5, 10, 20 mg capsules; 10 mg tablet.
Dose (adult—for anxiety): initially, 30 mg/day divided (range: 20–60 mg/day).
Start with 15 mg/day divided in aged or debilitated.
Elimination half–life of primary active metabolite desmethyldiazepam is 50–100 hr.

temazepam (Restoril)　　　Supplied as: 15, 30 mg capsules.
Dose (adult—to induce sleep): 30 mg PO at bedtime.
15mg may suffice and is the recommended initial dose in the aged or debilitated.
Note: Elimination half–life is 8–38 hr.

triazolam (Halcion)　　　　Supplied as: 0.125, 0.25 mg tablets.
Dose (adult—to induce sleep): 0.25–0.5 mg PO at bedtime.
Start with 0.125 mg in aged or debilitated.

BETA ADRENERGIC BLOCKERS:
acebutolol (Sectral), **atenolol** (Tenormin), **metoprolol** (Lopressor)
nadolol (Corgard), **pindolol** (Visken), **timolol** (Blocadren)
Find **propranolol** and **labetolol** elsewhere under seperate headings.

Action, contraindications, comments, cautions, side effects, treatment of overdose of beta blockers are as for propranolol.
Drug choice: All of the beta adrenergic blockers are equally effective in the treatment of hypertension and (if an indication) angina. Atenolol and metoprolol are relatively more selective beta–1–blockers and therefore may be useful when beta 2–blocking effects must be minimized—e.g. asthma, peripheral vascular disease, patient at risk of hypoglycemia (e.g. insulin–dependent diabetic). Selectivity is diminshed at higher doses. Atenolol and nadolol do not cross the blood–brain barrier as easily as other beta–blockers. The incidence of CNS side effects may therefore be reduced.

acebutolol (Sectral)　　　　Supplied as: 200, 400 mg capsules.
<u>Adult with hypertension</u> (alone or concurrent with other antihypertensives): Initially, 400 PO once daily or 200 mg twice daily. Usual dose is 400–800 mg/day. Range 200 once daily to 600 mg twice daily.
<u>Dose to reduce frequency of premature ventricular contractions in adult</u>: Initially, 200 mg PO twice daily. Increase gradually as needed to 300–600 mg twice daily. When discontinuing drug, do so gradually over a period of 2 weeks.
<u>Comments</u>: ●Acebutol is relatively more selective for beta–1 than for beta–2 receptors, but this selectivity is lost with increasing doses. ●Excretion is renal and nonrenal. Acebutolol is metabolized by the liver to the active metabolite diacetolol which is excreted by the kidneys. Elimination half–life of diacetolol but not acebutolol is increased in patients with renal failure.

atenolol (Tenormin)　Supplied as: 50, 100 mg tablets; IV preparation 5mg/10ml.
<u>Angina, adult</u>: Initially, 50 mg PO once daily. If necessary, increase the dose to 100 mg once daily after 1 week. Some patients require 200 mg once daily.
<u>Hypertension in adult</u> (alone or concurrent with diuretic): Initially, 50 mg PO once daily (full effect usually occurs within 1–2 wk). Increase dose if necessary. Maximum dose is 100 mg PO once daily.
<u>Acute myocardial infarction</u>: Administer 5 mg IV over 5 minutes, and then give another 5 mg IV 10 minutes later. Monitor blood pressure, heart rate, and EKG while

administering IV preparation. If the full IV dose (10 mg) is tolerated, give 50 mg PO 10 minutes after the last IV dose and 50 mg PO 12 hours later. Continue 50 mg PO bid (or 100mg PO qd) for another 6–9 days. The drug is stopped if bradycardia or hypotension requiring treatment, or other unacceptable side effect ensues. If IV administration is inadvisable, the patient may be started on oral therapy (unless there is a contraindication): 50mg PO bid (or 100mg PO qd) for at least 7 days.

Dose adjustment in renal failure: (1) creatinine clearance 15–35 ml/min/1.73 square meter: maximum dose is 50 mg/day PO; (2) creatinine clearance less than 15 ml/min/1.73 square meter: max dose is 50 mg every other day PO.

Comments: Atenolol is a beta–1 selective blocker at low doses, but both beta–1 and beta–2 sites are blocked at higher doses. Duration of action is at least 24 hours. Elimination half-life is about 6–7 hours. Atenolol is metabolized little if at all by the liver, and largely excreted unchanged by the kidneys.

metoprolol (Lopressor)   Supplied as: tablet (50, 100 mg); 5 ml ampul (1 mg/ml).

Angina: Adult dose is 50 mg PO twice daily initially. If necessary, increase dose at weekly intervals. Range: 100–400 mg/day.

Hypertension (alone or added to diuretic): Initial adult dose is 50 mg PO twice daily (or 100mg qd). Gradually increase at weekly intervals as needed. Range is 100–450 mg/day given as single daily dose or divided into 2 daily doses.

Myocardial infarction (long–term prophylaxis following infarct): After the patient is stabilized, start with three intravenous boluses of 5 mg each at 2 minute intervals while monitoring vital signs and EKG. If intravenous administration is tolerated, administer 50 mg PO q6h for 48 hours beginning 15 minutes after last intravenous bolus, and then 100 mg PO twice daily. Oral metoprolol is continued for at least 3 months. If the full IV dose (15mg) is not tolerated, administer 25 or 50 mg PO q6h (depending on the degree of intoleranace) beginning 15 minutes after the last IV dose or as soon as clinical condition permits. Stop the drug if there is severe intolerance.

Comments: Metoprolol is a beta–1 selective blocker at low doses, but both beta–1 and beta–2 sites are blocked at higher doses. Onset action PO is 1 hr; duration action is dose related. Metabolized by liver.

nadolol (Corgard)   Supplied as: 40, 80, 120, 160 mg tablets.

Hypertension (alone or concurrent with diuretic): Initial adult dose is 40 mg PO once daily. Increase gradually as needed by 40–80 mg increments to optimal blood pressure. Maximum: 240–320 mg PO once daily.

Angina: Initially, 40 mg PO once daily. Increase as needed every 3–7 days by 40–80 mg increments titrated to optimal therapeutic effect or pronounced slowing of heart rate. Range: 40–240 mg once daily.

Dose adjustment in renal failure (creatinine clearance : dose interval):
31–50 ml/min/1.73 sq. meter: 24–36 hr, 10–30 ml/min/1.73 sq. meter: 24–48 hr, less than 10 ml/min/1.73 sq. meter: 40–60 hr.

Comments: Nadolol is a nonselective beta–1 and beta–2 blocker. Half-life 20–24 hrs. Nadolol is not metabolized but is excreted unchanged, mostly by kidneys.

pindolol (Visken)   Supplied as: 5, 10 mg tablets.

Hypertension (alone or concurrent with other antihypertensive): Initial adult dose is 5mg PO twice daily. If necessary, increase dose by 10 mg/day increments at 3–4 week intervals up to maximum 60 mg/kg/day.

Comments: Pindolol is a nonselective beta–1 and beta–2 blocker. Half-life 3–4 hrs. Metabolized by liver and excreted mainly by kidney and to a small extent via the bile.

timolol (Blocadren)   Supplied as: 5, 10, 20 mg tablets.

Hypertension (alone or added to diuretic): Initial adult dose is 10 mg PO twice daily. Increase or decrease according to effect on heart rate and blood pressure. Increases should be made gradually at least 7 day intervals up to maximum 30 mg PO twice daily. Usual range: 10–20 mg twice daily.

Long term prophylaxis following myocardial infarction (to decrease mortality and risk of reinfarction): 10 mg PO twice daily.

Comments: Timolol is a nonselective beta–1 and beta–2 blocker. Half-life: 4 hr. Partially metabolized by liver and excreted by kidney.

BETHANECHOL (Urecholine, Myotonachol)

Action: Cholinergic. Primarily stimulates smooth muscle and glands (e.g. increased bladder tone, increased gastric motility, increased salivation).

Indications: ●Postoperative and postpartum nonobstructive urinary retention.

●Neurogenic bladder with retention.

Contraindications: hypersensitivity; hyperthyroidism; peptic ulcer; asthma; bradycardia; hypotension; vasomotor instability; coronary artery disease; AV conduction abnormalities; epilepsy; parkinsonism; mechanical obstruction of GI tract or bladder; detrussor–sphincter dyssynergia; questionable strength/integrity of GI tract or bladder (e.g. recent GI or bladder surgery, GI inflammation, peritonitis); concurrent use of ganglion blockers (e.g. trimethaphan). IM or IV administration contraindicated.

Caution: pregnancy, nursing mother.

Comments: Effects usually appear 5–15 minutes after subcutaneous administration.
After oral administration, effects appear within 60–90 minutes and persist for about 1 hour.

Side effects: salivation, lacrimation, nausea, vomiting, diarrhea, belching, abdominal discomfort/cramps, flushing, sweating, malaise, asthma, hypotension.

Supplied as: 5, 10, 25, 50mg tablet; 1 ml vial (5mg/ml) for SC injection.

Adult dose:

Oral: 5–10 mg initially. If necessary, repeat hourly up to cumulative total of 50 mg. Usual dose is 10–50 mg tid–qid.

Subcutaneous: 2.5 mg initially. If necessary, give additional 2.5 mg at 15–30 minute intervals up to maximum 4 doses given. Smallest effective dose may be given tid–qid as needed.

BLOOD and BLOOD COMPONENTS:

●**Blood: whole, fresh whole, packed red blood cells, leukocyte-poor red cells;**
●**platelets;**
●**fresh frozen plasma; plasma protein fraction; albumin;**
●**Rho (D) immune globulin;**
●**coagulation factors (cryoprecipitate, factor VIII, factor IX)**

General comments:

Choosing between whole blood and packed RBC's: Routine use of whole blood is expensive and wasteful. It should be reserved for massive acute blood loss with signs and symptoms of hypovolemia. Reconstituted whole blood (RBC's + FFP) is used for exchange transfusions in neonates. In order to avoid volume overload, patients with cardiac compromise or hypervolemia should ordinarily receive packed red cells rather than whole blood.

Massive acute blood loss may be treated with either (1) whole blood, or (2) packed RBC's in conjunction with crystalloid (isotonic normal saline or Ringers' lactate). Concurrent replacement of platelets and coagulation factors is usually necessary after the first 10 units of stored blood (whole or packed) have been transfused. One approach is to administer one unit of fresh whole blood (or one unit of packed RBC plus one unit FFP plus one unit platelets) for every 4 units of stored blood. ●An alternative to periodic platelet and FFP transfusion in a patient undergoing massive transfusion is to serially determine PT, PTT, fibrinogen, and platelet count; and administer blood components as indicated. FFP is administered if the PT and PTT are prolonged, and fibrinogen is given if the fibrinogen level falls to < 100mg/dl. Platelets are indicated if the count is < 50,000 and the patient is bleeding, or if the count is < 20,000 in the absence of bleeding. Platelet transfusion is also indicated in the absence of bleeding if the count is < 30,000 and the patient is to undergo surgery.

Method of blood administration: Needle size; RBC's should ordinarily be transfused thru an 18 gauge needle or larger. Smaller needles may be used but significantly prolong the transfusion. Furthermore, if a 23 gauge needle is used, hemolysis may occur if pressure is exerted in order to increase the rate of infusion. Isotonic normal saline; Blood should be infused with isotonic normal saline thru a Y set-up with normal saline in one limb and blood in the other. Cold blood should be warmed before and during massive transfusion, otherwise arrhythmias may occur. Macropore IV filters filter out platelet–fibrin aggregates and should be used when transfusing stored whole blood. Rate of infusion: Ordinarily, an unit of blood is infused in less than 2 hours to preclude bacterial growth at room temperature. Units should be split by the blood bank if the infusion rate/unit is greater than 4 hours.

Determining amount of blood required: One unit of whole blood (or packed RBC) will raise hematocrit of adult by about 3%. Use following formula for pediatric patient: required volume of

$$\text{blood transfusion} = \frac{80 \times (\text{weight in kg}) \times (\text{desired hct} - \text{actual hct})}{(\text{hct of transfused blood})}$$

Emergency transfusions: Type and crossmatch requires 45–60 minutes. Type and Rh requires about 5 minutes. It is best to at least wait until the patient's type and Rh is ascertained and then transfuse type specific blood. If a patient cannot tolerate even this delay, then unmatched O–negative blood may be transfused. If O–negative blood is unavailable, then males without prior history of transfusions may receive O–positive blood.

Investigation of transfusion reaction: Stop transfusion. Recheck identity of both patient and blood product. Centrifuge sample of patient's blood. Hemoglobin from hemolyzed RBC will result in red–tinged plasma if hemolysis is substantial. The urine may also be red–tinged. Laboratory: (1) Send untransfused blood product and sample of patient's blood for repeat type and cross-match, including direct and indirect Coombs' test of patient and donor serum. Pre–transfusion specimen should also be typed and crossmatched again. (2) Order hematocrit, platelet count, PT, PTT, hapatoglobin, fibrinogen level, quantitative fibrin split products, electrolytes, BUN, creatinine. (3) If bacterial contamination is suspected, obtain blood C&S of patient as well as gram stain and C&S of donor blood.

Transfusion reactions–clinical findings and treatment:

Febrile without hemolysis (common). Recipient leukoagglutinins react with donor WBC causing release pyrogens from WBC. Patient may experience fever and chills. *Treatment*: antipyretics.

Febrile with hemolysis (rare). Recipient antibodies react with donor RBC's resulting in hemolysis. Fever/chills may be the only clues. Patient may develop headache, chest pain, back pain, hypotension, tachycardia, weak pulse, cool clammy skin, disseminated intravascular coagulation. *Treatment*: Maintain diuresis until hemoglobinuria and hemoglobinemia resolves. Keep urine output at 1.5–2 ml/kg/hr with intravenous D5W. If diuresis is inadequate, administer furosemide or induce osmotic diuresis with 25 gram of 20% mannitol infused IV over 5 minutes. If BP falls; infuse normal saline, albumin, or fresh whole blood. Use vasopressor as last resort.

Allergic/immediate hypersensitivity (common). Usually due to unknown allergen in donor blood. IgA–deficient patients are prone to severe reaction. Patient may experience pruritits, urticaria, wheezing. Rarely, there is laryngeal edema, anaphylactic shock. *Treatment mild reaction*: diphenhydramine 50 mg IV/IM. *Treatment severe reaction*: epinephrine SC, diphenhydramine, and corticosteroids.

Bacterial contamination (rare). Signs and symptoms are secondary to bacterial pyrogens. Patient may experience high fever, chills, vomiting, diarrhea, hypotension. *Treatment*: obtain blood culture (also gram stain and culture donor blood) and administer antibiotic.

Blood and blood components:

whole blood (1 unit = about 500 ml) Indications: (1) acute massive blood loss with signs/symptoms of hypovolemia, (2) exchange transfusion. Comments: Storage life is up to 21 days. About 30% red blood cells lost over 3 weeks; platelet function is lost in 48 hours, factor VIII in 48 hours, factor V in 5 days, factor XI in 6–7 days.

fresh whole blood (whole blood less than 6–24 hours old). Indications: patient undergoing massive transfusion. Fresh whole blood is preferred for neonatal exchange transfusion because the increased levels of potassium in the plasma fraction of stored whole blood may cause hyperkalemia.

packed red blood cells is the most common form of red blood cell transfusion. One unit (200–350 ml) is prepared from 1 unit of whole blood. Hematocrit range: 60–90. Some plasma remains. Small amounts of platelets and leukocytes are also present. Advantages over whole blood: (1) relatively cheap compared to whole blood or other RBC preparations, (2) less risk of volume overload, (3) less risk of allergic reation since much of the allergenic potential has been removed (i.e. plasma, WBC, platelets).

leukocyte-poor red cells (leukopoor red cells). Indications: (1) patient requiring ongoing transfusions, (2) sensitized patient who has had prior transfusion reaction, (3) patient who has or anticipates having organ transplant. Washed RBC are leukopoor red cells with almost all WBC and plasma removed. "Washing" increases risk of bacterial contamination and so the product must be used within 24 hours of preparation if the blood is collected using an open system. This product is expensive. Filtered leukopoor red cells: An alternate way of providing leukopoor RBC's is to filter out the leukocytes with a special filter (Fenwal, Sepacell R500) as the blood is being transfused.

frozen red blood cells are used to store rare blood types, or store blood of patient for autotransfusion (e.g. patient anticipating elective surgery). Storage life is 3 yr. The risk of hepatitis is lower than whole blood or other RBC preparations. This product is "leukopoor" but not to the extent of washed RBC. If necessary, frozen RBC's can be further refined by "washing".

platelets 1 unit (1 pack) = platelets derived from 1 unit whole blood. Indications: (1) nonbleeding patient with platelet count less than 10–20 thousand, (2) thrombocytopenia with bleeding, (3) chemotherapy patient with platelet count less than 30 thousand, (4) prior to major surgery if platelet count is less than 50 thousand, (5) patient undergoing massive transfusion—i.e. transfusion of more than 10 units of stored blood. Comments: •Obtain platelet count 1 hour post transfusion. One unit will raise platelet count of adult by 5,000–12,000. Usually 4–8 units are needed to raise count significantly. •In presence of platelet destruction (e.g. immune thrombocytopenia) the platelet count may not increase. It is usually futile to administer platelets to patient undergoing immune–mediated hemolysis. •Storage life of platelets is 3–5 days. Viability after transfusion is normally 3–5 days. Single donor HLA matched platelets (usually from donor siblings) may be required in patient sensitized by prior transfusion who fails to realize an increase in platelet count, or in patient requiring ongoing platelet transfusions.

fresh frozen plasma (1 unit = 200–250 ml plasma). Blood typing should be performed prior to transfusing but crossmatching is not required. Indications: (1) patient undergoing massive transfusion—i.e. transfusion of over 10 units of stored blood; (2) thrombotic thrombocytopenic purpura; (3) bleeding secondary to oral anticoagulant; (4) coagulation deficiency due to liver disease (factor II, VII, IX, X are normally synthesized by the liver); (5) hereditary coagulation deficiencies (V, VII, IX, X, XI, von Willebrand's). All but minor bleeding due to factor IX deficiency requires factor IX concentrate. Factor VIII deficiency should be treated with cryoprecipitate or factor VIII concentrate.

plasma protein fraction (human) U.S.P. 5% (Plasma–Plex, Plasmatein, Protenate) is derived from pooled human plasma. Contains albumin, globulin, small amounts of gamma globulin. There is no risk of viral hepatitis. In contrast to fresh frozen plasma, this product does not contain coagulation factors. Indications: hypovolemic shock, hypoproteinemia. Administration: Solution is administered undiluted IV and must not be mixed in the same IV line with other IV solutions.
Adult dose: (1) hypovolemic shock: individualize according to patient needs,
(2) hypoproteinemia: infuse 1 liter and then reassess.
Pediatric dose: 10–20 ml/kg; repeat as needed.

albumin (Albutein, Buminate) is supplied as a 5% solution (isotonic, contains 5 gram albumin/100ml) and as a 25% solution (hypertonic, contains 25 gram albumin/100ml). The 25% solution is also referred to as salt–poor albumin. Albumin solution is heat–sterilized and carries no risk of hepatitis. Blood typing is not necessary.
Indications/Dose:
•Expand plasma volume (e.g. hypovolemic shock due to hemorrhage/burns)
   Adult: 25 gram (500 ml of 5% solution) administered rapidly IV. Give additional doses as needed.
   Pediatric: 15 ml of 5% solution/kg. Give additional doses as needed.
•Edema due to cirrhosis liver, nephrotic syndrome, malnutrition, idiopathic hypoproteinemia:
   Adult: 2 ml/kg of 25% solution IV at about 50 ml/hr. Repeat q24h as needed.

factor VIII concentrate Indication: factor VIII deficiency (hemophilia A).
Supplied as: Vials that state amount of factor VIII activity contained. One unit = amount of factor VIII activity in 1 ml of normal human plasma.
Dose for hemarthosis: 15–20 units/kg infused IV at about 10–15ml/min (sufficient to maintain factor VIII activity at 20–30% normal).
Dose for mild bleeding noncritical areas (muscles, soft tissue): 10 units/kg IV.
Dose for critical bleeding (CNS, retropharyngeal, retroperitoneal, severe trauma, bleeding into body cavity): Initially, 40–50 units/kg IV followed by 20–25 units/kg IV q12h until hemorrhage stops.
Preoperative dose: Sufficient to provide factor VIII activity 60% normal for 7–10 days.
Comments: •Administering 1 unit/kg will raise the patient's factor VIII level by 2%. •Factor VIII activity 5% of normal is generally sufficient to prevent spontaneous bleeding. •Testing patient for factor VIII inhibitors is recommended prior to factor VIII administration. •Blood typing is not necessary unless hemolysis occurs. If hemolysis does occur, administer cryoprecipitate from type and crossmatched donor, or cryoprecipitate derived from type O donors with low anti–A and anti–B titers.

cryoprecipitate contains factor VIII, fibrinogen, Von Willebrand's factor, fibronectin.
<u>Indications:</u> Factor VIII deficiency (hemophilia A), von Willebrand's disease, hypofi-brinogemia.
<u>Supplied as:</u> bag containing 60–125 units of factor VIII/bag and about 250mg fibrin-ogen (1 unit factor VIII = amount factor VIII activity in 1 ml of normal human plasma).
<u>Dose in Hemophilia A:</u> see units/kg dose guidelines under *factor VIII concentrate* above. Since the amount of factor VIII/bag is so variable, the patient's serum must subsequently be tested for factor VIII activity.
<u>Dose in Von Willebrand's disease and hypofibrinogemia</u> is individualized.

factor IX concentrate contains coagulation factors II, VII, IX, X.
<u>Indications:</u> (1) factor IX deficiency (Christmas disease, Hemophilia B); (2) treat-ment of patients with factor VIII deficiency who develop factor VIII inhibitors.
<u>Treatment of factor IX deficiency:</u> Treat minor bleeding with fresh frozen plasma. In other cases, use the lowest dose range (in units/kg) as indicated for *factor VIII concentrate* above. Factor IX concentrate also contains factors II, VII, X which may become activated and cause thrombosis. If large doses of factor IX concentrate are infused, it is advisable to add 5 units heparin/ml in order to preclude DIC.
<u>Treatment of patients with factor VIII inhibitors:</u> If bleeding is not life–threatening, administer 75 units factor IX concentrate/kg q8–12h as needed. Persistent or life–threatening hemorrhage is treated with anti–inhibitor coagulant complex (Autoplex).
<u>Contraindication:</u> suspected DIC or fibrinolysis in setting of liver disease.
<u>Comments:</u> ●Blood typing and crossmatch is not necessary. ●Oral anticoagulant–in-duced deficiencies of factors II, VII, IX, or X are treated with vitamin K or fresh frozen plasma, not factor IX concentrate.

Rho (D) immune globulin (RhoGam, HypRho–D) contains antibodies to Rho (D). Product carries no risk of hepatitis.
<u>Indications:</u> ●Postpartum, for the unsensitized Rh negative mother delivering an Rh + or Du + baby. ●Rh–negative woman at 28 week gestation and repeated post–par-tum if infant is Rh +. ●Rh–negative woman following abortion (spontaneous or in-duced), ectopic pregnancy, miscarriage, amniocentesis, abdominal trauma (if fetal blood enters maternal circulation). ●Rh–negative woman who receives transfusion Rh + blood.
<u>Dose/administration:</u> Product is administered IM, preferably within 72 hours of de-livery, miscarriage, etc. A standard vial can prevent iso–immunization of about 30 ml fetal blood and is sufficient for most situations after 13 weeks gestation. Low–dose preparations (MICRhoGAM, HypRho–D Mini–Dose) are indicated for abortion/ectopic pregnancy occuring at 12 weeks or less. ●If large fetal–maternal bleed occurs, the Kleihauer–Betke stain can distinguish fetal from maternal RBC's. Then, the number of standard vials of Rho (D) immune globulin administered =

$$2.3 \times (\text{\#fetal RBC/\#maternal RBC}) \times (\text{maternal ideal body weight in kg}).$$

BRETYLIUM (Bretylol)

Action: Lowers resting membrane potential thus reducing the threshhold for ventricular fibrillation. Increases duration action potential and refractory period. Automaticity and conduction velocity are unaffected.
Indications: ●ventricular fibrillation ●ventricular tachycardia ●ventricular arrhythmias not con-trolled by lidocaine or procainamide.
Caution: ●Bretylium initially releases endogenous norepinephrine and may thus cause transient hypertension, tachycardia, and increased ectopy. Arrhythmias secondary to digitalis toxicity may be exacerbated. ●Subsequent adrenergic blockade by bretylium may provoke postural hypotension (50% patients) and bradycardia (and there may be associated dizziness, vertigo, lightheadedness, syncope). Be prepared to give dopamine. Be aware that it may be particularly difficult for the patient with aortic stenosis or pulmonary hypertension to increase cardiac output sufficiently to maintain adequate blood pressure.
Side effects: (In addition to those noted in cautions above): nausea/vomiting (common with rapid IV infusion), diarrhea, hiccups, abdominal pain, angina, flushing, nasal congestion, sweating, conjunctivitis, rash, psychic disturbances.
Supplied as: 10 ml ampul/vial containing 500 mg for IV or IM administration.
Dose: Refer to appendix.

BUTOCONAZOLE (Femstat)

Indication: vulvovaginal candidiasis.
Contraindication: hypersensitivity to components of preparation, 1st trimester pregnancy.
Supplied as: 2% cream.
Dose: one applicatorful at bedtime for 3 consecutive nights.
For pregnant patients (2nd and 3rd trimester only):
one applicatorful at bedtime for 6 consecutive nights.

CALCITONIN, HUMAN (Cibacalcin)

Action: Synthetic polypeptide with same amino acid sequence as humans. Acts primarily on bone to reduce bone resorption and thus reduce serum calicium.

Indications: Paget's disease of bone.

Comments: ●Monitor therapeutic effect by relief of symptoms, and by measurement of serum alkaline phosphatase and 24 hour urinary hydroxyproline. These tests should be obtained before initiating therapy, during the first 3 months, and then every 3–6 months. ●Although calcitonin cannot cross placental barrier, it should be used with caution in pregnancy.

Side effects: nausea, vomiting, anorexia, diarrhea, abdominal discomfort/pain, flushing, urinary frequency. Rare side effects include mild tetany, chills, shortness of breath, chest pressure, headache, weakness, dizziness.

Supplied as: syringe containing 0.5 mg calcitonin.

Dose (adult): 0.5 mg once daily subcutaneously.

In some patients, 0.25 mg once daily or 0.5 mg 2–3 times/wk may suffice.

CALCITONIN, SALMON (Calcimar)

Action: Synthetic polypeptide identical in amino acid sequence to salmon calcitonin. Acts primarily on bone to reduce bone resorption and thus reduce serum calicium.

Indications: hypercalcemia, symptomatic Paget's disease of bone, postmenopausal osteoporosis.

Comments: ●Monitor therapeutic effect by periodic measurement of serum alkaline phosphatase and 24 hour urinary hydroxyproline (both of which should decrease) as well as by symptomatic relief. ●In hypercalcemic emergencies, calcitonin is initiated along with other measures (IV normal saline, furosemide, etc.). ●To rule out allergy consider skin testing first: withdraw 0.05 ml of preparation into Tb syringe; dilute to 1.0 ml with sodium chlorine injection USP and mix, discard 0.9 ml and inject 0.1 ml SC into volar aspect forearm. Wait 15 minutes. More than mild erythema or wheal constitutes positive response. ●Although calcitonin cannot cross placental barrier, it should be used with caution in pregnancy. ●Calcitonin inhibits lactation in animals. It is not known if drug is excreted in human milk.

Side effects: nausea, vomiting, rash, facial flushing, local inflammation.

Supplied as: 2 ml vial containing 200 IU for SC or IM injection.

Dose (adult):

Hypercalcemia: (1) Initially, 4 IU/kg SC or IM q 12 h. If after 2 days the response is inadequate, increase the dose to 8 IU/kg q12h; and if necessary after another 2 days to a maximum dose of 8 IU/kg q6h.

Paget's Disease: Initially, 100 IU (0.5 ml) once daily SC or IM.

Maintenance range: 50 IU once every other day to once daily. Maximum 100 IU once daily.

Postmenopausal osteoporosis (in conjunction with adequate calcium intake, vitamin D intake, and diet): 100 IU once daily SC or IM.

CALCIUM CHANNEL BLOCKERS:
diltiazem (Cardizem), nifedipine, (Procardia, Adalat), verapamil (Calan, Isoptin)

Action: ●Inhibits calcium influx into vascular smooth muscle. The reduced intracellular calcium concentration induces relaxation of vascular smooth muscle thereby dilating coronary arteries/arterioles (and so there is increased coronary blood flow) and peripheral arteries/arterioles (and so there is decreased afterload work of heart with consequent decreased myocardial oxygen consumption). The effect on venous vasculature is generally negligible. Nifedipine causes the most vasodilation, diltiazem the least. ●Inhibits calcium influx into myocardial contractile cells (slow calcium channel). The reduced intracellular calcium causes a decrease in myocardial contractility. ●Inhibits calcium influx (slow calcium channel) into the AV node thereby slowing AV node conduction. Verapamil exerts the greatest effect on AV conduction, nifedipine the least. ●Calcium channel blockers also depress the SA node.

Indications: ●chronic stable angina; ●unstable angina (i.e. increase in severity or frequency, or change in pattern of angina); ●Prinzmetal's variant angina (angina due to coronary vasospasm); ●Also, intravenous verapamil is indicated for (1) rapid conversion of paroxysmal supraventricular tachycardia to sinus rhythm, (2) temporary control of rapid ventricular rate in atrial flutter or atrial fibrillation.

Drug choice in the treatment of angina: ●Nifedipine exerts the greatest peripheral vasodilative effect but has negligible effect on SA and AV conducton. Consequently it finds greatest utility in angina that is associated with hypertension or cardiac conduction abnormalities. ●Verapamil causes less peripheral vasodilation than nifedipine but depresses the SA and AV nodes. It is therefore not a good choice for patients with sick sinus syndrome or AV block. It may, however, benefit patients with supraventricular arrhythmias (atrial flutter, atrial fibrillation, paroxysmal supraventricular tachycardia). ●Diltiazem causes the least peripheral vasodilation. It does depress the SA and AV nodes (but to a lesser extent than verapamil). Consequently, it should not be used in presence of sick sinus syndrome or AV conduction abnormalities. ●All calcium channel blockers have negative inotropic effects. They should be used cautiously in patients with borderline left ventricular reserve or patients receiving other myocardial depressants (e.g. beta blockers).

Comments: ●Calcium channel blockers decrease myocardial contractility (negative inotrope). Consequently, they should be used cautiously in patients with compromised left ventricular function. Beta blockers (e.g. propranolol) also have negative inotropic effects. Therefore, concurrent use of calcium channle blockers and a beta blocker may precipitate congestive heart failure in susceptible patients. ●Paradoxically, calcium channel blockers may induce angina. This may be because calcium channel blockers cause a decrease in diastolic pressure which in turn causes a decrease in coronary perfusion and a reflex increase in heart rate. ●Pregnancy: use only if clearly needed.

diltiazem (Cardizem)

<u>Supplied as:</u>   30, 60, 90, 120 mg tablet;
60, 90, 120 mg sustain release capsules (Cardizem SR)

<u>Adult dose for angina</u> (alone or concurrent with long or short–acting nitrates): Initially, 30mg PO qid before meals and bedtime. If necessary, increase dose gradually at 1–2 day intervals. Average dose is 180–240 mg/day.

For sustain release capsule: Start with 60–120 mg twice daily. Make dose adjustments as needed at 14 day intervals. Usual requirement is 240–360/day.

<u>Contraindications:</u> sick sinus syndrome, 2nd or 3rd degree AV block unless pacemaker is present, systolic blood pressure less than 90.

<u>Most common side effects:</u> edema, headache, nausea, dizziness, rash, asthenia.

nifedipine (Procardia, Adalat)

<u>Supplied as:</u>   10, 20 mg capsules;
30, 60, 90 mg extended release tablets (Procardia XL)

<u>Capsules, dose for angina</u> (alone or in conjunction with prn sublingual nitroglycerin): Initially 10 mg PO tid. Usual range 10–20 mg tid. Some patients require 20–30 mg tid–qid. More than 120 mg/day seldom required. Maximum 180 mg/day. Titration is usually carried out over a 1–2 week period. However, in more urgent circumstances, the dose may be increased from 10 mg tid to 20 mg tid and then to 30 mg tid over a 3 day period provided that the symptomatic response and blood pressure can be monitored frequently. The dose in hospitalized patients may be increased as needed by 10 mg increments every 4–6 hours but an individual dose should not ordinarily exceed 30 mg.

<u>Extended release tablets:</u>   Start with 30–60 mg once daily. Use caution in giving more than 90mg/day in angina patient. More than 120 mg/day is not advised.

<u>Contraindications:</u> hypersensitivity to drug. <u>Caution:</u> ●Angina may worsen when beta blocker therapy is discontinued, and taking nifedipine may in this circumstance occasionally aggravate angina. To preclude this development it is best to taper the beta blocker. Concurrent nifedipine and beta blocker therapy is not contraindicated. ●Nifedipine occasionally causes excessive hypotension, usually in a patient receiving a beta blocker concurrently. <u>Side effects:</u> peripheral edema, dizziness, lightheadedness, nausea, headache and flushing, weakness, transient hypotension, nasal congestion, chest congestion, dyspnea, diarrhea, constipation, cramps, flatulence, joint stiffness, muscle cramps, nervousness, sleep disturbances, blurred vision, difficulties in balance, dermatitis, pruritis, urticaria, fever, sweating, chills, sexual difficulties, syncope, allergic hepatitis, anemia, leukopenia, thrombocytopenia, purpura, gingival hyperplasia, erythromelalgia.

verapamil (Calan, Isoptin)

<u>Contraindications:</u> severe hypotension, cardiogenic shock, ventricular tachycardia, 2nd or 3rd degree AV block (unless functioning pacemaker present), sick sinus syndrome (unless functioning pacemaker present), severe congestive heart failure (unless due to supraventricular tachycardia treatable with verapamil), concurrent use with IV beta blocker, atrial flutter or fibrillation in patient with accessory bypass tract (e.g. Wolff–Parkinson–White, Lown–Ganong–Levine). <u>Side effects with IV administration:</u> symptomatic hypotension, bradycardia, tachycardia, dizziness, headache, nausea, abdominal discomfort. <u>Most common side effects with oral administration:</u> hypotension, peripheral edema, bradycardia, AV block, congestive heart failure, pulmonary edema, dyspnea, dizziness, headache, fatigue, nausea, constipation, rash, flushing.

<u>Supplied as:</u>   tablet (40, 80, 120 mg); sustain release tablets (180, 240 mg);
intravenous injection (2.5mg/ml).

<u>Intravenous dose for conversion paroxysmal supraventricular tachycardia including those associated with accessory bypass tracts (e.g. Wolff–Parkinson–White, Lown–Ganong–Levine):</u>

Adult: 5–10 mg (0.075–0.15 mg/kg) IV over 2 minutes (over at least 3 minutes in elderly). If adequate response does not occur after 30 minutes, administer additional 10 mg (0.15 mg/kg).

Pediatric: ●0–1 yr of age: 0.1–0.2 mg/kg IV over 2 minutes. Repeat after 30 minutes if necessary. ●1–15 yr of age: 0.1–0.3 mg/kg (maximum 5 mg) IV over 2

minutes. Repeat if necessary after 30 minutes (maximum 10 mg).
<u>Intravenous dose for temporary control of rapid ventricular rate in patient with atrial flutter/fibrillation:</u> same dosage as for conversion of paroxysmal supraventricular tachycardia. NOTE: Verapamil is contraindicated for this purpose when the patient is known to have a accessory bypass tract (e.g. Wolff–Parkinson–White syndrome, Lown–Ganong–Levine syndrome).
<u>Oral dose for angina</u> (alone or concurrent with short or long–acting nitrates): Initially, 80 mg PO tid. If necessary, increase dose weekly (or daily if angina unstable). In some cases, 40 mg tid may suffice. Maximum 480 mg/day.
<u>Oral dose for essential hypertension:</u> Initially, 80 mg PO tid. Consider starting with 40mg tid in those in whom an increased response is likely (e.g. small patient, elderly). Do not exceed 120 mg tid. ●If the sustain release tablets are used, the usual starting dosage is 180mg once daily in the morning. Consider starting with 120mg once daily in those in whom an increased response is likely (e.g. small patient, elderly). The antihypertensive effect is seen within a week. If the response to 180mg qd is inadequate, the dose may be increased to 240mg each morning. If yet another increase is needed, try 180mg morning and evening (or 240mg each morning and 120mg each evening). Up to 240mg q12h may be used. If the patient is being switched from the immediate release to the sustain release tablets, the total daily dose remains the same.
<u>Oral dose for prophylaxis repetitive supraventricular tachycardia:</u> 240–480 mg/day PO divided into 3–4 daily doses.
<u>Oral dose for control ventricular rate in patient with chronic atrial fibrillation/flutter</u> (in conjunction with digitalis): 240–480 mg/day PO divided into 3–4 daily doses.

CALCIUM CHLORIDE

Action: increases contractility of myocardium, increases automaticity of ventricles, increases depolarization threshold.
Indications: ●Adjunct in treatment of asystole and electromechanical dissociation.
●Severe hyperkalemia (e.g. potassium greater than 8 mEq/liter, changes in P wave or QRS).
Contraindications: ventricular fibrillation, hypercalcemia.
Caution: ●Allow interval between IV administration of calcium and sodium bicarbonate; otherwise calcium will precipitate as calcium carbonate. ●Bradycardia or cardiac arrest may occur if calcium is administered rapidly in presence of contracting heart. ●Calcium and digitalis are synergistic. The additive affects can precipitate digitalis toxicity (PVC's, ventricular fibrillation, asystole, etc.). ●Necrosis may occur at IV site if there is local infiltration.
Supplied as: 10 ml ampules of 10% calcium chloride
(10 ml = 1 gram calcium chloride = 13.6 mEq Ca ++).
Adult dose:
<u>Hyperkalemia:</u> 10 ml of 10% solution IV over 10 minutes with EKG monitor.
<u>Asystole/EM dissociation:</u> 2.5–5 ml 10% solution slow IV push. Repeat at 10 minute intervals if necessary.
Pediatric dose:
<u>Hyperkalemia:</u> 0.2 ml/kg (maximum 3 ml) IV over 10 minutes with EKG monitor.
<u>Cardiac arrest:</u> 0.2 ml/kg (maximum 3 ml) of 10% solution slow IV push.

CAPTOPRIL (Capoten)

Action: Inhibits angiotensin converting enzyme, the enzyme that converts angiotensin–1 to angiotensin–2 (a potent vasoconstrictor). Decreased levels of angiotensin–2 also lead to decreased aldosterone secretion with consequent small increases in serum potassium. Maximum blood pressure fall occurs 60–90 minutes after an individual dose. Duration of effect is dose related.
Indications: ●Hypertension.
●Heart failure insufficiently responsive to conventional diuretic and digoxin therapy.
Contraindications: hypersensitivity; nursing mother; pregnancy (unless benefit justifies risk); children (unless other regimens fail); potassium–sparing diuretics (e.g. spironolactone, triamterene) unless patient is hypokalemic.
Caution/comments: ●Captopril–treatment of hypertension in patient with renal impairment is advised only when multi-drug regimens have failed to control hypertension or have produced intolerable side effects. ●Elevation of BUN and creatinine following captopril–induced reduction in blood pressure in patient with renal disease (especially severe renal artery stenosis) may occur as a consequence of decreased renal perfusion. Discontinuation of diuretic or decreased captopril dosage is advised. However, in some patients captopril must be stopped because normotension cannot be achieved without compromising renal perfusion. ●Captopril–induced elevation of BUN and creatinine occurs in about 20% of heart failure patients. The elevations are usually stable. Captopril must be stopped in only a few cases (usually those with underlying renal disease) be-

cause of progressive increases in creatinine. ●Proteinuria in excess of one gram/day develops in 0.7 % patients, mostly patients with history of renal disease and/or patients receiving > 150 mg/day of captopril. Patients with these risk factors should therefore have dipstick checks for urinary protein before initiating captopril and then periodically. Patient should be advised to report edema (nephrotic syndrome ?). ●Neutropenia or agranulocytosis occasionally occurs. Patients with renal dysfuntion or autoimmune disease (e.g. lupus) are at greatest risk. In patients with renal dysfunction, obtain a WBC with differential before initiating and while receiving captopril (every 2 weeks for 3 months and then periodically). Consider risk versus benefits of captopril therapy in patient with autoimmune disease or in patient receiving drugs that may impair the immune system or leukocyte function, especially if there is renal dysfunction. Advise patient receiving captopril to report any signs of infection such as sore throat or fever in case neutropenia is developing. ●Hypotension is most likely to occur in the following settings: salt/volume depletion, diuretic therapy or salt-restriction, concurrent adrenergic–blocker (e.g. propranolol), ganglionic–blocking drug, concurrent vasodilator (e.g. nitroglycerin), heart failure. ●Surgery/anesthesia: If hypotension occurs, treat with normal saline to expand volume.
Side effects include: proteinuria, neutropenia, agranulocytosis, rash, fever, pruritis, eosinophilia, angioedema, hypotension, tachycardia, chest pain, myocardial infarction, Raynaud's syndrome, CHF, impaired taste.
Supplied as: 12.5, 25, 50, 100 mg tablets.

Adult dose (to be taken one hour before meals):

Hypertension: If possible, discontinue other antihypertensive drugs for 1 week before initiating captopril. Then administer 25 mg PO bid–tid. If response not adequate after 1–2 weeks, increase dose to 50 mg PO tid. If response still inadequate after another 1–2 weeks, add a thiazide diuretic at low dose and increase dose of thiazide as needed at 1–2 week intervals until patient is normotensive or maximum usual dose of diuretic is attained. If further blood pressure reduction is required, increase dose of captopril to 100 mg tid and then to 150 mg tid (the maximum dosage) while continuing the diuretic. ●NOTE: Patients receiving a diuretic may on rare occasions have precipitous fall in blood pressure within first 3 hours after inital dose of captopril. This is why discontinuation of other antihypertensive drugs 1 week prior to initiating captopril is advised. Alternatively (if other antihypertensives cannot be discontinued) monitor blood pressure carefully for 3 hours following initial dose. If hypotension occurs, place patient in supine position and infuse normal saline. Hypotension episode does not necessarily contradict further captopril therapy. Captopril may usually be continued once blood pressure is stablized with normal saline.

Severe hypertension (e.g. malignant or accelerated hypertension): Stop current antihypertensive drugs except for diuretics and start captopril promptly (25 mg PO bid–tid) with close medical supervision. Increase dose at 24 hour intervals as needed (maximum 450 mg/day). Furosemide may be added to this regimen.

Heart failure: In this setting, it is generally recommended that captopril be added to a regimen of digitalis plus a diuretic (unless digitalis is poorly tolerated or not possible), and that the patient be under close medical supervision. Start with 25 mg PO tid. If necessary, increase to 50 mg PO tid. Wait for 2 weeks to assess therapeutic effect before making further increases. Usual patient requires 50–100 mg PO tid (do not exceed 450 mg/day). ●NOTE: Hypotensive or normotensive heart failure patients who have been aggressively treated with diuretics and who may be hyponatremic or hypovolemic should be initiated at 6.25 or 12.5 mg PO tid in order to minimize hypotensive effect. Early in the treatment, about half the heart failure patients with normal to low blood pressure will have a transient BP decrease of > 20%. In most cases this temporary fall is tolerable and does not force discontinuation of captopril.

CARBAMAZEPINE (Tegretol)

Indications: Epilepsy; ●generalized tonic–clonic (grand mal) seizure disorder, ●partial seizures with complex symptomatology such as temporal lobe (psychomotor) epilepsy, ●mixed seizure disorders of the foregoing types. NOTE: Carbamazepine is not effective in treatment of absence (petit mal) seizures and does little to control atonic or myoclonic seizures.
Trigeminal or glossopharyngeal neuralgia may be controlled with carbamazepine.
Contraindications: hypersentivity to carbamazepine or to tricyclic antidepressants, history of bone marrow depression, concurrent use of MAO inhibitor. If possible, MAOI shoud be discontinued at least 2 weeks before initiating carbamazepine.
Caution: elevated intraocular pressure; history of cardiac, renal, hepatic, or hematologic abnormalities; pregnancy (consider risk vs benefit); nursing mother; children (safety not established); patient

who engages in hazardous activities (drowsiness and dizziness may occur).

Comments: ●Therapeutic level is 6–12 mcg/ml. ●Because of the risk of serious hematologic side effects; pretreatment CBC including platelet count, and possibly reticulocyte count and serum iron should be obtained. A CBC should be obtained every 2 weeks for first 2 months and then every 3 months. Patient should stop the drug and report to a physician if fever, sore throat, oral ulcers, easy bruising, petechiae, or other hematologic side effects occur. ●Also obtain pretreatment and periodic liver function tests, urinalysis, BUN. ●Perform pretreatment and periodic eye exam including tonometry and fundoscopy. ●Carbamazepine induces enzymes that decrease the serum levels of phenobarbital, phenytoin, primidone, valproic acid, ethosuximide, diazepam, clonazepam. Enzyme induction by carbamazepine may also speed degradation and therefore decrease the efficacy of other drugs—e.g. oral contraceptives, oral anticoagulants, quinidine, tetracycline, rifampin, chloramphenicol. Conversely; phenobarbital, phenytoin, primidone induce enzymes that decrease serum levels of carbamazepine.

Side effects: The most frequent side effects, especially during initial therapy, are in italics. _Blood_ (aplastic anemia, agranulocytosis, thrombocytopenia, leukopenia, leukocytosis, eosinophilia, lymphadenopathy) _Skin_ (rash, pruritis, urticaria, photosensitivity, altered skin pigmentation, erythema nodosum, erythema multiforme, Stevens–Johnson syndrome, exfoliative dermatitis, toxic epidermal necrolysis, worsening of systemic lupus, alopecia, diaphoresis) _Cardiovascular_ (congestive heart failure, worsening hypertension, hypotension, syncope, worsening of ischemic heart disease, arrhythmias, AV block, thrombophlebitis) _Pulmonary_ (hypersensitivity pneumonitis with fever and dyspnea) _Liver_ (abnormal liver function tests, hepatitis, cholestatic or hepatocellular jaundice) _GU_ (urinary frequency or retention, elevated BUN, oliguria with hypertension, renal failure, impotence, albuminuria, glycosuria, microscopic deposits in urine) _GI_ (_nausea, vomiting_, gastric distress, diarrhea, constipation, abdominal pain, anorexia, dry mouth, stomatitis, glossitis) _Neurologic_ (_dizziness, drowsiness, unsteadiness_, incoordination, dysphasia, involuntary movements, headache, fatigue, confusion, hallucinations, depression with agitation, paresthesias, peripheral neuritis, tinnitus) _Eye_ (blurred vision, transient diplopia, nystagmus, oculomotor disturbances, conjunctivitis, lens opacities) _Other_ (arthralgias, myalgias, leg cramps, fever, chills, SIADH).

Supplied as: 200 mg tablet, 100 mg chewable tablet,
oral suspension (100mg/5ml).

Dose, epilepsy:

Adult/child > 12 yr: Start with 200 mg twice daily. Increase daily dose as needed every 1–2 weeks by up to 200 mg/day increments. Divide the total daily dose into 3--4 doses. Adjust to smallest effective dose, usually 600–1200 mg/day. Usual maximum is 1200 mg/day for patient over 15 yr and 1000 mg/day in patient 12–15 yr.

Child 6–12 yr: Start with 100 mg twice daily. Increase daily dose as needed every 1--2 weeks by up to 100 mg/day increments. Divide the total daily dose into 3–4 doses. Adjust to smallest effective dose, usually 400–800 mg/day or 20–30 mg/kg/day. Usual maximum is 1000 mg/day.

Dose, trigeminal neuralgia: 100 mg twice on first day. Increase dose as needed by up to 100 mg every 12 hours until pain is relieved (maximum 1200 mg/day). Divide daily dose into 3–4 doses. Adjust to smallest effective dose, usually 400–800 mg/day.

CEPHALOSPORINS, FIRST GENERATION:

cefadroxil (Duricef, Ultracef); **cefazolin** (Ancef, Kefzol); **cephalexin** (Keflex); **cephradine** (Anspor, Velosef).

Spectrum: Gram–positive bacteria: First generation cephalosporins are more active against gram-positive bacteria than are the 2nd or 3rd generation. The first generation is active against staphylococci including penicillinase–producing strains, but not methicillin–resistant strains. They are active against streptococci (e.g. group A beta–hemolytic streptococci, S. pneumoniae, S. viridans, anaerobic streptococci) but are often inactive against enterococci (e.g. S. faecalis). The first generation will also cover some gram–positive bacilli (Clostridium perfringens, Corynebacterium diptheriae, Listeria monocytogenes). Gram–negative cocci (e.g gonococci, meningococci) are also sensitive to the first generation. Some gram-negative bacilli (e.g. E. coli, some klebsiella, some Proteus mirabilis) may be sensitive to first generation cephalosporins but the spectrum covered is narrower than the 2nd or 3rd generation.

Indications: Cephalosporins are not usually the antibiotic of first choice. They are expensive. ●Cephalosporins may be used to treat infections by susceptible bacteria in patients allergic to penicillins, unless there is a history of immediate hypersensitivity penicillin reaction. ●First generation cephalosporins are often used to treat staphylococcal infections. ●Although they are effective against most streptococci, it is best to rely on the effective and cheaper alternatives (penicillins, erythromycin) unless there is a contraindication to their use. ●First generation cephalosporins penetrate poorly into the CSF. Therefore, they should not be used to treat meningitis. ●A first generation cephalosporin may be used concurrently with an aminoglycoside to treat a life–threatening infection when the pathogen and/or its sensitivity is unknown.

Contraindications: cephalosporin hypersensitivity, history of severe hypersensitivity reaction to penicillins, treatment of meningitis. **Caution:** pregnancy, nursing mother.
Comments: ●Cefazolin causes less pain than other cephalosporins on IM injection. ●Monitor renal function if there is renal dysfunction. ●To preclude development of rheumatic fever or glomerulonephritis, treat group A beta–hemolytic streptococcal infection for at least 10 days. ●Cephalosporins may provoke pseudomembranous colitis by allowing overgrowth of Clostridium difficile. The condition may resolve with discontinuation of the cephalosporin may suffice although oral vancomycin may be required.
Side effects include: <u>gastrointestinal</u>; anorexia, nausea, vomiting, diarrhea, heartburn, abdominal bloating/cramping, pseudomembranous colitis; <u>hypersensitivity</u>; fever, rash, pruritis, urticaria, esosinophilia, joint pain or swelling, anaphylaxis; <u>blood</u>; neutropenia, leukopenia, thrombocytopenia, + Coombs test, hemolytic anemia, hypothrombinemia (the latter due to decreased GI bacterial vitamin K synthesis); <u>liver</u>; transient increases in SGOT, SGPT, and alkaline phosphatase; <u>neurologic</u>; headache, nervousness, dizziness; <u>renal</u>; Some cephalosporins (e.g. cefazolin, cefamandole, 3rd generation cephalosporins) may cause transient BUN elevation. Cephalosporins may contribute to nephrotoxic effects of concurrently administered aminoglycoside. <u>Overgrowth</u> nonsusceptible organisms—e.g. vaginal or oral candidiasis, pseudomonas, enterococcus; <u>local effects</u>—e.g. phlebitis with IV administration, pain on IM injection; <u>Antabuse reaction</u>; Certain cephalosporins (e.g. cefamandole, cefoperazone, moxalactam) may be associated with untoward effects following alcohol ingestion (e.g. flushing, fainting, sweating, nausea, vomiting, rash, tachycardia, increased blood pressure, shock). <u>False + test for glucose</u>—e.g. Clinitest, Fehling's, Benedict's. However, Clinistix or Tes–Tape are not affected.

cefadroxil (Duricef, Ultracef) like cephalexin is an orally administered cephalosporin whose greatest utility is in the treatment of mild to moderately severe staphylococcal infections (e.g. of skin and skin structures). It may be used to treat infections by other susceptible bacteria when cheaper drugs are contraindicated. <u>Sensitive bacteria</u> include staphylococci (including penicillinase–producing S. aureus but excluding methicillin–resistant strains), group A beta–hemolytic streptococci, pneumococcus, E. coli, Proteus mirabilis, klebsiella. <u>Resistant</u>; pseudomonas, Acinetobacter calcoaceticus, most enterococci (e.g. S. faecalis), most Proteus vulgaris, most P. morganii.
<u>Supplied as;</u> 500 mg capsule,   1000 mg tablet,
oral suspension (125, 250, 500mg/5ml).
<u>Dose (adult):</u>
●Uncomplicated lower UTI: 1–2 gram/day PO as single daily dose or divided into 2 doses. ●All other UTI: 1 gram PO twice daily.
●Skin & skin structures: 1 gram/day PO as single daily dose or divided into 2 doses.
●Pharyngitis: 1 gram once daily for 10 days or 500mg twice daily for 10 day.
<u>Dose adjustment renal failure:</u> 1 gram loading dose followed by 500 mg at following intervals (creatinine clearance—interval):
0–10 ml/min——36 hr,   10–25 ml/min——24 hr,   25–50 ml/min——12 hr.
●In a male the creatinine clearance is approximately = (wt in kg) x (140 – age) ÷ (72 x serum creatinine). Creatinine clearance in female = 0.9 x this figure.
<u>Pediatric dose;</u> 15 mg/kg PO q12h.

cefazolin (Ancef, Kefzol)
<u>Sensitive bacteria</u> include staphylococci (including penicillinase–producing staphylococci but excepting methicillin–resistant strains), streptococci (excepting enterococci—e.g. S. faecalis), pneumococcus, E. coli, Proteus mirabilis, klebsiella, Enterobacter aerogenes, Haemophilus influenza. <u>Usually resistant</u>; enterococci, Providencia rettgeri, Morganella morganii, indole + proteus (e.g. P. vulgaris). <u>Nearly always resistant</u>; pseudomonas, serratia, Acinetobacter calcoaceticus.
<u>Dose (adult):</u>
●Acute uncomplicated UTI: 1000 mg q12h IV or IM.
●Mild infection due to susceptible gram + cocci: 250–500 mg q8h IV or IM.
●Moderate to severe infection: 500–1000 mg q6–8h IV or IM.
●Life–threatening infection: 1000–1500 mg q6h IV or IM.
●Pneumonoccal pneumonia: 500 mg q12h IV or IM.
<u>Dose adjustment in adult with renal failure after usual initial dose</u>
(serum creatinine——dose):   1.6–3.0 mg/dl——full dose at least 8 hr interval,
3.1–4.5 mg/dl——half usual dose q12h,   > 4.5 mg/dl——half usual dose q18–24h.
●Dose adjustment based on creatinine clearance (creatinine clearance——dose):
35–54 ml/min——usual dose at at least 8 hr intervals, 11–34 ml/min——half usual dose q12h, less than 10 ml/min——half usual dose every 18–24 hr.
<u>Dose (child or infant > 1 mo);</u> 25–50 mg/kg/day IV or IM divided into 3–4 equal doses (maximum 100 mg/kg/day). Safety not established in premature infants or infants < 1 month.

Dose adjustment in child with renal failure after usual initial dose (creatinine clearance——dose):
    40–70 ml/min: 60% usual daily dose divided q12h,
    20–40 ml/min: 25% usual daily dose divided q12h,
    5–20 ml/min: 10% usual daily dose as single daily dose.

cephalexin (Keflex) is an orally administered cephalosporin whose greatest utility is in the treatment of mild to moderately severe staphylococcal infections (e.g. of skin and skin structures). It may be used to treat infections by other susceptible bacteria when cheaper drugs are contraindicated.
Sensitive bacteria include: staphylococci (except methicillin–resistant strains), beta–hemolytic streptococci, pneumococcus, E. coli, klebsiella, Proteus mirabilis, Haemophilus influenza, Neisseria catarrhalis. Resistant species include pseudomonas, herellea, most enterobacter, most Proteus vulgaris, most Morganella morganii, most enterococci (e.g. S. faecalis).
Supplied as: tablet (250, 500, 1000 mg);   capsule (250, 500 mg);
        oral suspension (125, 250 mg/5ml);   pediatric drops (100 mg/ml).
Adult dose: 250mg PO q6h (maximum 4 gram/day).
Pediatric dose: 6.25–12.5 mg/kg PO q6h.
●Double dose in serious infection.
●Treat beta–hemolytic streptococcal infections for 10 days.
Dose interval in renal failure (creatinine clearance——interval):
clearance 50–80 ml/min——interval 6 hr,   clearance 10–50 ml/min——interval 12 hr,
clearance < 10 ml/min——interval 24–48 hr.
In a male the creatinine clearance is approximately = (wt in kg) x (140 – age) ÷ (72 x serum creatinine). Creatinine clearance in female = 0.9 x this figure.

cephradine (Anspor, Velosef)
Sensitive bacteria: staphylococci (including penicillinase–producing strains but excepting methicillin–resistant strains), group A beta–hemolytic streptococci, pneumococcus, E. coli, Proteus mirabilis, klebsiella, Haemophilus influenza. Resistant: pseudomonas, Acinetobacter, Herellea. Usually resistant: enterococci, enterobacter, Proteus vulgaris, Proteus morganii.
Supplied as: capsule (250, 500 mg);   tablet (1000 mg);
        oral suspension (125, 250 mg/5ml);   IV or IM preparation.
Adult dose:
    IV or deep IM: 500–1000 mg q6h (up to max 8 gram/day in severe infection).
    Oral: ●Skin, soft tissue, and respiratory infections other than lobar pneumonia: 250mg PO q6h or 500 mg q12h.
        ●Pneumococcal lobar pneumonia and acute UTI (including prostatitis): 500 mg PO q6h (or 1 gram q12h).
Dose adjustment in adult with renal failure (creatinine clearance——dose):
20ml/min——500mg q6h, 5–20ml/min——250mg q6h, < 5 ml/min——250mg q12h.
●In a male the creatinine clearance is approximately = (wt in kg) x (140 – age) ÷ (72 x serum creatinine). Creatinine clearance in female = 0.9 x this figure.
Pediatric dose (not to exceed adult dose or 4 grams/day):
●IV or deep IM: 12.5–25 mg/kg q6h. Use with caution in infant < 1 yr. Safety not established in infant < 1 month or premature infant.
●PO: 25–100 mg/kg/day divided q6h or q12h. The effectiveness of twice daily administration is not established for infant < 9 months of age.

CEPHALOSPORINS, SECOND GENERATION:

cefaclor (Ceclor); **cefamandole** (Mandol); **cefonicid** (Monocid); **cefoxitin** (Mefoxin); **cefuroxime** (Kefurox, Zinacef).

Overview: The 2nd generation covers a wider spectrum of gram–negative bacteria than the first generation, but the 2nd generation is less active against gram–positive bacteria. With exception of cefuroxime, the 2nd generation cephalosporins (like the first generation) penetrate poorly into the CSF and therefore should not be used to treat meningitis.

cefaclor (Ceclor) is often used to treat otitis media due to suspected ampicillin–resistant strains of Haemophilus influenza. Sensitive bacteria include staphylococci (except methicillin–resistant strains), beta–hemolytic streptococci, pneumococcus, Haemophilus influenza (including ampicillin–resistant strains), gonococcus, Branhamella catarrhalis, E. coli, klebsiella, Proteus mirabilis, Citrobacter diversus, peptococci, peptostreptococci, bacteroides (except B. fragilis),

Propionibacteria acnes. Resistant bacteria; pseudomonas, Acinetobacter calcoaceticus, most enterobacter, most serratia, most indole + proteus, most enterococci (e.g. S. faecalis, group D strep), Bacteroides fragilis.

Supplied as: capsule (250, 500 mg); oral suspension (125, 250 mg/5ml).

Adult dose: 250 mg PO q8h. Use 500 mg q8h in more serious infections, Maximum 4 gram/day.

Pediatric dose: 20–40 mg/kg/day PO in equally divided doses q8h. Upper range is advised for more severe infection or otitis media. Maximum 1 gram/day.

Safety in infants < 1 month age not established.

Dose adjustment not necessary in renal failure.

cefamandole (Mandol) is most commonly used to treat serious infections (e.g. pneumonia, pyelonephritis, peritonitis, septicemia, osteomyelitis, septic arthritis) due to susceptible *gram-negative* bacteria not amenable to cheaper options. Sensitive bacteria include staphylococci, beta-hemolytic streptococci, pneumococcus, Haemophilus influenza, E. coli, klebsiella, proteus (except some P. vulgaris), peptococcus, peptostreptococcus, clostridia, fusobacterium, bacteroides (except most B. fragilis). Resistant bacteria; pseudomonas, most enterococci (e.g. S. faecalis), Bacteroides fragilis, Acinetobacter calcoaceticus, most serratia.

Adult dose: ●Skin infections, uncomplicated pneumonia: 500 mg q6h IV or IM.
●Uncomplicated UTI: 500 mg q8h IV or IM. ●Serious UTI: 1 gram q8h IV or IM.
●Severe infection: 1 gram q6h IV or IM (up to 2 g q4h in life-threatening infection).

Dose adjustment in adult with renal failure (creatinine clearance——maintenance dose):

creatinine clearance	maintenance dose
50–80 ml/min:	0.75–1.5 gram q6h (maximum 2 g q6h or 1.5 g q4h),
25–50 ml/min:	0.75–1.5 gram q8h (maximum 1.5 g q6h or 2 g q8h),
10–25 ml/min:	0.5–1.0 gram q8h (maximum 1g q6h or 1.25 g q8h),
2–10 ml/min:	0.5–0.75 gram q12h (maximum 0.67 g q8h or 1 g q12h,
< 2 ml/min:	0.25–0.5 gram q12h (max 0.5 g q8h or 0.75 g q12h).

●In a male the creatinine clearance is approximately = (wt in kg) x (140 – age) ÷ (72 x serum creatinine). Creatinine clearance in female = 0.9 x this figure.

Pediatric dose: 50–100 mg/kg/day IV or IM in equally divided dosed q4–6h (maximum 150 mg/kg/day or maximum adult dose of 12g/day whichever is least). Safety not established in premature infants or infants < 1 month age.

cefonicid (Monocid)

Sensitive bacteria include staphylococci (except methicillin-resistant strains), group A beta-hemolytic streptococci, group B strepotcocci (S. agalactiae), pneumococcus, Haemophilus influenza (including ampicillin-resistant strains), E. coli, Klebsiella pneumoniae, Proteus mirabilis and P vulgaris, Providencia rettgeri, Morganella morganii. ●In vitro sensitivity has also been demonstrated for gonococcus, Enterobacter aerogenes, Klebsiella oxytoca, Citrobacter freundii, C. diversus, Clostridium perfringens, Peptostreptococcus anaerobius, Peptococcus magnus, P. prevotii, Propionibacterium acnes, Fusobacterium nucleatum. Usually resistant; pseudomonas, serratia, enterococci, acinetobacter, Bacteroides fragilis.

Supplied as: 500 mg and 1000 mg vials for IV or IM injection.

Dose (adult):

●Uncomplicated UTI: 500mg once daily IV or IM.
●Other mild-moderate infections: 1000mg once daily IV or IM.
●Severe infections: 2 grams once daily IV or IM (divided at 2 sites).
●Surgical prophylaxis: 1 gram IV or IM one hour before operation.

cefoxitin (Mefoxin) may be used to treat serious infections (e.g. peritonitis, intra-abdominal abscess, septicemia, pelvic inflammatory disease, septic arthritis, osteomyelitis); particularly those due to susceptible *gram-negative* bacteria. It is effective against penicillinase-producing gonococci. It is also often used as a prophylactic in bowel and gynecologic surgery.

Sensitive bacteria include staphylococci (except methicillin-resistant strains), beta-hemolytic streptococci, pneumococcus, Haemophilus influenza, gonococcus (including penicillinase-producing strains), E. coli, klebsiella, Proteus mirabilis, P. vulgaris, providencia, Morganella morganii, clostridia, bacteroides (including B. fragilis), peptococcus, peptostreptococcus. Resistant; methicillin-resistant S. aureus, most Pseudomonas aeuruginosa, most enterococci, many Enterobacter cloacae.

Dose (adult):

●Uncomplicated infection: 1 gram q6–8h IV or IM (IM is painful).
●Moderate–severe infection: 1 gram IV q4h (or 2 gram IV q6–8h)
●Infections requiring large doses (e.g. gas gangrene): 2 gram IV q4h (or 3 gram IV q6h).

Dose adjustment in adult with renal failure (creatinine clearance——dose):

30–50 ml/min——1–2 gram q8–12h,   10–29 ml/min——1–2 gram q12–24h,
5–9ml/min——0.5–1.0 gram q12–24h,   < 5ml/min——0.5–1.0 gram q24–48h.
●In males the creatinine clearance is approximately = (wt in kg) x (140 – age) ÷ (72 x serum creatinine). Creatinine clearance in female = 0.9 x this figure.
Pediatric dose (> 3 month of age): 80–160 mg/kg/day divided into 4–6 equal daily doses (maximum 12 gram/day). Safety not established in infants < 3 month of age.

cefuroxime (Kefurox, Zinacef) enters the CSF (in contrast to other 2nd generation cephalosporins and to first generation cephalosporins). The parenteral form may therefore be used in treatment of meningitis due to susceptible bacteria. Like other 2nd generation cephalosporins, it is mostly used to treat serious infections due to susceptible *gram–negative bacilli* not amenable to cheaper options. Sensitive aerobes include staphylococci (excepting methicillin–resistant staph), streptococci (excepting enterococci– e.g. S. faecalis), pneumococcus, meningococci, gonococci (including penicillinase–producing strains), Haemophilus influenza (including ampicillin–resistant strains), H. parainfluenza, E. coli, klebsiella, salmonella, shigella, enterobacter (E. cloacae may be resistant), citrobacter (usually sensitive), proteus (e.g. P. mirabilis, P. inconstans); Morganella morganii (sometimes resistant), Providencia rettgeri. Sensitive anaerobes include peptococcus, peptostreptococcus, clostridia (C. difficile is resistant), fusobacterium, bacteroides (except most B. fragilis). Resistant bacteria include: methicilliin–resistant staphylococci, Clostridium difficile, Listeria monocytogenes, enterococci (e.g. S. faecalis), most Bacteroides fragilis, pseudomonas, campylobacter, Acinetobacter calcoaceticus, most serratia, most Proteus vulgaris.
Supplied as: vials containing 750 or 1500 mg for IV or IM injection.
Adult dose: 750–1500 mg q8h IV or IM. Upper range is advised for severe or complicated infections, or for bone or joint infections. Dose in life–threatening infections (e.g. meningitis) or infections due to less sensitive bacteria may be increased to 1500 mg IM or IV every 6 hr (maximum 3 gram q8h).
●Uncomplicated gonococcal infection: a single 1500 mg IM dose (divided into 2 sites) with 1 gram of probenecid PO.
●Surgical prophylaxis: 1.5 gram IV 30–60 minutes prior to surgery.
●For open–heart surgery, the recommended regimen is 1.5 gram at induction of anesthesia followed by 1.5 gram q12h x 3.
Dose adjustment in adult with renal failure: (creatinine clearance——dose):
> 20ml/min——750–1500mg q8h,   10–20ml/min——750mg q12h,
< 10ml/min——750mg q24h.
●In males the creatinine clearance is approximately = (wt in kg) x (140 – age) ÷ (72 x serum creatinine). Creatinine clearance in female = 0.9 x this figure. Hemodialysis patients should receive an additional dose following dialysis.
Pediatric dose (patient > 3 months of age): usual dose is 50–100 mg/kg/day IV or IM in equally divided doses every 6–8 hr not to exceed maximum adult dose. ●Bone and joint infections: 150 mg/kg/day in equally divided doses every 8 hr not to exceed maximum adult dose. ●Bacterial meningitis: 200–400 mg/kg/day IV in equally divided doses q6–8h but not to exceed 3 gram q8h.

CEPHALOSPORINS, THIRD GENERATION:
cefoperazone (Cefobid), **cefotaxime** (Claforan),
ceftazidime (Fortaz, Tazicef, Tazidime), **ceftizoxime** (Cefizox),
ceftriaxone (Rocephin), **moxalactam** (Moxam).

Overview: Third generation cephalosporins are more active and have a wider spectrum against gram–negative bacteria than 1st or 2nd generation cephalosporins, but they are less active against gram–positive bacteria. The fact that the 3rd generation is less active against gram-positive bacteria and also expensive argues against using the 3rd generation except for the treatment of infection by gram–negative bacilli. Some third generation cephalosporins (e.g. cefotaxime, ceftizoxime, moxalactam) have the advantage of being able to penetrate into the CSF and therefore may be used to treat meningitis due to susceptible gram–negative bacilli.

cefoperazone (Cefobid)
Sensitive bacteria include staphylococci (including penicillinase–producing staph but excepting methicillin–resistant strains), group A and group B beta–hemolytic streptococci, pneumococcus, enterococci, gonococcus, Haemophilus influenza, pseudomonas (including P. aeruginosa), E. coli, klebsiella, enterobacter, citrobacter, Proteus mirabilis, P. vulgaris, Morganella morganii,

Providencia rettgeri, P. stuartii, some Acinetobacter calcoaceticus, Serratia marcescens, clostridia, Bacteroides (including B. fragilis), Peptococcus, Peptostreptococcus. In vitro sensitivity (clinical significance unknown) is demonstrated by salmonella, shigella, Yersinia enterocolitica, Serratia liquefaciens, meningococcus, B. pertussis, Clostridium difficile, fusobacterium, eubacterium.

Dose (adult): 1–2 gram q8–12h IM or IV. Up to 12 gram/day divided into 2–4 doses may be required in severe infections or those due to less sensitive bacteria.

Dose adjustment not required in renal failure.

cefotaxime (Claforan)

Sensitive bacteria include staphylococci (including penicillinase–producing strains but excepting methicillin–resistant staph), group A and group B beta–hemolytic streptococci, pneumococcus, Haemophilus influenza (including ampicillin–resistant strains), gonococcus (including penicillinase–producing strains), meningococcus, E. coli, enterobacter, serratia, citrobacter, klebsiella, Proteus mirabilis, P. vulgaris, Providencia rettgeri, Morganella morganii, fusobacterium, peptococcus, peptostreptococcus, clostridia (excepting most C. difficile) ●Some Pseudomonas aeruginosa and some Bacteroides fragilis may be sensitive. In vitro sensitivity (unknown clinical significance) is demonstrated by salmonella, shigella, providencia. Resistance is seen with methicillin–resistant staphylococci, most enterococci, some Pseudomonas aeruginosa, most Clostridium difficile, some bacteroides.

Adult/child > 50 kg: 1–2 gram q6–8h IM or IV.
Up to 2 gram q4h IV in life–threatening infection (e.g. meningitis). Uncomplicated gonorrhea may be treated with a single 1 gram IM injection.

Pediatric 1 mo–12 yr (wt < 50 kg): 50–180 mg/kg/day divided into 4–6 equal doses.
Neonate 1–4 wk age: 50 mg/kg IV q8h.   Neonate 0–1 wk age: 50 mg/kg IV q12h.

Dose adjustment not required in renal failure unless creatinine clearance is less than 20ml/minute, at which point the dose is halved. In males the creatinine clearance is approximately = (wt in kg) x (140 – age) ÷ (72 x serum creatinine). Creatinine clearance in female = 0.9 x this figure.

ceftazidime (Fortaz, Tazicef, Tazidime)

Sensitive bacteria include Staph aureus (including penicillinase–produding strains but excepting methicillin–resistant strains), group A and group B streptococcus, pneumococcus, Haemophilus influenza (including ampicillin–resistant strains), meningococcus, E. coli, klebsiella, serratia, pseudomonas (including P. aeruginosa), enterobacter, citrobacter, Proteus mirabilis, P. vulgaris. In vitro sensitivity (clinical significance unknown) is seen with Staph epidermidis, gonococcus, H. parainfluenza, acinetobacter, providencia, Morganella morganii, salmonella, shigella, Yersinia enterocolitica, clostridia (excluding C. difficile), peptococcus, peptostreptococcus. Resistance is seen with methicillin–resistant S. aureus, many enterococci (including S. faecalis), Listeria monocytogenes, campylobacter, Clostridium difficile, many strains of Bacteroides fragilis.

Supplied as: vials containing 0.5, 1, and 2 grams for IV or IM injection.

Dose (adult): 1 gram q8–12h IV or IM.
In meningitis or other severe infections: 2 gram IV q8h.

Dose adjustment in adult with renal failure (creatinine clearance——dose):
31–50 ml/min——1 gram q12h,   16–30ml/min——1 gram q24h,
6–15ml/min——500 mg q24h,   less than 5ml/min——500 mg q48h.

●In a male the creatinine clearance is approximately = (wt in kg) x (140 – age) ÷ (72 x serum creatinine). Creatinine clearance in female = 0.9 x this figure.

Dose (child 1 month–12 yr): 30–50 mg/kg IV every 8 hours (maximum 6 gram/day).

Dose (neonate): 30 mg/kg IV every 12 hours.

ceftizoxime (Cefizox)

Sensitive bacteria; staphylococci (including penicillinase–producing staph but excepting methicillin–resistant staph); pneumococcus; Streptococcus pyogenes (group A beta–hemolytic); gonococci; meningococci; Haemophilus influenza (including ampicillin–resistant strains); E. coli; klebsiella; serratia; enterobacter; pseudomonas (including P. aerugenosa but many strains only moderately sensitive); Proteus mirabilis; Proteus vulgaris; Providencia rettgeri; Morganella morganii; bacteroides (including B. fragilis); anaerobic cocci (e.g. peptococci, peptostreptococci). Usually resistant; enterococci (e.g. S. faecalis), Clostridium difficile.

Dose (adult): 1–2 gram q8–12h IM or IV (severe infections: 6–12 gram/day IV).

Dose adjustment in adult with renal failure following initial dose of 0.5–1.0 gram IM or IV (creatinine clearance——dose):   50–79 ml/min——500–1500 mg q8h,
5–49 ml/min——250–1000 mg q12h,   0–4 ml/min——250–500 mg q24h.
The upper range is for life–threatening infection.

●In males the creatinine clearance is approximately = (wt in kg) x (140 – age) ÷ (72 x serum creatinine). Creatinine clearance in female = 0.9 x this figure.

Dose, child ≥ 6 months: 50 mg/kg q6–8h. Maximum 200 mg/kg/day or maximum adult dose whichever is least.

ceftriaxone (Rocephin)

Sensitive bacteria include staphylococci (including penicillinase–producing strains but excepting methicillin–resistant strains), Streptococcus pyogenes (group A beta–hemolytic), group B strepto-coccus, pneumococcus, meningococci, gonococci (including penicillinase–producing strains), Haemophilus influenza (including ampicillin–resistant strains), H. parainfluenza, E. coli, Proteus mirabilis, Proteus vulgaris, klebsiella, Enterobacter aerogenes, E. cloacae, Morganella morganii, Serratia marcescens, some Pseudomonas aeruginosa. Resistant: some strains of Pseudomonas aeruginosa; some enterococci (e.g. S. faecalis, group D strep), methicillin–resistant staphylococci, most C. difficile. In vitro sensitivity (clinical significance unknown) has been demonstrated for other bacteria—e.g. salmonella, shigella, providencia, bacteroides, clostridia (excepting C. difficile), Acinetobacter calcoaceticus, Citrobacter freundii, C. diversus.

Supplied as: vials containing 250, 500, 1000, and 2000 mg for IV or IM injection;
piggyback bottles containing 1 and 2 gram.

Adult dose: 1–2 gram/day IV or IM as a single daily dose or divided into 2 daily doses (maximum 4 gram/day).

●Uncomplicated gonococcal infection: single dose 250mg IM.
●Surgical prophylaxis: 1gram 1/2 to 2 hours prior to surgery.

Pediatric dose: 25–37.5 mg/kg q12h IV or IM (maximum 2 gram/day).
In meningitis the dose is 50 mg/kg q12h (maximum 4 gram/day).

Renal or hepatic failure: Dose adjustment not necessary. However, serum levels should be monitored in those with severe renal failure, or combined renal and liver dysfunction.

moxalactam (Moxam) like other 3rd generation cephalosporins has activity against both gram–positive and gram–negative bacteria. It is active against Bacteroides fragilis but is not consistently effective against Pseudomonas aeruginosa. Moxalactam does penetrate into the CSF and may be used to treat meningitis due to sensitive gram–negative bacilli.

Adult dose: 2–4 gram/day divided into equal doses q8–12h IM or IV.
Up to 12 gram/day in life–threatening infections.

Dose adjustment renal failure after initial loading dose of 1–2 gram:

creatinine clearance	dose	maximum dose
over 80ml/min	0.5–2 gram q8–12h	4 gram q8h
50–80ml/min	0.5–1 gram q8h	3 gram q8h
25–50ml/min	0.25–1 gram q12h	2 gram q8h or 3 gram q12h
2–25ml/min	0.25–0.5 gram q8h	1 gram q8h or 1.25 gram q12h
less than 2ml/min	0.25–0.5 gram q12h	1 gram q24h

●In a male the creatinine clearance is approximately = (wt in kg) x (140 – age) ÷ (72 x serum creatinine). Creatinine clearance in female = 0.9 x this figure.

Pediatric dose: ●child: 50 mg/kg q6–8h, ●infant > 1 month age: 50 mg/kg q6h, ●neonate 1–4 wk of age: 50 mg/kg q8h, ●neonate 0–1 wk of age: 50 mg/kg q12h. Do not exceed 200 mg/kg/day or maximum adult dosage of 12 gram/day.

CHARCOAL, ACTIVATED

Action: Adsorbent; thereby impedes gastrointestinal absorption of poisons.
Indication: acute poisoning.
Comments: ●Charcoal administration may need to be repeated every 2 hours if the ingested toxin undergoes enterohepatic circulation (e.g. phenobarbital, glutethimide, digitoxin, Amanita phalloides) or is secreted into the stomach after absorption (e.g. tricyclic antidepressants, phencyclidine). ●Charcoal adsorbs ipecac. Therefore, if ipecac is to be given, give it first and then give charcoal after emesis subsides. ●Mineral acids and alkalis are not absorbed to charcoal; ferrous sulfate and cyanide are poorly adsorbed to charcoal.
Contraindications/side effects: none.
Supplied as: oral suspension, powder (to be mixed with water).
Dose: Adult: 50–100 gram PO, Child: 20–50 gram PO.

CHLORAMPHENICOL (Chloromycetin)

Action: Inhibits bacterial protein synthesis by binding to 50s ribosome subunit.
Spectrum: <u>Sensitive:</u> streptcocci (S. Pneumoniae, S. pyogenes, S. viridans); meningococci; gonococci; haemophilus; listeria; Brucella; Pasterurella multocida; Corynebacterium diptheriae; anaerobes (including Bacteroides fragilis); treponemae; rickettsiae; chlamydia; mycoplasma. Most Staphylococcus aureus, salmonella, E. coli, klebsiella, and Proteus mirabilis are also covered. <u>Resistant:</u> most Pseudomonas aeruginosa, serratia, providencia, and Proteus rettgeri.
Indications include: <u>Typhoid fever</u> is one indication. However, note that the Salmonella typhii carrier state is treated with ampicillin or amoxicillin, and that cholecystectomy is indicated in patient with cholecystitis or cholelithiasis. <u>Serious infections (e.g. septicemia) caused by other salmonellae.</u> Note, however, that uncomplicated salmonellae-caused gastroenteritis does not require antibiotic therapy unless pathogen is S. typhii. <u>Meningitis in children</u> over 2 month of age is frequently due to H. influenza. However, H. influenza is not uncommonly resistant to ampicillin. Consequently, chloramphenicol is administered concurrently with ampicillin while awaiting culture & sensitivity results. <u>Meningitis in adults;</u> Chloramphenicol is an appropriate choice if CSF gram stain shows gram-negative rods. <u>Anaerobic intra-abdominal infections</u> may be treated with chloramphenicol (e.g. chloramphenicol covers Bacteroides fragilis).
Contraindications: chloramphenicol hypersensitivity.
Safety not established in pregnancy and nursing mothers.
Caution: ●Reserve chloramphenicol for serious infections when drugs less potentially dangerous are ineffective or contraindicated. ●Obtain CBC, platelet count, reticulocyte count at start of therapy and every 2 days while on therapy. Stop drug if signs of marrow suppression occur. ●Avoid repeat courses of drug if possible.
Side effects: <u>blood</u> (aplastic anemia, pancytopenia, thrombocytopenia, leukopenia, granulocytopenia, reticulocytopenia); <u>GI</u> (nausea, vomiting, diarrhea, stomatitis, colitis); <u>neurologic</u> (headache, confusion, depression, optic neuritis, peripheral neuritis); <u>allergic</u> (rash, fever, urticaria, angioedema, anaphylaxis); <u>vascular collapse</u> (gray syndrome in infants).

Supplied as: 250 mg capsule,   oral suspension 150 mg/5ml,
intravenous preparation.   IM not advised.

Dose:
<u>Adult or child:</u> 12.5 mg/kg q6h IV or PO. Up to 25 mg/kg q6h may be required for less sensitive bacteria or for severe infections (e.g. meningitis, bacteremia) but the dose should be reduced as soon as possible.
<u>Full term neonate > 2 week of age:</u> 6.25–12.5 mg/kg q6h IV or PO.
<u>Neonate < 2 weeks of age, premature infant, or child with immature metabolic processes:</u> 6.25 mg/kg q6h IV or PO.
NOTE: Monitor chloramphenicol blood levels in neonates, premature infants, and patients with hepatic or renal dysfunction. Adjust dose to therapeutic level of 5–20 mcg/ml.

CHLOROQUINE (Aralen)

Action: Acts against erythrocytic phase of plasmodium: P. vivax, P. malariae, P. ovale and sensitive strains of P. falciparum.
Indications: <u>Acute malarial attacks</u> due to Plasmodium: P. vivax, P. malariae, P. ovale, and *susceptible* strains of P. falciparum. <u>Suppression of malaria while in endemic areas.</u> Note, however, that some strains of P. falciparum are not suppressed by chloroquine. <u>Extraintestinal amebiasis.</u>
Contraindications: 4-aminoquinoline hypersensitivity, retinal or visual field changes due to any cause including 4-aminoquinoline compounds.
Caution: liver disease, alcoholism, G6PD deficiency, concurrent use of hepatotoxic drugs, psoriasis, porphyria, pregnancy. ●Children are very sensitive to chloroquine. Do not exceed recommended doses.
Comments: <u>Treatment of residual hepatic infection;</u> Since chloroquine is ineffectual against the exo-erythrocytic forms, relapses of P. vivax or P. ovale may occur unless the patient is subsequently treated with an 8-aminoquinoline (e.g. Primaquine) to eliminate the hepatic parasites. There are no persistent hepatic forms of P. falciparum or P. malariae. However, asymptomatic P. malariae erythrocytic infection may persist after chloroquine therapy. <u>Chloroquine-resistant strains of P. falciparum;</u> Adequate chloroquine therapy completely eliminates sensitive P. falciparum. If an attack by P. falciparum does not respond promptly to chloroquine therapy alone, chloroquine-resistance must be assumed and alternative therapy instituted (see "Malaria" chapter). With adequate chloroquine therapy, parasitemia should decline within 24–48 hours and asexual parasites should vanish within 5 days. <u>Treatment of person returning from endemic malarial region;</u> Although chloroquine will suppress malarial *attacks* (except for chloroquine-resistant strains of P. malariae), it will not by itself prevent infection. For this reason, a person (who does not have G6PD deficiency) returning from an endemic area may receive a course of primaquine in order to insure elimination of possible P. ovale or P. vivax, both of which may persist in the liver for up to 4 years. The alternative is to instruct the patient to report to a physician if fever develops

after returning from an endemic area. <u>Prolonged chloroquine therapy:</u> Perform periodic eye exams if patient is taking chloroquine for prolonged periods. Discontinue chloroquine if any of following ocular manifestations (not attributable to corneal opacities or impaired accomodation) occur: changes in visual acuity or visual field, retinal abnormalities, visual symptoms (e.g. light flashes, streaks). <u>Muscle weakness:</u> Discontinue chloroquine if muscle weakness occurs. <u>Blood dyscrasias</u> may occur with prolonged therapy. Perform periodic CBC.

Side effects: <u>eyes</u> (blurred vision, difficulty focusing, reversible corneal changes, irreversible retinal changes); <u>neurologic</u> (headache, psychic stimulation, etc.); <u>GI</u> (nausea, vomiting, diarrhea, anorexia, abdominal cramping); <u>cardiovascular</u> (hypotension, EKG changes); <u>skin</u> (pruritis, pigmentary changes, lichen planus–like eruptions); <u>other</u> (blood dyscrasias, tinnitus, impaired hearing).

Supplied as: 500 mg (= 300 mg base) tablets,
5 ml ampul containing 50mg/ml (= 40 mg/ml base) for intramuscular injection.

Dose (expressed as milligrams of base):

Uncomplicated acute attack of malaria:
<u>Adult:</u> (**1**) initial dose of 600 mg PO, (**2**) second dose is 300 mg PO taken 6 hours after initial dose, (**3**) then 300 mg PO once daily for next 2 days. Total dose over 3 days is 1500 mg base.
<u>Pediatric:</u> (**1**) first dose is 10 mg/kg base PO (maximum 600 mg), (**2**) second dose is 5 mg/kg base (maximum 300 mg) PO taken 6 hours after first dose, (**3**) third dose is 5 mg/kg base PO (maximum 300 mg) taken 18 hours after second dose, (**4**) fourth dose is 5 mg/kg PO (max 300 mg) taken 24 hours after third dose. NOTE: Complete cure is affected in cases of chloroquine–sensitive P. falciparum but chloroquine by itself will not prevent relapses of P. vivax, P. malariae, or P. ovale. In these cases, consequently, primaquine is administered in conjunction with chloroquine.

Severe malaria when oral administration not possible (change to PO as soon as possible):
<u>Adult:</u> 160–200 mg base IM initially, repeat same IM dose in 6 hours if necessary (maximum IM dose is 800 mg base/24h). Total dose IM + PO is 1500 mg base over 3 days.
<u>Pediatric:</u> 5 mg/kg base IM. Repeat same IM dose in 6 hours if necessary. Do not exceed 10 mg/kg/24 hr or 800 mg/24hr. Total dose IM + PO is 25 mg/kg base over 3 days but not to exceed total of 1500 mg base.

Suppression malaria in endemic area (begun 2 weeks before exposure and continued for 4 weeks after leaving endemic area):
<u>Adult:</u> 300 mg PO taken once a week on same day.
<u>Pediatric:</u> 5 mg/kg (maximum 300 mg) PO taken once a week on same day.

Extraintestinal amebiasis (adult): 600 mg base PO once daily for 2 days, then 300 mg base a day for minimum of 2–3 weeks. If PO administration is not possible, IM administration (160–200 mg base once daily) is permitted for 10–12 days or until PO administration is possible. Note: An intestinal amebicide (e.g. dehydroemetine, diiodohydroxyquin) is usually administered concurrently.

CIMETIDINE (Tagamet)

Action: Competitively binds to histamine H–2 receptors on gastric parietal cells. Thereby inhibits histamine–induced hydrochloric acid secretion.

Indications: ●Short–term treatment of active duodenal ulcer or active benign gastric ulcer. ●Hypersecretory conditions (e.g. Zollinger–Ellison syndrome, systemic mastocytosis). ●Prevention duodenal ulcer recurrence in patient who is poor surgical risk and who would otherwise require ulcer surgery.

Contraindication: cimetidine hypersensitivity, nursing mother. Do not use in pregnancy unless absolutely essential.

Comments: ●Antacids may be given as needed for pain relief. However, concomitant ongoing antacid therapy is not recommended since antacids may interfere with cimetidine absorption. ●Cimetidine may reduce hepatic metabolism of certain drugs: warfarin (monitor prothrombin time), phenytoin, propranolol, chlordiazepoxide, diazepam, lidocaine, theophylline. Dose adjustment of these drugs may be required. ●Symptomatic improvement in a gastric ulcer patient does not rule out a gastric malignancy. Post–treatment gastroscopy or upper GI is needed to exclude malignancy.

Side effects: diarrhea, dizziness, sleepiness, headache, anxiety, depression, agitation, confusion, hallucinations, gynecomastia (patients treated over 1 month), impotence (with high doses for at least 12 months), slightly elevated serum creatinine, increased serum transaminases, rash. ●<u>Rare:</u> joint or muscle pain, polymyositis, leukopenia, agranulocytosis, thrombocytopenia, aplastic anemia, fever, allergic reactions, interstitial nephritis, adverse hepatic effects, severe skin reactions, alopecia.

Supplied as: 200, 300, 400, 800 mg tablet;   300 mg/5ml oral liquid; 300 mg/2ml preparation for IM or IV administration.

Adult dose:

Oral: ●Active duedenal ulcer: (1) 800 mg PO at bedtime or
                                 (2) 300 mg PO qid with meals & at bedtime.
   Either regimen is continued for 4–6 wk unless endoscopy has shown healing.
   ●Active benign gastric ulcer: 800 mg PO at bedtime for up to 8 weeks,
                                  or 300 mg PO qid for up to 8 weeks.
   ●Hypersecretory conditions: 300 mg PO qid for as long necessary.
   Some patients require more frequent doses (maximum 2400 mg/day).

Intravenous: 300 mg (2ml) q6h. Dilute to 20 ml (e.g. with D5W, normal saline) and inject over minimum 2 minutes or dilute to 50–100 ml and infuse over 15–20 minutes.

NOTE: IM or IV route reserved for hypersecretory conditions, intractable ulcers, or when oral route not feasible.

Intramuscular: 300 mg (2ml) undiluted q6h.

Dose adjustment in adult with renal failure: 300 mg q12h PO or IV initially. Cautiously increase dose frequency as needed. Use smallest effective dose. Hemodialysis reduces cimetidine level; time dose to coincide with end of dialysis.

Pediatric dose: 20–40 mg/kg/day divided into 4 daily doses q6h PO, IM, or IV. Cimetidine is not generally recommended in child < 16 years of age.

CLINDAMYCIN (Cleocin)

Action/Spectrum: Bacteriostatic. Inhibits bacterial protein synthesis by binding to 50s ribosomal subunit. Sensitive bacteria; staphylococci (including penicillinase–producing S. aureus); streptococci (including S. pyogenes, S. pneumoniae, S. viridans, but not S. faecalis); bacteroides (including B. fragilis); fusobacterium; actinomyces; eubacterium; propionibacterium, peptococcus, peptostreptococcus, microaerophilic streptococci, most Clostridium perfringens, most C. tetani. Resistant; most aerobic gram–negative bacilli, many clostridia, Streptococcus faecalis, Nocardia, some Staph. aureus.

Indications: ●Serious anaerobic infections (including Bacteroides fragilis). ●Serious staphylococcal or streptococcal infection in penicillin–allergic patient (consider less toxic alternative such as erythromycin first).

Contraindications: clindamycin or lincomycin hypersentivity, treatment of meningitis (therapeutic levels are not achieved in the CSF). **Caution:** elderly, infants, history of GI disease (especially colitis), allergic diathesis, nursing mother, pregnancy (safety not established), severe renal or hepatic disease.

Comments: ●Discontinue clindamycin if significant diarrhea or abdominal cramps occur (emergence of pseudomembranous colitis ?). ●Periodically obtain CBC, and renal and liver function tests if patient is on prolonged therapy or is an infant. ●Monitor serum clindamycin levels if there is severe hepatic or renal disease, or if patient is receiving high doses. ●Clindamycin is not physically compatible with and should not be mixed in the same parenteral solution with ampicillin, phenytoin, barbiturates, aminophylline, calcium gluconate, magnesium sulfate.

Side effects: GI (nausea, vomiting, abdominal pain, diarrhea, pseudomembranous colitis, bitter taste); liver (abnormal liver function tests, jaundice); hypersensitivity (rash, urticaria, angioedema, erythema multiforme, exfoliative dermatitis, anaphylactoid reactions); blood (neutropenia, eosinophilia, thrombocytopenia)

Supplied as: 75, 150, 300 mg capsule;   oral suspension 75mg/5ml; injectable form.

Adult dose:

Oral: 150–300 mg q6h. Severe infection: 300–450 mg q6h.

Intravenous: 600–1200 mg/24hr in 2–4 equally divided dialy doses.
                Severe infection: 1200–2700 mg/24hr in 2–4 equally divided doses
Up to 4800 mg/24 hr has been used in life–threatening infection. IV infusion rate should not exceed 30 mg/min. Change to oral route when patient condition allows.

Intramuscular: Use intravenous dosage recommendations. Single IM injections greater than 600 mg not advised. Change to oral route as soon as possible.

Pediatric dose (not to exceed adult dose recommendations):

Oral: ●Capsule: 8–16 mg/kg/24hr divided q6–8h.
   In severe infection: 16–20 mg/kg/24hr divided q6–8h.
   ●Suspension: 8–12 mg/kg/24hr divided q6–8h. In severe infection: 13–16mg/kg/24hr divided q6–8h (maximum 25 mg/kg/24h). Minimum dose oral suspension in patient weighing ≤ 10 kg is 37.5 mg (1/2 tsp) tid.

<u>Intravenous:</u> ●Child/infant over 1 month age: 15–25 mg/kg/24hr divided q6–8h.
In severe infection: 25–40 mg/kg/24hr divided q6–8h.
●Infant < 1 month age: 15–20 mg/kg/24hr divided q6–8h.
<u>Intramuscular:</u> Follow intravenous dosage recommendations. Single IM injections greater than 600 mg are not advised.

CLONIDINE (Catapres)

Action: Stimulates alpha adrenergic receptors in the medulla thereby inhibiting the medullary sympathetic vasoconstrictor and cardioaccelerator centers. The consequent decrease in central sympathetic output causes a drop in peripheral vascular resistance and pulse rate.
Indications: mild to moderate hypertension.
Caution: severe coronary insufficiency, recent myocardial infarction, cerebrovascular disease, chronic renal failure, nursing mother, pregnancy (use only if clearly needed), children (safety not established).
Comments: ●Antihypertensive effect begins in 30–60 minutes, peaks in 2–4 hours, and lasts 6–8 hours. ●When discontinuing clonidine, do so over 2–4 days so as to preclude rebound hypertension. ●Clonidine may be sedating; use cautiously if patient engages in dangerous activities that require alertness. ●Periodic eye exams are advised in patients on long–term therapy.
Side effects include: <u>GI</u> (dry mouth, anorexia, nausea, vomiting, constipation, parotid gland pain, abnormal liver function test, hepatitis); <u>CNS</u> (sedation, headache, dizziness, insomnia, anxiety, depression, nervousness, restlessness, agitation, hallucinations); <u>cardiovascular</u> (orthostatic symptoms, tachycardia, bradycardia); <u>GU</u> (difficulty urinating, urinary retention, nocturia, decreased libido, impotence); <u>skin</u> (rash, itching, urticaria, angioedema, thinning hair); <u>other</u> (weakness, fatigue, arthralgias, myalgia, leg cramps, weight gain, gynecomastia, increased alcohol sensitivity, burning or itching eyes, dry nasal mucosa. transient elevation serum glucose or CPK).
Overdose: ●Empty stomach and administer activated charcoal. ●Symptomatic bradycardia with hypotension is treated with atropine. ●Hypotension in general is treated by placing patient in Trendelenberg position and administering IV fluids (e.g. normal saline). If hypotension persists, dopamine or dobutamine may be used to support blood pressure. Naloxone is also effective in reversing the hypotensive effects of clonidine. ●Massive overdose may cause paradoxic hypertension. This may require treatment with nitroprusside or diazoxide.
Supplied as: 0.1, 0.2, 0.3 mg tablet.
Dose (adult): Start with 0.1 mg PO twice daily. Gradually increase daily dose by 0.1 mg increments until response is adequate. Usual range is 0.2–0.8 mg/day. Maximum is 2.4 mg/day.

CLOTRIMAZOLE (Lotrimin, Gyne–Lotrimin, Mycelex, Mycelex–G)

Action: Fungicidal. Causes fungi to leak intracellular phosphorous with ensuing breakdown of intracellular nucleic acids.
Indications: ●Intradermal dermatophytes (Trichophyton, Epidermophyton, Microsporum) causing tinea pedis, tinea cruris, tinea corporis; ●Tinea versicolor; ●Candidal (monilial) infections of skin and vagina.
Contraindications: hypersensitivity to components, first trimester pregnancy.
Side effects: erythema, burning, blistering, pruritis, urticaria.
Supplied as: ●1% cream, 1% lotion, and 1% solution for the skin;
●1% vaginal cream (Gyne–Lotrimin, Mycelex–G);
●100 and 500 mg vaginal tablets (Gyne–Lotrimin, Mycelex–G).
Dose: ●<u>Fungal skin infectious:</u> massage into affected skin twice daily.
●<u>Vaginal candidiasis:</u> (**1**) One time dose at bedtime of 500 mg tablet intravaginally, (**2**) one 100 mg tablet intravaginally at bedtime for 7 days, (**3**) two 100 mg tablets intravaginally at bedtime for 3 days, or (**4**) one applicatorful of cream intravaginally for 7–14 days.

COLCHICINE

Action: By inhibiting normal leukocyte function, colchicine suppresses the inflammatory response to uric acid crystals deposited in joints.
Indication: treat or prevent acute attacks of gouty arthritis.
Contraindications: serious GI, renal, or cardiac disease; leukopenia; pregnancy (consider risk versus benefit); children.
Comments: ●Use colchicine cautiously in the elderly; the debilitated; nursing mother; and in presence of cardiac, renal, GI, or liver disease. ●Stop administration as soon as side effects occur (e.g. nausea, vomiting, diarrhea). ●Pain and inflammation usually controlled within 24–48 hours with oral administration and within 6–12 hours with IV administration. ●Because chronic therapy with allopurinol or probenecid by mobilizing uric acid may precipitate gouty attacks, prophylactic doses of colchicine should be continued for a year.

Side effects: ●Nausea, vomiting, diarrhea, and abdominal pain are common with oral route; and may also occur with IV route if dosage recommendations are exceeded. ●Overdose may cause marrow depression (agranulocytosis, thrombocytopenia, aplastic anemia); disseminated intravascular coagulation; hemorrhagic gastroenteritis; liver failure; anuria; peripheral neuritis; myopathy; hair loss. ●IV extravasation may result in skin and soft tissue necrosis.

Supplied as: 0.6 mg tablet; intravenous injection preparation.

Avoid SC or IM injection, severe local irritation may occur.

Dose (adult) in treatment acute gouty arthritis:

Oral: 0.6–1.2 mg at first warning of attack followed by 0.6 mg at 1–2 hour intervals until pain subsides or until GI distress (nausea, vomiting, or diarrhea) develops. GI distress usually occurs before a total of 8 mg has been administered. Administer no more than 9.6 mg (16 tablets) in 24 hours. After attack subsides, 0.6 mg tid may be given for a few days to maintain therapeutic effect. Switch to indomethacin if colchicine fails to control the attack.

Intravenous (when oral route not tolerated or contraindicated or when a faster response is needed): Initially, 2 mg IV. If necessary, administer an additional 1–2 mg IV in 4–6 hours (maximum 4 mg/24hr, maximum 4 mg/attack). Doses should be diluted in 20 ml sterile normal saline and administered slowly over 5 minutes. Do not dilute in D5W or bacteriostatic solutions.

Prevention gouty attacks: 0.6 mg PO 1–4 times/week. In stubborn cases, the dosage is 0.6 mg PO qd–bid.

CORTICOSTEROID preparations for systemic therapy and local parenteral therapy:

Indications include: ●adrenocortical insufficiency (use cortisone or hydrocortisone) ●congenital adrenal hyperplasia (e.g. use cortisone or hydrocortisone) ●neoplasias (e.g. leukemia, lymphoma, myelomas) ●collagen diseases–e.g. severe rheumatoid arthritis not responsive to nonsteroidal drugs, lupus, polymyositis, dermatomyositis, periarteritis nodosa. (However, corticosteroids are not effective in scleroderma.) ●severe asthma ●symptomatic sarcoidosis ●ulcerative colitis, Crohn's disease ●antenatal prophylaxis respiratory distress syndrome of newborn (e.g. use betamethasone) ●hypercalcemia due to neoplasia, sarcoidosis, hypervitaminosis D; (Not generally effective in hypercalcemia due to elevated parathyroid hormone or to neoplasms that secrete parathyroid hormone–like substances) ●shock secondary to sepsis or adrenal insufficiency (e.g. use hydrocortisone) ●cerebral edema (use dexamethasone) ●prevention/treatment transplant rejection ●chronic active hepatitis ●severe psoriasis, severe seborrheic dermatitis, pemphigus, severe erythema multiforme ●allergy (transfusion reactions, drug hypersensitivity, contact dermatitis, atopic dermatitis, etc).

Contraindications: hypersensitivity to components, systemic fungal infection.

Caution: GI ulcers, osteoporosis, hypertension, thromboembolism, ocular herpes simplex, myasthenia gravis, seizure disorder. ●Corticosteroids cross the placenta and high dosages may cause fetal adrenal hypoplasia. Monitor neonatal adrenal function (e.g. serum cortisol, cosyntropin test) and administer corticosteroid if indicated. ●Corticosteroids are secreted in breast milk. Breast feeding is contraindicated in mothers receiving large doses but may be permitted in mothers receiving small doses. ●Glucocorticoids are diabetogenic and may increase insulin requirements or unmask latent diabetes.

Comments: Pediatric dose may be less than adult dose but dose is generally dictated by clinical severity and response rather than by age or weight. Equivalent doses; 5 mg prednisone = 5 mg prednisolone = 4 mg methylprednisolone = 4 mg triamcinolone = 0.6 mg betamethasone = 0.75 mg dexamethasone = 20 mg hydorcortisone = 25 mg cortisone. Onset of action of systemic glucocorticoid is 4–6 hours. Local administration if effective (e.g. inhalation corticosteroid for stable asthmatic, intra–articular for monoarticular arthritis, topical skin preparations as indicated) is usually preferred because the systemic side effects of corticosteroids may be minimized. Hypothalamic–pituitary–adrenal axis suppression may be minimized by prescribing intermediate–acting glucocorticoid (prednisone, prednisolone, methylprednisolone) on alternate days in the AM. If this is not feasible, then a single daily AM dose is less suppressive than daily divided doses. Alternate day AM administration is less likely to cause growth suppression in children and osteopenia. Long–acting glucocorticoids (betamethasone, dexamethasone) are most likely to cause prolonged adrenal axis suppression. Stress (e.g. surgery, trauma, severe illness, severe emotional distress) increases the dosage requirement of systemic glucocorticoid for patient on chronic glucocorticoid therapy. Adrenal sluggishness may persist for up to 1 year following systemic corticosteroid discontinuation. Consequently, resumption of corticosteroids is advised during periods of stress (e.g. trauma, infection, surgery, psychologic distress). Glucocorticoids may mask infections (e.g. septicemia may occur without fever) and resistance to infections is compromised. Response to immunizations is blunted by corticosteroid administration. Alternate day administration will minimize immune suppression. Tuberculin sensitivity may be lost with corticosteroid therapy; consider tuberculin skin test prior to initiating glucocorticoids. Mineralocorticoid activity: Cortisone and hydrocortisone; and to a lesser extend prednisone, prednisolone, methylprednisolone possess mineralocorticoid activity which may induce hypokalemia, and sodium retention with edema. Monitor weight, blood pressure, and electrolytes—especially in patients with cardiac or renal dysfunction. Glucocorticoids inhibit GI calcium absorption. Consequently, chronic therapy may induce osteopenia. Alternate day administration may lessen this side effect. Vitamin D and calcium supplements may be required.

Side effects include: GI; peptic ulcer, bleeding, pancreatitis. Skin; acne, hirsutism, striae, poor wound healing, petechiae, ecchymoses. CNS; headache, seizures, pseudotumor cerebri, euphoria, depression, irritability, psychosis. Metabolic; protein catabolism, hyperglycemia, hypocalcemia, suppression hypothalamic–pituitary–adrenal axis, increased appetite, central obesity, weight loss, growth suppression in children, hypernatremia, edema, congestive heart failure, hypokalemia. The latter four are dependent on the mineralocorticoid activity of particular glucocorticoid. Eye; increased introcular pressure, glaucoma, cataracts, exophthalmos. Other; hypertension, menstrual irregularities, osteoporosis, fractures, aseptic necrosis femoral or humeral heads, mask infections, anorexia.

Discontinuing corticosteroids: Abrupt discontinuation or rapid tapering of glucocorticoid may precipitate withdrawal syndrome (fever, malaise, myalgia, arthralgia) and this may be confused with disease being treated. Therapy lasting 3 days or less; may discontinue abruptly. Therapy lasting 4–10 days; reduce dose by 25–30% daily. Therapy lasting 10–30 days; reduce dose by 25% decrements of initial dose at 4 day intervals. Therapy lasting over 1 month; First give daily dose as a single AM dose of intermediate–acting corticosteroid (prednisone, prednisolone, methylprednisolone, triamcinolone). Then reduce daily dose by 2.5–5 mg prednisone or equivalent at 3–7 day intervals until patient is receiving 10 mg/day of prednisone or equivalent. At this point, perform Cosyntropin (a corticotropin analog) test to assess adrenal function before stopping therapy. Cosyntropin test of adrenal function; Draw serum cortisol before and 30–60 minutes after administering cosyntropin (adult—0.25 mg IM, 1–5 yr age—0.15 mg IM, under 1 yr age—0.1 mg IM). Normal serum cortisol levels are: ≥ 10 mcg/dl before and > 18 mcg/dl after cosyntropin administration.

betamethasone (Celestone) Supplied as: 0.6 mg tablet, 0.6mg/5ml syrup.
Dose is individualized. Range is 0.6–7.2 mg/day PO initially. After clinical improvement occurs, adjust to smallest effective dose.

betamethasone sodium phosphate (Celestone phosphate)
Supplied as; 4 mg/ml for IV, IM, intralesion, or soft tissue injection.
Dose (IV or IM) is individualized: up to 9 mg/day initially (more in certain life–threatening cases). After clinical improvement occurs, adjust to smallest effective dose.

betamethasone sodium phosphate + betamethasone acetate
(Celestone Soluspan)
Supplied as: 3 mg betamethasone sodium phosphate + 3 mg betamethasone acetate per ml for IM, intra–articular, soft tissue, or intralesional injection.
●Intramuscular dose: 0.5–9.0 mg/day intially. Adjust to smallest effective dose.
●Intra–articular dose: 0.25–2.0 ml (1.5–12 mg) according to size of joint.
●Dermatologic lesion: 0.2 ml/square cm intradermally. Max 1 ml at weekly intervals.

cortisone acetate (Cortone Acetate)
Supplied as; 25 mg tablet; 25 and 50 mg/ml for IM injection.
Intramuscular; Individualize dose. Initial range: 20–300 mg/day.
Oral dose: Individualized dose.
●Chronic primary adrenocortical insufficiency (Addison's disease): 35–70 mg/day (32.5mg/square meter/24hr). Give 2/3 daily dose in AM upon awakening and 1/3 in afternoon.
●Salt–losing forms of congenital adrenal hyperplasia: 20–40 mg/square meter/24hr. Give 1/3 daily dose in AM upon awakening and 2/3 in afternoon.
●Anti–inflammatory: 25–300 mg/day initially.
Comment; In addition to glucocorticoid activity, both hydrocortisone and cortisone have weak mineralocorticoid activity. Consequently, they are not the corticosteroids of choice for chronic treatment of inflammatory conditions or for immune suppression where the sole requirement is a glucocorticoid. They are, however, drugs of choice in treatment of chronic primary adrenocortical insufficiency (Addison's disease) and salt–losing forms of congenital adrenal hyperplasia. In more severe cases and if the addition of a liberal amount of salt to the diet does not replenish salt loss or prevent orthostatic hypotension, a potent mineralocorticoid (e.g. desoxycorticosone or fludrocortisone) is administered in addition to hydrocortisone or cortisone.

dexamethasone (Decadron, Hexadrol)
Supplied as: 0.25, 0.5, 0.75, 1.5, 4, 6 mg tablet; 0.5mg/5ml elixir.
Dose: 0.75–9 mg/day PO divided into 2–4 doses initially (more or less may be required depending on situation). Gradually adjust to smallest effective dose after clinical improvement occurs.

dexamethasone sodium phosphate injection
(Decadron phosphate injection, Hexadrol phosphate injection)
Supplied as: ●4, 10, 20 mg/ml for IV, IM, intra–articular, intralesion, or soft tissue injection. ●24 mg/ml for IV injection only.
IV or IM dose: 0.5–9 mg/day initially. More or less may be required depending on situation. Gradually adjust to smallest effective dose after clinical improvement occurs.
  ●Cerebral edema: *Adult* : 10 mg IV followed by 4 mg q6h IM until symptoms subside. Response usually seen in 12–14 hours. Dose may be reduced after 2–4 days and gradually discontinued over 5–7 days.
  Child : 0.006–0.040 mg/kg IV or IM qd–bid.
  ●Shock: Adult, 40 mg IV q2–6h while shock persists.
  Child, 0.006–0.040 mg/kg IV or IM qd–bid.
  ●Prevention hyaline membrane disease: 4 mg IM tid to mother for two days prior to delivery.
Intra–articular, intralesion, or soft tissue injection: Dose depends on situation. Range: 0.2–6 mg. If necessary, the dose may be repeated at 3 day to 3 week intervals.

dexamethasone acetate (Decadron LA)
Supplied as: 8 mg dexamethasone equivalent/ml for IM, intra–articular, soft tissue, or intralesional injection. *Not* for IV injection.
Dose: ●IM: 1–2ml every 1–3 week as needed. ●Intra–articular/soft tissue: 0.5–2ml every 1–3 week as needed. ●Intralesion: 0.1–0.2ml per injection site.

hydrocortisone (Hydrocortone)
Supplied as: 10, 20 mg tablet; ●100mg/60ml retention enema (Cortenema).
Dose: ●Chronic adrenocortical insufficiency or congenital adrenal hyperplasia: 25–50 mg/day PO or 25–30 mg/square meter/day PO. Note: In adrenocortical insufficiency, give 2/3 of daily dose in AM and 1/3 in PM. Do the reverse in congenital adrenal hyperplasia (1/3 AM, 2/3 PM).
  ●Inflammatory conditions or immune suppression: 20–240 mg/day PO initially. Gradually adjust to smallest effective dose after clinical improvement occurs. Because of its mineralocorticoid effect (i.e. sodium and water retention), hydrocortisone is not the usual corticosteroid of choice for chronic treatment of inflammation or immune suppression.
  ●Retention enema (e.g. ulcerative colitis): 100 mg retained at least 30 minutes once or twice daily.

hydrocortisone acetate (Hydrocortone Acetate, Cort–Dome, Cortifoam)
Supplied as: ●25 mg/ml suspension for intra–articular or soft tissue injection.
  ●25 mg suppository (Cort–Dome), rectal foam (Cortifoam).
Intra–articular dose: 10–50 mg according to size of joint.
Soft tissue dose: 5–75 mg according to size of affected area.
Rectal dose: ●One suppository (Cort–Dome) twice daily. In more severe conditions: one suppository tid or two suppositories twice daily.
  ●One rectal application of foam (Cortifoam) once or twice daily.

hydrocortisone sodium phosphate (Hydrocortone phosphate)
Supplied as: 50 mg/ml for IV, IM, or SC injection.
Dose is individualized. Range: 15–240 mg/day initially depending on situation.

hydrocortisone sodium succinate (A–hydroCort, Solu–Cortef)
Supplied as: vials containing 100, 250, 500, 1000 mg for IV or IM injection.
Intravenous: 100–500 mg depending on condition. If necessary, the dose may be repeated at 2–6 hour intervals. Inject over a period of 30 seconds (for 100 mg) to 10 minutes (for 500 mg or more). Switch to oral therapy when feasible.
Intramuscular (when IV route not feasible): 100–250 mg initially; repeat if needed.

methylprednisolone (Medrol)   Supplied as: 2, 4, 8, 16, 24, 32 mg tablet.
Dose: 4–48 mg/day PO initially (more or less may be needed depending on situation). Gradually adjust to smallest effective dose after clinical improvement occurs.
methylprednisolone sodium succinate (Solu–Medrol, A–Methapred)
Supplied as: vials containing 40, 125, 500, 1000, 2000 mg for IV or IM injection.
Dose: Initial dose is 10–40 mg IV. Frequency of repeat IM or IV doses is gauged according to patient's response and condition.
●Treatment of shock: 30 mg/kg IV. Repeat as needed at 4–6 hour intervals for 48 hours.
methylprednisolone acetate (Depo–Medrol)
Supplied as: 20, 40, 80 mg/ml for IM and local injection. *Not for IV* administration.
Intramuscular dose: 40–120 mg. Repeat IM doses may be given weekly as needed. Weekly IM dose is equivalent to 7 times daily oral dose of methylprednisolone.
Intra–articular dose: 4–80 mg according to size of joint and severity of condition.
Soft tissue dose (e.g. bursitis, tendinitis): 4–30mg according to clinical situation.
Intradermal dose: 20–60 mg.

prednisolone   Supplied as: 5 mg tablet, 15 mg/ml syrup (Prelone).
Dose: 5–60 mg/day PO initially (more or less may be required depending on situation). Gradually adjust to smallest effective dose after clinical improvement occurs.
prednisolone sodium phosphate (Hydeltrasol)
Supplied as: 20 mg/ml for IV or IM injection.
Dose: 4–60 mg/day IV or IM initially (more or less may be needed depending on situation). Gradually adjust to smallest effective dose after clinical improvement occurs.
prednisolone acetate
Supplied as: 50 mg/ml for IM or local injection.
Intramuscular dose: 4–60 mg. Dose and interval must be individualized. Duration of effect is longer than prednisolone phosphate.
Intra–articular/intralesion/ soft tissue dose: 4–40 mg. Duration of effect is shorter than prednisolone tebutate.
prednisolone tebutate (Hydeltra T.B.A.)
Supplied as: 20 mg/ml for intra–articular, intralesion, or soft tissue injection.
Dose: 4–40 mg depending on the situation. May be repeated every 2–3 weeks. Weekly administration may be necessary in severe conditions.

prednisone (Deltasone, Liquid Pred Syrup)
Supplied as: 1, 2.5, 5, 10, 20, 25, 50 mg tablet;   5mg/5ml syrup.
Dose is individualized according to severity of condition and response.
    Adult: 50–60 mg/day PO initially for severe acute condition.
    Child: 0.5–2 mg/kg/day PO initially for severe acute condition.

triamcinolone (Aristocort, Kenacort)   Supplied as: 1, 2, 4, 8 mg tablet.
triamcinolone diacetate (Artistocort)   Supplied as: ●2mg/5ml syrup; ●40 mg/ml suspension (Aristocort Forte Parenteral) for IM, intra–articular, or intralesional injection; ●25 mg/ml suspension (Aristocort Intralesional) for intra–articular or intralesional injection.
triamcinolone acetonide (Kenalog 10, Kenalog 40) Supplied as: ●40 mg/ml suspension (Kenalog 40) for IM or intra–articular injection; ●10 mg/ml (Kenalog 10) for intra–articular, intradermal, or intrabursal injection.
triamcinolone hexacetonide (Aristospan)   Supplied as: ●5 mg/ml suspension for intralesional injection, ●20 mg/ml for intra–articular injection.
Dose of various triamcinolone preparations:
●Oral: (triamcinolone tablets, triamcinolone acetate syrup): Individualize dose. Usual range is 4–48 mg/day initially (more or less may be indicated depending on disease severity). Gradually adjust to smallest effective dose after clinical improvement occurs.
●Intramuscular (triamcinolone diacitate, triamcinolone acetonide) injection is usually used instead of or as a supplement to initial oral administration. Therapeutic effects may last 3–4 weeks. Individualize dose. Usual range is 20–80 mg depending on circumstances.

●<u>Intra–articular:</u> **(1)** triamcinolone diacetate, 5–40 mg depending on size of joint; duration of effect is 1–8 weeks. **(2)** triamcinolone acetonide, 2.5–15 mg depending on size of joint; **(3)** triamcinolone hexacetonide, 2–20 mg depending on size of joint; may repeat if needed in no sooner than 3–4 weeks.

●<u>Intralesion:</u> **(1)** triamcinolone diacetate, up to 12.5 mg depending on size of lesion; **(2)** triamcinolone acetonide, up to 1mg per injection site; **(3)** triamcinolone hexacetonide, up to 0.5 mg/square inch affected skin.

CORTICOSTEROIDS, TOPICAL SKIN

Indications include: psoriasis, sebborheic dermatitis, atopic dermatitis, contact dermatitis, discoid lupus, mummular eczema, lichen planus, granuloma annulare, pruritis ani.

Contraindications: hypersensitivity to components, ophthalmic application, viral skin infections, application of high–potency corticosteroids to face or genitalia.   **Caution:** pregnancy.

Drug choice: <u>Hydrocortisone</u> is the cheapest corticosteroid and is recommended when a corticosteroid of low potency will suffice; especially when prolonged use over wide area is required. <u>Creams</u> are suitable for most conditions including "weeping" lesions and moist areas such as skin folds. <u>Ointments</u> are useful if the skin lesion is dry. <u>Lotions</u> are indicated in hairy areas. <u>Facial application:</u> Because of the risks (e.g. thinning of skin, telangectsias, rosacea, acne); higher potency preparations should not be applied to the face. Hydrocortisone compounds and methylprednisolone are generally safe for facial application. <u>Scrotal application:</u> Higher potency preparations should not be applied to the scrotum.

Dose: Apply to affected skin bid–qid. Prescribe sufficient medication. For an adult a single application of cream or ointment to entire body requires about 30 gram (1oz). An adult leg requires 4 gram, an arm—3 gram, hands—2 gram, face—2 gram.

Side effects include: burning, itching, irritation, skin atrophy, striae, telangectasia, purpura, hypopigmentation, hypertrichosis, miliaria, folliculitis, acne, rosacea. ●Topical application of over 30 gram/wk of a high potency corticosteroid may cause systemic effects, and over 50 gram/wk may suppress hypothalamic–pituitary–adrenal axis.

Key to potency of the following preparations: high potency = ****, intermediate potency = ***, low potency = **, least potent = *.

Note: Relative potencies of corticosteroid preparations based in part on information from Robertson D.B. and Maibach H.I.: Topical Corticosteroids, International Journal Dermatology 21: 59;-67, 1982. Used with permission.

amcinonide (Cyclocort)
   0.1% cream, ointment**** (25, 30, 60 gram tube)
   0.1% lotion**** (20, 60 ml bottle)
betamethasone dipropionate (Alphatrex, Diprolene, Diprosone, Maxivate)
   0.05% cream or ointment**** (15 gram or 45 gram tube)
   0.05% lotion**** (20 ml or 60 ml bottle)
   0.1% aerosol**** (85 gram can)
Caution: None of these betamethasone dipropionate preparations should be used with occlusive dressings. Diprolene ointment, cream, and lotion are particularly potent preparations. No more than 45 gram of Diprolene ointment or cream, or 50 ml of Diprolene lotion may be applied per week, and treatment should not exceed 14 days.
betamethasone valerate (Valisone, Betatrex)
   0.01% cream** (15 or 60 gram tube)
   0.1% cream*** (15, 45, 110 gram tube or 430 gram jar)
   0.1% ointment*** (15 or 60 gram tube)
   0.1% lotion*** (20 or 60 ml bottle)
clobetasol propionate (Temovate)
   0.05% cream or ointment**** (15, 30, 45 gram tubes).
Caution: Temovate is a particularly potent preparation that should not be used with occlusive dressings, or for more than 14 days. Use no more than 50 gram/week.
desonide (Tridesilon)
   0.05% cream*** (15, 60 gram tube & 5 lb jar)
   0.05% ointment*** (15, 60 gram tube)
desoximetazone (Topicort)
   0.05% cream or gel*** (15, 60 gram tube)
   0.25% cream**** (15 gram, 60 gram, or 4 oz tube)
   0.25% ointment**** (15, 60 gram tube)
dexamethasone:
   0.1% gel in 30 gram tube* (Decaderm)
   0.01 % aerosol* (Aeroseb–Dex)
   aerosol* (10 mg per 25 gram container Decaspray)
dexamethasone sodium phosphate (Decadron phosphate)
   0.1% cream* (15, 30 gram tube)
diflorasone diacetate (Florone, Maxiflor)
   0.05% cream or ointment**** (15, 30, 60 gram tube)

fluocinolone acetonide (Synalar, Synemol)
    0.01% cream** (15, 30, 60 gram tube or 425 gram jar)
    0.01% solution** (20, 60 ml bottle)
    0.025% cream*** (15, 30, 60 gram tube or 425 gram jar)
    0.025% ointment*** (15, 30, 60, 120 gram tube or 425 gram jar)
    0.2% cream**** (12 gram tube)
fluocinonide (Lidex)
    0.05% cream, ointment, gel**** (15, 30, 60, 120 gram tube)
    0.05% solution**** (20, 60 ml bottle)
flurandrenolide (Cordran)
    0.025% cream or ointment***(30, 60 gram tube or 225 gram jar)
    0.05% cream or ointment***(15, 30, 60 gram tube or 225 gram jar)
    0.05% lotion*** (15, 60 ml bottle)
    4 mcg/sq. cm tape***(7.5 x 200 cm roll, 7.5 x 60 cm roll)
halcinonide (Halog)
    0.025% cream*** (15, 60 gram tube and 240 gram jar)
    0.1% cream or ointment**** (15, 30, 60 gram tube and 240 gram jar)
    0.1% solution**** (20, 60 ml bottle)
hydrocortisone
Supplied as 0.25, 0.5, 1.0, and 2.5 % preparations of cream, ointment and lotion. All are the least potent category. Preparations of 0.5% or less may be obtained without a prescription. Cream and ointment comes in tubes (usually 30 or 60 gram, or 1 oz). For patients requiring large volumes, there are 4 oz jars of cream (0.25%, 0.5%, 1.0%) and ointment (1%). Lotion is usually dispensed in bottles of 30 or 60 ml, or 2 or 4 fluid oz.
hydrocortisone acetate
    0.5% cream* in 1 oz tube (Corticaine)
    1% cream* in 1oz tube and 4oz jar (Carmol HC)
    1% and 2.5% ointment* (Cortef Acetate)
hydrocortisone valerate (Westcort)
    0.1% cream* (15, 45, 60, 120 gram tube)
    0.2% ointment*** (15, 45, 60 gram tube)
methylprednisolone acetate (Medrol)   0.25% and 1% ointment* (30 gram tube)
triamcinolone acetonide (Aristocort, Kenalog, Triamcinair, Trymex)
    0.025% cream** (15, 60, 80 gram tube; and 240 gram or 5.25 lb jar)
    0.025% ointment** (15, 60, 80 gram tube and 240 gram jar)
    0.025% lotion** (60 ml bottle)
    0.1% cream*** (15, 60, 80 gram tube; and 240 gram, 1lb, or 5.25 lb jar)
    0.1% ointment*** (15, 60, 80 gram tube; and 240 gram, 5 lb, or 5.25 lb jar)
    0.1% lotion*** (15, 60 ml bottle)
    0.5% cream**** (20 gram tube and 240 gram jar)
    0.5% ointment**** (15, 20 gram tube)
    aerosol* (Kenalog): up to 0.2mg/2 sec spray (23, 63 gram can)

CORTICOSTEROIDS, INHALED AEROSOLS:

beclomethasone (Beclovent, Vanceril); **flunisolide** (AeroBid), **triamcinolone** (Azmacort)

Indications: Bronchial asthma in patient who requires chronic corticosteroid therapy. These preparations are not indicated in patients: (**1**) whose asthma can be controlled with bronchodilators or other nonsteroidal drugs, (**2**) who require systemic steroids infrequently, (**3**) with nonasthmatic bronchitis.
Contraindications: ●hypersensitivity to components ●primary treatment of status asthmaticus or of acute asthmatic episodes requiring intensive therapy ●not recommended in child under 6 yr.
Caution: pregnancy, nursing mother.
Comments: ●Chronic systemic corticosteroid therapy may be replaced or significantly reduced by corticosteroid inhaler thrapy. Assuming that the patient has been stabilized with systemic corticosteroids, start corticosteroid inhaler therapy concurrently. After 1 week and every 1–2 weeks thereafter, reduce the daily systemic oral dose of corticosteroid by 2.5 mg prednisone or its equivalent. If signs of adrenal insufficiency occur (e.g. hypotension, weight loss) the oral corticosteroid dose should be temporarily increased. Since recovery of normal adrenal function of patients withdrawn from systemic corticosteroids may take up to 12 months, systemic corticosteroids will be required during periods of stress or severe asthma. ●If the patient is concurrently receiving bronchodilator inhaler therapy, the bronchodilator inhaler should be used prior to the corticosteroid inhaler in order to enhance penetration of the latter into the bronchial tree. Several minutes, however, should elapse between their use in order to reduce the risk of potential toxicity from the fluorocarbon propellants in the aerosols. ●Rinsing the mouth and gargling with water after inhalation will reduce systemic absorption. ●Therapeutic effects of the inhaled corticosteroids are usually seen within 1–4 weeks. ●At the recommended doses, beclomethasone does not suppress the hypothalamic–pituitary–adrenal axis. Although no significant axis suppression occurs with recommended dose of flunisolide, the manufacturer recommends periodic monitoring of adrenal function. Axis suppression has occurred with inhaled triamcinolone.

Side effects (the most common): hoarseness; dry mouth or throat; candida or aspergillus infections of mouth, pharynx, or larynx.

beclomethasone (Beclovent, Vanceril)
Supplied as: oral inhaler unit (42 mcg/inhalation).
Canister provides a minimum of 200 metered inhalations.
Adult/child > 12 yr: 2 inhalations tid–qid. Begin with total 12–16 inhalations/day divided in severe asthma. Maximum 20 inhalations/day.
Child 6–12 yr: 1–2 inhalations tid–qid. Maximum 10 inhalations/day.

dexamethasone sodium phosphate (Decadron Phosphate Respihaler)
Supplied as: aerosol container (84 mcg/inhalation).
Container provides minimum of 170 inhalations.
Adult: initially, 3 inhalations tid–qid. Max: 3 inhalations/dose, 12 inhalations/day.
Child: Initially, 2 inhalations tid–qid. Max: 2 inhalations/dose, 8 inhalations /day.

flunisolide (Aerobid)
Supplied as: oral inhaler system (250 mcg/inhalation).
Canister provides a minimum of 100 metered inhalations.
Adult: start with 2 inhalations twice daily. Maximum of 4 inhalations twice daily.
Child 6–15 yr: 2 inhalations twice daily.

triamcinolone (Azmacort)
Supplied as: oral inhaler unit (100 mcg/inhalation).
Canister provides minimum of 240 inhalations.
Adult: 2 inhalations tid–qid. Maximum 16 inhalations/day.
Child 6–12 yr: 2 inhalations tid–qid. Maximum 12 inhalations/day.

CROMOLYN SODIUM (Intal)

Action: Inhibits degranulation of sensitized mast cells thereby preventing the release of agents that cause bronchospasm (e.g. histamine, slow–reacting substance of anaphylaxis).
Indication: prevention of bronchial asthma.
Contraindications: cromolyn hypersensitivity, treatment of acute asthma attack.
Caution: renal or hepatic dysfunction.
Comments: ●Prior administration of a bronchodilator may prevent the bronchospasm–induced coughing that occurs in some patients following cromolyn inhalation. ●Improvement, if it occurs, is usually seen within first 4 weeks of therapy. Children are more likely to benefit than adults.
Side effects include: dry irritated throat, cough, wheezing, bad taste, nausea. ●Less common manifestations include substernal burning, headache, dizziness, dysuria, urinary frequency, parotid gland swelling, lacrimation, rash, urticaria, angioedema, anaphylaxis, eosinophilic pulmonary infiltrates, joint swelling/pain, myositis.
Supplied as: aerosol inhaler canister providing a minimum of 112 metered inhalations. ●Also supplied as capsule for inhalation via turbo–inhaler (Spinhaler) and ampul for inhalation via power–operated nebulizer.
Dose (adult or child ≥ 5 yr): Start with 2 inhalations of Intal Inhaler qid. This is also the maximum daily dose.
● If bronchospasm occurs following a known precipitant, try 2 inhalations 10–15 minutes before exposure (and no more than 60 minutes before exposure).
●Corticosteroid and/or bronchodilator therapy is continued as usual when beginning cromolyn. If asthma is well controlled, gradual tapering of bronchodilator and steroids may be attempted. Once the patient is no longer receiving concurrent asthma medications, gradually less frequent cromolyn administration may be tried.

CROMOLYN SODIUM NASAL SOLUTION

(Nasalcrom)
Action: see above.
Indication: prevention/treatment allergic rhinitis.
Contraindication: hypersensitivity to components. **Caution:** pregnancy, nursing mother.
Comments: ●Therapeutic effects may not become evident for 2–4 weeks. ●Antihistamines and/or nasal decongestant may be used concurrently with cromolyn. When full effect of cromolyn is seen, it may be possible to reduce or discontinue these concurrent medications.
Side effects: sneezing; nasal stinging, burning, or irritation; postnasal drip; nosebleed; headache; anaphylaxis.
Supplied as: 13 ml nasal spray bottle (provides minimum 100 sprays).

Dose (adults/child > 6 yr): one spray in each nostril tid—qid (max 6 treatments/day). May be of benefit when used prior to exposure to a known precipitant.

CROTAMITON (Eurax)

Contraindications: crotamiton hypersensitivity.
Caution: ●Avoid contact with eyes, mouth, or acutely inflamed or weeping skin. ●pregnancy.
Side effect: contact dermatitis.
Supplied as: cream (60 gram tube) or lotion (2 or 16 oz bottle).
Directions: <u>Scabies:</u> (1) bathe or shower and then dry; (2) then, thoroughly massage into skin from neck down; (3) repeat application in 24 hours; (4) bathe 48 hours after last application. Wash clothing and bed linen.
<u>Pruritis:</u> massage into affected skin as needed.

DIAZEPAM (Valium)

Action: Diazepam, a benzodiazepine, is a CNS depressant.
Indications: anxiety, tension, acute alcohol withdrawal, status epilepticus, skeletal muscle spasm.
Contraindications: diazepam hypersensitivity, treatment of psychosis, acute alcohol intoxication, acute narrow angle glaucoma, open angle glaucoma (unless patient is receiving adequate antiglaucoma therapy).
Caution: ●Limit use in first trimester pregnancy to status epilepticus. ●IV administration may cause apnea or cardiac arrest—particularly when patient is elderly, debilitated, has limited pulmonary reserve, or is receiving other CNS depressants. ●Chronic use may cause psychological and physical dependence. Therefore, diazepam should be discontinued gradually over 1–2 weeks because sudden withdrawal of diazepam in such patients may lead to tremor, vomiting, sweating, convulsions, etc. ●Warn patients about using diazepam or other benzodiazepines in dangerous settings that require alertness. Sedation is enhanced by alcohol and other CNS depressants. ●Depressed or suicidal patients may become further depressed with benzodiazepines. ●Benzodiazepines are metabolized in the liver, and should therefore be administered with caution to a patient with liver dysfunction or to the elderly.
Comments: ●The preferred parenteral route is intravenous. IM injection is painful and absorption is erratic. However, IM injection may be used if an IV line cannot be established. ●To preclude local irritation, thrombosis, or phlebitis; administer IV diazepam no faster than 5 mg/minute thru a large vein or as close as possible to insertion site of IV line. ●Diazepam is not very soluble. Do not mix with other solutions or drugs.
Side effects include: drowsiness, lethargy, fatigue, ataxia, dizziness, depression, confusion, amnesia, headache, blurred vision, diplopia, slurred speech, tremor, dry mouth, nausea, hiccups, constipation, jaundice, urinary retention or incontinence, changed libido, rash, urticaria. With IV administration: depressed respiration, apnea, hypotension, bradycardia, cardiac arrest. Paradoxical effects: anxiety, restlessness, hyperexcitability, rage, insomnia, vivid dreams, spasticity. Floppy infant syndrome (low Apgar, apnea, hypothermia, poor sucking) may occur if more than 30 mg is given IV to mother during last 15 hours of labor.
Supplied as: ●2, 5, 10 mg tablet
●5 mg/ml solution for injection (2 ml ampul or syringe, 10 ml vial).

Adult dose:
Status epilepticus: 5–10 mg slow IV push (5 mg/minute). If necessary, give repeat dose every 15 minutes up to total cumulative maximum of 30 mg.
Tension, anxiety, muscle spasm; ●PO: 2–10 mg 2–4 times a day;
●IV: 2–10 mg. Repeat as needed in 3–4 hr.
Severe muscle spasm/tetany: 5–10 mg IV. Dose may be repeated as needed in 3–4 hr. Larger dose may be required for treatment of tetany.
Acute alcohol withdrawal: (IV or PO depending on urgency)
●IV: 5–10 mg followed by 5 mg every 5–10 minutes until patient is sedated.
●PO: 10 mg tid—qid over first 24 hr, then 5 mg 3–4 times a day as needed.
Prior to procedure (e.g. endoscopy, cardioversion): Titrate to adequate sedation by giving 2.5–5 mg at 30 second intervals up to cumulative maximum of 20–30 mg.
Pediatric dose:
Status epilepticus:
●1month–5 yr: 0.2–0.5mg IV q2–5 min up to total 5mg. Repeat in 2–4 hr as needed.
●5 yr and older: 1mg IV q2–5 min up to total 10 mg. Repeat in 2–4 hr as needed.
Tetanus: ●1 month–5 yr: 1–2 mg IV q3–4h as needed.
●5 yr and older: 5–10 mg IV q3–4h as needed.

DIAZOXIDE (Hyperstat IV)

Action: Diazoxide is a thiazide derivative but is not a diuretic. It reduces blood pressure by relaxing peripheral arteriolar smooth muscle. Heart rate and cardiac output increase.
Indication: emergency reduction of blood pressure.
Contraindications: hypersensitivity to diazoxide, thiazides, or sulfonamide derivatives; pregnancy; pheochromocytoma–induced hypertension; dissecting aortic aneurysm–associated hypertension; compensatory hypertension (e.g. due to aortic coarctation, arteriovenous shunt).
Caution: compromised cardiac or cerebral circulation.
Side effects: effects of sodium and water retention (edema, congestive heart failure); vasodilative effects (hypotension, orthostatic effects, flushing, sweating); compromised coronary blood flow (myocardial ischemia, angina, arrhythmias, myocardial infarction); compromised cerebral blood flow (headache, dizziness, lightheadedness, sleepiness, weakness, anxiety, tinnitus, transient hearing loss, unconsciousness, seizures, paralysis, focal neurologic deficits, optic nerve infarction); gastrointestinal (nausea, vomiting, diarrhea, constipation, ileus, abdominal discomfort, pancreatitis, anorexia, abnormal taste, salivation, dry mouth, parotid swelling); respiratory (dyspnea, cough, choking); hypersensitivity (fever, rash, leukopenia); injection site extravasation (local pain, phlebitis, cellulitis); other (hyperglycemia, hyperuricemia, hirsutism, lacrimation).

Comments: (**1**) Keep patient supine for at least 1 hour following administration. Monitor blood pressure closely until stable. (**2**) If necessary, repeat IV injections may be given at 4–24 hour intervals until oral antihypertensive medication is started. (**3**) Diazoxide can cause sodium and water retention which may lead to edema and CHF. In fact, some patients unresponsive to diazoxide may be so on basis of increased extracellular fluid volume. Furosemide may be needed to prevent fluid overload and to optimize blood pressure reduction. (**4**) To preclude excessive hypotension, do not give IV diazoxide within 6 hours of administering hydralazine, reserpine, methyldopa, prazosin, minoxidil, beta–blocker, alphaprodine, nitrites or other papaverine–like compounds. (**5**) Thiazide diuretics potentiate the hyperglycemic and hyperuricemic effects of diazoxide.

Supplied as: 20 ml ampule (15mg/ml).

Dose (adult or child): 1–3 mg/kg (max 150 mg) undiluted and given IV via peripheral vein in 30 seconds or less with patient supine. If necessary, give repeat doses at 5–15 min intervals to achieve desired blood pressure. See first 4 comments above.

DIGOXIN (Lanoxin)

Action: Cardiac glycoside. ●Increases myocardial contractile force by increasing intracellular sodium (inhibition Na–K ATPase) and by increasing intracellular calcium. ●Shortens duration ventricular action potential (shortens QT interval). ●Slows AV node conduction and prolongs AV node refractory period (increase PR interval, AV block). ●ST segment depression, T wave inversion. ●Increased automaticity (i.e. increased rate diastolic depolarization) and shortened refractory period of atria and ventricles increase risk of ectopic rhythms.

Indications: ●Congestive heart failure. ●To slow ventricular rates in cases of atrial fibrillation, atrial flutter, or paroxysmal atrial tachycardia.

Contraindications: digoxin hypersensitivity, ventricular fibrillation, idiopathic hypertrophic subaortic stenosis, infiltrative myopathy (e.g. amyloidosis), atrial fibrillation in patient with Wolff–Parkinson–White syndrome, AV heart block more advanced than 2nd degree Mobitz II (unless pacemaker present), severe sick sinus syndrome (unless pacemaker present), pericardial constriction, cardiac tamponade.

Caution: pregnancy, carditis, glomerulonephritis, premature/immature infants, hypomagnesemia. Dose reduction may be necessary with hypothyroidism or renal insufficiency. Digoxin dose reduction may also become necessary with concurrent administration of certain drugs (e.g. quinidine, verapamil, amiodarone, propantheline, diphenoxylate) that may result in elevated serum digoxin level. Hypokalemic patient is at increased risk for digoxin–induced arrhythmias. Remember that diuretic therapy is a common cause of potassium depletion. Hypercalcemia aggravates digoxin toxicity. Calcium administration, particularly IV, may provoke arrhythmias in the patient on digitalis. Electrical cardioversion: Because cardioversion may precipitate ventricular arrhythmias in the patient on digitalis, digoxin should if possible be withheld prior to electrical cardioversion. If the patient cannot tolerate the delay, a bolus of lidocaine (75–100 mg in adult) is administered before attempting cardioversion. The initial cardioversion should be tried at 5–10 joules. Further attempts at electrical cardioversion are contraindicated if ventricular ectopy results.

Side effects include: gastrointestinal (anorexia, nausea, vomiting, diarrhea); neurologic (fatigue, sleepiness, weakness, headache, vertigo, confusion, restlessness, nightmares, psychiatric disturbances); ocular (yellow vision, halos, decreased visual acuity, mydriasis, photophobia); cardiac; Digitalis may provoke any type of heart block and virtually any arrhythmia. other: hypersensitivity reactions, gynecomastia.

Managing digitalis intoxication: ●EKG monitor. ●Stopping digoxin administration may be all that is needed with mild toxicity. ●Hypokalemia must be corrected. Mild hypokalemia may be treated with oral KCl (e.g. 40–80 mEq in divided doses). Administer KCl intravenously if hypokalemia is severe or associated with a dangerous arrhythmia (dilute 40 mEq KCl in 500 ml D5W and infuse thru peripheral vein no faster than 10–20 mEq/hr). Keeping the serum potassium in the high-normal range may help in the prevention/treatment of supraventricular and ventricular arrhythmias. ●Lidocaine or phenytoin is indicated in treatment of digoxin–related ventricular arrhythmias/ectopy. ●Hemodynamically unstable bradycardia is treated with intravenous atropine. Transvenous pacing may be needed. ●When toxicity is severe, intravenous injection of digoxin–specific antibody fragments (Digibind) will inactivate digoxin. ●Acute deliberate overdose: Empty the stomach and administer activated charcoal. Massive overdose may cause hyperkalemia which must be treated aggressively. Refer to "Hyperkalemia" in the clinical section for treatment of hyperkalemia.

Supplied as: ●0.125, 0.25, 0.5 mg tablet ●elixir (0.05 mg/ml)
●IV (0.1 or 0.25mg/ml).

Dose based on lean body weight and normal renal function:

Adult dose:

Intravenous digitalizing dose is 1 mg as follows: 0.25–0.5 mg initially, followed by two to three 0.25 mg doses at 4–6 hour intervals.

Oral digitalizing dose is 1.0–1.5 mg as follows: 0.5–0.75 mg initial dose followed at 6–8 hour intervals by 0.25–0.5 mg to cumulative total of 1.0–1.5 mg.

Maintenance: 0.125–0.5 mg once daily PO or IV. The usual maintenance range in the elderly is 0.125–0.25 mg once daily.

Estimated daily maintenance dose for adult with renal insufficiency and lean body weight of 70 kg = (digitalizing dose in mg) x (0.002) x (70 + creatinine clearance). If the creatinine clearance is unknown, it can be estimated as follows: creatinine clearance in male is approximately = (body weight in kg) X (140 – age) ÷ (72 X serum creatinine). Creatinine clearance in female = 0.85 X this figure.

Pediatric dose:
Oral digitalizing dose:
- Child > 10 yr: 0.010–0.015 mg/kg,
- Child 5–10 yr: 0.020–0.035 mg/kg,
- Child 2–5 yr: 0.030–0.040 mg/kg,
- Infant 1–24 month: 0.035–0.060 mg/kg,
- Fullterm neonate: 0.025–0.035 mg/kg,
- Premature neonate: 0.020–0.030 mg/kg.

Directions for oral digitalization: First dose is 1/2 oral digitalizing dose. Give 1/4 oral digitalizing dose 6–8 hours later and again in another 6–8 hours.
Directions for intravenous digitalization: Intravenous digitalizing dose is 80% of oral digitalizing dose (see above). First dose is 1/2 IV digitalizing dose. Give 1/4 IV digitalizing dose 6 hours later and again in another 6 hours.
Maintenance: The total daily PO or IV maintenance dose is 25–35% of the respective PO or IV digitalizing dose (20–30% in premature neonate). The daily IV or PO dose is administered as a single daily dose in child over 10 yr of age and divided into two equal doses at 12 hour intervals for those less than 10 yr.

Comments: ●IM route is very painful but may be used if IV or PO route is not possible. Dosage is as for IV. ●Therapeutic level, 0.8–2.0 nanograms/ml. ●Onset: 5–30 minutes IV, 1–2 hr PO. Peak effect: 1–4 hr IV, 2–6 hr PO.

DISOPYRAMIDE (Norpace)

Action: refer to quinidine; disopyramide has similar actions.
Indications: prevention/suppression of premature ventricular contractions and ventricular tachycardia.
Contraindications: disopyramide hypersensitivity, cardiogenic shock, uncompensated or marginally compensated congestive heart failure or hypotension, 2nd or 3rd degree heart block (unless pacemaker present), nursing mother, treatment of digitalis–induced arrhythmias. Disopyramide is also contraindicated in the following conditions unless appropriate treatment is assured: glaucoma, myasthenia gravis, urinary retention.
Caution: pregnancy (use only if essential), cardiomyopathy, history of heart failure, sick sinus syndrome, Wolff–Parkinson–White syndrome, bundle branch block, acute myocardial infarction.
Comments: Disopyramide in setting of atrial fibrillation or flutter; The anticholinergic (vagolytic) effect of disopyramide on the AV node may facilitate AV conduction and thus increase the ventricular rate in patients with atrial flutter or atrial fibrillation. To prevent this from happening, patients with these supraventricular arrhythmias should be digitalized before giving disopyramide. However, disopyramide should not be used if atrial fibrillation occurs in patient with Wolff–Parkinson–White syndrome because digitalization is not advisable in this syndrome. Heart block; Decrease dose if 1st degree heart block occurs. Consider discontinuing disopyramide if 1st degree block persists. Stop disopyramide (unless a ventricular pacemaker is present) if the patient develops 2nd or 3rd degree heart block; or fascicular block. QRS widening; Stop disopyramide if the QRS widens by > 25%. Consider stopping disopyramide if QTc widens by more than 25% and there is persistent ectopy. Patient with marginal cardiac reserve; Because of its negative inotropic effect, disopyramide may precipitate hypotension or congestive heart failure in patients with marginal cardiac reserve (e.g. cardiomyopathy, history of congestive heart failure). Concurrent administration of other antiarrhythmics; Because of the added risk of delayed conduction (e.g. widened QRS or QTc) and negative inotropic effect; concurrent therapy with other class 1 antiarrhythmic agents (e.g. quinidine, procainamide) or beta blockers (e.g. propranolol) is not advised unless there is a life-threatening arrhythmia that cannot be controlled with a single antiarrhythmic drug. Changing from quinidine or procainamide to disopyramide; 6–12 hours should elapse since the last quinidine dose or 3–6 hours since the last procainamide dose before commencing disopyramide. Do not give a loading dose of disopyramide in this setting.
Side effects include: cardiovascular; congestive heart failure; edema; weight gain; dyspnea; hypotension; syncope; angina; conduction abnormalities (heart block, wide QRS, etc); anticholinergic; dry mouth/throat/nose/eyes, blurred vision, constipation, urinary hesitancy/retention; GI; anorexia, nausea, vomiting, diarrhea, gas, bloating, pain, elevated liver enzymes, cholestatic jaundice; GU; urinary frequency/urgency, dysuria, impotence, elevated BUN/creatinine; neurologic; headache, dizziness, nervousness, depression, insomnia, numbness, acute psychosis (rare); skin; pruritis, rash or other eruptions; blood; decreased hemoglobin/hematocrit, thrombocytopenia (rare), agranulocytosis (rare); other; malaise, fatigue, muscle weakness, aches and pains, fever, hypokalemia, hypoglycemia, elevated cholesterol/triglycerides, gynecomastia (rare), lupus.
Overdose: Treatment is similar to quinidine. Resin hemoperfusion or hemodialysis may be necessary in severe cases requiring extracorporeal circulation—especially if there is renal failure.

Supplied as: immediate release capsule (100, 150 mg);
control release capsule (100, 150 mg Norpace CR).
Dose, immediate–release capsule: Dose must be individualized.

Most adults: 150 mg q6h (range 100–200 mg q6h). Give 300 mg loading dose if rapid control of ventricular arrhythmia is necessary.

Adult weighing < 50 kg: 100 mg q6h. Give 200 mg loading dose if rapid control of ventricular arrhythmia is necessary.

Hepatic insufficiency: 100 mg q6h.

Cardiomyopathy/possible cardiac decompensation: 100 mg q6h. Do not give loading dose.

Adult in renal failure with creatinine clearance:

> 40 ml/min:	100 mg q6h,	30–40 ml/min:	100 mg q8h,
15–30 ml/min:	100 mg q12h,	< 15 ml/min:	100 mg q24h.

Pediatric dose: ●< 1 yr: 10–30 mg/kg/day   ●1–4 yr: 10–20 mg/kg/day
●4–12 yr: 10–15 mg/kg/day   ●12–18 yr: 6–15 mg/kg/day.

Note: Pediatric dose is divided q6h or according to patient needs. Hospitalization is advised initially. Liquid suspension may be prepared by dissolving entire capsules in cherry syrup NF.

Dose, control–release capsule: usual adult: 300 mg q12h,
adult under 50 kg: 200 mg q12h,

adult with renal insufficiency but with creatinine clearance > 40 ml/min: 200 mg q12h. Note: Do not use control-release form if creatinine clearance is < 40ml/min. Also, this form must not be used for initial treatment if rapid control of ventricular arrhythmia is necessary.

DOBUTAMINE (Dobutrex)

Action: Acts principally on beta–1 receptors to increase myocardial contractility. Consequently, stroke volume and therefore cardiac output is increased. At usual doses, peripheral vasoconstriction and tachycardia does not occur. Increased renal blood flow results from increased cardiac output since renal dopaminergic receptors are unaffected.

Indications: ●Short–term treatment of cardiac decompensation due to decreased contractility (e.g. severe heart failure, cardiogenic shock, cardiac surgery). ●Septic shock.

Contraindication: Idiopathic hypertrophic subaortic stenosis.

Comments: ●Monitor EKG and blood pressure. If possible, also monitor pulmonary wedge pressure and cardiac output. ●Correct hypovolemia before starting dobutamine. ●Do not mix dobutamine with strongly alkaline solutions, including 5% sodium bicarbonate injection. ●Use dopamine with caution in setting of acute myocardial infarction, pregnancy, or childhood. ●Because dobutamine facilitates AV conduction, rapid ventricular rates may ensue in patients with atrial fibrillation.

Side effects: tachycardia, hypertension, increased ventricular ectopy, angina, headache, dyspnea, nausea.

Supplied as: 20 ml vials containing 250 mg.

Dose: see appendix.

DOPAMINE (Intropin)

Action: Naturally occurring catecholamine with alpha, beta, and dopamine receptor effects. At low doses (less than 2 mcg/kg/min) renal and mesenteric blood vessels are dilated without affecting blood pressure or heart rate. At 2–10 mcg/kg/min beta receptors respond and cardiac output is increased. At 10 mcg/kg/min peripheral vasoconstriction occurs as alpha receptors respond. At 20 mcg/kg/min alpha receptor response leads to decrease in renal and mesenteric blood flow.

Indications: cardiogenic shock (e.g. due to myocardial infarction, cardiac surgery/trauma); septic shock; severe congestive heart failure refractory to other measures.

Contraindications: pheochromocytoma.

Caution: Hypovolemia: Correct hypovolemia before using dopamine. Hypovolemic shock is treated with fluids not dopamine. Tachyarrhytmias: Dopamine may induce tachyarrhythmias and thus dictate reduction of dose or discontinuation of dopamine. Patients on monoamine oxidase inhibitor drugs require no more than a tenth the usual dopamine dose.

Side effects include: nausea, vomiting, ectopy, tachyarrhythmias, palpitations, angina, dyspnea, hypotension (at low dose), hypertension, gangrene of fingers and toes (after prolonged or high–dose infusion), local tissue necrosis due to extravasation (antidote to extravasation is local infiltration of phentolamine).

Supplied as: 5 ml vial/ampule/syringe containing 200, 400, or 800 mg.

Dose: refer to appendix.

DOXYCYCLINE (Vibramycin) is a tetracycline antibiotic. Refer to tetracy-
cline for action, indications, contraindications, additional comments, side effects.

Comments: ●In contrast to tetracycline, doxycycline: (**1**) requires only once or twice daily administration, (**2**) does not require dose adjustment in renal failure (**3**) serum half-life is not affected by hemodialysis, (**4**) is well absorbed orally when given with food (although antacids and iron may interfere with absorption), (**5**) causes diarrhea less frequently, (**6**) is more expensive. ●Since doxycycline is well absorbed orally and since IV therapy may cause thrombophlebitis, the oral route is preferred whenever possible. If IV administration is necessary, switch to PO therapy as soon as possible. ●Barbiturates, phenytoin, carbamazepine stimulate hepatic metabolism and decrease half-life of doxycycline.

Supplied as: capsule (50, 100 mg);   tablet (100 mg);
            oral suspension (25 or 50 mg/5ml);   vials (100, 200 mg) for IV injection.
Note: IM or SC not recommended.

Dose (adult/child over 8 yr and > 45 kg):
Intravenous: On first day, 200 mg as single infusion or divided into 2 infusions. Then, 100–200 mg/day in 1 or 2 infusions. Doxycycline is diluted and infused over 1–4 hours.

Oral:
Usual dosage is 100 mg q12h for 2 doses, then 100 mg once daily.
Primary/secondary syphilis: 300 mg/day PO in divided doses for minimum 10 days.
Uncomplicated gonococcal infection (but not for anorectal infection in men): Choice of 100 mg PO twice daily for 7 days or single visit regimen: 300 mg, wait one hour, give second 300 mg.
Acute epididymo–orchitis (gonococcal or chlamydial): 100 mg PO twice daily for minimum 10 days.
Nongonococcal urethritis (chlamydial or U. urealyticum): 100 mg PO twice daily for minimum 7 days.
Uncomplicated urethral, endocervical, or rectal infection due to chlamydia: 100 mg PO twice daily for minimum 7 days.
Prophylaxis traveler's diarrhea due to enteropathogenic E.coli: 100 mg PO once daily.

Dose (child over 8 yr but < 45 kg):
Oral: On first day, 2.2 mg/kg in two doses. Subsequently: 2.2 mg/kg/day as single dose, or for more severe infection 4.4 mg/kg/day divided into two daily doses.
Intravenous: 4.4 mg/kg on first day followed by 2.2–4.4 mg/kg/day. Daily dose may be given as a single infusion or divided into two infusions. Doxycycline is diluted and infused over 1–4 hours.

ECONAZOLE (Spectazole)

Indications: Tinea pedis, tinea cruris, or tinea corporis due to Microsporum (M. canis, M. audouini, M. gypseum); Trichophyton (T. rubrum, T. mentagrophytes, T. tonsurans); or Epidermophyton floccosum. ●Cutaneous candidiasis. ●Tinea versicolor.
Contraindications: hypersensitivity to any of ingredients.
Comments: ●Avoid using during 1st trimester of pregnancy unless essential to patient welfare. Use in 2nd or 3rd trimester only if clearly needed. ●Use with caution in the nursing mother.
Side effects: burning, itching, stinging, erythema.
Supplied as: 1% cream in 15, 30, and 85 gram tubes.
Dose: Apply to affected skin once daily. Twice daily for cutaneous candidiasis.

ENALAPRIL (Vasotek)

Action: Enalapril thru its metabolite enalaprilat inhibits angiotensin converting enzyme, the enzyme responsible for converting angiotensin–1 to angiotensin–2 (a potent vasoconstrictor). Decreased levels of angiotensin–2 also lead to decreased aldosterone secretion with consequent small increases in serum potassium. Following a single dose, the blood pressure begins to decrease in about an hour with maximum effect in 4–6 hours.
Indications: (1) hypertension, (2) adjunct in treatment of heart failure in patients inadequately responsive to diuretics and digitalis.
Contraindications: hypersensitivity to this product.
Comments: <u>Pregnancy:</u> Use enalapril only if possible benefit justifies risk. <u>Nursing mother:</u> Use enalapril with caution. <u>Children:</u> Enalapril safety and effectiveness not established. <u>Hyperkalemia:</u> By reducing aldosterone secretion, enalpril may induce hyperkalemia. Therefore; caution is advised if potassium supplements, potassium–containing salt substitutes, or potassium-sparing diuretics must be used. <u>Angiodema</u> has sometimes occurred in patients receiving enalapril. Enalapril must be discontinued if this occurs and may be all that is required. Antihistamines may help alleviate symptoms. Subcutaneous epinephrine is necessary if airway obstruction develops or is impending as a consequence of edema of the larynx, glottis, or tongue. <u>Enalapril–induced excessive hypotension</u> is treated by lying patient down. If necessary, intravenous isotonic saline may be administered. The risk of excessive hypotension is greatest in the following settings: heart failure, high–dose diuretic therapy, recently increased diuretic dose, recent vigorous diuresis, hyponatremia, severe water or salt depletion, dialysis. <u>Neutropenia:</u> Patients must immediately report symptoms of infection (e.g. fever, sore throat) since rare instances of enalapril–associated neutropenia have been observed.
Side effects: Adverse experiences reported in > 1% patients being treated for hypertension include orthostatic effects, fatigue, asthenia, nausea, diarrhea, headache, dizziness, cough, rash. ●Additional experiences reported in > 1% heart failure patients receiving enalapril include syncope, chest pain, abdominal pain, hypotension, postural hypotension, angina, MI, vertigo, headache, dyspnea, cough, bronchitis, pneumonia. ●Other reported adverse experiences include stroke, cardiac arrest, palpitations, arrhythmias, anorexia, dyspepsia, constipation, ileus, melena, pancreatitis, hepatitis, cholestatic jaundice, glossitis, altered taste, rhinorrhea, bronchospasm, URI, renal dysfunction or failure, oliguria, itching, photosensitivity, alopecia, flushing, hyperhidrosis, impotence, muscle cramps, tinnitus, blurred vision, paresthesias, ataxia, confusion, depression, confusion, nervousness, insomnia, somnolence, angioedema, neutropenia, thrombocytopenia, bone marrow depression, small decreases in hemoglobin and hematocrit, hyperkalemia, elevated liver enzymes and serum bilirubin.
Supplied as: 2.5, 5, 10, 20 mg tablets; 2 ml vial (1.25 mg/ml) for IV injection.
Dose (adult):

<u>Hypertension:</u> Start with 5 mg PO once daily. Titrate to acceptable blood pressure. Usual range is 10–40 mg/day as a single dose or divided into 2 daily doses. ●If the patient is on a diuretic, the diuretic should if possible be discontinued before starting enalapril. If this is not possible, start with 2.5 mg PO once daily. ●When oral therapy is not practical, enalepril may be administered intravenously: 1.25 mg given over 5 minutes every 6 hours.

<u>Heart failure:</u> Start with 2.5 mg PO once daily. Following the initial dose, monitor the patient for at least 2 hours and until the blood pressure is stable for at least another hour. The usual therapeutic range is 5–20 mg/day, maximum 40 mg/day.

EPINEPHRINE (Adrenalin, Sus–Phrine)

Action: Naturally occurring catecholamine with both alpha and beta receptor stimulating properties which at the usual pharmacologic doses results in: increased heart rate (beta–1), increased contractility (beta–1), and peripheral vasoconstriction (alpha) with consequent increases in blood pressure and myocardial oxygen consumption. Bronchodilation results from relaxation of bronchial smooth muscle (beta–2) and from vasoconstriction in the bronchial mucosa (alpha).
Contraindications: relative to gravity of patients condition.
Caution: patient over 40, pulse > 140, hypertension, cardiovascular disease, cerebrovascular disease, narrow–angle glaucoma, hyperthyroidism, diabetes mellitus, pregnancy, patient receiving

monoamine oxidase inhibitor.
Comments: ●Epinephrine is potentiated by tricyclics and some antihistamines (e.g. diphenhydramine, chlorpheniramine). ●Arrhythmias may occur if epinephrine is administered during general anesthesia with halogenated hydrocarbons or cyclopropane.
Side effects: headache, anxiety, restlessness, tremor, pallor, nausea, vomiting, dizziness, weakness, palpitations, arrhythmias, angina.
Supplied as:

1:10,000 solution (1mg/10ml) for IV, endotracheal, or intracardiac administration;
1: 1000 solution (1mg/ml) for subcutaneous administration;
1: 200 suspension (5mg/ml) [Sus–Phrine] sustained–action preparation for subcutaneous administration;
racemic epinephrine 2.25% solution for nebulization.
Dose: refer to appendix.

ERGOTAMINE (Ergomar, Ergostat, Medihaler Ergotamine)
ERGOTAMINE plus CAFFEINE (Cafergot, Wigraine)

Action: ●Ergotamine constricts cranial blood vessels. ●Caffeine is also a vasoconstrictor.
Indications: prevent or abort vascular headaches. (e.g. migraine, cluster).
Contraindications: hypersensitivity to components, coronary artery disease, peripheral vascular disease, hypertension, kidney or liver disease, pregnancy, nursing mother, sepsis, malnutrition.
Caution: High doses or prolonged use may cause severe vasoconstriction and gangrene of extremities.
Side effects: nausea, vomiting, diarrhea, epigastric distress, tachycardia, bradycardia, itching, localized edema. Vasoconstrictive phenomena include: pulselessness, weakness, myalgia, paresthesias of limbs, chest pain/distress.

Cafergot
Supplied as: Cafergot or Wigraine tablet (1mg ergotamine plus 100mg caffeine)
           Cafergot suppository (2mg ergotamine plus 100mg caffeine).
Oral dose (adult): Two tablets at first sign attack. One additional tablet every half hour as needed. Maximum 6 tablets/attack, 10 tablets/week.
Rectal dose (adult): One suppository at first sign attack. If necessary, one additional suppository in one hr. Maximum 2 suppositories/attack, 5 suppositories/week

Ergomar, Ergostat   Supplied as: 2 mg sublingual tablet.
Dose (adult): 1 tablet sublingual at first sign attack followed by 1 additional tablet sublingual at half hour intervals up to maximum 3 tablets/attack.
Maximum 3 tablets/24 hr or 5 tablets/week.

Medihaler Ergotamine   Supplied as: aerosol (0.36 mg ergotamine/inhalation).
Dose (adult): 1 inhalation at first sign of attack. Repeat inhalation as needed. Wait at least 5 minutes between each inhalation.
Maximum 6 inhalations/24hr or 15 inhalations/week.

ERYTHROMYCIN (E–mycin, Eryc, Ery–Tab, Ilotycin).
ERYTHROMYCIN ETHYL SUCCINATE (E.E.S., Ery–Ped, Pediamycin, Wyamycin E)
ERYTHROMYCIN ESTOLATE (Ilosone)
ERYTHROMYCIN STEARATE (Erythrocin Stearate, Wyamycin S)
ERYTHROMYCIN GLUCEPTATE (Ilotycin Gluceptate)
ERYTHROMYCIN LACTOBIONATE (Erythrocin Lactobionate)

Action: Macrolide antibiotic. Inhibits bacterial protein synthesis by binding to 50s ribosome.
Spectrum: streptococci (e.g. S. pneumoniae, S. pyogenes, S. viridans, some S. faecalis); many staphylococci; gram–positive bacilli (Listeria monocytogenes, Clostridium tetani, Clostridium welchii, diptheria); gram–negative bacteria (Brucella, yersinia, neisseria, campylobacter); other (syphilis, Legionella, Mycoplasma pneumonia, Actinomyces israeli, chlamydia, Ureaplasma urealyticum rickettsiae). Resistant organisms include: some Staph aureus; some Staph epidermidis; some H influenza; Bacteroides fragilis; most aerobic gram–negative bacilli (e.g. Pseudomonas, E coli, Proteus), some Nocardia.
Indications include: Legionnaire's disease, Mycoplasma pneumoniae, B. pertussis, Chlamydia trachomatis. ●Alternative antibiotic in penicillin–allergic patient with infection by streptococci (e.g. S. pneumoniae, S. pyogenes); or anthrax. ●Because tetracyclines are contraindicated in pregnancy, erythromycin is an alternative treatment for syphilis or gonorrhea in penicillin–allergic pregnant patient.
Contraindications: erythromycin hypersensitivity, history of liver disease (erythromycin estolate).

Caution: pregnancy, hepatic dysfunction (erythromycin is metabolized by the liver). ●Patient on theophylline who takes erythromycin may have to reduce theophylline dosage because erythromycin may cause the serum theophylline level to rise.

Side effects: nausea; vomiting; diarrhea; cholestatic jaundice (most frequently with erythromycin estolate); hypersensitivity (rash, urticaria, anaphylaxis); phlebitis with IV administration.

Supplied as:

erythromycin:	capsule (250 mg);	tablet (250, 333, 500 mg);
erythromycin estolate:	capsule (250 mg);	tablet (125, 250, 500 mg);
	oral suspension (125, 250 ml);	pediatric drops (100 mg/ml).

erythromycin ethyl succinate: tablet (200, 400 mg); oral susp. (200, 400 mg/5ml).
erythromycin stearate: 250, 500 mg tablet;
erythromycin gluceptate and erythromycin lactobionate for IV administration.

Oral dose:
- ●Adult: 250–500 mg q6h. Up to 1000 mg q6h for serious infections including Legionella.
- ●Child: 30–50 mg/kg/day divided q6h. Maximum 4 gram/day.

Note: The total daily PO dose may be divided q8–12h if desired.

Intravenous dose (adult or child): 15–20 mg/kg/day by continuous infusion preferably or in divided doses q4–6h. Higher doses may be administered in very severe infection. Maximum 4 gram/day.

ESTROGENS, CONJUGATED U.S.P. (Premarin)

This product is derived from natural sources and is similar in composition to the estrogen sulfates (mostly estrone and equilin) found in the urine of pregnant mares.

Contraindications: pregnancy; breast cancer (except in selected patients with metastatic disease); estrogen–dependent neoplasia; undiagnosed abnormal vaginal bleeding; active thrombophlebitis or thromboembolism. Unless the patient is being treated for breast or prostatic cancer, estrogen therapy is also contraindicated if past estrogen administration has been associated with thrombophlebitis, thrombosis, or thromboembolism.

Caution: liver dysfunction; history of jaundice during pregnancy; hypercalcemia–associated metabolic bone disease; child/adolescent (estrogen therapy may impair bone growth); conditions that may be adversely affected by fluid retention (e.g. cardiac/renal dysfunction, migraine, epilepsy, asthma); uterine fibroids.

Comments: Perform pretreatment and periodic physical exam which includes blood pressure check, breast/abdominal/pelvic exam, and pap smear.

Side effects: refer to "Oral Contraceptives".

Supplied as: ●tablet (0.3, 0.625, 0.9, 1.25, 2.5 mg);
- ●vaginal cream (0.625 mg conjugated estrogens/gram) in 42.5 gram tube;
- ● vial containing 25 mg for IV or IM injection.

Oral dose:

Menopausal symptoms (e.g. vasomotor symptoms, atrophic vaginitis, kraurosis vulvae): give just enough to provide symptomatic relief but not so much as to cause recurrence of menses. As a rule, patients in early menopause require less since the ovary may still be producing some estrogens. The usual range is 0.625–1.25 mg PO once daily given cyclically (e.g. 3 wk on and 1 wk off). During the last 7 days of estrogen administration it is common practice to give medroxyprogesterone acetate (Provera) 10mg PO once daily along with the estrogen. Neither estrogen nor progestin is given during the 4th week and then the cycle is begun again.

Osteoporosis (to retard progression): same regimen as above.

Replacement therapy in female castration and primary ovarian failure: 0.625–1.25 mg PO once daily for first thru 25th day of each month. Medroxyprogesterone acetate (Provera) 10 mg PO once daily is added from 16th to 25th day of each month.

Inoperable progressing breast cancer in postmenopausal women and selected men: 10 mg PO tid for at least 3 months.

Inoperable progressing prostatic cancer: 1.25–2.5 mg PO tid. Therapeutic effect is gauged by symptomatic response and serum acid phosphatase.

Dysfunctional uterine bleeding due to atrophic or denuded endometrium: 7–10 day regimen consisting of once daily PO administration of 2.5–3.75 mg conjugated estrogens plus 10 mg medroxyprogesterone acetate (Provera). Bleeding should stop and then be followed by withdrawal bleeding which may be heavy. A combination oral contraceptive is then begun and is usually continued for 1 year.

Intravenous dose (emergency treatment of dysfunctional uterine bleeding due to atrophic or denuded endometrium): 25 mg IV q4h for 3 doses. Subsequently, start oral therapy as outlined above for this condition.

Vaginal dose (atrophic vaginitis and kraurosis vulvae): 2–4 gram (1/2 to 1 applicatorful) per day intravaginally or topically, 3 wk on 1 wk off. Try to taper or discontinue therapy at 3–6 month intervals.

ETHAMBUTOL (Myambutol)

Action/indications: Bacteriostatic. Inhibits metabolism of mycobacteria including M. tuberculosis, M. bovis, some M. kansasii.
Contraindications: ethambutol hypersensitivity, optic neuritis.
Caution/comments: ●pregnancy. ●Not recommended in patient less than 13 years of age. ●To preclude emergence of resistant strains, concurrent adminstration of at least one other antituberculous drug is mandatory. Common regimens are isoniazid + ethanbutol and isoniazid + ethambutol + streptomycin. ●In retreatment regimens, combine ethambutol with another drug not previously used to which there is demonstrated in vitro sensitivity. ●Patient should report any changes in vision. Periodically check visual acuity. Optic neuritis is most likely to occur in patient with decreased renal function or in patient receiving prolonged high–dose therapy. Monthly checks of fundus, color discrimination, and perimetry are advised. ●Periodically check blood count, and renal and liver function when therapy prolonged. ●In renal failure, reduce dose as indicated by serum ethambutol measurements.
Side effects: optic neuritis (e.g. decreased visual acuity, decreased visual field, altered color vision); peripheral neuritis (numbness/tingling extremities); headache; dizziness; confusion; anorexia, nausea; vomiting; abdominal pain; fever; dermatitis; itching; arthritis; anaphylactoid reactions; elevated serum uric acid; abnormal liver function tests.
Supplied as: 100, 400 mg tablet.
Dose:
No prior antituberculous treatment: 15 mg/kg as single daily dose.
Retreatment: 25 mg/kg as single daily dose. Decrease to 15 mg/kg after 60 days.

ETHOSUXIMIDE (Zarontin)

Action: Suppresses the paroxysmal 3 cycle/second spike and wave EEG pattern that is associated with lapses of consciousness in petit mal epilepsy.
Indication: absence (petit mal) epilepsy.
Contraindication: hypersensitivity to succinimides.
Caution: pregnancy, nursing mothers, liver or renal disease.
Comments: ●Because of possibility of blood dyscrasias, periodic blood counts are advised. ●Periodic urinalysis and liver function tests are also advised. ●Because ethosuximide may be sedating, it should be used cautiously in patients who engage in dangerous activities that require alertness. ●Ethosuximide may be used with other anticonvulsants if petit mal epilepsy is accompanied by other types of epilepsy. Ethosuximide as the sole anticonvulsant may in some cases actually lead to an increase in grand mal seizures in a patient with mixed seizure disorder.
Side effects include: GI: anorexia, stomach upset, nausea, vomiting, diarrhea, abdominal pain, weight loss; neurologic: sleepiness, lethargy, fatigue, headache, dizziness, hiccough, incoordination, impaired concentration, sleep disturbances, irritability, euphoria, hyperactivity, aggressiveness; blood: leukopenia, agranulocytosis, thrombocytopenia, pancytopenia, aplastic anemia, eosinophilia; skin: urticaria, itchy rash, Stevens–Johnson syndrome, lupus; other: gum hypertrophy, swollen tongue, hirsutism, vaginal bleeding, myopia.
Supplied as: 250 mg capsule, 250 mg/5 ml syrup.
Dose adult or child > 6 yr: 500 mg/day initially. Increase daily dose by 250 mg every 4–7 days until there is adequate control of seizures or unacceptable side effects develop. Optimum dose for children is usually 20 mg/kg/day. Adjust dose according to response and serum therapeutic range of 40–100 mcg/ml. Doses greater than 1000 mg/day seldom enhance efficacy and dosages greater than 1500 mg/day must be cautiously administered in divided doses with careful physician monitoring.
Dose child 3–6 yr: 250 mg/day intially. Increase daily dose as needed as outlined above.

FERROUS SULFATE, FERROUS FUMARATE, FERROUS GLUCONATE

Indications: •treatment of iron deficiency anemia •prevention of iron deficiency anemia in patient with increased requirements (e.g. pregnancy, lactation, heavy menses, child receiving iron-deficient diet). <u>Note:</u> Iron is avidly retained by the body. Therefore, under normal circumstances, iron supplements are not advised in men or postmenopausal women. In any case, prolonged supplementation is not advised unless there is chronic blood loss or persistently increased requirements. Iron overload and possible hemosiderosis may occur—especially in patients who absorb increased amounts of iron (e.g thalassemia, chronic hemolysis, sideroachrestic anemia, Laennec's cirrhosis).

Contraindications: anemia other than iron deficiency anemia.

Comments •Iron salts are best absorbed on an empty stomach. They may be taken with food if GI upset occurs. However, they should not be taken with antacids since they will markedly impair iron absorption. Ferrous gluconate or fumarate may be better tolerated than ferrous sulfate. •Avoid enteric-coated or time-release pills because iron absorption is not reliable. •Obtain baseline hemoglobin, hematocrit, and reticulocyte count before initiating treatment of iron deficiency anemia. Reticylocyte count should rise in one week followed by a gradually increasing hemoglobin after 2 weeks. •Iron salts may interfere with absorption of tetracycline. Allow a 2 hour interval to elapse between their administration.

Side effects: nausea; vomiting; diarrhea; constipation; black stools; heartburn; abdominal cramps; exacerbation of GI disease (e.g. peptic ulcer, inflammatory bowel disease).

Overdose: •Young children are especially susceptible to toxicity. Manifestations may include nausea, vomiting, shock, gastric necrosis, hepatic necrosis. •Toxicity may occur if > 20 mg/kg of elemental iron has been ingested. Ingestion of > 60 mg/kg may be lethal. •Lavage or induce emesis. •Sodium bicarbonate is then administered PO in order to form nonabsorbable iron salts Before administration, dilute standard sodium bicarbonate ampuls 1: 4 in normal saline. •Chelation therapy with deferoxamine is indicated if the patient is in shock or if the serum iron level 3–6 hours following ingestion is > 500 mcg/dl.

Supplied as (amount of elemental iron is in parenthesis):
<u>Ferrous sulfate</u>: •pills,   100 (20)mg, 195 (39)mg, 300 (60)mg, 325 (65)mg
             •elixir,   300 (60) mg/5ml, 220 (44) mg/5ml, 90 (18) mg/5ml
             •pediatric drops, 75 (15) mg/0.6 ml .
<u>Ferrous fumarate</u>: •pills, 100 (33)mg, 325 (108)mg;
              •suspension, 100 (33) mg/5ml;
              •pediatric drops, 45 (15)/0.6ml.
<u>Ferrous gluconate</u>: •pills, 435 (50)mg, 320 (37) mg;
              •elixir, 300 (35) mg/5ml.

Treatment iron deficiency anemia (to replenish iron stores).
Treatment is continued for 4–6 months after hemoglobin returns to normal.
<u>Adult</u>: 50–100 mg elemental iron PO 3 times a day.
     (e.g. 300 mg ferrous sulfate supplies 60 mg elemental iron).
<u>Pediatric</u>: 2 mg elemental iron/kg PO 3 times a day.
Prevention iron deficiency:
<u>Pregnancy</u>: 30–60 mg/day elemental iron (e.g. 150–300 mg/day ferrous sulfate).
<u>Lactation</u>: 25 mg/day elemental iron.
<u>Menstruating female</u>: 20 mg/day elemental iron (more if menses heavy).
<u>Infant—10 yr</u>: 1 mg/kg/day elemental iron (up to 15 mg/day).
<u>Adolescent</u>: 20 mg/day elemental iron.

FLECAINIDE (Tambocor)

Action: Automaticity is decreased in the ventricles and sinus node. Conduction is slowed thru the atrium, AV node, His–Purkinje system, and ventricular tissue. The PR, QRS, and QT intervals are increased. Left ventricular function is depressed.

Indicatons: suppression of life-threatening ventricular arrhythmias.

Contraindications: hypersensitivity to drug, cardiogenic shock, 2nd or 3rd degree AV block (unless artificial pacemaker present), bifascicular block (unless artificial pacemaker present).

Caution: sick sinus syndrome, patient with pacemaker, history of congestive heart failure or myocardial dysfunction, complex arrhythmias, sustained ventricular tachycardia, liver dysfunction, concurrent administration with negative inotropes (e.g. beta blocker, verapamil, disopyramide); concurrent administration of amiodarone; pregnancy.

Side effects: <u>cardiovascular</u> (dizziness, lightheadedness, faintness, near syncope, palpitation, chest pain, new or worsening CHF, edema, dyspnea, new or worsening ventricular arrhythmias, unresuscitatable ventricular tachycardia or ventricular fibrillation, 2nd or 3rd degree AV block, sinus bradycardia, sinus pause, sinus arrest, tachycardia, angina, hypertension, hypotension); <u>gastrointestinal</u> (nausea, constipation, abdominal pain, vomiting, diarrhea, dyspepsia, anorexia, flatulence); <u>neurologic</u> (headache, tremor, somnolence, vertigo, tinnitus, syncope, paresthesias, hypoesthesia, paresis, ataxia, impaired speech, twitching, seizures, stupor, flushing, impotence, increased sweating, altered taste, dry mouth); psychiatric (anxiety, depression, confusion, amnesia, apathy, decreased libido, euphoria, morbid dreams, depersonalization); eyes (visual disturbances, eye pain/irritation, photophobia, nystagmus); skin (rash, itching, urticaria, exfoliative dermatitis); urinary system (polyuria, urinary retention); other (fatigue, asthenia, malaise, fever, swollen lips/mouth/tongue, bronchospasm, arthralgia, myalgia).

Supplied as: 50, 100, 150 mg tablet.

Dose: Start with 100 mg q12h. If necessary, increase the dose by 50mg bid every 4 days. Maximum 200 mg q12h. Dose titration in patient with renal failure should be guided by serum level determinations.

FLUOXETINE (Prozac)

Action: Antidepressant action is presumably due to the drug's inhibition of serotonin uptake by neurons of the CNS.

Indication: major depression.

Contraindications: hypersensitivity to the fluoxetine.

Comments: ●Discontinue fluoxetine if rash, urticaria, respiratory distress, or other possibly allergic incident occurs that cannot be attributed to another cause. ●Because depressed patients are at increased risk for suicide, try to minimize the chance of overdose by prescribing no more than is sufficient for effective patient management. ●The dosage of insulin or oral hypoglycemic drug may need to to be adjusted if fluoxetine is administered concurrently. ●Avoid concurrent administration with MAO inhibitor. ●Caution is advised if certain other drugs are taken concurrently with fluoxetine: tryptophan, lithium (monitor lithium level), other anti-depressants, diazepam, or other CNS-active drugs, coumadin. ●Because fluoxetine may impair motor function, judgment, or thinking; patients should be warned to avoid hazardous activities such as driving until the effects of the drug are known. ●Unless there is a clear need, fluoxetine should not be used in pregnancy. ●Since fluoxetine and metabolites are excreted in milk, the drug should be administered with caution to nursing women. ●Safety and efficacy in children not established.

Side effects: The most common side effects not occuring at equivalent incidence in patients receiving placebo are anxiety, nervousness, insomnia, drowsiness, fatigue, asthenia, tremor, dizziness, lightheadedness, sweating, anorexia, nausea, diarrhea.

Supplied as: 20mg pulvule.

Dose: Start with a single 20mg dose each morning. The daily dose should be divided bid (i.e. morning and noon) if more than 20mg/day is required. It may take 4 weeks before the full anti-depressant effect is realized. Do not exceed 80mg/day. Dosage may need to be reduced if there is liver or renal impairment, in the elderly, in those with concurrent disease, or in those on multiple medications.

FUROSEMIDE (Lasix)

Action: Potent diuretic. Inhibits sodium and chloride reabsorption—primarily in ascending loop of Henle, but also in proximal and distal tubules. Excretion of potassium, calcium, magnesium, bicarbonate is also increased.

Indications: ●acute pulmonary edema ●edema that is associated with congestive heart failure, liver cirrhosis, or renal disease (including nephrotic syndrome) ●hypertension ●hyperkalemia ●hypercalcemia.

Contraindications: furosemide hypersensitivity, anuria, pregnancy (except for life-threatening situations), nursing mother, hepatic coma, concurrent lithium administration, concurrent cephaloridine administration, concomitant administration of ethacrynic acid.

Caution/comments: Onset/peak/duration of action; Intravenous onset of action within 5 min, peak within 1/2 hr, duration 2 hr. Oral onset of action within 1 hr, peak 1–2 hr, duration 6–8 hr. Monitor electrolytes frequently when patient is undergoing rapid diuresis, and periodically if patient is on chronic therapy. Potassium chloride supplements may be administered to prevent hypokalemia. Overly aggressive diuresis may precipitate shock in patient with pulmonary edema and hypotension secondary to myocardial infarction. Aggressive diuresis may precipitate hypotension in patient with acute pulmonary edema who is not volume overloaded. Cirrhosis; Treat cirrhotic edema/ascites very cautiously since abrupt changes in plasma volume and electrolytes may precipitate shock and/or hepatic coma. Treatment of these patients is usually initiated with a potassium-sparing diuretic (e.g. spironolactone), and furosemide or a thiazide diuretic is added cautiously if diuresis is inadequate. Caution: severe renal disease, diabetes mellitus, gout, lupus. Concurrent administration with certain drugs: Use furosemide cautiously in patient receiving indomethacin, digitalis, high-dose salicylates, aminoglycosides (furosemide may potentiate ototoxic effects), other antihypertensive medications, corticosteroids.

Side effects include: Consequences of excessive diuresis: dehydration, reduced blood volume, hypotension, shock, thrombosis, embolism, hyponatremia, hypokalemia, hypocalcemia, hypochloremic alkalosis; gastrointestinal; anorexia, nausea, vomiting, diarrhea, constipation, cramping, jaundice, pancreatitis; neurologic; dizziness, vertigo, tinnitus, deafness, headache, blurred vision, paresthesias, restlessness; blood; anemia, leukopenia, thrombocytopenia, agranulocytosis; hypersensitivity/skin; rash, itching, urticaria, photosensitivity, erythema multiforme, exfoliative dermati-

tis, angitis; _other;_ weakness, muscle spasm, hyperglycemia, hyperuricemia.
Supplied as: tablet (20, 40, 80 mg); oral solution (10 mg/ml); injection (10 mg/ml).

Adult dose:

Acute pulmonary edema (adjunct to oxygen, morphine, etc.); 40 mg IV over 1–2 minutes. If adequate diuresis has not occurred within an hour, give additional 80 mg IV over 1–2 minutes.

Edema:

●Oral: 20–80 mg. Repeat as needed in 6–8 hours. If the initial dose does not induce adequate diuresis, the dose may be increased by 20–40 mg increments, Wait at least 6–8 hours between doses. The maximum allowable daily dose is 600 mg. The smallest effective dose is given once daily or is divided into 2 daily doses. Alternate day or 2–4 consecutive days/wk dosing is recommended.

●IV/IM (when oral route not feasible): 20–40 mg IM or IV over 1–2 minutes. Repeat as needed in 2 hours. If the initial dose does not induce adequate diuresis, the dose may be increased by 20 mg increments. Wait at least 2 hours between doses. The smallest effective dose is given once daily or is divided into 2 daily doses.

Hypertension:

●Oral: 40 mg twice daily initially. Adjust to smallest effective dose. Up to 600 mg/day may be required in setting of renal insufficiency. NOTE: (1) Reserve oral furosemide for treatment of chronic hypertension with creatinine clearance less than 30 ml/min. (2) Hypertension that cannot be controlled with thiazides will probably not respond to furosemide alone.

●Intravenous (adjunct in hypertensive emergency): 40–80 mg IV over 1–2 minutes.

Hypercalcemia (preceded by and concurrent with IV isotonic normal saline to maintain adequate extracellular fluid volume): 80–100 mg IV q1–2h in severe hypercalcemia; smaller doses q2–4h in less urgent cases.

Pediatric dose:

Intravenous/intramuscular (when prompt diuresis required): 1 mg/kg. If the initial dose does not induce adequate diuresis, the dose may be increased by 1mg/kg increments. Wait at least 2 hours between doses. Maximum dose 6 mg/kg. The smallest effective dose is given once daily or is divided into 2 doses.

Oral: 2 mg/kg. Repeat as needed in 6–8 hours. If the initial dose does not induce adequate diuresis, the dose may be increased by 1–2 mg/kg increments. Wait at least 6–8 hours between doses. Maximum dose is 6 mg/kg. Use smallest effective maintenance dose.

GLUCAGON

GLUCAGON

Action: Naturally occurring hormone produced by alpha cells of pancreatic islets. Raises blood glucose by promoting breakdown of hepatic glycogen.
Indication: severe hypoglycemia in comatose patient when IV dextrose cannot be administered.
Supplied as: vial for IV, IM, or SC injection.
Dose (adult or child): 0.5–1.0 mg SC or IM as needed at 15–20 min intervals x 2–3.
Comments: ●Response time is 5–20 minutes. ●Glucagon is not effective when liver glycogen is depleted (e.g. starvation, chronic hypoglycemia, adrenal insufficiency). ●Juvenile–onset diabetics generally do not respond as well as adult–onset diabetics. ●Glucagon by releasing catecholamines may exacerbate hypertension in patient with pheochromocytoma. ●Glucagon by promoting hyperglycemia may stimulate insulin release and result in rebound hypoglycemia in patient with insulinoma.

GRISEOFULVIN

Microcrystalline form (Fulvicin–U/F, Grifulvin V, Grisactin).
Ultramicrocrystalline form (Fulvicin P/G, Gris–PEG, Grisactin Ultra).
Action/Indications: Griseofulvin incorporates into the skin, hair, and nails where it exerts a fungistatic effect by inhibiting mitosis of dermatophytes of the species Epidermophyton, Microsporum, Trichophyton. It is of no value against bacteria or other genera of fungi (e.g. Candidiasis, tinea versicolor, histoplastmosis, coccidioidomycosis, cryptococcosis, sporotrichosis, etc). It is not recommended in minor dermatophytic infections responsive to topical agents alone. It is indicated for infections of the scalp, beard, nails, palms, soles, or widespread skin infections by susceptible fungi.
Contraindications: griseofulvin hypersensitivity, porphyria, hepatic failure, pregnancy.
Comments: ●Duration of treatment is a function of the time needed for infected skin, hair, or nails to grow out. Tinea corporis is treated for 2–4 wk, tinea capitis 4–6 wk, tinea pedis 4–8 wk, fingernails at least 4 months, toenails 6–15 months or longer. Nail infections may be resistant. ●Concurrent application of topical antifungal agents (e.g. miconazole) is usually required for effective treatment and prevention of recurrences, particularly when treating tinea pedis. ●Periodic tests: Periodically obtain CBC, liver and renal function tests if patient is on prolonged therapy. ●Drug interactions: Griseofulvin by inducing hepatic enzymes decreases the activity of warfarin–type anticoagulants; adjust anticoagulant dose accordingly. Phenobarbital decreases the activity of griseofulvin; griseofulvin dose increase may be required. ●Avoid undue exposure to sunlight.
Side effects include: hypersensitivity (rash, urticaria, angioedema, photosensitivity); neurologic (headache, dizziness, fatigue, confusion, insomnia, paresthesias); GI (nausea, vomiting, diarrhea, epigastric distress, thrush); other (liver toxiciy, proteinuria, leukopenia).
Supplied as:
Microcrystalline form: tablet (125, 250, 500 mg);   capsule (125, 250 mg);
                        oral suspension (125 mg/5 ml).
Ultramicrocrystalline form: 125, 165, 250, 330 mg tablets.

Dose of microcrystalline form:
  Adult: 500 mg PO once daily (1gram once daily for tinea pedis or tinea unguium).
  Child 2 yr or older: approximately 2.3 mg/kg (5 mg/lb) PO once daily.
  Dose not established for child under 2 years of age..
Dose of ultramicrocrystalline form: Use 2/3 of dose of microcrystalline form.

GUANETHIDINE (Ismelin)

Action: Guanethidine is transported into adrenergic neurons causing: (1) adrenergic blockade (2) catecholamine release and depletion.
Indication: moderate to severe essential hypertension; renal hypertension (e.g. hypertension due to renal artery stenosis, renal amyloidosis). NOTE: Use of this drug is generally reserved for treatment of severe hypertension not amenable to the usual combination antihypertensive drug regimens. It is usually added to multiple drug regimens already in place. In particular, concurrent therapy with a diuretic (e.g. thiazide) is recommended both to potentiate the antihypertensive effect of guanethidine, and to prevent guanethidine–induced sodium and fluid retention.
Contraindications: guanethidine hypersensitivity, pheochromocytoma, severe heart failure, concurrent MAO inhibitor therapy (or within 1 week of discontinuation). Use guanethidine in pregnancy only if essential.
Caution/comments: Postural hypotension; Warn patient of postural hypotension—e.g. avoid abrupt or prolonged standing. Postural hypotension may be aggravated by exercise, hot weather, fever, alcohol. Surgery: Discontinue guanethidine 2 weeks before surgery if feasible. If emergency surgery is necessary, reduce dose of pre–anesthetics and anesthetics, and use vasopressors with great caution. Caution: peptic ulcer disease, cartiac failure, coronary artery disease, recent myocardial infarction, cerebrovascular disease, severe renal disease, bronchial asthma. Drug in-

teractions: Following drugs may oppose antihypertensive effect of guanethidine: sympathomimetics (e.g. amphetamines, ephedrine); methylphenidate; tricyclic antidepressants; phenothiazines; MAO inhibitors; oral contraceptives. Concurrent reserpine therapy may cause undue mental depression, bradycardia, and/or orthostatic hypotension.

Side effects: Common side effects: (**1**) effects secondary to sympathetic blockade: postural or exertional hypotension (manifests as dizziness, weakness, syncope); interference with ejaculation; (**2**) effects secondary to unopposed parasympathetic action (e.g. bradycardia, diarrhea); (**3**) sodium and fluid retention unless patient is also on a diuretic. Other side effects: fatigue, depression, tremor, ptosis, blurred vision, nocturia, urinary incontinence, nausea, vomiting, dry mouth, parotid gland tenderness, nasal congestion, dyspnea, asthma, dermatitis, hair loss, myalgia, angina, weight gain.

Supplied as: 10, 25 mg tablet.

Adult dose:

  Ambulatory patient: 10 mg PO once daily. Increase dose as needed at 5–7 day intervals (usual requirement is 25–50 mg once daily). In assessing the drug's effect on blood pressure; take blood pressure supine, after standing 10 minutes, and if possible immediately following mild exercise. Decrease dose if the supine blood pressure is normal, if there is an exessive fall in blood pressure when standing, or if there is severe diarrhea. Increase dose only if the standing blood pressure is not less than a prior measurement of standing blood pressure.

  Hospitalized patient: 25–50 mg PO once daily. Increase as needed by 25–50 mg increments daily or every other day. Check standing blood pressure regularly if feasible and especially prior to discharge.

Pediatric dose: 0.2 mg/kg/day. Increase dose at 7–10 day intervals as needed.

HEPARIN SODIUM

Action: Inhibits several steps of the coagulation cascade thereby leading to prolongation of partial thromboplastin time, thrombin time, and clotting time. The prothrombin time is generally not prolonged with continuous IV infusion. Heparin prevents formation or extension of a clot but has no effect on established clots.

Indications: To prevent further clotting in the following circumstances: deep venous thrombosis, pulmonary thromboembolism, atrial fibrillation with thromboembolism, coronary occlusion–associated acute myocardial infarction (as adjunctive measure), peripheral arterial thromboembolism (as adjunctive measure), thrombotic stroke in evolution, disseminated intravascular coagulation. To prevent clotting during open heart surgery with extracorporeal circulation, and during hemodialysis. Low–dose heparin for the prevention of deep venous thrombosis and pulmonary thromboembolism in the following situations: post myocardial infarction, sedentary or bedridden patient, patient over 40 undergoing major abdominal or thoracic surgery.

Contraindications: same as warfarin.

Caution: hepatic or renal disease, women over 60, pregnancy, immediately postpartum, concurrent administration of medications that inhibit platelet aggregation (e.g. aspirin, indomethacin).

Comments: Measurement of prothrombin time: With continuous IV heparin, the PT is little affected. However, intermittent IV or SC heparin prolongs the prothrombin time (PT). To obtain a valid PT (which is necessary to monitor warfarin therapy) in a patient receiving intermittent IV or SC heparin, wait at least 5 hours after the last IV dose or 24 hours after the last SC dose. Treatment of bleeding due to heparin therapy: Half–life of heparin is short (heparin will normally disappear from the patient's plasma in 4 hr) so just stopping heparin usually suffices. In urgent situations, the antidote is protamine sulfate (1mg of 1% protamine sulfate IV will neutralize each 100 unit of heparin). If heparin is being given by continuous IV infusion, the assumption is that half of the preceding hourly dose of heparin has disappeared (e.g. patient on 1000 unit heparin/hr is given enough protamine sulfate to neutralize 500 unit heparin—i.e. 5 mg protamine sulfate). If the patient is receiving intermittent IV injections and has just received a heparin bolus, 1mg protamine is needed to neutralize each 100 unit of that bolus while 0.5 mg protamine/100 unit heparin given will suffice if the bolus was injected 30 minutes ago. Administer protamine sulfate intravenously (no faster than 5 mg/min, maximum of 50 mg per dose). Assess PTT immediately after giving protamine. Pregnancy: Although heparin does not cross the placenta, there is an increased risk of maternal hemorrhage, stillbirth, and prematurity. Breast feeding is safe because heparin is not excreted in milk. Following conditions may increase heparin requirements: certain clinical states (fever, thrombosis, thrombophlebitis, myocardial infarction, cancer); certain drugs (digitalis, tetracyclines, antihistamines).

Side effects: blood (bleeding; thrombocytopenia); subcutaneous injection site complications (ecchymoses, hematoma, irritation, skin necrosis); hypersensitivity (fever, chills, urticaria, rhinitis, asthma, anaphylactoid reaction); consequences of prolonged therapy (osteoporosis, bone pain, myalgia); other (alopecia, priapism, elevated serum transaminases, suppression aldosterone synthesis, rebound hyperlipidemia on cessation of heparin).

Adult dose (administer IV or SC; *avoid IM injection*):

Continuous IV infusion (the preferred method): Undiluted 5000 unit initial IV bolus via established IV line. Then dilute 20,000 unit in 1 liter of D5W or normal saline and start continuous IV infusion at 1000 unit/hr (50 ml/hr). Adjust rate of infusion so that the PTT is 1.5-2.5 times the control. Obtain PTT every 4 hours initially, and daily once a steady state is achieved. Continuous IV infusion is the preferred method of administering heparin because bleeding complications are fewer and the PT (which is necessary to monitor warfarin therapy) is little affected by heparin. The transition to oral anticoagulation therapy is thus facilitated.

Intermittent IV injection: 5,000–10,000 unit IV bolus every 4 hours. In the early stages of heparin therapy, the PTT is measured just before each injection and the heparin dose is adjusted so that PTT is 1.5-2.5 x control.

Deep subcutaneous intrafat injection (using a 25 gauge needle and using different site for each injection): 8,000–12,000 unit at 8 hr intervals, or 15,000–20,000 unit at 12 hr intervals. In the early stages of therapy, the PTT is measured just before each injection and the heparin dose adjusted so that PTT is 1.5-2.5 x control.

Dose child/infant:

Continuous IV infusion: 50 ml/kg initial IV bolus followed by 20 unit/kg/hr continuous IV infusion. Adjust rate of infusion to achieve PTT 1.5-2.5 x control as in adult.

Intermittent IV injection: 50 unit/kg initial IV bolus followed by 50–100 unit IV bolus at 4 hour intervals with dose adjustments according to PTT as in adult.

Minidose for prevention of deep venous thrombosis and pulmonary embolism: 5000 unit SC every 12 hours until patient is fully ambulatory or leaves the hospital. In patients about to undergo major surgery, the first dose is given 2 hours prior to surgery. With low–dose heparin, ongoing monitoring of PTT or clotting time in not necessary if the patient has a normal coagulation profile.

HETASTARCH (Hespan)

Action: Hetastarch (hydroxyethylstarch) expands the plasma volume by exerting a colloid osmotic pressure about equal to human albumin.
Indications: adjunct in restoration of plasma volume in patient in shock due to hemorrhage, sepsis, or burns. Hetastarch is not a blood or plasma substitute.
Contraindications: severe bleeding disorders, severe congestive heart failure, severe renal failure with anuria or oliguria.
Caution: renal insufficiency, history of liver disease, pregnancy, patient at risk for congestive heart failure or pulmonary edema.
Comments: ●Large volumes may alter coagulation with prolongation of prothrombin time, partial thromboplastin time, clotting time, and possibly bleeding time. ●By a dilutional effect, large volumes may decrease the hematocrit and plasma protein concentrations.
Side effects: vomiting; mild fever; chills; itching; salivary gland enlargement; flu–like symtoms; headache; myalgias; leg edema; anaphylactoid reactions.
Dose (adult): Total dose and rate of IV infusion depends on the extent of plasma volume depletion. The usual dose is 500–1000 ml IV. The typical 70 kg patient does not usually receive more than 1500 ml or 20 ml/kg. However, larger doses may be needed in severe hypovolemic shock. The rate of infusion in severe hemorrhagic shock may approach 20 ml/kg/hr.

HYDRALAZINE (Apresoline)

Action: Directly relaxes arteriolar smooth muscle, and the smooth muscle of veins to a lesser extent. The consequent vasodilation causes the blood pressure to fall. In the absence of concurrent beta–blocker therapy, there is a reflex increase in heart rate and stroke volume. Consequently, cardiac output and myocardial oxygen consumption are increased. In the absence of a diuretic, sodium and water retention occurs. Renal, cerebral, coronary, splanchnic, and uterine blood flow generally increase.
Indications: ●Essential hypertension. Hydralazine is not a drug of intial choice in the treatment of chronic essential hypertension. It is usually added to a diuretic and a beta–blocker when additional antihypertensive effect is required. ●Parenteral hydralazine may be used in hypertensive emergencies (e.g. malignant hypertension, preeclampsia/eclampsia–associated hypertension).
Contraindications: hydralazine hypersensitivity, coronary artery disease, rheumatic mitral valve disease, dissecting aortic aneurysm.
Caution: cerebrovascular disease, renal disease, concurrent MAO inhibitor administration, pregnancy, nursing mother.
Comments: Onset/peak/duration of action: Intravenous onset/peak/duration: 10–20 min/20–40 min/3–8 hr. Intramuscular onset/peak/duration: 20–40 min/40–60 min/3–8 hr.
PO onset/peak/duration: 30–60 min/1.5–2 hr/6–8 hr. Monitor blood pressure very carefully if patient is receiving other parenteral antihypertensive drugs concurrently. Reflex increase in heart rate and cardiac output engendered by the hypotensive effect of hydralyzine may be controlled with a beta–blocker (e.g. propranolol) or clonidine for example. Sodium and water retention is controlled with diuretic. Lab tests: Obtain pretreatment and periodic CBC and ANA during prolonged therapy. Lupus–like syndrome may occur (usually in those receiving > 200 mg/day) and requires discontinuation of hydralazine. However, a positive ANA in the absence of lupus manifestations does not require cessation of hydralazine. The lupus–like syndrome is usually reversible but corticosteroids may be needed. Peripheral neuritis (paresthesias, numbness, tingling) may be an antipyridoxine side effect of hydralazine. It can be treated with pyridoxine.
Side effects (common side effects in italics): gastrointestinal; *anorexia, nausea, vomiting, diarrhea*, constipation, ileus; cardiovascular; *palpitations, tachycardia, angina*, hypotension, paradoxical pressor response; blood; anemia, leukopenia, agranulocytosis, purpura, eosinophilia; neurologic; *headache*; dizziness; tremor; depression; anxiety; confusion; peripheral neuritis (paresthesias, numbness, tingling); lupus–like syndrome; + ANA, + LE prep, fever, rash, myalgias, arthralgias, splenomegaly, lymphadenopathy, edema; hypersensitivity; itching, urticaria, rash, eosinophilia, hepatitis; other; sodium and water retention, dyspnea, nasal congestion, lacrimation, conjunctivitis, flushing, muscle cramps, difficult micturition.
Overdose: Empty stomach of any remaining drug and administer activated charcoal. If hypotension occurs, place patient in Trendelenberg position and if necessary give IV isotonic fluids. Administer dobutamine or dopamine if hypotension persists.
Supplied as: tablet (10, 25, 50, 100 mg);
1ml ampul (20mg/ml) for IV or IM administration.

Adult dose:

     <u>Oral:</u> 10 mg 4 times/day Initially. If necessary after 2–4 days, increase dose to 25 mg 4 times/day. If necessary, increase after first week to 50 mg 4 times/day. The daily maintenance requirement may be divided into 2–4 daily doses. Maximum 300 mg/day.

     <u>Intravenous:</u> 10–20 mg every 30 minutes until blood pressure controlled. Give additional doses at 2 to 4 hour intervals if necessary. Change to oral route as soon as possible.

●In preeclampsia/eclampsia, the following protocol may be used: 5 mg initial IV dose; 20 mg IV in 20 minutes if adequate blood pressure reduction has not occurred. Judiciously administer additional doses as needed.

     <u>Intramuscular:</u> 10–20 mg initially. Repeat if no effect seen within 30–40 minutes Usual range 10–40 mg at 3–6 hour intervals. Change to oral route as soon as possible.

Pediatric dose:

     <u>Oral:</u> 0.75 mg/kg/day divided q6h initially. Gradually increase the dose as needed over 3–4 weeks up to maximum 7.5 mg/kg/day or 200 mg/day whichever is least.

     <u>Intravenous/intramuscular:</u> 0.1–0.2mg/kg as needed at 4–6 hour intervals. Maximum initial dose is 20 mg.

IMIPENEM–CILASTATIN (Primaxin)

Spectrum includes <u>streptococci</u>: S. pneumoniae, S. pyogenes, S. viridans, group D including enterococci (e.g. S. faecalis); group B, C, and G streptococci; <u>staphylococci</u>; S. aureus, S. epidermidis; <u>gram-negative bacteria</u>; H. influenzae, H. parainfluenza, Pseudomonas aeruginosa, E coli, Klebsiella (including K. pneumoniae), Proteus mirabilis, Proteus vulgaris, Providencia rettgeri, Providencia stuartii, Citrobacter, Serratia, Morganella morganii, Acinetobacter, Gardnerella vaginalis; <u>Anaerobes</u>; Clostridia, Peptococcus, Peptostreptococcus, Bacteroides (including B. fragilis), Fusobacteria, Eubacterium, Propionibacterium.

   <u>Resistant bacteria</u> include Strep. faecium, many strains of methicillin–resistant staphylococci. Some strains of Pseudomonas aerugenosa may develop resistance during imipenem therapy. Imipenem and an aminoglycoside may act synergistically against Pseudomonas aerugenosa.

Indications: serious infections due to susceptible bacteria involving lower respiratory tract, urinary tract, gynecologic structures, bones, joints, skin and skin structures.

Contraindications: hypersensitivity to any of components. This drug must not be used to treat meningitis since safety and efficacy is unknown.

Comments: ●CNS side effects (e.g. confusion, myoclonic activity, convulsions) may occur, especially if maximum dosage is exceeded. ●Probenecid should not be given concurrently with this drug. ●This drug must not be physically mixed with other antibiotics, although other antibiotics (e.g. aminoglycosides) may be used concurrently. ●Risk to fetus is unknown. Use drug in pregnancy only if potential benefit justifies potential risk. ●Safety and efficacy of this drug in children < 12 yr is unknown.

Side effects: <u>Local effects</u>; phlebitis/thrombophlebitis, injection site pain/erythema, vein induration or infection. <u>Most common systemic effects</u> in decreasing order are nausea, vomiting, diarrhea, rash, fever, hypotension, seizures, dizziness, pruritus, urticaria, somnolence. Other systemic effects have been reportered in < 0.2% of patients.

Supplied as preparation for IV administration only.

Dose recommendations presented below are based on body weight of 70kg. In a patient weighing less than 70kg, multiply the selected dose by patient's weight/70. The maximum total daily dosage is 50mg/kg/day or 4 grams/day whichever is least. The dose may need to be reduced if there is renal impairment (see product insert).

	fully susceptible organism	moderately susceptible (primarily some strains of P aerugenosa)
Mild infection	250mg q6h	500mg q6h
Moderate infection	500mg q6–8h	500mg q6h or 1 gram q8h.
Severe infection	500mg q6h	1 gram q6–8h
Uncomplicated UTI	250mg q6h	250mg q6h
Complicated UTI	500mg q6h	500mg q6h

INSULIN

Action: Lowers plasma glucose by stimulating glucose transport into muscle, fat, leukocytes. Inhibits hepatic glucose production. Inhibits lipolysis in adipose tissue.

Indications: symptomatic diabetes mellitus not responsive to diet, weight reduction, or exercise; and including diabetic crises (diabetic ketoacidosis, hyperosmolar nonketotic coma).

Comments: <u>Insulin requirements may be increased</u>; weight gain; decreased activity; pregnancy; infection; stress; hyperthyroidism; Cushing's syndrome; excessive growth hormone (e.g. acromegaly), immune resistance (i.e. elevated level insulin–binding antibodies), certain drugs (e.g. glucocorticoids, thiazides, estrogens, phenobarbital, phenytoin). <u>Insulin requirements may be decreased</u>; weight loss; increased activity; adrenal or pituitary insufficiency; malabsorption; certain drugs (e.g. ethanol, anabolic steroids, MAO inhibitor, guanethidine, salicylates in large doses, phenylbutazone, beta blockers such as propranolol). Beta blockers may mask symptoms of hypoglycemia with exception of sweating. "<u>Human insulins</u>" (Humulin, Novolin, VeLosulin Human) are identical to naturally occurring human insulin. Humulin is synthesized by E. coli bacteria that have had DNA that codes for human insulin introduced in their genomes. Velosulin Human and Novolin are produced by enzymatic substitution of a single amino acid in the amino acid sequence of porcine insulin. Human insulin may be particularly useful in presence of insulin allergy, insulin resistance, or insulin lipodystrophy. Furthermore, administration of human insulin to patient who only ocassionally requires insulin (e.g. infection, surgery, pregnancy) will preclude allergic sensitization. <u>Dose adjustments may be necessary when switching from one product to another.</u> For instance, switching to human insulin may require a reduction in dose. <u>Selecting the concentration of insulin for subcutaneous administration</u>; To preclude dose error, U 100 (100 unit/ml) is the only concentration that should ordinarily be prescribed. U 40 (40 mg/ml) may be used in children. U 500 (500 mg/ml) regular insulin is available for patients with insulin resistance (i.e. patients requiring > 200 units/day) so as to allow smaller volume subcutaneous injection. <u>Kinetics following subcutaneous injection of insulin</u>; Reported time of onset, peak, and duration of various preparations after SC administration are approximate. Sources of variation include: patient differences, injection depth and site (absorption faster from abdomen than from limbs), activity (exercising injection site hastens absorption).

Side effects: Hypoglycemia may manifest as fatigue, lethargy, sweating, nervousness, tremor, tachycardia, nausea, hunger, headache, confusion, nightmares, seizures, coma, hypothermia. Patient should carry candy or sugar in case hypoglycemic symptoms develop, should not skip meals, and should snack before exercise. Glucagon (1 mg SC or IM) should be available to close associates in event of insulin shock. Somogyi effect (post–hypoglycemia hyperglycemia): Patients receiving too much insulin become hypoglycemic. This may be followed by hyperglycemia and frequently ketonuria as counterregulatory hormones (glucagon, epinephrine, cortisol, growth hormone) exert their influence. Diagnosis: (**1**) wide swings in serum glucose or urine ketones over a 4–6 hr period. Since the hypoglycemic phase is frequently nocturnal, blood and double–void urine must also be tested during sleeping hours. (**2**) nightmares, morning headache and hypothermia reflect hypoglycemia. Treatment: gradually decrease insulin dose (e.g. 5 unit decrements). Insulin resistance (patient requires > 200 unit/day for 1 week). Causes: obesity, infection, ant–iinsulin antibodies, glucocorticoid or growth hormone excess, hemochromatosis, acanthosis nigricans, Werner's Syndrome, lipoatrophic diabetes. If anti–insulin antibodies are the cause, switch to human or purified porcine insulin (U 500 regular may be necessary so that a smaller volume can be injected). An alternative is to give prednisone (40–50 mg/day) concurrent with the insulin regimen and decrease prednisone as insulin requirement decreases. Systemic allergic reaction including generalized pruritis, urticaria, or anaphylaxis is rare. After treating the acute reaction, the treatment of insulin allergy consists of desensitization with either human insulin or purified porcine insulin. Injection site complications: ●Local allergic reaction (pain, erythema, swelling, pruritis) usually resolves spontaneously. If not, try human or purified porcine insulin and/or avoid insulins containing protein additives (i.e. NPH, globin, PZI). ●Lipoatrophy (absorption of SC fat at injection site) may respond to daily injection of human or purified porcine insulin into atrophic area. ●Lipohypertrophy (accumulation of fat at injection site) is remedied by rotating injection sites.

Regular insulin is the only insulin preparation that can be administered IV and IM as well as SC. All other preparations are suspensions for SC administration only. Regular insulin is commonly mixed in the same syringe with NPH or lente for subcutaneous injection. However, the mixture of regular insulin and NPH is preferred since the excess zinc present in lente binds to regular insulin retarding its effect. Intravenous kinetics: Following a bolus IV injection there is rapid onset of action with a peak effect in 15–30 minutes. The duration of effect is dose dependent with a waning effect within 2 hr. Intramuscular kinetics: onset in 10–30 min, peak effect 30–60 min, duration 1–3 hr. Subcutaneous kinetics: onset in about 30 min, peak effect 2–5 hr, duration 8 hr.

Unless otherwise stated the products listed below come in U 100 (100 units/ml) concentrations only.

Regular Insulin USP (Pork) by Novo Nordisk.
Regular Purified Pork Insulin USP.
Regular Iletin I is a bovine–porcine insulin mixture available as U 100 or U 40.
Regular Iletin II (Beef) and Regular Iletin II (Pork) are purified preparations.
Velosulin is a purified pork insulin.
Velosulin Human, Novolin R , and Humulin R preparations contain insulin that is identical to naturally occurring human insulin. See "Comments" above.
Humulin BR is a buffered Humulin preparation reserved for use in patients with external infusion pumps.
Regular (Concentrated) Iletin II, U 500 is a concentrated (500 unit/ml) porcine insulin preparation intended for IM or SC administration in diabetics with insulin resistance (i.e. diabetics requiring over 200 unit insulin/day) so that a smaller volume can be administered.
Semilente (prompt insulin zinc suspension) is for subcutaneous injection only. Onset of action is 1.5 hr, peak effect 5–10 hr, duration 16 hr.
Semilente USP (Beef) by Novo Nordisk comes as U100 concentration.
Semilente Iletin I is a bovine–porcine insulin mixture that is available in both U 100 and U 40 concentrations.
NPH (neutral protamine hagedorn) = isophane insulin suspension is for subcutaneous injection only. It may be mixed in the same syringe with regular insulin. Onset of action is 1.5 hr, peak effect 4–12 hr, duration 24 hr. With the exception of NPH Iletin I which is available in both U 100 and U 40 concentrations, the products listed come only in U 100 concentration.
NPH Iletin I is a bovine–porcine insulin mixture.
NPH Iletin II (Pork) or NPH Iletin II (Beef) are purified preparations.
NPH insulin USP (Beef) by Novo Nordisk.
Insulatard NPH Human is a purified pork insulin.
NPH Purified Pork Insulin USP.
Humulin N and Novolin N preparations contain insulin that is identical to naturally occurring human insulin. See "Comments" above.
70% NPH + 30% regular is for subcutaneous injection only. The regular fraction gives it a rapid onset (≈ 1/2 hour) while the NPH portion provides a duration of up to 24 hours. According to the manufacturers, the maximal effect following the injection of either of the first two products presented below is 4–8 hours and the peak range of the third product is 2–12 hours. These products come only in U 100 concentration.
Mixtard 70/30 is a purified pork preparation.
Mixtard Human 70/30 *
Humulin 70/30 *
*Contains insulin identical to naturally occurring human insulin. See "Comments" above.

Lente (70% ultralente + 30% semilente) is for subcutaneous injection only. It may be mixed in the same syringe with regular insulin. Onset of action is 2–5 hr, peak effect 7–15 hr, duration about 24 hr. With the exception of Lente Iletin I which is available in both U 100 and U 40 concentrations, the products listed come only in U 100 concentration.

    <u>Lente Iletin I</u> is a bovine–porcine insulin mixture.
    <u>Lente Iletin II (Pork)</u> and <u>Lente Iletin II (Beef)</u> are purified preparations.
    <u>Lente insulin USP (Beef)</u> by Novo Nordisk.
    <u>Lente Purified Pork Insulin USP.</u>
    <u>Humulin L and Novolin L</u> preparations contain insulin that is identical to naturally occurring human insulin. See "Comments" above.

Ultralente (extended insulin zinc suspension) is for subcutaneous injection only. Onset of action is 4 hr, peak effect 10–30 hr, duration about 36 hr. Ultralente is seldom used because the peak effect occurs at night when there is no food intake. Consequently, the risk of nocturnal hypoglycemia is increased. With the exception of Ultralente Iletin I which is available in both U 100 and U 40 concentrations, the products listed come only in U 100 concentration.

    <u>Ultralente Iletin I</u> is a bovine–porcine insulin mixture.
    <u>Ultralente insulin USP (Beef)</u> by Novo Nordisk.
    <u>Humulin U</u> preparation contains insulin that is identical to naturally occurring human insulin. See "Comments" above.

PZI (protamine zinc insulin) is for subcutaneous injection only. PZI must not be mixed in the same syringe with regular insulin. Onset of action is 4–6 hr, peak effect 14–24 hr, duration about 36 hr. Like ultralente, PZI is seldom used because there is an increased risk of nocturnal hypoglycemia. This is because the peak effect occurs at night when there is no food intake.

    <u>Protamine, Zinc & Iletin I</u> is a bovine–porcine insulin mixture available in U 100 and U 40 concentration.
    <u>Protamine, Zinc & Iletin II (Pork)</u> and <u>Protamine, Zinc & Iletin II (Pork)</u> are purified preparations that come in U 100 concentration.

INTRAVENOUS SOLUTIONS

	Na	Cl	K	Ca	lactate	glucose	cal/L	mOsm/kg
	(mEq/liter)					(gram/L)		
5 % dextrose in water (D5W)						50	170	252
10 % dextrose in water (D10W)						100	340	505
0.9 % NaCl (isotonic/normal saline)	154	154						308
3 % NaCl	513	513						1026
0.45% NaCl (half normal saline)	77	77						154
5% dextrose + 0.2 % NaCl (D5-1/4 NS)	34	34				50	170	348
5% dextrose + 0.45% NaCl (D5-1/2 NS)	77	77				50	170	434
5% dextrose + 0.9 % NaCl (D5 NS)	154	154				50	170	584
Ringer's lactate (RL)	130	109	4	3	28		< 10	272
5% dextrose + Ringer's lactate (D5 RL)	130	109	4	3	28	50	80	552

Selecting appropriate IV solution: Use clinical judgment based on patient history, physical exam, and laboratory data. Suggested regimens follow.
Maintenance fluids: Use D5-1/4 NS (5% dextrose plus 0.2% NaCl).
For the first 10 kg of body weight: 100 ml/kg/24 hr is required.
For the second 10 kg of body weight: 50 ml/kg/24 hr is required.
For body weight over 20 kg: 20 ml/kg/24 hr is required.
For example, the 24 hr maintenance fluid requirements for a 35 kg patient would be (10 kg x 100 ml/kg) + (10 kg x 50 ml/kg) + (15 kg x 20 ml/kg) = 1800 ml/24 hr. Assuming that renal function is normal, 20 mEq of KCl is usually added to each liter of fluid if the patient receives intravenous maintenance fluid for more than 24–48 hr.
Intravenous fluid therapy for blood loss:
<u>Percent blood loss in an adult may be estimated as follows:</u>
●less than 15% blood loss (slight elevated pulse rate).
●20–25% blood loss (pulse rate over 100, pulse pressure down to 30, slow capillary refill, urine output 25–30 ml/hr, respiratory rate 20–30)
●30–35% blood loss (pulse rate over 120, BP 70–90 systolic/50–60 diastolic, pulse pressure 20–30, slow capillary refill, urine output 5–15 ml/hr, resp rate 30–40).
●50% blood loss (pulse rate over 140, systolic BP less than 50–60, pulse pressure 10–20, slow capillary refill, anuria, respiratory rate over 35).
<u>Using estimated percent of blood lost, calculate the volume of blood lost :</u> Normal adult blood volume in liters is about 7% of ideal body weight in kg. So an adult with an ideal body weight of 70 kg with 10 % blood loss has lost about 70 kg x 7 % x 10 % = 0.49 liter. Normal pediatric blood volume is about 80 ml/kg.
<u>Replace blood volume lost with Ringer's lactate 3: 1.</u> That is to say, administer 3 liters Ringer's lactate for each liter of blood that is lost.

Blood transfusion will also be necessary if blood loss is 30% or more.

Burns: Use lactated Ringer's. Volume required in ml = 3 ml/kg x percent of body surface with 2nd and 3rd degree burns. Give 1/2 of this calculated amount in the first 8 hours and the remaining 1/2 over the following 16 hours. Remember to give the daily mainenance requirement as well. Adjust rate so that urine output does not fall below 50 ml/kg/hr in adult and 1ml/kg/hr in child.

Emesis/nasogastric suction: Patient loses Na, K, H, Cl with consequent hypokalemic hypochloremic alkalosis. Initial replacement is with D5–1/4 NS or D5–1/3 NS. Add 20 mEg KCl per liter fluid (assuming renal function is normal). Use electrolyte measurements of gastric secretions and serum to guide further therapy. Remember to add maintenance requirements.

Diarrhea: Patient loses Na, K, Cl, and bicarbonate. If acidosis present, administer D5W or D5–1/4 NS with added KCl and NaCO3. If acidosis not present, administer D5–NS with added KCl. In either case use electrolyte determinations of stool and serum to guide therapy. Remember to add maintenance requirements.

IPECAC, Syrup of

Action: Ipecac alkaloids induce vomiting by stimulating chemoreceptor trigger zone in the medulla and by a local effect on gastric mucosa.

Indication: poisoning due to orally ingested drugs or chemicals.

Contraindications: ●Coma, significant depression of consciousness, loss of gag reflex, seizures. ●Ingestion of caustic acid/alkali; petroleum distillate (e.g. kerosene, gasoline, fuel oil, coal oil, paint thinner, cleaning fluid).

Dose:

Adult/child over 1 yr: 1 tablespoon (15 ml) PO followed by 1–2 full glass water in adult and older child and preceded by 10 ml water/kg in younger child.

Infant 6–12 months of age: 1–2 teaspoon (5–10 ml) preceded by 10 ml water/kg.

Less than 6 months of age: not recommended.

Comments/caution: ●Dose may be repeated in 20–30 minutes if emesis does not occur. Gastric lavage if emesis does not occur after second dose. ●Ambulation promotes emesis. ●Activated charcoal (since it will inactivate ipecac) is withheld until emesis has occurred. ●Emesis may recur within first 2 hr if additional PO fluid is given. ●Phenothiazine overdose may not respond to ipecac since phenothiazines supress emesis. ●Do not use fluid extract of ipecac (a concentrated form of ipecac).

IPRATROPIUM BROMIDE (Atrovent)

Action: Anticholinergic bronchodilator chemically related to atropine. Bronchodilation is chiefly a local site-specific effect.

Indication: maintenance therapy of bronchospasm due to chronic obstructive pulmonary disease. This medication is not for treatment of acute attack of bronchospasm when a rapid response is necessary.

Contraindication: hypersensitivity to atropine or derivatives.

Caution: narrow-angle glaucoma, prostatic hypertrophy, bladder neck obstruction, pregnancy.

Side effects: palpitations, dizziness, headache, nervousness, tremor, rash, nausea, vomiting, GI distress, blurred vision, dry mouth, oropharyngeal irritation from aerosol, cough, aggravation of respiratory symptoms.

Supplied as: metered dose inhaler, 14 gram vial delivers 200 inhalations.

Dose: 2 inhalations qid. Maximum 12 inhalations per 24 hr.

IRON DEXTRAN (Imferon)

Indications: treatment of iron deficiency anemia when oral iron replacement is not tolerated (e.g. inflammatory bowel disease) or is insufficient (e.g. ongoing blood loss > 500 ml/wk), or when iron stores must be replenished quickly (e.g. severe anemia in 3rd trimester pregnancy).

Contraindications: iron dextran hypersensitivity, all anemias except iron deficiency anemia. Not recommended in infant < 4 months. Do not administer during acute stage of kidney infection.

Caution: asthma; allergic tendency; serious liver dysfunction; pregnancy (animal studies show increased fetal anomalies, stillbirths, and decreased neonatal survival); nursing mother. Large IM doses have been associated with sarcomas in animals.

Comments: Measurement of hemoglobin; In iron deficiency anemia, the hemoglobin should increase by 1gram/dl within 2 weeks of iron administration. The diagnosis of iron deficiency anemia is questionable if it does not. Serum ferritin measurement may be used to assess adequacy of iron stores. However, colorimetric serum iron measurement obtained within 3 weeks of iron dextran administration may not be reliable. Bone marrow exam; Small amounts of iron dextran complex may persist in the reticuloendothelial system for 3–4 months. Consequently, bone marrow samples may show stainable iron even though iron stores are depleted. Iron overload and possible hemosiderosis may occur if patient is overtreated, or treated inappropriately for anemia other than iron deficiency anemia.

Side effects include: anaphylactic shock; dyspnea; bronchospasm; chest pain; hypotension; flushing; tachycardia; urticaria; itching; rash; purpura; arthralgias; arthritis; myalgia; seizures; headache; dizziness; paresthesias; malaise; fever; chills; sweating; leukocytosis; lymphadenopathy; nausea; vomiting; diarrhea; abdominal pain; hematuria; phlebitis at IV site; IM injection site effects (soreness, inflammation, sterile abscess, brown skin discoloration).

Supplied as: 50 mg elemental iron/ml
(2 ml ampul for IV or IM injection, 10 ml vial for IM only).

Intravenous administration (the preferred route):
Stop oral iron before administering iron dextran.
Calculate the dose:
Total amount of elemental iron required in mg =
66 X wt in kg X (normal hemoglobin – patient hemoglobin)
(normal hemoglobin)
where the normal hemoglobin is 11 g/dl at 1 month–1yr, 13 g/dl at 2–15 yr, 14–18 g/dl in adult male, 12–16 g/dl in adult nonpregnant female, 10–14 g/dl in late pregnancy.

Administration: First give test dose: 0.5 ml IV. Wait 1 hour. If no reaction occurs, give the balance of that day's dose IV. The total elemental iron requirement is divided into single daily doses if the total requirement exceeds the maximum recommended daily dose of: 0.5 ml (25 mg) in infants under 5 kg, 1 ml (50 mg) in child under 10 kg, and 2 ml (100 mg) in others. The daily intravenous dose is administered undiluted and slowly (not to exceed 1ml/min).

Intramuscular administration: Use this route only if intravenous administration is not possible. Calculate total requirement as above. Administer 0.5 ml IM test dose. Wait 1 hour and if no reaction occurs, administer balance of that day's dose. Daily dose should not exceed 0.5 ml in infants under 5 kg, 1 ml in child under 10 kg, or 2 ml in others. Note: Inject deep IM into upper outer quadrant of buttock using Z–track technique (i.e. displace skin laterally prior to injection).

ISOPROTERENOL (Isuprel)

Action: Potent beta–receptor stimulant with following consequences: (1) Increased heart rate, (2) increased myocardial contractility, (3) decreased peripheral vascular resistance, (4) bronchodilation. Net effect of 1 and 2 is to increase cardiac output and to increase the work of the heart, and thus leads to increased myocardial oxygen consumption. Decreased vascular resistance may cause a fall in diastolic pressure. Systolic pressure remains the same or is increased.

Indications: As inhalant in treatment of bronchospasm—asthma, bronchitis, or emphysema. Intravenous infusion: (1) temporary treatment of bradycardia due to sinus bradycardia or AV block that is hemodynamically significant and refractory to atropine, (2) low cardiac output due to cardiac failure (consider dopamine first).

Contraindications: hypertension, tachyarrhythmias (particularly those resulting from digitalis toxicity), myocardial infarction (except in setting of ventricular asystole). Isoproterenol is generally contraindicated in the setting of myocardial infarction because isoproterenol increases the work of the heart (and therefore oxygen consumption) and may thus lead to extension of the infarct.

Caution: hypokalemia, ventricular ectopy, concurrent use with epinephrine or other sympathomimetics, hyperthyroidism, diabetes mellitus, coronary insufficiency, pregnancy.

Comments: ●Because isoproterenol is a nonselective beta agonist, it is liable to cause untoward cardiac stimulation (tachycardia, arrhythmias) in a patient being treated for bronchospasm. Consider more selective bronchodilators (see "Adrenergic Bronchodilators"). ●Isoproterenol may lose its effectiveness or even cause paradoxic bronchospasm if it is used too frequently.

Side effects: tachycardia, arrhythmias, palpitations, tremor, dizziness, weakness, sweating, skin flushing, nervousness, headache, angina, arrhythmias, nausea, vomiting, tachyphylaxis, paradoxic bronchospasm with too frequent administration.

Supplied as: Intravenous: 0.2 mg/ml in 1 ml and 5 ml ampul;
solution for nebulization: 1: 200 and 1: 100 dilution;
aerosol inhalers: Isuprel Mistometer (0.131 mg/inhalation),
Medihaler–Iso (0.08 mg/inhalation),
Norisodrine Aerotrol (0.12 mg/inhalation).

Intravenous dose:
Adult: Add 1 mg isoproterenol to 250 ml D5W. Start infusion at 2–10 mcg/min (30–150 ml/hr rate) and titrate to effect. Infusion must not cause heart rate to exceed

160.
Pediatric (for treatment of respiratory failure due to asthma): Add 0.6 mg to 100 ml of D5W. Then 1 ml/kg/hr delivers 0.1 mcg/kg/min. The infusion is started at 0.1 mcg/kg/min and titrated to effect by increasing the rate of infusion by 0.1 mcg/kg/min increments every 5–15 minutes. The infusion should not exceed 1.5 mcg/kg/min or cause the heart rate to go above 180.

Inhalation dose in treatment of bronchospasm:

Aerosol inhalers (adult or child): 1 inhalation. Repeat in 1–5 minutes if necessary. Treatment may be repeated up to 5 times in 24 hr. Maximum 2 inhalations/treatment. Maximum 6 inhalations in any given hour.

Hand–bulb nebulizer (adult or child): 5–15 inhalations of 1: 200 solution. Adult with severe attack may be treated with 3–7 inhalations of 1: 100 solution. ●In asthma, the treatment may be repeated once after 5–10 minutes if necessary (maximum of 5 treatments/day). ●In COPD, the treatment may be repeated at not less than 3–4 hour intervals.

Via air/oxygen nebulizer or IPPB: 0.5 ml of 1: 200 solution (diluted with 2 ml water or isotonic saline). Maximum 5 treatments/day.

ISONIAZID (INH, Laniazid)

Action: Bactericidal against intra and extracellular Mycobacterium tuberculosis and some other mycobacteria (e.g. M. kansasii, M. bovis).

Indications:

Treatment of active tuberculosis, in conjunction with other antituberculosis drugs (e.g. rifampin, ethambutol, streptomycin).

As a single drug in treatment of active disease in certain patients with subclinical infection (i.e. + tuberculin skin test but no active disease seen on chest x-ray): (**1**) patient with positive tuberculin test and evidence of prior disease on chest x-ray; (**2**) patient with positive tuberculin test who is at high risk of developing active disease (e.g. diabetes mellitus, silicosis, gastrectomized patient, leukemia, Hodgkins, receiving adrenocorticoids or other immunosuppressants; (**3**) patient of any age with negative to positive conversion of tuberculin skin test within past 2 yr; (**4**) patient less than 35 yr with positive tuberculin skin test. Treatment of patients 21–35 yr is controversial.

NOTE: Patients over 35 yr with subclinical infection are not treated with isoniazid because of the increased risk of hepatitis. They may be treated with rifampin but this is controversial.

As a single drug in prevention of infection in intimate or household contact of patient with active tuberculosis.

Contraindications: acute liver disease, history of isoniazid hepatotoxicity or hypersensitivity, pregnancy (unless active tuberculosis is present).

Caution/Comments: Hepatoxicity: Risk of isoniazid–induced hepatitis is age–dependent (under 20 yr—rare, over 50 yr—2.3%). Daily alcohol intake or combined use with rifampin may potentiate hepatoxicity. 10–20% patients receiving isoniazid will have elevated transaminases which usually return to normal even with continued therapy. Isoniazid need not be discontinued unless: (**1**) symptomatic hepatitis occurs (e.g. fatigue, weakness, malaise, anorexia, nausea, vomiting); (**2**) serum transaminases (SGOT, SGPT) rise to 3–5 times normal; or (**3**) there is any elevation in transaminases concurrent with rise in serum bilirubin or alkaline phosphatase. Isoniazid is contraindicated in acute liver disease and must be used with caution in patient with chronic liver disease or severe renal disease. Pregnancy and nursing: Isoniazid crosses placenta and is excreted in breast milk. In pregnancy, isoniazid is reserved for patient with active disease. Monitor neonates and breast fed infants of isoniazid–treated mothers for side effects. Isoniazid inhibits phenytoin metabolism. Phenytoin dose may need to be reduced.

Side effects: In contrast to rapid inactivators (most orientals, eskimos, latin americans, american indians); low inactivators (50% blacks and whites, elderly) maintain higher isoniazid blood levels and are at greater risk for side effects. Liver: anoxeria, nausea, vomiting, malaise, fatigue, elevated serum transaminases (SGPT or SGOT), elevated bilirubin, jaundice; neurologic: peripheral neuritis, optic neuritis, seizures, toxic encephalopathy/psychosis; gastrointestinal: nausea, vomiting, epigastric discomfort; blood: anemia (hemolytic, sideroblastic or aplastic); thrombocytopenia; agranulocytosis; eosinophilia; hypersensitivity: fever, skin eruptions, vasculitis, lymphadenopathy; other: pyridoxine deficiency/pellagra, metabolic acidosis, hyperglycemia, gynecomastia, rheumatic or lupus–like syndromes.

Overdose: ●Empty stomach and administer administer activated charcoal. A cathartic (e.g. magnesium citrate) is then administered PO. ●Administer IV pyridoxine hydrochloride—1 mg for every 1 mg of isoniazid ingested (prepare a 5–10% solution with water and infuse over 30 minutes). ●Pyridoxine together with IV diazepam are the drugs of choice for controlling seizures. ●Administer IV sodium bicarbonate if there is acidosis.

Supplied as: tablet (50, 100, 300 mg); syrup (50 mg/5ml).

Dose (active disease requires combined drug regimens):

Adult: 5 mg/kg PO as single daily dose (maximum 300 mg/day).

Note: To preclude peripheral neuritis, pyridoxine 50 mg/day PO is commonly given.

Pediatric:
- Active tuberculosis: 10–20 mg/kg/day PO as single daily dose (maximum 300–500 mg/day).
- Prevention: 10 mg/kg/day PO as single daily dose (maximum 300 mg/day).

KETOCONAZOLE cream (Nizoral)

Indications: tinea cruris, tinea corporis, tinea versicolor, and cutaneous candidiasis. ●Seborrheic dermatitis.
Contraindications: hypersensitivity to any of ingredients.
Comments: Use in pregnancy only if potential benefit justifies potential risk to fetus.
Side effects: irritation, itching, stinging.
Supplied as: 2% cream in 15, 30, and 60 gram tubes.
Dose: <u>Fungal infection</u>: apply to affected skin once daily.
     <u>Seborrheic dermatitis</u>: apply twice daily for 4 weeks or until clinical clearing.

KETOCONAZOLE tablets (Nizoral)

Indications: systemic fungal infections due to blastomycosis, coccidioidomycosis, histoplasmosis, chromomycosis, paracoccidioidomycosis.
●Candida: systemic candidiasis, chronic mucocutaneous candidiasis, candiduria, oral thrush.
●Severe recalcitrant cutaneous dermatophyte infections that are unresponsive to to topical treatment or oral griseofulvin, or when patient is unable to take griseofulvin.
Contraindications: hypersensitivity to drug.
Comments: ●Drug may be hepatoxic. Liver function tests (e.g. SGPT, SGOT, alkaline phosphatase) are obtained prior to treatment and frequently during treatment. Discontinue drug if symptoms of liver dysfunction develop (e.g. unusual fatigue, anorexia, nausea, vomiting, jaundice, dark urine, pale stools); and/or if liver function test abnormalities occur (unless they are mild and transient). ●Use in pregnancy only if potential benefit justifies potential risk to fetus. ●Breast feeding is not allowed during therapy with ketoconazole. ●Use in pediatric patient only if potential benefit outweighs risks. ●Ketoconazole requires acidity for dissolution. Consequently, if the patient is taking agents that oppose gastric acidity (antacids, H2–blockers, anticholinergics); ketoconazole should be taken at least 2 hours after these agents. In patients with achlorhydria, ketoconazole is dissolved in 4 ml aqueous 0.2N HCl and then ingested via a straw so as to avoid contact with teeth. ●Ketoconazole may enhance anticoagulant effect of coumarin–like drugs. ●Ketoconazole should not be taken concurrently with INH or rifampin. ●Ketoconazole increases the blood level of concurrently administered cyclosporin A. Monitor the blood level of the latter if the drugs are given concurrently. ●Monitor ketoconazole and phenytoin if they are given concurrently because concurrent administration may affect the metabolism of either or both.
Side effects: nausea, vomiting, abdominal pain, and pruritis are the most common complaints. The following have been reported in < 1% patients: headache, dizziness, somnolence, fever, chills, photophobia, diarhea, gynecomastia, impotence, thrombocytopenia, leukopenia, hemolytic anemia, bulging fontanelles. Hypersensitivity reactions (urticaria, anaphylaxis) have been reported in patients taking ketoconazole. Neuropsychiatric abnormalities (e.g. severe depression, suicidal tendency) are rare.
Supplied as: 200 mg tablet.
Dose: 200 mg once daily. The dose may be increased to 400mg once daily in severe infections or if the clinical response is inadequate in the expected time. Treatment should be continued for at least 1–2 weeks for candidiasis. Chronic mucocutaneous candidiasis usually requires maintenance treatment. Treatment should be continued for at least 6 months for other systemic mycoses. Treatment of recalcitrant dermatophyte infections is for at least 4 weeks.

LABETALOL (Normodyne, Trandate)

Action: Labetalol has both selective alpha-1 blocking effect and nonselective beta-blocking action. Consequently, it induces a dose–related reduction in blood pressure without reflex tachycardia or a significant fall in heart rate.

Indication: hypertension.

Contraindications: bronchial asthma, overt cardiac failure, greater than 1st degree heart block, cardiogenic shock, severe bradycardia.

Caution: ●Use with caution in patient with cardiac failure or history thereof. ●Use in pregnancy only if potential benefit justifies potential risk to fetus. ●Breast feeding is not allowed during therapy with ketoconazole. ●Safety and efficacy in children not established. ●Drug may be hepatoxic. Liver function tests (e.g. SGPT, SGOT, alkaline phosphatase) are obtained if symptoms of liver dysfunction develop (e.g. unusual fatigue, anorexia, nausea, vomiting, jaundice, dark urine, pale stools). The drug is stopped and not restarted if there is there is jaundice if liver function test abnormalities. ●Abrupt withdrawal of a beta-blocker may result in angina (but has not been reported with labetolol), particularly in those with ischemic heart disease. Consequently, if labetolol is to be discontinued in a patient on chronic labetolol treatment, it should be tapered and discontinued over 1–2 weeks. ●Beta-blockade may mask symptoms of hypoglycemia. ●Beta-blockade may inhibit release of insulin in response to hyperglycemia. Consequently, the dosage of antidiabetic drugs may have to be adjusted. ●Labetolol may alleviate hypertension and symptoms in pheochromocytoma. However, caution must be exercised because paradoxical hypertension has occurred. ●Consider discontinuing labetolol prior to major surgery because beta-blockers may cause prolonged hypotension and problems starting or sustaining heart beat.

Side effects include dizziness, fatigue, drowsiness, headache, asthenia, paresthesias, nasal stuffiness, ejaculation failure, impotence, increased sweating, edema, postural hypotension, dyspnea, rash, vertigo, vision abnormality, nausea, vomiting, dyspepsia, diarrhea, abdominal pain, abnormal taste.

Supplied as: 100, 200, and 300 mg tablet. IV preparation (5mg/ml concentration).

Dose (adult):

Oral: Start with 100mg twice daily whether used alone or in addition to concurrent diuretic therapy. Guided by the standing blood pressure response, increase the dosage as needed every 2–3 days in increments of 100mg bid. The usual required range is 200–400mg twice daily. Up to 1200–2400mg/day (± diuretic) may be needed in severe hypertension.

Intravenous: Blood pressure should be monitored during and after intravenous administration in order to avoid a rapid or excessive fall in pressure. With patient supine, labetol may be administered as a slow continuous infusion or as repeated injections. As an example of slow continuous infusion: add 40 ml of labetolol injection preparation to 250ml of IV solution and infuse at 3ml/min (approx 2mg/min). The rate may be titrated according to the blood pressure response. If labetolol is to be given by repeated injections, start with 20mg administered slowly over 2 minutes. Check blood pressure immediately after injection and again in 5 and 10 minutes. If necessary, additional 40–80mg injections can be given every ten minutes or until total 300mg given. Starting oral therapy: When the supine diastolic pressure has begun to increase, give 200mg PO. Depending on blood pressure response, give additional 200–400mg PO in 6–12 hours. In inpatients, further titration to optimum blood pressure may proceed at one day intervals as follows: 200mg bid → 400mg bid → 800mg bid → 1200mg bid.

LAXATIVES

Bulk forming laxatives psysllium (Effersyllium, Konsyl, Metamucil); methylecellulose (Cologel); malt soup extract (Maltsupex)

Stool softeners: docusate calcium (Surfak); docusate potassium (Dialose, Kasof); docusate sodium (Colace, Disonate, Doxinate)

Lubricant: mineral oil (Agoral Plain, Kandremul, Petrogalar Plain, Fleet Oil Enema)

Stimulants: bisacodyl (Dulcolax); senna (Senokot); phenolphthalein (Ex–Lax, Prulet); danthron (Modane); castor oil (Fleet flavored castor oil, Neoloid); glycerin (Babylax)

Saline laxatives: magnesium citrate, magnesium hydroxide (Milk of Magnesia)

Other: lactulose (Chronulac, Cephulac).

Note: ●By absorbing water, the bulk forming agents may be useful in lessening watery diarrhea even though total water loss is not reduced. ●Lactulose (Cephulac) is also used to treat hepatic encephalopathy. ●Magnesium hydroxide is also used as an antacid.

psyllium (Effersyllium, Fiberall, Metamucil)
Action: Psyllium, a nondigestible and nonabsorbable fiber, absorbs water thereby increasing the water content and bulk of stool. Onset of action is in 24–72 hr.
Indication: Safe for longterm use in chronic constipation, anorectal conditions (e.g. hemorrhoids), irritable bowel. Because it absorbs water, psyllium may also be useful in lessening nonspecific watery diarrhea. However, total water loss is not reduced.
Contraindications: GI obstruction, fecal impaction.
Supplied as: powder.
Adult dose: 1 round tsp (or packet) in 8 oz glass water/juice qd–tid.
Child 6–12 yr: 1/2 adult dose.
Comment: In order to preclude inspissation of psyllium and possible GI impaction/obstruction, an adequate amount of fluid should be taken with psyllium.

methylcellulose (Cologel)
Action: bulk–forming agent (mixes with water forming a colloid that makes the stool bulkier and softer). Onset of action is 1–3 days.
Indications: chronic constipation, anorectal conditions (e.g. hemorrhoids). Also, because it decreases the fluidity of stool, methylcellulose may be of use in alleviating nonspecific watery diarrhea.
Adult dose: 1–4 tsp of liquid with glass water 3 times a day.

malt soup extract (Maltsupex)
Action/indication: bulk forming agent. Same action/indications as psyllium.
Supplied as: tablet, powder, liquid.
Adult:
  Tablet: 4 tablets with glass water qid, with meals and at bedtime.
          Adjust dosage according to response.
  Powder or liquid: 2 tbsp twice daily with glass water for 3–4 days or until relief.
Child: 1 – 2 tbsp powder or liquid in 8 oz. glass liquid once to twice daily.
Infant: 1/2 to 2 tbsp powder or liquid in day's total formula, or 1–2 tsp with single feeding.

docusate calcium [= dioctyl calcium sulfosuccinate] (Surfak)
Action: Promotes fecal water absorption by a surface action. Stools are softer and bulkier.
Indications: constipation, painful anorectal conditions, reduce strain of defecation (e.g. cardiac conditions).
Supplied as: 50, 240 mg capsule.
Adult: 240 mg PO qd until bowel movements normal. 50–150 mg/day may suffice.
Child over 6 yr: 50–150 mg/day PO.

docusate potassium [= dioctyl potassium sulfosuccinate] (Dialose, Kasof)
Action/indications: see docussate calcium.
Supplied as: Dialose 100 mg capsule,   Kasof 240 mg capsule.
Adult: 100–300 mg/day PO (e.g. one 240 mg capsulse once daily, 100 mg capsule qd–tid).
Child over 6 yr: 100 mg PO at bedtime.

docusate sodium [= dioctyl sodium sulfosuccinate] (Colace, Disonate)
Action/indications: see docussate calcium.
Supplied as: capsule (50,   100 mg); syrup (20 mg/5ml);   drops (10 mg/ml).
Dose:•adult: 50–240 mg/day; •6–12 yr: 40–120 mg/day; •3–6 yr: 20–60 mg/day;
      •under 3 yr: 10–40 mg/day.

mineral oil
Action: Mixes with feces thereby softening and lubricating.
Indications: reduce strain of defecation (e.g. cardiac conditions), painful anorectal conditions (e.g. hemorrhoids), rectal administration to aid in expelling impacted or hard feces.
Comments: Bulking agents (e.g. psyllium) or docusate salts are generally safer and more convenient for the patient than PO mineral oil (see side effects). Onset of action PO is 6 hours.
Side effects from PO administration: lipid pneumonia if aspirated; anal leakage of mineral oil; interferes with absorption of fat–soluble vitamins A, D, E, K.
Oral dose: •Adult: 15–30 ml (1–2 tbsp)/day;
           •Child over 6 yr: 5–15 ml (1–3 tsp) at bedtime.
Rectal dose: •Adult: 120 ml;   •Child over 2 yr: 30–60 ml.

bisacodyl (Dulcolax, Fleet Bisacodyl Enema)
Comments: ●Bisacodyl stimulates sensory nerves of colonic mucosa resulting in reflex peristalsis.
●Contraindicated in acute surgical abdomen. ●Side effects: abdominal cramps, allergic reaction (due to tartrazine in tablets).
Supplied as: 5 mg tablet, 10 mg suppository, enema.
Adult dose:
   ●Oral: 2–3 tablet (up to 6 tablets in preparation for special procedure). Tablet must be swallowed whole and must not be taken within 1 hour of antacids or milk. Onset is usually within 6 hours.
   ●Rectal: 1 suppository or enema as needed. Onset 15–60 minutes.
Child dose: ●Oral: 5–10 mg (do not give to child too small to swallow tablet whole);
           ●Rectal: 1 suppository as needed (1/2 suppos if under 2 yr); or enema.
           Enema contraindicated if < 2 yr of age.

senna (Senokot)
Action: Induces peristalsis by stimulating intestinal mucosa. Onset of action is 8–10 hours.
Indication: short term use for constipation.
Contraindication: acute surgical abdomen.
Comment: Senna is best administered at bedtime.
Supplied as: tablet, granules, syrup.
Dose of tablets/granules:
●Adult: Initially, 2 tablets or 1 level tsp. Maximum 4 tablet (or 2 level tsp) twice daily.
●Elderly/debilitated/Ob–Gyn patient: start with 1/2 usual initial adult dose.
●Child over 27 kg: Initially 1 tablet or 1 level tsp (maximum 2 tab or 1 level tsp bid).
Note: Dose of tablets above is for Senokot tablet. Two Senokot Tablet is equal to one Senokot X–tra Tablet.
Dose of syrup:
   ●Adult: Initially 2–3 tsp (maximum 2–3 tsp twice daily). In the elderly, de
            bilitated, or Ob–Gyn patient; the initial dose is 1/2 the usual adult dose.
   ●5–15 yr: Initially 1–2 tsp (maximum 2 tsp bid).
   ●1–5 yr: Initially 1/2 to 1 tsp (maximum 1 tsp bid).
   ●1month–1yr: Initially 1/4–1/2 tsp (maximum 1/2 tsp bid)

phenolphthalein (Ex–Lax, Prulet)
Indication: short term treatment constipation.
Side effects: pink color to urine or feces, dermatitis, pruritus.
Contraindications: nausea, vomiting, abdominal pain.
Comments: ●Onset 6–8 hr. ●Due to enterohepatic circulation, the effects may last for 3–4 days.
Supplied as: 60, 90 mg tablet.
Adult dose: 30–270 mg/day; Child ≥ 6 yr: 30–60 mg/day; 2–5 yr: 15–20 mg/day.

castor oil (Fleet Flavored Castor Oil, Neoloid plain or flavored castor oil)
Action: In the small intestine, castor oil is hydrolyzed to the fatty acid ricinoleic acid. This agent alters mucosal transport of water and electrolytes such that watery stools ensue in 2–6 hours.
Indications: when a complete bowel evacuation is required (e.g. prior to radiologic or endoscopic procedure). Castor oil is not for routine treatment of constipation.
Contraindications: nausea, vomiting, abdominal pain. Caution: pregnancy.
Comments: ●Best result if taken on empty stomach followed by glass water. ●Prolonged use may lead to laxative dependence, and excessive loss of water and electrolytes.
Adult dose: ●Purgative: 6 tbsp (90 ml). ●Laxative: 3 tbsp (45 ml).
 2–12 year of age: 1 tbsp (15 ml); Up to 2 yrear of age: up to 1 tsp (5ml).

glycerin (Fleet Babylax)
Action: (1) softens and lubricates stools; (2) stimulates rectal contraction, probably by an irritant effect. Usually acts within 15–30 minutes.
Contraindications: nausea, vomiting, abdominal pain.
Dose child 1–6 yr: 1 rectal applicator (4 ml glycerin).

magnesium hydroxide (Milk of Magnesia), **magnesium citrate**
Action: These agents are hypertonic solutions which by osmotic effect retain water in the intestinal lumen. The resulting increased intestinal volume stimulates peristalsis. Onset of action is 2–6 hr.
Indications: short–term treatment constipation; bowel prep (e.g. prior to surgery, x–ray procedure, or rectal exam); rapid purge following toxic ingestion.
Contraindications: renal insufficiency, GI obstruction.
Dose (drink full glass water with each dose):
   Magnesium citrate: ●adult: 120–240 ml PO.   ●pediatric: 4 ml/kg PO.
   Magnesium hydroxide: ●adult: 15–60 ml (1–4 tbsp) PO.   ●pediatric: 0.5 ml/kg PO.

lactulose (Cephulac, Chronulac)

Action: Lactulose is converted by colonic bacteria to acidic metabolites thus creating an acidic environment which traps ammonium ions within the GI lumen. The osmotically active metabolites also exert a laxative effect which also hastens excretion of ammonia.

Indications: constipation, treatment/prevention hepatic encephalopathy.

Contraindications: patient requiring low galactose diet.   Caution: diabetes mellitus, pregnancy.

Comments: ●Encephalopathy may improve within 2 hours of first enema. Via oral route, improvement may occur within 24 hours but may take 48 hours. ●In the treatment of hepatic encephalopathy, other laxatives must not be administered concurrently since the appearance of loose stools is used to assess the adequacy of lactulose dosage. ●Soap suds enemas or other alkaline cleansing enemas should not be administered prior to lactulose retention enema.

Side effects: gaseous distention, flatulence, belching, abdominal cramps, nausea, vomiting.

Supplied as: syrup contaning 10 gram lactulose/15ml. Per 15ml, the preparation contains < 2.2 g galactose, < 1.2 g lactose, and < 1.2 g other sugars.

Dose for treatment constipation (Chronulac):

●Adult: 1–2 tbsp/day (15–30 ml/day) PO. Increase to 60 ml/day as needed. Laxative effect may not be seen for 24–48 hours.

●Children's dose not established.

Dose for treatment/prevention hepatic encepalopathy (Cephulac):

●Adult:

Oral: 2–3 tbsp (30–45 ml) tid–qid. Adjust dose to produce 2–3 soft stools daily. If encephalopathy present, hourly doses may be given until laxative effect noted.

Enema (when treatment is urgent or oral route is not feasible): 300 ml lactulose plus 700 ml water retained 30–60 minutes. Repeat as needed at 4–6 hr intervals.

●Older child/adolescent: 40–90 ml/day PO in divided doses. Adjust dose to produce 2–3 soft stools a day.

●Infant: 2.5–10 ml/day PO in divided doses. Adjust dose to produce 2–3 soft stools a day.

LEVOTHYROXINE [T4] (Synthroid, Levothroid)

Action: synthetic T4 with same effect as endogenous T4. Onset of action is 6–8 hr IV and 1–3 days PO. Half-life is 6–7 days in euthyroid patient and 8–9 days in hypothyroidism.

Indications: hypothyroidism, simple (nontoxic) goiter.

Contraindications: acute myocardial infarction, uncorrected adrenal insufficiency, thyrotoxicosis.

Comments: Laboratory tests: Before starting thyroid hormone therapy for hypothyroidism, it is essential that blood be obtained for serum TSH level. In addition, blood should be obtained for measurement of T4, and T3 uptake. Furthermore, save enough serum for cortisol, FSH, and LH should those tests become necessary. An elevated TSH is to be expected when hypothyroidism is due to primary thyroid failure, while a low or normal TSH indicates hypothyroidism secondary to pituitary or hypothalamic malfunction. If immediate treatment is not imperative, it may be best to await the serum TSH result before starting thyroid hormone therapy. If serum TSH is not elevated, the patient needs a workup for panhypopituitarism, and a glucocortcoid must be administered along with levothyroxine. Monitor ongoing therapy by clinical observation and by periodically obtaining TSH and free T4 index. Diabetes mellitus: Hypothyroidism may mask or lessen signs and symptoms of diabetes mellitus. The patient may require an increase in insulin or oral hypoglycemic medication as hypothyroidism is corrected. Diabetes insipidus may be aggravated as hypothyroidism is corrected. Patient on oral anticoagulant generally requires less anticoagulant as hypothyroidism is corrected. Monitor prothrombin time. Digitalis requirements may be increased as hypothyroidism is corrected because digitalis will be metabolized more quickly. Cholestyramine must not be given within 4–5 hours of oral levothyroxine. Cholestyramine binds to levothyroxine in the intestinal lumen and thus interferes with levothyroxine absorption.

Side effects are due to overdose, and are the signs and symptoms of hyperthyroidism.

Supplied as: 25, 50, 100, 150, 175, 200, 300 microgram tablets;
vials containing 200 or 500 micrograms for IV or IM injection.

Adult dose:

Otherwise healthy young to middle–aged adult: Start with 50–100 mcg PO once daily. The dose is increased as needed by 25–50 mcg every 2–3 weeks based on clinical response, and results of serum TSH and free T4 index. The usual maintenance dose is 100–200 mcg PO once daily.

Patient who is elderly, has cardiovascular disease, or has longstanding hypothyroidism: Start with 25 mcg PO once daily. The dose is increased as needed by 25 mcg every 3–4 weeks based on clinical response and results of serum TSH and free T4 index.

Myxedema coma/stupor: Give an initial dose of 200–500 mcg IV followed by 100 mcg/day. Switch to oral medication when feasible and adjust PO dose (usually 100–200 mcg PO once daily) according to clinical response, and results of serum TSH and free T4 index. Use the smaller dose recommendations and proceed cautiously if there is severe cardiac disease. Because hypothyroidism may mask adrenal insufficiency; thyroid hormone therapy alone will raise metabolic rate and may thus engender acute adrenal insufficiency. For this reason, IV hydrocortisone (100 mg q8h) is also administered concurrently, and then discontinued if serum cortisol is found to be normal.

Parenteral dose (for patient who is unable to take PO medication): Start with a daily IM or preferably IV dose that is half of the recommended daily oral dose and subsequently adjust dose according to clinical response and thyroid function tests.

Pediatric dose (congenital hypothyroidism):

Oral dose: Initial dose for patient 0–6 months is 8–10 mcg/kg/day, for patient 6–12 months is 6–8 mcg/kg/day, for patient 1–5 yr is 5–6 mcg/kg/day, for 6–12 yr is 4–5 mcg/kg/day. Subsequently, adjust dose according to clinical response and thyroid function tests.

Parenteral dose (for patient who is unable to take PO medication): Start with a daily IM or preferably IV dose that is half of the recommended daily oral dose, and subsequently adjust dose according to clinical response and thyroid function tests.

LIDOCAINE

Action: ●Decreases automaticity of ventricles by slowing rate of diastolic depolarization. ●Suppresses reentrant arrhythmias by decreasing conduction velocity thru ischemic myocardium.
Indications: ●Supression of premature ventricular contractions with any of the following characteristics: more than 6/min, two or more consecutively, multifocal, falls on preceding T wave. ●Ventricular tachycardia or ventricular fibrillation. ●Prevention of ventricular arrhythmias in setting of acute myocardial infarction. ●Control rapid ventricular response to atrial fibrillation/flutter in patient with accessory pathway (e.g. Wolff–Parkinson–White syndrome).
Contraindications: hypersensitivity to local anesthetics; heart rate less than 50; severe sinoatrial, AV, or intraventricular heart block; Adams–Stokes syndrome.
Side effects (usually at toxic levels): neurologic: drowsiness, confusion, slurred speech, paresthesias, muscle twitching, seizures, respiratory depression; cardiovascular: reduced myocardial contractility, hypotension, sudden cardiovascular collapse, impaired AV conduction, sinus arrest, increased ventricular rate in presence of atrial fibrillation/flutter.
Supplied as:
for direct IV bolus Injection: 5 ml syringe containing 50 mg (10 mg/ml),
　　　　　　　　　　　　　　　5 ml syringe or ampul containing 100 mg (20 mg/ml).
for dilution: vials or additive syringes containing 1 or 2 grams.
for IM Injection: 5 ml ampul containing 500 mg (100 mg/ml).
Dose: refer to appendix.

LINDANE [gamma benzene hexachloride] (Kwell, Scabene)

Action: induces convulsions in and thereby kills arthropods.
Indications: head lice, pubic lice (crabs), scabies.
Contraindications: lindane sensitivity.
Caution: ●Lindane penetrates skin and has potential for CNS toxicity. Therefore, do not apply other creams, ointments, or oils simultaneously with this product because skin absorption will be enhanced. ●Avoid contact with eyes, face, mucous membranes, and open wounds. ●Use with caution in pregnancy or in young children (less toxic options are available). In lice infestations, the shampoo preparation is preferred since there is less risk of systemic absorption.
Side effects: eczema, CNS toxicity.
Supplied as (2 oz or 16 oz units): 1% cream, 1% lotion, and 1% shampoo.
Directions:

　　Scabies (cream or lotion): If there are crusted lesions, first bathe with soap and warm water, dry, and allow skin to cool. Rub in a thin layer of cream or lotion to entire body from neck down. Leave on for 8–12 hours. Bathe. Repeat in 1 week if living mites are demonstrated. Continued pruritus alone is not an indication of treatment failure.

　　Head lice (cream, lotion, or shampoo): Rub cream or lotion into hair and scalp. Leave on for 8–12 hours. Bathe. Repeat in 7 days if living lice are seen. ●Alternatively, work shampoo thoroughly into infested hair adding small amounts of water as necessary to produce lather. Leave in place for 4 minutes. Rinse and dry. Remove nits with fine tooth comb or tweezers. Repeat in 7 days if living lice are seen. Treatment failures are greater with shampoo than with cream or lotion.

Pubic lice (cream, lotion, or shampoo)**:** Apply to pubic area in same manner as for head lice. In addition to pubic area, apply lindane as needed to infested thighs, trunk, and axilla. Treat sex contacts at the same time.

LISINOPRIL (Privinil, Zestril)

Action: angiotensin–converting enzyme inhibitor. See captopril.
Indication: hypertension.
Contraindication: hypersensitivity to product. Discontinue immediately if angioedema occurs.
Caution: salt or volume depletion, severe congestive heart failure, renal artery stenosis, pregnancy, nursing mother.
Comments: ●Concurrent use of potassium–sparing diuretics, potassium supplement, or potassium–containing salt substitutes may lead to hyperkalemia. ●Captopril, another angiotensin–converting enzyme inhibitor, has been known to cause bone marrow suppression with agranulocytosis. This occurs most frequently in patients with renal failure (particularly those with collagen vascular disease). Periodic assessment of WBC count is justified. Patients should immediately report symptoms of infection since this may signal neutropenia. ●Patient should report lightheadedness and should discontinue the drug if syncope occurs. ●Warn patient that conditions that lead to volume depletion (e.g. excessive sweating, vomiting, diarrhea) may provoke fall in blood pressure.
Side effects seen in > 1% patients treated with lisinopril, or lisinopril plus hydrochlorothiazide: dizziness, vertigo, headache, fatigue, asthenia, diarrhea, upper respiratory symptoms, nasal congestion, cough, nausea, vomiting, dyspepsia, hypotension, orthostatic effects, chest pain, impotence, decreased libido, muscle cramps, back pain, rash, paresthesia.
Supplied as: 5, 10, 20, 40 mg tablets.
Dose:
Uncomplicated essential hypertension in patient not receiving diuretic: Start with 10 mg PO once daily. Increase dose if necessary. The usual requirement is 20–40 mg once daily. Add a diuretic (e.g. hydrochlorothiazide 12.5 mg/day) if lisinopril alone is inadequate. Be especially cautious when making dose adjustments in older patients.
Patient who is receiving diuretic: If possible, stop diuretic for 2–3 days before starting lisinopril and then proceed as above. If the diuretic cannot be stopped, give a 5 mg initial dose and keep the patient under close medical supervision for 2 hours and until the blood pressure has stabilized for another hour.
Initial dosage in renal failure:

creatinine clearance > 30 ml/min:	10 mg once daily
creatinine clearance 10–30 ml/min:	5 mg once daily

In patient with creatinine clearance < 10 ml/min (usually a dialysis patient), start with 2.5 mg once daily and then titrate dosage or dose interval according to blood pressure response.

LITHIUM CARBONATE (Eskalith, Lithane, Lithobid)
LITHIUM CITRATE (Cibalith–S Syrup)

Indications: treatment/prevention of mania in manic–depressive illness.
Contraindications: dehydration, sodium depletion, profuse sweating, prolonged diarrhea or vomiting, severe debility, severe infection, nursing mother. Avoid in pregnancy (especially first trimester) if at all possible. Relative contraindications: significant renal or cardiovascular disease, child < 12 years of age.
Comments: Concurrent diuretic administration increases risk of lithium toxicity because diuretic–induced sodium depletion leads to increased lithium reabsorption by renal tubules. Profuse sweating, diarrhea, or salt–deficient diet also lead to sodium depletion and predispose to lithium toxicity. Other drugs that may increase lithium blood levels: metronidazole; nonsteroidal anti–inflammatory drugs (e.g. indomethacin, piroxicam). Advise patient and family of symptoms of lithium toxicity: vomiting, diarrhea, tremor, ataxia, drowsiness, muscle weakness. Lithium may impair mental/physical performance. Avoid hazardous activities until drug effect is known. Infection with fever may dictate that lithium be discontinued or the dose reduced. Laboratory tests: Obtain thyroid and renal function tests every 6–12 months. Assess renal function if polyuria or nocturia occurs. Neuromuscular–blocking drug effects may be prolonged by lithium. Avoid concurrent administration of iodides.
Side effects: Incidence is dose–related. Most common: thirst, polyuria, nausea, vomiting, diarrhea, fine hand tremor, incoordination. Other: The list is long and includes sedation, confusion, restlessness, dizziness, vertigo, tinnitus, ataxia, slurred speech, blurred vision, nystagmus, hyperactive deep tendon reflexes, choreoathetosis, seizures, muscle weakness, EKG changes, arrhythmias, hypotension, abnormal taste, salivation, swelling salivary glands, hyperglycemia, goiter, hypothyroidism, oliguria, incontinence, diabetes insipidus, itching, rash, hair thinning/loss, vasculitis, leukocytosis.

Overdose: ●Empty stomach if the ingestion is acute. Activated charcoal is not effective. ●Cessation of lithium administration may suffice in mild cases. ●Alkalinizing the urine will enhance urinary excretion. ●Diuresis (e.g. acetazolamide, mannitol) will also enhance excretion. ●Hemodialysis may be necessary in severe cases.

Supplied as: 300 mg capsule or tablet,
450 mg control–release tablet (Eskalith CR),
300 mg slow–release tablet (Lithobid),
lithium citrate syrup (8 mEq lithium/5ml where 8 mEq lithium citrate is equivalent to 300 mg lithium carbonate).

Dose (adult):

<u>Acute episode</u>: usual dose is 600 mg PO tid.

<u>Maintenance</u>: usual dose is 300 mg PO tid (or 450 mg twice daily for control–release tablet).

<u>Note</u>: Adjust dose according to therapeutic response and serum lithium level. The serum lithium level should be measured twice weekly during acute psychiatric episode and at least every 2 month when receiving maintenance dose. The desired therapeutic level during an acute psychiatric episode is 1.0–1.5 mEq/l, and during maintenance therapy is 0.6–1.2 mEq/l. Blood sample should be drawn just before the next dose (8–12 hours after the last dose). 1–3 weeks may elapse fefore therapeutic effects are noted.

MAGNESIUM SULFATE

Action: Exerts anticonvulsant effect by inhibiting release of acetylcholine at myoneural junction. Uterine contractions are inhibited. There is a small decrease in blood pressure.

Indications: ●Treatment or prevention of seizures associated with pre–eclampsia or eclampsia. ●Seizures, particularly when associated with magnesium deficiency. ●Hypomagnesemia or magnesium depletion (e.g. due to alcoholism, malabsorption, diabetic ketoacidosis, hyperthyroidism, hypothyroidism, total parenteral nutrition, prolonged diarrhea or nasogastric suction). ●Atrial fibrillation or ventricular tachycardia due to digitalis toxicity.

Caution/comments: ●Caution: renal insufficiency, heart block, patient receiving digitalis. ●Therapy may be gauged by a decrease in the patella reflex. Discontinue magnesium if the patella reflex disappears. ●The newborn of a mother who received magnesium sulfate prior to delivery may exhibit magnesium toxicity and require ventilatory assistance. Calcium gluconate is the antidote. ●Succinylcholine and nondepolarizing muscle relaxants are potentiated by magnesium sulfate.

Side effects (due to hypermagnesemia): hyporeflexia, muscle weakness, flaccid paralysis, hypotension, increased QT interval, AV block, cardiac arrest, coma, respiratory depression.

Supplied as: 10% solution (1 gram magnesium sulfate/10ml),
  50% solution (1 gram magnesium sulfate/2ml).
  One gram magnesium sulfate = 8.1 mEq.

Dose for eclampsia/severe pre–eclampsia:
  Loading: 4 gram 10% solution IV over 20 minutes,
    or dilute 4 grams in 100 ml D5W and administer IV over 20 minutes.
  Maintenance: Add 10 gram to 1000 ml D5W and infuse IV via constant infusion pump at 100 ml/hr (approximately 1 gram/hr).
●Alternative but less preferred IM maintenance regimen: 10 gram 50% solution deep IM (5 gram in each buttock) followed by 5 gram (10 ml of 50% solution) deep IM q4h alternating buttocks.

Dose for magnesium depletion/hypomagnesemia:
  Adult: If patient is seizing, administer 2 gram 10% solution IV over 2 minutes. If necessary, give additional 1–2 gram 10% solution IV over next 15–20 minutes. Then proceed to maintenance infusion as for eclampsia above. In less urgent circumstances, therapy may begin with the maintenance infusion or intramuscular injections. If IM therapy is chosen, a suggested regimen is a loading dose of 5 gram of 50% solution IM followed by 1 gram of 50% solution q6h until hypomagnesemia resolves.
  Pediatric: 25–50 mg/kg IV or IM at 4–6 hour intervals until hypomagnesemia resolves.

MANNITOL

Action: Generalized intracellular dehydration occurs because intracellular water is drawn by the osmotically active mannitol into the intravascular space. Osmotic diuresis occurs because mannitol is filtered at glomeruli (but less than 10% is reabsorbed by the tubules) and water is excreted along with mannitol.

Indications: Temporary measure in management of increased intracranial pressure (e.g. intracranial bleed/tumor/abcess, pseudotumor cerebri). Increased intraocular pressure (e.g. glaucoma). Prevention of acute renal failure (e.g. hemolytic transfusion reaction, myoglobinuria).

Contraindications: hypovolemia, anuria, mannitol hypersensitivity.

Caution/comments: ●In order to remove crystals, mannitol should be administered thru an inline IV filter. ●Monitor blood pressure, urine output, body weight, central venous pressure, electrolytes, BUN, creatinine. ●Mannitol infusion must be stopped or reduced if the CVP increases without a significant increase in urinary output. ●Because mannitol mobilizes intracellular water, there may be an acute rise is intravascular volume with ensuing CHF and pulmonary edema. This is most likely to occur if urine output is inadequate, if too much mannitol is given over too short a period, or if there is limited cardiac reserve. ●By shrinking the brain, mannitol may increase intracranial blood flow and thus increase bleeding in the patient with intracranial bleeding. ●A rebound increase in intracranial pressure may occur after mannitol diuresis. ●Use mannitol cautiously in presence of cirrhosis of liver, pregnancy, pelvic or GU trauma.

Side effects: dehydration/hypovolemia with consequent hypotension, tachycardia, polydipsia); electrolyte abnormalities (especially hyponatremia); acidosis; chest pain; congestive heart failure; pulmonary edema; nausea; vomiting; chills; headache; confusion; dizziness; lethargy; thrombophlebitis; hypersensitivity reactions.

Supplied as: 5, 10, 15, 20, 25% solutions for IV administration.
  The 20% solution contains 100 gram/500 ml.

Dose to reduce intracranial or intraocular pressure (adult or child): 1–2 gram/kg (5–10 ml/kg of 20% solution) IV over 30–60 minutes. If necessary, the dose may be repeated twice at 6 hour intervals.

Dose to induce diuresis (e.g. hemoglobinuria, myoglobinuria, oliguria):

Adult: If the patient is markedly oliguric or if there is doubt concerning adequacy of kidney function, first administer a test dose: 0.2 gram/kg IV over 5 minutes. If kidney function is adequate, the urine output should be at least 30 ml/hr over the next 2–3 hours. If the response is inadequate, further mannitol administration is not advisable. ●Dose varies according to clinical circumstances and the response to mannitol infusion. The range is from 50 gram to a maximum of 200 gram per 24 hr. The daily requirement may be divided into periodic IV infusions at 4–6 hour intervals or given as a continuous infusion. The goal is to maintain an urine output of at least 30 ml/hr. In a hemolytic transfusion reaction, the urine output should be maintained at at least 100 ml/hr for 18–24 hours. Hypovolemia should be avoided before and during therapy, and electrolyte and fluid losses should be replenished.

Child: 0.75 gram/kg IV over 5 minutes. If adequate diuresis ensues (i.e. ≥ 0.5 ml/kg/hr over next 2–3 hours), additional mannitol may be administered to keep urine output > 0.5 ml/kg/hr. Dose range is 0.5–2.0 gram/kg q4–6h not to exceed 200 gram/day. Hypovolemia should be avoided before and during therapy, and electrolyte and fluid losses should be replenished.

MEBENDAZOLE (Vermox)

Indications: pinworm (Enterobius vermicularis), roundworm (Ascaris lumbricoides), whipworm (Trichuris trichiura), hookworm (Ancyclostoma duodenale and Necator americanus).
Contraindications: pregnancy.   **Caution:** patient < 2 years of age.
Side effects: nausea, vomiting, diarrhea, abdominal pain.
Supplied as: 100 mg tablet.
Dose (adult or child): 1 tablet PO morning and evening for 3 consecutive days. Tablet may be chewed or crushed and mixed with food. Treatment may be repeated in 3 weeks if needed. Fasting or purging are not required.
Pinworm: 1 tablet PO once.
Hydatid disease due to Echinococcus granulosus may respond to mebendazole with regression of cysts (50 mg/kg/day for 3 months).
Tapeworm: Although not the treatment of choice, mebendazole may be used to treat tapeworm infestations (300 mg tid for 3 days).

METHENAMINE MANDELATE (Mandelamine)
METHENAMINE HIPPURATE (Hiprex, Urex)

Action/spectrum: Methenamine is hydrolyzed in an acid urine to ammonia and formaldehyde. The latter agent is effective against both gram–positive and gram–negative bacteria, and some fungi. Resistant bacteria do not emerge. Effectiveness depends on an acid urine. It should only be used when an acid urine (pH less than 6) can be assured (see first comment). The mandelate or hippurate components contribute to urinary acidification and are themselves antibacterial.
Indications: prevention/suppression of recurrent urinary tract infections.
Note; Methenamine activity is largely restricted to the bladder because not enough formaldehyde is generated in the kidney to suppress/treat upper urinary tract infections. If acute urinary tract infection develops (upper and/or lower) while on methenamine, it should be treated with other antimicrobial drugs but not a sulfonamide (see contraindications).
Contraindications: hypersensitivity to any of components, dehydration, severe renal or hepatic insufficiency, gout, concurrent sulfonamide administration (formaldehyde may form insoluble precipitates with sulfonamides), concurrent acetazolamide (because this drug alkalinizes the urine).
Comments: ●Safety in pregnancy not established. ●Patient should test urine with pH paper and maintain a pH of 5.5 or less with a high–protein diet, cranberry juice, prune juice, and if necessary with vitamin C (500–1000 mg PO qid). Discontinue drug if a pH less than 6 cannot be maintained. ●Urea–splitting bacteria (proteus, some pseudomonas) interfere with antibacterial activity by alkalinizing the urine. ●Drinking large volumes of fluid decreases the effectiveness of methenamine (the urine is less acidic, formaldehyde is diluted and less is generated). ●Aspiration of oral suspension may cause lipid pneumonia. For this reason, methenamine mandelate suspension should be administered cautiously in the elderly or debilitated. ●Formaldehyde may interfere with assessment of urinary catecholamines, VMA, 5HIAA, estriol, 17–hydroxycorticosteroids.
Side effects: nausea, vomiting, upset stomach, rash, dysuria, hematuria.

methenamine mandelate

Supplied as: tablets (500, 1000 mg); granules (1000 mg packets); oral suspension (250, 500 mg/5ml)

Dose: Adult: 1000 mg PO 4 times a day (after meals and at bedtime).
Child 6–12 year of age: 500 mg PO qid (after meals & at bedtime).
under 6 year of age: 50 mg/kg/day PO divided into 3 daily doses.

methenamine hippurate

Supplied as: 1000 mg tablet.

Dose: Adult/child over 12 year: 1 tablet PO twice daily.
Child 6–12 year: 1/2 to 1 tablet PO twice daily.

METHOHEXITAL SODIUM (Brevital)

Indications: ●to produce anesthesia for procedure lasting 15 min or less (e.g. cardioversion, intubation, minor surgery, reduce fracture); ●to induce anesthesia or supplement other anesthetics.

Contraindications: barbiturate hypersensitivity, porphyria, status asthmaticus.

Caution: severe cardiac disease, hypotension, shock, asthma, myasthenia gravis, myxedema, Addison's disease, hepatic/renal dysfunction, elevated blood urea, severe anemia, excessive premedication, pregnancy.

Comments: ●Methohexital should be prepared with one of following diluents: sterile water injection USP, D5W, 0.9% saline. ●Drug is not compatible with Ringers lactate and should not be mixed with acid solutions (e.g. atropine, succinylcholine).

Side effects: respiratory or cardiac depression, cardiorespiratory arrest, bronchospasm, laryngospasm, hiccups, salivation, nausea, vomiting, headache, emergence delirium, muscle twitching, allergic reactions. ●Accidental intra–arterial injection may lead to arteritis, thrombosis, vasospasm, gangrene. ●Extravasation may cause neuritis or skin sloughing.

Supplied as: vials containing 0.5, 2.5, 5 gram for dilution.

Dose (adult) of 1% solution: First administer 2 ml IV test dose.
To induce anesthesia, administer 5–12 ml (50–120 mg).
To maintain anesthesia, administer 2–4 ml doses as needed.

METHYLDOPA (Aldomet)

Action: Antihypertensive mechanism is uncertain. Methyldopa is metabolized to alpha–methyl-norepinephrine which in turn probably stimulates inhibitory alpha–adrenergic receptors in the CNS. The consequent reduction in sympathetic outflow from the CNS decreases total peripheral resistance and hence blood pressure (both supine and standing). Heart rate and cardiac output are little affected, and there is usually no change in renal blood flow or glomerular filtration rate.

Indications: Moderate to severe hypertension. A diuretic is usually prescribed concurrently for the additional antihypertensive effect, and to counteract the sodium and water retention that may occur with methyldopa therapy.

Contraindications: hypersensitivity; active liver disease or history of methyldopa–associated liver disorder, hypertensive encephalopathy, hypertension with intracranial bleeding.

Caution: pregnancy, nursing mother, renal failure, history of liver disease.

Comments: Coombs testing and hemolytic anemia; A positive direct Coombs test develops in 10–20% patients on prolonged therapy and may persist for several months after discontinuing methyldopa. A positive Coombs test per se is not a contraindication to continued methyldopa treatment. Rarely, however, a Coombs–positive hemolytic anemia develops which does mandate discontinuation of methyldopa. Hemolytic anemia usually resolves promptly after methyldopa is stopped. Sometimes a + indirect Coomb's test develops and this may interfere with crossmatching for transfusion. As a precaution, it is advisable to obtain a direct Coombs test (pretreatment and at 6 and 12 months), and a pretreatment and periodic CBC. Hepatic complications; Periodic liver function testing is recommended (especially during first 6–12 wk) to rule out development of drug–induced hepatitis. Discontinue methyldopa if abnormal liver function tests, jaundice, or unexplained fever develops. Tolerance to antihypertensive effects may develop This can usually be remedied by adding a diuretic or increasing the dose. Edema and weight gain may occur and usually responds to diuretics. Renal failure; Methyldopa is excreted by kidney. Reduce dose in renal failure. Dialysis removes methyldopa.

Side effects include: blood (+ Coombs test, hemolytic anemia, leukopenia, granulocytopenia, thrombocytopenia, bone marrow depression); liver (abnormal liver function tests, hepatitis, fever, jaundice, hepatic necrosis); gastrointestinal (nausea, vomiting, diarrhea, constipation, distention, flatus, colitis, dry mouth, sialadenitis, sore or black tongue, pancreatitis); neurologic (sedation, asthenia, headache, lightheadedness, dizziness, depression, decreased mental acuity, nightmares, mild psychosis, paresthesias, choreoathetosis, parkinsonism, Bell's palsy); cardiovascular (worsening angina, postural hypotension, sodium and water retention with edema, bradycardia, carotid sinus hypersensitivity, myocarditis, pericarditis); endocrine/genital (hyperprolactinemia, lactation, breast enlargement, gynecomastia, amenorrhea, impotence, decreased libido); other (drug fever, + ANA, + LE prep, + rheumatoid factor, lupus–like syndrome, arthralgia, myalgia, rash, toxic epidermal necrolysis, nasal congestion, increased BUN).

Overdose: ●Emesis or gastric lavage followed by administration of activated charcoal. ●Monitor blood pressure. Trendelenberg position and administer isotonic fluids IV if the patient is hypotensive. Dopamine or dobutamine may be used if hypotension persists. ●Hemodialysis may be required in severe cases.

Supplied as: tablet (125, 250, 500 mg); oral sususpension (250mg/5ml); IV injection (250 mg/5ml)

Oral dose:

Adult: 250 mg bid–tid initially. Increase or decrease dose as needed by 250 mg every 2–3 days. Usual range is 500–2000 mg/day divided into 2–4 daily doses. Maximum 3000 mg/day. NOTE: ●To minimize daytime sedation make initial dose increases in the evening. ●If other antihypertensives are administered concurrently, the initial dosage of methyldopa must not exceed 500 mg/day. This restriction does not apply to thiazides.

Pediatric: 10 mg/kg/day divided into 2–4 daily doses.
Maximum 65 mg/kg/day or 3000 mg whichever is least.

Intravenous dose: Intravenous methyldopa is seldom used in hypertensive emergencies because there is a delay of 4–6 hr before antihypertensive effect is seen.

Adult: 250–500 mg q6h. Maximum 1000 mg q6h. Doses are dissolved in 100 ml D5W and infused over 30–60 minutes.

Pediatric: 5–10 mg/kg q6h. Maximum 65 mg/kg/day or 3000 mg/day whichever is least. Doses are dissolved in D5W and infused over 30–60 minutes.

METHYLERGONOVINE MALEATE (Methergine)

Action: induces uterine contractions.
Indications: prevent/control hemorrhage following delivery of placenta or following abortion.
Contraindications: hypersensitivity, hypertension, pregnancy, toxemia of pregnancy.
Caution: sepsis, obliterative vascular disease, heart disease, mitral valve stenosis, hepatic or renal disease.
Comments: ●Onset of action IV/IM/PO: immediate/2–5 min/5–10 min respectively. ●Duration: several hours. ●Because of the risk of precipitating hypertension and cerebrovascular accident, intravenous administration is reserved for emergencies.
Side effects: hypertension, nausea, vomiting, headache, blurred vision. ●Rare reactions include tinnitus, dizziness, diaphoresis, palpitations, chest pain, dyspnea, diarrhea.
Supplied as: 0.2 mg tablet; 1 ml ampul (0.2 mg/ml) for IV or IM injection.
Dose:

Intramuscular: 0.2 mg following delivery placenta or during puerperium. Repeat as needed at 2–4 hour intervals.

Oral: 0.2mg tid–qid for 1–2 days (maximum 1 week).

Intravenous (in emergency only): 0.2 mg over no less than 60 seconds while monitoring blood pressure.

METRONIDAZOLE (Flagyl, Metric 21, Protostat)

Spectrum/Indications: Protozoa (Trichomonas vaginalis, Entamoeba histolytica, Giardia lamblia); Obligate anaerobic bacteria (Bacteroides including B. fragilis, clostridia, fusobacterium, Peptococcus, Peptostreptococcus); Gardnerella (Haemophilus) vaginalis; Dranunculus medinensis (Guinea worm).
Contraindications: metronidazole hypersensitivity, first trimester pregnancy. ●Administer in 2nd and 3rd trimester only when absolutely essential, and avoid single–dose therapy. ●Nursing should be discontinued while taking drug.
Caution: CNS disease, history of blood dyscrasia, severe liver disease (metronidazole may accumulate). ●Avoid indiscriminate use (carcinogenicity has been shown in rats). ●Avoid alcohol during therapy because Antabuse reaction may occur (headache, flushing, nausea, vomiting, abdominal cramps). ●Discontinue metronidazole if neurologic side effects occur.
Drug interactions: ●Metronidazole by potentiating oral anticoagulants may further prolong the prothrombin time. ●Drugs that stimulate hepatic metabolism (e.g. phenobarbital, phenytoin) may hasten elimination of metronidazole thereby decreasing plasma metronidazole level. ●Cimetidine inhibits liver enzyme activity and thus elevates the plasma metronidazole level.
Side effects: gastrointestinal (anorexia, nausea, vomiting, diarrhea, epigastric distress, abdominal cramps, constipation, proctitis, abnormal taste, Candidal overgrowth with "furry" tongue, glossitis, stomatitis); neurologic (seizures, peripheral neuropathy, dizziness, vertigo, incoordination, depression, irritability, insomnia, confusion, weakness); blood (neutropenia, thrombocytopenia); hypersensitivity (fever, rash, urticaria, flushing, nasal congestion, dry mouth/vagina); renal (dark urine, dysuria, cystitis, polyuria, incontinence); other (joint pains, decreased libido, dyspareunia, vaginal Candidal overgrowth, flattening T wave EKG).

Supplied as: 250, 500 mg tablet;   IV preparation.
Dose:
Trichomonas
>   Adult: 250 mg PO tid for 7 days, or single 2 gram PO dose.
>   Child: 5 mg/kg PO tid for 7 days.

Giardia
>   Adult: 250 mg PO tid for 7 days.
>   Child: 5 mg/kg PO tid for 7 days.

Amebiasis (E. histolytica)
>   Adult: 750 mg PO tid for 5–10 days.
>   Child: 35–50 mg/kg/day divided into 3 daily doses PO for 10 days.

Dranunculus medinensis (Guinea worm)
>   Adult: 250 mg PO tid for 10 days.
>   Child: 25 mg/kg/24 hr divided into 3 daily doses PO for 10 days
>   (maximum 750 mg/24hr).

Gardnerella (Haemophilus) vaginalis Adult: 500 mg PO twice daily for 7 days.
Serious anaerobic infections Adult: 15 mg/kg IV loading dose followed by 7.5 mg/kg IV q6h. Intravenous dose is infused over 1 hour. Change to oral therapy when feasible, 7.5 mg/kg PO q6h. Maximum 4 gram/24 hr.

MEXILETINE (Mexitil)

Action: Orally active structural analog of lidocaine with similar electrophysiologic/antiarrhythmic properties. Like lidocaine, mexiletine depresses ventricular automaticity. Normally, mexiletine does not affect the sinus node or AV conduction. However, mexiletine may (1) depress the sinus node and cause bradycardia in the sick sinus syndrome, and (2) can cause AV block when there is disease of His–Purkinje network.
Indications: suppression of symptomatic ventricular arrhythmias—e.g. frequent PVC's, ventricular tachycardia.
Contraindications: cardiogenic shock,
                    2nd or 3rd degree AV block in absence of artificial ventricular pacemaker.
Caution: preexisting sinus node dysfunction or intraventricular conduction abnormalities, liver disease, hypotension, severe congestive heart failure.
Side effects: <u>cardiovascular</u> (palpitations, chest pain, increased PVC's/ventricular arrhythmias, AV block/conduction abnormalities, bradycardia, atrial arrhythmias, syncope, hypotension, hypertension, cardiogenic shock, edema, hot flashes); <u>neurologic</u> (dizziness, lightheadedness, tremor, nervousness, incoordination, sleep disturbance, paresthesias, weakness, fatigue, confusion, depression, headache, tinnitus, blurred vision, short–term memory loss, psychosis, seizures, loss of consciousness); <u>gastrointestinal</u> (nausea, vomiting, heartburn, diarrhea, constipation, abdominal discomfort/cramps/pain, altered appetite, dysphagia, dry mouth, altered taste, upper GI bleed, esophageal perforation, hiccups, abnormal liver function tests); <u>blood</u> (thrombocytopenia, neutropenia, agranulocytosis, myelofibrosis); <u>skin</u> (rash, dry skin, sweating, hair loss); <u>other</u> (dyspnea, fever, malaise, pharyngitis, urinary hesitancy/retention, impotence, decreased libido, arthralgia, positive ANA, SLE syndrome).
Supplied as: 150, 200, 250 mg tablets.
Dose (adult): 200–300 mg q8h is the usual requirement. Arrhythmia control should be verified clinically and with EKG monitoring (e.g. Holter). Take the drug with food or antacid. If necessary, the dose may be increased to 400 mg q8h provided lesser dose is tolerated. The daily dose may be divided q12h in those patients who have been stabilized on 300mg q8h or less (up to 450 mg may be given q12h). Continued arrhythmia control should be verified. If rapid control of ventricular arrhythmia is essential, a 400mg intial dose may be given followed by a 200mg dose 8 hours later.

MICONAZOLE (Monistat, Micatin)

Action: Inhibits synthesis of ergosterol and in so doing disrupts normal fungal cell membrane permeability.
Indications: <u>Dermatologic preparation</u> is indicated in treatment of (1) cutaneous candidiasis; (2) tinea cruris, cruris, or corporis due to intradermal dermatophytes (Trichophyton, Epidermophyton); (3) tinea versicolor due to Malassezia furfur. <u>Intravaginal preparation</u> is used to treat candidal vaginitis. <u>Injectable form</u> (as alternative to amphotericin B) is reserved for severe systemic fungal infections (coccidioidomycosis, paracoccidioidomycosis, cryptococcosis, candidiasis, petriellidiosis) and for treatment of chronic mucocutaneous candidiasis.
Contraindications: miconazole hypersensitivity.
Caution: IV miconazole; pregnancy; nursing mother; infant < 1 yr old; concurrent administration of certain drugs (coumarin drugs, oral hypoglycemics, rifampin, cyclosporin A, phenytoin, carbam-

azepine). Intravaginal; first trimester pregnancy, nursing mother. Dermatologic; avoid eye contact.
Side effects: with IV use; itching, rash, phlebitis, flushing, nausea, vomiting, diarrhea, anorexia, drowsiness, fever, chills, anaphylaxis, hyperlipemia, transiently decreased serum sodium and hematocrit, thrombocytopenia, RBC aggregation/rouleau formation on blood smears; with dermatologic use; irritation, burning, maceration, allergic contact dermatitis; with vaginal use; vulvovaginal effects (burning, irritation, itching); skin rash; urticaria; pelvic cramps; headache.

Supplied as:
dermatologic: 2% skin cream or lotion;
vaginal: 2% vaginal cream (Monistat 7),   100 mg vaginal suppository (Monistat 7),
   200 mg vaginal suppository (Monistat 3);
injection (Monistat IV): ampul containing 200 mg for intravenous or intrathecal injection, or bladder instillation.

Dose, dermatologic (Micatin, Monistat–Derm): apply cream or lotion twice daily for 2 weeks. Note: ●Reconsider diagnosis if not improved after 1 month. ●Treat tinea pedis for 2 month. ●Once daily application suffices in tinea versicolor. ●The lotion is preferred for intertriginous regions.

Dose, intravaginal: One applicatorful Monistat 7 vaginal cream at bedtime for 7 days, or one Monistat 7 vaginal suppository at bedtime for 7 days. Alternative: Monistat 3 vaginal suppository at bedtime for 3 days.

Dose, intravenous:
   Adult: ●Candidiasis: 600–1800 mg/day for 1 wk to over 20 wk.
      ●Cryptococcosis: 1200–2400 mg/day for 3 wk to over 12 wk.
      ●Coccidioidomycosis: 1800–3600 mg/day for 3 wk to over 20 wk.
      ●Petriellidiosis: 600–3000 mg/day for 5 wk to over 20 wk.
      ●Paracoccidioidomycosis: 200–1200 mg/day for 2 wk to over 16 wk.
   Child; 20–40 mg/kg/day divided into 3 daily doses. An individual dose must not exceed 15 mg/kg.
Comments concerning intravenous administration; ●Divide daily dose into 3 equal doses. ●Each 200 mg ampul is diluted in 200 ml of normal saline or D5W and infused over over 2 hr (rapid infusion may cause arrhythmias). Of course, more rapid infusion is necessary if the patient requires more than 2400 mg/day. ●IV miconazole–associated nausea/vomiting may be alleviated by giving antiemetics before infusion, decreasing rate or dose of infusion, avoiding infusion at mealtime. ●Monitor hemoglobin, hematocrit, and serum electrolytes and lipids. ●Fungal meningitis must be treated with both intravenous and intrathecal miconazole. ●Bladder infections must be treated both intravenously and with bladder instillation. ●Miconazole does not require dose adjustment in renal failure. ●Do not use IV miconazole in trivial infections. ●Amphotericin B is more effective (but more toxic) than miconazole in the treatment of severe systemic fungal infections. Miconazole is therefore reserved for cases in which amphotericin B is not effective or is not tolerated.

Dose, intrathecal (as adjunct to intravenous miconazole in treatment of fungal meningitis): 20 mg undiluted solution given at 3–7 day intervals. Rotate between lumbar, cervical, and cisternal punctures.

Dose, bladder instillation (as adjunct to IV therapy for fungal cystitis): 200 mg diluted.

MIDAZOLAM (Versed)
Action: short–acting benzodiazepine CNS depressant.
Contraindications: hypersensitivity to drug, acute narrow–angle glaucoma, open–angle glaucoma (unless patient is receiving appropriate treatment), shock, coma, acute alcohol intoxication with depressed vital signs.
Caution/comments: ●Because IV administration may cause respiratory depression/apnea; competent personnel with oxygen and equipment to maintain patent airway and ventilation must be immediately on hand. ●COPD patients are particularly prone to respiratory depression with this drug. ●Narcotics and other CNS depressants add to midazolam's sedative and respiratory depressant effects. ●The elimination half–life is increased in patients with CHF or chronic renal failure. ●Caution: pregnancy.
Side effects include: respiratory; decreased tidal volume and/or resp rate, apnea, dyspnea, tachypnea, hyperventilation, laryngospasm, bronchospasm, wheezing, airway obstruction; cardiovas-

cular; PVC's, bigeminy, tachycardia, nodal rhythm, vasovagal episode; <u>gastrointestinal</u>; hiccups, nausea, vomiting; <u>neurologic</u>; headache, drowsiness, retrograde amnesia, euphoria, dysphoria, nervousness, anxiety, restlessness, emergence delirium or agitation, prolonged emergence from anesthesia, insomnia, nightmares, dizziness, lightheadedness, paresthesias, impaired balance, ataxia, slurred speech, dysphonia, athetoid movements; <u>eyes</u>; blurred vision, difficulty focusing, diplopia, nystagmus, pinpoint pupils, cyclic movements of eyelids; <u>skin</u>; itching, hives, rash; <u>injection site effects</u>; pain, redness, induration, muscle stiffness with IM, phlebitis with IV.

Supplied as: 1 mg/ml concentration (2, 5, 10 ml vials);
5 mg/ml concentration (1, 2, 5, 10 ml vials and 2 ml disposable syringe).

indications/adult dose:
<u>Intravenously for conscious sedation just prior to short diagnostic or endoscopic procedure:</u>
●Healthy adult < 60 yr: Titrate to desired level of sedation starting with 1 mg to up to maximum of 2.5 mg over at least 2 minutes. Observe the patient for at least 2 minutes. Then, if further sedation is needed, administer additional small amounts with at least a 2 minute pause between doses. No more than a total of 5 mg is usually necessary for initial sedation. Patients receiving narcotics or other CNS depressants will need about 30% less. Additional doses (25% of the initial dose) may be administered as needed to maintain sedation.
●Debilitated, chronicallly ill, or adult > 60 yr: Titrate to desired level of sedation starting with 1 mg to up to maximum of 1.5 mg over at least 2 minutes. Observe the patient for at least 2 minutes. Then, if further sedation is needed, administer additional small amounts (no faster than 1 mg/2 min) with at least a 2 minute pause between doses. No more than a total of 3.5 mg is usually necessary for initial sedation. Patients receiving narcotics or other CNS depressants will need less. Additional doses (25% of the initial dose) may be administered as needed to maintain desired level of sedation.
<u>Intramuscular for preoperative sedation:</u> 0.07–0.08 mg/kg IM (5 mg IM in usual adult) about 1 hour before surgery. Onset within 15 minutes, peak 30–60 minutes. Atropine, scopolamine, or reduced dose of narcotic may be given concomitantly.
<u>Induction of general anesthesia before administration of other anesthetics:</u>
●Average <u>unpremedicated</u> adult < 55 yr receives 0.30–0.35 mg/kg IV over 20–30 seconds initially. Additional doses (25% of the initial dose) may administered as needed. Maximum total dose is 0.6 mg/kg IV. Initial dose in good risk patient over 55 yr is 0.3 mg/kg IV. Inititial dose in debilitated/poor risk patient is 0.2–0.25 mg/kg IV.
●Average premedicated adult < 55 yr receives 0.25 mg/kg IV over 20–30 seconds. Good risk patient over 55 receives 0.2 mg/kg IV. 0.15 mg/kg IV may suffice in debilitated/poor risk patient.

MINOXIDIL (Loniten)
Action: Reduces both diastolic and systolic BP by directly dilating peripheral arterioles. The hypotensive effect causes a reflex increase in sympathetic output with ensuing tachycardia and increased cardiac output. Renal compensation with fluid retention also occurs.
Indication: hypertension that cannot be controlled with maximum therapeutic doses of a diuretic plus two other antihypertensive drugs.
Contraindications: pheochromocytoma.
Caution: pregnancy, nursing mother, renal failure, dialysis patient.
Comments: <u>To prevent tachycardia</u>, propranolol 80–160 mg/day in divided doses (or some other beta blocker) must usually be given concurrently. If beta blockers are contraindicated, start one of the following alternatives: methyldopa 250–750 mg twice daily (begun at least 24 hr before starting minoxidil) or clonidine 0.1–0.2 mg twice daily. <u>To prevent sodium and fluid retention</u>, a diuretic must be given concurrently (e.g. furosemide 40 mg twice daily and increased as needed). <u>Pericardial effusion</u>, sometimes with tamponade develops in about 3% patients. Aggressive diuresis and/or stopping minoxidil may suffice but dialysis, pericardiocentesis, or even surgery may be needed. <u>Guanethidine</u> must be stopped before starting minoxidil because severe orthostatic hypotension may occur. Patient must be hospitalized if this cannot be done.
Side effects: sodium and water retention; pericardial effusion ± tamponade; hirsutism (occurs in 80% patients, may persist 1–6 months after discontinuation); EKG changes (flattening or inversion T waves, increased QRS voltage); breast tenderness; nausea; vomiting; allergic reaction (rash, bullae, Stevens–Johnson syndrome); thrombocytopenia; leukopenia.
Overdose: Empty stomach and then administer activated charcoal. If the patient is hypotensive, place in trendelenberg position and administer isotonic fluids IV. Administer dopamine or dobutamine if hypotension persists.
Supplied as : 2.5, 10 mg tablets.

Dose (in conjunction with a diuretic and a beta blocker):

Patient over 12 yr: Initially, 5 mg PO once daily. Increase the dose in steps as needed: 10, 20, and then 40 mg/day as single daily dose or divided into 2 daily doses (usual range 10–40 mg/day, maximum 100 mg/day). Normally, one should allow at least 3 days between dose increases. However, in urgent cases dose increases can be made every 6 hours with careful monitoring. Note: If supine blood pressure has decreased by less than 30 mm Hg, give a single daily dose. If supine blood pressure has decreased by more than 30 mm Hg, divide daily dose into two equal doses.

Patient under 12 yr: Initially 0.2 mg/kg once daily. If necessary, gradually increase by 50–100% increments. Usual requirement is 0.25–1.0 mg/kg/day. Maximum 50 mg/day.

MORPHINE SULFATE

Action: Opium alkaloid. Therapeutic actions: (1) <u>analgesia</u> due to reaction with opioid receptors of central and peripheral nervous system; and (2) <u>vasodilation</u> with consequent increased venous capacitance (decreased cardiac preload) and decreased peripheral vascular resistance (decreased cardiac afterload). Decreased preload and afterload reduce the work of the heart and alleviate acute pulmonary edema of cardiac etiology.

Indications: severe pain, acute pulmonary edema of cardiac etiology, preoperative sedation/analgesia.

Contraindications: morphine hypersensitivity, hypotension, severe bronchospasm, post biliary tract surgery.

Caution: ●IV morphine must be administered in small increments to preclude hypotension or respiratory depression. Use with great caution, if at all, in patient who is hypovolemic. ●asthma (morphine contracts bronchial smooth muscle); ●prostatic hypertrophy (because urinary tract smooth muscle tone is increased and urinary retention may result); ●abdominal pain of undetermined cause (because clinical signs may be masked); ●head injuries, intracranial lesions, or increased intracranial pressure (because clinical signs may be masked and because morphine may depress respirations leading to CO_2 retention with ensuing cerebral vasodilation and increased intracranial pressure); ●respiratory, hepatic, renal, or adrenal compromise; ●delirium tremens; ●hypothyroidism; ●patient who engages in activities that require alertness.

Side effects include: drug dependence, respiratory depression, sedation, headache, confusion, euphoria, dysphoria, anxiety, hallucinations, lightheadedness, dizziness, ataxia, nausea, vomiting, constipation, biliary spasm, supraventricular tachycardia (due to vagolytic effect on AV node), hypotension, syncope, bradycardia, urinary retention, sweating, miosis, allergic reaction.

Supplied as: injection (2, 8, 10, 15 mg/ml);   tablet (10, 15, 30 mg);
oral solution (10 mg/5ml, 20 mg/5ml, 20 mg/ml).

Adult dose:

Intravenous (acute pulmonary edema of cardiac etiology; immediate pain relief): 2 mg IV push. Repeat every 5 minutes as needed up to cumulative total of 15 mg. Titrate according to therapeutic effect—blood pressure and respiratory status allowing.

Subcutaneous/intramuscular: 2–15 mg as needed at 4 hour intervals.

Oral: 20–75 mg or more as needed at 4 hour intervals. Because of rapid hepatic metabolism, PO dose requirements vary considerably from patient to patient.

Pediatric dose: 0.1–0.2 mg/kg IV or SC as needed at 2–4 hour intervals. Maximum of 15 mg/dose.

NALIDIXIC ACID (NegGram)

Action: Bactericidal against gram–negative bacteria over whole range of urinary pH.

Indications: Lower urinary tract infections due to susceptible gram–negative bacteria (e.g. E. coli, Enterbacter, Klebsiella, Proteus). ●Pseudomoas is usually resistant. ●Gram–positive bacteria are resistant. ●Nalidixic acid is not the drug of first choice in treatment of lower urinary tract infection. Furthermore, it is not effective in systemic infection or upper UTI such as pyelonephritis.

Contraindications: nalidixic hypersensitivity, infant < 3 months of age, first trimester pregnancy.

Caution: renal failure, liver failure, history of seizure disorder, nursing mother, prepubertal children (erosion of cartilage is observed in immature animals), concurrent oral anticoagulant administration (nalidixic acid enhances the anticoagulant effect), excessive exposure to sunlight (photosensitivity may result).

Comments: ●Bacterial resistance may emerge rapidly (usually within 48 hr) especially if initial dosage is inadequate. ●Perform CBC, renal and liver function tests periodically if treatment extends beyond 2 weeks. ●Glucoronic acid, a by–product of nalidixic acid metabolism, may result in a false + test for glucose with certain glucose tests but not with enzyme–based colorimetric tests (e.g. Tes-Tape, Clinistix).

Side effects: gastrointestinal; nausea, vomiting, diarrhea, abdominal pain, cholestasis; allergic; fever, rash, urticaria, eosinophilia, photosensitivity, arthralgias, anaphylaxis; blood; hemolytic anemia (particularly in those with G6PD deficiency), leukopenia, thrombocytopenia; neurologic; headache, drowsiness, confusion, weakness, dizziness, vertigo, convulsions, paresthesias, toxic psychosis; visual; blurred vision, diplopia, 6th nerve palsy, photophobia, altered color vision; other; metabolic acidosis, increased intracranial pressure with papilledema and bulging anterior fontanelle in infants.

Supplied as: tablet (250, 500, 1000 mg); oral suspension (250mg/5ml).

Dose: Adult: 1000 mg PO four times a day for 1–2 week.
Reduce to 500 mg qid if therapy prolonged.
Child under 12 yr: 55 mg/kg/day PO divided into 4 equal daily doses.
Reduce to 33 mg/kg/day if therapy prolonged.

NALOXONE (Narcan)

Action: Reverses the effects of opiate/opoid drugs (respiratory depression, coma, sedation, analgesia, pupillary constriction, hypotension, etc) by competing for opiate receptor sites.

Indications: reversal of respiratory depression or coma caused by opiate/opioid drugs including morphine; codeine; heroin; hydromorphone (Dilaudid); hydrocodone (Hycodan); oxycodone (component of Tylox, Percodan, Percocet); meperidine (Demerol); methadone (Dolophine); butorphanol (Stadol), propoxyphene (Darvon), pentazocine (Talwin). Other indications: clonidine overdose, alcoholic coma.

Comments: Onset is 1–2 minutes IV and 3–5 minutes IM or SC. Duration is 1–4 hours. ●Sudden reversal of narcotic depression may result in nausea, vomiting, tachycardia, hypertension. Rarely, cardiac arrhythmias (e.g. ventricular tachycardia, ventricular fibrillation) or pulmonary edema results. ●In physically–dependent patient, abrupt reversal may induce withdrawal syndrome (nausea, vomiting, sweating, tremulousness, tachycardia, hypertension, convulsions).

Supplied as: concentrations of 0.02 mg/ml, 0.4 mg/ml, and 1 mg/ml.

Adult dose:

Opiate/opioid overdose: 2 mg IV. Repeat every 2–3 minutes if no response. Reconsider diagnosis if there is no response after giving 10 mg. However, large doses may be required in propoxyphene overdose. ●Since naloxone has a short half-life, repeat boluses may be necessary or a continuous IV infusion may be started: add 2 mg naloxone to 500 ml D5W or normal saline and titrate to effect. ●Administer IM or SC if unable to administer IV. May also be given via endotracheal tube.

Postoperative narcotic depression: Give 0.1–0.2 mg IV at 2–3 minute intervals as needed to achieve desired effect. Titrate carefully because sudden reversal may, in addition to reversing analgesia and sedation, have untoward effects (see comments above).

Pediatric dose:

Overdose: 0.01mg/kg IV is initial dose. If no response, give 0.1 mg/kg IV every 3–5 minutes until there is a response or 5 doses given. May also be given IM or SC.

Postoperative narcotic depression: Give 0.005–0.01 mg/kg IV at 2–3 minute intervals as needed to achieve desired effect.

Neonatal dose (for narcotic depression): 0.01 mg/kg IV, IM, or SC. Repeat as needed.

NARCOTIC ANALGESICS: butorphanol (Stadol), codeine, hydromorphone (Dilaudid), meperidine (Demerol), levorphanol (Levo–Dromeran), methadone (Dolophine), nalbuphine (Nubain), oxycodone, oxymorphone (Numorphan), pentazocine (Talwin), propoxyphene (Darvon).

Find **morphine** under separate heading.

Action/Indications: Narcotics exert analgesic effect by reacting with opiate receptors of central and peripheral nervous system. The medullary cough center is suppressed (codeine is a commonly used antitussive). Methadone is indicated for treatment of narcotic addiction.

Contraindications: hypersensitivity to drug, meperidine in patient receiving MAO inhibitor.
●Because they increase the work of the heart, butorphanol or pentazocine are not recommended in setting of acute myocardial infarction, coronary insufficiency, or left ventricular dysfunction.

Comment: Naloxone will reverse the effects of all the opioid drugs (respiratory depression, sedation, hypotension, etc). However, the duration of action of naloxone may be shorter than the opioid being reversed (e.g. half–life of methadone is about 24 hr). Consequently, repeated administration of naloxone may be required. Keep in mind that too rapid a reversal in patient physically dependent on narcotics may induce acute abstinence syndrome.

Caution: Intravenous narcotic must be injected slowly and in small increments to preclude hypotension, respiratory depression, circulatory collapse, or cardiac arrest. Respiratory disorders (e.g. asthma, COPD, respiratory insufficiency): Narcotics may cause respiratory depression, bronchospasm, and depress the cough reflex. Prostatic hypertrophy: Narcotics may increase urinary tract smooth muscle tone and thus lead to urinary retention. Abdominal pain of unknown cause: Narcotics may mask clinical signs. Intracranial lesion or increased intracranial pressure: Narcotics may mask the clinical signs associated with these conditions. Furthermore, narcotics may cause respiratory depression which in turn may lead to CO_2 retention with consequent cerebral vasodilation and increased intracranial pressure. Patient who engages in activities that require alertness should be warned that mental and physical performance may be compromised by narcotics. Supraventricular tachyarrhythmias: In this setting, the vagolytic effect of certain opiates (e.g. meperidine) on the AV node may increase the ventricular rate. Biliary tract disorder: Narcotics may induce spasm of sphincter of Oddi. Meperidine is vagolytic and is therefore less likely to be associated with this side effect. Seizure disorder may be exaxerbated by narcotics. Administration during labor: Following delivery, neonatal respiratory depression may occur. Neonate may require naloxone. Use caution and reduce initial dose in the following settings: elderly; debilitated; hepatic, renal, or adrenal compromise; hypothyroidism. Caution is advised if patient is concurrently receiving other CNS depressants—e.g. other narcotics, phenothiazines, tricyclic antidepressants, benzodiazepines, barbiturates, alcohol, general anesthetics. Postoperative patient, hypovolemic patient, patient receiving phenothiazine or certain anesthetics: Narcotics may precipitate hypotension in these patients.

Side effects include: drug dependence, sweating; respiratory (respiratory depression, apnea, bronchospasm, laryngospasm); gastrointestinal (anorexia, nausea, vomiting, constipation, diarrhea, dry mouth, biliary tract spasm); neurologic (sedation, lightheadedness, dizziness, confusion, headache, euphoria, dysphoria, nervousness, anxiety, agitation, insomnia, hallucinations, ataxia, tremor, paresthesias, miosis, blurred vision, diplopia, nystagmus, elevated intracranial pressure); GU (ureteral spasm, urinary retention); cardiovascular (hypotension, syncope, bradycardia, tachycardia, palpitations, circulatory collapse and cardiac arrest after rapid IV injection, flushing); hypersensitivity (itching, rash, urticaria, anaphylactoid reactions).

butorphanol (Stadol)
Supplied as: 1mg/ml or 2 mg/ml for IM or IV injection.
Dose (adult):
    Intramuscular: 2 mg q3–4h (range: 1–4 mg q3–4h).
    Intravenous: 1 mg q3–4h (range: 0.5–2 mg q3–4h).
Note: ●Not recommended in patient less than 18 yr. ●Butorphanol increases the work of the heart. Consequently, it should not be used in setting of acute myocardial infarction, coronary insufficiency, or left ventricular dysfunction unless other strong narcotics are contraindicated. ●Butorphanol is a narcotic agonist–antagonist. The antagonistic effect contraindicates its use in patients physically dependent on narcotics. ●2 mg butorphanol has about same analgesic effect as 10 mg morphine. ●Intramuscular onset/peak/duration : within 10 min/30–60 min/3–4 hr. ●Intravenous onset/peak/duration : very rapid/within 30 min/3–4 hr.

codeine
Supplied as: tablets (15, 30, 60 mg); injection (30, 60 mg/ml).
Dose:
    Adult: Pain: 30–60 mg q4–6h PO, IM, or SC.
              Antitussive: 10–20 mg q4–6h. Maximum 120 mg/24hr.

Child: Pain: 0.5 mg/kg q4–6h PO, IM, or SC.
         Antitussive: 1mg/kg/24hr divided q4–6h, maximum 60 mg/24hr.
Note: ●65 mg PO codeine has about same analgesic effect as 650 mg aspirin or acetaminophen.
●120 mg IM codeine has about same analgesic effect as 10 mg morphine.

codeine combinations:

Empirin #2 (15 mg codeine + 325 mg aspirin):   Adult dose, 1–2 tablet q4h.
Empirin #3 (30 mg codeine + 325 mg aspirin):   Adult dose, 1–2 tablet q4h.
Empirin #4 (60 mg codeine + 325 mg aspirin):   Adult dose, 1 tablet q4h.
Tylenol #1 (7.5 mg codeine + 300 mg acetaminophen):   Adult dose, 1–2 tablet q4h.
Tylenol #2 (15 mg codeine + 300 mg acetaminophen):   Adult dose, 1–2 tablet q4h.
Tylenol #3 (30 mg codeine + 300 mg acetaminophen):   Adult dose, 1–2 tablet q4h.
Tylenol #4 (60 mg codeine + 300 mg acetaminophen):   Adult dose, 1 tablet q4h.
Tylenol with Codeine elixir (12mg codeine + 120mg acetaminophen/5ml):
●Adult: 15ml (1 tbsp) q4h ●7–12 yr: 10ml (2tsp) tid–qid ●3–6 yr: 5 ml (1tsp) tid–qid.

hydromorphone (Dilaudid)
Supplied as: tablet (1,2,3,4 mg);   rectal suppository (3 mg);
              injection (1,2,4,10 mg/ml).
Dose (adult):
    IV, IM, or SC: Initially, 1–2 mg q4–6h.
    PO: Initially, 2 mg q4–6h.
    Rectal: 3 mg q6–8h.
Note: IV injection should take place over at least 2–3 minutes. ●Safety not established in children
●1.5 mg parenteral hydromorphone has about same analgesic effect as 10 mg parenteral morphine. ●Parenteral onset: within 15 minutes; duration of effect: up to 5 hours. ●PO onset: within
30 minutes; duration of effect: 4–6 hours.

levorphanol (Levo–Dromeran)
Supplied as: 2 mg tablet,   2 mg/ml for SC injection.
Dose (adult): 2–3 mg PO or SC.
Note: ●Duration of effect is up to 6–8 hours. ●1.25–2.5 mg parenteral levorphanol has about
same analgesic effect as 10 mg morphine.

meperidine (Demerol)
Supplied as: tablet (50, 100 mg),   syrup (50 mg/5ml);
              injection (25, 50, 75, 100 mg/ml).
Dose
    Adult: 50–150 mg q3–4h IM, SC, or PO.
            If IV administration is necessary—reduce dose, dilute, and inject slowly.
    Child: 1.0–1.5 mg/kg q3–4h SC, IM, or PO (maximum 150 mg/dose).
Note: ●60–80 mg parenteral meperidine has about same analgesic effect as 10 mg morphine.
●IM administration is preferred over SC administration when repeated doses are given.
●Intramuscular onset/peak effect/duration: 10 min/30–50 min/2–4 hr. ●Because of its vagolytic
effect, equivalent analgesic doses of meperidine may cause less biliary tract spasm and constipation than morphine or other narcotics. ●Vagolytic effect may also result in increased ventricular
rate in patient with supraventricular tachyarrhythmias.

methadone (Dolophine)
Supplied as: tablet (5, 10 mg);   40 mg tablet for treatment narcotic addiction;
              oral solution (5, 10 mg/5ml);   injection (10 mg/ml).
Dose (for pain):   Adult: 2.5–10 mg q3–4h PO, IM, or SC.
Note: ●Methadone has a long half–life (about 24 hr) and accumulates after several doses.
Consequently, the dose and interval may need to be adjusted if therapy is prolonged. ●IM adminis-
tration is preferred over SC when repeated doses are given. ●Safety in pregnancy not established.
Inadvisable for obstetric analgesia. ●Concurrent rifampin administration may decrease blood level
of methadone. ●8–10 mg of parenteral methadone has about the same analgesic effect as 10 mg
of parenteral morphine.

morphine sulfate: find under individual heading "Morphine Sulfate".

nalbuphine (Nubain)
Supplied as: 10, 20 mg/ml for IV, IM, or SC injection.
Dose (adult): 10 mg q3–6h IV, IM or SC. Maximum 20 mg/dose and 160 mg/24 hr.
Note: ●Analgesic potency of 10 mg nalbuphine is about equivalent to 10 mg morphine. ●Onset is
within 2–3 minutes IV and within 15 minutes IM or SC. Duration of effect is 3–6 hours.

●Nalbuphine is a narcotic agonist–antagonist. The antagonistic effect may induce withdrawal syndrome if patient is physically addicted to narcotics.

oxycodone combinations:

Roxicet   Adult: 1 tablet PO q6h.
(5 mg oxycodone HCl + 325 mg acetaminophen)
Roxicet oral solution   Adult: 1 tsp PO q6h.
(5mg oxycodone HCl + 325mg acetaminophen per 5 ml)
Tylox   Adult: 1 tab PO q6h.
(4.5 mg oxycodone HCl + 0.38 mg oxycodone terephthalate + 500 mg acetaminophen)
Percocet   Adult: 1 tablet PO q6h.
(5 mg oxycodone HCl + 325 mg acetaminophen)
Percodan, Roxiprin   Adult: 1 tablet PO q6h.
(4.5mg oxycodone HCl + 0.38mg oxycodone terephthalate + 325mg aspirin)
Percodan–demi
2.355mg oxycodone HCl + 0.19mg oxycodone terephthalate + 325mg aspirin)
● Adult: 1–2 tablet PO q6h.   ●Over 12 yr: 1/2 tab q6h.   ●6–12 yr: 1/4 tab q6h.

oxymorphone (Numorphan)
Supplied as: rectal suppository (5 mg), injection (1, 1.5 mg/ml).
Dose (adult): ●IV: 0.5 mg initially. ●IM or SC: 1.0–1.5 mg q4–6h.
                     ●Rectal: 1 suppository q4–6h.
Note: ●Parenterally, 1mg oxymophone has about same analgesic effect as 10 mg morphine.
●Onset within 5–10 minutes; duration of effect 3–6 hours. ●Safe use in child under 12 yr not established.

pentazocine (Talwin)
Supplied as: ●Talwin Nx (50 mg tablet, also contains 0.5 mg naloxone to discourage IV drug abuse); ●injection (30 mg/ml).
Dose (adult):
    Oral: Initially 50 mg q3–4h. If necessary, give 100mg q3–4h (max 600 mg/24hr).
    IV: 30 mg q3–4h (maximum 30 mg/dose and 360 mg/24 hr).
    IM or SC: 30 mg q3–4h (maximum 60 mg/dose and 360 mg/24 hr).
Note: ●Ulceration (sloughing) and severe sclerosis of skin and subcutaneous tissue (and rarely underlying muscle) may occur after repeated IM or SC doses at same site. IM route is preferred to SC if injections are frequent. Injection sites must be rotated. ●Not recommended in child under 12 yr. ●Pentazocine is a narcotic agonist–antagonist. The antagonistic effect may induce withdrawal syndrome if patient is physically addicted to narcotics. ●30 mg parenteral pentazocine has about same analgesic effect as 10 mg parenteral morphine, and 30 mg PO pentazocine is equivalent to 60 mg PO codeine. ●Oral onset/peak effect/duration: 15–30 min/1–3 hr/3 hr or longer.
●IM onset/peak effect/duration: within 15–20 min/30–60 min/2–3 hr. ●Onset IV is within 1–2 min.

propoxyphene HCl (Darvon): 32, 65 mg capsules.
Dose (adult): 65 mg PO q4h as needed for pain (maximum 390 mg/day).
Note: ●Not recommended in child under 12 yr. ●65 mg propoxyphene provides about same analgesic effect as 650 mg of aspirin or acetaminophen.

NEOMYCIN, oral
Indications: Aminoglycoside antibiotic. Administered orally so as to sterilize the bowel in (1) patients with hepatic encephalopathy, (2) preparation for abdominal surgery.
Contraindications: bowel obstruction, neomycin hypersensitivity.
Caution: ●About 3% of PO neomycin is absorbed from GI tract. Consequently, reduce the dose or use other modalities if there is renal insufficiency. ●Neomycin may interfere with vitamin K absorption. Use neomycin cautiously in patients receiving oral anticoagulants.
Side effects: nausea, vomiting, diarrhea, malabsorption. ●In patients with renal failure, systemic aminoglycoside side effects may occur if there is sufficient GI absorption. (see "Aminoglycosides").
Supplied as: 500mg tablet, liquid (125mg/5ml).
Dose (adult):
Hepatic coma: 1 gram q4–6h PO or via nasogastric tube.
Preoperative bowel prep: In conjunction with mechanical bowel prep, the patient is given 1 gram of neomycin PO plus 1 gram erythromycin PO at 1, 2, and 11 PM the day before surgery .

NITRATES

Action: Relaxes vascular smooth muscle resulting in: (1) <u>systemic venous dilation</u> leading to peripheral venous pooling and thus decreased cardiac return with decreased preload; (2) <u>systemic arterial dilation</u> leading to decreased peripheral resistance and thus decreased afterload, (3) <u>coronary artery dilartion.</u> The effect of 1 and 2 is to decrease work of the heart and thereby decrease myocardial oxygen consumption.

Side effects: The vasodilative effects of nitrates may precipitate headache and postural hypotension. ●Hypotension may provoke cerebral ischemia with weakness, dizziness, or fainting. ●Other possible consequences of vasodilation with hypotension include tachycardia, pallor, sweating, nausea, vomiting, collapse. ●Hypotension with decreased coronary perfusion may cause worsening of angina. ●Other observed side effects include paradoxical bradycardia, cutaneous vasodilation with flushing, nausea, vomiting, abdominal pain, tolerance, rash, dermatitis. <u>Note;</u> Alcohol ingestion may aggravate the hypotensive effects of nitrates.

Sublingual nitroglycerin tablet (Nitrostat)

<u>Indication;</u> treatment or prevention of anginal attack.
Onset of action is 1–2 minutes, duration 30 minutes.
<u>Contraindications;</u> hypersensitivity to nitrates or nitrites, increased intracranial pressure, postural hypotension, hypovolemia, severe anemia, acute myocardial infarction, hypertrophic cardiomyopathy.
<u>Caution;</u> ●As a precaution against dizziness and falling, it is advisable that the patient be seated when taking tablet. ●Concurrent administration of certain drugs (e.g. alcohol, beta blockers, calcium channel blockers, phenothiazines) may enhance hypotensive effect of nitrates.
<u>Supplied as;</u>   0.15 mg (1/500 gr),   0.3 mg (1/200 gr),   0.4 mg (1/150 gr),
          0.6 mg (1/100 gr).
<u>Dose in angina;</u> 0.15–0.6mg as needed at 5 min. intervals. Max. 3 tablets/15 min.
<u>To prevent angina;</u> take tablet 5–10 min. prior to activity that provokes an attack.

Nitroglycerin lingual aerosol (Nitrolingual Spray)

<u>Indication;</u> treatment or prevention of anginal attack.
<u>Contraindications/caution;</u> see sublingual nitroglycerin tablet above.
<u>Supplied as;</u> container delivers 200 metered doses.
<u>Dose in angina;</u> 1 or 2 metered doses sprayed onto tongue preferably. The spray should not be inhaled. Maximum 3 doses within 15 minutes.
<u>To prevent angina;</u> take dose 5–10 min prior to activity that might provoke angina.

Intravenous nitroglycerin (Nitro–Bid IV, Nitrostat IV, Tridil)

<u>Indications;</u> angina, treatment of acute myocardial infarction–associated congestive heart failure, to produce controlled hypotension during surgery, control of perioperative hypertension.
<u>Contraindications;</u> hypersensitivity to nitrates or nitrites, hypotension, hypovolemia, constrictive pericarditis, pericardial tamponade, increased intracranial pressure, inadequate cerebral circulation, hypertrophic cardiomyopathy. <u>Caution;</u> severe renal or liver disease, pregnancy.
<u>Dose;</u> Dilute 25 mg nitroglycerin in glass bottle containing 250 ml D5W or normal saline for a concentration of 100 mcg/ml. Start infusion at 5 mcg/min (3 ml/hr) via infusion pump. Increase every 3–5 min in 5 mcg/min increments until blood pressure change occurs. If the blood pressure still does not change with 20 mcg/min (12 ml/hr), increase rate of infusion by 10 mcg/min or if needed 20 mcg/min increments. Once blood pressure response is noted, further dose increases must be made gradually. On occasion, patients have received 200 mcg/min or more.

Nitroglycerin oral sustain release capsule

(Nitrocine Timecaps, Nitroglycerin SR, Nitrong, Nitrospan)
<u>Indication;</u> prevention of angina.
<u>Contraindications;</u> hypersensitivity to nitrates or nitrites, acute myocardial infarction, severe anemia, orthostatic hypotension, hypovolemia, increased intracranial or intraocular pressure, hypertrophic cardiomyopathy.
<u>Caution;</u> ●In order to avoid withdrawal reaction, nitroglycerin therapy should be discontinued gradually if patient has been on prolonged therapy. ●Alcohol or calcium channel blockers enhance the hypotensive effects of nitrates.
<u>Supplied as;</u> 2.5, 2.6. 6.5, 9 mg.
<u>Dose;</u> Start with 2.5 mg PO tid–qid. If needed, increase daily dose over days to weeks by 5–10 mg/day increments (divide the total daily dose into 3–4 doses). Up to 26 mg qid has been used. Onset of action is about 60 minutes and duration is 8--12 hr. Capsules are to be swallowed. They are not to be chewed and are not for sublingual administration.

Nitroglycerin topical ointment 2% (Nitro–Bid, Nitrol, Nitrong, Nitrostat)

Indication: prevention of angina. Not indicated for treatment of acute anginal attack. Onset of action is about 15 minutes.

Contraindications: hypersensitivity to nitrates or nitrites, hypertrophic cardiomyopathy, increased intracranial pressure, severe anemia, hypovolemia, low systolic blood pressure.

Caution: ●Monitor patient carefully in setting of congestive heart failure or acute myocardial infarction. ●In order to avoid withdrawal reaction, nitroglycerin therapy should be discontinued gradually if patient has been on prolonged therapy. ●Alcohol or calcium–channel blockers enhance the hypotensive effects of nitrates.

Dose: Start with 1/2 inch q8h. Increase by 1/2 inch increments as needed to prevent angina while not inducing headache. If angina only occurs several hours after an application, try decreasing the interval between applications to every 3–6 hr. Usual dose is 1/2 to 2 inches q4–6h. Rarely, up to 5 inches may be required.

Nitroglycerin skin patches

(Deponit, Nitrodisc, Nitro–Dur, Minitran, Transderm–Nitro)

Indication: prevention of angina.

Contraindications/caution: as for ointment, see above.

Comment: Patches become ineffective if they are applied daily for 24 hours. Patches delivering 10 mg or more per 24 hour can retain their effectiveness if there is a 10–12 hour daily hiatus during which they are not used.

Supplied as (available strengths in terms of amount of nitroglycerin delivered per 24 hr is in parenthesis following the product name):

Deponit (5 or 10 mg/24hr); Minitran (2.5, 5, 10, or 15 mg/24hr);
Nitrodisc (5, 7.5, or 10 mg/24 hr); Nitro–Dur (2.5, 5, 7.5, 10, or 15 mg /24 hr);
Transderm–Nitro (2.5, 5, 10, or 15 mg/24 hr).

Dose: Apply one patch daily. Do not apply to distal extremities or hairy areas. Change patch after bathing. Rotate sites.

isosorbide dinitrate (Isordil, Sorbitrate)

Supplied as: sublingual tablet (2.5, 5 10 mg); chewable tablet (5, 10 mg); regular swallow tablet (5, 10, 20, 30, 40 mg); sustain release tablet or capsule (40 mg).

Dose (for prevention of angina):
●Sublingual: 5–10 mg q2–3h (onset 2–5 minutes, duration 1–2 hr).
  Chewable tablet: 5–10 mg q2–3h.
●Swallow tablet: 5–20 mg initially, 10–40 mg q6h maintenance.
  (onset 15–30 minutes, duration 4 hr).
●Sustain release tablet/capsule: 40 mg initially, 40–80 mg q8–12h maintenance.
  (onset 2 hr, duration 6–12 hr).

erythrityl tetranitrate (Cardilate)

Supplied as: 10 mg tablet for sublingual administration or for swallowing.

Dose (for prevention of angina):
Oral/sublingual tablet: Initially, 5–10 mg sublingual prior to angina–inducing situations. Increase dose as needed. If swallowed, start with 10 mg before meals, between meals, and at bedtime (up to 100 mg/day has been used).
Note: ●Swallowed—onset/peak/duration: 15–30 min/60 min/6 hr.
  ●Sublingual—onset/peak/duration: 5 min/15 min/up to 3 hr.

pentaerythritol tetranitrate (Duotrate, Peritrate)

Supplied as: tablet (10, 20, 40 mg); sustain release capsule (30, 45, 80 mg).

Dose (for prevention of angina): Start with 10–20 mg PO four times a day (1/2 hr before or 1 hr after meals, and at bedtime). Maintenance 10–40 mg four times a day. Tablet may be chewed or swallowed.
●Sustain release form: 30–80 mg PO q12h. Take on empty stomach. Do not chew.

NITROFURANTOIN (Furadantin, Macrodantin)

Action: Bacterial enzyme inhibitor. Bacteriostatic at low concentrations and bactericidal at higher concentrations. Sensitive bacteria include E.coli, enterococci (e.g. S. faecalis), S. aureus, most klebsiella, most enterobacter. ●Pseudomonas (including P. aeruginosa) are resistant as are most proteus and serratia.

Indications: treatment and prophylaxis of urinary tract infections (e.g. cystitis, pyelonephritis) due to susceptible bacteria. ●Nitrofurantoin is not indicated for treatment of systemic infections, or for renal cortical or perinephric abscesses.

Contraindications: nitrofurantoin hypersensitivity, anuria, oliguria, creatinine clearance < 40 ml/min, pregnancy at term, neonates.

Caution: ●Be alert for development of pulmonary hypersensitivity reactions (see side effects below). ●G6PD–deficient patient may develop hemolytic anemia. ●Severe and/or irreversible peripheral neuropathy may occur, particularly in setting of diabetes mellitus, anemia, electrolyte abnormalities, vitamin B deficiencies, or renal failure with creatinine clearance less than 40 ml/min.

Side effects include: <u>gastrointestinal</u>: anorexia, nausea, vomiting, diarrhea, abdominal pain; <u>blood</u>: hemolytic anemia in G6PD–deficient patient, megaloblastic anemia, granulocytopenia, leukopenia, thrombocytopenia; <u>neurologic</u>: headache, drowsiness, dizziness, vertigo, peripheral neuropathy; <u>acute pulmonary hypersensitivity</u> (usually occurs within first week therapy and resolves after discontinuing drug): fever, chills, cough, dyspnea, chest pain, pulmonary infiltrate with consolidation or pleural effusion, eosinophilia; <u>chronic pulmonary hypersensitivity</u> (usually occurs after 6 mo therapy and sometimes results in permanent pulmonary dysfunction even after cessation of drug): cough, malaise, dyspnea or exertion, interstitial pneumonitis and/or pulmonary fibrosis; <u>other hypersensitivity reactions</u>: asthma attack in asthmatic patient, fever, chills, rash, itching, urticaria, angioedema, anaphylaxis, arthralgias, myalgia, hepatitis, cholestatic jaundice, pancreatitis, lupus–like syndrome; <u>skin</u>: transient alopecia, exfoliative dermatitis, erythema multiforme, eczema.

Supplied as: tablet (50, 100 mg); capsule (25, 50, 100 mg); oral suspension (25mg/5ml).

Adult dose:

<u>Urinary tract infection</u>: 50–100 mg qid with food (50 mg qid for uncomplicated UTI). Continue treatment for at least 1 week and for at least 3 days after urine is sterile.
<u>Prevention of recurrent UTI</u>: 50–100 mg PO at bedtime may suffice.

Pediatric dose:

<u>Urinary tract infection</u>: 5–7 mg/kg/24 hr PO in 4 equal doses.
<u>Prevention of recurrent UTI</u>: 1 mg/kg/day may suffice. May be given as single daily dose or divided into 2 daily doses.

NITROPRUSSIDE (Nipride, Nitropress)

Action: Dilates both arteries and veins by a direct action on vascular smooth muscle. An almost immediate reduction in blood pressure results. The effect ends when the IV infusion is stopped.

Indications: ●hypertensive crisis ●temporary treatment of severe refractory heart failure in hypertensive or normotensive patient ●during surgery, to produce controlled hypotension in order to reduce bleeding (but only to be used if patient has adequate cerebral circulation).

Contraindications: compensatory hypertension (e.g. arteriovenous shunt, coarctation of aorta).

Caution: pregnancy, nursing mother, hepatic or renal insufficiency, hypothyroidism, elderly.

Supplied as : vial containing 50 mg for dilution in D5W.

Dose (adult or child): refer to appendix.

Comments: <u>Infusion rate must be precisely controlled (e.g. infusion pump, microdrip regulator) and blood pressure must be closely monitored</u>. Too rapid a reduction in blood pressure may cause nausea, vomiting, sweating, headache, dizziness, apprehension, restlessness, substernal discomfort, palpitations, muscle twitching, or abdominal pain. These symptoms resolve when infusion is stopped or reduced. <u>Preparing and protecting solution</u>: Dilute nitroprusside in D5W. Do not mix other drugs in nitroprusside solution. Nitroprusside is light sensitive. Cover the IV solution with aluminum or paper bag (cover IV tubing at very slow infusion rates). The solution is stable for up to 24 hours if properly protected from light. <u>Begin oral antihypertensive drug</u> while the hypertensive crisis is being controlled with nitroprusside. <u>Toxicity</u>: The toxic metabolites cyanide and thiocyanate may accumulate with excessive or prolonged infusion. Patients with renal or hepatic dysfunction are particularly susceptible. Do not exceed 10 mcg/kg/min infusion. ●Cyanide toxicity is manifested as metabolic acidosis (the earliest sign), tolerance to the drug, dyspnea, headache, vomiting, dizziness, unconsciousness, imperceptible pulse, distant heart sounds, shallow breathing, pink color, widely dilated pupils. Treatment of cyanide toxicity: (1) discontinue nitroprusside (2) if there is massive overdose, administer sodium nitrite and sodium thiosulfate. ●Thiocyanate toxicity (tinnitus, blurred vision, delirium, hypothyroidism). It is advisable to obtain daily thiocyanate levels if the infusion is continued longer than 72 hours. A level > 10 mg/dl is considered toxic.

NIZATIDINE (Axid)

Action: Decreases gastric acid secretion by inhibiting histamine at H–2 receptors (especially those on gastric parietal cells).
Indications: treatment of active duodenal ulcer, maintenance after duodenal ulcer has healed.
Contraindications: hypersensitivity to drug. Use with caution if there is history of hypersensitivity to other H-2 receptor antagonists.
Caution: moderate to severe renal insufficiency, pregnancy, nursing mother.
Side effects: sweating, urticaria, somnolence. Other observed events for which a causal relationship has not been established include liver injury with elevated liver enzymes, ventricular tachycardia, impotence, decreased libido, rash, exfoliative dermatitis, hyperuricemia.
Supplied as: 150, 300 mg capsules.
Dose:

  Active duodenal ulcer: 150 mg PO twice daily (or 300 mg PO once daily at bedtime) for up to 8 weeks if necessary. Healing usually occurs within 4 weeks. Reduce dosage to 150 mg once daily if there is renal insufficiency with creatinine clearance 20–50 ml/min, and to 150 mg every other day if the creatinine clearance is < 20 ml/min.

  Maintenance for healed duodenal ulcer: 150 mg PO at bedtime.
Reduce dosage to 150 mg every other day if there is renal insufficiency with creatinine clearance 20–50 ml/min, and to 150 mg every 3 days if the creatinine clearance is < 20 ml/min.

NONSTEROIDAL ANTI-INFLAMMATORY DRUGS (NSAID): fenoprofen (Nalfon), ibuprofen (Motrin, Advil, Nuprin, Rufen), indomethacin (Indocin), ketoprofen (Orudis), meclofenamate (Meclomen), naproxen (Naprosyn), naproxen sodium (Anaprox), piroxicam (Feldene), sulindac (Clinoril), tolmetin (Tolectin).

Note: See also "Aspirin" and "Other Salicylates and Derivatives".

Action: Inhibitors of prostaglandin synthesis with analgesic, antipyretic, and anti–inflammatory properties.
Contraindications: history of aspirin or other nonsteroidal anti–inflammatory drug-induced hypersensitivity reaction (e.g. nasal polyps–associated asthma, rhinitis, urticaria, or angioedema); pregnancy; nursing mother; children (except for tolmetin which may be used in children over 2 yr).
Caution: GI effects: Use with caution in patient with active peptic ulcer or history of upper GI disease because NSAID may lead to GI bleeding/ulceration/perforation. Platelet effects: NSAID inhibit platelet function and must therefore be used cautiously in patients with bleeding disorders or in patients receiving anticoagulants. Interaction with warfarin: Plasma protein–binding by NSAID may competitively displace warfarin and thus enhance the anticoagulant effect of warfarin. Monitor prothrombin time. Note, however, that ibuprofen and sulindac do not significantly effect warfarin anticoagulation, and tolmetin does not effect warfarin anticoagulation. Hepatic effects: NSAID may cause elevation of liver function tests (SGOT, SGPT, alkaline phosphatase); jaundice; hepatitis. Stop NSAID if significant abnormalities occur. Use NSAID cautiously if there is liver disease. Renal effects: NSAID may cause renal injury (e.g. nephrotic syndrome, interstitial nephritis, cystitis). Therefore, monitor renal function if there is renal compromise, and avoid using NSAID if there is a prior history of renal side effects. Fluid retention and edema may occur. Therefore, use NSAID cautiously in presence of hypertension or cardiac compromise. Visual effects: Nonsteroidal anti–inflammatory drugs may cause visual impairment. Stop drug if visual side effects occur. Perform eye exams periodically if patient is on chronic NSAID therapy. NSAID may mask signs of infection as a consequence of their antipyretic and anti–indlammatory properties.

fenoprofen (Nalfon)   Supplied as: 200, 300 mg capsule;   600 mg tablet.
Dose (adult): ●Mild to moderate pain: 200 mg PO q4–6h.
●Rheumatoid arthritis/osteoarthritis: 300–600 mg PO 3–4 times a day.
Note: Maximum 3200 mg/day.   Absorption is decreased when given with food.
Most common side effects: dyspepsia, constipation, nausea, vomiting, diarrhea, abdominal pain, anorexia, flatulence, occult blood in stool, dry mouth, headache, somnolence, dizziness, tremor, nervousness, insomnia, confusion, fatigue, malaise, tinnitus, decreased hearing, blurred vision, pruritis, rash, urticaria, increased sweating, palpitations, tachycardia, dyspnea.

ibuprofen (Advil, Motrin, Nuprin, Rufen)
Supplied as: ●capsule (200 mg); ●tablet (200, 300, 400, 600, 800 mg).
Dose (adult):
- ●Mild to moderate pain: 200–400 mg PO q4–6h.
- ●Rheumatoid arthritis/osteoarthritis: 1200–3200 mg/day divided into 3–4 doses.
- ●Dysmenorrhea: 400 mg PO q4h as needed.

Note: ●Administer with meals or milk if GI side effects occur. ●Maximum 3200 mg/day.
Most common side effects: nausea, epigastric pain, heartburn, diarrhea, vomiting, abdominal discomfort/cramps/pain/bloating, indigestion, anorexia, dizziness, headache, nervousness, tinnitus, edema.

indomethacin (Indocin)
Supplied as: capsule (25, 50 mg);   sustain release capsule (75 mg);
             oral suspension (25mg/5ml);   suppository (25 mg).
Dose (adult):
- ●Moderate to severe cases of rheumatoid arthritis, osteoarthritis, or ankylosing spondylitis: 25 mg PO bid–tid initially. Increase as needed by 25–50 mg/day increments at weekly intervals. Maximum 150–200 mg/day. The 75 mg sustain release tablet may be substituted as a single daily dose in patient requiring 25 mg tid, or twice daily for patient taking 50 mg tid.
- ●Acute gouty arthritis: 50 mg PO three times a day until pain abates; then taper and stop drug over 1 week.

Note: Take indomethacin with or after meals, or with antacids.
Most common side effects: nausea, vomiting, dyspepsia, diarrhea, abdominal distress/pain, constipation, headache, dizziness, vertigo, somnolence, fatigue, malaise, tinnitus.

ketoprofen (Orudis)   Supplied as: 25, 50, 75 mg capsules.
Dose (adult):
- ●Rheumatoid arthritis, osteoarthritis: 200 mg/day divided into 3–4 doses.
                                          Maximum 300 mg/day.
- ●Mild–moderated pain or dysmenorrhea: 25–50 mg q6–8h.

Note: Reduce dose in smaller patients, patients with renal insufficiency, and in the elderly. Ketoprofen may be taken with antacids or food; but food may interfere with absorption.
Most common side effects: anorexia, nausea, vomiting, diarrhea, constipation, flatulence, abdominal pain, stomatitis, headache dizziness, CNS inhibition (e.g. somnolence, depression, malaise); CNS excitation (e.g. nervousness, insomnia, dreams); tinnitus, visual abnormalities, rash, increased BUN, edema, signs and symptoms of urinary tract irritation.

meclofenamate (Meclomen)   Supplied as: 50, 100 mg capsules.
Dose (adult) for rheumatoid arthritis, osteoarthritis: 200–400 mg/day divided into 3–4 equal doses. Maximum 400 mg/day.
Note: ●May be given with meals or milk. ●Optimum therapeutic effect may not be seen for 1–2 weeks.
Most common side effects: diarrhea, nausea, vomiting, abdominal discomfort or pain, heartburn, flatulence, constipation, peptic ulcer, anorexia, stomatitis, edema, rash, itching, urticaria, headache, dizziness, tinnitus.

naproxen (Naprosyn)
Supplied as: tablet (250, 375, 500 mg);   oral suspension (125mg/5ml).
Dose (adult):
- ●Rheumatoid arthritis, osteoarthritis, ankylosing spondylitis: 250–500 mg PO bid.
- ●Juvenile arthritis: 5 mg/kg twice daily.
- ●Acute gout: 750 mg initial dose followed by 250 mg q8h until attack subsides.
- ●Mild to moderate pain, primary dysmenorrhea, acute tendonitis, acute bursitis: 500 mg initial dose followed by 250 mg q6–8h as needed. Max. 1500 mg/day.

Most common side effects: constipation, heartburn, abdominal pain, nausea, diarrhea, dyspepsia, stomatitis, itching, rash, sweating, bruising, purpura, headache, drowsiness, lightheadedness, dizziness, vertigo, tinnitus, hearing or visual abnormalities, palpitations, dyspnea, edema, thirst.

naproxen sodium (Anaprox)   Supplied as: 275, 550 mg tablet.
Dose (adult):
- ●Rheumatoid arthritis, osteoarthritis, ankylosing spondylitis: 275–550 mg twice daily. Maximum 1650 mg/day.
- ●Acute gout: 825 mg initial dose followed by 275 mg q8h until attack subsides.
- ●Mild–moderate pain, primary dysmenorrhea, acute tendonitis and acute bursitis: 550 mg initial dose followed by 275 mg q6–8h as needed. Max 1375 mg/day.

Most common side effects : see naproxen.

piroxicam (Feldene)   Supplied as: 10, 20 mg capsules.

<u>Dose (adult):</u> Rheumatoid arthritis, osteoarthritis: 20 mg once daily. Full therapeutic effect may not be felt for 2 weeks.

<u>Most common side effects:</u> nausea, epigastric distress, indigestion, abdominal discomfort/pain, flatulence, diarrhea, anorexia, stomatitis, decrease in hemoglobin and hematocrit, anemia, leukopenia, eosinophilia, itching, rash, headache, somnolence, dizziness, vertigo, tinnitus, malaise, edema, increased BUN and creatinine.

sulindac (Clinoril)   Supplied as: 150, 200 mg tablets.

<u>Dose (adult):</u>   Note: Do not exceed 400 mg/day.

●<u>Rheumatoid arthritis, osteoarthritis, ankylosing spondylitis;</u> 150 mg PO twice daily with food.

●<u>Acute gouty arthritis;</u> 200 mg bid PO with food (7 days therapy usually suffices).

●<u>Bursitis, tendonitis;</u> 200 mg bid PO with food (7–14 days therapy usually suffices).

<u>Most common side effects;</u> abdominal pain/cramping, dyspepsia, nausea, vomiting, diarrhea, constipation, flatulence, anorexia, itching, rash, headache, nervousness, dizziness, tinnitus, edema.

tolmetin (Tolectin)   Supplied as: 200 mg tablet, 400 mg capsule.

<u>Rheumatoid arthritis;</u>

●Adult: 400 mg PO three times a day initially. Adjust dose according to response. Range is 600–1800 mg/day divided into 3–4 daily doses.

●Child 2 yr or older: initially, 20 mg/kg/day divided into 3–4 doses. Adjust dose according to response. Range is 15–30 mg/kg/day divided into 3–4 daily doses.

<u>Osteoarthritis (adult);</u> 400 mg PO three times a day initially.

Adjust dose according to response. Range is 600–1600 mg/day in 3–4 doses.

<u>Note:</u> May be taken with aluminum/magnesium hydroxide antacids if GI side effects occur. Food or milk may interfere with absorption.

NYSTATIN (Mycostatin, Nilstat, Nystex)

Action: Fungistatic and fungicidal. Binds to sterols in fungal cell membrane, and by so doing leads to leakage of fungal cell contents.

Indicatons: Candidal (monilial) infections of skin, mucous membranes, oral cavity (thrush), vagina, and GI tract.

Contraindications: hypersensitivity to nystatin or associated components. Oral tablets contain tartrazine. Tartrazine may cause allergic reaction, particularly in those with aspirin hypersensitivty.

Side effects: Rarely, irritation occurs with topical forms. Although generally very little is absorbed systemically, large oral doses may cause nausea, vomiting, and/or diarrhea.

Supplied as: <u>Creams or ointment</u> (100,000 unit/gram),
<u>topical powder</u> (100,000 unit/gram),
<u>oral suspension</u> (100,000 unit/ml),
<u>oral tablet</u> (500,000 unit/tablet),
<u>oral pastille</u> (200,000 unit),
<u>vaginal tablet</u> (100,000 unit/tablet).

Dose:

<u>Skin or mucous membranes;</u> apply topical form twice daily.

<u>Thrush:</u> Treatment is continued until at least 48 hours after clinical cure.

Adult or child: 2–3 ml oral suspension 4 times a day in each side of mouth and retained as long as possible before swallowing. Alternatively, 1–2 pastilles dissolved in mouth 4–5 times/day.

Infants: 2 ml suspension in each side of mouth 4 times a day.

<u>Vaginal candidiasis:</u> 1 vaginal tablet daily for two weeks.

<u>Intestinal candidiasis;</u> 1–2 oral tablets three times a day. Continue medication for at least 48 hours after clinical cure.

OPHTHALMIC ANTIBIOTICS

chloramphenicol (Chloromycetin Ophthalmic solution or ointment) has a broad anti-bacterial spectrum (e.g. staph, strep, neisseriae, H. influenza, klebsiellae, enterobacter, E. coli, moraxella) but is not effective against Pseudomonas aerugenosa or Serratia marcescen.

Dose: 2 drops or small amount of ointment in affected eye every 3 hr for 48 hr and then less often. Continue treatment for at least 48 hr after the eye appears normal.

erythromycin (Ilotycin Ophthalmic Ointment) is active against gram–positive bacteria (e.g. streptococci, some staphylococci) and chlamydia.

Treatment of ocular infection: Apply once daily or more frequently as needed.

Prophylaxis of neonatal gonococcal or chlamydial conjunctivitis: One application in each conjunctival sac.

gentamycin (Garamycin Ophthalmic) is active against both gram–positive bacteria: staphy-lococci (including coagulase–postitive forms), streptococci, pneumococci; and gram–negative bacteria: neisseriae (including gonococci), H. influenza, moraxellae, Pseudomonas aeruginosa, proteus, klebsiella, E. coli.

Solution: 1–2 drops every 4 hours (2 drops every hour in severe infections).

Ointment: Small amount affected eye 2–3 times daily.

silver nitrate 1%

To prevent neonatal gonococcal conjunctivitis: 1 drop in each eye.

tetracycline (Achromycin Ophthalmicc)

Trachoma: 1% ointment tid–qid for 30 days along with oral tetracycline 250 mg qid. Substitute oral erythromycin for oral tetracycline when treating child less than 8 yr.

Inclusion conjunctivitis: 1–2 drops in effected eye 2–4 times daily.

COMBINATION OPHTHALMIC ANTIBIOTICS:

NOTE: Bacitracin is active against gram + bacteria (e.g. staph., strep.) as well as Haemophilus in-fluenza, gonococci, meningococci. Gramicidin is active against gram + cocci (e.g. staph., strep.); gram + bacilli. Neomycin is active against a wide range gram–negative bacteria (e.g. E. coli, Enterobacter, Klebsiella, Proteus, Haemophilus influenza) but not Pseudomonas. Sensitization may occur, especially if neomycin use is prolonged over 5 days. Moreover, the subsequent allergic conjunctivitis may suggest continuing infection. Polymyxin B spectrum: gram–negative aerobic ba-cilli (e.g. E. coli, klebsiella, enterobacter, Pseudomonas aeruginosa). However, proteus and providencia are resistant to polymyxin B.

Neosporin Ophthalmic Ointment (bacitracin + neomycin + polymyxin B)

Dose: Apply small amount ointment to affected eye every 3–4 hours for 7–10 days.

Neosporin ophthalmic solution (gramicidin + neomycin + polymyxin B)

Dose: 1–2 drops 2–4 times daily or more often if needed. In acute infection, begin therapy with 1–2 drops every 15–30 minutes, and then reduce frequency as infection controlled.

Polysporin Ophthalmic (bacitracin + polymyxin B)   Adult: Apply every 3–4 hours.

ANTIVIRAL OPHTHALMIC AGENTS:

idoxuridine (Dendrid, Stoxil)

Ointment 0.5%: Apply to lower conjunctival sac 5 times/day (every 4 hours with last dose at bedtime). Continue therapy for 3–5 days after healing seems complete. Limit treatment to 21 days.

Solution 0.1%: 1 drop every hr during day and every 2 hr at night. Continue therapy for 3–5 days after healing seems complete (1 drop q2h during day & 1 drop q4h at night). Limit treatment to 21 days.

vidarabine [adenosine arabinoside] (Vira–A ophthalmic ointment 3%)

Dose: 1/2 inch ointment 5 times/day at 3 hour intervals. Consider other therapy if there is no improvement in 7 days. Continue therapy at reduced frequency (e.g. 2 times/day) for another 7 days after healing seems complete. Limit treatment to 21 days.

trifluridine 1% solution (Viroptic)

Indication: primary keratoconjunctivitis or recurrent keratitis due to herpes simplex type 1 or type 2.

Dose: 1 drop every 2 hours while awake (maximum 9 drops/day). After healing seems complete, apply 1 drop every 4 hours while awake for additional 7 days (mini-mum 5 drops/day). Limit treatment to 21 days.

ORAL CONTRACEPTIVES

Action: ●Ovulation is suppressed by the following mechanism: (1) the estrogen component inhibits pituitary FSH secretion via negative feedback inhibition on the hypothalamus. (2) the progestin component (potentiated by the estrogen) similarly inhibits pituitary LH secretion. ●The progestin component also: (1) produces a scant and thick cervical mucus which prevents normal sperm transport, (2) alters the endometrium so that implantation of the fertilized ovum cannot occur. Progestin-only pills (minipill) frequently do not suppress LH sufficiently to prevent ovulation (40% ovulate regularly, 20% ovulate intermittently). Contraception depends on the effects on the cervical mucus and endometrium.

Key to abbreviations:
PROGESTIN: norgestrel = NG, ethynodiol diacetate = ED, norethindrone = N, norethynodrel = ND norethindrone acetate = NA, levonorgestrel = L.
ESTOGREN: ethinyl estradiol = EE, mestranol = M.

Combination pills containing < 50 mcg estrogen:

	progestin per active pill/per month	estrogen per active pill/per month
Loestrin 1/20	1 mg/21 mg NA	20 mcg/420 mcg EE
Loestrin 1.5/30	1.5 mg/31.5 mg NA	30 mcg/630 mcg EE
Levlen	0.15 mg/3.15 mg L	30 mcg/630 mcg EE
Nordette	0.15 mg/3.15 mg L	30 mcg/630 mcg EE
Lo/Ovral	0.3 mg/6.3 mg NG	30 mcg/630 mcg EE
Brevicon	0.5 mg/10.5 mg N	35 mcg/735 mcg EE
Modicon	0.5 mg/10.5 mg N	35 mcg/735 mcg EE
Ovcon 35	0.4 mg/8.4 mg N	35 mcg/735 mcg EE
Ortho–Novum 1/35	1 mg/21 mg N	35 mcg/735 mcg EE
Norethin 1/35	1 mg/21 mg N	35 mcg/735 mcg EE
Norinyl 1+35	1 mg/21 mg N	35 mcg/735 mcg EE
Demulen 1/35	1 mg/21 mg ED	35 mcg/735 mcg EE

	progestin	estrogen
Biphasic combination pill: Ortho-Novum 10/11		
days 1–10	0.5 mg N	35 mcg EE
days 11–21	1.0 mg N	35 mcg EE
total/month	16 mg N	735 mcg EE
Triphasic combination pills: Tri–Norinyl		
days 1–7	0.5 mg N	35 mcg EE
days 8–16	1.0 mg N	35 mcg EE
days 17–21	0.5 mg N	35 mcg EE
total/month	15 mg N	735 mcg EE
Triphasil, Tri-Levlen		
days 1–6	0.05 mg L	30 mcg EE
days 7–11	0.075 mg L	40 mcg EE
days 12–21	0.125 mg L	30 mcg EE
total/month	1.925 mg L	680 mcg EE
Ortho-Novum 7/7/7		
days 1–7	0.5 mg N	35 mcg EE
days 8–14	0.75 mg N	35 mcg EE
days 15–21	1.0 mg N	35 mcg EE
total/month	15.75 mg N	735 mcg EE

Combination pills containing 50 mcg estrogen:

Norethin 1/50	(1 mg N+50 mcg M)	Ovral	(0.5 mg NG+50 mcg EE)
Ortho–Novum1/50	(1 mg N+50 mcg M)	Ovcon 50	(1 mg N+50 mcg EE)
Norinyl 1+50	(1 mg N+50 mcg M)	Norlestrin 1/50	(1 mg NA+50 mcg EE)
Demulen 1/50	(1 mg ED+50 mcg EE)	Norlestrin 2.5/50	(2.5 mg NA+50 mcg EE)

Combination pills containing > 50 mcg estrogen are reserved for special circumstances. See comments below.

Ortho-Novum 1/80	(1 mg N+80 mcg M)	Ortho-Novum 2mg	(2 mg N+100 mcg M)

prrogestin–only pill (Mini Pill):

Nor Q.D.	(0.35 mg norethindrone)	Micronor	(0.35 mg norethindrone)
		Ovrette	(0.075 mg norgestrel)

Choosing a pill:

Note: ●The combination pills are available as 21 day or 28 day packs with the exception of Ortho--Novum 2 (21 day only). ●The 28 day packs contain 21 hormonally active pills and 7 inert pills. ●The 7 "inert" pills of the 28 day packs of Loestrin 1/20, Loestrin 1.5/30, and Norlestrin 2.5/50 contain 75 mg ferrous fumerate. Norlestrin 1/50 28 day pack is available with or without ferrous fumerate. A ombination pill containing 30 or 35 mcg estrogen is the usual oral contraceptive pill of first choice. Combination pills containing > 50 mcg estrogen are reserved for special circumstances. Progestin–only pill may be useful for women over 35 yr or for women with history of hypertension, migraines, chloasma, symptoms of fluid retention. Spotting, irregular menses, or amenorrhea commonly occurs with progestin–only pills. However, total blood loss is reduced. Postpartum considerations: Because of the risk of thromboembolism, combination pills should not be started until 2 weeks postpartum. However, a progestin–only pill may be prescribed immediately postpartum and is the pill of choice if the mother is breast–feeding.

Instructions for taking combination pills: There are 3 acceptable ways to start combination pills: (**1**) take first pill on first day of menses, (**2**) take first pill on 5th day of menses, or (**3**) take first pill on Sunday following start of menses or on Sunday if menses begins on a Sunday. Patient using 28 day pack takes one pill each day and begins following pack without interruption. Patient using 21 day pack waits seven days after finishing one pack before starting another (i.e. 21 days on—7 days off regimen). For the first month, an additional means of contraception is advised. Take the pill at the same time each day (this helps maintain more even level of hormones). Missed pills: (**1**) Miss one pill: Take missed pill as soon as you remember and another at usual time. (**2**) Miss two pills: Take two pills as soon as you remember. The next day take two pills at usual time. Use an additional means of contraception until that pack is completed. (**3**) Miss three pills: Discard pack; start new pack next Sunday bleeding or not; and use additional means of contraception until two weeks into the new pack. If any pills are missed and menses subsequently fail to occur, obtain a sensitive pregnancy test. Intentionally delaying menses: Occasionally, a woman using a combined pill may for convenience delay her menses for a few days. After finishing the 21 active pills in the current pack, the woman starts a new pack the next day and discontinues this pack at her convenience. A third new pack is then begun after a 7 day hiatus and continued in the usual manner.

Instructions for taking progestin–only pills: Take first pill on first day of period and take one pill a day at the same time. Begin the next pack without interruption. Using an additional means of contraception during first two months and during midcycle will reduce failure rate which is about 2.5%. Missed pills: (**1**) Miss one pill: Take one pill as soon as you remember and another at usual time. Use additional means of contraception until next period. (**2**) Miss two pills: Take one pill as soon as you remember and another at usual time. The next day, take two pills at usual time. Use additional means of contraception until next period. Irregular periods and spotting between periods is common with progestin–only pills. However, pregnancy testing is advised if a period has not occurred in 45 days.

Managing common pill complaints: Nausea. Use pill with low estrogen potency (e,g, Loestrin 1/20, Lo/Ovral, Demulen 1/35, Demulen 1/50, or progestin–only pill). Taking pill with food at bedtime may help. Oily skin, acne, or hirsutism: Try pill with low androgen potency (Brevicon, Modicon, Ovcon–35, Demulen). Depression may be due to cyclical fluid retention (see below). Depression may be a progestin effect and may therefore respond to a reduction in progestin potency (e.g. Ortho–Novum 10/11, Ortho–Novum 7/7/7, Tri–Norinyl, Ortho–Novum 1/50, Norinyl 1+50, Ovcon 35, Modicon, Brevicon, Ortho–Novum 1/35, Norinyl 1+35). Sometimes an increase in estrogen potency helps (e.g. Ovcon 50). Pyridoxine (vitamin B6) 25 mg PO once daily may also possibly alleviate pill–related depression. Cyclical fluid retention is an estrogenic and/or progestin effect that may result in a number of complaints—e.g. premenstrual tension (headache, irritability); breast tenderness; cyclical weight gain. These symptoms may be alleviated by using a pill with low estrogen and/or progestin potency—e.g. Loestrin 1/20, Norinyl 1+50, Ortho–Novum 1/50. The progestin–only pills (Micronor, Nor Q.D., Ovrette) have no estrogen potency and low progestin potency. Weight gain due to increase in subcutaneous fat (mainly of breasts, hips, thighs) and not associated with increased appetite may respond to a pill with low estrogen potency. Loestrin 1/20 has the least of estrogen potency of the combination pills followed by Norinyl 1+50 and Ortho–Novum 1/50. The progestin–only pills (Micronor, Nor Q.D., Ovrette) have no estrogen potency. Noncyclic weight gain due to increased appetite: Use combination pill with low androgen potency (Brevicon, Modicon, Ovcon–35, Demulen) or progestin–only pill (Micronor, Nor Q.D., Ovrette). Breakthrough bleeding or spotting is common with pills containing < 50 mcg estrogen. Occasional spotting is well tolerated in most cases and may be minimized by taking the pill at the same time each day. Troublesome breakthrough bleeding may be managed by switching to a pill with greater progestin and/or estrogen potency. Amongst the pills containing 30 mcg estrogen; Lo/Ovral, Levlen, and Nordette have the greatest progestin potency. Demulen 1/35 is a step higher in progestin potency and has a little more estrogen potency. Demulen 1/35, Ovral, and Demulen 1/50 have the same progestin potency but the latter two have greater estrogen potency. Absence of withdrawal bleeding (missed menses) is common with pills containing < 50 mcg estrogen. The pill may be continued on schedule but a pelvic exam and a sensitive pregnancy test (e.g. serum beta–HCG) is advised before the next anticipated menses. If missed menses are a persistent problem, switch to a pill with greater progestin and/or estrogen potency (see recommendations for breakthrough bleeding above).

Comments: Important warning symptoms; Since oral contraceptives have potentiallly dire side effects; the patient should be told to report severe leg pain (? deep venous thrombosis); chest pain (? pulmonary thromboembolism, ? coronary thrombosis); headache or visual symptoms (? stroke, ? hypertension, ? migraine); abdominal pain (? mesenteric thrombosis, ? hepatic adenoma, ? cholecystitis, ? pancreatitis). Hypertension; Oral contraceptives increase risk of hypertension. The risk increases with duration of use and with age (particularly in women over 35 yr). Blood pressure should therefore be checked initially, 3 months later, and every 6–12 months thereafter; especially if there is a history of hypertensive renal disease. Pill must be stopped if there is moderate to severe hypertension. If mild hypertension develops, a sub–50 mcg pill may be tried if patient is not already using one. A progestin–only pill may be prescribed if hypertension persists after 3 months, or may be prescribed when hypertension is first noted. Discontinue pill if hypertension continues. Elective surgery; Because of the risk of thromboembolic phenomena, the pill should be discontinued 4 weeks prior to elective surgery. Smoking increases risk of serious cardiovascular side effects, particularly in older women. Noncontraceptive benefits of oral contraceptives; Oral contraceptives relieve menstrual cramps, mittelschmerz, and reduce bleeding days and blood/iron loss. There is reduced risk of pelvic inflammatory disease, functional ovarian cysts, fibrocystic breast, fibroadenomas of the breast, rheumatoid arthritis, and possibly uterine and ovarian carcinomas. Endometriosis may improve. Premenstrual tension syndrome may be relieved. Frequency of refills; Having the patient return frequently simply for refills may discourage pill use. Assuming no complications arise, a reasonable approach is to prescribe a 3 month supply initially and then refills every 6 months.

Absolute contraindications: past or present thromboembolic disorder (e.g. thrombophlebitis, pulmonary embolism); cerebrovascular disease; coronary artery disease; known or suspected breast cancer or estrogen dependent neoplasia; pregnancy; undiagnosed abnormal vaginal bleeding; liver dysfunction; past or present hepatic adenoma.

Relative contraindications: hypertension, migraines, cardiac or renal disease, diabetes mellitus or history gestational diabetes, sickle cell anemia, elective surgery, major leg trauma, prolonged immobilization of a limb, varicose veins, history of hepatic disorders, gallbladder disease, acute mononucleosis, over 35 and smoker, uterine fibroma, history of annovulation/infertility, epilepsy, hyperlipidemia. Relative contraindications to combination pills but acceptable conditions for use of progestin–only pills; mild hypertension, migraines, chloasma, nursing mother, less than 14 days postpartum. Relative contraindication to progestin–only pill but not to combination pill; history of ectopic pregnancy.

Side effects (partial list): thrombophlebitis; thromboembolism (e.g. pulmonary embolism, mesenteric/cerebral/retinal thrombosis); hypertension; coronary thrombosis; mesenteric thrombosis; cerebral thrombosis/bleeding; varicose veins; telangectasias; erythema multiforme; hemorrhagic skin eruptions; headaches including vascular headaches; altered appetite; weight gain or loss; fluid retention; edema; breast tenderness; breast secretion; increased or decreased breast size; hepatic adenoma; cholestatic jaundice; gallbladder disease; menstrual irregularities (e.g. spotting, breakthrough bleeding, missed menses); oily skin; acne; hirsutism; loss of scalp hair; chloasma; melasma; depression; irritability; nervousness; altered libido; fatigue; nausea/vomiting; abdominal cramps/bloating; dizziness; vaginal candidiasis; atrophic vaginitis; decrease glucose tolerance; aggravation of porphyria; increase size of fibromyomata; cystitis–like syndrome; change in cervical erosion, change in amount of cervical secretion. Fluid retention may alter corneal curvature so that contact lens may not fit.

OTIC DRUGS for topical application

acetic acid 2 % solution (Otic Domeboro, VoSol)
Action; Acetic acid is both antibacterial and antifungal (e.g. Candida, Pseudomonas). Resistant species do not emerge.
Indication; otitis externa.
Contraindications; hypersensitivty to components, perforated eardrum.
Dose: Instill 4–6 drops in ear at 2–8 hour intervals. For the first 24 hours, a cotton wick that has been saturated with the solution may be inserted into the external ear canal and kept moist by adding solution as necessary.

chloramphenicol 0.5% solution (Chloromycetin Otic)
Indication; otitis externa due to susceptible bacteria—e.g. staphylococci, H. influenza, E. coli, Pseudomonas aerugenosa, Klebsiella pneumoniae, Aerobacter aerogenes, proteus.
Side effects; overgrowth of non–susceptible bacteria or fungi; bone marrow hypoplasia and aplastic anemia has been reported after topical application.
Dose: 2–3 drops into affected ear 3 times a day. Add appropriate systemic antibiotic if infection is more than superficial.

polymyxin B + neomycin + hydrocortisone (Cortisporin Otic Solution or susp.)
Indication; Otitis externa due to susceptible gram–positive and gram–negative bacteria. The suspension is also indicated for infections of mastoidectomy and fenestration cavities.
Contraindications; hypersensitivity to components; herpes simplex, varicella, or vaccinia infection.
Caution: Because of the ototoxicity of neomycin, this product should be used with caution if there is uncertainty as to the integrity of tympanic membrane.
Side effect; overgrowth non–susceptible bacteria or fungi.
Dose: Clean and dry external auditory canal. Instill 4 drops into affected ear 3–4 times a day for up to 10 days (3 drops infant/child). Lie with affected ear upward when instilling and maintain position for 5 minutes.

colistin + neomycin + hydrocortisone + thonzonium bromide (Coly–Mycin S Otic).
Indication; Otitis externa due to susceptible bacteria—e.g. pseudomonas, E. coli, klebsiella–aerobacter, proteus, Staphylococcus aureus.
Dose/contraindications/caution/side effects; as for Cortisporin Otic (see above).

glycerol with carbamide peroxide (Debrox)
Indication; soften and remove earwax.
Contraindications; tympanic injury/perforation, ear discharge/pain/irritation/rash.
Dose: 5–10 drops retained in ear for several minutes. If necessary, continue treatment twice daily for 4 days. Flush with warm water to facilitate wax removal.

triethanol polypeptide oleate (Cerumenex)
Indication; removal of earwax.
Contraindications; prior adverse reaction, perforated eardrum, otits media.
Caution; otitis externa, allergic history, dermatologic idiosyncrasies.
Directions: Fill ear canal with head tilted at 45 degrees; insert cotton plug and wait 15–30 minutes; gently flush ear canal with lukewarm water using rubber syringe. Limit periaural skin contact and wash exposed skin with soap and water.

antipyrine + benzocaine + glycerin (Auralgan)
Indication; pain associated with otitis media. Glycerin component softens earwax to facilitate removal..
Contraindication; perforated ear drum or ear discharge, hypersensitivity to components.
Comment; systemic analgesics may be required since a topical agent may not relieve pain.
Dose: Fill ear canal with solution and then insert cotton pledget moistened with solution. Repeat every 1–2 hour as needed to ease pain.

OXTRIPHYLLINE (Choledyl)

Action: like theophylline but with less gastric irritation and more easily absorbed.
Indications: bronchial asthma, bronchitis–associated or emphysema–associated bronchospasm.
Caution, side effects: see "Theophylline".
Supplied as: tablet (100, 200 mg); elixir (100mg/5ml);
sustained action tablet (400, 600 mg).
Dose: Adult: 200 mg four times a day. Once total daily dose is established, the daily dose may be divided into 2 equal doses using the sustained action tablet.
Child 2–12 yr: 100 mg/27 kg body weight 4 times a day not to exceed adult dose.

OXYGEN

Indications include hypoxemia, shock, myocardial infarction, angina, carbon monoxide toxicity, pulmonary edema. Hyperbaric oxygen may be indicated in treatment of carbon monoxide or cyanide poisoning, gas gangrene, pneumonitis secondary to smoke inhalation, Meleney's ulcer, skin grafts.
Caution: <u>Atelectasis with consequent shunting</u> may occur at high FI O_2 because nitrogen is washed out of the lungs. Not exceeding an FI O_2 of 90% if possible will help reduce incidence of atelectasis. <u>Chronically hypoxic patients</u> may lose their ventilatory drive if they receive too much oxygen. Thus, such patients should generally receive oxygen via nasal cannula at 1–2 liters/min (or via venturi mask for more precise oxygen delivery). However, if the patient needs more oxygen, give what is necessary and be ready to assist ventilation or intubate. <u>Oxygen toxicity:</u> FI O_2 of 50 % can be tolerated for long periods. An FIO_2 of ≥ 60% for prolonged periods may cause lung damage. Acutely, however, a high FIO_2 is safe. Manifestations of oxygen toxicity may include sore throat, cough, nasal congestion, substernal discomfort, pulmonary congestion, nervousness, tinnitus, vertigo, facial twitch, myoclonus, convulsions. <u>Oxygen administration in neonates;</u> Premature neonates receiving FIO_2 greater than 30% may develop retrolental fibroplasia and blindness. To prevent this development, adjust dose to achieve PaO_2 of 50–60.

Methods of oxygen delivery and percent oxygen inspired:

<u>Mouth–to–mouth resuscitation</u> (expired air) delivers FI O_2 of 16 %.
<u>Breathing room air:</u> FI O_2 21 %.
<u>Nasal cannulae (prongs);</u> Generally, a 1 liter/minute increment in oxygen flow rate increases the FI O_2 by 2–3%. Thus, a 1 liter/minute oxygen flow rate should result in a FI O_2 of approximately 24%, and a flow rate of 4 liter/minute should generally yield an FI O_2 of about 30%. However, the actual FI O_2 is uncertain because it depends not only on the flow rate but also on the patient's minute ventilation, and on the duration of inspiration and expiraton. Nasal cannulae at a flow rate 5 liter/minute or greater is uncomfortable.
<u>Face mask without reservoir bag;</u> 100% oxygen at 6–10 liter/minute results in an FI O_2 of 50–60%. The FI O_2 is influenced by the flow rate, fit of the mask, minute ventilation, and duration of inspiration and expiration.
<u>Nonrebreathing oxygen reservoir mask</u> with a good fit at 10–12 liter/min will result in a FI O_2 of about 90 %.
<u>Venturi mask</u> is designed to deliver oxygen at a controlled FI O_2. This is important for patients who are chronically hypoxic because they may lose their ventilatory drive if they receive too much oxygen. By this method an FI O_2 of 24, 28, 31, 35, 40, or 50 % can be achieved.
<u>Bag–valve–mask at room air:</u> FI O_2 21%.
<u>Bag–valve–mask with oxygen reservoir bag and high flow:</u> FI O_2 greater than 90% may be achieved.
<u>Tents:</u> With an oxygen flow rate of 6–10 liter/minute; the maximum FI O_2 attainable with canopy tent is 50%, and with a face tent is 70%.
<u>Hood (head box);</u> maximum attainable FI O_2 at 6–10 liter/min is 95%.
<u>Incubator:</u> maximum FI O_2 attainable is 40%.

OXYTOCIN (Pitocin, Syntocinon)

Action: Naturally occuring hormone; synthesized in hypothalamus and stored in posterior pituitary. Induces and enhances uterine contractions. Uterus is relatively insensitve to oxytocin during first and second trimester. Responsiveness markedly increases during third trimester, especially at term.
Indications: <u>Induction and/or augmentation labor;</u> Specific indications include uterine inertia or poor progress of labor, amnionitis, premature rupture of membranes with delivery indicated, mild preeclampsia at term, fetal demise, erythroblastosis fetalis, gestation > 42 wk.
<u>To control postpartum bleeding/atony.</u>
Contraindications: oxytocin hypersensitivity, fetal distress, malpresentation, unengaged head, severe toxemia, prior C–section or uterine surgery, active genital herpes, complete placenta previa, vasa previa, presenting or prolapsed umbilical cord, premature separation placenta, obstetric emergencies requiring C–section, grand multipara, uterine overdistension.
Caution: ●Use IV infusion pump for precise control of infusion rate. ●Carefully monitor vitals, fetal heart rate, uterine contractions. ●Discontinue if uterine tetany occurs.
Side effects: anaphylaxis, fetal bradycardia/arrhythmias, uterine spasm/tetany/rupture, nausea/vomiting, maternal hypertension/arrhythmias. ●Because of its ADH activity, excessive oxytocin may induce water intoxication. ●Excessive oxytocin may provoke vasodilation and hypotension.
Supplied as: 0.5 and 1 ml containers (10 unit/ml).

Dose:

Induction/stimulation of labor: Add 10 units (1 ml) oxytocin to 1000 ml normal saline or Ringer's lactate for a concentration of 10 milliunit/ml. Using constant infusion pump, start IV infusion at 1–2 milliunit/minute (at this concentration each 1 milliunit/minute increment is equivalent to an increase of 6 ml/hr). Increase rate at 1–2 milliunits/minute increments every 15–30 minutes until adequate response is achieved (8–10 milliunits/minute is the average required rate).

Control postpartum bleeding/uterine atony: Add 10 units (1 ml) to 500 ml normal saline or Ringer's lactate. Infuse IV at 20–40 milliunit/minute (i.e. 60–120 ml/hr at this concentration). Note: If IV route not available, administer 10 unit (1 ml) undiluted IM after delivery of placenta.

Incomplete or inevitable abortion: Add 10 units (1 ml) to 500 ml normal saline or Ringer's lactate. Infuse IV at 10–20 milliunits/minute (30–60 ml/hr).

PANCRELIPASE

(Entolase, Cotazym, Ku–zyme HP, Pancrease,Viokase, Zymase)

Action: Pork pancreas extract. Provides digestive enzymes (proteases, lipase, amylase).
Indications: Exocrine pancreatic insufficiency. Examples: cystic fibrosis, chronic pancreatitis, pancreatic duct obstruction, pancreatectomized patient.
Contraindication: pork protein hypersensitivity.
Side effects: Acute toxicity does not occur. Very large doses may cause GI upset, diarrhea, hyperuricemia, and hyperuricosuria. Inhalation of Viokase powder may irritate respiratory tract and precipitate asthma in sensitive patients.
Supplied as capsules containing:

	lipase (USP units)	protease (USP units)	amylase (USP units)
Entolase*	4,000	25,000	20,000
Entolase HP*	8,000	50,000	40,000
Cotazyme	8,000	30,000	30,000
Cotazyme-S*	8,000	30,000	30,000
Ku-zyme HP	8,000	30,000	30,000
Pancrease*	4,000	25,000	20,000
Pancrease MT 4*	4,000	12,000	12,000
Pancrease MT 10*	10,000	30,000	30,000
Pancrease MT 16*	16,000	48,000	48,000
Zymase*	12,000	24,000	24,000
Viokase	8,000	30,000	30,000
Viokase powder (1/4 tsp)	16,800	70,000	70,000

* designates enteric coated preparations that resist gastric inactivation.
Dose: The dose must be individualized according to response (i.e. improvement of steatorrhea or nutritional status). Expressed in terms of the lipase component; 4000–16,000 USP units with meals may suffice. In more severe cases of pancreatic deficiency, a dose may need to be taken with meals and also 1 hour before and after a meals.

PENICILLIN

Action: Bactericidal by interfering with bacterial cell wall synthesis.
Indications: <u>gram–positive cocci</u>; non–penicillinase–producing staphylococci, pneumococcus, aerobic and anaerobic streptococci (enterococci may be resistant); <u>gram–negative cocci</u>: meningococci, gonococci (except penicillinase–producing gonococci); <u>gram–positive bacilli</u>: anthrax; diptheria; clostridia (C. perfringens, C. tetani); Listeria monocytogenes; <u>gram–negative bacilli</u>: bacteroides (except B. fragilis), Leptotrichia buccalis (Vincent's infection), Pasteurella multocida, Spirillum minor (rat bite fever), Streptobacillus moniliformis (rat bite fever); <u>actinomycetes</u> (A. israeli, A. bovis); <u>spirochetes</u>: treponema (syphilis, yaws, pinta, bejel); Leptospira; Borrelia recurrentis.
Contraindications: penicillin hypersensitivity, procaine penicillin G in patient allergic to procaine.
Caution/comment: ●Caution: asthma, multiple allergies, cephalosporin hypersensitivity. ●In order to preclude development of rheumatic fever or poststreptococcal glomerulonephritis, group A streptococcal infections should be treated for at least 10 days.
Side effects: <u>hypersensitivity</u>: fever; chills; urticaria; angioedema; laryngeal edema; rhinitis; asthma; anaphylaxis; dermatologic (e.g. maculopapular rash, exfoliation, Stevens–Johnson syndrome); vasculitis; interstitial nephritis (with hematuria, proteinuria); serum sickness (fever, chills, edema, arthralgia); Coombs + hemolytic anemia; thrombocytopenia; eosinophilia; <u>gastrointestinal</u>: nausea, vomiting, epigastric distress, diarrhea, black hairy tongue, pseudomembranous colitis; <u>neurologic</u>: Large IV doses, especialy when renal clearance is low (renal insufficiency, infants), may result in hyperreflexia, delirium, convulsions. <u>Other</u>: neutropenia, bone marrow supression, IV administration–associated thrombophlebitis, syphilis–associated Herxheimer reaction, hyperkalemia with high–dose IV penicillin G potassium.

acqueous penicillin G potassium or sodium

<u>Supplied as:</u> injection (IV or IM). PO form is not recommended because it is not stable in gastric acid.
<u>Dose & duration therapy</u> varies according to pathogen, and site and severity of infection.
●<u>Adult:</u> Severe pneumococcal pneumonia is treated with 1–2 million units IV q4h. Pneumococcal or meningococcal meningitis is treated with 2 million units IV q2h. Endocarditis due to Strep Viridans is treated with 2 million units IV q4h for 4 weeks.
●<u>Child:</u> 25,000–100,000 unit/kg/24hr IV or IM divided q4–6h. Life threatening infection/meningitis: 200,000–400,000 unit/kg/24 hr IV divided q2–4h.
●<u>Neonate 1–4 wk age:</u> 75,000 unit/kg/24hr IV or IM divided q8h.
   Meningitis: 150,000–250,000 unit/kg/24 hr IV divided q6–8h.
●<u>Neonate < 1 wk age:</u> 25,000 unit/kg IV or IM divided q12h.
   Meningitis: 100,000–150,000 unit/kg/24 hr divided q8–12h.

Comments; ●400,000 unit = 250 mg. ●IM route is painful but may be used when IV route is not feasible. IM route should not be used when more than 10 million units/24 hr is required. ●Aqueous penicillin G potassium IV is the usual form and route of choice when high blood levels of penicillin are required (e.g. meningitis, septicemia, peritonitis, empyema, endocarditis, septic arthritis, severe pneumonia). Since renal excretion is rapid, severe infections may require q2h administration initially. Probenecid may be given to delay renal excretion. ●Penicillin G potassium contains 1.7 mEq potassium/million units. Therefore, in order to preclude hyperkalemia, caution is advised if very large IV doses are given to a patient with renal insufficiency. Penicillin G sodium is an alternative in these patients. ●Dose adjustment in severe renal failure (GFR < 10ml/min): maximum 24 hr dose is 1/3 of the usual maximum. Hemodialysis patients require a dose after dialysis.

procaine penicillin G (Pfizerpen–AS, Wycillin)
Supplied as; intramuscular injection only (300,000 or 600,000 units/ml).
　　　　　Avoid IV adminstration.
Adult dose: 600,000 unit IM q12h, or 1.2 million units IM once daily. Uncomplicated gonorrhea is treated with a single dose of 4.8 million units (2.4 million units injected in each buttock) with 1 gram probenecid PO.
Pediatric dose: 300,000–1.2 million unit IM once daily. Uncomplicated gonorrhea is treated with a single dose 100,000 units/kg IM along with probenecid PO (25 mg/kg, maximum 1 gram).
Comments; ●When high serum levels of penicillin G are required (meningitis, bacteremia, peritonitis, endocarditis, pericarditis, septic arthritis) aqueous penicillin G is preferred. Procaine penicillin G is suitable for less severe infections or when lower blood levels of penicillin suffice (e.g. syphilis, uncomplicated gonorrhea, pneumococcal pneumonia). ●Procaine penicillin G is for IM use only. Accidental IV administration may be cardiotoxic; fatalities have occurred. ●The procaine component mitigates the pain of IM injection. ●Procaine penicillin G is contraindicated in patient allergic to procaine. ●Procaine pen G is absorbed slowly after IM injection. Therefore once or twice daily administration will suffice. A plateau–like blood level is seen at 4 hrs which then falls gradually over next 15–20 hours. ●In infants < 3 months of age, sustained therapeutic levels are achieved with aqueous penicillin G and is preferred over procaine penicillin G.

penicillin G benzathine (Bicillin L–A)
Supplied as; IM injection only (300,000 or 600,000 units/ml). Avoid IV injection.
Adult dose:
●Prevention of rheumatic fever and poststreptococcal glomerulonephritis: 1.2 million unit IM once a month.
●Group A streptococcal pharyngitis: single dose 1.2 million unit IM.
●Yaws, bejel, pinta: single dose 1.2 million unit IM.
●Syphilis: refer to "Syphilis" in clinical section.
Child > 27 kg (indications and interval as in adult): 900,000 unit IM.
Child < 27 kg (indications and interval as in adult): 300,000–600,000 unit IM.
Comment; Benzathine penicillin G provides low serum levels of penicillin for up to 4 weeks. It is suitable for the treatment of syphilis, streptococcal pharyngitis, and for the prophylaxis of rheumatic fever and glomerulonephritis.

Ccmbined benzathine and procaine penicillin G
(Bicillin C–R, Bicillin C–R 900/300)
Supplied as (IM only): Bicillin C–R contains equal amounts of benzathine and procaine forms. Bicillin C–R 900/300: 2ml contains 900,000 units benzathine form and 300,000 units procaine form.
Comment; Combined benzathine and procaine penicillin G may be used to treat group A streptococcal infections (e.g. pharyngitis) and pneumococcal infections (except meningitis), but it is usually best to use the individual preparations. This combination preparation must not be used to treat syphilis, yaws, pinta, bejel, gonorrhea.

penicillin V potassium [phenoxymethyl penicillin]
(Betapen–VK, Pen–Vee K, Veetids)
Supplied as; tablet (125, 250, 500 mg); oral solution (125, 250 mg/5ml). (250 mg = 400,000 unit penicillin G).
Adult dose: 250–500 mg PO q6h.
Child dose: 6.25–12.5 mg/kg PO q6h. Neonate: 25 mg/kg PO q6h.
Comment; Penicillin V potassium is relatively stable in gastric acid and is the preferred oral form. It is less active than penicillin G against gram–negative bacteria (e.g. gram–negative anaerobes, haemophilus) and it must not be used in treatment of gonorrhea, severe pneumonia, empyema, bacteremia, pericarditis, meningitis, or septic arthritis.

PENICILLINASE–RESISTANT PENICILLINS

(antistaphylococcal penicillins): cloxacillin (Cloxapen, Tegopen)**, dicloxacillin** (Dynapen, Pathocil)**, methicillin** (Staphcillin)**, nafcillin** (Nafcil, Unipen)**, oxacillin** (Prostaphlin)
Spectrum: staphylococci (both penicillin G resistant & nonresistant), streptococci, pneumococcus.
Indications: penicillinase–producing (penicillin G resistant) staphylococci, suspected staph.
Drug choice
 Parenteral choice: Nafcillin is the usual choice for parenteral administration. In neonates, methicillin is preferred over nafcillin. Nafcillin does not require dose adjustment in renal failure.
 Oral choice: Cloxacillin, dicloxacillin, or oxacillin are the usual drugs of choice for oral administration. Dose adjustment is not required in renal failure.
Contraindications: hypersensitivity to penicillins.
Caution: pregnancy, significant allergies, cephalosporin hypersensitivity.
Comments: ●Bacterial strains resistant to one of the penicillinase–resistant penicillins are presumed resistant to all, and may be resistant to cephalosporins as well. ●Oral administration should be 1 hour before or 2 hours after meals.
Side effects: refer to penicillin.

cloxacillin (Cloxapen,Tegopen)
Supplied as: capsule (250, 500 mg); oral solution (125mg/5ml).
Adult and child over 20 kg: 250–1000 mg PO q4–6h depending on severity of infection.
Child less than 20 kg: 12.5–25 mg/kg PO q6h.

dicloxacillin (Dynapen, Pathocil)
Supplied as: capsules (125, 250, 500 mg); oral suspension (62.5mg/5ml).
Adult and child over 40 kg: 250–1000 mg PO q4–6h.
Child less than 40 kg: 6.25–25 mg/kg PO q6h.

methicillin (Staphcillin) Supplied as: preparation for IM or IV injection.
Adult: IV dose is 1–2 gram q4–6h. IM dose is 1 gram q4–6h.
Dose interval in renal failure: creatinine clearance 50–80ml/min—dose interval 6hr, clearance 10–50 ml/min—interval 8 hr, clearance < 10 ml/min—interval 12 hr.
Child: 25–75 mg/kg q6h IV or IM.
Neonate over 1 wk age: 25 mg/kg q6–8h IV or IM.
Neonate less than 1 wk age: 25 mg/kg q8–12h IV or IM

nafcillin (Nafcil, Unipen)
Supplied as: 250 mg capsule, 500 mg tablet, oral solution (250mg/5ml), preparation for IM or IV injection.
Adult: ●IV: 500–2000 mg q4h. ●IM: 500 mg q4–6h. ●PO: 250–1000 mg q4–6h.
Child: ●IV or IM: 150 mg/kg/day divided q6h. ●PO: 12.5–25 mg/kg q6h.
Neonate: ●IM: 10 mg/kg q12h. ●PO: 10 mg/kg q6–8h.

oxacillin (Prostaphlin)
Supplied as: capsule (250, 500 mg); oral solution (250mg/5 ml); injection IV or IM.
Adult/child over 40 kg: ●PO: 500–1000 mg q6h.
 ●IV or IM: 250–1000 mg or more q4–6h depending on severity of infection.
Child less than 40 kg: ●PO: 12.5–25 mg/kg q6h.
 ●IM/IV: 50–100 mg/kg/day divided q4–6h.

PENICILLINS–ANTIPSEUDOMONAL

azlocillin (Azlin) **mezlocillin** (Mezlin)
piperacillin (Pipracil) **ticarcillin** (Ticar)

Indications: Although these antibiotics show in vitro activity against a wide spectrum of gram-positive and gram-negative bacteria, their principal use is against susceptible gram-negative organisms—mainly Pseudomonas aerugenosa. They are usually administered in conjunction with an aminoglycoside to prevent emergence of resistant strains. Azlocillin is chiefly indicated for infections due to susceptible strains of Pseudomonas aerugenosa. It is also effective against E. Coli, Proteus mirabilis, Haemophilus influenza, and Strep. faecalis. Mezlocillin and piperacillin have been shown to be clinically effective against Pseudomonas aerugenosa as well as H. influenza, Klebsiella, Proteus, E. coli, Enterobacter, Serratia, Bacteroides, Peptococcus, Peptostreptococcus, Strep. faecalis, gonococcus. Ticarcillin is active against Pseudomonas aerugenosa. It is also clinically effective against Proteus and E. Coli.
Contraindications: hypersensitivity to penicillins.

Caution: pregnancy, significant allergies, cephalosporin hypersensitivity.
Side effects: refer to penicillin.

azlocillin (Azlin)

Dose (adult): In serious infections the usual dose is 3 gram IV q4h. The dose may be increased to 4 gram iv q4h for life–threatening infection. For uncomplicated UTI 2 gram q6h will suffice while complicated UTI is ually treated with 3 grams q6h.

Dose adjustment in renal failure patient with serious systemic infection: creatinine clearance > 30ml/min: usual dosage, creatinine clearance 10–30ml/min: 2 gram q8h, creatinine clearance < 10ml/min: 3 gram q12h. Hemodialysis patients receive 3 gram after each dialysis and then 3 gram q12h.

mezlocillin (Mezlin)

Dose, adult: Usual dose is 3 gram IV q4h or 4 gram q6h. Up to 4 gram IV q4h may be used in life–threatening infections. Mezlocillin may be given IM. However, the IV route is advised if there is a serious infection and no more than 2 gram/dose may be given IM.

Dose adjustment in renal failure patient with serious systemic infection: creatinine clearance > 30ml/min: usual dosage, creatinine clearance 10–30ml/min: 3 gram q8h, creatinine clearance < 10ml/min: 2 gram q12h. Hemodialysis patients receive 3–4 gram after each dialysis and q12h. Peritoneal dialysis patient may be given 3 gram q12h.

Dose from > 1 month to 12 yr of age): 50mg/kg q4h.

Dose, neonate ≤ 7 days of age: 75mg/kg q12h.

Dose, neonate > 7 days of age: 75mg/kg q8h if ≤ 2kg in weight and q6h if > 2kg.

piperacillin (Pipracil)

Dose (adult): The usual dose is 3–4 gram IV q4–6h. Maximum 24 gram/day. Piperacillin may be given IM (e.g. for uncomplicated urinary tract infection, uncomplicated gonorrhea). However, no more than 2 gram per IM injection site is permitted.

Dose adjustment in renal failure: For patient with serious systemic infection: creatinine clearance > 40ml/min: usual dosage, creatinine clearance 20–40ml/min: 4 gram q8h, creatinine clearance < 20ml/min: 4 gram q12h. The maximum dosage in hemodialysis patient is 2 gram q8h. An additional 1 gram is given following each dialysis.

ticarcillin (Ticar)

Dose, adult: The usual dosage for serious urinary tract and systemic infection is 3 gram IV q4h or 4 gram IV q6h.

Dose adjustment in renal failure:

creatinine clearance > 60ml/min: usual dosage, creatinine clearance 30–60ml/min: 2 gram q4h, creatinine clearance 10–30ml/min: 2 gram q8h,

creatinine clearance < 10ml/min: 2 gram q12h,

creatinine clearance < 10ml/min with hepatic dysfunction: 2 gram q24h. Hemodialysis patients receive 3 gram after each dialysis and then 2 grams q12h. Peritoneal dialysis patient is given 3 gram q12h.

Dose, child < 40kg: The usual dose for serious infections is 200–300mg/kg/day not to exceed adult dosage.

Neonate > 7 days: 75mg/kg q8h if < 2kg in weight and 100mg/kg q8h if > 2kg.

Neonate ≤ 7 days: 75mg/kg q12h if < 2kg in weight and 75mg/kg q8h if > 2kg.

PHENAZOPYRIDINE (Pyridium)

Action: Produces anesthesia of urinary tract mucosa as it is excreted in the urine.
Indications: lower urinary tract pain, burning, urgency, frequency.
Contraindication: renal insufficiency.
Side effects: orange discoloration urine, GI upset, headache. Following side effects usually only occur with overdose, or when there is accumulation of the drug due to renal insufficiency: methemoglobinemia, hemolytic anemia, renal or hepatic toxicity, yellow discoloration of skin and sclerae.
Supplied as: 100 and 200 mg tablets.
Adult dose: 200 mg PO 3 times a day after meals.
Pediatric dose (6–12 yr): 100 mg PO 3 times a day after meals.

PHENOBARBITAL

Action: CNS depressant.
Indications: epilepsy, sedation, to induce sleep.
Contraindications: porphyria; severe pulmonary, renal, or hepatic disease.
Caution/comments: ●Serum therapeutic level: 15–40 mcg/ml. ●Sedation may interfere with performance of hazardous activities. Concurrent alcohol ingestion and other CNS depressants increase CNS depression. ●Caution: hyperthyroidism, diabetes mellitus, anemia, elderly, debilitated. ●Seizures and other withdrawal symptoms may be precipitated if phenobarbital is suddenly withheld from a patient receiving chronic high doses.
Side effects: headache, dizziness, confusion, paradoxical excitement, hangover, nausea, vomiting, rash, respiratory depression, hypotension, impotence.

Supplied as: tablet (8,15,16,30,32,60,65,100 mg);   capsule (16 mg); drops (16 mg/ml);   elixir (20 mg/5 ml);   injection (30, 60, 65, 130 mg/ml). Note: 1 grain = approximately 65 mg.

Adult dose:

  Status epilepticus not controlled by diazepam or phenytoin: 15 mg/kg IV at 25–50 mg/minute while carefully monitoring for signs of respiratory depression or hypotension. Administration may be facilitated by diluting the total amount of phenobarbital in 100 ml normal saline and infusing IV piggyback with an infusion pump to control the rate of infusion. Brain concentrations reach a peak about an hour after the infusion. If there is still no response after 15 mg/kg, an additional 5 mg/kg may be administered. Use intramuscular route if IV route not available.
  Maintenance anticonvulsant: 50–100 mg PO 2–3 times daily. Serum therapeutic level is 15–40 mcg/ml. A steady state plasma level is not achieved until 14–21 days after initiating therapy.
  Sedation: 30–120 mg/day divided into 2–3 daily doses IM or PO.
  To induce sleep: 100–320 mg IM or PO.

Pediatric dose:

  Status epilepticus: While monitoring carefully for signs of respiratory depression or hypotension, give 2–3 mg/kg at 5–10 minute intervals IV until 10 mg/kg has been administered. Wait 20 minutes. If still no response, an additional 5–10 mg/kg may be administered. Use intramuscular route if IV route not available.
  Maintenance anticonvulsant: 3–5 mg/kg/day PO divided into 2–3 daily doses.
  Sedation: 2–3 mg/kg q8h IM or PO.
  To induce sleep: 6–10 mg/kg IM or PO.

PHENOTHIAZINES AND DRUGS WITH SIMILAR PHARMACOLOGY

PHENOTHIAZINES: chlorpromazine (Thorazine)**, fluphenazine** (Prolixin, Permitil)**, mesoridazine** (Serentil)**, perphenazine** (Trilafon)**, prochlorperazine** (Compazine)**, thioridazine** (Mellaril)**, trifluoperazine** (Stelazine).
THIOXANTHENES: chlorprothixene (Taractan)**, thiothixene** (Navane).
BUTYROPHENONE: haloperidol (Haldol).
DIHYDROINDOLONE: molindone (Moban).
DIBENZOXAZEPINE: loxapine (Loxitane).

Action: Psychiatric effects: Alters the mood, thinking, and behavior of psychotic patients, perhaps by blocking CNS adrenergic and dopaminergic receptors. Antiemetic by blunting the medulla's chemoreceptor trigger zone. However, these drugs are not generally effective when nausea or vomiting is secondary to motion sickness or vestibular disease. Anticholinergic effects. Antihistaminic. effects.
Indications: psychosis (including schizophrenia, manic–depressive illness, organic brain syndrome–associated psychosis); severe agitation (e.g. Haldol, Thorazine); nausea/vomiting (e.g. Compazine); Intractable hiccups (Thorazine); suppress shivering (Thorazine).
Drug choice: A sedating drug would usually be the drug of choice in psychosis with excitement as a prominent feature. The more sedating antipsychotics have the advantage of having a lower incidence of extrapyramidal side effects (excepting tardive dyskinesia which is equally common in the antipsychotics presented here). Of the more sedating antipsychotics, thioridazine (Mellaril) and mesoridazine (Serentil) have the lowest incidence of extrapyramidal side effects followed by chlor-

prothixene (Taractan), and then chlorpromazine (Thorazine). A disadvantage of the more sedating antipsychotics is that they tend to have a greater incidence of autonomic side effects (e.g. orthostatic hypotension). See 'side effects' below. Of the four antipsychotics just mentioned, the incidence of autonomic side effects is greatest with chlorpromazine and least with mesoridazine. A less sedating antipsychotic such as haloperidol (Haldol) or thiothixene (Navane) would be advantageous in a withdrawn schizophrenic. Furthermore, autonomic side effects are less common with these drugs. However, extrapyramidal side effects are more likely.

Contraindications: hypersensitivity; coma; severe CNS depression; marrow depression; blood dyscrasia (Navane, Prolixin, Stelazine, and Thorazine are contraindicated); liver disease (Stelazine and Prolixin are contraindicated); pregnancy; nursing mothers.

Caution: liver or cardiac disease, chronic respiratory disorders, glaucoma, urinary retention, the elderly or debilitated, concurrent use of CNS depressants, patient who engages in activities that require alertness.

Comments: Increase dose gradually to achieve optimal therapeutic effect. After patient is stable, reduce dose gradually to the smallest effective maintenance dose. Avoid abrupt discontinuation if possible because GI symptoms and/or tremor may ensue. Stop medication 1–2 time/yr to evaluate therapeutic effect and to judge whether dose reduction or discontinuation is indicated. Stop medication if tardive dyskinesia occurs. Fine worm-like movements of the tongue may be an early warning sign. To minimize risk of hypotension patient should be kept recumbent for at least 1/2 hr after IM injection. Antiemetic action of these drugs may obscure diagnosis of: overdose of other drugs, intestinal obstruction, brain tumors, encephalopathy. Reduce dose in elderly or debilitated.

Overdose: Empty the stomach and administer charcoal: Ipecac may used in the alert patient. However, it may not be effective because phenothiazines suppress the medullary vomiting center. Because the phenothiazines inhibit gastric motility, gastric lavage is indicated in the comatose patient no matter how long has elapsed since ingestion. A cathartic may also be administered. In severe overdose, charcoal is administered every 2 hours until stool turns black. Hypotension is treated by supine or Trendelenberg position, and if necessary by administering isotonic saline. A vasoconstrictor (norepinephrine or phenylephrine) is sometimes needed. EKG monitor; Phenothiazine overdose frequently causes arrhythmias but death seldom occurs. Lidocaine or phenytoin may be used to control ventricular tachycardia or ventricular fibrillation. Transvenous pacing has also been used. Acute dystonic reactions are treated with diphenhydramine (Benadryl): 50 mg IV or IM in adult, 2mg/kg in child. The culpable drug is discontinued and additional doses of diphenhydramine are administered PO over the next 2–3 days to prevent recurrence. Ineffective measures; Phenothiazines are highly protein-bound. Consequently, forced diuresis and dialysis are not effective.

Side effects include: Extrapyramidal; *Tardive dyskinesia* (involuntary and repetitive lip smacking, tongue movements, grimacing, and/or limb movements) occurs with long-term therapy and generally does not subside even after the drug is stopped. *Pseudoparkinsonism* (tremor, rigidity, mask-like faces, akinesia) may develop. However, prolonged use of anti–Parkinson drugs to deal with this side effect is not recommended. *Acute dystonias* (involuntary spasms such as oculogyric crisis, torticollis, etc.) is managed with diphenhydramine (Benadryl). *Akathisia* (motor restlessness) may require dose reduction or addition of a barbiturate. Other CNS side effects; sedation, fatigue, agitation, headache, confusion, dizziness/vertigo, grand mal seizures, abnormal CSF analysis, hyperreflexia, catatonia, cerebral edema. Autonomic nervous system; Anticholinergic—e.g. dry mouth, constipation, urinary retention, impotence, blurred vision, mydriasis, tachycardia; Antiadrenergic—e.g. postural hypotension (usually with parenteral administration), inhibition of ejaculation. Blood dyscrasias; leukopenia, agranulocytosis (rarely), thrombocytopenia, pancytopenia. Blood dyscrasia is an indication for discontinuing the drug. Be suspicious if patient complains of sore throat or mouth, and/or respiratory infection. Obtain CBC. Hypersensitivity; cholestatic jaundice, rash, urticaria, photosensitivity, eosinophilia. Endocrine; galactorrhea, gynecomastia, menstrual aberrations, false + pregnancy test, hyperglycemia, hypoglycemia. Ophthalmic; lens and corneal depositis, pigmentary retinopathy, epithelial keratopathy. Other; skin pigmentation, lupus–like syndrome, fever, arrhythmias.

chlorpromazine (Thorazine)

Supplied as: tablet (10, 25, 50, 100, 200 mg); oral concentrate (30, 100 mg/ml); syrup (10mg/5ml); suppository (25, 100 mg);IM injection (25mg/ml).

Adult dose:

Nausea/vomiting: Oral: 10–25mg q4–6h.   Rectal: 50–100mg q6–8h.
Intramuscular: 25 mg initial dose. If hypotension does not result, give 25–50 mg IM q3–4h until vomiting ceases.

Intractable hiccups: 25–50 mg PO tid–qid. If hiccups persist after 2–3 days, give 25–50 mg IM. If still no effect, add 25–50 mg to 500–1000 ml of normal saline and infuse IV slowly with patient supine and while monitoring blood pressure.

Psychosis:
•Intramuscular route is used if rapid control of symptoms is necessary. Initial dose is 25 mg. Then, if needed, give 25–100 mg IM in 1 hour provided that hypotension has not occurred. Repeat IM injections 25–100 mg q1–4h may be administered until there is adequate control (500–1000 mg/24 hr usually suffices). Elderly or debilitat-

ed patients should be started on lower doses with more gradual increases.

●Oral administration: In severe cases, start with 200–600 mg/day divided into 3 daily doses. If necessary, increase the daily dose (usual effective range is 500–800 mg/day, maximum 2000 mg/day). In less severe cases, start with 25 mg PO tid for 1–2 days and then if necessary gradually increase daily dose by 25–50 mg increments. Elderly or debilitated patients should be started on lower doses with more gradual increases. Use the smallest effective dose in all patients.

Tetanus (usually in conjunction with barbiturates): 25–50 mg IM tid–qid. Increase dose gradually as needed. May be given IV if necessary; dilute to at least 1mg/ml and infuse at 1mg/minute.

Pediatric dose: (Contraindicated in child under 6 months.)

Nausea/vomiting: oral—0.5 mg/kg q4–6h;   rectal—1mg/kg q6–8h;
                 IM—0.5 mg/kg q6–8h.

Psychosis: same dose as for nausea/vomiting. Increase dose if needed. In severe cases, 50–100 mg/day may be required, and 200 mg/day or more may be needed in older children. Do not exceed 40 mg/day IM in child under 5 yr (or under 23 kg) or 75 mg/day IM in child 5–12 yr (or 23–45 kg).

Tetanus: 0.5 mg/kg q6–8h IM or IV (dilute IV dose to at least 1 mg/ml and infuse at 1 mg/min).

chlorprothixene (Taractan)

Supplied as: tablet (10, 25, 50, 100 mg);   oral concentrate (100mg/5ml);
             IM injection (25mg/2ml).

Adult: Initially, 25–50 mg PO tid–qid (10–25 mg PO tid–qid if elderly or debilitated). Increase dose as needed. More than 600 mg/day is seldom needed. ●Acutely agitated patient: 25–50 mg IM up to tid–qid. Use oral route as soon as possible.

Child over 6 yr: 10–25 mg PO tid–qid. Use smallest effective dose.

Note: Safety not established for PO administration in child under 6 yr, or for IM administration in child under 12 yr.

flunephazine hydrochloride (Prolixin, Permitil)

Supplied as: tablet (1, 2.5, 5, 10 mg);   elixir (2.5mg/5ml);
             oral concentrate (5mg/ml);   IM injection (2.5mg/ml).

Dose (adult):

Oral: Initially, 2.5–10 mg/day divided into 3–4 doses. Start with 1.0–2.5 mg/day in elderly. Less than 20 mg/day often suffices but some patients may require up to 40 mg/day. After symptoms controlled, gradually reduce to smallest effective dose (this is particularly important in aged or debilitated patients). The usual maintenance range is 1–5 mg/day which can often be given as a single daily dose.

Intramuscular (when oral route not feasible): Initial dose is 1.25 mg IM. Usual range is 2.5–10 mg/day divided q6–8h. Use smallest effective dose. Doses > 10 mg/day should be used cautiously. Elderly or debilitated patients should be started on lower doses with more gradual increases. Start PO therapy as soon as possible.

fluphenazine decanoate (Prolixin Decanoate) and fluphenazine enanthate (Prolixin Enanthate) are a long–acting depot forms for IM or SC injection. They are especially useful when there is noncompliance with oral medication.

Supplied as: 25 mg/ml.

Dose (adult): Start with 12.5–25 mg IM or SC every 2 weeks. Increase dose as needed but limit dose increases to 12.5mg increments after 50mg dose is reached. Max. dose is 100mg every 2–6 wk. The interval between injections is usually every 2 wk but some patients will require a single injection every 4 wk or even every 6 wk.

haloperidol (Haldol)

Supplied as: tablet (0.5, 1, 2, 5, 10, 20 mg);   oral concentrate (2mg/ml);
             IM injection (5mg/ml).

Adult/child over 12 yr: Initially, 0.5–2 mg PO bid–tid (3–5 mg PO bid–tid if symptoms severe). Increase dose as needed. Usual maintenance range is 2–8 mg/day divided into 2–3 doses. However, in rare instances up to 100 mg/day has been used. Use the smallest effective dose (this is particularly important in aged or debilitated patients).

●Prompt control of acutely agitated patient: 2–5 mg IM. Repeat as needed at 1–8 hour intervals.

Child 3–12 yr: 0.05–0.15 mg/kg/day PO divided into 2–3 daily doses. Start with 0.5 mg/day and increase by 0.5 mg increment at 5–7 day intervals until optimal response achieved.

haloperidol decanoate (Haldol Decanoate) is a long-acting depot form.

Supplied as: intramuscular injection (50 mg haloperidol/ml).

Dose: The initial injection is 10 to 15 times the daily maintenance dose of oral haloperidol up to maximum of 100 mg. The usual dose interval is monthly. Clinical experience with injections greater than 300 mg is limited.

loxapine (Loxitane)

Supplied as: capsule (5, 10, 25, 50 mg); oral concentrate (25mg/ml); IM injection (50mg/ml).

Dose (adult/16 yr and older):

Oral: Start with 10 mg twice daily (up to 50 mg/day if severely disturbed). If needed, the dose may be increased rapidly over the next 7–10 days. Usual requirement is 60–100 mg/day divided into 2–4 daily doses. Use the smallest effective dose (this is particularly important in aged or debilitated patients). Maximum is 250 mg/day. Use smallest effective maintenance dose; 20–60 mg/day divided into 2–4 doses will often suffice.

Intramuscular (acutely agitated patient or when PO not feasible): 12.5–50 mg q4–6h or longer. Titrate dose and interval up or down according to patient response. Two daily doses may suffice. Titrate with especial care in elderly or debilitated patient. Administer via oral route as soon as possible.

mesoridazine (Serentil)

Supplied as: tablet (10, 25, 50, 100 mg); oral concentrate (25mg/ml); IM injection. (25mg/ml).

Dose adult/child over 12 yr:

Oral: Initially, 50 mg PO tid. Usual requirement is 100–400 mg/day. Use the smallest effective dose (this is particularly important in aged or debilitated patients).

Intramuscular (when oral route not feasible or prompt control required): Initially, 25 mg. Repeat in 30–60 minutes if needed. Usual requirement is 25–200 mg/day. Lower range in elderly or debilitated patients.

molindone (Moban)

Supplied as: tablet (5, 10, 25, 50, 100 mg); oral concentrate (20 mg/ml).

Dose (adult): Start with 5–15 mg PO tid–qid. Increase gradually as needed. Use the smallest effective dose (this is particularly important in aged or debilitated patients). Usual maintenance range is 5–25 mg PO tid–qid. Up to 225 mg/day in divided doses may be needed in severe cases.

perphenazine (Trilafon)

Supplied as: tablet (2, 4, 8, 16 mg); oral concentrate (16mg/5ml); IM or IV injection (5mg/ml).

Dose (adult):

Oral: 4–8 mg tid (8–16 mg bid–qid in hospitalized psychotic). Reduce to smallest effective dosage as soon as possible (this is particularly important in aged or debilitated patients). Maximum 64 mg/day. Prolonged administration of doses greater than 24 mg/day reserved for hospitalized patient.

Intramuscular (when prompt control is necessary or oral route not feasible): 5 mg and repeated q6h as needed. An initial dose of 10 mg may be needed if patient is severely agitated. Titrate dose carefully in aged or debilitated patients. Usual maximum 15 mg/day in ambulatory patient or 30 mg/day in hospitalized patient. Switch to PO route as soon as possible; this is usually possible within 24 hours.

For treatment of severe nausea/vomiting the dose is 5 mg IM (10 mg IM rarely), or 8–16 mg/day PO divided into 3 daily doses.

prochlorperazine (Compazine)
Supplied as: tablet (5, 10, 25 mg);   syrup (5mg/5ml);
            suppository (2.5, 5, 25 mg);   IM injection (5 mg/ml).
Adult dose:
Nausea/vomiting;   ●Intramuscular: 5–10 mg q3–4h (maximum 40 mg/day),
       ●Oral: 5–10 mg 3–4 times a day, or ●rectal: 25 mg suppository twice daily.
Psychosis: Initially, 5–10 mg PO tid–qid. If needed, increase in small increments
every 2–3 days. 15–40 mg/day may suffice in mild conditions; severe cases may re-
quire 100–150 mg/day. Use the smallest effective dose (this is particularly impor-
tant in aged or debilitated patients). For prompt control of severe symptoms: 10–20
mg q1–4h IM. More than 3–4 IM injections is seldom required. Titrate carefully in
aged or debilitated patients.
Dose child 2–12 yr: Contraindicated for child under 9 kg or < 2 yr.
Nausea/vomiting;
      weight 9–13 kg: 2.5 mg qd–bid PO or PR (maximum 7.5 mg/day).
      weight 14–18 kg: 2.5 mg bid–tid PO or PR (maximum 10 mg/day).
      weight 18–39 kg: 2.5 mg tid PO or PR (maximum 15 mg/day).
Intramsucular: 0.13 mg/kg. One dose usually suffices.
Psychosis: Initially, 2.5 mg bid–tid PO or PR. Increase if needed. Usually, dose is
not > 20 mg/day in child 2–5 yr, or > 25 mg/day in child 6–12 yr.
Intramuscular: 0.13 mg/kg. One dose usually suffices. Switch to PO as soon as
possible.

thiothixene (Navane)
Supplied as: capsule (1, 2, 5, 10, 20 mg);   oral concentrate (2mg/ml);
            IM injection (2 or 5mg/ml).
Dose (adult):
Oral; Initially, 2 mg PO tid (5 mg PO twice daily in more severe cases). If needed,
increase dose gradually. Use smallest effective dose (particularly important in aged
or debilitated patients). Usual requirement is 20–30 mg/day. Up to 60 mg/day is
sometimes required. Larger dosage seldom brings further benefit.
Intramuscular (acute symptoms when oral route not feasible): 4 mg bid–qid. Increase or decrease dosage as needed. Use smallest effective dose (particularly important in aged or debilitated patients). Usual requirement is 16–20 mg/day.
Maximum is 30 mg/day.

thioridazine (Mellaril)
Supplied as: tablet (10, 15, 25, 50, 100, 150, 200 mg);
     oral concentrate (30 or 100 mg/ml);   oral suspension (25 or 100 mg/5ml).
Adult: Initially, 50–100 mg PO tid. If needed, increase gradually up to maximum 800
mg/day. Once psychosis is under control, reduce gradually to smallest effective
dosage. This is particularly important in aged or debilitated patients. Range is 200–
800 mg/day divided into 2–4 daily doses.
Child over 2 yr: ●Moderate disorder, start with 10 mg PO bid–tid. ●Severe disorder,
start with 25 mg PO bid–tid. Titrate gradually to smallest effective dosage. Range
is 0.5 to maximum 3 mg/kg/day.

trifluoperazine (Stelazine)
Supplied as: tablet (1, 2, 5, 10 mg);   oral concentrate (10mg/ml);
            IM injection (2mg/ml).
Adult: Start with 2–5 mg PO twice daily. Usual requirement is 15–20 mg/day.
Sometimes ≥ 40 mg/day is needed. Dose in aged and debilitated patients is 1/3 to
1/2 the usual dose. ●Intramuscular (when prompt control severe symptoms is nec-
essary): 1–2 mg IM q4–6h as needed. Seldom is more than 6 mg/24 hr required.
Titrate dose and interval cautiously in aged or debilitated patient.
Child 6–12 yr: Initially, 1 mg PO once or twice daily. Increase gradually as needed.
More than 15 mg/day PO is seldom required, except perhaps in an older child with
severe symptoms. ●Intramuscular (experience limited): 1mg once or twice daily.

PHENOXYBENZAMINE (Dibenzyline)

Action: Exerts vasodilative influence by binding to alpha adrenergic receptors thus blocking the effects of catecholamines on blood vessels. Consequently, there is increased blood flow to skin, mucosa, and abdominal viscera (skeletal muscle blood flow is not affected). There is a fall in both supine and erect blood pressure.

Indications: ●Control hypertension and sweating due to pheochromocytoma.
●Reduce Raynaud's phenomenon–associated vasoconstriction.

Contraindications: conditions in which a drop in blood pressure is inadvisable.

Caution: marked cerebral or coronary arteriosclerosis, renal disease. ●Alpha blockers leave beta receptors unopposed. Consequently, concurrent administration of an agent that acts on both receptors (e.g. epinephrine) may cause a marked fall in blood pressure and tachycardia.

Comments: ●Excessive tachycardia may be controlled with a beta blocker. ●Symptoms of respiratory infection may be aggravated by phenoxybenzamine.

Side effects: postural hypotension, reflex tachycardia, nasal congestion, miosis, or inhibition of ejaculation are due to alpha blockade and tend to decrease with continued therapy. Other side effects are drowsiness, fatigue, nausea, vomiting, diarrhea.

Supplied as: 10 mg tablet.

Dose (adult):

Pheochromocytoma; 10 mg PO twice daily initially. Increase dose every other day until blood pressure controlled or side effects troublesome. Usual requirement is 20–40 mg bid–tid.

Raynaud's phenomena: Start with 10 mg/day. Increase daily dose by 10 mg every fourth day until relief obtained or side effects troublesome. Usual requirement is 20–60 mg/day divided.

PHENTOLAMINE (Regitine)

Action: Competitively binds to alpha–adrenergic receptors on vascular smooth muscle thereby preventing catecholamine–induced vasoconstriction.

Contraindications: coronary artery disease (e.g. angina, myocardial infarction or history thereof); pregnancy (consider risk versus benefit).

Caution: Myocardial infarction and cerebrovascular spasm/occlusion have resulted from phentolamine administration, particularly when marked hypotension has been induced.

Side effects: acute and prolonged hypotension, postural hypotension, tachycardia, arrhythmias, flushing, dizziness, weakness, nasal stuffiness, nausea, vomiting, diarrhea.

Supplied as: vials containing 5 mg for IV or IM injection.

Indications/dose:

Control pheochromocytoma–induced hypertension: 5 mg IV in adult and 1 mg IV in child. Repeat if necessary. Dose may also be given IM.

Phenylephrine overdose: Dosage is same as above.

Control hypertension resulting from interaction of catecholamines and monoamine oxidase inhibitor: Dosage is same as above.

Diagnosis pheochromocytoma (Regitine blocking test). Urinary and plasma assay of catecholamines and their metabolites is the preferred method of diagnosis. However, Regitine blocking test may be used if diagnosis is still in doubt and the risk of using phentolamine is considered. A drop in systolic BP > 35 and a drop in diastolic BP > 25 following administration of 5 mg phentolamine in adult and 1 mg in child is consistent with pheochromocytoma.

Treatment of dermal necrosis and sloughing following extravasation of norepinephrine or dopamine; 5–10 mg in 10 ml normal saline injected into region of extravasation.

Prevention of dermal necrosis and sloughing in patient receiving intravenous norepinephrine: Add 10 mg phentolamine per liter of norepinephrine–containing solution.

PHENYTOIN (Dilantin)

Indications: ●Grand mal and psychomotor seizures.
●Arrhythmias, particularly those related to digitalis or tricyclic toxicity.

Contraindications: phenytoin hypersensitivity, nursing mother. IV administration is contraindicated in patients with sinus bradycardia, sino–atrial block, 2nd or 3rd degree AV block, Stokes–Adams syndrome, hypotension.

Caution: hepatic dysfunction, elderly, debilitated, pregnancy.

Comments: ●Serum therapeutic level is 10–20 mcg/ml. ●Rapid IV administration may cause bradycardia, hypotension, AV block, etc. ●Because phenytoin precipitates easily, it must not be added to intravenous solutions for administration as a continuous IV infusion. ●To reduce venous irritation, flush IV with normal saline after administering each phenytoin. ●If phenytoin is to be discontinued and the patient has been maintained on phenytoin, the drug should be discontinued gradually in order to preclude precipitating seizures.

Side effects: nystagmus, ataxia, slurred speech, motor twitching, sedation, confusion, headache, nausea, vomiting, constipation, gingival hyperplasia, hirsutism, rash, dermatitis, lupus, Stevens–Johnson syndrome, marrow suppression, folic acid depletion with consequent megaloblastic anemia, osteomalacia due to altered vitamin D metabolism, lymphadenopathy.

Supplied as: extended capsule (30,100 mg); chewable flavored tablet (50 mg), oral suspension (30 or 125 mg/5ml); IV injection preparation (50 mg/ml).

Dose in treatment of status epilepticus (adult or pediatric): 15–18 mg/kg IV. With the IV running with normal saline, administer phenytoin directly and close to the IV catheter insertion site at no faster than 50 mg/min in adult nor faster than 0.5 mg/kg/min in child. Phenytoin must not be administered as a continuous IV infusion. Monitor blood pressure, respirations, and EKG when administering phenytoin IV.

Dose as maintenance anticonvulsant:

Adult: 100 mg PO tid of any of the oral preparations (extended capsule, chewable tablet, or oral suspension). The usual requirement is 300–400 mg/day. If necessary, increase up to maximum 200 mg PO tid. Those patients whose seizures are controlled with 100 mg PO tid may try taking a single daily dose of three 100 mg extended capsules at bedtime. ●An initial loading dose may be administered if a therapeutic level must be attained quickly. The loading dose is 1000 mg divided into 3 doses at 2 hour intervals: 400, 300, 300 mg. Do not use loading dose in patient with renal or hepatic disease.

Pediatric: 5 mg/kg/day PO divided into 2–3 doses.
　　　　　(range: 4–8 mg/kg/day, maximum 300 mg/day).

Dose in treatment of arrhythmia:

Adult: 100 mg IV every 5 minutes until arrhythmia controlled, side effects develop, or maximum of 1000 mg given. With the IV running with normal saline, administer phenytoin directly and close to the IV catheter insertion site at no faster than 25–50 mg/minute. 250 mg is usually sufficient to control a digitalis–induced arrhythmia. Monitor blood pressure, respirations, and EKG.

Pediatric: 2–4 mg/kg at no faster than 0.5 mg/kg/minute. Repeat if necessary. Stop if side effects develop. Usual requirement is 20–30 mg/kg.

POTASSIUM CHLORIDE, intravenous

Indications: hypokalemia, prevent potassium depletion.
Contraindications: hyperkalemia.
Caution/comments: ●Administer with particular caution to those in renal failure. ●Be certain that urine output is adequate before administering IV potassium. ●Administer potassium requirements orally if possible. ●NEVER administer intravenous potassium undiluted or IV push. ●Central venous or intracardiac administration is dangerous and should be avoided. ●Potassium infusion rate must not exceed 40mEq/hr. ●Concentration of potassium solution must not exceed 60mEq/liter. ●Concentrations > 40mEq/liter should not be given via a small vein because venous irritation with phlebitis may ensue. ●Take following precautions when administering intravenous KCl at high rates (10 mEq/hr or greater) or high concentrations (greater than 40 mEq/liter): use a constant infusion pump, continuous EKG monitoring, frequent serum potassium determinations. ●Concurrent administration of IV glucose may oppose correction of hypokalemia because glucose causes potassium to move intracellularly and thus decrease plasma potassium.
Side effects are those of hyperkalemia: arrhythmias/EKG abnormalities (e.g. peaked T waves, short QT interval, wide QRS, increased PR interval, absence of P wave and finally sine wave, ventricular fibrillation, asystole); hypotension; muscle weakness; paralysis; confusion.

Adult dose:

Maintenance: Adding 20 mEq KCl to each liter of maintenance solution usually suffices. The 24 hour potassium requirement is 50–100 mEq. Do not forget to take into account additional sources of potassium (e.g. oral potassium supplements, potassium–rich foods) or administration of potassium–sparing diuretic.

Hypokalemia:
　●Nonurgent cases (i.e. serum potassium > 2.5 mEq/liter, absence of muscle weakness or EKG changes): Infuse IV thru peripheral vein at no greater than 10 mEq/hr using a concentration no greater than 40 mEq/liter. See comments.
　●Emergency (i.e. serum potassium below 2.0 mEq/liter, profound muscle weakness, paralysis, arrhythmias): Infuse intravenously at no greater than 20–40 mEq/hr using a concentration no greater than 60 mEq/liter. See comments.

Pediatric dose:

Maintenance: 20 mEq KCl per liter of maintenance solution ususally suffices. To be more precise, calculate total 24 hour potassium requirement as follows:
(2.5 mEq/kg for first 10 kg body weight) + (1.25 mEq/kg for 2nd 10 kg body weight) + (0.5 mEq/kg for weight over 20 kg).
Using 25 kg patient as ecample: (2.5 mEq/kg) (10 kg) + (1.25 mEq/kg) (10 kg) + (0.5 mEq/kg) (5 kg) = 40 mEq KCl/24hr.

Hypokalemia:
- In nonurgent cases, infuse at 0.25 mEq/kg/hr using concentration no greater than 40 mEq/liter.
- In emergencies (i.e. serum potassium below 2.0 mEq/liter, profound muscle weakness, paralysis, arrhythmias): 0.5–1.0 mEq/kg/hr may be administered using constant infusion pump with continuous EKG monitoring and frequent serum potassium determinations.

POTASSIUM, oral supplements

Indications: hypokalemia, prevention potassium depletion.
Contraindications: hyperkalemia, severe renal dysfunction, untreated Addison's disease, dehydration, heat cramps, familial periodic paralysis, concurrent administration potassium–sparing drugs (e.g. spironolactone, triamterene).
Additional contraindications to use of slow–release tablet: Any condition impairing passage of tablet such as GI obstruction, decreased GI motility, esophageal compression from enlarged left atrium.
Caution: To preclude hyperkalemia, periodically monitor serum potassium. EKG signs of hyperkalemia include: peaked T, ST depression, loss of P wave, prolonged QT, wide QRS.
Side effects: hyperkalemia may lead to arrhythmias, cardiac arrest, muscle weakness, paralysis, confusion, hypotension, nausea, vomiting, diarrhea, abdominal discomfort, GI obstruction, GI bleeding, GI perforation.
Comments: Potassium–rich foods: Potassium supplements may not be necessary if potassium–rich foods are ingested: 1 orange = 8–10 mEq potassium, 1 banana = 20–22 mEq potassium, 1 tomato = 16–22 mEq potassium, 8 oz glass orange juice = 11 mEq potassium, 8 oz glass prune juice = 15 mEq potassium. Choosing appropriate supplement: Potassium chloride is the usual oral supplement for treating/preventing hypokalemia. However, hypokalemia in the presence of hyperchloremia is treated with a preparation that does not contain chloride—e.g. potassium gluconate, potassium bicarbonate/citrate. Method of administration: To preclude gastric irritation; the oral solutions, powders, granules, or dissolving tablets should all be mixed in a glass of water or juice, and administered after meals if possible. Slow–release (time–release) tablets are reserved for non-compliant patients or for patients who cannot tolerate other oral potassium supplements.

Adult dose: ●Hypokalemia: 20–40 mEq 2–3 times a day.
●Prevent potassium depletion (e.g. patient on thiazide diuretic): 10–20mEq 1–4 times a day depending on requirements.
Pediatric dose: 1–2 mEq/kg/day or more as required divided into 2–3 daily doses.

Oral Potassium Solutions:
5% KCl solution (10mEq KCl/15ml).
10% KCl solution (20mEq KCL/15ml):
    KAY CIEL Oral Solution (sugar-free, contains saccharin);
    Kaochlor (contains sugar, saccharin);
    Kaochlor S–F (sugar–free; contains saccharin);
    Klorvess 10% liquid (contains sucrose and saccharin).
15% KCl solution (30mEq KCl/15ml): Rum K (sugar and alcohol free).
20% KCl solution (40mEq KCL/15ml): Kaon–Cl 20% (sugar-free, contains saccharin).
Potassium gluconate (20mEq K/15ml): Kaon Elixir (sugar–free).
Potassium powder/granules:
Potassium chloride (mEq KCl per packet is in parenthesis):
    KATO (20mEq, tomato flavored),   KAY CIEL Powder (20mEq),
    K–Lor (15 or 20mEq),   KLOR–CON Powder (20mEq),
    KLOR–CON/25 Powder (25mEq),   K–Lyte/Cl powder (25mEq/scoop),
    K+ Care (20mEq).
Potassium chloride, K bicarbonate, L–lysine mono HCl: Klorvess Effervesent Granules (contains 20mEq potassium per packet).
Rapidly dissolving tablets:
Potassium chloride/ bicarbonate/citrate, L–lysine HCl (mEq potassium per tablet in parenthesis): Klorvess Effervescent Tablet (20mEq); K–Lyte/CL (25mEq), K–Lyte/CL 50 (50mEq).
Potassium bicarbonate/citrate (mEq potassium per tablet in parenthesis):
    K–Lyte (25mEq),   K–Lyte DS (50mEq),   KLOR–CON EF (25mEq).
Potassium bicarbonate: K+ Care ET (contains 25mEq potassium/tablet).

Slow–release tablet/capsule (reserve for patient who is non-compliant or who cannot tolerate potassium solution). Unless otherwise indicated, the pill must be swallowed whole and not crushed or chewed. No more than 20 mEq should be taken at one time. Should be taken with glass of water at mealtime.

Potassium chloride (mEq KCl per pill is in parenthesis):

Kaon–Cl (6.7 mEq),	Kaon–Cl 10 (10mEq),	Slow K (8mEq),
Klotrix (10mEq),	K–tab (10 mEq),	K+ 10 (10mEq),
KLOR–CON 8 (8mEq),	KLOR–CON 10 (10mEq),	K–Norm (10mEq),

Micro–K Extencaps (8mEq, contents of capsule may be sprinkled on food),
Micro–K 10 Extencaps (10mEq, contents of capsule may be sprinkled on food),
Ten–K (10mEq, tablet may be crushed),
K–DUR (10 or 20 mEq, tablet may be dissolved in water before ingestion).

PRAZOSIN (Minipress)

Action: Blocks postsynaptic alpha–adrenergic receptors of vascular smooth muscle. The consequent dilation of veins and arterioles leads to reduction in blood pressure.
Indications: mild to moderate hypertension. Prazosin is usually used as a step 3 drug (e.g. added to a thiazide diuretic and a beta blocker) when further reduction in blood pressure is required.
Caution: nursing mother. Safety not established in pregnancy and children.
Side effects: most common; dizziness, headache, drowsiness, lack of energy, weakness, palpitations, nausea; 1–4% patients; orthostatic hypotension, syncope, edema, dyspnea, urinary frequency, vomiting, diarrhea, constipation, dry mouth, nasal congestion, epistaxis, nervousness, vertigo, depression, blurred vision, reddened sclera, rash; less than 1%; tachycardia, abdominal discomfort/pain, liver function abnormalities, pancreatitis, hallucinations, paresthesias, tinnitus, itching, lichen planus, alopecia, arthralgias, + ANA, sweating, fever.
Supplied as: 1, 2, 5 mg capsule.
Dose (adult): 1 mg 2-3 times a day. Increase gradually as needed up to 20 mg/day in divided doses. Usual requirement is 6–15 mg/day. Orthostatic hypotension with dizziness, lightheadedness, tachycardia, and/or syncope may occur 30–90 minutes following the initial dose, after rapid dose increases, or following the addition of another antihypertensive drug. Therefore: (**1**) start with 1 mg doses (syncope occurs in about 1% in patients whose initial dose is 2 mg or more), (**2**) gradually increase dose as needed, (**3**) reduce dose to 1-2 mg 3 times a day and retitrate when adding another antihypertensive drug.

PRIMIDONE (Mysoline)

Action: Barbiturate derivative. Converted to the active metabolites phenobarbital and phenylethylmalonamide, both of which raise seizure threshold by unknown mechanism.
Indications: Alone or in combination with other anticonvulsants (e.g. phenytoin) for treatment of gran mal, psychomotor, or focal seizures. Primidone is not effective for treatment absence (petit mal) epilepsy.
Contraindications: porphyria, hypersensitivty to primidone or phenobarbital.
Caution: pregnancy, nursing mother (discontinue if infant becomes unusually drowsy).
Comments: ●Full therapeutic effect may not be realized for several weeks. ●Serum therapeutic level is 5-12 mcg/ml. ●To preclude neonatal hemorrhage, pregnant women receiving primidone should receive prophylactic vitamin K for 1 month prior to and during delivery. ●Discontinuing primidone in patient on maintenance regimen: in order to preclude precipitating status epilepticus, taper and withdraw the drug over at least 2 weeks. ●CBC and panel 12 is recommended every 6 months.
Side effects: ataxia, vertigo, nystagmus, diplopia, fatigue, drowsiness, irritability, emotional disturbances, anorexia, nausea, vomiting, impotence, rash, folate–responsive megaloblastic anemia.
Supplied as: tablet (50, 250 mg); oral suspension (250mg/5ml).
Dose:

Adult/child over 8 yr:
●day 1–3: 100–125 mg at bedtime, ●day 4–6: 100–125 mg twice daily,
●day 7-9: 100–125 mg tid, ●day10–maintenance: 250mg tid. Maximum is 500 mg qid.

Child under 8 yr:
●day 1–3: 50 mg at bedtime, ●day 4–6: 50 mg twice daily,
●day 7-9: 100 mg twice daily, ●day 10–maintenance: 125–250 mg tid
(or 10–25 mg/kg/day divided into 3 daily doses).

PROBENECID (Benemid)

Action: ●Increases urinary excretion of uric acid by inhibiting renal tubular reabsorption. ●Blocks renal tubular secretion of penicillins, thereby increasing plasma levels of penicillins.

Indications: ●Hyperuricemia that is associated with gout and gouty arthritis. ●To inhibit excretion of penicillin, ampicillin, methicillin, oxacillin, cloxacillin, dicloxacillin, nafcillin, or cephalosporins.

Contraindications: probenecid hypersensitivity, under 2 yr of age, history of uric acid kidney stones, history of blood dyscrasias, concurrent salicylate administration, uric acid excretion > 800 mg/24 hr.

Caution: pregnancy, peptic ulcer disease, G6PD deficiency.

Comments: Uric acid stones: Risk of precipitating uric acid stones may be reduced by maintaining a high fluid intake and an alkaline urine. Gout: If a gouty attack occurs while taking probenecid, continue probenecid without changing dose and treat attack with indomethacin or colchicine. Do not start probenecid during gouty attack. The dose of probenecid may be reduced when gout attacks have not occurred for 6 months. Adjust dose to maintain serum uric acid within normal limits. Drug interactions: Probenecid inhibits excretion of indomethacin and certain other nonsteroidal anti-inflammatory drugs as well as methotrexate, sulfonamides, sulfonylureas, and rifampin. Consequently, the dose of these drugs may need to be reduced. Excretion of penicillins is also inhibited. Consequently, concurrent administration of probenecid with penicillins is not recommended in setting of renal failure. Avoid concurrent administration of salicylates and probenecid because salicylates interfere with probenecid's uricosuric effect.

Side effects: neurologic (headache, dizziness); gastrointestinal (anorexia, nausea, vomiting)—may be alleviated by taking dose with food; urinary tract (urinary frequency, exacerbation of gout and uric acid stones, nephrotic syndrome); hypersensitivity (itching, dermatitis, urticaria, anaphylaxis, fever); blood: anemia, hemolytic anemia (may be associated with G6PD deficiency), aplastic anemia, leukopenia; other (sore gums, flushing, hair loss, hepatic necrosis).

Supplied as: 500 mg tablet.

Dose in treatment of gout (adult):

250 mg PO twice daily for one week followed by 500 mg PO twice daily.

Renal failure: Probenecid is of no use in gout therapy if GFR is less than 30 ml/minute. In less severe renal failure, larger daily doses of probenecid may be needed. Increase the daily dose as needed by 500 mg every 4 weeks up to maximum 2000 mg/24 hr.

Dose to inhibit urinary excretion of penicillins:

Adult or child over 50 kg: 500 mg PO 4 times a day. Patients receiving single dose therapy for uncomplicated gonorrhea should receive a single 1 gram dose of probenecid prior to IM administration of aqueous procaine penicillin G, or simultaneously with oral ampicillin or amoxicillin.

Child 2–14 yr: Initial dose of 25 mg/kg PO followed by 10 mg/kg PO 4 times a day. Children receiving single dose therapy for uncomplicated gonorrhea should receive a single 25 mg/kg (maximum 1 gram) dose of probenecid prior to IM administration of aqueous procaine penicillin G, or simultaneously with oral ampicillin or amoxicillin.

PROCAINAMIDE (Pronestyl, Pronestyl–SR, Procan SR)

Action: ●decreases automaticity of myocardium including ectopic foci (i.e. decreases rate of spontaneous diastolic depolarization); ●decreases myocardial excitability (i.e. increases depolarization threshold); ●prolongs AV node refractory period and slows AV conduction (increase PR interval); ●slows conduction thru His–Purkinje and ventricular muscle (widens QRS); ●prolongs repolarization (prolongs QT interval); ●decreases myocardial contractility. ●Anticholinergic (vagolytic) effect may facilitate AV conduction and consequently paradoxically increase the ventricular rate (rationale for digitalizing first when treating atrial flutter or atrial fibrillation).

Indications:

Ventricular tachycardia, ventricular fibrillation, or premature ventricular contractions refractory to lidocaine; give procainamide intravenously.

Chronic suppression of premature ventricular contractions or ventricular tachycardia; give procainamide PO. However, PO quinidine is usually preferred (see comment 2).

To convert atrial flutter and atrial fibrillation to normal sinus rhythm (see comment 1 and 2). Intravenous procainamide may be used but DC cardioversion is preferred. Oral procainamide prevents recurrence but oral quinidine is usually preferred (see comment 2).

Paroxysmal supraventricular tachycardia. Procainamide not drug of choice.

Premature atrial contractions. However, PAC's usually do not require treatment. And furthermore, quinidine is preferred if PAC's must be suppressed.

Contraindications: procainamide, procaine, and related drug hypersensitivity; myasthenia gravis; 2nd, 3rd, or complete heart block; prolonged QT interval; Torsades de Pointes.

Caution: pregnancy, nursing mother, renal insufficiency, patient over 50 yr of age.

Comments: (1) Procainamide has a vagolytic effect on the AV node. Therefore, a sudden increase in ventricular rate may ensue if procainamide is given to patient with atrial flutter or atrial fibrillation. Consequently, prior digitalization is required to control the ventricular response if such supraventricular tachyarrhythmias are present. However, digitalis should not be given and therefore procainamide should be avoided if there is atrial fibrillation in setting of Wolff-Parkinson-White syndrome. (**2**) Quinidine is usually preferred to procainamide when chronic oral therapy is required. Up to 75% of patients receiving long-term oral procainamide develop a + ANA and a third of these develop a lupus-like syndrome. Periodically obtain CBC and ANA test if patient is on long-term procainamide therapy. (**3**) Prior to correction of atrial fibrillation, heparin or warfarin anticoagulation is required to preclude embolization of a mural thrombus. (**4**) Reduce procainamide dosage if there is CHF, renal dysfunction, or liver dysfunction. (**5**) Hyperkalemia may enhance toxicity and hypokalemia may reduce effectiveness of procainamide.

Side effects: <u>cardiovascular</u> (usually with IV use): hypotension, bradycardia, prolonged QT interval, AV block, ventricular fibrillation, asystole; <u>gastrointestinal</u>: anorexia, nausea, bitter taste, diarrhea, elevated liver enzymes, hepatomegaly; <u>neurologic</u>: weakness, depression, hallucinations, psychosis; <u>hypersensitivity</u>: fever, rash, urticaria, angioedema, nephrotic syndrome; <u>blood</u>: thrombocytopenia, Coomb's + hemolytic anemia, neutropenia, agranulocytosis, pancytopenia; <u>lupus-like syndrome</u>: arthralgias, arthritis, myalgia, skin lesions, pleuritic pain/effusion, pericarditis, etc.

Overdose: Treatment is similar to quinidine. Resin hemoperfusion or hemodialysis may be necessary in cases requiring extracorporeal circulatory assistance or in patients in renal failure.

Supplied as: capsule or tablet (250, 375, 500 mg);
sustain release tablet (250, 500, 750 mg);
IV or IM injection (100, 500 mg/ml).

Adult dose:
<u>Intravenous:</u>
●Initially, 100 mg q 5 minutes (no faster than 50 mg/min) until arrhythmia suppressed or until maximum of 1000 mg given. Stop if hypotension occurs or if QRS widens by 50%. To facilitate control of rate of infusion, dilute procainamide in D5W.
●Follow with maintenance infusion of 1–4 mg/minute. Example: 1 gram procainamide added to 250 ml D5W and running at 30 ml/hr delivers 2 mg/minute.
<u>Oral:</u> 50 mg/kg/day divided q3–6h is the usual maintenance dose. A loading dose of 1000–1250 mg may be given, and an additional 750 mg may be given in 1 hour if arrhythmia persists. After the arrhythmia is controlled, the daily dose may be divided q6h using sustain release tablets.
<u>Intramuscular</u> (when oral route not feasible): 500–1000 mg q6h.

Pediatric dose:
<u>Intravenous:</u> 2 mg/kg (maximum 100 mg) diluted in D5W and administered slowly over 5 minutes. Repeat at 10–15 minute intervals until arrhythmia controlled. Stop if hypotension occurs or if QRS widens by 50%, and do not infuse more than 1000 mg. Maintenance: continuous IV infusion 0.020–0.080 mg/minute. Total 24 hr IV dose should not exceed 2 gram.
<u>Oral:</u> 50 mg/kg/day divided q3–6h. (maximum 4 gram/day).
<u>Intramuscular</u> (when oral route not feasible): 20–30 mg/kg/day divided q6h (maximum 4 gram/day).

PROGESTINS: medroxyprogesterone acetate (Amen, Cycrin, Depo-Provera, Provera), megestrol acetate (Megace), norethindrone acetate (Aygestin, Norlutate)

Contraindications: hypersensitivity to drug, pregnancy, undiagnosed vaginal bleeding, missed or threatened abortion, liver disease, thrombophlebitis, thromoembolic disorders, stroke, history of latter 3 conditions. **Caution:** nursing mother.

Comments: ●Progestogens may cause fluid retention. Therefore, they must be used cautiously in conditions that may be adversely effected by fluid retention (e.g. migraine, asthma, epilepsy, cardiac or renal dysfunction). ●Discontinue progestin at first sign of thrombotic disorder (e.g. thrombophlebitis, pulmonary embolism, cerebrovascular disorder, retinal thrombosis). ●Discontinue progestin if there is sudden onset of partial or complete loss of vision, migraine, diplopia, proptosis. Do not start or restart therapy in presence of papilledema or vascular retinopathy. ●Discontinue progestin if serious psychic depression occurs.

Side effects: congenital anomalies in infants of mothers given progesterone during pregnancy, fluid retention, breast tenderness, galactorrhea, thromboembolic phenomena, breakthrough bleeding, spotting, change in menstrual flow, amenorrhea, changes in cervical erosion or cervical secretions, cholestatic jaundice, anaphylactoid reactions or anaphylaxis, allergic rash (with or without pruritis), fever, insomnia, somnolence. ●Refer to "Oral Contraceptives" for additional side effects which are seen with estrogen-progestin combinations and which may possibly be due to progestins.

progesterone in oil   Supplied as: 50 mg/ml for IM injection.

<u>Diagnostic evaluation of amenorrhea</u>: 200 mg IM once. Withdrawal bleeding should occur in 2–7 days if the ovaries are at least capable of secreting estrogen to prime the endometrium.

<u>Dysfunctional uterine bleeding</u>: 100 mg IM. Bleeding should stop and then be followed in a few days by withdrawal bleeding. The discussion on dysfunctional uterine bleeding under medroxyprogesterone acetate below is pertinent.

medroxyprogesterone acetate

<u>Supplied as:</u>   10 mg tablet (Provera, Amen, Cycrin);
           100 or 400 mg/ml for IM injection (Depo–Provera).

<u>Dysfunctional uterine bleeding</u> (abnormal uterine bleeding due to hormonal imbalance that is unassociated with organic pathology): 10mg PO once daily for 5 days. Withdrawal bleeding should occur within 3–7 days after discontinuing the drug if the endometrium has been adequately primed by endogenous estrogen. The regimen of 10 mg PO once daily for 5 days may be repeated every 2 months if spontaneous menses fail to occur because of anovulation, and the patient does not want contraception. Use an oral contraceptive instead if the patient does not wish to become pregnant (oral contraceptive is started on the 5th day of withdrawal bleeding).

NOTE that the initial therapy for dysfunctional uterine bleeding usually consists of (**1**) combined estrogen–progestin therapy (any of the combination oral contraceptives 1 pill 4 times a day for 5–7 days); or (**2**) if bleeding has been prolonged and heavy, with high–dose estrogen (e.g. 25 mg Premarin IV q4h until bleeding is alleviated or a total 6 doses given).

<u>Secondary amenorrhea</u>: 5–10 mg PO once daily for 5–10 days. Withdrawal bleeding should begin within 3–7 days of stopping therapy.

<u>Endometriosis</u>: 150 mg Depo–Provera IM every 3 months. An alternative is 30 mg PO once daily which may be continued for a few months or until annoying breakthrough bleeding occurs.

<u>Palliation endometrial carcinoma</u>: 400–1000 mg Depo–Provera IM once a week initially. As little as 400 mg once a month may suffice once patient is stable.

megestrol acetate (Megace)   Supplied as: 20, 40 tablet.

Palliation advanced breast cancer: 40 mg PO 4 times a day.
Palliation advanced endometrial cancer: 40–320 mg/day in divided doses.

Norethindrone acetate (Aygestin, Norlutate)   Supplied as: 5 mg tablet.

<u>Dysfunctional Uterine Bleeding</u>: (abnormal uterine bleeding due to hormonal imbalance that is unassociated with organic pathology): 2.5–10 mg PO once daily for 5–10 days. The discussion for dysfunctional uterine bleeding under medroxyprogesterone acetate is pertinent.

<u>Secondary amenorrhea</u>: 2.5–10 mg PO once daily for 5–10 days.

<u>Endometriosis</u>: Initially, 5 mg PO once daily for 2 weeks. Increase daily dose by 2.5 mg every 2 weeks until patient is receiving 15 mg once daily. This dosage may be continued for 6–9 months or until annoying breakthrough bleeding indicates temporary termination.

PROPRANOLOL (Inderal)

Action: Competitively binds to beta–adrenergic receptor sites thereby blocking the effects of catecholamines.

Cardiac effects are due to blockade of beta–1 receptors; ●There is a decrease in heart rate and contractility which has 2 consequences: (1) decreased cardiac output and therefore decreased myocardial oxygen consumption, (2) decrease in both standing and supine blood pressure. The reduction in blood pressure is due to a combination of effects—e.g. decreased cardiac output, inhibition of renin release, effect on adrenergic receptors in CNS. ●Blockade of beta–1 receptors also causes slowed AV conduction and suppression of automaticity.

Blockade of beta–2 receptors may result in bronchospasm, inhibition of peripheral vasodilation (e.g. blockade of beta receptors of vascular smooth muscle may provoke Raynaud's phenomenon), inhibition of glycogenolysis with possible adverse effects (e.g. potentiation of insulin–induced hypoglycemia, risk of hypoglycemia during prolonged exercise).

Indications: hypertension (propranolol is usually prescribed concurrently with thiazide diuretic); to control angina (propranolol usually used in conjunction with nitrates); myocardial infarction (as long–term therapy to reduce mortality following acute phase of myocardial infarction); cardiac arrhythmias including: (**1**) paroxysmal supraventricular tachycardias—particularly those due to catecholamines or digitalis, or associated with Wolff–Parkinson–White syndrome); (**2**) rapid ventricular rate due to atrial fibrillation or flutter that is not slowed with digitalis or digitalis is contraindicated, (**3**) digitalis–induced tachyarrhythmias which are not associated with high–degree AV block and which persist after discontinuing digitalis, correcting electrolytes abnormalities, and a trial of phenytoin; (**4**) ventricular tachycardia due to catecholamine excess; (**5**) ventricular tachycardia refractory to conventional treatment; <u>other indications:</u> hypertrophic subaortic stenosis, migraine prophylaxis, pheochromocytoma, hyperthyroidism.

Contraindications: sinus bradycardia, heart block greater than first degree, cardiogenic shock, right ventricular failure due to pulmonary hypertension, CHF (unless CHF is due to tachyarrhythmia treatable with propranolol), bronchial asthma, allergic rhinitis during pollen season, patient who has received adrenergic–augmenting psychotropic drugs (e.g. MAO inhibitor) during last 2 weeks.

Caution: ●Beta blockers may precipitate heart failure in patient with limited cardiac reserve. ●Abrupt discontinuation of beta blocker in patient with ischemic heart disease may aggravate angina, or even precipitate myocardial infarction or sudden death. ●Use beta blockers cautiously in insulin–dependent diabetic; the warning signs of hypoglycemia may be masked. ●Beta blockers may mask signs of hyperthyroidism and alter thyroid function tests. Abrupt discontinuation may worsen symptoms of hyperthyroidism or precipitate thyroid storm. ●Beta blockers may need to be discontinued prior to major surgery. ●Use beta blockers cautiously in following circumstances: renal or liver dysfunction; pregnancy; nursing mother; children; nonallergic bronchospasm (e.g. bronchitis, emphysema).

Side effects: <u>cardiovascular</u> (bradycardia, congestive heart failure, worsening AV block, hypotension, Raynaud–type arterial insufficiency); <u>respiratory</u> (bronchospasm); <u>blood</u> (agranulocytosis, thrombocytopenic or nonthrombocytopenic purpura); <u>gastrointestinal</u> (nausea, vomiting, diarrhea, constipation, cramps, epigastric distress, mesenteric arterial thrombosis, ischemic colitis); <u>neurologic</u> (lethargy, fatigue, weakness, lightheadedness, mental depression, catatonia, insomnia, vivid dreams, hallucinations, visual disturbances, disorientation, short–term memory loss, emotional lability, clouded sensorium, impaired neuropsychometric performance, paresthesias); <u>allergic</u> (fever with sore throat and aching, pharyngitis with agranulocytosis, erythematous rash, laryngospasm and respiratory distress); <u>other</u> (alopecia, rash, dry eyes, lupus–like reactions, impotence, Peyronie's disease).

Treatment of overdose or exaggerated or unwanted response: If an overdose is is recent, empty stomach and administer charcoal. <u>Bradycardia and hypotension:</u> Clinically significant bradycardia is first treated with IV atropine, and then if necessary IV isoproterenol. A pacemaker may be necessary. IV glucagon may be used to help overcome the negative inotropic influence of propranolol. Hypotension may respond to challenge of IV normal saline, and insertion of a Swan–Ganz catheter will help guide further fluid administration (a wedge pressure < 12 mm Hg is an indication for administering additional fluid). Persistent hypotension may require IV infusion of a vasopressor (e.g. epinephrine). Cardiogenic shock refractory to the foregoing measures is an indication for an intra–aortic balloon pump. <u>Arrhythmias:</u> ●AV block with junctional or ventricular bradycardia requires a pacemaker. Atropine, isoproterenol, and if necessary glucagon are administered until the pacemaker can be inserted. ●PVC's (unassociated with bradycardia) or ventricular tachycardia are treated with lidocaine. Phenytoin is the 2nd choice. Bretylium or overdrive pacing may be tried if necessary. Countershock may be used for ventricular tachycardia refractory to the foregoing measures. <u>Hypoglycemia</u> is treated with intravenous glucose.

Supplied as:

tablets (10, 20, 40, 60, 80, 90 mg); oral solution (20 and 40 mg/5ml);
long–acting capsules (60, 80, 120, 160 mg); intravenous preparation (1mg/ml).

Dose (adult):

<u>Arrhythmias:</u>
●Intravenous (for emergency treatment): 1 mg at 5 minute intervals up to maximum of 0.15 mg/kg. Do not administer faster than 1 mg/minute. Monitor blood pressure and EKG.
●Oral: requirements vary. Range is 10–80 mg PO 3–4 times a day.

<u>Hypertension</u> (usually in combination with thiazide diuretic). Start with 40 mg PO twice daily, and then titrate to appropriate blood pressure. Usual requirement is 160–240 mg/day divided.

<u>Angina</u> : Start with 10–20mg PO 3–4 times a day. Titrate to effect up to maximum of 320 mg/day.

<u>Myocardial infarction:</u> 180–240 mg/day divided into 3–4 doses.

<u>Hypertrophic subaortic stenosis:</u> 20–40 mg PO 3–4 times a day.

<u>Pheochromocytoma:</u> (in conjunction with an alpha–adrenergic blocking agent which must be started before adding propranolol): 60 mg/day PO for 3 days prior to surgery. If the tumor is inoperable, chronic therapy is 30 mg/day PO in divided doses.

<u>Hyperthyroidism:</u> In the case of a thyrotoxic crisis, propranolol may be administered intravenously as for arrhythmias. Otherwise, treatment is begun with oral doses titrated to relief of symptoms and tachycardia. Start with 10–20 mg PO q6h. Usual requirement is 80–320 mg/day divided.

Migraine prophylaxis: 80 mg PO daily in divided doses. Propranolol will not allevi-ate migraine in progress.

Indications/dose long–acting capsules:

Hypertension: Start with 80 mg once daily, increase as needed. Usual requirement is 120–160 once daily.

Angina: Start with 80 mg once daily, increase as needed at 3–7 day intervals. Usual requirement is 160 mg once daily.

Hypertrophic subaortic stenosis: 80–160 mg once daily.

Migraine prophylaxis: Start with 80 mg once daily. Usual requirement is 160–240 mg once daily.

PROPANTHELINE BROMIDE (Pro–Banthine)

Action: Anticholinergic. Inhibits GI motility and decreases gastric acid secretion by competitively blocking acetylcholine at visceral effector site (antimuscarinic effect). The antimuscarinic effect also inhibits detrusor muscle contraction thereby increasing bladder capacity.

Indications: neurogenic bladder, adjunct in treatment of peptic ulcer.

Contraindications: glaucoma, urinary obstruction, GI obstruction, elderly or debilitated patients with intestinal atony, severe ulcerative colitis, myasthenia gravis, acute hemorrhage with unstable cardiovascular status.

Caution: congestive heart failure, tachyarrhythmias, coronary artery disease, hypertension, auto-nomic neuropathy, liver or kidney disease, ulcerative colitis, hiatal hernia with reflux esophagitis, hyperthyroidism, high environmental temperature (since in this setting decreased sweating may provoke fever and heat stroke), patient who engages in hazardous activities (drowsiness and blurred vision may occur), nursing mother, elderly.

Comments: ●Concurrent administration of other drugs with anticholinergic properties may provoke excessive cholinergic blockade (e.g. belladonna alkaloids, meperidine, antihistamines, phenothiaz-ines, tricyclic antidepressants, quinidine, procainamide, disopyramide). ●Phenothiazines potenti-ate sedative effect of propantheline.

Side effects: ocular (blurred vision, mydriasis, cycloplegia, increased introcular pressure); urinary (retention, hesitancy); cardiac (tachycardia, palpitations); neurologic (headache, drowsiness, weak-ness, dizziness, confusion, nervousness, insomnia, loss of taste); gastrointestinal (nausea, vomit-ing, constipation, bloated feeling); allergic (anaphylaxis, urticaria or other skin reactions); other (dry mouth, decreased sweating); impotence, suppression of lactation).

Overdose: (**1**) empty stomach, (**2**) physostigmine 0.5–2 mg IV (repeat if necessary up to cumula-tive total of 5 mg), (**3**) cooling measures if fever present, (**4**) IV Valium if patient is agitated.

Supplied as: 7.5, 15 mg tablet.

Dose:

Uninhibited neurogenic bladder: ●Adult: 15 mg PO q4–6h initially.
●Child: 7.5 mg PO q4–6h initially.

Reflex neurogenic bladder (to prevent incontinence between catheterizations): ●Adult: 15–30 mg PO q4–6h. ●Child: 7.5–15 mg PO q4–6h.

Peptic ulcer (adult): Start with 15 mg half hour before each meal and 30 mg at bedtime (total 75 mg/day). Subsequently adjust dose according to response and tolerance. 7.5 mg 3 times a day may suffice.

PROPYLTHIOURACIL [PTU]

Action: Inhibits two steps in thyroid gland synthesis of T4 and T3: (**1**) oxidation and incorporation of iodide into tyrosine residues of thyroglobulin to form monoiodotyrosine (MIT) and diiodotyrosine (DIT); (**2**) Linking of DIT + DIT to form T4 or MIT + DIT to form T3. In the peripheral tissues, PTU also inhibits conversion of T4 to T3.

Indications: hyperthyroidism, preparation for thyroid surgery or radioiodine therapy.

Contraindication: hypersensitivity to PTU. **Caution:** nursing mother, pregnancy.

Comments: Course of therapy: Since PTU does not curtail the effects of existing thyroid hor-mone, PTU–related relief of hyperthyroidism manifestations with decrease in serum T4 does not occur for 2–4 weeks. The dosage is tapered to maintenance requirements after the patient becomes euthyroid (usually in about 6 weeks). The serum T4 should not be allowed to fall below normal since the serum TSH may increase, and this in turn may result in further thyroid enlargement and aggravation of ophthalmopathy. After 12–18 months, about half the patients will have permanent remission. However, some will require therapy for years. Assessment of remission should be done by gradually reducing dosage. Pregnancy: PTU crosses the placenta and can cause fetal goi-ter and cretinism. Use smallest effective dose to maintain the mother slightly hyperthyroid. Hyperthyroidism often improves in pregnancy thus allowing dose reduction. Marrow suppression (agranulocytosis, granulocytopenia, thrombocytopenia) is a rare consequence of PTU therapy. The patient must report any illness (sore throat, fever, adenopathy, headache, malaise, rash) and a CBC must be obtained promptly. Particular caution is advised if patient is receiving other drugs with potential for causing agranulocytosis. Be aware that hyperthyroidism itself may cause leuko-penia. In addition, the patient should report any bleeding abnormality (e.g. easy bruisability, bleeding gums); a prothrombin time should be obtained.

Side effects: <u>blood</u> (granulocytopenia, agranulocytosis, thrombocytopenia); <u>skin</u> (rash, pruritis, urticaria, alopecia, pigmentation); <u>gastrointestinal</u> (nausea, vomiting, epigastric distress, hepatitis, jaundice); <u>CNS</u> (headache, vertigo, drowsiness, neuritis, paresthesias); <u>other</u> (lupus–like syndrome, drug fever, periarteritis, lymphadenopathy, salivary gland enlargement, loss of taste, edema, myalgia, arthralgia).

Supplied as: 50 mg tablet.

Dose

<u>Adult:</u> 100–150 mg q8h is the usual starting dose but up to 400 mg q8h may be required if hyperthyroidism is severe. Maintenance 50–100 mg 2–3 times a day.

<u>Child >10 yr:</u> Start with 150–300 mg/day divided into 3 equal doses q8h. Maintenance: adjust according to response.

<u>Child 6–10 yr:</u> Start with 50–150 mg/day divided into 3 equal doses q8h. Maintenance: adjust according to response.

PYRANTEL PAMOATE (Antiminth)

Action: Paralyzes worms by neuromuscular blockade thereby allowing peristalsis to eliminate worms from GI tract.

Indications: pinworm (Enterobius vermicularis); roundworm (Ascaris lumbricoides); hookworm (Necator americanus, Ancyclostoma duodenale).

Caution: pregnancy (safety not established), child under 2 yr, liver disease.

Side effects: <u>gastrointestinal</u> (anorexia, nausea, vomiting, diarrhea, abdominal cramps, tenesmus); <u>liver</u> (transient SGOT elevation); <u>neurologic</u> (headache, dizziness, drowsiness, insomnia); <u>rash.</u>

Supplied as: oral suspension 50 mg/ml.

Dose (adult or child):

<u>Pinworm, roundworm:</u> 11mg/kg PO (maximum 1000 mg) as single PO dose.

<u>Hookworm:</u> 11 mg/kg/day (maximum 1000 mg) PO once daily for 3 days.

Comments: Fasting or purgatives are not required. May be taken with milk or juice at any time relative to meals.

QUINIDINE SULFATE (Quinora, Quinidex Extentabs)
QUINIDINE GLUCONATE (Duraquin, Quinaglute Dura-Tabs)
QUINIDINE POLYGALACTURONATE (Cardioquin)

Action: decreases automiticity of myocardium including ectopic foci (i.e. decrease rate of spontaneous diastolic depolarization); decreases myocardial excitability (i.e. increases depolarization threshold); prolongs AV node refractory period and slows AV conduction (increase PR interval); slows conduction thru His–Purkinje and ventricular muscle (widens QRS); prolongs repolarization (prolongs QT interval); anticholinergic (consequent vagolytic effect facilitates AV conduction which may cause increased ventricular rate, see comment 2); decreases myocardial contractility.

Indications: ●Conversion and prevention of atrial fibrillation and atrial flutter (see comment 2). ●Treatment and prevention of symptomatic premature atrial contractions. ●Prevention of premature ventricular contractions or ventricular tachycardia. ●Prevention of paroxysmal supraventricular tachycardia.

Contraindications: ●hypersensitivity, ●history of quinidine–associated thrombocytopenia purpura, ●complete AV block with AV nodal or idioventricular pacemaker, ●complete bundle branch block, or other severe intraventricular conduction abnormality that is associated with wide or bizarre QRS complexes, ●ectopy and rhythms due to escape mechanisms, ●arrhythmias or AV conduction abnormalities due to digitalis intoxication.

Caution: incomplete AV block, severe CHF, renal or hepatic insufficiency, asthma, hyperthyroidism, hyperkalemia, myasthenia gravis, pregnancy, nursing mother.

Drug interactions: Caution is advised when quinidine is administered concurrently with certain drugs—e.g. digoxin (digoxin levels may be increased); neuromuscular blockers (blocking effect enhanced by quinidine); drugs with anticholinergic properties (vagolytic effect is additive to quinidine's); coumarin anticoagulants (PT increased and bleeding may occur); other antiarrhythmic drugs (additive cardiac depression may occur); drugs that alkalize urine (quinidine excretion is decreased); other drugs that increase quinidine half–life (cimetidine, verapamil, amiodarone); drugs that may lead to decreased quinidine levels (e.g. phenobarbital, phenytoin, rifampin, nifedipine); phenothiazines or reserpine (additive cardiac depression may occur).

Comments: (1) Plasma quinidine level determinations and continuous EKG monitoring are required if > 2 gram/day of quinidine sulfate or > 2.5 gram/day of quinidine polygalacturonate is administered. Quinidine must be discontinued if QRS widens by 50% or if frequent PVC's occur. **(2)** To preclude a rapid ventricular response (because of quinidine's vagolytic effect), the patient with atrial flutter or atrial fibrillation must first be digitalized before starting quinidine. Furthermore, because of the risk of arterial embolization, patients who have had atrial fibrillation for more than 7 days must be anticoagulated for 30 days (e.g. warfarin) prior to attempting cardioversion with quinidine or other means. **(3)** Periodically obtain CBC, and liver and kidney function tests if quinidine therapy is prolonged.

Side effects: Cinchonism (tinnitus, vertigo, headache, nausea, disturbed vision) may occur after single dose in sensitive patient. Gastrointestinal side effects are the most common: nausea, vomiting, diarrhea, abdominal pain. Cardiovascular: wide QRS, wide QT, ST depression, U wave, PVC's, ventricular dysrhythmias (e.g. ventricular tachycardia and fibrillation); asystole, bradycardia, paradoxical tachycardia, SA or AV block, worsening CHF, hypotension, arterial embolism). Blood: hemolytic anemia, thrombocytopenia, purpura, agranulocytosis, hypoprothrombinemia, neutropenia, leukocytosis. Neurologic: headache, depression, confusion, apprehension, excitement, delirium, ataxia, vertigo, tinnitus, decreased hearing, mydriasis, blurred vision, photophobia, abnormal color vision, night blindness, diplopia, scotoma, optic neuritis. Hypersensitivity: urticaria, angioedema, bronchospasm, respiratory arrest, hepatoxicity. Skin: pruritis with flushing, rash, eczema, exfoliative eruption, psoriasis, abnormal pigmentation); Other: fever, lupus, arthralgia, myalgia, elevated CPK.

Overdose: Empty stomach and then administer activated charcoal. Acidification of the urine may hasten urinary excretion. Hypotension may be the consequence of vasodilation, decreased myocardial contractility, and/or bradycardia. Administration of isotonic saline and a sympathomimetic (e.g. dopamine, dobutamine) is recommended. Insertion of a Swam-Ganz catheter to monitor wedge pressure will help guide therapy. An intra-aortic balloon pump may be necessary if the foregoig measures fail to prevent shock. Ventricular arrhythmias may respond to lidocaine, bretylium, phenytoin, or electrical cardioversion. Isoproterenol or overdrive pacing may be necessary. Other measures: Intravenous sodium lactate may help relieve cardiotoxicity but should not be administered if there is alkalosis. Resin hemoperfusion may be used to remove the drug in patients with liver failure or those requiring extracorporeal circulatory assistance.

Supplied as:
quinidine sulfate: 100, 200, 300 mg tablet; 300 mg extended–release tablet;
quinidine gluconate:
    330mg tablet (Duraquin) equivalent to 248mg quinidine sulfate;
    324mg tablet (Quinaglute Dura-Tabs, Quinidine Gluconate S–R) equivalent to
    243mg quinidine sulfate;
quinidine polygalacturonate: 275 mg tablet (Cardioquin) equivalent to 200 mg
    quinidine sulfate.

DOSE: Test dose quinidine sulfate should be given first to rule out idiosyncrasy: adult 200 mg PO, child 2 mg/kg PO.

Quinidine sulfate (Quinora):
Adult:
Premature atrial contractions/premature ventricular contractions: 200–300 mg PO 3–4 times a day.
Paroxysmal supraventricular tachycardia: 400–600 mg PO q2-3h until arrhythmia terminates (see comment 1 above).
Conversion atrial flutter: Individualize dose (see comments 1 and 2 above).
Conversion atrial fibrillation (see comments 1 and 2 above): 200 mg PO q2-3h for 5–8 doses until arrhythmia terminated. Assuming toxicity does not develop, further increases in the daily dose may be tried if atrial fibrillation persists. Maximum 3–4 gram/day.
Maintenance: 200–300 mg PO 3–4 times a day is the usual requirement.
Child: 6 mg/kg PO q6h.

Quinidine sulfate extended–release tablet (Quinidex):
Adult, 1–2 tablets (300–600 mg) PO q8–12h.

Quinidine polygalacturonate (Cardioquin):
To terminate arrhythmia (adult): 1–3 tablets (275–825 mg) q3–4h until arrhythmia terminated or 3–4 doses given. If arrhythmia persists, increase dose by 1/2 to 1 tablet (137.5–275mg) and administer q3–4h until arrhythmia terminated or 3 doses given. Further dose increases may be tried if necessary (see comment 1 above).
Maintenance (adult): 1 tablet (275 mg) 2–3 times a day.

Quinidine gluconate (adult dose for 324 or 330 mg tablet):
Prevention premature atrial, nodal, or ventricular contractions: 1–2 tab q8–12h.
Maintenance of normal sinus rhythm following conversion of paroxysmal tachycardia: 2 tablets q12h, or 1.5 to 2 tablets q8h.

Intravenous quinidine gluconate is available but this route is dangerous (e.g. severe hypotension) and is seldom used. 200–400 mg is diluted in D5W and infused at approximately 10 mg/minute with continuous EKG and BP monitoring.

RAMOTIDINE (Pepcid)

Action: Competitively binds to histamine H2 receptors on gastric parietal cells. Thereby inhibits histamine–induced hydrochloric acid secretion.
Contraindication: hypersensitivity to any component.
Caution: pregnancy, nursing mother, children. Reduce dose in severe renal insufficiency (creatinine clearance < 10ml/minute).
Side effects: Most common side effects are headache (4.7%), dizziness (1.3%), diarrhea (1.7%), constipation (1.2%). Infrequent side effects of uncertain causal relationship; nausea, vomiting, abdominal discomfort, anorexia, dry mouth, abnormal taste, asthenia, fatigue, depression, anxiety, decreased libido, insomnia, somnolence, paresthesias, seizures, tinnitus, arthralgia, musculoskeletal pain, palpitations, bronchospasm, orbital edema, conjunctival injection, alopecia, rash, acne, itching, dry skin, flushing, liver enzyme abnormalities, thrombocytopenia.
Supplied as: tablet (20, 40 mg); oral suspension (40mg/5ml);
IV injection (10mg/ml).
Indications/dose (adult):
Active duodenal ulcer: 40 mg PO once daily at bedtime, or 20 mg PO twice daily. Treatment is usually for 4 weeks; treatment for more than 6–8 weeks is seldom required.
Maintenance therapy after healing of duodenal ulcer: 20 mg PO at bedtime.
Benign gastric ulcer: 40 mg PO once daily at bedtime.
Hypersecretory conditions (Zollinger–Ellison syndrome, systemic mastocytosis): Start with 20 mg PO q6h. Up to 160 mg q6h has been used.
Intravenous (for intractable ulcer, hypersecretory condition, or when oral route not possible): 20 mg q12h.

RANITIDINE (Zantac)

Action: Competitively binds to histamine H2 receptors on gastric parietal cells. Thereby inhibits histamine–induced hydrochloric acid secretion.

Contraindications: hypersensitivity to the drug.

Caution: renal or liver dysfunction, pregnancy, nursing mother, children.

Comments: In active duodenal ulcer or hypersecretory conditions, antacids may be used concurrently to relieve pain. Food or antacids does not significantly interfere with ranitidine absorption.

Side effects are uncommon and a causal relationship is often unclear. Patients may complain of headache, nausea, vomiting, diarrhea, constipation, abdominal discomfort/pain. Increases in SGPT over pretreatment levels are not uncommon after 5–7 days IV administration. Infrequently or rarely reported phenomena include CNS complaints (e.g. malaise, dizziness, vertigo, confusion, depression, insomnia); arrhythmias; blood dyscrasias; hepatitis; pancreatitis; rash; hypersensitivity reactions (e.g. bronchospasm, angioedema, anaphylaxis, eosinophilia, rash, slightly elevated serum creatinine); impotence, gynecomastia.

Supplied as: tablet (150, 300 mg), syrup (1ml equivalent to 15mg), 2ml vial (25mg/ml) for IV or IM injection.

Indications/oral dose (adult):

<u>Active duodenal ulcer:</u> 150 mg PO twice daily or 300 mg at bedtime. Healing usually occurs within 4 weeks.

<u>Maintenance therapy after healing of duodenal ulcer:</u> 150 mg PO at bedtime.

<u>Benign gastric ulcer:</u> 150 mg PO twice daily. Healing usually occurs within 6 weeks.

<u>Esophageal reflux:</u> 150mg twice daily.

<u>Hypersecretory conditions</u> (e.g. Zollinger–Ellison Syndrome): 150 mg PO twice daily for as long as necessary. More frequent doses may be required in severe cases. Up to 6 gram/day has been used.

Parenteral administration is reserved for pathologic hypersecretory conditions, intractable duodenal ulcer, or when oral route not feasible.

<u>Intramuscular (adult):</u> 50 mg (2ml) undiluted q6–8h.

<u>Intravenous (adult):</u> 50 mg (2 ml) q6–8h. Dose may be diluted in 20 ml of compatible solution (e.g. isotonic saline, D5W) and injected over not less than 5 minutes; or diluted in 100 ml compatible solution and infused over 15–20 minutes. Some patients may require more frequent 50 mg doses but no more than 400 mg/day is generally allowed.

RESERPINE (Serpasil)

Action: Depletes catecholamines from the CNS and from nerve endings of peripheral sympathetic neurons. Thereby leads to decreased peripheral vasoconstriction, and decreased cardiac rate and cardiac output.

Indication: hypertension. Reserpine is usually added to a thiazide diuretic when an additional antihypertensive agent is required.

Contraindications: reserpine hypersensitivity, history of depression, active peptic ulcer, ulcerative colitis, patient receiving electroconvulsive therapy or MAO inhibitor, nursing mother. Reserpine should not be used in pregnancy unless absolutely essential.

Caution: children, renal insufficiency, patient receiving digitalis or quinidine, history of peptic ulcer or gallstones, epilepsy. Discontinue reserpine at first sign of despondency, early morning insomnia, loss of appetite, or impotence.

Side effects: <u>CNS</u> (depression, drowsiness, anxiety, nervousness, nightmares, headache, dizziness, dull sensorium, deafness, rare parkinson syndrome and other extrapyramidal effects); <u>ophthalmic</u> (glaucoma, uveitis, optic atrophy, conjunctival injection); <u>cardiovascular</u> (bradycardia, arrhythmia, angina–like symptoms, syncope, edema); <u>gastrointestinal</u> (anorexia, nausea, vomiting, diarrhea, hypersecretion, dry mouth); <u>respiratory</u> (nasal congestion, epistaxis, dyspnea); <u>skin</u> (purpura, rash, pruritis); <u>GU/endocrine</u> (impotence, decreased libido, breast engorgement, pseudolactation, gynecomastia, dysuria); <u>other</u> (myalgia, weight gain).

Overdose: Empty stomach and administer activated charcoal. Antacids may also be administered. If there is hypotension, place in Trendelenberg position and give isotonic fluids IV. Give dobutamine or dopamine if hypotension persists.

Supplied as: 0.1, 0.25 mg tablet.

Dose (adult or child): 0.1–0.25 mg PO once daily. Maximum 0.25 mg/day.

RIFAMPIN (Rifadin, Rimactane)

Action: Inhibits bacterial DNA–dependent RNA polymerase. Bactericidal against intra and extracellular Mycobacterium tuberculosis, M. bovis, most M. kanasii.

Indications:
- Treatment pulmonary tuberculosis. Rifampin is administered in combination with at least one other antituberculosis drug.
- Asymptomatic meningococcus carrier.

Contraindications: rifampin hypersensitivity.

Caution: liver disease (obtain liver function tests periodically), pregnancy (consider risk versus benefit), nursing mother.

Comments: ●Rifampin may induce hepatic enzymes that hasten the metabolism of certain drugs (e.g. oral hypoglycemics, oral contraceptives, corticosteroids, digitalis, quinidine, methadone). Increased dosages of these drugs may be required. ●Oral anticoagulant dose (e.g. warfarin) may also need to be increased. Make dose adjustments according to prothrombin time. ●Aminosalicyclic acid may decrease the absorption of rifampin. Take these 2 drugs 4 hours apart.

Side effects: gastrointestinal; anorexia, nausea, vomiting, diarrhea, heartburn, cramps, pseudomembranous colitis (rare); liver; elevated transaminases, bilirubin, and alkaline phospotase, jaundice, hepatitis; neurologic; headache, drowsiness, dizziness, confusion, fatigue, ataxia, visual disturbances, muscle weakness, generalized numbness; hypersensitivity; pruritis, urticaria, rash, pemphigoid reaction, eosinophilia, sore mouth/tongue, conjunctivitis. A serious hypersensitivity reaction sometimes occurs, particularly when the patient is treated intermittently or when treatment is resumed. Manifestations may include dyspnea, wheezing, leukopenia, thrombocytopenia, purpura, hemolysis, hemoglobinuria, hematuria, renal insufficiency. other; fever, menstrual irregularities, leg cramps, muscle or joint pain, elevated BUN and serum uric acid, orange discoloration of urine, tears, sweat, and feces.

Supplied as: 150, 300 mg capsule; ●Intravenous preparation.

Dose: Adult: 600 mg PO once daily 1 hour before or 2 hours after a meal.
Child: 10–20 mg/kg PO once daily (maximum 600 mg/day).
Asymptomatic meningococcus carrier receives above dose for 4 consecutive days.
*Rifampin may be given intravenously in the same dosage when the drug cannot be given PO.

SCOPOLAMINE, TRANSDERMAL (Transderm–Scop)

Action: Scopolamine (an anticholinergic) is absorbed transdermally from a disc applied to the skin behind the ear. Scopolamine is believed to prevent motion sickness by inhibiting vestibular input to the CNS. One disc delivers 0.5 mg scoplamine at an uniform rate over 72 hours.

Indication: prevention of motion sickness in adults.

Contraindications: hypersensitivity to scopalamine or components of disc, glaucoma, children.

Caution: pregnancy, nursing mother, elderly, pyloric or intestinal obstruction, bladder neck obstruction; impaired metabolic, kidney, or liver function; concurrent use of alcohol and other drugs with CNS effects (particularly those with anticholinergic effects). Because scopolamine may cause drowsiness, patients should be warned against using this product if they are to be engaged in dangerous activities that require alertness.

Side effects: dry mouth, drowsiness, blurred vision, mydriasis. Infrequent effects include confusion, impaired memory, restlessness, hallucinations, dizziness, glaucoma, difficulty urinating, rash and erythema; dry, itchy, or red eyes.

Dose (adult): One disc applied to hairless area behind the ear 4 hours before required antiemetic effect. Wear only one disc at a time. The disc may be replaced by another in 72 hours. <u>Note</u>: Wash hands with soap after handling disc to prevent traces of scopolamine coming into contact with eyes.

SODIUM BICARBONATE

Indications: ●Metabolic acidosis due to: cardiac arrest, shock, dehydration, diabetic ketoacidosis (only if pH < 7), methanol or salicylate poisoning. ●Treatment hyperkalemia. ●Renal tubular acidosis. ●Overdose of certain drugs—e.g. tricyclic antidepressants; hasten excretion of phenobarbital or aspirin.

Caution: ●Whenever possible, use arterial blood gas measurements to guide intravenous sodium bicarbonate therapy. ●Avoid simultaneous administration in same IV line with catecholamines (they are inactivated) or calcium (it is precipitated). ●In ventilatory arrest or insufficiency, use ventilation (not $NaHCO_3$) to correct respiratory acidosis. ●A paradoxical CSF <u>acidosis</u> may ensue from bicarbonate administration. This is because an elevated pH reduces the ventilatory drive which in turn leads to an increase in CO_2. CO_2 then diffuses into the CSF producing CSF acidosis. ●Excessive bicarbonate may cause: (1) hypernatremia and hyperosmolar state with consequent volume overload; (2) hypokalemia (due to a shift of potassium into cells); (3) metabolic alkalosis. Metabolic alkalosis may in turn lead to arrhythmias and/or impair oxygen delivery to the tissues. Alkalosis impairs oxygen delivery because there is a shift of oxygen dissociation curve.

Supplied as:

intravenous injection: 1 mEq/ml (10 or 50 ml syringe),
      0.9 mEq/ml (50 ml syringe containing 44.6 mEq),
      0.5 mEq/ml (5 or 10 ml syringe);
tablets: 325 mg (= 3.9 mEq HCO_3), 650 mg (= 7.7 mEq HCO_3);
powder;

Dose (adult or pediatric):

Life–threatening metabolic acidosis: 1 mEq/kg initial IV bolus. If necessary, give an additional 0.5 mEq/kg IV bolus at 10 minute intervals. NOTE: If possible obtain arterial blood gas and calculate bicarbonate requirements as follows:
amount of sodium bicarbonate needed in mEq =
$$0.4 \times (\text{weight in kg}) \times (25 \text{ mEq/l} - \text{arterial } HCO_3 \text{ mEq/l}).$$
Give half this amount and then reassess.

Hyperkalemia: 1–2 mEq/kg initial IV bolus over 1–2 min. Monitor effect with EKG.

Distal renal tubular acidosis: 1–3 mEq/kg/24hr PO in 4–5 divided doses. Adjust dose so as to correct acidemia. Children require larger doses per kg.

Proximal renal tubular acidosis: 4–5 mEq/kg/24hr or more PO in 4–5 divided doses. Part of the bicarbonate requirement is given as potassium bicarbonate.

To enhance diuresis of certain drug overdoses: Start with 1–2 mEq/kg IV bolus. Administer additional sodium bicarbonate (and/or hyperventilate) as needed to maintain arterial pH at about 7.5 and an alkaline urine. Akaline diuresis may be accomplished by adding 44–100 mEq sodium bicarbonate to each liter of 0.45% saline and running the IV at 200–500 ml/hr in adult (assuming normal cardiac and renal status) so as to maintain urine output of 3–6 ml/kg/hr.

SODIUM POLYSTYRENE SULFONATE (Kayexalate)

Action: Nonabsorbable cation exchange resin. In the GI lumen the resin-bound sodium is released and replaced by potassium.

Indication: treatment of hyperkalemia.

Comments: ●Approximately 0.5–1.0mEq of potassium is removed for each gram of resin administered. ●Additional measures to treat hyperkalemia must be used in urgent cases since resin therapy may take hours to days to reduce serum potassium (e.g. IV calcium and IV bicarbonate, glucose and insulin infusion, dialysis). ●Hypokalemia may result from overtreatment. Besides the serum potassium, evidence of hypokalemia may include EKG findings (widened QT, flat or inverted T, U wave, etc.) and clinical abnormalities (confusion, muscle weakness, paralysis, etc.). ●Constipation: Sorbitol is added to counteract constipating effect of the resin. If constipation does occur, give 10–20 ml of 70% sorbitol PO q2h to produce 1–2 watery stools/day. ●Sodium overload may occur because sodium is released from the resin in exchange for potassium. Use caution in conditions in which sodium excess is detrimental (e.g. severe congestive heart failure, severe hypertension, marked edema). ●Avoid concurrent administration of nonabsorbable cation-donating antacids (e.g. magnesium hydroxide, aluminum carbonate) because the potassium exchange effectiveness of the resin is lessened and systemic alkalosis may result. In addition, aluminum hydroxide concretions may result and lead to GI obstruction.

Side effects: gastric irritation, anorexia, nausea, vomitting, hypokalemia, hypocalcemia, sodium retention, constipation, fecal impaction.

Supplied as:
powder containing approximately 15 gram/4 level teaspoons;
ready-to-use suspension for rectal or oral administration contains 15 gram sodium polystyrene sulfonate and 14.1 gram sorbitol per 60 ml.

Adult dose:
Oral: 15–30 gram 1–5 times per day as needed. When preparing a suspension from the powder, also add sorbitol to prevent constipation. Example: 15–30 gram Kayexalate + 20 gram sorbitol in 100 ml water. Dose may also be given via nasogastric tube.
Retention enema: 30–50 gram q6h. When preparing a suspension from the powder, also add sorbitol to prevent constipation. Example: 30–50 gram Kayexalate + 20 gram sorbitol + 100 ml water at room temperature. An initial cleansing enema is advised, and then Kayexalate is administered through a French 28 tube advanced approximately 20 cm. The tube is then clamped and the suspension is retained for a few hours. The resin is removed by irrigation with non-sodium-containing solution.

Dose, infant or small child (oral or retention enema): 0.25–0.5 gram/kg q6h. When preparing a suspension from the powder, mix 1 gram Kayexalate per 4 ml of 20% sorbitol.

SPECTINOMYCIN (Trobicin)

Action: Inhibits bacterial protein synthesis by binding to bacterial 30s ribosome subunit.

Indications: Acute gonococcal urethritis and proctitis in males.
Acute gonococcal cervicits and proctitis in females.

Comments: ●Ceftriaxone ((250 mg IM once) is currently the therapy of choice for outpatient treatment of gonorrhea. It is effective at all mucosal sites. Spectinomycin is an alternative. ●Spectinomycin is not effective for pharyngeal gonococcal infection. ●Spectinomycin is not effective for treatment of PID, epididmitis, disseminated gonococcal infection, gonococcal ophthalmia. ●Spectinomycin is not effective in the treatment of syphilis or Chlamydia trachomatis. When the diagnosis of uncomplicated gonorrhea is made, the patient is also treated presumptively for syphilis and chlamydial infection: a 10 day course of doxycycline or tetracycline is recommended provided the patient is not a pregnant female or a child < 8 yr. A serologic test for syphilis is obtained and again in 3 months.

Contraindications: spectinomycin hypersensitivity.

Side effects: injection site soreness, fever, chills, nausea, dizziness, insomnia, urticaria, anaphylaxis.

Supplied as: 2 and 4 gram vials for intramuscular injection only.

Dose:
Adult: 2 gram IM once. In areas where resistant strains of gonorrhea are prevalent, the dose is 4 gram IM divided between two gluteal sites.
Child: 40 mg/kg IM once.

SPIRONOLACTONE (Aldactone)

Action: Structural analog of aldosterone. Competitively binds to aldosterone receptor sites in the distal convoluted renal tubule. This results in increased sodium and water excretion as well as potassium retention.

Contraindications: anuria, renal insufficiency, hyperkalemia, nursing mother.

Caution: Hyperkalemia (with risk of arrhythmias) may result from spironolactone therapy. Avoid concurrent administration of potassium supplements or excessive intake of potassium-rich foods. Monitor serum potassium. Hyponatremia may occur, expecially if patient is receiving thiazides concurrently or ingesting excessive water. Hepatic cirrhosis: Patient with hepatic cirrhosis is at risk of developing hyperchloremic acidosis. Monitor serum bicarbonate and potassium. Pregnancy: Diuretics are not indicated in the physiologic edema that occurs with pregnancy. If for other reasons a diuretic must be used, a thiazide diuretic is preferred. Chronic high doses of spironolactone cause tumors in rats. Drug interactions: Half-life of concurrently administered digoxin may be prolonged leading to digoxin toxicity. Spironolactone may potentiate the effects of diuretics and antihypertensives. Concurrent administration of captopril or indomethacin has been associated with hyperkalemia.

Side effects: electrolyte: hyperkalemia, hyponatremia, hyperchloremic metabolic acidosis (usually in association with hyperkalemia); gastrointestinal: nausea, vomiting, diarrhea, abdominal pain, gastritis, ulceration, bleeding; neurologic: headache, drowsiness, confusion, ataxia; GU/endocrine: gynecomastia, impotence, hirsutism, menstrual irregularities, breast carcinoma (causal relationship not established); other: drug fever, rash, urticaria.

Supplied as: 25, 50, 100 mg tablet.

Dose, adult:

Primary hyperaldosteronism: smallest effective dose.

Edema due to cirrhosis of the liver: Treatment consists of bed rest, sodium/fluid restriction, and spironolactone. Start with 100 mg/day in single or divided doses. When taken as the sole diuretic, diuresis may not become apparent for 5 days. A thiazide diuretic may be added if adequate diuresis has not occurred after 5 days. Usual spironolactone range is 25–100 mg/day, maximum 50 mg qid.

Edema due to nephrotic syndrome or congestive heart failure: same dosage regimen as above.

Essential hypertension: In the treatment of essential hypertension, spironolactone is usually added to a thiazide diuretic (e.g. hydrochlorothiazide) to counteract the potassium-depleting effects of the thiazide in a patient who cannot or will not take oral potassium supplements, or who must avoid hypokalemia (e.g. patient subject to arrhythmias or taking digitalis). Start with 50–100 mg/day as a single dose or divided into 2 doses. Wait 2 weeks before adjusting dose since it may that long before the full effect is realized. Maximum dosage is 200 mg/day in divided doses.

Hypokalemia (e.g. to control thiazide-induced hypokalemia when potassium supplementation is not feasible): 25–100 mg/day.

Pediatric dose: Edema: 3 mg/kg/day as single or divided doses. Adjust to smallest effective dosage after 5 days.

SPIRONOLACTONE + HYDROCHLOROTHIAZIDE
(Aldactazide)

Supplied as: tablet containing 25 mg spironolactone + 25 mg hydrochlorothiazide, tablet containing 50 mg spironolactone + 50 mg hydrochlorothiazide.

Adult dose:

Essential hypertension: usual requirement is 50–100 mg/day of each component as single daily dose or in divided doses.

Edema (due to hepatic cirrhosis, nephrotic syndrome, congestive heart failure): usual requirement is 100 mg/day of each component as a single daily dose or in divided doses. Range is 25–200 mg/day of each component.

Pediatric dose: Edema: 1.65–3.3 mg/kg/day of each component.

Additional information: see individual drugs.

STREPTOKINASE (Kabikinase, Streptase)

Action: Streptokinase leads to conversion of plasminogen to plasmin. The latter is a proteolytic enzyme that breaks down fibrin and fibrinogen.

Indications: Used to lyse thrombi/emboli in the following conditions: acute evolving transmural myocardial infarction, pulmonary embolism, deep vein thrombosis, arterial thrombosis/embolism.

Contraindications: active internal bleeding; ●history of stroke, or intracranial or intraspinal surgery within the last 2 months; ●intracranial neoplasm; ●severe uncontrolled hypertension, ●history of severe allergic reaction to this product.

Caution/comments: Ascertain hemostatic status prior to starting streptokinase infusion; Order hematocrit, platelet count, aPTT, PT, TT. Use with caution in conditions that would increase the risk of streptokinase-associated bleeding; For instance, the occurrence of any of the following within the past ten days should compel caution: major surgery or trauma, organ biopsy, cardiopulmonary resuscitation, obstetric delivery, GI or GU bleeding, puncture of noncompressible blood vessel (e.g. subclavian or internal jugular puncture). Other conditions dictating caution because of possible bleeding or attendant complications include: cerebrovascular disease, blood pressure ≥ 180 systolic or ≥ 110 diastolic, hemostatic abnormalities, oral anticoagulant therapy, high probability of left heart thrombus (e.g. atrial fibrillation), acute pericarditis, subacute bacterial endocarditis, septic thrombophlebitis, obstructed AV cannula at seriously infected site, hemorrhagic ocular condition (e.g. hemorrhagic diabetic retinopathy), significant hepatic dysfunction, pregnancy, age > 75 yr. Arterial or venous puncture; Puncture of noncompressible vessels is contraindicated (e.g. subclavian or internal jugular puncture) in patient receiving streptokinase. Furthermore, arterial or venous puncture in general should be minimized. If arterial puncture must be performed, use an upper extremity and apply pressure to the puncture site for at least 30 minutes following the procedure. Intramuscular injections must be avoided in patients receiving streptokinase. Heparin may be considered to prevent re-thrombosis in patient with deep venous thrombosis, pulmonary thromboembolism, and possibly in patient with acute myocardial infarction. If heparin is to be used following streptokinase therapy, it should not be started until the PTT and thrombin time are less than twice the normal control times. Moreover, the usual loading dose of heparin is omitted. Be alert for bleeding. The effects of streptokinase on PTT and TT usually wane within 3–4 hr after completing streptokinase infusion. Oral anticoagulants and anti-platelet drugs (aspirin, dipyridamole) administered after streptokinase infusion increases the risk of bleeding. Arrhythmias may ensue from coronary thrombolysis with reperfusion. The arrhythmias are treated in the usual manner. If uncontrollable bleeding occurs, discontinue streptokinase immediately. Resistance to streptokinase (due to antistreptokinase antibodies) may occur if the patient has had a streptococcal infection or received streptokinase from 5 days to 6 months previously.

Side effects: bleeding and its complications; allergic reactions (e.g. anaphylactic/anaphylactoid reactions, bronchospasm, angioedema, urticaria, itching, headache, flushing, nausea); fever; noncardiogenic pulmonary edema, arrhythmias following reperfusion of thrombosed coronary artery.

Dose:

Acute evolving myocardial infarction; Streptokinase should be administered as soon as possible, preferably within an hour of the onset of symptoms. There is a statistically significant reduction in mortality if streptokinase is administered within 6 hours of the onset of symptoms. Streptokinase may be infused intravenously or by intracoronary infusion. By the intravenous route, 1,500,000 units is infused within 60 minutes. By the intracoronary route, a 20,000 unit bolus is followed by a 2000 unit/minute infusion for 60 minutes.

Pulmonary embolism, deep venous thrombosis, or arterial thrombosis/embolism; The patient receives an IV loading dose of 250,000 units over 30 minutes followed by an IV infusion of 100,000 units/hour. The infusion is continued for 72 hr for deep venous thrombosis, 24 hr for pulmonary embolism (72 hr if concomitant deep venous thrombosis is suspected), and 24–72 hr for arterial thrombosis/embolism.

STREPTOMYCIN

Action/spectrum: Bactericidal against Mycobacterium tuberculosis, Francisella tularensis (tularemia), Yersinia pestis (plague), Pseudomonas mallei (glanders), Brucella, Haemophilus ducreyi (chancroid), Calymmatobacterium granulomatis (granuloma inguinale), Spirillum minor (rat bite fever), Streptococcus viridans, nonhemolytic streptococci. Resistant bacteria include anaerobes, rickettsia, many gram–negative aerobic bacilli (e.g. Pseudomonas aeruginosa), most gram–positive bacteria (including many enterococci).

Indications: plague, tularemia, adjunct in treatment of tuberculosis, adjunct to tetracycline in treatment of brucellosis and glanders, adjunct to penicillin in treatment of endocarditis due to Streptococcus viridans or nonenterococcal group D streptococci.

Contraindications: aminoglycoside hypersensitivity, first trimester pregnancy. Do not exceed total of 20 gram in last half of pregnancy.

Caution: elderly; renal dysfunction; neuromuscular disorders (e.g. Parkinsonism, myasthenia gravis); concurrent of sequential administration of other potentialy nephrotoxic or ototoxic drugs (e.g. furosemide, ethacrynic acid, other aminoglycosides, vancomycin, cephaloridine, polymyxin B); concurrent administration of neuromuscular blocking drugs or anesthetics.

Side effects include: <u>otoxicity</u> (deafness, vertigo ± nausea and vomiting); <u>other neurologic</u> (headache, paresthesias, peripheral neuritis, muscular weakness, amblyopia); <u>hypersensitivity</u> (fever, rash, exfoliative dermatitis, urticaria, angioedema, anaphylaxis, eosinophilia); <u>blood</u> (neutropenia, agranulocytosis, thrombocytopenia, hemolytic anemia, aplastic anemia).
Supplied as: IM preparation only.
Adult dose:
<u>Tuberculosis:</u> Streptomycin is reserved for complicated cases requiring a 3rd antituberculous drug (usually added to isoniazid and rifampin). Start with 15 mg/kg IM once daily (up to 1 gram/day) for 2–3 weeks. In most cases, the interval can then be changed to 1 gram 3 times/wk and finally 1 gram 2 times/wk. Smaller doses are used in patients with renal dysfunction, the elderly, or small adults.
<u>Plague or tularemia:</u> 15 mg/kg q12h for 10 days.
<u>Endocarditis due to Streptococcus viridans or nonenterococcal group D streptococci with penicillin MIC > 0.1 mcg/ml:</u> Treatment is in conjunction with penicillin G (2 million units q4h for 4 wk). Streptomycin is stopped after 2 wk of therapy. For adults under 60 yr, the dose is 1 gram IM q12h for the first wk and 0.5 gram IM q12h for the 2nd wk. Patients over 60 receive 0.5 gram IM for 2 wk.
<u>Brucellosis:</u> Treatment is in conjunction with tetracycline (500 mg PO qid for 4–6 wk). Streptomycin is administered for 2 wk, 500 mg q12h IM.
Pediatric dose: 10–15 mg/kg q12h.   <u>Neonate:</u> 5–10 mg/kg q12h.

SUCRALFATE (Carafate)

Action: Sucralfate is a complex of sulfated sucrose and aluminum hydoxide that acts locally at the ulcer site. The mechanism of action is uncertain but it is believed that, by adhering to proteinaceous exudate at the ulcer site, it acts as a protective barrier against acid, pepsin, and bile acid. Sucralfate does not inhibit gastric acid secretion nor does it significantly neutralize stomach acid. Only a small amount is absorbed.
Indication: short-term treatment of duodenal ulcer.
Contraindications: none. **Caution:** pregnancy, nursing mother, children.
Comments: ●Antacids may be used concurrently for relief of pain. However, because antacids may interfere with action of sucralfate, they should be taken at least a half hour apart. ●Sucralfate may interfere with the absorption of tetracyclines, phenytoin, and cimetidine. Allow 2 hours to elapse between administration of these drugs and sucralfate.
Side effects: constipation, diarrhea, nausea, gastric discomfort, indigestion, dry mouth, rash, pruritis, back pain, dizziness, vertigo, drowsiness.
Supplied as: 1 gram tablet.
Dose: 1 tablet PO 4 times a day for 4–8 weeks or less if ulcer healing is demonstrated by endoscopy or x-rays. Take sucralfate on an empty stomach.

SULFASALAZINE (Azulfidine)

Action: Sulfonamide derivative. Mode of action unknown.
Indications: <u>Ulcerative colitis:</u> (1) alone in the treatment of mild to moderate ulcerative colitis, (2) in conjunction with corticosteroid for treatment of severe ulcerative colitis, (3) to reduce frequency of exacerbations for ulcerative colitis in remission.
   <u>Crohn's disease:</u> Exacerbations of Crohn's disease involving the colon. Sulfasalazine is not effective in Crohn's disease limited to small bowel nor is it effective in maintaining remissions.
Contraindications: sulfonamide or salicylate hypersensitivity, intestinal or urinary obstruction, infant under 2 yr, nursing mother, porphyria.
Caution/comments: ●Use in pregnancy only if clearly needed. Avoid in pregnancy at term. ●See also caution/comments under "Sulfonamides".
Side effects: headache, anorexia, nausea, vomiting, fever, rash, itching, urticaria, hemolytic anemia, Heinz body anemia, impaired digoxin and folic acid absorption, reversible decrease in sperm count and infertility. ●See also side effects under "Sulfonamides".
Supplied as: 500 mg tablet,   250mg/5ml oral suspension,
   500 mg enteric coated tablet (to reduce GI side effects).
Dose, adult:
<u>Active disease:</u> 3–4 gram/day PO in four divided doses.
<u>Maintenance:</u> usually, 500 mg PO 4 times a day. Some patients require up to 3 gram/day divided.
Dose, child > 2yr:
<u>Active disease:</u> 40–60 mg/kg/day PO divided into 3–6 daily doses.
<u>Maintenance:</u> 30 mg/kg/day PO divided into 4 daily doses.

SULFAMETHOXAZOLE + TRIMETHOPRIM
(Bactrim, Septra)

Action: Sulfamethoxazole and trimethoprim inhibit consecutive steps in the bacterial synthesis of tetrahydrofolic acid, an essential factor that bacteria must synthesize. This combination is often bactericidal even though the components by themselves are bacteriostatic.

Spectrum includes staphylococci, streptococci, gonoccocci, meningococci, E. coli, proteus, klebsiella, enterobacter, Serratia marcescens, Providencia stuartii, salmonella, shigella, cholera, H. influenza, H. ducreyi, Gardnerella vaginalis, Bordetella pertussis, Brucella, Yersinia pestis, Y. enterocolitica, Nocardia, Chlamydia trachomatis, Pneumocystis carinii.

Indications:
- Urinary tract infection due to E. coli, klebsiella, enterobacter, proteus, or M. morganii.
- Acute otitis media due to H. influenza or pneumococcus.
- Acute exacerbations of chronic bronchitis due to H. influenza or pneumococcus.
- Treatment/prophylaxis of Pneumocystis carinii pneumonia.
- Shigellosis.
- Alternative in treatment of brucellosis, whooping cough, cholera, salmonella, Mycobacterium marinum, melioidosis, chancroid, granuloma inguinale, chlamydia, gonorrhea.
- Other possible indications: prostatitis, chronic sinusitis, osteomyelitis in sickle cell patient.

Contraindications: hypersensitivity to components, pregnancy at term, nursing mother, less 2 months of age, treatment streptococcal pharyngitis.

Caution: G6PD deficiency, hepatic or renal insufficiency, elderly, patient with severe allergies or bronchial asthma, malnourished patient who might have folate deficiency, AIDS patient (at greater risk for side effects). <u>Blood dyscrasias:</u> Be alert for signs of drug-induced blood dyscrasia (e.g. fever, sore throat, pallor, purpura, jaundice). Periodically obtain CBC if patient is on prolonged therapy. <u>Drug interactions:</u> Sulfonamides may enhance the effects of certain drugs—e.g. oral hypoglycemics, warfarin, phenytoin, methotrexate.

Side effects: Refer to "Sulfonamides" for side effects of sulfamethoxazole. Side effects attributable to trimethoprim include fever, itching, rash, glossitis, epigastric distress, nausea, vomiting, thrombocytopenia, leukopenia, neutropenia, megaloblastic anemia, methemoglobinemia, elevated serum transaminases, elevated BUN or serum creatinine.

Supplied as:

<u>regular tablet</u>	(400 mg sulfamethoxazole + 80 mg trimethoprim),
<u>double-strength tablet</u>	(800 mg sulfamethoxazole + 160mg trimethoprim),
<u>oral suspension</u>	(200mg sulfamethoxazole + 40mg trimethoprim per 5ml),
<u>intravenous</u>	(80mg sulfamethoxazole + 16mg trimethoprim per ml).

Adult dose:

<u>Urinary tract infection:</u> Acute uncomplicated lower UTI may be treated with single dose therapy consisting of 1600 mg sulfamethoxazole/320 mg trimethoprim (e.g. two double-strength tablets). Otherwise, the standard dosage is 800 mg sulfamethoxazole/160 mg trimethoprim (e.g. one double-strength tablet) q12h for 10 days. If intravenous therapy is necessary, the dosage based on the trimethoprim component is 8–10 mg/kg/24h divided q6–12h for up to 14 days.

<u>Shigellosis:</u> 800 mg sulfamethoxazole/160 mg trimethoprim (e.g. one double-strength tablet) q12h for 5 days. If intravenous therapy is necessary, the dosage based on trimethoprim component is 8–10 mg/kg/24h divided q6–12h for 5 days (maximum 60 ml/day).

<u>Acute exacerbation chronic bronchitis:</u> 800 mg sulfamethoxazole/160 mg trimethoprim (e.g. one double-strength tablet) q12h for 14 days.

<u>Pneumocystis carinii pneumonia</u> dosage based on trimethoprim component is 20 mg/kg/24h PO divided q6h for 14 days or 15–20 mg/kg/24h IV divided q6–8h for up to 14 days.

Pediatric dose (based on trimethoprim component):

<u>Urinary tract infection/ acute otitis media:</u> 4 mg/kg q12h for 10 days.

<u>Shigellosis:</u> 4 mg/kg q12h for 5 days.

<u>Pneumocystis carinii:</u> same as adult.

Comments: <u>Dose adjustment in renal failure:</u> normal dose if creatinine clearance > 30 ml/min, half dose if clearance 15–30 ml/min, do not use if clearance < 15 ml/min. <u>Crystalluria:</u> Encourage generous fluid intake in order to avoid crystalluria and its consequences. <u>Intravenous administration:</u> Dilute in D5W and infuse dose over 60–90 minutes. Do not mix with other drugs or other IV solutions.

SULFONAMIDES: sulfamethizole (Thiosulfil),

sulfamethoxazole (Gantanol), sulfizoxazole (Gantrisin), sulfadiazine.
See also sulfamethoxazole–trimethoprim (Bactrim, Septra).

Action: Folate is an essential factor that some bacteria must synthesize. Sulfonamides are structurally similar to para–aminobenzoic (PABA) and exert their bacteriostatic effect by competitively inhibiting synthesis of folate from PABA.

Spectrum includes: S. pneumonia, S. pyogenes, anthrax, diptheria, E. coli, Klebsiella, Proteus mirabilis, H. influenza, H. ducreyi (chancroid), Pseudomonas pseudomallei, Brucella, vibrio, Yersinia pestis, Nocardia, actinomyces, chlamydia. Resistant bacteria include Pseudomonas aeruginosa, enterobacter, proteus, shigella, meningococci, gonococci, syphilis, rickettsia, tularemia.

Indications:
● Acute uncomplicated lower urinary tract infection (cystitis, urethritis) due to susceptible bacteria (e.g. E. coli, Klebsiella, Proteus mirabilis).
● Norcardiosis.
● Adjunct in treatment of malaria due to chloroquine–resistant Plasmodium falciparum.
● Adjunct in treatment of toxoplasmosis.
● Alternative in treatment of: chancroid; lymphogranuloma venereum; melioidosis; certain chlamydial infections (trachoma, inclusion conjunctivitis, pneumonia).

Contraindications: sulfonamide hypersensitivity, last 3 months pregnancy, infant < 2 months of age, nursing mother, treatment of group A beta–hemolytic streptococci infection. Concurrent administration of the urinary antiseptic methenamine is contraindicated because methenamine releases formaldehyde which may precipitate with sulfonamides to cause crystalluria.

Caution: renal or liver dysfunction, G6PD deficiency, severe allergies, bronchial asthma.

Comments: Crystalluria and nephrolithiasis may occur if the patient fails to maintain generous fluid intake (1–2 liter/day). Crystalluria is uncommon with sulfisoxazole and sulfamethizole. The risk is greater with sulfamethoxazole and greatest with sulfadiazine. Photosensitivity reaction may occur if there is undue exposure to sunlight or other ultraviolet source. Drug interactions: Sulfonamides may enhance the effects of certain drugs—e.g. oral hypoglycemics, warfarin, phenytoin, methotrexate. Sulfonamide–induced blood dyscrasia; Stop sulfonamide and obtain CBC if fever, sore throat, jauncice, and/or purpura develops. Rash; Discontinue sulfonamide if rash develops.

Side effects: gastrointestinal; anorexia, nausea, vomiting, diarrhea, abdominal pain, stomatitis, pancreatitis, hepatitis; blood; hemolytic anemia (G6PD deficient patient at greatest risk), agranulocytosis, leukopenia, aplastic anemia, methemoglobinemia, thrombocytopenia, hypoprothrombinemia, purpura, eosinophilia; neurologic; headache, depression, confusion, drowsiness, weakness, insomnia, dizziness, vertigo, tinnitus, ataxia, peripheral neuritis, hallucinations, convulsions; renal; (1) crystalluria possibly leading to hematuria, proteinuria, stones, and/or obstructive oliguria/anuria; (2) toxic nephrosis with oliguria or anuria in absence of crystalluria; skin/allergic: itching, urticaria, anaphylaxis, photosensitivity, rash, generalized skin eruptions, erythema multiforme, Stevens–Johnson syndrome, epidermal necrolysis, exfoliative dermatitis, serum sickness, arthralgias, myocarditis, periorbital edema, scleral/conjunctival injection; other: fever, chills, goiter, hypoglycemia, periarteritis nodosa, lupus.

sulfamethizole (Thiosulfil Forte)   Supplied as; 500 mg tablet.
Adult dose: 500–1000 mg PO 3–4 times a day..
Pediatric (> 2 month of age): 30–45 mg/kg/24hr divided q6h.

sulfamethoxazole (Gantanol)
Supplied as: tablet (500 mg); oral suspension (500mg/5ml).
Adult dose: 2 gram PO initial dose, then 1 gram PO q12 h (or q8h in severe infection).
Pediatric (> 2 month of age): 50–60 mg/kg initial dose, then 25–30 mg/kg q12h. Maximum 75mg/kg/24hr.

sulfixoxazole (Gantrisin)
Supplied as: tablet (500 mg), syrup or suspension (500 mg/5ml).
Adult dose: 2–4 gram PO initial dose, then 4–8 gram/24 hr divided q4–6h.
Pediatric (> 2 month of age): 75 mg/kg PO initial dose, then 150 mg/kg/day divided q4–6h not to exceed 6 grams/24hr.

sulfadiazine   Supplied as; tablet (300, 500 mg);   IV injection preparation.
Adult dose: PO: 2–4 gram initial dose, then 1 gram q4–6h.
IV: 100 mg/kg (max 5 gram) initial dose, then 30–50 mg/kg q6–8h.
Pediatric (> 2 mo age): 75 mg/kg initial dose, then 150 mg/kg/day divided q4–6h not to exceed 6 gram/24 hr.
Note: Because of the risk of crystalluria, sulfadiazine is generally reserved for treatment of Nocardiosis, Toxoplasmosis, or as adjunct in treatment of malaria due to

chloroquine–resistant Plasmodium falciparum. In order to prevent crystalluria, PO fluid intake should be sufficient to maintain urine output at at least 1.5 liter/day. Alkalizing the urine is also recommended.

SULFONYLUREAS:

chlorpropamide (Diabinese)
glipizide (Glucotrol)   **glyburide** (DiaBeta, Micronase)
tolazamide (Tolinase)   **tolbutamide** (Orinase)

Action: Exert hypoglycemic effect by stimulating release of insulin from pancreatic islet beta cells. Sulfonylureas are not effective if the pancreas ie unable to secrete insulin. The insulin secretory stimulus may decline with chronic administration. However, extrapancreatic effects may persist in contributing to a hypoglycemic response (e.g. enhanced insulin–induced glucose transport into adipose tissue and skeletal muscle, decreased hepatic release of glucose, possible increase in insulin receptors).

Indication: Mild non–ketotic non–insulin–dependent diabetes mellitus (type II diabetes) that is not responsive to exercise, diet, weight reduction.

Contraindications: ●When insulin is required—e.g. type I diabetes (juvenile onset diabetes); diabetic keotacidosis; diabetic coma; severe or unstable diabetes; severe stress (e.g. major surgery/trauma, infection). ●Not recommended in pregnancy or while nursing. ●Safety not established in children. ●Sulfonylureas are not generally advisable in those with renal or liver disease.

Caution/comments: Risk of hypoglycemia: Sulfonylureas, particularly chlorpropamide, may cause severe and prolonged hypoglycemia requiring hospitalization. Blood and urine glucose should be tested periodically. The elderly, debilitated, or malnourished are particularly prone to hypoglycemia. Patients with hepatic, renal, adrenal, or pituitary dysfunction are also susceptible. Alcohol ingestion, decreased caloric intake, or prolonged exercise may provoke hypoglycemia. The hypoglycemic effects of sulfonylureas are potentiated by nonsteroidal anti–inflammatory drugs, salicylates, sulfonamides, chloramphenicol, probenecid, coumarins, MAO inhibitors, beta–adrenergic blockers, guanethidine, clofibrate, anabolic steroids. Drugs that oppose hypoglycemic effects of sulfonylureas: The glucose lowering effect of sulfonylureas may be opposed by agents that tend to induce hyperglycemia (e.g. thiazides and other diuretics, corticosteroids, estrogens, oral contraceptives, phenothiazines, phenytoin, phenobarbital, sympathomimetics, calcium channel blocker). Relative effectiveness of sulfonylureas: Reduction of blood glucose is more rapidly achieved with a short–acting sulfonylurea (e.g. tolbutamide). Otherwise, one sulfonylurea is in general no more effective in lowering blood glucose than any other. Occasionally however, a different sulfonylurea may be successfully substituted for a sulfonylurea that is no longer effective. Congestive heart failure: Chlorpropamide and rarely tolbutamide may cause water retention and should therefore be used cautiously in those with heart failure. Tolazamide and glyburide on the other hand are mildly diuretic. Gout: Acetohexamide is uricosuric and may be preferred is diabetics with gout.

Side effects: hypoglycemia; gastrointestinal: (1) *acetohexamide* (nausea, epigastric fullness, heartburn); (2) *chlorpropamide* (anorexia, nausea, vomiting, diarrhea, hunger, proctocolitis); (3) *glipizide* (nausea, diarrhea, constipation, gastralgia); (4) *glyburide, tolazamide, and tolbutamide* (nausea, epigastric fullness, heartburn); skin: photosensitivity, porphyria cutanea tarda, allergic skin reactions (pruritis, urticaria, eczema, erythema, skin eruption); blood: leukopenia, agranulocytosis, thrombocytopenia, hemolytic anemia, aplastic anemia, pancytopenia; hepatic: elevated SGOT, elevated alkaline phosphotase, hepatic porphyria (chlorpropamide, glipizide, tolazamide, tolbutamide); cholestatic jaundice (tolazamide, tolbutamide); mixed cholestatic–hepatic jaundice (acetohexamide); other: elevated BUN, elevated creatinine; elevated LDH, SIADH (chlorpropamide); disulfiram–like reaction after alcohol ingestion (e.g. facial flashing).

chlorpropamide (Diabinese)   Supplied as: 100, 250 mg tablet.
Dose (adult): Initially, 250 mg PO as single daily dose (100–125 mg once daily in elderly) with breakfast. Increase or decrease by 50–125 mg at 5–7 day intervals based on blood glucose response. Usual requirement: less 100 mg in mild diabetics to 500 mg/day in more severe cases. Maximum 750 mg/day.
Duration of action is 72–96 hr.

glipizide (Glucotrol)   Supplied as: 5, 10 mg tablet.
Dose (adult): Initially, 5 mg PO before breakfast. (2.5 mg if elderly or if liver disease present). If needed, increase dose gradually by 2.5–5 mg increments based on blood glucose response up to maximum 40 mg/day. Divide daily dose into 2 doses if receiving > 15 mg/day. Duration of action is 24 hr.

glyburide (DiaBeta, Micronase)   Supplied as: 1.25, 2.5, 5 mg tablet.
Dose (adult): Initially, 2.5–5 mg before breakfast or first main meal. Increase daily dose as needed at weekly intervals by no more than 2.5 mg increments based on blood glucose response up to a maximum 20 mg/day. Dose may be given as single daily dose but patients receiving over 10 mg/day may benefit by dividing daily dose into 2 doses. Duration of action is 24 hr.

tolazamide (Tolinase)   Supplied as: 100, 250, 500 mg tablet.

<u>Dose (adult)</u>: Initially, 100 mg PO as single daily dose if fasting blood glucose is less than 200 mg/dl (or if patient malnourished, underweight, elderly) and 250 mg as single daily dose if fasting glucose over 200 mg/dl. Subsequently, adjust daily dose by 100–250mg increments at weekly intervals based on blood glucose response. Range: 100mg to maximum 1000mg/day, average 250–500mg/day. Daily dose is taken in 2 doses if receiving > 500 mg/day. <u>Duration of action</u> is 12–24 hr.

tolbutamide (Orinase)   <u>Supplied as</u>: 250, 500 mg tablet.

<u>Dose (adult)</u>: Initially, 500 mg PO twice daily. Adjust dose at 5–7 day intervals based on blood glucose response. Maintenance: 250–3000 mg/day but seldom > 2000 mg/day. Daily dose may be given as single morning dose or divided doses. <u>Duration of action</u> is 6–24 hr.

TARS

Action/Indications: Derivatives of coal tar inhibit reproduction of epidermal cells thereby alleviating hyperplastic eczemas (e.g. psoriasis, seborrheic dermatitis, atopic dermatitis, lichen simplex chronicus).

Contraindications: coal tar sensitivity. Do not apply to acutely inflamed, open, or infected skin.

Side effects: folliculitis, possibility of epidermal carcinomas with prolonged use.

Supplied as:

Cream (e.g. Alphosyl, Tarbonis, Tegrin): apply to affected skin as needed.

Gel: Estar is applied qd—bid (massage into affected skin & remove excess after 5 minutes. See individual instructions for other tar gels (e.g. T-Gel, PsoriGel).

Lotion: Alphosyl is applied to affected skin bid—qid at first, and then 2–3 times/week when control achieved. Other lotions include Tar–Doak, Tegrin, T/Derm.

Bath preparations (e.g. Balnetar, Lavatar, Polytar, Zetar): add to bath and soak for 10–20 minutes. Preparation may be used once daily to once every third day.

Shampoo (e.g. Denorex, Pentrax, Sebutone, T/Gel, Tegrin, Zetar, DHS Tar).

TERCONAZOLE (Terazol)

Indication: vulvovaginal candidiasis.

Contraindication: hypersensitivity to components of preparation.

Comments: ●Avoid using during 1st trimester of pregnancy unless essential to patient welfare. ●In the nursing mother, consider temporarily suspending nursing while taking the drug. ●Safety and efficacy in children not established. ●Avoid concomitant use with a diaphragm because the preparation may interact with rubber latex found diaphragms. ●Discontinue and do not retreat if there is sensitization, irritation, fever, chills, or flu–like symptoms associated with use of preparation.

Supplied as: 80mg vaginal suppositories, vaginal cream (20mg/applicatorful).

Dose: One vaginal suppository at bedtime for 3 consecutive nights _or_ one applicatorful at bedtime for 7 consecutive nights.

TETRACYCLINE (Achromycin, Sumycin)

Action: Bacteriostatic. Inhibits bacterial protein synthesis by binding to bacterial 30S ribosomal subunit.

Spectrum/Indications: rickettsiae; Rocky Mountain spotted fever, typhus group, Q fever, rickettsialpox; chlamydia; lymphogranuloma venereum, psittacosis/ornithosis, C. trachomitis (e.g. inclusion conjuctivitis, nongonococcal uretheritis/endocervicitis/rectal infection); Mycoplasma pneumoniae; Ureaplasma urealyticum; certain gram–negative bacilli; brucellosis, granuloma inguinale, cholera, melioidosis (Pseudomonas pseudomallei), glanders (Pseudomonas mallei); relapsing fever (Borrelia recurrentis); acne.

Alternative in treatment of: H. influenza, chancroid, syphilis, yaws, Legionella, plague, tularemia, Pasteurella multocida, clostridia (C. tetani, C. perfringens), anthrax, Listeria monocytogenes, bacteroides, Campylobacter, Fusobacterium fusiforme (Vincent's infection), Actinomyces israeli, rat bite fever.

Resistance is common with: gonococcus, staphylococci, streptococci, E. coli, klebsiella, enterobacter, proteus, Pseudomonas aeruginosa, acinetobacter, shigella.

Contraindications: tetracycline hypersensitivity, renal failure (use doxycycline if a tetracycline is indicated), pregnancy, nursing mothers, children < 8 yr (except in urgent cases where alternative drugs are contraindicated or are not effective). Note: Tetracycline may be hepatotoxic in pregnant and postpartum women; cause retarded skeletal growth of fetus and young children; and cause permanent staining of teeth if administered during tooth development (i.e. last half pregnancy to up to 8 yr of age).

Comments: ●Be aware that concurrent use of tetracyclines (which are bacteriostatic) may interfere with bactericidal antibiotics (e.g. penicillins, cephalosporins) because bactericidal antibiotics require actively dividing bacteria to exert their effect. ●Periodically obtain CBC, BUN, creatinine and liver function tests during long–term administration of tetracycline. ●Tetracyclines may potentiate the effect of oral anticoagulants (and be reflected in an increased prothrombin time) so that the oral anticoagulant dosage may need to be reduced.

Side effects: gastrointestinal; anorexia, nausea, vomiting, diarrhea, stomatitis, glossitis, black tongue, dysphagia, colitis, anogenital inflammation, (GI effects are often due to overgrowth resistant organisms—e.g. candida; skin (rash, exfoliative dermatitis), photosensitivity); hypersensitivity (urticaria, angioedema, anaphylaxis, anaphylactoid purpura, pericarditis, aggravation systemic lupus); blood (hemolytic anemia, thrombocytopenia, neutropenia, eosinophilia); renal (elevated BUN); liver (acute fatty liver—especially in pregnant or postpartum patient with renal dysfunction or pyelonephritis); neurologic (pseudotumor cerebri rarely); local (thrombophlebitis with IV use).

Supplied as: capsule (250, 500 mg); syrup/oral suspension (125mg/5ml), IV injection preparation.

●IM injection is very painful and is not advised.

Dose, adult:

Oral: 250–500 mg q6h. Food, antacids, and iron supplements interfere with absorption. Take tetracycline one hour before or 2 hours after meals.

Specific oral regimens:

Early syphilis (primary, secondary, latent less than 1 yr): 500 mg PO q6h for 15 days, late syphilis: 500 mg PO q6h for 30 days,
pelvic inflammatory disease: 500 mg PO q6h for 10 days,
nongonoccal urethritis: 500 mg PO q6h for at least 7 days,
acute epididymo–orchitis: 500 mg PO q6h for at least 10 days,
chlamydial infection of urethra, cervix, or rectum: 500 mg PO q6h for at least 7 days,
lymphogranuloma venereum: 500 mg PO q6h for at least 14 days.

Intravenous: 250–500 mg q6–12h (diluted and infused over 2 hr). Switch to oral route as soon as possible.

Dose, child > 8 yr:

Oral: 6.25–12.5 mg/kg q6h one hour before or 2 hours after meals. Do not to exceed adult dose.

Intravenous: 10–20 mg/kg/day divided q8–12h. Do not to exceed adult dose. Dilute doses and infuse over 2 hours.

THEOPHYLLINE

Action: Methylxanthine. Inhibits phosphodiesterase, the enzyme that breaks down cyclic AMP. Consequently, the level of cyclic AMP is increased within bronchial smooth muscle cells. This leads to smooth muscle relaxation with consequent bronchodilation.

Indications: ●bronchial asthma; ●bronchospasm that is associated with emphysema, chronic bronchitis, or pulmonary edema; ●Cheynes–Stokes respiration; ●neonatal apnea.

Contraindications: theophylline hypersensitivity, infants < 6 months of age (treatment of neonatal apnea excepted).

Caution: severe cardiac disease, acute myocardial infarction, hypertension, hyperthyroidism, liver or renal failure, COPD, cor pulmonale, pregnancy, nursing mother, peptic ulcer disease. Half-life of theophylline is prolonged, and consequently smaller doses generally suffice in the following settings: alcoholism, liver or renal dysfunction, congestive heart failure, chronic obstructive pulmonary disease, neonates, high fever, active influenza infection or following influenza immunization, patient over 55 yr of age. Concurrent administration of certain drugs may lead to increased serum theophylline level—e.g. erythromycin, cimetidine, beta blockers, furosemide, oral contraceptives, high–dose allopurinol. Concurrent treatment with sympathomimetic bronchodilators increases risk of side effects (e.g. CNS stimulation, cardiovascular effects).

Comments: Serum theophylline therapeutic level is 10–20 mcg/ml. Assuming theophylline has been taken properly for past 48 hours, the serum sample is obtained 2 hours after last oral dose (4 hr after last oral dose if sustain release pills are being used). Sustain release pills are best prescribed after the total daily theophylline requirements have been establised with the rapidly–absorbed preparations. Sustain–release pills are especially useful for asthmatics who experience exacerbation of symptoms during sleeping hours. Smokers metabolize theophylline faster and require larger maintenance doses. This effect may last up to 2 yrs after cessation of smoking. Drugs that may lower serum theophylline level: phenobarbital (enhances hepatic metabolism theophylline), phenytoin, rifampin. Taking theophylline with food reduces gastric irritation; absorption is complete but prolonged.

Side effects (usually at serum level greater than 20 mcg/ml): gastrointestinal : nausea, vomiting, diarrhea, epigastric pain, hematemesis; neurologic: headache, dizziness, nervousness, insomnia, restlessness, agitation, muscle twitching, seizures; respiratory: tachypnea; cardiovascular: palpitations, tachycardia, extrasystoles, arrhythmias, flushing, hypotension, shock; renal: albuminuria, diuresis, urinary retention in males; other: hyperglycemia, SIADH, rash, fever (in child), diaphoresis (in child).

Supplied as:

Capsules:	Bronkodyl (100,200mg);	Elixophyllin (100,200mg);
Tablets:	Slo–phyllin (100,200mg);	Theolair (125,250mg);
Liquid:	Aerolate (150mg/15ml);	Elixophyllin (80mg/15ml);
	Slo–phyllin (80mg/15ml);	Theoclear–80 (80mg/15ml);
	Theolair (80mg/15ml);	Theon (50mg/5ml);
	Theostat (80mg/15ml);	

Sustained/controlled release pills:

Constant T (200,300mg);	Aerolate (65,130,260mg);
Elixophyllin SR (125, 250mg);	Duraphyl (100,200,300mg);
Slo–phyllin Gyrocap (60,125,250mg);	Slo–bid Gyrocaps (50,100,200,300mg);
Theobid Duracap (130,260mg);	Sustaire (100,300mg);
	Theoclear LA (130,260mg);

Theo–Dur (100,200,300,450mg);   Theolair–SR (200,250,300,500mg);
Theospan SR (130,260mg);   Theovent (125, 250mg).

DOSE (based on ideal body weight):

(1) Acute asthma attack NOT requiring IV therapy in patient NOT currently receiving theophylline/aminophylline medication (use rapidly absorbed preparations only):

6 month–9 yr: 5 mg/kg PO initial dose* followed by maintenance dose of 4 mg/kg q6h. Maximum 24 mg/kg/day unless serum theophylline level is available to guide dose adjustments to therapeutic level (10–20 mcg/ml).

9–16 yr or smoker: 5 mg/kg PO initial dose* followed by maintenance dose of 3 mg/kg q6h. Unless serum theophylline level is available to guide dose adjustments to therapeutic level (10–20 mcg/ml); do not exceed the lesser of 900 mg/day or the following: 20 mg/kg/day in patient 9–12 yr, 18 mg/kg/day in patient 12–16 yr, 13 mg/kg/day in patient over 16 yr.

Otherwise healthy nonsmoking adult: 5 mg/kg PO initial dose* followed by maintenance dose of 3 mg/kg q8h. Unless serum theophylline level is available to guide dose adjustments to therapeutic level (10–20 mcg/ml), do not exceed 13 mg/kg/day or 900 mg/day whichever is less.

Older adult or patient with cor pulmonale: 5 mg/kg PO initial dose* followed by maintenance dose of 2 mg/kg q8h. Use serum theophylline level to guide dose adjustments to therapeutic level (10–20 mcg/ml).

Patient with congestive heart failure or liver disease: 5 mg/kg PO initial dose* followed by maintenance dose of 1–2 mg/kg q12h. Use serum theophylline level to guide dose adjustments to therapeutic level (10–20 mcg/ml).

*NOTE: If an adequate response is not noted 1 hour following the initial oral loading dose, then an IV loading dose of 2.5 mg/kg aminophylline may be given (diluted and infused over 15–20 min) followed by maintenance IV aminophylline infusion. See "Aminophylline".

(2) Acute asthma attack NOT requiring IV therapy in patient who IS currently receiving theophylline medication (use rapidly absorbed preparations only):

Loading dose: 2.5 mg/kg PO. The alternative, if a stat serum theophylline level is available, is to give a sufficient oral loading dose to raise the serum theophylline to therapeutic level (10–20 mcg/ml): each 0.5 mg/kg theophylline will raise serum theophylline by 1 mcg/ml.

Maintenance: Use maintenance doses stated above according to age, clinical status, and/or serum theophylline level.

(3) Chronic asthma/non–urgent cases (adult or pediatric):

Initially: 16 mg/kg/24hr or 400 mg/24hr whichever is less divided into 3–4 daily doses q6–8h. If sustain–release pills are prescribed, the daily dose is given in 2–3 divided doses q8–12h.

Subsequently: If necessary, increase dose by 25% at 3 day intervals. However, (unless serum theophylline level is available to guide dose adjustments to therapeutic level of 10–20mcg/ml) do not exceed the lesser of 900 mg/day or the following: 13 mg/kg/day in patient over 16 yr, 18 mg/kg/day in patient 12–16 yr, 20 mg/kg/day in patient 9–12 yr, 24 mg/kg/day in patient 6 months–9 yr.

THIAZIDE DIURETICS & sulfonamide diuretics with similar pharmacology

Action: <u>Diuretic</u> by inhibiting renal sodium reabsorption.
<u>Antihypertensive</u> possibly by relaxing vascular smooth muscle.

Indications: <u>hypertension;</u>,
<u>edema</u> due to congestive heart failure, cirrhosis, or corticosteroid or estrogen therapy.

Contradindications: anuria, thiazide or sulfonamide derivative hypersensitivity. Concurrent administration of lithium is not advised (thiazides decrease renal excretion of lithium).

Caution: renal or hepatic disease, hyperuricemia, gout, diabetes mellitus.

Comments: <u>Electrolyte abnormalities:</u> Monitor serum and urine electrolytes periodically; particularly in presence of vomiting, diarrhea, or parenteral fluid intake. Be alert to evidence of fluid or electrolyte abnormalities (e.g. thirst, lethargy, restlessness, muscle cramps/weakness, hypotension, tachycardia, oliguria). <u>Hypokalemia:</u> Thiazides increase the urinary excretion of potassium (as well as sodium, chloride, magnesium, bicarbonate). The risk of hypokalemia is lessened by adding a potassium–sparing diuretic (e.g. triamterene, spironolactone), potassium supplementation, or encouraging potassium–rich foods. Hypokalemia is aggravated by vomiting, diarrhea, or high sodium intake. Hypokalemic patient receiving digitalis is at increased risk for cardiac arrhythmias. Hypokalemia may precipitate hepatic coma in cirrhotic patient. <u>Dilutional hyponatrenia</u> may occur, particularly in the edematous patient and especially during hot weather when water intake is increased. Dilutional hyponatrenia is treated by restricting fluid intake.

Side effects: <u>gastrointestinal;</u> anorexia, nausea, vomiting, diarrhea, constipation, gastric irritation, cramps, cholestatic jaundice, pancreatitis, sialadenitis; <u>neurologic;</u> headache, dizziness, vertigo, restlessness, weakness, paresthesias, xanthopsia, blurred vision; <u>blood;</u> leukopenia, agranulocytosis, thrombocytopenia, aplastic anemia, hemolytic anemia; <u>hypersensitivity;</u> rash, urticaria, vasculitis, purpura, photosensitivity, fever, pneumonitis, pulmonary edema, anaphylaxis; <u>cardiovascular;</u> postural hypotension; <u>other;</u> hyperglycemia, hyperuricemia/gout, muscle spasm.

bendroflumethiazide (Naturetin)　　　　<u>Supplied as;</u> 5, 10 mg tablet.
<u>Hypertension (adult);</u> Initially, 5–20 mg/day. Maintenance: 2.5–15 mg/day
<u>Edema (Adult);</u> Initially: 5–20mg/day in 1–2 doses. Maintenance:2.5–5mg once/day.
<u>Onset/peak/duration;</u> 1–2 hr/6–12 hr/18–24 hr.

benzthiazide (Exna)　　　　　　　　　<u>Supplied as;</u> 25, 50 mg tablet.
<u>Hypertension (adult);</u> Initially, 25–50 mg bid. Maintenance: up to 50 mg qid.
<u>Edema (adult);</u>　　Initially, 50–200 mg/day (divide into 2 doses if ≥ 100 mg/day).
　　　　　　　　　　Maintenance: 50–150 mg/day.
<u>Onset/peak/duration;</u> 2 hr/4–6hr/12–18hr.

chlorothiazide (Diuril)
<u>Supplied as;</u> tablet (250, 500 mg); oral suspension (250mg/5ml); IV preparation.
<u>Adult dose:</u>　●Hypertension: 250–500 mg PO one or two times per day.
　　　　　　　　●Edema: 500–1000 mg PO once to twice daily.
<u>Pediatric dose:</u>　●Hypertension: 5–10 mg/kg PO twice daily.
　　●Edema: 11 mg/kg PO bid. Infant < 6 month, up to 33 mg/kg/day in 2 doses.
<u>Onset/peak/duration;</u> 2 hr/4 hr/6–12 hr.

hydrochlorothiazide (Esidrix, HydroDIURIL, Oretic)
<u>Supplied as;</u> 25, 50 mg tablet.
<u>Adult dose:</u>
　●Hypertension: 25–50 mg qd–bid. Rarely, up to 200 mg/day divided.
　●Edema: 50–100 mg qd–bid. Intermittent therapy may suffice—e.g. alter
　nate day administration, 3–5 days a week administration.
<u>Pediatric dose:</u> ●Hypertension: 0.5–1.0 mg/kg twice daily.
●Edema: 1 mg/kg twice daily. Infant < 6 mo. may need up to 1.5 mg/kg twice daily.
<u>Onset/peak/duration;</u> 2 hr/4 hr/6–12 hr.

hydroflumethiazide (Diucardin, Saluron)　　<u>Supplied as;</u> 50 mg tablet.
<u>Adult dose:</u>　Hypertension: 50–100 mg/day.　　Edema: 25–200 mg/day divided.
<u>Pediatric dose:</u> 1 mg/kg/day initially.
<u>Onset/peak/duration;</u> 1–2 hr/3–4 hr/18–24 hr.

methyclothiazide (Aquatensen, Enduron)　　<u>Supplied as;</u> 2.5, 5 mg tablet.
<u>Adult dose:</u>　Hypertension: 2.5–5 mg once daily.　　Edema: 2.5–10 mg once daily.
<u>Pediatric dose;</u>　0.05–2.0 mg/kg once daily.
<u>Onset/peak/duration;</u> 2 hr/6 hr/24 hr.

polythiazide (Renese)　　　　　　　　<u>Supplied as;</u> 1, 2, 4 mg tablet.
<u>Adult dose:</u>　Hypertension: 2–4 mg/day.　Edema: 1–4 mg/day.
<u>Pediatric dose;</u>　individualize dosage, 0.02–0.08 mg/kg/day.
<u>Onset/peak/duration;</u> 2 hr/4 hr/24–36 hr.

trichlormethiazide (Naqua) Supplied as: 2, 4 mg tablet.
Adult dose: Hypertension: 2–4 mg/day. Edema: 1–4 mg/day.
Pediatric dose (edema or hypertension): 0.07 mg/kg/24 hr initially.
Onset/peak/duration: 2 hr/6 hr/24 hr.

SULFONAMIDE DIURETICS WITH PHARMACOLOGY SIMILAR TO THIAZIDES:
chlorthalidone (Hygroton) Supplied as: 25, 50, 100 mg tablet.
Adult dose: Hypertension: 25–50 mg once daily. Edema: 50–100 mg once daily or
100 mg every other day (maximum 200 mg/day).
Onset: 2 hr, Duration: 24–72 hr.
metolazone (Diulo, Zaroxolyn) Supplied as: 2.5, 5, 10 mg tablet.
Dose (adult): Hypertension: 2.5–5 mg once daily. Edema: 5–20 mg once daily.
Onset/peak/duration: 1 hr/2 hr/12–24 hr.
quinethazone (Hydromox) Supplied as: 50 mg tablet.
Dose (adult): Hypertension: 50–100 mg once daily.
        Edema: 50–100 mg once daily (maximum 200 mg/day).
Onset/peak/duration: 2 hr/6 hr/18–24 hr.

THIOPENTAL SODIUM (Pentothal)

Refer to methohexital sodium (Brevital) for indications, contraindications, cautions,
and side effects.
Supplied as: 2.5% solution (25mg/ml) for IV injection.
Preparation/compatibility: Thiopental should be prepared with the following di-
luents: sterile water injection USP, sodium chloride injection USP, or 5% dextrose in-
jection USP. Thiopental must not be mixed with acid solutions (e.g. atropine, succi-
nylcholine, tubocurarine).
Adult dose: Test dose is given first, 50 mg IV.
Induction: 50–75 mg IV. Repeat at 20–40 second intervals until adequate response.
Maintenance: 25–50 mg IV whenever patient moves.
Pediatric dose (5–15 yr of age):
Induction: inject 2.5% solution slowly IV. Repeat as needed at 30 second intervals.
A total dose of 4–5 mg/kg is the usual induction dose.
Maintenance (child 30–50 kg): 25–50 mg IV as needed.

TISSUE PLASMINOGEN ACTIVATOR:
Alteplase, recombinant (ACTIVASE)

Action: Alteplase is a tissue plasminogen activator—i.e. a proteolytic enzyme that converts plasminogen (a protein found in blood clots and circulating blood) to plasmin. Because alteplase binds
to fibrin, its activity is primarily directed locally at the clot (systemic proteolytic activity is limited).
Plasmin (itself a proteolytic enzyme) in turn reduces clots by lyzing fibrin. Plasmin also lyzes the fibrin precursor, fibrinogen.
Indication: lysis of thrombi occluding coronary arteries in adult undergoing acute myocardial infarction.
Contraindications: active internal bleeding, history of cerebrovascular accident, intracranial or intraspinal trauma or surgery within past 2 months, intracranial neoplasm, intracranial AV malformation, intracranial aneurysm, bleeding diathesis, severe uncontrolled hypertension.
Caution: Conditions which increase the risk of t–PA–associated bleeding: For instance, the occurrence of any of the following within the past ten days should compel caution: major surgery,
trauma, obstetric delivery, GI or GU bleeding, puncture of noncompressible blood vessel (e.g. subclavian or internal jugular puncture). Other conditions dictating caution because of possible
bleeding or attendant complications include: cerebrovascular disease, blood pressure $\geq$ 180 systolic or $\geq$ 110 diastolic, hemostatic abnormalities, oral anticoagulant therapy, high probability of
left heart thrombus (e.g. atrial fibrillation), acute pericarditis, subacute bacterial endocarditis, septic thrombophlebitis, obstructed AV cannula at seriously infected site, hemorrhagic ocular condition
(e.g. hemorrhagic diabetic retinopathy), significant hepatic dysfunction, pregnancy, over 75 yr of
age. Arterial or venous puncture: Puncture of noncompressible vessels (e.g. subclavian or internal jugular puncture) is contraindicated in patient receiving t–PA. Furthermore, arterial or venous
puncture in general should be minimized. If arterial puncture must be performed, it should be
done in an upper extremity and pressure should be applied to the puncture site for at least 30
minutes following the procedure. Intramuscular injections must be avoided while receiving t–PA.
Heparin has been infused concurrently with and after t–PA administration in order to decrease the
risk of a clot reforming. Be alert for bleeding. Oral anticoagulants and anti–platelet drugs (aspirin, dipyridamole) administered before or during t–PA infusions may increase the risk of bleeding.
Arrhythmias: Coronary thrombolysis with reperfusion may result in arrhythmias—which are treated

in the usual manner. <u>Discontinue t-PA and heparin immediately if serious bleeding occurs</u>.
Side effects: bleeding and its complications, mild allergic reactions. Other associated effects of uncertain causal relationship: nausea, vomiting, hypotension, fever.
Supplied as: vials containing 20 or 50 mg for reconstitution.
Dose (adult):   The usual regimen is 100mg administered over 3 hours:
<u>first hour:</u> give 60 mg with the first 6–10 mg given as an IV bolus over 1–2 minutes;
<u>second and third hour:</u> administer 20 mg/hr.
  •Patients weighing less than 65 kg receive 1.25 mg/kg over 3 hours.

TOCAINIDE (Tonocard)

Action: An orally active structural analog of lidocaine with similar electrophysiologic/antiarrhythmic properties. Like lidocaine, tocainide (**1**) shortens the duration of action potential; (**2**) shortens effective refractory period of atrium, AV node, and right ventricle; (**3**) does not prolong ventricular depolarization—i.e. QRS duration unchanged; (**4**) does not prolong ventricular repolarization—i.e. QT interval unchanged; (**5**) does not significantly affect sinus node—i.e. cardiac rate unchanged; (**6**) does not affect AV conduction or significantly alter intracardiac conduction in general.
Indications: life–threatening ventricular arrhythmias primarily.   Because of potential toxicity, tocainide is usually reserved for patients in whom other agents are ineffective. It is often effective in the prevention/treatment of ventricular arrhythmias refractory to other antiarrhythmics (e.g. quinidine, disopyramide, propranolol).   Arrhythmias responsive to lidocaine will usually respond to tocainide; and lidocaine–unresponsive arrhythmias will usually not respond to tocainide.
Contraindications: hypersensitivity to drug,
                       2nd or 3rd degree AV block in absence of artificial ventricular pacemaker.
Caution: <u>Blood dyscrasias</u> (sometimes fatal) is reported in 0.18% patients. This usually occurs within the first 12 weeks therapy. Consequently, a CBC including differential and platelet count is advised weekly for the first 12 weeks and periodically thereafter. Patient should report any symptoms of infection (e.g. fever, chills, sore throat); or bruising or bleeding. <u>Pulmonary reactions</u> (e.g. pulmonary fibrosis, interstitial pneumonitis, fibrosing alveolitis, pulmonary edema) is reported in 0.11% patients.   Patient should report dyspnea, cough, wheezing. <u>Liver or kidney disease</u> may impair elimination of the drug and necessitate dose reduction. <u>Heart failure or marginal cardiac reserve;</u> Tocainide does not markedly depress the left ventricle but caution is advised.
Side effects: <u>blood</u> (bone marrow depression, agranulocytosis, leukopenia, neutropenia, hypoplastic anemia, anemia, thrombocytopenia); <u>pulmonary</u> (pulmonary fibrosis, interstitial pneunonitis, fibrosing alveolitis, pneumonia, pulmonary edema, dyspnea, respiratory arrest, hiccups); <u>cardiovascular</u> (hypotension, palpitations, bradycardia, tachycardia, chest pain, extension of acute MI, left ventricular failure, CHF/worsening CHF, cardiogenic shock, sinus arrest, AV block, widenened QRS, prolonged QT, right bundle branch block, ventricular fibrillation, vasovagal episodes, syncope, orthostatic hypotension, cold extremities, vasculitis); <u>gastrointestinal</u> (anorexia, nausea, vomiting, diarrhea, constipation, abdominal discomfort/pain, dyspepsia, dysphagia, stomatitis, dry mouth, thirst, hepatitis, jaundice, abnormal liver function tests, pancreatitis); <u>skin, hypersensitivity, or immune effects</u> (sweating, fever, arthralgias, eosinophilia, positive ANA, lupus syndrome, rash, itching, urticaria, erythema multiforme, Stevens–Johnson syndrome, exfoliative dermatitis, alopecia, pallor/flushed face); <u>neurologic/psychiatric</u> (dizziness, vertigo, paresthesias, tremor, altered mood/awareness, confusion, disorientation, hallucinations, headache, nervousness, anxiety, unsteadiness, incoordination, ataxia, seizures, coma, myasthenia gravis, dysarthria, slurred speech, increased stuttering, disturbed sleep, insomnia, dream abnormalities, depression, psychic abnormalities, agitation, psychosis); <u>special senses</u> (blurred vision, nystagmus, diplopia, altered taste/smell, earache); <u>urogenital</u> (urinary retention, polyuria); <u>other</u> (malaise, asthenia, muscle cramps/spasm/twitching, cinchonism, edema).
Supplied as: 400, 600 mg tablet.
Dose (adult): Start with 400 mg q8h. Clinical exam and EKG (including Holter monitor if necessary) are used to gauge antiarrhythmic effectiveness and to direct dose titration. Usual requirement is 1200–1800 mg/day in 3 doses. Twice daily dosing may be tried if tid dosing is tolerated. Less than 1200 mg/day may suffice in some patients (e.g. renal or hepatic dysfunction). Tocainide may be taken with food since bioavailability will not be lessened.

TRIAMTERENE + HYDROCHLOROTHIAZIDE

(Dyazide, Maxide)

Action: Triamterene is a diuretic which acts directly at the distal renal tubules to inhibit the process by which sodium is reabsorbed in exchange for porassium and hydrogen. Thus, while promoting sodium loss, triamterene conserves potassium, hydrogen, and chloride thereby offsetting the hydrocholorothiazide–induced loss of the latter three ions. Triamterene may also have a weak antihypertensive effect. Hydrochlorothiazide, in addition to promoting sodium diuresis, has a antihypertensive effect.

Indications: Treatment of hypertension or edema in patient (1) who becomes hypokalemic while on thiazide diuretic alone, or (2) for whom a thiazide diuretic is indicated but hypokalemia cannot be risked. As a diuretic, this drug combination may be used as an adjunct in the treatment of edema due to congestive heart failure, cirrhosis, nephrotic syndrome, or corticosteroid or estrogen--induced edema.

Contraindications: hypersensitivity to components or sulfonamide derivatives; hyperkalemia; anuria; renal insufficiency/impairment; increasing renal or hepatic dysfunction while on drug (e.g. oliguria, azotemia); concurrent administration of potassium supplements (unless hypokalemia is present or potassium intake is markedly impaired); concurrent administration of other potassium–sparing drugs (spironolactone, amiloride); concurrent lithium administration; nursing mother.

Caution: pregnancy (use only if clearly needed); liver dysfunction; history of kidney stones; gout; respiratory or metabolic acidosis; hypochloremia; concurrent use of certain drugs (e.g. nonsteroidal anti–inflammatory drug, angiotensin–converting enzyme inhibitor, oral anticoagulant, chlorpropamide).

Comments: Pregnancy: Diuretics must not be used for the physiologic edema that occurs with pregnancy but may be indicated if a pathologic cause exists. Concurrent potassium supplementation is contraindicated unless hypokalemia is present. Close monitoring of serum potassium is required if potassium supplements are necessary. Fluid/electrolyte/renal abnormalities: Periodically monitor serum electrolytes. This may be crucial in certain circumstances (e.g. cirrhosis, kidney disease, congestive heart failure, considerable vomiting or diarrhea, parenteral fluid therapy). Be alert to possible manifestations of fluid or electrolyte abnormalities (e.g. hypotension, tachycardia, oliguria, thirst, lethargy, restlessness, weakness, muscle pain/cramps/fatigue, GI disturbances). Dyazide may cause a decrease in intravascular volume or glomerular filtration, and thus lead to elevated BUN and/or serum creatinine. BUN and creatinine usually correct folllowing cessation of Dyazide. Periodically monitor BUN and serum creatinine, especially in elderly or in presence of renal dysfunction.

Side effects (see also "Thiazide Diuretics"): muscle cramps, weakness, dizziness, headache, dry mouth, rash, urticaria, photosensitivity, anaphylaxis, nausea, vomiting, diarrhea, constipation, postural hypotension.

Supplied as/adult dose:

Dyazide (capsule contains 50 mg triamterene and 25 mg hydrochlorothiazide):
Dose is 1–2 capsules twice daily. One capsule a day or every other day may suffice. Maximum 4 capsules/day. Adjust dose according to serum potassium level and clinical response.

Maxide (tablet contains 75 mg triamterene + 50 mg hydrochlorothiazide):
Dose is 1 tablet daily.

Maxide–25 MG (tablet contains 37.5 mg + 25 mg hydrochlorothiazide):
Dose is 1–2 tablets given once daily.

TRICYCLIC ANTIDEPRESSANTS: amitriptyline (Elavil, Endep); amoxapine (Asendin); desipramine (Norpramin, Pertofrane); doxepin (Adapin, Sinequan); imipramine (Tofranil, Janimine); nortriptyline (Pamelor); protriptyline (Vivactil); trimipramine (Surmontil).

Action: Tricyclics possibly exert their antidepressant effect by blocking norepinephrine reuptake by adrenergic neurons; or perhaps by influencing central adrenergic, dopaminergic, and serotonergic receptors.

Indications: ●Depression, particularly endgenous depression.
　　　　　　　●Enuresis in children over 6 years of age (imipramine only).

Contraindications: hypersensitivity to drug, concurrent administration of MAO inhibitor, recovery phase myocardial infarction, pregnancy, nursing mother, children (except imipramine for enuresis).

Caution: cardiovascular disease, history of glaucoma or urinary retention, hyperthyroidism, seizure history, elderly, debilitated, patient who engages in activities requiring alertness.

Comments: Sedation: Desipramine, protriptyline, amoxapine, are the least sedating while amitriptyline, doxepine, trimipramine are the most sedating. Imipramine and nortriptyline are intermediate. Optimizing maintenance dosage: Typically, mood improves over several weeks. After a stable therapeutic response is achieved, the dose may be gradually titrated down to the smallest effective dose. Discontinuing tricyclic: After approximately 20 weeks of sustained therapeutic effect, the drug may be discontinued to assess whether continued therapy is advised. Withdrawal symptoms (excitement, nausea, vomiting, etc.) can be avoided by gradually reducing dose over several weeks. Schizophrenia: Tricyclics may precipitate/aggravate psychosis in schizophrenics. If this occurs, antipsychotic medication (a phenothiazine) may be given concurrently or the dose of tricyclic decreased. Tricyclic medication should not be used while the patient is agitated. Manic-depressive disorders: Tricyclics may precipitate mania or hypomania. Suicidally-inclined patients are often most vulnerable to suicide as the tricyclic effects emerge and the depressed patient becomes more active. Since tricyclic overdose is a common means of suicide, it is best to avoid prescribing more than a gram of medication until the patient is stabilized.

Drug interactions: Anticholinergics (e.g. antihistamines) add to the anticholinergic effect of tricyclics and may thus potentiate dry mouth, constipation, urinary retention, blurred vision, acute glaucoma, etc. Alcohol and other CNS depressants potentiate sedative effects of tricyclics. Monoamine oxidase inhibitor: Avoid concurrent MAOI administration because untoward effects may result (e.g. fever, excitability, convulsions, death). Allow 2 weeks to elapse after stopping MAOI before initiating tricyclic therapy, and 1 week conversely. Guanethidine: Tricyclics, by blocking the uptake of guanethidine by adrenergic neurons, make guanethidine ineffectual in controlling blood pressure. Clonidine: Tricyclics decrease the antihypertensive effect of clonidine. Sympathomimetics: Concurrent administration with tricyclic may cause fever, hypertension, arrhythmias. Barbiturates, by unknown mechanism, may cause the patient to be unresponsive to tricyclic therapy. Barbiturates also hasten hepatic metabolism of tricyclics.

Side effects: cardiovascular: orthostatic hypotension, hypertension, stroke, myocardial infarction, tachycardia, arrhythmias, heart block; neurologic/psychiatric: sedation, weakness, fatigue, headache, dizziness, tinnitus, excitement, insomnia, nightmares, anxiety, agitation, confusion, delusions, hallucinations, aggravated psychosis, paresthesias, peripheral neuropathy, tremor, incoordination, seizures, extrapyramidal symptoms; anticholinergic: dry mouth, constipation, paralytic ileus, urinary retention, blurred vision, mydriasis, increased intraocular pressure; blood: marrow depression, agranulocytosis, thrombocytopenia, eosinophilia; gastrointestinal: anorexia, nausea, vomiting, diarrhea, epigastric distress, abdominal cramps, paralytic ileus, stomatitis, black tongue, peculiar taste, parotid swelling, altered liver function, jaundice; endocrine: altered libido, gynecomastia, testicular swelling, impotence, breast enlargement and galactorrhea in females, increased or decreased blood sugar, SIADH; allergic: rash, pruritis, urticaria, facial/lingual edema, photosensitivity, petechiae; other: flushing, sweating, urinary frequency, alopecia, weight gain/loss.

Overdose: Empty the stomach and administer charcoal: Since patients may deteriorate rapidly, it is usually best to empty the stomach by gastric lavage (even if the patient is alert) rather than wait for ipecac to work and the additional delay before charcoal can be administered. Give a dose of charcoal via the lavage tube before beginning lavage. If the patient is comatose, charcoal is administered every 4–6 hours because tricyclics and their metabolites undergo enterohepatic circulation. Administer charcoal even if 24 hours has elapsed since ingestion. Alkalinize the blood: This is very important and can be accomplished by hyperventilation and by administering sodium bicarbonate (1–3mg/kg IV push initially) The blood pH should be maintained above 7.45. Alkalinizing the blood increases tricyclic protein–binding thereby preventing/treating tricyclic–induced arrhythmias, hypotension, and possibly convulsions. Lidocaine may be used to treat arrhythmias. Phenytoin may be of use for either arrhythmias or seizures. Physostigmine (refer to "Anticholinesterases") is reserved for critical cases (e.g. seizures refractory to usual anticonvulsants, refractory severe hypotension). The dose is 1–2mg slow IV in adult and 0.5mg slow IV in child. Additional doses may be needed because of physostigmine's short half life. Forced diuresis, dialysis, or hemoperfusion are not useful.

amitriptyline (Elavil, Endep)
Supplied as:　tablet (10, 25, 50, 75, 100, 150 mg);
　　　　　　　intramuscular injection (10mg/ml).

Adult outpatient: Initially 50–100 mg PO at bedtime. If necessary, increase dose gradually by 25–50 mg increments up to total 150 mg PO at bedtime. Alternative is to start with 25 mg PO tid, and then gradually increase the bedtime dose as needed until patient is receiving up to 150 mg/day.

Maintenance: usually, 50–100 mg at bedtime (40mg PO at bedtime may suffice).

Elderly/adolescent: Start with 10 mg PO 3 times during day plus 20 mg PO at bedtime. A single maintenance dose of 40mg at bedtime may suffice.

Hospitalized patient may need 100 mg/day initially. If necessary, increase gradually to 200 mg/day (maximum 300 mg/day).

Intramuscular: 20–30mg 4 times a day. Switch to PO as soon as possible.

amoxapine (Asendin)   Supplied as: 25, 50, 100, 150 mg tablet.

Adult: Initially, 50 mg PO tid. Tolerance allowing, the dosage may be increased to 100mg PO bid–tid by end of first week. If necessary, increases above 300 mg/day may be made after 3 weeks of therapy if the patient has been receiving 300 mg/day for at least 2 weeks. Patients requiring more than 300 mg/day should have the daily dose divided. The maximum allowable daily dose is 400 mg in outpatient and 600 mg in inpatient. Maintenance: give smallest effective dose as a single bedtime dose if the requirement is 300 mg/day or less.

Elderly: Initially, 25 mg PO bid–tid. Tolerance allowing, dose may be increased to 50 mg PO tid by end of first week. Maintenance: Give smallest effective dose as a single bedtime dose. Maximum 300mg/day.

desipramine (Norpramin: 10, 25, 50, 75, 100, 150 mg tablet)
                            (Pertofrane: 25, 50 mg capsule).

Adult: Initially, 75 mg/day as divided or single bedtime dose. Increase stepwise to 150 mg/day in divided doses by end of first week. If a satisfactory response has not been achieved after 2 weeks, the dose may be increased as needed at weekly intervals by 50 mg/day increments up to maximum of 300 mg/day in divided doses. Titration to 300 mg/day should be done in hospital setting with EKG's. Maintenance: Use smallest effective daily dosage (as divided daily dose or as single bedtime dose). Usual maintenance requirement is 75–150 mg/day.

Elderly/adolescent: Initially, 25–50 mg/day. Increase gradually as needed to 100 mg/day. Use smallest effective daily dosage (as divided daily dose or single bedtime dose). Maximum 150 mg/day.

doxepin (Sinequan, Adapin)

Supplied as: capsule (10, 25, 50, 75, 100, 150 mg); oral concentrate (10mg/ml).

Adult: Initially, 25mg PO tid. Increase or decrease according to response. Usual maintenance requirement is 75–150 mg/day which may be given as a single bedtime dose. 25–50 mg/day may suffice in mild cases. In severe cases, one may start with 50 mg tid, and if necessary increase gradually up to maximum 300 mg/day (divide daily dose if > 150mg/day is required).

imipramine (Tofranil, Janimine)

Supplied as: tablet (10, 25, 50 mg); IM injection (25mg/2ml).

Adult, outpatient: Initially, 75 mg/day in divided doses. Increase to 150 mg/day in divided doses. If the response is not satisfactory after 2 weeks, the dose may be increased to 200 mg/day divided. Maintenance: 50–150 mg/day which may be given as a single bedtime dose.

Adult, hospitalized: Start with 100 mg/day in divided doses. If necessary, increase gradually to 200 mg/day in divided doses. If response is still inadequate after 2 weeks, the dose may be increased gradually to 250–300 mg/day in divided doses.

Elderly/adolescent: Initially, 30–40 mg/day PO. Increase gradually as needed up to 100 mg/day. Maintenance requirement may be given as a single bedtime dose.

Intramuscular: Initially, up to 100 mg/day in divided doses. Switch to PO as soon as possible.

Enuresis in child 6 yr or older: Initially, 25 mg PO 1 hour before bedtime. If no response in 1 week, increase dose to 50 mg PO before bedtime in child under 12 yr, and up to 75 mg PO before bedtime in child over 12 yr.

nortriptyline (Pamelor)
Supplied as: capsule (10, 25, 75 mg); oral solution (10mg/5ml).
Adult: Start with low dose and increase as needed. Usual requirement is 25 mg PO tid–qid. Daily requirement may also be given as a single daily dose. Use smallest effective dose. Maximum 150 mg/day. Patients requiring > 100 mg/day should have dose adjusted to maintain serum level of 50–150 ng/ml.
Elderly/adolescent: 30–50 mg/day in divided doses or as single bedtime dose.

protriptyline (Vivactil)   Supplied as: 5, 10 mg tablet.
Adult: 15–40 mg/day PO divided into 3–4 doses. Increase as needed up to maximum 60 mg/day by increasing the morning dose. Use smallest effective dose.
Elderly/adolescent: Initially, 5 mg PO tid. Monitor cardiovascular system in elderly patient requiring more than 20 mg/day.

trimipramine (Surmontil)   Supplied as: 25, 50, 100 mg tablets.
Adult outpatient: Initially, 75 mg/day in divided doses. Increase gradually as needed to 150 mg/day (maximum 200 mg/day). Maintenance: 50–150 mg/day which may be given as single bedtime dose.
Adult inpatient: Initially, 100 mg/day in divided doses. Increase gradually as needed to 200 mg/day. If no response after 2–3 weeks, increase up to maximum of 250–300 mg/day in divided doses.
Elderly/adolescent: Initially 50 mg/day. If necessary, increase the dose gradually up to 100 mg/day. Maintenance: use smallest effective dose. This may be given as single bedtime dose.

TRIMETHOBENZAMIDE (Tigan)

Action: Suppresses nausea and vomiting perhaps by acting on the chemoreceptor trigger zone of the medulla.
Indication: Control of nausea and vomiting (e.g. postoperative nausea/vomiting, radiation sickness, gastroenteritis). Note: This drug is *not* useful for controlling vertigo or motion-sickness.
Contraindications: hypersensitivity to drug, administration of suppository to patient sensitive to benzocaine or similar local anesthetics, suppository in premature or newborn infants, intramuscular administration in children.
Caution: Pregnancy or nursing mother; safety not established. Children; Antiemetics are not recommended for uncomplicated vomiting in children. Reserve use for prolonged vomiting of *known* cause because (1) there is concern that antiemetics may contribute to development of or adversely affect the course of Reye's syndrome, (2) this drug may cause extrapyramidal side effects and thus suggest that vomiting is due to an undiagnosed disorder associated with CNS effects (e.g. Reye's syndrome or other encephalopathy). Acute febrile illness, encephalitides, gastroenteritis, dehydration, electrolyte imbalance: Because of concern of possibly precipitating CNS reactions (e.g. extrapyramidal symptoms, seizures, coma) in these patients; this drug or other antiemetics should be administered cautiously—especially to children, the aged, the debilitated, or those receiving other CNS–acting drugs (e.g. phenothiazines, barbiturates). Patients who will be engaged in hazardous activities requiring alertness: Caution is advised since drowsiness is a possible side effect.
Side effects: drowsiness, headache, dizziness, disorientation, depression, blurred vision, extra pyramidal symptoms, seizures, coma, muscle cramps, diarrhea, jaundice, hypersensitivity reactions, blood dyscrasias.
Supplied as: capsule (100, 250 mg);
            suppository (100mg pediatric and 200mg adult);
            IM injection (100 mg/ml).
Adult dose: 250 mg tid–qid PO, or 200mg tid–qid IM or suppository.
Pediatric dose: 4–5 mg/kg PO or PR q6–8h. Note: IM contraindicated in children.

VALPROIC ACID (Depakene)

Indications: ●Sole or adjunctive therapy of simple absence (petit mal) seizures or complex absence seizures. ●Multiple seizure types which include absence seizures.

Contraindications: valproic acid hypersensitivity, hepatic disease or significant hepatic dysfunction.

Caution: pregnancy (use only if clearly needed, drug may be teratogenic); nursing mother; history of hepatic disease.

Comments: Usual therapeutic level is 50–100 mcg/ml. Hepatic complications: Fatal hepatic failure has resulted from valproic acid therapy, usually during first 6 months treatment. Patients < 2 yr of age are at increased risk. Liver function tests are advised before beginning therapy and frequently thereafter, especially during first 6 months of therapy. Manifestations of liver toxicity may include loss of seizure control, anorexia, vomiting, malaise, weakness, lethargy, facial edema. Valproic acid should be stopped immediately if there is known or suspected liver dysfunction, or if clinically significant hyperammonemia develops. Hyperammonemia may be present in absence of lethargy, coma, or abnormal liver function tests. Platelet and coagulation effects: Valproic acid inhibits platelet aggregation and thrombocytopenia occurs occasionally. Platelet count and coagulation tests are therefore recommended prior to starting treatment and then periodically. Dose reduction or discontinuation is advised if bruising, hemorrhage, or abnormal coagulation/hemostasis occur. Use caution if other drugs affecting coagulation are administered concurrently. Sedation/CNS depression; Until the sedative effects are assessed, valproic acid must be used cautiously in patients who engage in hazardous activities. Sedation is potentiated by other CNS depressants—e.g. alcohol, phenobarbital, primidone. Concurrent administration of phenobarbital or primidone (which is partially metabolized to phenobarbital) has been associated with severe CNS depression. Monitoring of phenobarbital levels and neurologic status is advised. Phenytoin may interact adversely with valproic acid—e.g. phenytoin toxicity may occur, seizures may recur. Clonazepam administered concurrently with valproic acid has been associated with absence status epilepticus in a few patients.

Side effects: Note: Because valproic acid is often prescribed in combination with other antiepileptics, it is usually impossible to ascribe a particular side effect solely to valproic acid or to the combination of antiepileptics. gastrointestinal; nausea, vomiting, indigestion, diarrhea, abdominal cramps, constipation, anorexia with weight loss, increased appetite with weight gain; neuro/psychiatric; sedation, headache, dizziness, tremor, ataxia, dysarthria, asterixis, weakness, nystagmus, diplopia, "spots before eyes", depression, emotional upset, hyperactivity, aggression, behavioral deterioration, psychosis; skin; itching, rash, erythema mulitforme, transient alopecia; blood; thrombocytopenia, alterered bleeding time, petechiae, bruising, hematoma, hemorrhage, hypofibrinoginemia, relative lymphocytosis, leukopenia, anemia, bone marrow depression; liver; elevated transaminases, elevated bilirubin; other; pancreatitis, hyperglycemia, irregular menses, secondary amenorrhea, breast enlargement, galactorrhea, hyperammonemia, abnormal thyroid function tests.

Supplied as: 250 mg capsule, 250 mg/5ml syrup.

Dose (adult or child): 15 mg/kg/day PO initially. Increase daily dose by 5–10 mg/kg/day at weekly intervals until seizures controlled or side effects occur. Maximum dose 60 mg/kg/day. Divide daily dose into 2–3 doses if greater than 250 mg/day is required. Usual requirement is 1000–3000 mg/day in adult and 15–60 mg/kg/day in child.

VANCOMYCIN (Vancocin)

Action: Glycopeptide antibiotic. Bactericidal spectrum includes staphylococci (including methicillin--resistant strains), beta–hemolytic streptococci, Streptococcus viridans, S. bovis, pneumococcus, enterococcus, gonococcus, diphtheria, clostridia, actinomyces, Listeria monocytogenes, anthrax. Resistance: Vancomycin is not active against gram–negative bacilli.

Indications: ●Severe staphylococcal infections resistant to penicillins (including penicillinase–resistant penicillins) or cephalosporins. ●Patient with serious infection due to staphylococci or enterococci who is allergic to both penicillins and cephalosporins. ●Adjunct to aminoglycoside in treatment of enterococcal endocarditis. ●Orally administered vancomycin is used in treatment of staphylococcal enterocolitis or pseudomembranous colitis due to Clostridium difficile.

Contraindications: vancomycin hypersensitivity.

Caution: renal dysfunction, hearing impaired, elderly, infants, concurrent or sequential use of other nephrotoxic or neurotoxic/ototoxic drugs, pregnancy (use only if clearly needed).

Comments: Nephrotoxicity and ototoxicity: Because vancomycin is potentially nephrotoxic and ototoxic, care should be taken not to exceed dosage recommendations. Serial renal function testing is advised if there is renal impairment, if the patient is receiving other nephrotoxic/ototoxic drugs (e.g. aminoglycoside), or if therapy is continued for over a week. Serial hearing testing is also recommended. Reversible neutropenia sometimes occurs. Periodic WBC count is advised if therapy is prolonged. Avoid rapid intravenous administration because hypotension or cardiac arrest may result. Doses are to be diluted and infused over at least 60 minutes. Staphylococcal endocarditis shoud be treated for at least 3 weeks.

Side effects: fever, chills, thrombophlebitis, nephrotoxicity, ototoxicity, rash, urticaria, anaphylaxis, eosinophilia, neutropenia.

Supplied as: intravenous injection preparation; capsule (125, 250mg); oral solution.
Adult dose:
  Intravenous: 500 mg q6h or 1000 mg q12h. Infuse over at least 60 minutes.
  ●Dose adjustment , renal failure: <u>creatinine clearance</u> : <u>dosage</u>

50–80 ml/min:	1 gram q24–72h
10–50 ml/min:	1 gram at 3–7 day intervals
less than 10 ml/min:	1 gram at 7 day intervals

  Oral (for treatment of enterocolitis): 500 mg q6h.
Pediatric dose: 40 mg/kg/24hr IV divided q6–12h.
  Neonate ≤ 7 days of age: 30 mg/kg/day divided q12h.

VASOPRESSIN (Pitressin)
DESMOPRESSIN (DDAVP, Stimate)
LYPRESSIN (Diapid)

Action: ●Induces a cyclic AMP–mediated increase in the permeability of renal collecting tubules to water. Consequently, there is an increase in the reabsorption of solute–free water and thus an increase in urine osmolality. ●Induces constriction of smooth muscle of blood vessels, intestine, and uterus. ●Desmopressin stimulates release of coagulation factor VIII–C and von Willebrand factor from endothelial cells.
Indications: ●central diabetes insipidus (these agents are not effective in nephrogenic diabetes insipidus), ●mild hemophilia A (desmopressin), ●mild von Willebrand's disease (desmopressin), ●prevention/treatment of postsurgical abdominal distension (vasopressin), ●to dispel interfering gas shadows in abdominal roentgenography (vasopressin).
Contraindications: hypersensitivity to components. ●For restrictions on use of desmopressin in particular, see "Dose, hemophilia A or mild to moderate von Willebrand's disease" below.
Caution: vascular disease (especially coronary artery disease), hypertensive cardiovascular disease, pregnancy. ●These agents can cause water intoxication and hyponatremia. This is especially true in patients not being treated for diabetes Insipidus. If this is the case, the patient should ingest only enough fluid to satisfy thirst. Urine volume, urine osmolality, and plasma osmolality may be used to monitor patient. Drowsiness, lethargy, and headache are early warnings of water intoxication.
Side effects: <u>vasopressin</u>; tremor, sweating, vertigo, circumoral pallor, "pounding" in head, abdominal cramps, flatus, nausea, vomiting, urticaria, bronchial constriction, anaphylaxis; <u>desmopressin acetate injection</u>; headache, nausea, abdominal cramps, vulva pain, facial flushing, slight increase blood pressure; <u>desmopressin acetate intranasal</u>; nasal congestion, rhinitis, flushing, headache, nausea, abdominal cramps; <u>lypressin</u>; nasal congestion; rhinorrhea; irritation and itching of nasal passages; nasal ulceration; headache; abdominal cramps and increase in bowel movements; conjunctivitis; periorbital edema with itching; heartburn (due to excessive nasal administration with drippage into pharynx); inadvertant inhalation with substernal tightness, cough, and/or dyspnea.
Supplied as:
<u>vasopressin injection</u> (Pitressin): 0.5 and 1 ml ampule containing 20 pressor units/ml for IM or SC injection;
<u>vasopressin tennate in oil</u> (Pitressin Tannate in oil): 1 ml ampule containing 5 pressor units/ml for IM injection;
<u>desmopressin acetate Injection</u> (DDAVP injection, Stimate): 1 ml ampule (DDAVP) and 10 ml multiple dose vial (Stimate) both containing 4 mcg/ml for IV or SC injection;
<u>desmopressin acetate intranasal</u> (DDAVP): 2.5 ml vial;
<u>lypressin nasal solution</u> (Diapid) : 8 ml plastic bottle (0.185 mcg/ml = 50 pressor units/ml).

Dose, central diabetes insipidus (deficiency of endogenous antidiuretic hormone):
<u>Vasopressin tannate injection;</u> Individualize dosage, 5–10 units (0.25–0.5 ml) 2–3 times a day IM or SC.
<u>Vasopressin tannate in oil injection;</u> Individualize dosage, 1.5–5 units (0.3–1ml) IM at 1–4 day intervals.
<u>Lypressin nasal spray</u> (adult or child): Individualize dosage. 1–2 sprays in each nostril qid is usual dosage; give an additional dose at bedtime if nocturia is present. Patients needing more than 2 sprays/nostril q4–6h should receive additional doses at shorter intervals rather than increasing the number of sprays/dose (more than 2–3 sprays/nostril results in wastage).

Desmopressin acetate (intranasal via plastic tube): Individualize dosage. Usual adult dosage is 0.1–0.4 ml/day as single dose or divided into 2–3 doses. For children 3 months–12 yr, the usual dosage is 0.05–0.3 ml/day as single daily dose or divided into 2 doses.

Desmopressin acetate Injection: Individualize dosage. Usual adult dosage is 0.5–1 ml/day IV of SC usually divided into 2 doses. Adjust AM and PM doses separately for optimum effect.

Dose, hemophilia A or mild–moderate von Willebrand's disease (type I):

Desmopressin acetate injection: 0.3 mcg/kg diluted in sterile hypotonic saline and infused slowly over 15–30 minutes while monitoring blood pressure and pulse. Use 50 ml of diluent if patient over 10 kg and 10 ml if less than 10 kg. If desmopressin is given preoperatively, it should be given 30 minutes before the procedure. NOTE: **(1)** Uses for desmopressin: to provide hemostasis during surgical procedures; and to provide hemostasis in the setting of spontaneous or traumatically–induced hemarthrosis, intramuscular hematomas, or mucosal bleeding. **(2)** In hemophilia A, desmopressin is indicated only if factor VIII coagulant activity is > 5%, and it is not indicated in a patient with factor VIII antibodies. **(3)** Desmopressin is not indicated for treatment of Hemophilia B. **(4)** Desmopressin is contraindicated in Von Willebrand's type II–B and pseudo von Willebrand's disease. It is not indicated for treatment of severe von Willebrand's type I or if there is an abnormal molecular form of factor VIII antigen. **(5)** In infants < 3 months of age, desmopressin is contraindicated in treatment of coagulation defects/deficiencies.

VITAMIN D and ANALOGS:

Vitamin D2 [ergocalciferol] (Calciferol)
dihydrotachysterol (DHT)
calcitriol (Rocaltrol, Calcijex)

Action: ●The metabolites of vitamin D and the vitamin D analogs promote intestinal absorption of calcium, phosphorus, and magnesium. Large amounts of Vitamin D or therapeutic doses of the analogs also mobilize calcium from bone and thus exert a hypercalcemic effect similar to parathyroid hormone. ●Vitamin D2 (ergocalciferol) is derived by the ultraviolet irradiation of the plant sterol ergosterol. Vitamin D3 (cholecalciferol) occurs naturally (e.g. fish liver oils), and is formed by ultraviolet irradiation of 7–dehydrocholesterol in the subcutaneous tissue. Both Vitamin D2 and D3 undergo hypdroxylation (on the 25 position in the liver and the 1 position in the kidney) to form the active metabolite 1, 25 dehydroxy Vitamin D. ●Dihydrotachysterol is a synthetic Vitamin D analog. It undergoes hydroxylation in the liver (but not in the kidney) to form the active metabolite. ●Calcitriol is the synthetic preparation of 1, 25 dehydroxy vitamin D3. It acts rapidly since it does not require renal or hepatic activation.
Contraindications: hypercalcemia, hypervitaminosis D.
Caution: pregnancy, nursing mother.
Comments: An adequate dietary intake of calcium must be assured since the function of vitamin D metabolites and vitamin D analogs is to promote the intestinal absorption of calcium and bone mineralization. Laboratory testing including monitoring of serum calcium: Check serum calcium periodically to preclude development of hypercalcemia. This should be done twice weekly at first and then periodically after the serum calcium has been stabilized. Dosage should be titrated to achieve a serum calcium of 9–10 mg/dl. Also check following periodically: serum phosphorus, magnesium, serum alkaline phosphatase, and (with the exception of renal dialysis patient) 24 hr urinary calcium and phosphate. Serum alkaline phosphatase is an useful indicator of impending hypercalcemia because it usually decreases prior to development of hypercalcemia. Renal dialysis patients and patients with hyperphosphatemia should take aluminum hydroxide antacids (e.g. Amphogel) and restrict dietary phosphorus in order to control serum phophate level and thereby prevent ectopic calcification. Magnesium–containing antacids should be avoided in chronic renal dialysis patients because of risk of hypermagnesemia. Time course of pharmacologic activity: With ergosterol, the blood calcium elevating effect becomes evident 10–24 hours following initiation of therapy (although the therapeutic effectiveness may not be apparent for 2 wk or so); the peak effect with daily administration is seen in 4 weeks; and the duration of effect may be 2 months or more. Dihydrotachysterol acts more quickly and the duration of effect is shorter. Calcitriol has the most rapid onset of activity and the shortest duration of action (3–5 days). The practical significance of these differences is that in the case of the rapid onset–short duration form calcitriol: (1) hypocalcemia is corrected quickly, (2) hypercalcemia can develop rapidly if care is not taken, (3) hypercalcemia resolves quickly upon discontinuing calcitriol. In the case of the slow onset–long duration form ergosterol, the therapeutic effectiveness may not become apparent for weeks and toxicity should it occur may be prolonged (2–3 months or more). Dihydrotachysterol–induced hypercalcemia will resolve within 1–3 weeks after the drug is stopped.

Supplied as:
vitamin D2 [ergocalciferol] (Calciferol):   50,000 IU (1.25 mg) tablet;
    8,000 IU/ml oral solution;   500,000 IU/ml (12.5 mg/ml) for IM injection;
Vitamin D3 (cholecalciferol) is found in cod liver oil, and in fish liver oil–containing
OTC vitamin capsules.
dihydrotachysterol: tablet (0.125, 0.2, 0.4 mg);   oral solution (0.2mg/ml);
calcitriol: capsules (0.25, 0.5 mcg);   IV injection (1 mcg/ml, 2 mcg/ml).

Dietary vitamin D maintenance requirements under normal conditions:
400 IU Vitamin D/day.

Dose, rickets: rickets secondary to vitamin D deficiency: Start with 1000–4000
IU/day ergocalciferol. Maintenance dose is 400 IU/day. genetic vitamin D–dependent rickets; 5000—50,000 IU/day ergocalciferol; vitamin D–resistant rickets:
50,000–500,000 IU/day ergocalciferol. NOTE: Treatment of rickets should also include a good diet with high intake of phosphorous and also calcium supplements.

Dose, familial hypophosphatemia: 10,000–80,000 IU/day ergosterol plus 1–2
gram elemental phosphorous/day.

Dose, osteomalacia: secondary to vitamin D deficiency: start with 1000–2000
IU/day ergocalciferol. Maintenance dose is 400 IU/day. secondary to malabsorption: 10,000–50,000 IU/day ergocalciferol in adult and 10,000–25,000 IU/day in
child; secondary to anticonvulsant medication: 1000 IU/day ergocalciferol in adult
or child. NOTE: A good diet including adequate calcium intake should be assured
when treating osteomalacia.

Dose, hypoparathyroidism: With dihydrotachysterol (DHT): Start with 0.8–2.4
mg/day for several days. Adjust dose to maintain serum calcium at 8.5–9.0
mg/100ml. Usual maintenance dose is 0.2–1.0 mg/day. With vitamin D2
[ergocalciferol] (Calciferol): Start with 20,000 IU/day. Increase dose gradually allowing serum calcium to reach a steady level before each increase. Up to 400,000
IU/day may be required. Usual requirement is 40,000–120,000 IU/day. With
calcitriol: Start with 0.25 mcg/day PO. Increase dose as needed at 2–4 week intervals. Determine serum calcium twice weekly during titration period. Stop calcitriol
immediately if hypercalcemia develops and do not resume drug until there is
normocalcemia. Usual PO range is 0.25–2 mcg/day in patients 6 yr and older, and
0.25–0.75 mcg/day in patients 1–5 yr.

Control hypocalcemia in chronic renal dialysis patient: Calcitriol; Start with
0.25 mcg/day PO as a single morning dose. If necessary, titrate upward by 0.25
mcg/day increments at 4–8 week intervals. Determine serum calcium twice weekly
during titration period. Stop calcitriol immediately if hypercalcemia develops and do
not resume drug until there is normocalcemia. Usual PO requirements range from
0.25 mcg every other day to 1.0 mcg once daily. ●If the IV injection form (Calcijex) is
used, start with 0.5 mcg three times per week. If necessary, titrate upward by 0.25–
0.5 mcg increments at 2–4 week intervals. Determine serum calcium and phosphorus at least twice weekly while titrating. Stop calcitriol immediately if hypercalcemia
develops and do not resume drug until there is normocalcemia. Usual IV requirement is 0.5–3.0 mcg (0.01–0.05 mcg/kg) three times per week.

VITAMIN K 3 derivative
[menadiol sodium diphosphate] (Synkayvite)

Action: Water-soluble synthetic vitamin K. Promotes hepatic synthesis of coagulation factors II, VII, IX, and X.

Indications: ●treatment/prevention of hypoprothrombinemia due to impaired GI bacterial synthesis of vitamin K or due to impaired GI absorption of vitamin K (e.g. as a consequence of antibacterial therapy, intestinal resection, inflammatory bowel disease, cystic fibrosis, sprue, celiac disease); ●hypoprothrombinemia due to salicylates.

Contraindications: hypersensitivity to components, prevention/treatment of hemorrhagic disease of newborn, last few weeks of pregnancy, oral anticoagulant–induced hypoprothrombinemia. Also, not recommended in patients with G6PD deficiency, obstructive jaundice, or biliary fistula.

Comments: Prothrombin time: The efficacy of and need for vitamin K administration is gauged by the prothrombin time. Contrasts between menadiol sodium diphophate and phytonadione (vitamin K1): **(1)** In contrast to vitamin K1 (phytonadione), oral anticoagulant–induced hypoprothrombinemia is not reversed by vitamin K3 (menadione). **(2)** Vitamin K3 (menadione) may cause hemolysis in patients with G6PD deficiency or in neonates. Therefore, it should be avoided during last few weeks of pregnancy, in neonates, and in patients with G6PD deficiency. In contrast, vitamin K1 (phytonadione) does not cause hemolysis in patients with G6PD deficiency, and it is less likely to cause hemolysis and hyperbilirubinemia in neonates. **(3)** Menadiol sodium diphosphate is water-soluble, a property that may facilitate GI absorption in conditions in which GI absorption is impaired.

Side effects: prolonged prothrombin time, rash, urticaria, hemolysis in G6PD-deficient patient, further depression of liver function in patient with severe liver disease. Furthermore, this drug may provoke hemolysis, hyperbilirubinemia and/or kernicterus in neonate.

Supplied as: 5 mg tablet; injection (5mg/ml, 10mg/ml, 75mg/2ml).

Dose: Adult: 5–15 mg once to twice daily PO, SC, IM, or IV.
Child: 5–10 mg once to twice daily PO, SC, IM, or IV.

VITAMIN K 1 [PHYTONADIONE]
(AquaMEPHYTON, Mephyton, Konakion)

Action: Naturally occurring vitamin K. Promotes hepatic synthesis of coagulation factors II, VII, IX, and X.

Indications: Treatment/prevention of hypoprothrombinemia secondary to: **(1)** oral anticoagulants; **(2)** impaired GI absorption/synthesis Vitamin K (e.g. as a consequence of antibacterial therapy, intestinal resection, inflammatory bowel disease, cystic fibrosis, obstructive jaundice); **(3)** hyperalimentation; **(4)** hemorrhagic disease of newborn.

Contraindication: hypersensitivity to any of components.

Caution/comments: **(1)** If reversal of hypoprothrombinemia is urgent (eg CNS bleed, severe hemorrhage); fresh frozen plasma or fresh whole blood should also be given. Factor IX concentrate may also be used but there is increased risk of hepatitis. **(2)** The onset of action (as reflected by shortened prothrombin time) after IV administration is 1–2 hours. Bleeding is usually controlled within 3–6 hours; the prothrombin time may return to normal in 12–24 hours. Duration of effect, 1-4 days. **(3)** If anticoagulation is essential (e.g. prosthetic heart valve), use the smallest effective dose of vitamin K. Fresh frozen plasma may be a better alternative since the prolonged effect of vitamin K may delay restoration of effective oral anticoagulation. If vitamin K is used, interim heparin anticoagulation may be required until effects of vitamin K diminish. **(4)** Vitamin K will not reverse the effects or control bleeding due to heparin administration. **(5)** Because of the risk of severe reactions (shock, cardac/respiratory arrest); IV administration of vitamin K should be limited to urgent cases or to cases in which other routes of administration are not possible. **(6)** Vitamin K is not effective in hypoprothrombinemia due to liver disease, and repeated large doses are not justified if an initial therapeutic response is not seen. Furthermore, vitamin K is not effective in hereditary hypoprothrombinemia; or in hereditary defects in the synthesis of factors VII, IX, or X. **(7)** Vitamin K is effective in hypoprothrombinemia secondary to salicylates, sulfonamides, quinidine, or antibiotics.

Side effects: flushing sensation, peculiar taste, dizziness, sweating, brief hypotension, rapid and weak pulse, dyspnea, cyanosis; injection site effects: pain, swelling, tenderness, hematoma; in neonates: hemolysis with ensuing hyperbilirubinermia; with IV administration: shock, cardiac and/or respiratory arrest.

Supplied as: 5 mg tablet (Mephyton);
1mg/0.5ml and 10mg/ml for IV, IM, SC injection (AquaMEPHYTON);
1mg/0.5ml and 10mg/ml for IM injection only (Konakion).

Dose:
Adult: The dose depends on the circumstance. Range is 2.5–25 mg (rarely 50 mg). For instance, a small dose might be adequate therapy for management of minor bleeding due to oral anticoagulant therapy (or simply skipping 1–2 oral anticoagulant doses may suffice). The adequacy of treatment and the need for further doses is

gauged by the prothrombin time which should be shortened within 6–8 hours. Oral or subcutaneous administration is preferred in nonurgent situations. Intramuscular administration may result in a hematoma if coagulation deficiency is marked. The IV route may have to be used if there is serious bleeding (dilute the dose in D5W or normal saline and inject very slowly, no faster than 1mg/min). Also administer 2–3 units of fresh frozen plasma if there is life–threatening hemorrhage.

<u>Pediatric:</u> depending on circumstances, 2.5–10 mg (2 mg infants). See adult dose above regarding route of administration.

<u>Neonate</u> (prevention/treatment of hemorrhagic disease newborn):

Prophylaxis: 1mg IM or SC.

Treatment: 1mg administered IM, SC, or IV depending on circumstances.

WARFARIN (Coumadin, Panwarfin)

Action: Vitamin K is required for the hepatic synthesis of coagulation factors II, VII, IX, X. Warfarin acts by interfering with vitamin K activity. Warfarin prevents formation or extension of clots but has no effect on established clots.

Indications: ●prophylaxis/treatment of venous thrombosis and pulmonary thromboembolus; ●prevention/treatment atrial fibrillation–associated thromboembolization; ●prevention of systemic thromboembolization following myocardial infarction.

Contraindications include: <u>patient who cannot be monitored</u> e.g. unreliable patient, inadequate laboratory; <u>bleeding or bleeding risk</u> e.g. CNS bleeding, active GI ulcer, hemophilia or other blood dyscrasias, dissecting aortic aneurysm, pericarditis, bacterial endocarditis, severe renal or liver disease, pregnancy, threatened abortion, eclampsia, preeclampsia, malignant hypertension, spinal puncture/anesthesia, recent or anticipated CNS or eye surgery, traumatic surgery resulting in large open surface.

Caution/comments: <u>Use warfarin with caution in the following circumstances:</u> moderate–severe renal or hepatic disease, severe diabetes mellitus, trauma with risk of internal bleeding, surgery, moderate–severe hypertension, vasculitis, protein C deficiency, nursing mother, elderly or debilitated patient. <u>Prothrombin time:</u> Obtain PT before starting warfarin and daily for first week. Then (if the PT is stable) weekly for one month, and monthly thereafter. <u>Switching from heparin to warfarin anticoagulation:</u> Since there is a delay of 24–48 hours before the PT begins to increase and 6–7 days before warfarin exerts its full effect, it is common practice to start heparin and warfarin together and discontinue heparin when the PT is adequately prolonged. *Continuous* IV heparin is preferred because fewer bleeding complications occur and because the PT (which is necessary to monitor warfarin therapy) is little affected. On the other hand, SC or *intermittent* IV heparin administration significantly prolongs the PT so that at least 5 hours must elapse after last IV heparin dose (24 hr after last SC dose) before a valid PT can be obtained. <u>Drug interactions:</u> A variety of diseases and numerous drugs enhance or suppress the activity of warfarin. Therefore, be alert for abnormal bleeding, petechiae, etc. And periodically monitor PT, hematocrit, urine for hematuria, and stool for occult blood. <u>IM injections</u> should be avoided in an anticoagulated patient. <u>Nursing infant of an anticoagulated mother</u> must have PT checked regularly. <u>Antidote to warfarin:</u> In urgent situations, 1–3 units of fresh frozen plasma will usually quickly reverse warfarin anticoagulation. Fresh frozen plasma is also the antidote of choice if the patient requires immediate reinstitution of warfarin anticoagulation. Vitamin K1 (AquaMEPHYTON) will also reverse warfarin effects but bleeding may not be controlled for 4–6 hours.

Side effects: bleeding. <u>Uncommon side effects</u> include fever, urticaria, dermatitis, alopecia, nausea, diarrhea, abdominal cramps, cholestasis, elevated transaminases, necrosis of skin or other tissues, purple toes syndrome.

Supplied as: 2, 2.5, 5, 7.5, 10 mg tablets.

Dose (adult): Start with 10 mg PO once daily for 3 days. Adjust dose to achieve prothrombin time of 1.5 times the control. Usual requirement is 2–10 mg once daily.

Drug Index

Drug Index

Drug Index

Drug Index

Drug Index

Drug Index

Drug Index

Drug Index

Drug Index

References:

Alpert, JS and Francis, GS.: Manual of Coronary Care, 4th edition, Boston, Little Brown and Company, 1987.
Ali Jameel et al: Advanced Trauma Life Support Course for Physicians, Committee on Trauma American College of Surgeons, Chicago, 1989.
Andreoli TE, Carpenter CCJ, Plum F, Smith Jr LH: Cecil Essentials of Medicine, Phila., W.B. Saunders Company, 1986.
Arndt, KA with collaboration Bernhardt, MS: Manual of Dermatologic Therapeutics, 4th edition, Boston, Little Brown and Company, 1988.
Barkin, Roger M. editor: Emergency Pediatrics, St Louis, C.V. Mosby Company, 1984.
Behrman, RE et al editors: Nelson Textbook of Pediatrics, 12th edition, Philadelphia, W.B. Saunders Company, 1983.
Behrman, RE et al editors: Nelson Textbook of Pediatrics, 13th edition, Philadelphia, W.B. Saunders Company, 1987.
Benitz, WE and Tatro, DS: The Pediatric Drug Handbook, 2nd edition, Chicago, Year Book Medical Publishers 1988.
Bennett, Donald R.: editor-in-chief: AMA Drug Evaluations, 5th edition, American Medical Association, Chicago, 1983.
Centers for Disease Control: Health Information for International Travel 1988, U.S. Department of Health and Human Services, Atlanta, Georgia.
Centers for Disease Control: 1989 Sexually Transmitted Diseases Treatment Guidelines; MMWR 1989; 38 (No.S-8); Atlanta, Georgia.
Cunningham, Gary F. et al: Williams Obstetrics, 18th edition, Norwalk, Conn., Appleton and Lange, 1989.
Dornbrand L, Hoole AJ, Fletcher RH, Pickard Jr CG: Manual of Clinical Problems in Adult Ambulatory Care, Boston, Little Brown and Company, 1985.
Davis, Bernard D.: Microbiology, 3rd edition, Philadelphia, JB Lippincott, 1980.
DeMyer, William: Technique of the Neurologic Examination a Programmed Text, 2nd edition, New York, McGraw-Hill Book Company, 1974.
Fishman, Mark C et al: Medicine, Philadelphia, J.B. Lippincott Company 1985.
Gangeness, DE and White, RD: Emergency Pharmacology, Bowie, Maryland, Robert J. Brady Company, 1984.
Ganong, William F.: Review of Medical Physiology, 6th edition, Los Altos, California, Lange Medical Publications 1973.
Goldberg, Stephen: Clinical Neuroanatomy Made Ridiculously Simple, Miami, Florida, MedMaster Inc, 1979.
Gomella, LG editor: Clinician's Pocket Reference, 4th edition, Norwalk, Connecticut, Appleton-Century-Crofts, 1983.
Harper, HA: Review of Physiological Chemistry, 14th edition, Los Altos, California, Lange Medical Publications, 1973.
Harris, JH and Harris, WH: The Radiology of Emergency Medicine, Baltimore, Williams and Wilkins Company, 1975.
Harvey, AM et al editors: Principles & Practice of Medicine, 21st ed, Norwalk, Conn., Appleton-Century-Crofts 1984.
Hatcher RA et al: Contraceptive Technology 1988-89, 14th revised edition, New York, Irvington Publishers Inc, 1988.
Havens, Carol et al editors: Manual of Outpatient Gynecology; Boston; Little, Brown, and Company; 1986.
Hershman, JM editor: Endocrine Pathophysiology: A Patient-Oriented Approach, 3rd ed, Phila., Lea & Febiger, 1988.
Jaffe, Allan S. et al, Textbook of Advanced Cardiac Life Support, American Heart Association, 1987.
Johns Hopkins Hospital Staff: The Harriet Lane Handbook, 11th edition, Chicago, Year Book Medical Publishers, 1987.
Julian, Desmond G.: Cardiology, 2nd edition, London, Bailliere Tindal, 1973.
Junqueira LC, Carneiro J, Contopoulos AN: Basic Histology, Los Altos, California, Lange Medical Publications 1975.
Kase NG and Weingold AB: Principles and Practice of Clinical Gynecology, New York, John Wiley and Sons, 1983.
Lampe, Kenneth F. editor-in-chief: Drug Evaluations, 6th edition, American Medical Association, Chicago, 1986.
Landow, Kenneth R.: Handbook of Dermatologic Treatment, Greenbrae, California, Jones Medical Publications, 1983.
Manual for Staging of Cancer, 3rd edition, American Joint Committee on Cancer, Philadelphia, JB Lippincott Company, 1988.
Marriott, Henry J. L.: Practical Electrocardiography, 6th edition, Baltimore, Williams and Wilkins Company, 1977.
Mazza, Joseph J. editor: Manual of Clinical Hematology, Boston, Little Brown and Company, 1988.
Jones Jr, HW et al: Novak's Textbook of Gynecology, 11th edition, Baltimore, Williams and Wilkins Company, 1988.
Markell, Edward K. et al: Medical Parasitology, 6th edition, Philadelphia, W.B. Saunders Co, 1986.
McEvoy, Gerald K. editor: American Hospital Formulary Service Drug Information; Bethesda, Maryland, American Society of Hospital Pharmacists, 1989.
National Cancer Institute, PDQ State-of-the-Art Cancer Treatment Information, 1988-1989.
Newell, Frank W.: Ophthalmology Principles and Concepts, 6th edition, St Louis, C.V. Mosby Company, 1986.
Niswander, Kenneth R. editor: Manual of Obstetrics, 3rd edition; Boston; Little, Brown & Co; 1987.
Orland, MJ and Saltman, RJ: Manual of Medical Therapeutics, 25th edition, Boston, Little Brown and Company, 1988.
Physicians Desk Reference, 44th edition, Medical Economics Company Inc., Oradell, New Jersey 1990.
Physicians Desk Reference, 45th edition, Medical Economics Company Inc., Oradell, New Jersey 1991.
Physicians Desk Reference for Nonprescription Drugs, 10th edition, Medical Economics Company Inc., Oradell, New Jersey 1989.
Roth CS, Weaver DT: Pocket Manual of Emergency Medical Therapy, 4th edition, Toronto, B.C. Decker Inc., 1987.
Sauer, Gordon C.: Manual of Skin Diseases, 5th edition, Philadelphia, J.B. Lippincott Company, 1986.
Schrier, Robert W. editor: Manual of Nephrology, 3rd edition; Boston; Little, Brown & Co; 1990.
Snell, Richard S.: Clinical Anatomy for Medical Students, Boston, Little Brown and Company, 1973.
Speroff, L. et al: Clinical Gynecologic Endocrinology & Infertility, 4th ed, Baltimore, Williams & Wilkins Company, 1988.
Franklin, Stanley S editor.: Practical Nephrology, New York, John Wiley & Sons, 1981.
Taber, Ben-Zion: Manual of Gynecologic & Obstetric Emergencies 2nd ed, Phila., W.B. Saunders Company, 1984.
Tietz, Norbert W.: Clinical Guide to Laboratory Tests, Philadelphia, W. B. Saunders Company, 1983.
Tintinalli, JE., Krome RL, Ruiz E Editors, Emergency Medicine -A Comprehensive Study Guide, 2nd edition, New York, McGraw-Hill Book Company, 1988.
Waterbury, Larry: Hematology for the House Officer 3rd edition, Baltimore, Williams and Wilkins Company, 1988.
Way, Lawrence W.: Current Surgical Diagnosis and Treatment, Norwalk, Conn., Appleton and Lange, 1988.
Weiner, Howard L. et al: Neurology for the House Officer, 4th edition, Baltimore, Williams and Wilkins Company, 1989.
Wyngaarden, JB & Smith, LH editors: Cecil Textbook of Medicine 17th ed, Phila., W.B. Saunders Company, 1985.
Wallach, Jacques: Interpretation of Diagnostic Tests, A Handbook Synopsis of Laboratory Medicine third edition; Boston; Little, Brown and Company, 1978.
Wynn, Ralph M.: Obstetrics and Gynecology, 4th edition, Philadelphia, Lea & Febiger, 1988.
Zagelbaum GL and Paré JAP: Manual of Acute Respiratory Care, Boston, Little Brown and Company, 1982.

Temperature conversion:

35.5 C = 96.0 F		39.0 C = 102.2 F	
36.1 C = 97.0 F		40.0 C = 104.0 F	
37.0 C = 98.6 F		41.0 C = 105.8 F	
38.0 C = 100.4 F		43.3 C = 110.0 F	

Estimated weight by age:

term newborn	3–4 kg	2 yr	12–14 kg	8 yr	26–30 kg
6 month	7–8.5 kg	4 yr	16–18 kg	10 yr	about 35 kg
1 year	10–11 kg	6 yr	20–24 kg	12 yr	about 45 kg.

Vital Signs:

	systolic BP	heart rate	resp rate
newborn	50–70	70–190	~ 40
1 month	64–96	80–160	24–30
6 month	60–118	80–160	
1 yr	66–126		20–24
2 yr	80–112	80–130	
4 yr	80–112	80–120	14–20
6 yr	80–115		
8 yr	85–120	70–110	12–20
10 yr	90–130		
12 yr	95–130	65–110	12–20

Normal Adult Resting Cardiac Values:

Right atrial pressure: 1.0–7.5 mm Hg.

Right ventricle pressure (mm Hg): systolic 15–32, diastolic 0–8.

Pulmonary artery wedge pressure (mm Hg): systolic 15–32, diastolic 4–15, mean 10–20.

Pulmonary capillary wedge : 4.5–13 mm Hg.

Left atrial pressure: 1–21 mm Hg.

Left ventricle pressure (mm Hg): systolic 90–140, diastolic 5–12.

Cardiac output: 4–8 liters/minute.

Cardiac index: 2.5–3.5 liters/minute/sq. meter.

Hematology/Coagulation:

	hemoglobin (gram/dl)	hematocrit (percent)	WBC Count (x 1000/cu mm)
1 day +	17.0–21.0	57–68	7–35
1–4 wk	15.0–20.0	46–62	5–20
2 month	9.0–14.0	28–42	6–18
6 mo–6 yr	10.5–14.0	33–42	6–15
6–12 yr	11.0–16.0	35–45	4.5–13.5
adult female	12.0 ± 2.0	41 ± 5	4–11
adult male	14.0 ± 2.0	47 ± 6	4–11

Mean corpuscular volume (MCV) is normally 80–100 cu micron in adult. From 6 to 12 yr of age, the normal range is 77–95. In infants the normal range is 70–86. Normal neonates have MCV of 107–129.

Mean corpuscular hemoglobin concentration (MCHC) is normally 31–36 in adults and children.

Reticulocyte count: 0.2–2.0 %.

Platelet count: 150,000–400,000/cu mm.
In the first wk of life, the normal range is 84,000–478,000.

Erythrocyte sedimentation rate (mm/hr):

	child	adult male	adult female
Wintrobe method:	0–13	0–9	0–20
Westergren method:	0–10	0–15*	0–20*

*0–20 in male > 50 yr, 0–30 in female > 50 yr.

Bleeding time (Ivy): 2–7 minutes.
Partial thromboplastin time, activated (aPTT): 25–35 seconds.
Prothrombin time (one stage): 11–15 seconds.
Thrombin time: ± 2 seconds of control time with control time of 11–13 seconds.
Fibrinogen: 200–400 mg/100ml.

Arterial blood gas:

pH	7.35–7.45	
pCO2	35–45 mm Hg	
pO2	75–105 mm Hg	(decreases with age and altitude)
oxygen saturation	95–100%	
carbon dioxide content	22–31 mEq/liter	
carboxyhemoglobin (COHb)	normally < 2% in nonsmoker.	
	May be 5–20% in smoker.	

Serum chemistries:

osmolality		270–295 mOsm/kg
anion gap [Na - (Cl + HCO3)]		7–14 mmole/liter.
sodium		135–145 mEq/liter
potassium		3.5–5.0 mEq/liter
chloride		95–105 mEq/liter
bicarbonate		22–30 mEq/liter
calcium	adult	8.4–10.3 mg/100ml
	child	8.8–10.8 mg/100ml
magnesium		1.5–2.5 mEq/liter
phosphorus		
	adult	2.5–4.5 mg/100ml
	child	4.5–5.5 mg/100ml
ammonia		11–35 μ mol/liter
		(may be higher in neonates)
creatinine		
	adult	0.5 –1.2 mg/100ml
	child	0.3–0.7 mg/100ml
urea nitrogen (BUN)		7–25 mg/100ml

(1) The higher levels expected following high protein intake.
(2) Lower limit is 5 mg/100ml in infant or child.

bilirubin, direct		0.0–0.2 mg/100ml
bilirubin, total		0.2–1.0 mg/100ml

Higher total bilirubin may normally occur in first few days
of life. However, in fullterm newborn, the serum level
should normally be < 6 mg/100ml in the first 24 hr and
< 12 mg/100ml on days 3–5. Premature infants
commonly have yet higher levels. The presence of
jaundice implies a total bilirubin ≥ 5 mg/100ml.

cholesterol, total		
	child	120–200 mg/100ml
	adult	130–300 mg/100ml
		(< 220 desirable in adult)
albumin (adult)		3.5–5.0 gram/100ml
protein, total (adult)		6.0–8.5 gram/100ml
uric acid		3.0–8.0 mg/100ml

Normal levels selected drugs:

digoxin	0.5–2.0 ng/ml
lithium	0.6–1.2 mmol/liter
phenobarbital	15–40 mg/liter
phenytoin	10–20 mg/liter
primidone	
primidone	5–15 mg/liter
phenobarbital	15–40 mg/liter
quinidine	1.3–5.0 mg/liter
salicylate	15–30 mg/dl (toxic > 30 mg/dl)
theophylline	10–20 mg/liter
valproic acid	50–100 mg/liter

Suggested format hospital admission orders:

<u>Date and time</u>:
<u>Admit to</u>:   ward ?   physician ?
<u>Diagnosis</u>:
<u>Condition</u>: (e.g. critical, serious, satisfactory).
<u>Allergies</u>:
<u>Vital signs</u> taken every (e.g. 15 minute, hour, 8hr).
  *Notify physician if blood pressure, pulse rate, or temperature are not within ac
  ceptable limits and state those limits according to the clinical circumstances.
  *Also include here whether you want other important parameters monitored and
  how often (e.g. urine output, neurologic status).
<u>Activity</u>: e.g. bed rest ?, bed rest with commode priviliges ?, bathroom priviliges ?,
  sit in chair ?, ad lib ?
<u>Nursing</u>: e.g. oxygen (? liters/minute, nasal catheter ? mask ?), Foley catheter ?,
  daily weight ?, record input/output ?, instructions for wound care ?, etc.
<u>Diet</u>: e.g. NPO ?; clear liquid ?; soft diet ?; bland diet ?; regular diet ?; salt restric
  tion (e.g. no added salt, 2 gram sodium) ?; fluid restriction ?; caloric restriction
  (e.g. 1500 calorie diabetic diet) ?
<u>Intravenous fluid orders</u>:
<u>Medications</u>:
<u>Laboratory tests</u>: Tests commonly ordered include CBC, urinalysis, blood chemistry
  panel. chest x-ray, EKG.
<u>Additional tests/procedures</u> to be arranged according to circumstances: e.g. CAT
  scan or other special radiologic tests, echocardiogram, EEG, treadmill,
  endoscopy, etc.
<u>Specialized personnel to be contacted</u> (e.g. surgeon, physical therapist, respiratory
  therapist) as circumstances dictate.
<u>Consent</u> for surgery or other invasive procedures.

Post-operative note:

Preoperative diagnosis:
Postoperative diagnosis:
Operation:
Surgeon: Assistant: Anesthesiologist:
Type anesthesia (general, local, spinal).
Complications:
Estimated blood loss:
Fluids:
Drains (location):
Specimens obtained and result of frozen section.
Patient condition:

Post-partum note:

<u>Time labor began</u>; spontaneous or oxytocin-induced ?
<u>Rupture of membranes</u>: time ? spontaneous or artificially ruptured ?
<u>Medications</u> administered during labor and delivery:
<u>Anesthesia</u> (e.g. local, epidural, pudental)
<u>Time of delivery</u>:
<u>Delivery description</u>: pesentation (vertex, breech ?); forceps ? midline episiotomy ?
<u>Infant</u>: sex, weight, APGAR. See that gonococcal eye prophylaxis (e.g. silver nitrate,
erythromycin) and vitamin K (1 mg IM) are administered and so state.
<u>Placenta</u>: time of delivery ? intact ? cord with one vein and 2 arteries ?
<u>Pitocin administered post-partum</u> ?
<u>Episiotomy or laceration</u>: If lacerated, to what extent (1st, 2nd, or 3rd degree) ?
                  Repair (simple ?, type of suture ?).
<u>Fluids given to mother</u>:
<u>Estimated maternal blood loss</u>:
<u>Condition of mother and infant</u> upon leaving for recovery room:
<u>Rh immune status</u>: Mother Rh negative or positive ? Verify that specimen of mater-
nal blood and cord blood has been sent to lab for antibody screen and so state.

Routine Postpartum Orders:

<u>Allergies:</u>

<u>Vital signs:</u>
- ❑ Immediate postpartum: Check signs every 15 minutes for one hour or until stable.
- ❑ Subsequently, check vitals q 8 hours or according to usual routine.

<u>Intravenous fluids:</u>
- ❑ Discontinue if patient is stable.
- ❑ Other.

<u>Postpartum bleeding:</u>
- ❑ Methergine 0.2mg PO q4h for excessive bleeding (provided patient is normotensive).
- ❑ Notify physician if bleeding unusually heavy or vital signs abnormal.

<u>Activity:</u>
- ❑ Bed rest immediately postpartum.
- ❑ Then, ambulate ad lib if stable.

<u>Diet:</u>
- ❑ house.
- ❑ other:

<u>Perineal care:</u>
- ❑ Ice pack to perineum immediate postpartum.
- ❑ Sitz baths 3 times/day and prior to bedtime prn perineal pain or swelling.
- ❑ Tucks and Dermoplast to perineum if there is pain/discomfort from episiotomy or hemorrhoids.

<u>Stool softener and/or laxative:</u>
- ❑ Docusate calcium (Surfak) 240mg, one capsule per day.
- ❑ Milk of magnesia, 30ml PO qhs prn constipation.

<u>Urinary retention:</u>
- ❑ Catheterize at 4–6 hour intervals.
- ❑ Insert Foley catheter for 24 hours.

<u>Analgesia:</u>
- ❑ Tylenol #3, 1–2 tablets PO q3–4 hours prn mild to moderate pain.
- ❑ Meperidine (Demerol) 50–100mg q3–4 hours prn severe pain.

<u>Nausea/vomiting:</u>
- ❑ Promethazine (Phenergan) 12.5–25mg q4–6 hours IM.

<u>Insomnia:</u>
- ❑ Flurazepam (Dalmane) 15–30 mg PO prn sleep.
- ❑ Other:

<u>Lactation suppression:</u>
- ❑ Breast binder and ice packs.
- ❑ Bromocriptine (Parlodel) 2.5mg PO twice daily for 14 days.

<u>Iron/vitamins:</u>
- ❑ Ferrous sulfate 300mg PO twice daily.
- ❑ Multivitamin PO once daily.

<u>Laboratory:</u>
- ❑ Obtain CBC on the morning of the day following delivery.
- ❑ Type and screen. Administer RhoGam provided that mother is Rh–negative and antibody screen is negative.

Dose, Emergency Drugs

<u>Note</u>: These drugs are also presented in the main drug section if additional information is needed.

Aminophylline (dose based on ideal body weight):

Intravenous loading dose for patient who has NOT received theophylline medication in last 24 hr: 6 mg/kg. Administer no faster than 25 mg/minute.
Loading dose is usually diluted in 50–250 ml D5W or normal saline and administered over 15–20 minutes but may also be given undiluted via syringe.

Intravenous loading dose in patient who IS currently receiving or has received theophylline medication in last 24 hr: 3 mg/kg.
If a stat serum theophylline level can be obtained, give a sufficient loading dose to raise serum theophylline to therapeutic level (10–20mcg/ml). A 3.1 mg/kg dose will raise serum theophylline by 5 mcg/ml.

Intravenous maintenance dose must be individualized.
The serum theophylline therapeutic level is 10–20 mcg/ml.
Suggested maintenance infusion rate:

<u>6 month–9 yr</u>: 1.0 mg/kg/hr	<u>9–16 yr</u>: 0.8 mg/kg/hr
<u>adult smoker < 50 yr</u>: 0.8 mg/kg/hr	<u>adult nonsmoker</u>: 0.5 mg/kg/hr
<u>elderly</u>: 0.3 mg/kg/hr	<u>cor pulmonale</u>: 0.3 mg/kg/hr
<u>cardiac or liver insufficiency</u>: 0.1–0.2 mg/kg/hr	

<u>Example of IV maintenance infusion</u>:
Dilute 1:1 with D5W or normal saline (e.g. 250 mg aminophylline in 250 ml D5W).
Then the infusion rate in ml/hr = (desired mg/kg/hr) X (ideal body weight in kg).

Bretylium

Ventricular fibrillation or hemodynamically unstable ventricular tachycardia:
After unsuccessful electrical cardioversion, give 5 mg/kg by rapid IV push. Then attempt cardioversion again.
If response is inadequate, increase dose to 10 mg/kg and (in conjunction with electrical cardioversion) repeat every 15 minutes as necessary or until maximum allowed cumulative bolus total of 30 mg/kg has been given.

Life-threatening ventricular arrhythmias not controlled by lidocaine or procainamide: Administer 5–10 mg/kg IV over 8–10 minutes after diluting contents of one ampule to 50 ml (this is to avoid nausea and vomiting).
May repeat in 1–2 hours for persistent arrhythmias. Dose may be given IM.

Maintenance suppression of ventricular arrhythmia:
(1) 1–2 mg/minute constant infusion, or
(2) 5–10 mg/kg IV given over > 8 minutes at 6 hour intervals.
May also be given IM: 5–10 mg/kg q6h.

Calcium chloride

Adult dose:
<u>Hyperkalemia</u>: 10 ml of 10% solution IV over 10 minutes with EKG monitor.
<u>Asystole/EM dissociation</u>: 2.5–5 ml of 10% solution slow IV push. If necessary, the dose may be repeated every 10 minutes.

Pediatric dose:
<u>Hyperkalemia</u>: 0.2 ml/kg (maximum 3 ml) IV over 10 minutes with EKG monitor.
<u>Cardiac arrest</u>: 0.2 ml/kg (maximum 3 ml) of 10% solution slow IV push.

Diazepam

Adult dose:

<u>Status epilepticus:</u> 5–10 mg slow IV push (5 mg/min). If necessary, dose may be repeated every 15 min or until maximum cumulative total of 30 mg has been given.

<u>Acute alcohol withdrawal:</u> 5–10 mg followed by 5 mg every 5–10 minutes until patient is sedated. Over 200 mg has been used to control severe agitation.

Pediatric dose:

<u>Status epilepticus:</u>
- 1month–5 yr: 0.2–0.5 mg IV q2–5 min up to total 5 mg. Repeat in 2–4 hr prn.
- 5 yr and older: 1 mg IV q2–5 minute up to total 10 mg. Repeat in 2–4 hr prn.

Diazoxide (adult or child): 1–3 mg/kg (max 150 mg) undiluted and given

IV via peripheral vein in 30 seconds or less with patient supine.
Repeat at 5–15 minute intervals as needed to achieve desired blood pressure.

Dobutamine

Titrate to effect. Usual range is 2.5–10 mcg/kg/min (rarely up to 40 mcg/kg/min).

Adult:

If 250 mg dobutamine is diluted in D5W or normal saline to make 250 ml of solution; then 0.6 X (desired rate of infusion in mcg/kg/min) X (patient weight in kg) = rate of infusion in ml/hr.

EXAMPLE: 70 kg patient and you wish to deliver 5 mcg/kg/min: 0.6 X 5 X 70 = 21 ml/hr (assuming 250 mg dobutamine is diluted to make 250 ml of solution).

Pediatric:

If 60 mg dobutamine is added to D5W or normal saline to make 100 ml of solution; then an infusion rate of 0.25 ml/kg/hr delivers 2.5 mcg/kg/minute, 0.5 ml/kg/hr delivers 5 mcg/kg/minute, 1 ml/kg/hr delivers 10 mcg/kg/minute.

Dopamine Using infusion pump, start at 2–5 mcg/kg/minute and ti-

trate to adequate blood pressure and urine output. Rates less than 20 mcg/kg/min are usually sufficient. If necessary, gradually increase up to 50 mcg/kg/min. If diastolic blood pressure rises yet pulse pressure drops, significant vasoconstriction may be occuring. Try reducing rate of infusion. Dopamine must not be mixed with alkaline solutions (e.g. sodium bicarbonate injection) because it will be inactivated.

Adult: If 200 mg dopamine is diluted in D5W or normal saline to make 250 ml IV solution; the rate of infusion may be calculated as follows:

0.075 X (desired mcg/kg/minute) X (weight in kg) = rate of infusion in ml/hr.

EXAMPLE: 70 kg patient and you wish to deliver dopamine at rate of 5 mcg/kg/min: 0.075 X 5 X 70 = 26 ml/hr (assuming 200 mg dopamine is diluted to make 250 ml of IV solution).

Pediatric: Dilute 60 mg dopamine to make 100 ml of IV solution.
Then an infusion rate of 0.25 ml/kg/hr delivers 2.5 mcg/kg/minute, 0.5 ml/kg/hr delivers 5 mcg/kg/minute, 1 ml/kg/hr delivers 10 mcg/kg/minute.

Epinephrine

Adult dose:

Asystole, ventricular fibrillation, electromechanical dissociation:
5–10 ml (0.5–1.0 mg) of 1: 10,000 solution IV. If necessary, the dose may be repeated every 5 minutes. Dose may be administered via endotracheal tube (or intracardiac as last resort) if IV route is not available.

Asthma/anaphylaxis:
0.3–0.5 ml (0.3–0.5 mg) of 1:1000 solution subcutaneous. If necessary, the same dose may be repeated twice at 20 minute intervals.
●If respiratory failure is imminent or patient is in shock, use the intravenous route :
3–5 ml (0.3–0.5 mg) of 1: 10,000 solution. If necessary, the dose may be repeated every 5–10 minutes.

Pediatric dose:
Cardiac arrest: 0.1ml/kg (0.01mg/kg) of 1: 10,000 solution given by intravenous, intraosseous, or endotracheal route. Repeat every 5 minutes if necessary.

Asthma/anaphylaxis: 0.01 ml/kg (0.01 mg/kg) of 1:1000 solution subcutaneous. If necessary, repeat twice at 15–20 minute intervals.
●If patient responds to 1:1000 subcutaneous injection, the sustain-action 1: 200 suspension (Sus-Phrine) may be used: 0.005 ml/kg subcutaneous. Maximum dose child under 30 kg is 0.15 ml. Repeat no more frequently than every 6 hour
●In life-threatening cases unresponsive to subcutaneous injection, intravenous epinephrine is used: 0.1 ml/kg of 1: 10,000 solution. May repeat every 5–15 minutes if necessary.
●Depending on the circumstances, a continuous IV infusion may be started to support the blood pressure. Add 0.6 mg epinephrine to 100 ml D5W. At this dilution, 1ml/kg/hr delivers 0.1mcg/kg/minute. Starting at this rate, titrate to effect up to maximum of 1.0 mcg/kg/minute.

Croup: 0.5 ml of 2.25% racemic epinephrine diluted in 3.5 ml normal saline and inhaled via nebulized mist.

Furosemide (Lasix)

Adult dose:
Acute pulmonary edema (adjunct to oxygen, morphine, etc.): 40 mg IV over 1–2 minutes. If adequate diuresis has not occurred within an hour, give additional 80 mg IV over 1–2 minutes.
Hypertension (adjunct in hypertensive emergency): 40–80 mg IV over 1–2 minutes.
Pediatric dose:
Intravenous/intramuscular (when prompt diuresis required): 1 mg/kg. If the initial dose does not induce adequate diuresis, the dose may be increased by 1mg/kg increments after intervals of at least 2 hr between doses (maximum dose 6 mg/kg).

Isoproterenol (Isuprel)

Adult: Add 1 mg isoproterenol to 250 ml D5W. Start infusion at 2–10 mcg/min (30–150 ml/hr rate) and titrate to effect while not allowing heart rate to exceed 160.
Pediatric (for treatment of respiratory failure due to asthma):
Add 0.6 mg to 100 ml of D5W. Then 1 ml/kg/hr delivers 0.1 mcg/kg/minute.
The infusion is started at 0.1 mcg/kg/min and titrated to effect by increasing the rate of infusion by 0.1 mcg/kg/min increments every 5–15 minutes. The infusion should not exceed 1.5 mcg/kg/min or cause the heart rate to go above 180.

Lidocaine

Adult dose:

<u>Loading:</u> 1 mg/kg initial IV bolus. If arrhythmia not suppressed, give 0.5 mg/kg every 2–5 minutes until arrhythmia controlled or until maximum allowed cumulative bolus total of 3 mg/kg has been given.

<u>Maintenance:</u> Immediately (as bolus therapy underway) begin constant IV infusion at 2–4 mg/minute. For example: 2 grams lidocaine added to D5W to make total of 500 ml of solution results in a lidocaine concentration of 4 mg/ml. Then 15 ml/hr infusion delivers 1 mg/minute, 30 ml/hr infusion delivers 2 mg/minute, etc.

<u>Note:</u> Reduce loading dose by half and the maintenance infusion to 1–2 mg/minute in the presence of CHF, shock, liver dysfunction, or if the patient is over 70.

Pediatric dose:

<u>Loading:</u> 1 mg/kg initial IV bolus. If necessary, repeat twice at 5–10 min intervals.

<u>Maintenance:</u> Immediately begin IV maintenance infusion at 20–50 mcg/kg/min as follows: 120 mg is added to D5W to make 100 ml of solution.

Then 1.0–2.5 ml/kg/hr delivers 20–50 mcg/kg/min.

Mannitol   To reduce intracranial or intraocular pressure.

<u>Dose (adult or child);</u> 1–2 gram/kg (5–10 ml/kg of 20% solution) IV over 30–60 minutes. Dose may be repeated twice at 6 hour intervals if necessary.

Morphine

Adult

<u>Intravenous</u> (acute pulmonary edema of cardiac etiology, immediate pain relief): Titrate to therapeutic effect by giving 2mg IV push every 5 minutes (blood pressure and respiratory status allowing). Range: up to 15 mg cumulative total.

<u>Subcutaneous/intramuscular:</u> 2–15 mg q4h.

Pediatric: 0.1–0.2 mg/kg q2–4h IV or SC (maximum 15 mg/dose)

Naloxone (Narcan) for treatment of narcotic overdose:

Adult dose: 2 mg IV. Repeat every 2–3 minutes if no response. Reconsider diagnosis if there is no response after giving 10 mg (large doses may be required in propoxyphene overdose).

● Since naloxone has a short half-life, repeat boluses may be necessary or a continuous IV infusion may be started: add 2 mg naloxone to 500 ml D5W or normal saline and titrate to effect.

● Administer IM or SC if unable to administer IV. May also be given via endotracheal tube.

Pediatric dose: 0.01mg/kg IV initial dose. If no response, give 0.1 mg/kg IV every 3–5 minute until there is a response or 5 doses given. May also be given IM or SC.

Nitroprusside

Adult or child: Start infusion at 0.5–1.5 mcg/kg/minute and titrate slowly to desired effect. Average dose is 3 mcg/kg/minute. Range is 0.5 mcg/kg/minute up to maximum 10 mcg/kg/minute.

<u>Note:</u> In heart failure much lower doses may suffice. Start with 10 mcg/minute (note: not 10 mcg/kg/minute).

Calculating the infusion rate (assuming nitroprusside is diluted in 250 ml D5W): rate of infusion in ml/hr =

$$\frac{15 \times (\text{desired rate in mcg/kg/min}) \times (\text{patient weight in kg})}{(\text{number of mg of nitroprusside in 250 ml of D5W})}$$

<u>Example;</u> 70 kg patient and you wish to deliver nitroprusside at 0.5 mcg/kg/min : Add 50 mg nitroprusside to 250 ml D5W;

$$\text{then } \frac{15 \times 0.5 \text{ mcg/kg/min} \times 70 \text{ kg}}{50 \text{ mg}} = 10.5 \text{ ml/hr.}$$

Phenobarbital

Adult dose:

Status epilepticus not controlled by diazepam or phenytoin; While carefully monitoring for signs of respiratory depression or hypotension, give 15 mg/kg IV at 25–50 mg/minute. ●Administration may be facilitated by diluting the total amount of phenobarbital in 100 ml normal saline and infusing IV piggyback with an infusion pump to control the rate of infusion.

●Brain concentrations reach a peak about an hour after the infusion.
●If no response after 15 mg/kg, an additional 5 mg/kg may be administered.
●Use intramuscular route if IV not available.

Pediatric dose:

Status epilepticus; While monitoring carefully for signs of respiratory depression or hypotension, give 2–3 mg/kg every 5–10 minutes IV until 10 mg/kg has been administered. Wait 20 minutes. If still no response, an additional 5–10 mg/kg may be administered. Use intramuscular route if IV not available.

Phenytoin

●Monitor blood pressure, respirations, and EKG when administering phenytoin IV.
●Phenytoin must not be administered as a continuous IV infusion.
●With the IV running with normal saline, administer phenytoin directly and close to the IV catheter insertion site

Status epilepticus (adult or pediatric): 15–18 mg/kg IV.

Administer no faster than 50 mg/minute in adult or 0.5 mg/kg/minute in child.

Arrhythmia:

Adult: 100 mg IV every 5 minutes until arrhythmia controlled, side effects develop, or maximum of 1000 mg given. Administer no faster than 25–50 mg/minute. 250 mg is usually sufficient to control a digitalis-induced arrhythmia.

Pediatric: 2–4 mg/kg IV at no faster than 0.5 mg/kg/minute. Repeat if necessary. Stop if side effects develop. Usual requirement is 20–30 mg/kg.

Procainamide

Adult dose:

Initially, 100 mg IV every 5 minutes (at no faster than 50 mg/minute) until arrhythmia suppressed or until maximum of 1000 mg given.

●Stop if hypotension occurs or if QRS widens by ≥ 50%.
●Monitor blood pressure, respirations, and EKG when administering phenytoin IV.
●To facilitate control of rate of infusion, dilute procainamide in D5W.

Follow with continuous maintenance infusion at 1–4 mg/minute. Example: 1 gram procainamide added to 250 ml D5W and running at 30 ml/hr delivers 2 mg/minute.

Pediatric dose:

Initially: 2 mg/kg (max 100 mg) diluted in D5W and administered IV slowly over 5 minutes. May repeat every 10–15 minute until arrhythmia controlled, but do not infuse more than 1000 mg total. Stop if hypotension occurs or if QRS widens by ≥ 50%.

Maintenance; continuous IV infusion 0.020–0.080 mg/kg/minute. Total 24 hr IV dose should not exceed 2 gram.

Sodium bicarbonate

Dose in life-threatening metabolic acidosis (adult or pediatric):

1 mEq/kg initial IV bolus.

If necessary, give additional 0.5 mEq/kg IV bolus every 10 minutes.

NOTE: If possible obtain arterial blood gas and calculate bicarbonate requirements as follows: amount of sodium bicarbonate needed in mEq =

$$0.4 \times (\text{weight in kg}) \times (25 \text{ mEq/l} - \text{arterial HCO3 mEq/l}).$$

Give 1/2 this amount and then reassess.

Emergency Protocols:

Anaphylaxis:

Airway maintenance: Be prepared to intubate should severe respiratory compromise occur. Hoarseness or stridor suggests laryngeal edema which may make intubation impossible. Therefore, also be prepared to perform tracheostomy. If tracheostomy cannot be immediately performed, a 16—18 gauge needle inserted between the tracheal rings may provide a temporary route for ventilation.

Treatment of bronchospasm or angioedema in the absence of shock:
If respiratory failure is imminent or patient is in shock, administer epinephrine by intravenous route:
- Adult IV dose: 3—5 ml (0.3—0.5 mg) of 1: 10,000 dilution. If necessary, give repeat dose at 5—10 minute intervals.
- Pediatric IV dose: 0.1 ml/kg of 1: 10,000 dilution. If necessary, give repeat dose at 5—10 minute intervals.

Otherwise, administer epinephrine 1:1000 dilution by subcutaneous injection:
- Adult: 0.3—0.5 ml. If necessary, give repeat dose in 15 minutes. If anaphylaxis is the consequence of an injection or an insect sting in a limb, place a tourniquet proximal to the site and inject an additional 0.1 ml of 1: 1000 epinephrine at the site.
- Pediatric: 0.01 ml/kg. If necessary, give repeat dose in 15 minutes.

If there is persistent bronchospasm, administer IV aminophylline and nebulized bronchodilators–e.g. metaproterenol [Bronkosol], isoetharine [Alupent].

Diphenhydramine (Benadryl) is given as an adjunct to epinephrine.
- Adult dose: 50 mg IV. To help prevent recurrent urticaria-angioedema and bronchospasm, administer 50 mg IM or PO every 4—6 hour for a minimum of 24 hr.
- Pediatric dose: 1mg/kg. To help prevent recurrent urticaria-angioedema and bronchospasm, administer 1mg/kg IM or PO every 4—6 hour for a minimum of 24 hr.

In the presence of shock or vascular collapse:
Administer epinephrine intravenously,
- Adult: Mix 0.1 mg epinephrine in 10 ml of normal saline and inject IV over 5—10 minutes.
- Child: Mix 1 mg in 250 ml D5W (4 mcg/ml concentration) and start infusion at 0.1 mcg/kg/minute (1.5 mcg/kg/hr). Increase rate of infusion if necessary. Maximum rate is 1.5 mcg/kg/minute.

Other measures to be used in hypotensive patients: Trendelenberg position, intravenous normal saline, MAST trousers (if hypotension severe).

Dopamine drip may be needed if hypotension persists.

Urticaria and angioedema:
Anaphylactic reaction confined to mild angioedema, urticaria, and/or itching may be treated with diphenhydramine (Benadryl) alone.
- Adult: 50 mg IV or IM. If necessary, give repeat doses IM or PO at 4–6 hr intervals.
- Pediatric: 1mg/kg IV or IM. If necessary, give repeat doses IM or PO at 4–6 hr intervals.

Severe urticaria or angioedema requires subcutaneous epinephrine 1:1000 dilution.
- Adult dose: 0.2—0.4 ml subcutaneous epinephrine 1:1000 dilution. If necessary, repeat in 30 minutes.

To help prevent recurrent urticaria-angioedema, administer diphenhydramine 50mg IM or PO every 4—6 hours for a minimum of 24 hr.
- Pediatric: 0.01 ml/kg. If necessary, repeat in 30 minutes.

To help prevent recurrent urticaria-angioedema, administer diphenhydramine 1mg/kg IM or PO every 4—6 hours for a minimum of 24 hr.

Corticosteroids have no immediate effect but may also be administered to prevent recurrence.

Carefully monitor patients who have a severe reaction (shock, airway obstruction) for a minimum of 24 hr.

Prophylaxis: • Selected patients at risk for anaphylaxis may need to carry epinephrine for injection with them (e.g. EpiPen, Ana-Kit). • Desensitization injections are indicated in patients who develop anaphylactic reactions after insect stings. • Patients receiving horse serum (e.g. snake bite antivenom) should be skin tested first.

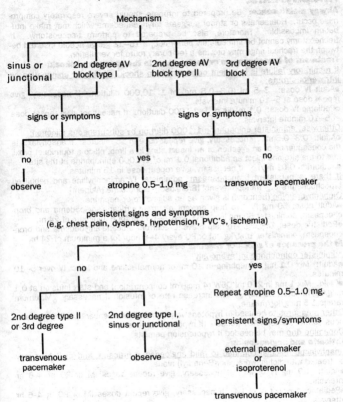

Bradycardia*
(< 60 beats/minute)

Mechanism

- sinus or junctional
- 2nd degree AV block type I
- 2nd degree AV block type II
- 3rd degree AV block

signs or symptoms

signs or symptoms

no → observe

yes → atropine 0.5–1.0 mg

no → transvenous pacemaker

persistent signs and symptoms
(e.g. chest pain, dyspnea, hypotension, PVC's, ischemia)

no

- 2nd degree type II or 3rd degree → transvenous pacemaker
- 2nd degree type I, sinus or junctional → observe

yes

Repeat atropine 0.5–1.0 mg.

persistent signs/symptoms

external pacemaker or isoproterenol

transvenous pacemaker

*Algorithm is from JAMA 1986; 255(21):2945.

Paroxysmal Atrial Tachycardia (PAT) is characterized

by atrial tachycardia (140–250/minute) that usually begins suddenly, lasts variably (seconds to hours), and ends abruptly. The QRS complexes occur regularly and generally have a normal appearance. If there is QRS widening due to an associated intraventricular block, PAT may be confused with ventricular tachycardia. A 2:1 AV block may be present if the atrial rate exceeds 200. The P waves are usually not visible since they are buried in the preceding T wave.

Treatment of unstable patient (e.g. hypotension, pulmonary edema):
●<u>Electrical cardioversion</u> First sedate conscious patient (e.g. intravenous Valium, Brevital). Attempt cardioversion with less than 100 joules in synchronized mode. If unsuccessful, attempt cardioversion successively at 200 and then 360 joules. Electrical cardioversion is generally contraindicated if PAT is due to digitalis toxicity.
●<u>If PAT persists, administer verapamil</u> 5 mg IV push. If still not converted, give additional 10 mg 15–20 minutes later.
●<u>Electrical cardioversion</u> may be tried again if necessary.
●<u>In refractory or recurrent cases, digoxin or propranolol</u> may be administered to control the ventricular response and may terminate PAT.
●<u>Drug prophylaxis</u> (e.g. verapamil, digoxin, beta blocker, quinidine, procainamide) may benefit patients who experience recurrent episodes of PAT.

Treatment of stable patient:
●Measures to increase vagal tone may be attempted first (e.g. Valsalva maneuver, carotid sinus massage).
●If this fails, administer 5 mg verapamil IV push. If PAT persists, give additional 10 mg 15–20 min later.
●Drug prophylaxis (e.g. verapamil, digoxin, beta blocker, quinidine, procainamide) may benefit patients who experience prolonged or frequent attacks of PAT.

Atrial Flutter (aberrant atrial depolarization occurring at a rate of 220–

350 that sually results in a "sawtooth" wave that is best seen in leads 2, 3, and aVF). Except at slower rates, the AV node is not usually capable of conducting all the flutter waves and consequently every 2nd, 3rd, ..., wave is conducted to the ventricles producing atrial-ventricle conduction ratios of 2:1, 3:1, etc. The most common situation is a 2:1 AV block with an atrial rate of about 300 and a ventricular response of about 150. The QRS complexes are generally normal. The T waves are not usually visible since they are buried within the flutter waves. ●Alarmingly high ventricular rates may ensue when certain drugs (e.g. quinidine, procainamide, disopyramide) are administered and the atrial rate slows to about 200 because then the AV node is capable of conducting all the atrial impulses (i.e. 1:1 AV conduction). ●Carotid sinus massage may slow AV conduction and thereby increase the atrial-ventricle conduction ratio so that the flutter waves may be clarified. However, carotid sinus massage does not convert atrial flutter and the effect lasts only while pressure is applied. Atrial flutter often spontaneously converts to normal sinus rhythm or to atrial fibrillation.

Treatment unstable patient (e.g. CHF, pulmonary edema, hypotension, myocardial ischemia): Synchronized cardioversion. Less than 50 joules usually suffices.

Treatment stable patient: <u>Intravenous verapamil, digoxin, or propranol</u> are administered to slow the ventricular response, and may restore normal sinus rhythm or convert to atrial fibrillation. <u>If atrial flutter persists, add another drug once the ventricular rate has been slowed sufficiently</u> e.g. IV or PO procainamide, PO quinidine, or PO disopyramide. <u>Synchronized cardioversion</u> is indicated if drug therapy fails. <u>Overdrive pacing</u> of the atria may be necessary if electrical cardioversion is contraindicated (e.g. digitalis toxicity).

Atrial Fibrillation   Treat underlying contributing disorder if possible (e.g. thyrotoxicosis, hypertension, mitral stenosis, pulmonary embolism). Anticoagulants are administered to prevent thromboembolism.

Patient made unstable by rapid ventricular response (e.g. pulmonary edema, hypotension, angina): Anticoagulate with IV heparin first. Then attempt synchronized cardioversion starting at 50 joules. Quinidine is administered to prevent recurrence. Electrical cardioversion of digitalized patients may be hazardous: hypokalemia must be corrected first. Oral or heparin anticoagulation is continued for 2–3 wk.

Stable patient with recent onset atrial fibrillation (i.e. onset < 12 months) and with normal left atrium: Patient is anticoagulated for 2–3 weeks before and after cardioversion. Also, the ventricular response rate must first be controlled with digoxin, propranol, or verapamil. Conversion is then carried out with PO quinidine, PO or IV procainamide, or PO disopyramide. Electrical cardioversion may be tried if drug therapy fails.

Patient with chronic atrial fibrillation and/or enlarged left atrium: Cardioversion is not attempted since successful conversion to and/or maintenance of normal sinus rhythm is unlikely.

Premature Ventricular Contractions (PVC's)

are depolarizations that originate in the ventricles. They usually produce wide (> 0.12 sec) and bizarre QRS complexes that are generally followed by a T wave that points in direction away from the main QRS component. <u>PVC's may be confused with supraventricular impulses with aberrant intraventricular conduction.</u> The usual but not infallible way of distinguishing the two is to note that PVC's: (1) are not preceded by a P wave and (2) are usually followed by a full compensatory pause (interval between the QRS that precedes the PVC and the QRS that follows the PVC is exactly twice the normal QRS to QRS interval). The compensatory pause occurs because the PVC does not usually disturb the sinus node and therefore the next P wave appears on schedule. **Etiology:** PVC's commonly occur in normal persons. They are also associated with myocardial ischemia/infarction, cardiomyopathy, hypertensive cardiac disease, acute rheumatic fever, hypokalemia, hypocalcemia, hypoxia, acidosis. Drugs may be responsible: caffeine; catecholamines (epinephrine, amphetamines, isoproterenol, etc); tricyclic antidepressants; digitalis; quinidine; procainamide; tobacco. **Criteria for treatment:** Asymptomatic patients without evidence of cardiac disease do not require therapy. Patients with heart disease receive drug therapy if PVC's: are more frequent than 5 times/minute, occur in runs of 2 or more in row, are multifocal, or fall on the preceding T wave.

*Following algorithm based on JAMA 1986; 255(21):2945.

Determine whether suppressive therapy is necessary.
Exclude treatable causes.
Atropine may abolish PVC's due to bradycardia.
Are any of the following possibly to blame: electrolyte disturbance
(e.g. abnormal serum potassium), drugs (e.g. digitalis), acid–base
disturbance, hypoxemia ?

|

Lidocaine 1mg/kg IV bolus.

|

If PVC's persist, give lidocaine 0.5 mg/kg IV bolus every 2–5 minutes until PVC's disappear or until cumulative total of 3 mg/kg given (count the initial 1mg/kg bolus given above in the total).

If PVC's persist, give procainamide 20 mg/min until PVC's disappear or up to 1000 mg given.

|

If PVC's persist: unless contraindicated give bretylium 5-10 mg over 8-10 minutes.

|

If PVC's persist, consider overdrive pacing.

Maintenance rates once PVC's controlled:

After lidocaine 1mg/kg	→	lidocaine 2 mg/min drip.
After lidocaine 1–2 mg/kg	→	lidocaine 3 mg/min drip.
After lidocaine 2–3 mg/kg	→	lidocaine 4 mg/min drip.

After procainamide → 1–4 mg/min drip. Rate is subsequently adjusted to achieve optimal serum therapeutic level.

After bretylium → bretylium 2 mg/min drip.

Chronic PVC's may be treated with PO drugs (e.g. quinidine, disopyramide, propranolol, tocainide).

Ventricular Tachycardia (3 or more consecutive ventricular ec-
topic beats occurring at a rate of > 100—usually 150—220 beats/minute). Rate is
generally regular. The complexes are wide with a bundle branch pattern (usually left
bundle branch pattern). This arrhythmia is often a complication of heart disease (especially myocardial infarction) but may also be due to drugs (e.g. digoxin, quinidine,
procainamide, tricyclics). Ventricular tachycardia may be confused with supraventricular tachycardia with aberrant conduction. The latter can be excluded if the
EKG discloses P waves that are dissociated from the QRS complexes. Carotid sinus
massage may help reveal the P waves and may terminate supraventricular tachycardia. However, carotid sinus massage has no effect on ventricular tachycardia. Two
other findings that may be observed with ventricular tachycardia include irregular cannon waves in the jugular veins and variation in intensity of the first heart sound while
the patient holds his breath.

***Treatment of ventricular tachycardia in absence of pulse:** treat as for ventric-
ular fibrillation.

***Treatment of ventricular tachycardia with pulse in unstable patient** (e.g. hy-
potension, pulmonary edema, chest pain)**:**
● Sedate if the patient is conscious (e.g. intravenous Valium, intravenous Brevital).
● Attempt synchronized cardioversion. Start at 50 joules. If ventricular tachycardia
persists; attempt to cardiovert successively at 100, 200, and then up to 360 joules.
● If cardioversion fails or ventricular tachycardia recurs, administer lidocaine
1mg/kg IV bolus and again attempt electrical cardioversion as just outlined or at a
previously successful energy level.
● Start an intravenous lidocaine infusion at 2–4 mg/minute.
● If arrhythmia persists, additional lidocaine bolus therapy is indicated along with
attempts at electrical cardioversion. Give 0.5 mg/kg lidocaine bolus every 5
minutes until arrhythmia controlled or cumulative bolus total of 3 mg/kg given (count
the initial 1mg/kg bolus given above in the total).
● If arrhythmia persists, administer bretylium 5 mg/kg IV push and again attempt
synchronized cardioversion (200—360 joules or previously successful energy level).
● If arrhythmia persists, additional bretylium bolus therapy is indicated along with
attempts at synchronized cardioversion at 200—360 joules. Give bretylium 10
mg/kg IV bolus every 15 minutes until arrhythmia controlled or until cumulative bolus
total of 30 mg/kg given (count the intial 5mg/kg in the total). If successful, start IV
bretylium infusion at 1—2 mg/minute.
● Overdrive pacing may be tried if the above measures fail or if ventricular tachycardia recurs.

***Treatment of ventricular tachycardia in stable patient** (i.e. asymptomatic, nor-
motensive)**:**
● Lidocaine 1mg/kg IV bolus. Then, immediately start IV infusion of lidocaine at 2–4
mg/minute.
● If ventricular tachycardia persists, give lidocaine 0.5 mg/kg IV bolus every 5—8
minutes until arrhythmia controlled or cumulative bolus total of 3 mg/kg has been
given (count the initial 1mg/kg bolus in the total).
● If lidocaine fails to restore normal rhythm, administer procainamide 20
mg/minute until ventricular tachycardia resolves or total of 1000 mg has been given.
● If ventricular tachycardia persists, attempt synchronized electrical
cardioversion. Sedate first if the patient is conscious (e.g. IV Valium or Brevital).
Start at 50 joules. If unsuccessful, try to cardiovert successively at 100, 200, and
then up to 360 joules.
● Overdrive pacing may be tried if the above measures fail.

*Above protocols based on JAMA 1986; 255(21):2945.

Ventricular Fibrillation*

witnessed arrest | unwitnessed arrest

Check pulse.
If no pulse, precordial thump.

Check pulse.
If no pulse

Check pulse.
If no pulse

Start CPR
Verify ventricular fibrillation on monitor.
Defibrillate 200 joules

In children, the intial
defibrillation dose is
2 joules/kg; doubled
if no response.

If no pulse, defibrillate 200–300 joules.

If no pulse, defibrillate 360 joules.

If no pulse, resume CPR and start IV line.

Epinephrine, 1:10,000 solution
Adult dose: 5–10 ml IV push.
Pediatric dose: 0.1 ml/kg.
Dose may be repeated every 5 minutes as needed.
Epinephrine may be given via endotracheal tube if no IV access.

Intubate if possible.

Defibrillate 360 joules.

If no pulse, resume CPR and give lidocaine 1 mg/kg IV push.

Defibrillate 360 joules.

If no pulse, resume CPR.
Give bretylium 5 mg/kg IV push.

Alternative to bretylium:
Give lidocaine 0.5mg/kg
every 8 minutes as needed
up to cumulative total
3mg/kg (count the initial
1mg/kg lidocaine bolus
given above in the total).

Defibrillate 360 joules.

If no pulse, resume CPR.
Give bretylium 10 mg/kg IV push.

Defibrillate 360 joules.

If no pulse, resume CPR and repeat bretylium or lidocaine.

Defibrillate 360 joules.

*Algorithm based on JAMA
1986; 255(21):2945.

Ventricular Asystole*

CPR

|

If tracing is unclear and possibly ventricular fibrillation,
countershock as for ventricular fibrillation.

|

Confirm asystole in two leads.

|

Continue CPR.
Start IV line.

|

Epinephrine 1: 10,000 solution.
Adult dose: 5–10 ml IV push.
Pediatric dose: 0.01 ml/kg IV push.
Dose may be repeated prn every 5 minutes.
Dose may be given endotracheally.

|

Intubate when possible.

|

Atropine
Adult dose: 1 mg IV push.
Pediatric dose: 0.01–0.03 mg/kg   (minimum of 0.1mg).
If necessary, dose may be repeated once in 5 min.

|

Consider bicarbonate.
Dose: 1 mEq/kg IV.
An additional 0.5 mg/kg may be given every 10
minutes but it is best to use arterial blood gas
measurement as a guide.

|

Consider external or transvenous pacemaker.

*Algorithm based on JAMA 1986; 255(21):2945.

Electromechanical Dissociation (EMD)*

CPR

|

Start IV line.

|

Epinephrine 1: 10,000 solution.
Adult dose: 5–10 ml (0.5–1.0 mg) IV push.
Pediatric dose: 0.01 ml/kg IV push.
Dose is repeated every 5 minutes as needed.
Dose may be given endotracheally.

|

Intubate when possible.

|

Consider bicarbonate.
Dose: 1 mEq/kg.
Half initial dose may be repeated every 10 minutes
as needed, guided preferably by arterial blood gas.

|

<u>Consider causes of EMD for which there may be a specific remedy</u>: hypovolemia (administer fluids), cardiac tamponade (perform pericardiocentesis), tension pneumothorax (perform needle decompression), acidosis or hypoxemia (perform effective CPR, ventilation, oxygenation). Distended neck veins may signal the presence of tension pneumothorax or cardiac tamponade.

<u>Causes of EMD that are often unresponsive to treatment</u> include extensive myocardial injury, massive pulmonary embolism, prolonged myocardial ischemia.

*Algorithm based on JAMA 1986; 255(21):2945.

*Guidelines for Face Mask, Laryngoscope,

Patient age	Face Mask	Laryngoscope
premature infant	0 Rendell-Baker 1 Vital Signs	Miller 0*
Term infant	1 Rendell-Baker 2 Vital Signs	Miller 1* Wis–Hipple 1 Robertshaw 0
6 months		
1 year	2 Rendell–Baker	Wis–Hipple 1-1/2 Robertshaw 1
2 years	3 Vital Signs	Miller 2 Flagg 2
4 years	3 Rendell–Baker	
6 years	4 Vital Signs	
8 years	Small Trimar	Miller 2 MacIntosh 2
10 years		
12 years	Ohio 2 or 3 5 Vital Signs	MacIntosh 3
Adolescent	Ohio 3 or 4	MacIntosh 3 Miller 3

Oxyscope modifications are available for Miller 0 and 1 blades. They may reduce the likelihood of hypoxemia during laryngoscopy in infants.

*Reproduced with permission. ©Textbook of Advanced Cardiac Life Support, 1987, Copyright American Heart Assn.

and Tracheal Tube Sizes.

Endotracheal Tube Size		
Internal Diameter (mm)	Length (cm) Midtrachea to Teeth	Suction Catheter (Fr)
2.5, 3.0 Uncuffed	8	5 or 6
3.0, 3.5 Uncuffed	10	6
3.5, 4.0 Uncuffed	12	8
4.0, 4.5 Uncuffed	12	8
4.5 Uncuffed	14	8
5.0 Uncuffed	16	10
5.5 Uncuffed	16	10
6.0 Cuffed or Uncuffed	18	10
6.5 Cuffed or Uncuffed	18	12
7.0 Cuffed	20	12
7.0, 8.0 Cuffed	22	12

Usual adult female: Use 8.0 or 8.5 mm cuffed endotracheal tube.
Usual adult male: Use 8.5 or 9.0 mm cuffed endotracheal tube.

Comments:
- A rough estimate of tube size is that the outside diameter of the tube is approximately the diameter of the patient's little finger. After 1 yr of age the tube size in children may also be estimated by the formula (age + 16)/4.
- Before intubating, ventilate with 100% oxygen using bag-valve mask.
- Cuffed tubes are inflated with just enough air to provide air seal: 5–10 ml in adult, and up to 5 ml in children ≥ 8 yr.
- Check for position of tube by listening for bilateral breath sounds over the chest and the absence of breath sounds over the stomach.
- Obtain chest x-ray to verify proper tube position.